Occupational Therapy

for Children

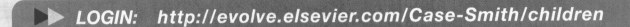

Occupational Therapy

for Children

fifth edition

Jane Case-Smith, EdD, OTR/L, FAOTA

Professor
Division of Occupational Therapy
The Ohio State University
School of Allied Medical Professions
Columbus, Ohio

With 28 Contributing Authors

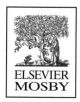

ELSEVIER
MOSBY

ELSEVIER
MOSBY

11830 Westline Industrial Drive
St. Louis, Missouri 63146

OCCUPATIONAL THERAPY FOR CHILDREN
Copyright © 2005, Elsevier Inc.

Previous editions copyrighted 1985, 1989, 1996, 2001

ISBN-13: 978-0-323-02873-8
ISBN-10: 0-323-02873-X

Acquisitions Editor: Kathy Falk
Developmental Editor: Melissa Kuster Deutsch
Publishing Services Manager: Linda McKinley
Project Manager: Rich Barber
Designer: Teresa McBryan

Printed in the United States

Last digit is the print number: 9 8 7 6 5 4 3 2

Contributors

Susan J. Amundson, PhD, OTR/L, FAOTA
Executive Director
OT Kids, Inc.
Homer, Alaska

Beth Ann Ball, MS, OTR/L
Occupational Therapist
Columbus Public Schools
Columbus, Ohio

Laura Crooks, OTR/L
Manager, Department of Occupational Therapy,
  Physical Therapy, Theraputic Recreation
Children's Hospital and Regional Medical Center
Seattle, Washington

Debora A. Davidson, MS, OTR
Associate Professor
Occupational Therapy Program
School of Health Professions
Maryville University
St. Louis, Missouri

Brian J. Dudgeon, PhD, OTR, FAOTA
Assistant Professor, Division of Occupational Medicine
Department of Rehabilitation Medicine
University of Washington
Seattle, Washington

Charlotte E. Exner, PhD, OTR, FAOTA
Professor, Department of Occupational Therapy and
  Occupational Science
Dean, College of Health Professions
Towson University
Towson, Maryland

Ruth Humphry, PhD, OTR/L
Professor, Division of Occupational Science
University of North Carolina
Chapel Hill, North Carolina

Jan G. Hunter, MA, OTR
Neonatal Clinical Specialist, Infant Special Care Unit
Assistant Professor, Occupational Therapy, School of
  Allied Health
University of Texas Medical Branch
Galveston, Texas

Susan H. Knox, PhD, OTR/L, BCP, FAOTA
Director of Education and Research
Therapy in Action
Tarzana, California

Mary Law, PhD, FCAOT
Professor and Associate Dean, School of Rehabilitation
  Science
Co-Director, CanChild Centre for Childhood
  Disability Research
McMaster University
Hamilton, Ontario, Canada

Zoe Mailloux, MA, OTR, FAOTA
Director of Administration
Pediatric Therapy Network
Torrance, California

Patricia S. Nagaishi, PhD, OTR/L, BCP
Part-time Lecturer
Division of Health Sciences, Occupational Therapy
  Program
California State University—Dominguez Hills
Carson, California
Pediatric Occupational Therapy Consultant
Clinical Services
South Central Los Angeles Regional Center
Los Angeles, California
Special Education—Infant/Preschool
Pasadena Unified School District
Pasadena, California

Deborah S. Nichols, PT, PhD
Director, Associate Professor
Physical Therapy Division
The Ohio State University
Columbus, Ohio

Susan O'Daniel, OTR
Case Manager, Occupational Therapist
Transition Services
Littleton Public Schools
Littleton, Colorado

L. Diane Parham, PhD, OTR, FAOTA
Associate Professor
Department of Occupational Science and Occupational
　Therapy
University of Southern California
Los Angeles, California
Director of Research and Education
Pediatric Therapy Network
Torrance, California

Pamela K. Richardson, PhD, OTR, FAOTA
Assistant Professor of Occupational Therapy
San Jose State University
San Jose, California

Jan Rogers, MS, OTR/L
Occupational Therapist
Private Practice
Pickerington, Ohio

Sandra Rogers, PhD, OTR
Assistant Professor
Occupational Therapy
Pacific University
Forest Grove, Oregon

Elizabeth Russel, PhD, OTR/L
Therapy Consultant
Department of Health Services
Children's Medical Services
Los Angeles, California

Colleen M. Schneck, ScD, OTR/L, FAOTA
Professor
Department of Occupational Therapy
Eastern Kentucky University
Richmond, Kentucky

Winifred Schultz-Krohn, PhD, OTR/L, BCP, FAOTA
Associate Professor of Occupational Therapy
San Jose State University
San Jose, California

Jayne T. Shepherd, MS, OTR/L
Associate Professor
Occupational Therapy
Virginia Commonwealth University
Richmond, Virginia

Karen C. Spencer, PhD, OTR
Associate Professor
Occupational Therapy
Colorado State University
Fort Collins, Colorado

Linda C. Stephens, MS, OTR/L, FAOTA
Director and Owner
Atlanta Children's Therapy, Inc.
Atlanta, Georgia

Katherine B. Stewart, MS, OTR/L, FAOTA
Occupational Therapist
Boyer Children's Clinic
Seattle, Washington

Yvonne Swinth, PhD, OTR/L, FAOTA
Associate Professor
School of Occupational Therapy and Physical Therapy
University of Puget Sound
Tacoma, Washington
Occupational Therapist
Special Education
University Place School District
University Place, Washington

Susan Rooder Tauber, MEd, OTR/L
Founder and Executive Director
Adaptive Learning Center for Infants and Children,
　Inc.
Atlanta, Georgia

Barbara Marin Wavrek, MHS, OTR/L
Private Practice
Columbus, Ohio

Christine Wright-Ott, MPA, OTR/L
Occupational Therapist
Private Practice and Consultation
Cupertino, California

CONTRIBUTORS TO THE FOURTH EDITION:

Cheryl Missiuna

Nancy Pollock

Debra Stewart

Foreword

One measure of civilization is the value it places on its children. Jane Case-Smith, EdD, OTR/L, FAOTA, the editor of the fifth edition of *Occupational Therapy for Children*, has combined her expertise with that of colleagues to create a comprehensive introduction to pediatric occupational therapy that reflects this valuing of children. The book, although designed specifically as a pediatric text for entry-level students, is equally useful as a resource for practicing therapists.

The strengths of this text include its comprehensiveness, its emphasis on participation, and its recognition of the importance of content grounded in research. The book lays the foundation for occupational therapy practice and identifies the broad knowledge base required for this endeavor. Building on this foundation, the book progresses logically from assessment through intervention with specific foci on postural control, hand function, visual perception, psychosocial and emotional development, feeding and oral motor skills, self-care and adaptation for independent living, play, handwriting, augmentative communication and computer access, and mobility. Specific strengths in content that merit emphases are the attention to the psychosocial development and needs of children, the use of technology to increase function, the importance of families and others in the child's system through the continuing process of adaptation, and the legislation that is relevant to children with disabilities and their families.

The book's concluding section on arenas of pediatric occupational therapy practice is addressed from a developmental perspective. This section provides integrative function, facilitating understanding of the therapy process starting in the neonatal intensive care unit, progressing through early intervention and preschool and school programs, and appropriately concluding with the transitioning from school to adult life. For pediatric therapists, this longitudinal perspective assists with understanding a child's program within the context of the child's past, present, and future.

Understanding of the needs of students when using a textbook is reflected in the logical organization of the text and the editor's careful inclusion of study aids in each chapter. Key terms, chapter objectives, and study questions are strategically offered to guide learning and provide opportunities to apply and integrate knowledge.

The editor has coordinated the efforts of an impressive group of authors, reflecting a broad range of expertise in pediatric practice. The diverse and rich contributions of these individuals are organized logically and meaningfully so that this knowledge can be used by students and therapists who work daily to facilitate the potential of children to play, to care for themselves, and to work. The fifth edition of *Occupational Therapy for Children* reflects caring, empowering, and respect. It is a treasure for occupational therapists and for children with disabilities and their families.

Jean Deitz, PhD, OTR/L, FAOTA
Professor and Graduate Program Coordinator
Department of Rehabilitation Medicine
University of Washington

Preface

Since the first edition of *Occupational Therapy for Children* was published, the practice of occupational therapy has experienced tremendous growth and change. In the first two editions of this book, Pratt and Allen described the roles and functions of pediatric occupational therapists, the core knowledge of the profession, and the occupational therapy process as it existed in the 1980s. During that time, assessment tools and intervention techniques were limited and theoretic rather than empirically tested. Most of the children who received occupational therapy had physical disabilities such as cerebral palsy. Occupational therapists primarily worked in hospitals and rehabilitation centers, often in one-on-one sessions with a child.

In the 1990s the field of occupational therapy expanded, and its leaders, scholars, and researchers refined core theories and practices. External forces, including new legislation and federal programs, brought about some of the changes in the profession. Amendments to the Individuals with Disabilities Education Act (IDEA, 1990, 1997) had significant impact on service delivery by increasing services to infants and young children and their families, improving access to assistive technology in schools, and encouraging inclusion. Our mandated presence in the schools fueled the development of classroom-based interventions and technologies designed to enable children to fully participate in the school environment. The types of children who receive our services expanded to include those with a range of functional limitations that included learning and behavioral difficulties.

In addition to legislative changes that have expanded our roles in early intervention and schools, the research base supporting pediatric occupational therapy practices has increased in recent years. Many of the revisions in this edition of *Occupational Therapy for children* reflect recent findings from research studies and interpretations of those findings.

The current edition has four sections with complementary purposes. Section I describes foundational knowledge that forms the basis for pediatric practice. This section uses theories of human development and occupation as it relates to performance and participation. The influence of caregivers, culture, and community on children's acquisition of occupations and social roles is explained. Researched theories from fields such as psychology, sociology, physics, human ecology, medi-

cine, family, and cultural studies have influenced our models of practice. These theories and models form the basis for making clinical decisions and for designing occupational therapy programs. The theories and models presented in Section I form the basis for the intervention methods described throughout the text. When available, research studies that have examined the effectiveness of these theories are discussed to further the reader's understanding of how interventions are most appropriately applied.

Current revisions also reflect the growing consensus about our focus in enhancing a child's occupational performance and participation in home, school, and community environments. Because occupational therapy services are now often provided in a child's natural environment, their relevance and importance has increased; at the same time we are challenged to implement services that accommodate to the complexity and diversity of natural environments. Although practice in the child's natural environment may require travel and can be logistically difficult, working in the child's daily environment provides us with new insights into the child's daily routines; interactions with caregivers, family, and peers; and participation in home/school activities. Family-centered and child-centered philosophies are core to the practices described, with emphasis on assessing and embracing family and child priorities.

Section II includes two chapters on occupational therapy assessment of children. Evaluation is explained as a process in Chapter 7, focusing on analysis of functional performance and participation within natural contexts. Chapter 8 describes how to administer standardized tests and interpret the findings. Recently developed instruments are described in both chapters, and measures of function and participation are emphasized.

Child occupations, performance limitations, and interventions to enhance performance and/or accommodate to limitations are described in Section III. These chapters have been updated in the fifth edition to include information on revised models of practice, advocated service delivery models, recently developed intervention methods, and new technology. Each chapter presents research findings that support occupational therapy theories and practices. Descriptive studies help to improve our understanding of children's occupations, instruments to assess performance, and ways that disability affects participation. Efficacy studies help to clarify with whom an intervention should be applied and what performance outcomes can be expected. The evolution and refinement of our theoretical approaches are documented in this third section.

Section IV describes arenas of occupational therapy practice. This section was developed in recognition of the importance of the environment to the child's occupations and ability to participate. The environment also directly influences occupational therapy practice by defining the constraints within we must work. Current practice has shifted from an emphasis on the individual to the individual within his or her social and physical environments. Therefore the performance areas addressed in therapy must always consider the demands and resources of the child's environment. In many cases, the goals of occupational therapy shift from changing the individual to modifying the environment, enabling therapy to support the child's performance and functional independence. This section explains how the selection of intervention approaches and service delivery models relate to the systems in which the occupational therapist practices. Contrasting examples of therapy in medical, community, early intervention, and educational environments illustrate the varying roles of occupational therapists. A developmental framework (birth to adulthood) organizes chapters in Section IV. This life-span perspective helps promote understanding of how occupational therapists manage the functional problems imposed by disabilities at different ages and in different contexts. For example, early intervention services with infants are essentially different from school-based services. Developmental theories, although critical for young children, are less important as the child enters school and develops compensatory strategies for functioning in the classroom.

The text also emphasizes cultural competence. The case studies exemplify children of different cultures and emphasize cultural sensitivity in evaluation and intervention. Case studies that emphasize the child's social and physical context have greater potential to teach clinical reasoning than those studies that emphasize clinical information.

We have maintained the primary purpose of the book as a text for professional programs; however, we recognize that some of the content is beyond entry level. For example, the chapter on practice in the neonatal intensive care setting reflects advanced knowledge and skill required to work with preterm infants. Chapters on mobility and assistive technology also contain information relevant to specialized areas of practice. Reference and resource lists provide helpful information to practitioners who may continue to use the text. In the interest of manageable book size, information on low incidence conditions is presented only when illustrating a frame of reference, intervention approach, or practice setting.

I acknowledge with gratitude those who have contributed to this book and have guided its development. Many clinicians, too many to list, helped inspire the authors and me to present information that is helpful in developing professional skills. Clinicians and faculty who have guided me and assisted in developing the chapters include Beth Ball, Mary Stover, Debora Davidson, Jan Rogers, Lori Schoeppner, Cathy Tela, Dale Deubler, Diane Sainato, and Becky Selegue. I also acknowledge the original editors of the book, Pat Pratt and Anne Allen, who established a comprehensive text that described pediatric occupational therapy using theories and philosophies of the profession in combination with examples of clinical practice. Mosby/Elsevier editors have been resourceful and helpful in developing this edition. In particular, I appreciate the expertise and support of Kathy Falk, Melissa Kuster, and Rich Barber. Finally, I acknowledge my family, Greg, David, and Stephen, for their ongoing support, love, and patience. They have donated many "family hours" that have allowed me to complete this text.

Jane Case-Smith, EdD, OTR/L, FAOTA

Contents

SECTION IV

Areas of Pediatric Occupational Therapy Services

Occupational Therapy
for Children

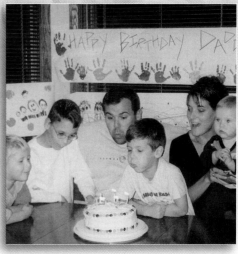

Knowledge Base of Occupational Therapy in Pediatrics

1 An Overview of Occupational Therapy for Children

Jane Case-Smith ■ Pamela Richardson ■ Winifred Schultz-Krohn

KEY TERMS

Clinical reasoning
Participation
Performance/activity
Client factors/
 impairment
Contextual factors

Assistive technology
Natural environments
Cross-cultural
 competence
Evidence-based practice

CHAPTER OBJECTIVES

1 Explain how occupational therapists use clinical reasoning in providing services to children.
2 Apply the International Classifications of Functioning, Disability, and Health to evaluation and intervention planning.
3 Define and illustrate occupational therapy intervention goals and strategies
4 Discuss models of service delivery used in a child's natural environment.
5 Describe elements of cross-cultural competence.
6 Discuss efficacious use of assistive technology.
7 Illustrate evidence-based occupational therapy practice with children.

Occupational therapists develop interventions from analysis of the interactions among a child's skills, activities and occupations, and the context for those occupations. When evaluating a child's performance, the therapist determines how limitations in performance relate to the child's innate ability, to external factors in the environment, or to discrepancies between the child's abilities and activity demands. Analysis of the interrelationships among environments, occupations, persons, and the goodness-of-fit of these elements is the basis for sound clinical decisions. At the same time that occupational therapists systematically analyze the child's occupational performance and social participation, they acknowledge that the spirit of the child determines who he or she is and will become.

This text presents theories, principles, and strategies that are used in occupational therapy with children. Its pages present intervention strategies to help children and families cope with disability and master occupations that have meaning to them. Although this theoretical and technical information is important to occupational therapy practice with children, it is childhood itself that creates meaning for the practitioner. Childhood is hopeful, joyful, and ever new. The spirit, the playfulness, and the joy of childhood create the context for occupational therapy with children.

The first section of this chapter describes how occupational therapists use clinical reasoning in evaluation and intervention planning. The process of evaluating participation, performance, client factors, and contextual factors is described. Interventions are presented that (1) improve performance and participation, (2) compensate for performance limitations through activity adaptations and assistive technology, (3) modify environments, or (4) promote children's participation and prevent disability through education. The second section of this chapter discusses best-practice concepts in pediatric occupational therapy.

CLINICAL REASONING

Occupational therapists use clinical reasoning to assess, plan, and provide intervention for children. This reasoning process enables occupational therapists to think broadly and deeply about their clients and to develop interventions that are holistic and effective. Six aspects of clinical reasoning have been identified (Fleming, 1994; Mattingly, 1994; Schell, 2003); although each is discrete, different aspects of clinical reasoning are used together. Table 1-1 illustrates each type of reasoning.

TABLE 1-1 Types of Clinical Reasoning

Scientific	Narrative	Pragmatic	Interactive	Ethical	Conditional
How is the disability affecting performance?	What story is this child in?	What practical issues are affecting service delivery?	How do I interact with this child and family?	What is the ethical action given a situation of competing interests?	What is the long-term vision for this child and family?
Given this condition, what assessment tools should be used?	What are the family's priorities?	Are resources available?	What is important to the child and family?	What are the benefits and risks to the child? Do the benefits warrant the risks?	What outcomes can I expect?
What practice model should be used to improve performance?	What family resources are available?	What are the practical concerns regarding where therapy services should be delivered?	What interests the child? What is fun?	When resources are limited, how should I prioritize services?	What outcomes are desired by the family?
What intervention strategies will improve performance?	What are family concerns?	What are the limitations in the time available for services?	What are the child's favorite play activities?	What action should I take when observing a situation that is unfair or poor treatment?	Given the resources and environments available to the child, what can be achieved?
What activities can be implemented to promote higher level function?	What are cultural considerations?	Is space available for intervention services?	What sensory systems should be primarily used in interaction?		How can therapy help the family achieve its dreams for their child?
What is developmentally appropriate and functionally desired for this client?	What routines and environments should be the focus of intervention?		How can I build a relationship with this child?		

Scientific Reasoning

This type of reasoning includes *diagnostic* and *procedural reasoning*. In scientific reasoning, occupational therapists use research evidence as well as their own experience and training. When given information about a child's diagnosis, the occupational therapist engages in diagnostic reasoning to plan what type of assessment to administer. For example, a child with autism is effectively assessed using structured observation in a natural setting and parent interview. It is not realistic to think that a child with autism can follow instructions and complete items on a standardized test. In comparison, when asked to evaluate a child with developmental coordination disorder, the therapist selects a standardized test knowing that he or she probably has the cognitive skills to follow multistep instructions during testing. Following interpretation of the assessment data, the occupational therapist uses scientific reasoning to select

the most appropriate intervention approaches and strategies.

Specific techniques and activities are selected based on the performance problems that the child exhibits or the issues inherent in the diagnosis. For example, Aaron with arthrogryposis has limited upper extremity range of motion and difficulty holding utensils or opening packages. He is unable to carry his books during school transitions. Using scientific reasoning, the therapist selects a compensatory/adaptation approach, recognizing that the condition, arthrogryposis, presents with fixed deformities and no significant improvements in range of motion and strength over time. In the case of Claire, who has a diagnosis of dyspraxia and poor handwriting, the occupational therapist selects a remedial approach to improve functional performance. The therapist reasons that with systematic practice and enhanced kinesthetic feedback from Claire's hand movements, her handwriting legibility and speed will improve.

Narrative Reasoning

Through narrative reasoning, the occupational therapist takes a broader view of the child, placing him or her into the context of family and community. When using narrative reasoning, the therapist asks, what story is the child in? Understanding the family context is important in narrative reasoning because it helps to determine the priorities for intervention and the outcomes that are most valued. All aspects of the context are considered, including the family's cultural background, composition, resources, and supports. For example, Teresa has Down syndrome, and her parents, who are both lawyers, are high achieving with financial resources and strong family supports. They are very motivated to implement therapeutic activities at home and request weekly home programs. The occupational therapist designs weekly home programs that meet the family's priorities and can be implemented on equipment available in the home.

Jack, who has cerebral palsy, is placed in a foster home with six other children. Despite the foster mother's best intentions, her full, hectic, and chaotic days prevent daily implementation of exercises designed to improve Jack's motor coordination. The occupational therapist reasons that any recommendations must be easily implemented in the foster parents' daily routines. The occupational therapist helps the family focus on one priority goal at a time. She lends the family toys for Jack to play with to reach the priority goal.

Pragmatic Reasoning

In pragmatic reasoning, the occupational therapist considers the practical resources available and problem-solves when resources do not seem adequate for ideal solutions. Pragmatic reasoning is needed when the family's health insurance will not pay for an adapted car seat and the occupational therapist finds an agency that lends adapted car seats. Pragmatic reasoning is also used when the parents cannot attend therapy sessions and the occupational therapist must problem-solve the best form of service delivery and communication. A child's intervention program is always influenced by pragmatic concerns. Resourceful practical reasoning helps the occupational therapist problem-solve through barriers of time constraints, limited financial resources, limited space, or limited personnel. Compromise and negotiation may be required in this type of reasoning.

Interactive Reasoning

Interactive reasoning is critical to therapeutic use of the self. The occupational therapist analyzes how to connect with the child. What interests the child? What does the child attend to most? What is play and fun? Interactive reasoning is used to establish a relationship with the child and family. By engaging the child, his or her participation in the intervention program increases. Zach loves fire trucks and his face lights up at the mention of one. To engage Zach, therapeutic activities are designed so that he climbs in, over, and on imaginary fire trucks. Graded activities to improve his skills were embedded in scenarios of racing to and putting out imaginary fires.

Cory is diagnosed with autism and is easily overwhelmed by sensory stimulation. He is hypersensitive to touch and auditory input. The occupational therapist uses a soft, low voice when communicating with him. In interaction, she carefully applies a firm touch and only touches him after she has prepared him for the stimulus. She coaches his teacher to implement these same interaction methods; this close attention to appropriate interaction helps to improve Cory's engagement and attention to the classroom activities.

Ethical Reasoning

Ethical reasoning can involve weighing the risks and benefits of a specific intervention approach or strategy (Schell, 2003). Occupational therapists use ethical reasoning to prioritize care when time or other resources are limited or when the occupational therapist observes actions of other team members that are in conflict with the program's values or the client's goals. The occupational therapist may need to use ethical reasoning more when resources are scarce. Ethical reasoning may have priority over other types of reasoning when a child is at risk or the therapist is in a moral dilemma. Ethical dilemmas may be experienced when a program's therapeutic resources and services do not meet a family's need. When children need very specialized services or assistive technology, the therapist engages in ethical reasoning to decide the boundaries of her or his role and the role of the agency and to make appropriate referrals to help the family gain additional resources. When insurance has lifetime caps on reimbursement, a long-term plan for using the family's coverage is needed and may require that the child receive less than optimal intensity and duration of occupational therapy services. Careful use of a family's resources is both a pragmatic and ethical concern.

Conditional Reasoning

Conditional reasoning (Fleming, 1994; Mattingly, 1994) enables the occupational therapist to view the big picture. Through conditional reasoning, the occupational therapist assimilates his or her understanding of the client, the context, the anticipated activities, the family's priorities, and the envisioned future to make optimal intervention decisions. An intervention activity that seems helpful at the moment may not be useful when the long-term outcome is considered. For example, learning to trace letters is not a functional goal for a child who will never be able to handwrite legibly. If a child will be using the computer for testing and written assignments, focusing occupational therapy on teaching keyboarding skills rather than handwriting performance becomes important. When parents have limited intellectual skills and did not graduate from high school, obtaining high-end technology devices for the child that require programming and frequent troubleshooting may not be appropriate.

Summary

In clinical reasoning an occupational therapist considers multiple perspectives of the child and family including their values, interests, priorities, and contexts. Through this reasoning process, the occupational therapist analyzes the relevant dimensions of a situation to arrive at an optimal solution. Most decisions in services for children are made by teams, adding to the complexity of how decisions are made and what perspectives are used when making decisions. Mattingly and Fleming (1994) explained that occupational therapists reason by considering all of these dimensions simultaneously. For example, in the case of an eight-year-old with ataxia, intervention strategies are selected by analyzing the clinical problem (e.g., poor balance), the child's priority (e.g., riding a bike), and pragmatic contextual concerns (the home suitability for bike riding and the family's resources for purchasing a bicycle).

In another example, the occupational therapist uses pragmatic and conditional reasoning to recommend a service delivery schedule for a preterm infant in a home-based early intervention program. The therapist decides that once-a-month monitoring versus direct services is appropriate because the infant was healthy during her neonatal intensive care unit (NICU) stay (scientific reasoning), has attentive parents in a home with resources and supports in place (conditional and narrative reasoning), and the therapist knows that the home-based specialist will implement the suggestions for therapeutic activities (conditional reasoning). A different decision about service delivery may have been made if only one aspect of clinical reasoning were applied.

OCCUPATIONAL THERAPY EVALUATION

Evaluation involves systematic data collection and analysis to guide development of an intervention plan. Standardized and nonstandardized instruments are used to gain relevant information about a child's abilities, performance, contexts, and the interaction between the child's abilities and the demands of the environment. Evaluation should focus on the issues identified by parents, teachers, physicians, or through observations, but also should be comprehensive in order for the therapist to gain a thorough understanding of the problem(s) and its effects of the child's performance and participation. Occupational therapy evaluation is described in depth in Chapters 7 and 8. The evaluation process is briefly described in the following sections.

Participation in Occupations

Using a top-down approach (Trombly, 1995), the occupational therapist begins to assess the child by gaining an understanding of the child's *level of participation in daily occupations and routines* with family, other caregiving adults, and peers (Figure 1-1). Initially, the therapist surveys multiple sources to acquire a sense of the child's performance and to form a picture of the child. This initial picture is based on (1) concerns of the parents, (2) concerns of other adults who interact with the child, (3) informal observations of the child in his or her natural environment, (4) administration of a screening instrument, and (5) review of evaluation reports written about the child by other professionals. This background information helps the occupational therapist target specific occupations and performance patterns to further assess.

Participation in occupation

Play

ADL

IADL

School

Performance skills, activities, activity limitations, activity demands

Motor

Process

Interaction

Client factors, body functions and structures, impairments

Sensory responsiveness

Sensory integration

Range of motion

Strength

Eye-hand coordination

Manipulation

Praxis

Visual perception

Contextual factors

Cultural

Physical

Social

FIGURE 1-1 Occupational therapy evaluation of children.

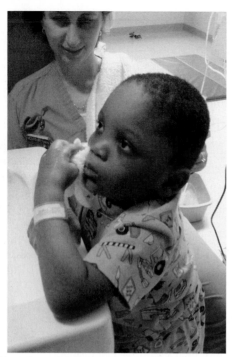

FIGURE 1-2 Evaluation of the child's participation in activities of daily living includes observation in naturally occurring scenarios to assess the child's performance, the natural content for performance, and the supports available. (Courtesy of Jayne Shepherd and Sheri Michael.)

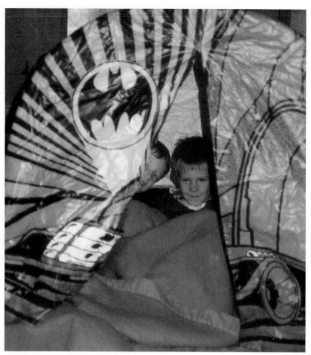

FIGURE 1-3 Special places and favorite play partners have high significance to young children.

Identifying levels of participation involves assessing the child's ability to participate in multiple environments and in various social roles. In occupational therapy with children, participation in *play, activities of daily living (ADL), instrumental ADL, and school occupations* is of greatest interest (Figure 1-2). Initial assessment of the child's participation also involves evaluating the environment to identify problems or potential problems that appear to affect the child's participation. Assessment of the environment helps to determine the discrepancy between the child's performance and expected performance.

To assess a child's participation in his or her natural environments, the occupational therapist uses narrative reasoning—that is, the therapist identifies which story he or she is in with the child. Over time, the story unfolds as the therapist gains understanding of the child, family, and context. Mattingly (1994) explains that prospective stories are useful because they give the therapist a starting point for evaluation; however, the therapist willingly adjusts and adapts the story as new information becomes known. This unique story assists the occupational therapist in identifying what is significant and meaningful to the child (Figure 1-3). The occupational therapist uses the story to create meaningful experiences that engage the child and are valued by the child and his or her family. For example, the child who loves to go fishing with a grandfather may be highly motivated by a pretend fishing

expedition in a "rocking boat" in the preschool's gross motor room. Narrative reasoning helps to establish intervention priorities through an understanding of what the family values, and it allows the therapist to orient further evaluation and planning to those priorities. For example, a rural family who owns a farm may want to focus on their child's physical skills and mobility, hoping that, as a youth, he or she can contribute to the farm chores. Parents who are teachers may primarily be interested in the child's literacy, believing that reading skills will contribute most to their child's vocational potential.

Performance of Activities

With an understanding of the child's participation and the context, the therapist continues the evaluation process to define *specific abilities and limitations in performance of activities*. Therapists use quantitative and qualitative observational assessments to judge performance. In addition to documenting whether expected activities for the child's age are missing, delayed, or deficient, occupational therapists note whether the performance becomes possible or moves to a higher level when the child is given assistance. Is the child able to perform the activity with adapted equipment or assistive technology? When the child performs well with adapted equipment or environmental accommodations, the activity is not considered limited and is probably not an appropriate focus of intervention. Another consideration is that children perform differently in different environments and when possible skills should be assessed in each of their primary environments. For example, a child with physical disabilities and high distractibility is independent in self-feeding at home; however, because of the noise level, physical arrangement, and time restrictions, this child requires assistance to eat in the school cafeteria.

Performance areas of greatest interest to occupational therapists are *motor, process,* and *communication/ interaction skills.* To identify missing or delayed performance skills, the therapist can administer a standardized test, such as the Peabody Developmental Motor Scales (2nd edition, Folio & Fewell, 2000), Developmental Test of Visual Perception–2 (Hammill, Pearson, & Voress, 1993), or the Evaluation Tool for Children's Handwriting (Amundson, 1996). Standardized tests are helpful for analyzing the basis for activity limitations and impairments in client factors (described in the following section).

Activity and participation limitations can be measured by quality of performance, degree of assistance required, safety, and developmental level (Holm, Rogers, & James, 2003). Occupational therapists observe children playing or performing in the classroom and at home as part of this evaluative process. Careful observation allows the therapist to understand the qualitative aspects of performance and to determine the relative influence of the environment and the innate abilities of the child. The therapist uses scientific reasoning to analyze discrepancies between the child's performance and activity demands. Using pragmatic reasoning, the therapist identifies supports that would enable the child to achieve higher-level performance and greater participation.

After a period of observing the child, the therapist may provide facilitation or cues to determine how therapeutic methods of assistance influence the child's performance. Assessing the quality of assisted performance helps the therapist judge how the child may respond to social, sensory, or physical assistance, support, or accommodations. Interpreting the child's response to assistance or adaptation of the activity allows the therapist to refine her ideas about which interventions and environmental modifications to apply and what outcomes are realistic.

Interactive reasoning is used at this stage of evaluation to discover what interests and motivates the child (Figure 1-4). The therapist gathers information about the child's temperament and personality that may be helpful in building a relationship with the child. The therapist seeks to understand the child's interests to build an alliance with the child. Clues from parents and teachers are sought to determine which sensory systems are preferred for learning, which play interests are favored, and how the child's temperament influences his or her actions.

As the occupational therapist analyzes performance, she or he uses narrative reasoning to continue to refine the child's story. The therapist seeks to identify activities

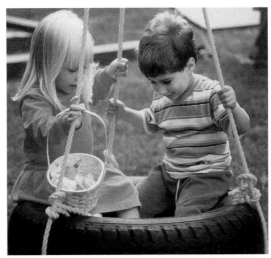

FIGURE 1-4 The interests of the child are influenced by siblings and his or her physical surroundings.

that have the greatest meaning to the child and those that relate to the child's perceived self-esteem. Generally, qualitative social or sensory aspects of an activity become most important in developing an intervention plan. What motivates the child to perform, and to what does he or she attend? Does the child exert more effort when music is played? Does the child demonstrate greater skill and motivation with peers or adults involved in the activity? Does the child enjoy animals? Would including a pet in therapeutic activities elicit the child's optimal participation? *Narrative reasoning* helps the therapist identify what outcomes the family desires. As in the initial assessment of participation, the family's values and the activities that are most important to the child become the priorities of the program that is developed.

Client Factors

With an explicit understanding of performance patterns and activity limitations, the therapist seeks to uncover the impairments associated with these limitations. The International Classification of Functioning, Disability, and Health (ICF) (World Health Organization [WHO], 2001) defines impairment as a loss or a deficit of body structure or body function (including physiological and psychological). At this level of evaluation, the therapist identifies client factors that are impaired or missing, thus limiting performance and participation. Examples of factors measured at this level of performance are *range of motion (passive or active), strength, muscle tone, balance, sensory responsiveness, sensory integration, praxis, manipulation, eye-hand coordination, and visual perceptual skills. Sensory processing and preferences* are assessed to determine how sensory responsiveness is affecting behaviors. The occupational therapist also identifies the underlying factors that are strengths and those on which the child relies to perform an activity. The therapist explores the associations between client factors and activity demands that may explain the performance problems and identifies the client factors that have the greatest potential to improve the level of participation in age-appropriate, desired occupations.

Scientific reasoning is used when assessing client factors and linking the identified impairments to the performance and participation limitations. The therapist asks, how are impairments causing the activity limitations, and if client factors improve, would performance improve? When client factors are fixed or unlikely to change, the focus of therapy becomes compensation and modifying the environment to improve the child's participation with the impairment.

Contextual Factors

Occupational therapists evaluate the contexts in which the child learns, plays, and interacts. The child's natural environment is the context for his or her learning and development and should be the context for assessment. Evaluating performance in multiple contexts (e.g., home, school, daycare, and other relevant community settings) allows the therapist to appreciate how different contexts affect the child's performance and participation.

Contexts important to consider when evaluating children include *physical, social, and cultural factors*. The physical space available to the child can facilitate or constrain exploration and play. Family is the primary social context for the young child, then peers become important aspects of the social context at preschool and school ages. Tools have been developed (e.g., the Nursing Child Assessment Feeding and Teaching Scales [Sumner & Spietz, 1994]) to assess parent-child interaction in the young child. The interaction between parents and infants is known to have a powerful effect on development and personality (McCollum, 2002; McCollum & Hemmeter, 1997) and should be assessed, at least informally, in infant evaluation.

The occupational therapist evaluates physical and social contextual factors using the following questions:

- Does the environment allow physical access?
- Are materials to promote development available?
- Does the environment provide an optimal amount of supervision?
- Is the environment safe?
- Are a variety of spaces and sensory experiences available?
- Is the environment conducive to social interaction?
- Are opportunities for exploration, play, and learning available?
- Is positive adult support available and developmentally appropriate?

The family's cultural background has a multitude of implications for evaluation and intervention. Cultural values that are important to the occupational therapy perspective include how the family (1) values independent versus interdependent performance, (2) has a sense of time and future versus past orientation, (3) is forward thinking versus lives for the moment, (4) makes decisions that influence family members, (5) defines health, wellness, disability, illness, and (6) practices customs related to dress, food, traditions, and religion (Lynch & Hanson, 1997). Often these values vary by cultural group; they also vary in individuals within a cultural group, depending on level of acculturation—that is, the degree to which a family has assimilated into the dominant culture (Garcia Coll & Magnuson, 2000).

The occupational therapist uses scientific reasoning to assess how the environmental and activity demands facilitate or constrain the child's performance. Interactive and narrative reasoning are used to gain an understanding and appreciation of the family's culture, lifestyle, parenting style, and values. These contextual factors have a profound influence on the child's development and need to be considered in the intervention program.

Summary

Through comprehensive evaluation, the therapist analyzes the discrepancies between performance and activity demands. She or he identifies potential outcomes that fit the child and family's story. By moving from assessment of participation to analysis of performance, client factors and contexts, the therapist gains a solid understanding of the strengths, concerns, and problems of the individuals involved (e.g., child, parent, or caregiver; family members; teachers). The occupational therapist also understands how to interact with the child to build a trusting and a positive relationship.

INTERVENTION PLANNING

Interpreting the information gained from the evaluation to plan intervention requires that the therapist further analyze the child's occupational performance and participation from the perspective of a future orientation. The following questions guide the therapist's development of an intervention plan.

Guiding Questions

What are the priorities of the family and the child? Which areas of occupation are of greatest concern and value to the family? Families frequently respond that they are more concerned about a child's participation in social activities and interaction with family members than with performance of activities of daily living.

What skills does the child need to meet occupational roles? What skills does the child currently possess and what skills will allow the child to successfully meet his or her environment's demands? A child who is transitioning from elementary to middle school may need to develop strategies for organizing materials and assignments from several different classes, as well as for moving from class to class in an efficient manner. Organizational skills would become the focus of the therapist's intervention.

What developmental trajectory does this child demonstrate? The child's rate of development is a good predictor of future development. A 5-year-old child who displays gross motor skills commensurate to a 7-month-old infant may never reach age-appropriate skills of walking, running, or hopping. The occupational therapist must consider what modifications will allow this child to compensate for limited gross motor skills instead of focusing the intervention plan solely on the development of a specific skill.

What are influences of the performance contexts? How does the environment affect the child's engagement in activity and performance? For example, adaptive positioning and mobility strategies may differ in the home, classroom, and playground. Use of adaptive equipment may also vary according to the child, parent, and teacher preferences in various environments.

Which theoretical models of practice or frames of reference guide the intervention? Selection and application of the practice model guide the planning process. Behavioral approaches may be combined with visual cueing to structure the routines and environments of a child with autism. A therapist may use social learning strategies to support the child's social and play interactions with peers (Vygotsky, 1978; Wolfberg, 2003). Use of the sensory integration practice model guides the therapist in modifying the child's environment, implementing an adapted routine with a balance of sensory activities, and adapting specific activities to meet the child's sensory needs.

What is the nature of the disability? By understanding how client factors affect performance limitations, intervention strategies can focus on the constraining factors. A child with autism may have difficulty processing auditory language or may have auditory hypersensitivity. This necessitates a focus on modeling activities and use of visual rather than verbal cues as the primary avenue for interacting with the child. A child with strong sensory seeking behaviors may need to have these sensory needs met before sedentary tasks that require focused attention.

What adult support is needed to sustain improvements in the child's performance? Generally other adults in the child's environment spend more time with the child than the therapist. The therapist coaches parents and teachers to implement the intervention strategies designed to help the child reach agreed-upon outcomes. These training and consultation activities involve modeling for and instructing parents and teachers, then encouraging and reinforcing their efforts. For the family who brings home a medically fragile infant from the NICU, the therapist will emphasize collaborative consultation and training roles, teaching family members holding and positioning techniques to facilitate feeding, sleeping, play, and socialization (Richardson, 2003).

The next step in intervention planning is to formulate child outcome statements. Child goals or outcome statements are generally written in collaboration with an interdisciplinary team of professionals and family members.

Writing Collaborative Outcome Statements

Performance limitations are often the basis for establishing short-term goals and objectives, and participation restrictions are often the basis for establishing long-term outcomes. Outcome statements concerning the activities the child will perform include the environmental conditions, environmental modifications, and activity assistance (e.g., adaptive equipment) to ensure the child's optimal participation. To formulate outcome statements, the occupational therapist, interdisciplinary team, and family members envision how the child can participate in new social roles and how he or she can more fully participate in current ones. For example, which interventions will enable the child to play independently on the playground, to participate in a regular education classroom for a full day, or to make new friends? The occupational therapist contributes to the vision because he or she understands the possibilities and has experiences with similar children.

To establish meaningful outcomes with the family, the occupational therapist uses conditional and pragmatic reasoning (see Table 1-1). In conditional reasoning, the therapist assimilates all the information about the child and his or her occupations and environments to create a future picture of the child. Fleming (1994) defined conditional reasoning as forming an image of future life possibilities for the person. The child's impairments are understood, as are the constraints of the environment. The use of adaptive equipment, compensatory techniques, and environmental accommodations are all considered in developing a vision for the child and an outcome of increased participation.

Pragmatic reasoning is also important in intervention planning (Schell, 2003). Potential outcomes may not be feasible, depending on funding, time, and system constraints. Certain outcomes may be more practical, more realistic, or more appropriate when considering these constraints. For example, will the family support the child's use of an augmentative communication device? Will family members be able to physically manage a power wheelchair weighing 40 pounds? Is the parent interested in and does he or she have the time to implement a therapeutic program at home? Through pragmatic reasoning, the therapist, in collaboration with the team, identifies the most practical ways to reach meaningful outcomes.

Scientific reasoning to plan intervention also involves the application of research evidence related to the child's diagnosis, identified problem, or described outcomes. Research evidence (i.e., findings from clinical trials and experimental studies) guides the therapist's selection of an intervention approach or practice model. The therapist also uses empirical evidence to analyze the probability that a specific intervention approach will be successful and to estimate how much benefit can be expected when a specific approach is used.

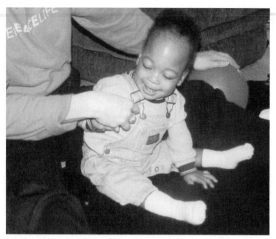

FIGURE 1-5 Goal-directed activity engages the child and elicits a higher level performance. (Courtesy of Jayne Shepherd and Audrey Kane.)

INTERVENTION: PURPOSES AND STRATEGIES

With goals established, the occupational therapist continues to use clinical reasoning to design and implement therapeutic activities. Almost all intervention activities with children have playful qualities, because play is an occupation of high relevance and importance to a child. The child who is playing is active, goal directed, and intrinsically motivated (Bundy, 2002; Rubin, Fein, & Vandenberg, 1983) (Figure 1-5). During play a child exhibits an internal sense of control (Bundy, 1997). With a play goal established through collaboration of the occupational therapist and child, the child is given choices about the activity to further motivate him or her. Play within a therapy session begins with the child's current skills level, then the therapist guides the activity to a point at which it becomes challenging for the child, with the goal of eliciting a higher level response. The therapist grades the task to focus on specific skills and supports performance through modeling, cueing, physical assistance, and reinforcement. The therapist may

need to adapt or modify the activity to enable the child to accomplish it.

Intervention focuses on enhancing a child's ability to perform everyday activities and to participate in multiple environments. Intervention includes the following aims:

1 Improving functional performance
2 Adapting activities or providing assistive technology
3 Modifying environments
4 Promoting children's participation and preventing disability through education (Table 1-2)

Improving Functional Performance
Using Occupation as Means

The focus of most occupational therapy interventions with children is to improve performance and participation. Childhood is a period of great change, and occupational therapists guide that change in positive directions. Various practice models or frames of reference guide how the occupational therapist approaches

---

TABLE 1-2   Intervention Purposes and Strategies

Intervention Purpose	Strategies
Improving performance	Using occupation as means
	Graded activities: the "just right" challenge
	Preparation for activities
	Augmented and individualized sensory cueing and feedback
	Therapeutic use of self
	Caregiver and teacher education and consultation
Adapting activities or providing assistive technology	Compensatory strategies
	Concurrent developmental and functional goals
	Educating adults who support the use of compensatory strategies
Environment modifications	Improving the fit between child and environment
	Consultation and negotiation with adults in the child's environment
Promoting participation and preventing disability through education	Educating other professionals and administrators
	System change in the child's community

intervention to improve occupational performance. The authors of this text in (e.g., Chapters 3, 11, and 16) and others (e.g., Kramer & Hinojosa, 1999) explain these practice models. To establish new skills, the therapist uses occupation as means. An activity is selected that has meaning for the child and successfully engages the child. The activity generally has a purpose or goal that is valued by the individual child. The therapist often entices the child into an activity by defining its purpose. "Let's build a castle." "Would you like to make a bracelet?" "Can you swing to the edge of the mat and pick up some dog bones to feed our hungry dog?" The theme must have meaning to the child to enhance and sustain the child's efforts (Trombly, 1995). Humphry (2002) explained that young children are more inclined to imitate activities that seem to have purpose. Humphry's perspective implies that eliciting children's imitations of actions is more successful when that action has a clear purpose and meaning (i.e., is embedded in an occupation such as play).

In addition, for the child to effectively learn a skill, the activity needs to be integrated into his or her daily routines. If first learned and practiced in a clinic setting with the occupational therapist, the skill must then be integrated into the child's daily routine through extended practice in natural environments. Skills that are first learned within the child's natural environment can easily become part of the child's daily behavior and generalize to a variety of situations and contexts (Cripe & Venn, 1997; McCollum, 2002).

Graded Activities: The "Just Right" Challenge

An activity that is a child's "just right" challenge has the following elements: (1) the activity engages and motivates the child, (2) it challenges the child's current skills, and (3) it can be mastered with the child's focused effort. Occupational therapists select highly adaptable activities and, as a result, can carefully raise or lower the task's difficulty level based on the child's performance. To promote change in the child, the activity must be challenging and create a degree of stress. The stress is meant to elicit a higher level of response. The therapist's interactions with the child are similar to those of a dance: the therapist poses a problem or challenge to the child, who is then motivated by that challenge and responds. The therapist facilitates or supports the child's action so that he or she successfully responds at a higher level. The therapist then gives feedback regarding the action and presents another problem of greater or lesser difficulty, based on the success of the child's response. Cognitive, sensory, motor, perceptual, or social aspects of the activity may be made easier or more difficult (Box 1-1). By precisely assessing the adequacy of the child's response, the occupational therapist finds the just right challenge.

BOX 1-1   Grading an Activity: Challenging and Eliciting Full Participation

Aaron, a 10-year-old child with autism, participated in a cooking activity with the occupational therapist and three peers. The children were proceeding in an organized manner—sharing cooking supplies and verbalizing each step of the activity. As they proceeded, Aaron had great difficulty participating in the task; the materials were messy, and the social interaction was frequent and unpredictable. He performed best when the activity was highly structured, the instructions were very clear, and the social interaction was kept at a minimum. To help him participate at a comfortable level, the occupational therapist suggested that his contribution to the activity be to put away supplies and retrieve new ones. The other children were asked to give him specific visual and verbal instructions as to what they needed and what should be replaced in the refrigerator or cupboard. With this new rule in place, the children gave simple and concrete instructions that Aaron could follow. Importantly, this strategy included the support of his peers to elicit an optimal level of participation and could be generalized to other small-group activities involving Aaron and his peers.

Preparation for Activities

At times, the therapist focuses on the body functions and structures that appear to be limiting performance. For example, a child with cerebral palsy may experience tightness in the shoulder girdle. Certain passive techniques may be used to elongate and relax the muscles around the shoulder to improve range of motion and freedom of movement. This increased range can allow the child to participate in a reaching or weight-bearing activity, which also helps to elongate tight muscles and can improve shoulder range of motion. An activity designed to increase range of motion should be purposeful and meaningful to gain the child's participation and effort. The biomechanical goal (increased range of shoulder motion) can be achieved when the child perceives the activity as a cognitive goal (e.g., placing magnetic letters on a vertical board to spell words), a playful goal (e.g., lining up toy bears on the top shelf), or a psychosocial goal (e.g., participating in a contest to see who can stack blocks highest). A number of studies have demonstrated that exercises embedded in goal-directed, purposeful activity are more effective that rote exercise (Lin, Wu, Tickle-Degnen, & Coster, 1997; Nelson et al., 1996).

Occupational therapists often intervene when children have difficulties with sensory responsivity and modulation that interferes with occupational performance. Children with hypersensitivity may need calming or help in organizing responses before they can engage in an activity. The therapist may begin a session by applying linear, rhythmic vestibular input or deep pressure to calm the child and improve his or her focus and attention. Sensory preparation is a well-accepted therapeutic principle (Koomar & Bundy, 2002; Miller & Heaphy, 1998; Miller, Reisman, McIntosh, & Simon, 2001). Although the benefits of vestibular, tactile, and proprioceptive input related to a child's performance lack empirical evidence, practitioners testify to the immediate and powerful effects of these proximal senses (Kimball, 1999; Koomar & Bundy, 2002).

Augmented and Individualized Sensory Cueing and Feedback

To promote the individual child's performance during an activity, the therapist uses a variety of techniques. The techniques are selected based on the child's learning style and patterns of performance. The therapist uses the child's preferred sensory systems to support performance that appears deficient. The therapist may use a multisensory approach to cue and guide performance and to provide augmented feedback about performance. For example, the child with visual perceptual problems may benefit from manipulating cutout wooden letters to learn manuscript handwriting. For the child in the autism spectrum, visual cueing or modeling are preferred strategies for teaching new skills. The child with autism often demonstrates more appropriate and higher-level behaviors when presented with a picture card demonstrating the behaviors expected in an activity (Schopler, 1994; Schopler, Mesibov, & Hearsey, 1995). The child with low muscle tone and a poor sense of his or her body's movements in space can use heavy objects or a weighted vest to enhance sensory feedback from movement.

Examples include finger rings that can be worn during a keyboarding activity to enhance the child's awareness of individual finger movements. The rings add weight to a child's fingers and can enhance proprioceptive feedback with movement. The therapists can also apply Herzog keys (e.g., key inserts with small bumps to help the child identify the home row keys). These keys give tactile cueing to help the child identify where to place his or her fingers. Sensory feedback is also used to reinforce action; for example, the occupational therapist can set up a block tower that can be knocked over when the child reaches beyond his or her baseline upper extremity range. Sensory feedback can help the child compensate for limited perception and delayed performance by augmenting the sensory systems that are used most in learning new skills. For instance, if a child is a visual learner and has difficulty processing auditory information, the therapist may emphasize visual input during an activity by providing pictures of what comes next and what action is an appropriate response.

Therapeutic Use of Self

The occupational therapist establishes a relationship with the child that encourages and motivates. The therapist becomes invested in the child's success and makes evident to the child the importance of his or her efforts. The therapist first establishes a relationship of trust (Bundy & Koomar, 2002; Tickle-Degnen & Coster, 1995) (Figure 1-6). Although the therapist presents challenges and asks the child to take risks, the therapist also supports or facilitates the performance so that the child succeeds or feels okay when he or she fails. This trust enables the child to feel safe and willing to take risks. The occupational therapist shows interest in the child, enjoys his or her personality, and values his or her preferences and goals. The child's unique traits and behaviors become the basis for designing activities that will engage the child and provide the just right challenge. By individualizing activities so that the child feels important and by grading the activity to match the child's abilities, the child achieves mastery and a sense of accomplishment.

A child's self-esteem and self-image are influenced by skill achievement and the child's success in mastering tasks. Generally, the intrinsic sense of mastery is a stronger reinforcement to the child than external rewards, such as verbal praise or other contingent reward systems. The occupational therapist vigilantly attends to the child's performance during an activity to provide precise levels of support that enable the child to succeed in the activity.

The occupational therapist remains highly sensitive to the child's emerging self-actualization and helps the team and family provide activities and environments that support the child's sense of self as an efficacious person.

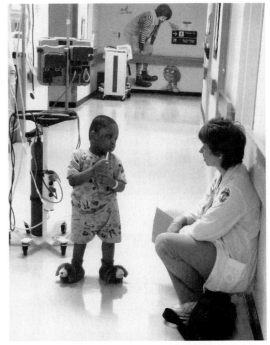

FIGURE 1-6 A hallway conversation helps to establish the therapist's relationship with the child. (Courtesy of Jayne Shepherd and Sheri Michael.)

Self-actualization, as defined by Fidler and Fidler (1978), occurs through successful coping with problems in the everyday environment. It implies more than the ability to respond to others; self-actualization means that the child initiates play activities, investigates problems, and initiates social interactions. A child with a positive sense of self seeks experiences that are challenging, responds to play opportunities, masters developmentally appropriate tasks, and forms and sustains relationships with peers and adults.

Caregiver and Teacher Education and Consultation

Children acquire skills through practice. The high-level responses that a child demonstrates in a therapy session must be practiced and reinforced in the child's natural environments to become part of his or her repertoire. Often the child's performance continues to require some cueing or assistance from an adult (Figure 1-7). It also may require specific materials that offer the just right challenge. The occupational therapist may suggest that a student use a slant board in the classroom to improve posture (i.e., it helps to encourage upright posture), wrist extension and grasping pattern (i.e., wrist extension is required to write on a slanted surface), and eye tracking (i.e., eye tracking is generally easier when the eyes are oriented straight ahead). In an example in a preschool classroom, the occupational therapist suggests that the teacher implements a calming sensory strategy for a very active, distractible 4-year-old boy during the sedentary story time. The therapist suggests that the child be provided with deep pressure by wearing a weighted vest during story time (Fertel-Daly, Bedell, & Hinojosa,

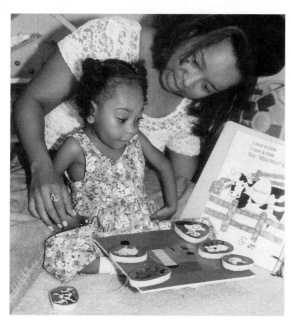

FIGURE 1-7 Verbal, physical, and visual cueing are used to elicit the child's full participation in the activity.

2001; Vanderberg, 2001). This successful sensory strategy is then implemented on a daily basis to encourage the child to attend and listen during story time. Soon he requests the vest on his own when he feels disorganized, which signifies an improved ability to self-regulate according to his sensory needs.

Consultation with teachers, parents, assistants, child-care providers, or any adults who spend a significant amount of time with the child is an essential ingredient of service delivery. The therapist helps to develop solutions that fit into the child's natural environment and promote the child's transfer of new skills into a variety of environments. Yet the skills demonstrated in a therapy session within the preschool classroom with the support of the therapist do not automatically generalize to other environments. It is important that the child feels supported to try new skills in other environments. Sometimes simply informing caregivers and teachers about an emerging skill or a new activity is sufficient for others to encourage and support practice in other environments. It is most helpful for the therapist to share the level of support or type of facilitation and cueing that the child needs to perform at a higher level. As the therapist teaches other adults how to implement activities with the child, the therapist adjusts to the adult's learning style and learning preferences. The therapist uses pragmatic reasoning to judge how much time and effort the teacher or parent will be able to give to an individualized activity with a child.

Pragmatic reasoning is also used to determine when it is appropriate to teach strategies that involve some risk to the child when implemented improperly. If a highly specific, technical activity is needed to elicit a targeted response, then teaching others may not be appropriate, and a less complex and less risky strategy should be transferred to the caregivers to implement. For example, therapists often use therapy balls to help children develop balance reactions and postural stability. However, when a child has difficulty maintaining postural alignment without the therapist's handling, teaching others to implement balance activities with the child on a therapy ball is not advised. Teaching parents, teachers, and assistants to work on the child's balance using a stable surface can provide a similar benefit and present less risk to the child. Teachers and caregivers need to feel confident about and successful in applying a strategy recommended by the therapist in order to implement that strategy on a routine basis.

Adapting Activities or Providing Assistive Technology
Compensatory Strategies

Occupational therapists help children compensate for delays or deficits in performance by adapting activities or applying assistive technology (Figure 1-8). Compensatory approaches allow a child to accomplish an activity

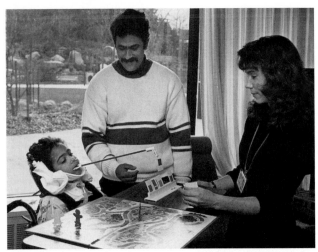

FIGURE 1-8 The occupational therapist designed a mouth stick and game board setup so that the child can play the game with his father.

in an adapted way or with the use of technology. Adapted techniques for play activities include switch toys, battery-powered toys, enlarged handles on puzzle pieces, or magnetic pieces that can easily fit together. In activities of daily living, adapted techniques may be used when the child first learns to dress. For example, the therapist may suggest that children with poor balance dress while sitting in the bedroom's corner or lying in bed. A child with hemiparesis is taught to how to stabilize his shirt to button. (Chapter 15 offers many examples of adapted techniques to increase a child's independence in self-care.)

Adapted techniques are also used at school to help the child successfully participate in school occupations such as managing and manipulating materials, transitioning between classes, moving within the classroom, and eating independently in the cafeteria. Examples of adapted techniques used to increase function at school are methods to grasp pencils or scissors or one-handed techniques for eating, for handling books and papers, and for writing.

Generally, most compensatory methods incorporate adapted equipment or assistive technology. Technology is pervasive throughout society and has become increasingly versatile so that it is easily adaptable to a child's individualized needs. (Technology solutions are described throughout this text and are the focus of Chapters 15, 18, and 19.) Appropriate use of assistive technology involves thorough assessment of the activity to be performed, the individual's abilities, and the environmental constraints and supports.

Low-technology solutions are often applied to enhance self-care performance or to increase a child's independence in self-care. Examples include built-up handles on utensils, weighted cups, elastic shoelaces, and electric toothbrushes. High-technology solutions are often used to increase mobility or functional communi-

cation. Examples include power wheelchairs, augmentative communication devices, and computers.

High technology is becoming increasingly available and typically involves computer processing and switch or keyboard access (e.g., augmentative communication devices). Occupational therapists frequently support the use of assistive technology by identifying the most appropriate device or system and features of the system. They often help to obtain funding to purchase the device, set up or program the system, train others to use it, monitor its use, and make themselves available to problem-solve the inevitable technology issues that arise. High technology for children is carefully selected so that it can grow with the child. For example, the size of the wheelchair is adjustable, or the number of keys on the augmentative communication device can be increased. Assistive technology is further addressed in the section on best practices.

Concurrent Developmental and Functional Goals

The role of assistive technology with children is not simply to compensate for a missing or delayed function; it is also used to promote development in targeted performance areas. Research (e.g., Butler, 1986, 1988; Campos & Bertenthal, 1987) has demonstrated that increased mobility with the use of a power wheelchair increases social and perceptual skills (see Chapter 19). The use of an augmentative communication device can enhance language and social skills and may prevent behavioral problems common in children who have limited means of communicating. Therefore the occupational therapist selects compensatory methods that not only enable the child to participate more fully in functional or social activities but also enhance the development of skills related to a specific occupational area. For example, when a child has a physical disability with motor impairments, the therapist may set up a computer game as a play activity. The computer game simulates reading a book to promote preliteracy skills and uses an expanded keyboard to promote computer skills (Figure 1-9).

Educating Adults Who Support the Use of Compensatory Strategies

The application of technology involves educating parents, care providers, and teachers. This education needs to include how to use the technology, how to adapt or adjust it, and how to troubleshoot when it does not work. The therapist can model its use and walk the parents or teachers through different scenarios of how the device can be used.

Assistive technology solutions continually change as devices become more advanced and more versatile.

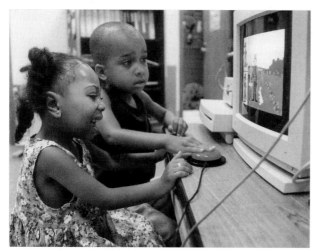

FIGURE 1-9   A switch activates the computer program that simulates a storybook.

Current technology offers an array of choices in devices with varying levels of complexity. The occupational therapist needs to be sensitive to the learning needs of those who will support the use of this technology. Often, it is important to talk through and model each step in the use of the technology and to remain available and supportive to others when the technology is first implemented. Strategies for integrating the technology into a classroom or home environment (i.e., discussing the ways the device can be used throughout the day) help to derive the greatest benefit. All team members need to update their skills continuously so that they have a working knowledge of emerging technology. (See the following section of this chapter.)

Summary

Compensatory methods promote a child's functional performance and developmental skills across domains. The following statements guide the occupational therapist in the use of compensatory approaches and assistive technology.

- Compensatory strategies should be selected according to the child's individual abilities (intrinsic variables), expected or desired activities, and environmental constraints (extrinsic variables).
- Techniques and technology should be adaptable and flexible so that devices can be used across environments and over time as the child develops.
- Technology should be selected with a future goal in mind and a vision of how the individual and environment will change.
- The strategy should be selected in consultation with caregivers, teachers, and other professionals and all adults who support its use.
- Extensive training and follow-up should accompany the use of assistive technology.

Environmental Modifications
Improving the Fit between the Child and the Environment

To succeed in a specific setting, a child with disabilities often benefits from adaptations to the environment. Environmental modifications include temporary or permanent adaptations that enhance a child's performance, increase safety or sense of safety, and improve comfort. Children with physical disabilities may require specific environmental adaptations to increase accessibility or safety. For example, although a school's bathroom may be accessible to a child in a wheelchair, the therapist may recommend the installation of a bar beside the toilet so that the child can safely perform a standing pivot transfer. Ramps may need to be installed or desk heights and chairs may need to be adjusted for the child in a wheelchair. Many of the physical accommodations to improve accessibility are in place as schools and community facilities comply with the Americans with Disabilities Act (ADA) (1990).

Often the role of the occupational therapist is to recommend adaptations to the sensory environment that accommodate children with sensory processing problems (Haack & Haldy, 1998; Miller & Heaphy, 1998). Preschool and elementary school classrooms usually have high levels of auditory and visual input. Classrooms with visual clutter may be overwhelmingly disorganizing to a child who does not filter visual input. Young children who need proprioceptive input or quiet times during the day may need a beanbag chair placed in a pup tent in the corner of the room. The therapist may suggest that a preschool teacher implement a quiet time or turn down the lights for a period (Haack & Haldy, 1998). Sitting on movable surfaces (e.g., liquid-filled cushions) can help a child's posture and improve arousal and attention (Schilling, Washington, Billingsley, & Deitz, 2003). The intent of recommendations regarding the classroom environment is often to maintain a child's arousal and level of alertness without overstimulating or distracting him or her. Modifications should enhance the child's performance, make life easier for the parent or teachers, and have a neutral or positive effect on siblings, peers, and others in the environment. Due to the dynamic nature of the child and the environment, adaptations to the environment may require ongoing assessment of the goodness of fit between the child and the modified environment with adjustments made throughout the year.

Consultation and Negotiation with Adults in the Child's Environment

Environmental adaptations can only be accomplished through consultation with the adults who manage the environment. High levels of collaboration are needed to create optimal environments for the child to attend and learn at school and at home.

Environmental modifications often affect everyone in the room, so they must meet the needs of and be appropriate for all children in that environment. The therapist articulates the rationale for the modification and negotiates the changes to be made by considering what is most appropriate for all, including the teacher and other students. Through discussion, the occupational therapist and teacher reach agreement as to what the problems are. With consensus regarding the problems and desired outcomes, often the needed environmental modification logically follows. It is essential that the therapist follow through by evaluating the impact of the modification on the targeted child and others.

Promoting Participation and Preventing Disability through Education
Educating Other Professionals and Administrators

Therapists provide education to improve accessibility to recreational, school, or community activities; modify curriculum materials; develop educational materials; or help improve attitudes toward disabilities. By participating in curriculum revision or course material selection, therapists can help establish a curriculum with sufficient flexibility to meet the needs of children with disabilities. Often a system problem that negatively affects one child is problematic to others as well. The occupational therapist needs to recognize which system problems can be changed and how these changes can be encouraged. For example, if a child has difficulty reading and writing in the morning, he or she may benefit from physical activity before addressing deskwork. The occupational therapist cannot change the daily schedule and move recess or physical education to the beginning of the day, but she or he may convince the teacher to begin the first period of the day with warmup activities. Even if the teacher cannot allot warmup time, she or he may allow the student to hold and handle "fidgets" during reading. Sometimes a crunchy snack can increase arousal and alertness. The occupational therapist can work with the teacher to establish a policy that allows children to eat a snack in the morning and then encourage parents to pack a crunchy snack.

To effectively educate professionals within a system, the occupational therapist must become part of the system (Case-Smith, 1998; Hanft & Place, 1996). This has not always occurred in schools or childcare centers; often therapists with health care backgrounds and medical-based education feel like visitors in the classrooms. It has been difficult for occupational therapists to become integral parts of the educational system because

of their limited understanding of the system. Similarly, teachers and principals do not always understand occupational therapy. To become part of the system, occupational therapists need to make conscious efforts to (1) define their profession and their roles, (2) determine the roles of school and childcare personnel, and (3) learn the rules, both overt and unspoken, that govern the system. Importantly, the occupational therapist needs to spend time with teachers, care providers, and administrators and develop relationships with them. By participating in school routines (e.g., helping at recess, lunch, or assembly time), the occupational therapist demonstrates his or her interest in supporting the work of teachers and the school's overall operation. Participating in school activities also gives the therapist insight into the child's ability to cope with the routine and to participate in all school functions. The therapist also gains insight in how to establish working relationships with teachers and how to approach problems that may be primarily an issue of difficult interaction between a child and teacher.

System Change in the Child's Community

To change the system on behalf of all children or children with disabilities requires communication with stakeholders or persons who are invested in the change (Case-Smith, 1998). The occupational therapist needs to confidently share the rationale for change and negotiate when needed. When a change in the system (e.g., curriculum) is considered, inevitably many points of view are expressed and need to be considered. A system change is most accepted when the benefits appear high and the costs are low. Can all children benefit? Which children are affected? If administrators and teachers in a childcare center are reluctant to enroll an infant with a disability, the occupational therapist can advocate for accepting the child by explaining specifically the care that the child would need, the resources available, behaviors and issues to expect, and the benefits to other families.

Convincing a school to build an accessible playground is one example of how education can create system change. Occupational therapists are frequently involved in designing playgrounds that are accessible to all and promote the development of sensory motor skills. Another example is helping school administrators select computers that are accessible to children with disabilities. The occupational therapist can also serve on the school committee that selects computer software for the curriculum and can advocate for software that is easily adaptable for children with physical or sensory disabilities. A third example is helping administrators and teachers select a handwriting curriculum to be used by regular and special education students. The occupational therapist may advocate for a curriculum that emphasizes prewriting skills or one that takes a multisensory approach to teaching handwriting. The occupational therapist may also advocate for adding sensory-motor-perceptual activities to an early childhood curriculum. These examples of system change suggest that occupational therapists become involved in helping educational systems improve occupational performance and prevent disability among children at risk, as well as increase participation for children with specific diagnoses.

BEST PRACTICES WITH CHILDREN

Inclusion and Services in Natural Environments

Legal mandates and best practice guidelines require that services to children with disabilities be provided in environments with children who do not have disabilities. The Individuals with Disabilities Education Act (IDEA, 1997) requires that services to infants and toddlers be provided in "natural environments" and that services to preschool and school-aged children be provided in the "least restrictive environment." The infant's natural environment is most often his or her home, but it may include a childcare center. The family defines the child's natural environment. (See further discussion in Chapter 21.) This requirement shifts when the child reaches school age, not in its intent but with recognition that community schools and regular education classrooms are the most natural and least restrictive environments for services to children with disabilities. School-aged children with severe medical or behavioral problems sometimes receive services in the home, but this environment is considered restrictive. Inclusion in natural environments or regular education classrooms only succeeds when specific supports and accommodations are provided to children with disabilities. Occupational therapists are often important team members in making inclusion successful for children with disabilities. (This concept is further discussed in Chapter 22.)

A recent focus of educators and related health care service providers, such as occupational therapists, is the inclusion of children with disabilities as not only a physical arrangement but also an opportunity for optimal learning and a method for reaching educational outcomes on par with those expected from all students. Therefore the goal of inclusion of students with disabilities is full participation in the school's curriculum and activities. This goal requires that teachers work closely with related service personnel to design course materials for the child with disabilities and to adapt learning experiences to ensure that he or she can achieve many of the same learning goals as do his or her peers.

Goals and Strategies

With the team focused on inclusion, its goals, strategies, and methods lean toward outcomes that make inclusion successful (e.g., children functioning and learning with their peers in regular education classrooms). Inclusion of all children encompasses the following outcomes:

- Children with disabilities are full participants in school, preschool, and childcare center activities.
- Children with disabilities have friends and relationships with their peers.
- Children with disabilities learn and achieve with the general educational curriculum to the best of their abilities.
- All children learn to appreciate individual differences in people.
- Children with disabilities participate to the fullest extent possible in their communities.

Occupational therapists contribute in meaningful ways to all these outcomes. Often the primary reason children fall short of reaching their goals is social or behavioral problems. Teachers can adapt the curriculum for specific learning issues, but behavioral problems are more difficult to manage because they disrupt the entire class and can negatively affect other children's ability to learn. Children who are extremely active, aggressive, impulsive, loud and boisterous, or oppositional are disruptive to classes and are a great concern of teachers.

Occupational therapists routinely address specific goals that are essential to a child's ability to function in a regular education classroom and promote the teacher and peers' acceptance of the child (Table 1-3). Occupational therapists approach these goals with important insight into the student's ability to respond to sensory input and to self-regulate (e.g., inhibit impulsive reactions). By sharing their understanding of the reasons a child responds in certain ways, the occupational therapist may help teachers, parents, aides, and other professionals reframe the problem. Often, reframing the problem is an important step in developing the most appropriate solutions to the student's problems.

Occupational therapists also participate in comprehensive behavioral programs designed by the team, and they apply behavioral strategies to help manage the child's behaviors. These approaches are effective when they are consistently applied across situations and environments. Therefore it is important to gain consensus and support for a behavioral program from all adults working with a child. With his or her understanding of the child's sensory, motor, and cognitive skills and social function, the occupational therapist can contribute insights as to which behavioral strategies have a high probability for success.

Service Delivery Models

The goal that children should participate to the fullest extent possible in their natural environment also suggests that occupational therapists adopt certain methods of service delivery. The occupational therapist needs to

TABLE 1-3   Occupational Therapy Goals for Promoting Inclusion

Goals	Examples of Strategies
Decrease student's disruptive behaviors	Promote calming
	Decrease sensory-seeking behaviors by providing appropriate outlet for sensory seeking (e.g., break for jumping on trampoline or for applying deep pressure)
Increase student's time management	Give strategies for completing tasks on time
	Give method for cueing transition to new activities
Decrease student's aggressive behaviors	Decrease frustration by simplifying challenging activities
	Meet sensory needs throughout day
Improve student's interpersonal skills	Help child initiate and sustain interaction with peers
	Increase understanding of social norms
Improve student's responsiveness and self-regulation	Facilitate arousal, using appropriate but enhanced sensory input
Improve student's attention span and decrease distractibility	Provide materials that enhance visual focus
Improve student's ability to organize and manage materials	Teach compensatory methods for locating and assembling correct materials

work within the classroom, childcare center, or other natural environments. To be invited into the classroom or home environment, the occupational therapist must learn the classroom rules and routines and have an appreciation for the adults who manage the environment (Hanft & Place, 1996). To work within the classroom, the occupational therapist needs to be familiar with the curriculum and the expected behaviors and performance levels for all students. Strong skills in consultation and collaboration are needed to help children function effectively in their natural environments. To become part of the system, the occupational therapist acknowledges the importance of educator roles and the skills of the adults who teach and work with the child. With trust and respect between the therapist and teaching staff established, the therapist can recommend modifications and accommodations to the environment and curriculum that will be implemented and appreciated.

This process is similar for therapists who provide services in the home. Before making recommendations to implement specific strategies, the occupational therapist needs to understand the family's routines, the rules and expectations, as well as the resources available in the home. Then the intervention strategies recommended can fit easily into the daily routine and are more likely to become part of the family daily activities.

To transfer intervention activities to other adults who care for or teach the child, an occupational therapist uses collaborative consultation. Hanft and Place (1996) described the critical elements of effective consultation as the following: (1) dynamic interaction over time, (2) respectful relationships, and (3) collaborative efforts to reach common ground. With collaborative consultation, the occupational therapist commits to developing and sustaining relationships with parents and other professionals to solve the problems incurred by a student. When the occupational therapist suggests solutions, he or she is sensitive to the needs of these adults

and offers practical solutions that recognize time constraints, environmental restrictions, and learning priorities. All suggestions involve follow-up and adaptations to the approach to ensure that the most workable and effective strategy is implemented.

Occupational therapists also attend to the style in which they provide consultation. As much as possible, the therapist should match the learning and interaction styles of those being consulted (e.g., the teacher). For example, if the teacher is a visual learner, the therapist should provide pictures or handouts of positions and activities to use with a student. If the teacher is a kinesthetic learner, the occupational therapist may suggest that the teacher practice a movement or handling technique to build confidence before applying it with a child. When the person being consulted has an interaction style reflecting that she or he is an achiever, the occupational therapist must also recognize that recommendations need to produce short-term effects. If the person has an analytic style, details and specificity are important when making recommendations (Deboer, 1986).

Summary

Occupational therapists support inclusion by (1) focusing on goals that enable the child to be successful in inclusive environments, (2) providing services in the least restrictive environment or in the child's natural environment, and (3) using consultation and education as primary methods of service delivery. Helping students function in inclusive settings implies that occupational therapists integrate their services into these settings and they become an integral part of the system.

Cross-Cultural Competence

Cross-cultural competence can be defined as "the ability to think, feel, and act in ways that acknowledge, respect, and build upon ethnic, [socio]cultural, and linguistic diversity" (Lynch & Hanson, 1993, p. 50). Cultural competence in health care refers to behaviors and attitudes that enable an individual to function effectively with culturally diverse clients (Rorie, Paine, & Barger, 1996). Occupational therapists with cultural competence can respond optimally to all children in all sociocultural contexts. Chan (1990) identified its three essential elements: self-awareness, knowledge of information specific to each culture, and interaction skills sensitive to cultural differences. The following reasons, described in this section, support the importance of cross-cultural competence to occupational therapists:

- Cultural diversity of the United States continues to increase.
- A child's development of occupations is embedded in the cultural practices of his family and community.

Cultural Diversity in the United States

The diversity and heterogeneity of American families continues to increase each year. In 2002, 32.5 million Americans were foreign born, representing 11.5% of the population (U.S. Census Bureau, 2002). This percentile has increased from 8.7% in 1994 and 4.8% in 1970. Of these, 52% are from Latin America and 25.5% are from Asia. Of the families who immigrated to the United States, 25% have family households of five or more people, compared to 12% of native-born Americans. Sixteen percent of immigrants live below the poverty level, compared to 11.5% of native-born Americans.

Children in minority groups are increasing in number at a much faster rate than increases in the general population. The general population increased by 13.2% from 1990 to 2000; in comparison, the Hispanic population increased 60%, from 22.4 million to 35.3 million (U.S. Census Bureau, 2002). Diversity of ethnicity and race can be viewed as a risk or as a resource to child development (Garcia Coll & Magnuson, 2000). A risk or potential barrier to services for people of color is continued segregation in certain regions of the country despite the laws and litigation supporting integration. Low birthrate, preterm delivery, and infant mortality are higher in African American families, suggesting that these families frequently need early childhood intervention programs. Race can also be a resource; for example, African American families are well supported by their communities and focused on their children (Figure 1-10). Parents often perceive discipline and politeness as positive attributes and instill these in their children (Willis, 1997). Occupational therapists who work with African American and Hispanic families find many positive attributes in their family interactions and parenting styles.

Poverty has a pervasive effect of children's developmental and health outcomes (Children's Defense Fund, 2003). The number of American children who live in poverty remains significant. Families in poverty often have great need for, yet limited ability to access, health care and educational services. Many families who are served by early intervention and special education systems are of low socioeconomic status. When families lack resources (e.g., transportation, food, and shelter), their priorities and concerns orient to these basic needs. Responsive therapists provide resources to assist with these basic needs, making appropriate referrals to community agencies. They also demonstrate understanding of the family's priorities, which may not include their children's occupational performance goals.

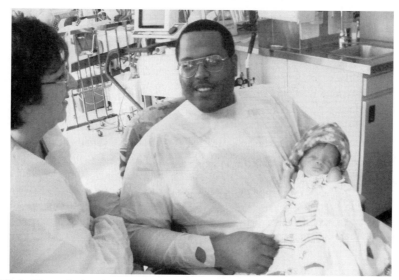

FIGURE 1-10   A father bonds with his just-born son. (Courtesy of Jayne Shepherd and Patti Cooper.)

Influence of Cultural Practices on a Child's Development of Occupations

To impact a child's occupational development, it is critical for the therapist to understand how cultural practices influence skill development. Table 1-4 lists the cultural values that may influence the child's development of occupations. Goals for independence may not be appropriate at certain ages for children of certain cultures. For example, Middle Eastern families often do not emphasize early independence in self-care; therefore, skills such as self-feeding may not be a family priority until ages well beyond the normative expectations (Sharifzadeh, 1997). In Hispanic cultures, holding and cuddling is highly valued, even in older children (Zuniga, 1997). Mothers hold and carry their preschool children. Recommending a wheelchair for a young child may be unacceptable to families who value close physical contact and holding. In some cultures (e.g., Polynesian), parents delegate childcare responsibilities to older siblings. Therefore in established families, siblings care for the infants. Young children in Polynesian cultures tend to rely on their older siblings rather than their parents for structure, assistance, and support. Being responsible for a younger sibling helps the older sibling mature quickly by learning responsibility and problem solving (Rogoff, 2003). Sibling care may present as a problem when the young child has a disability and needs additional or prolonged care. The literature is replete with examples of the influence of culture on children's occupations (Deater-Deckard, Dodge, Bates, & Petit, 1996; Jarrett, 1996; Rogoff, 2003; Rogoff & Morelli, 1989). The occupational therapist's appreciation of the influence of culture on children's occupations facilitates the development of appropriate priorities and the use of strategies that are congruent with the family's values and lifestyle.

Because the focus of occupational therapy is to enhance a child's ability to participate in his or her natural environment and everyday routines, the therapist must appreciate, value, and understand those environments and routines. Recommendations that counter a family's cultural values probably will not be implemented and may be harmful to the professional-family relationships. To assimilate the family's values, the therapist uses

TABLE 1-4 Cultural Values and Styles That Influence Children's Development of Occupations

Value or Style	Guiding Questions
Family composition	Who are the members of the family?
	How many family members live in the same house?
	Is there a hierarchy in the family based on gender or age?
Decision making	Who makes the decisions for the family
Primary caregiver	Who is the primary caregiver?
	Is this role shared?
Independence/interdependence	Do family members value independence?
	Is reliance on each other more important than independence?
Feeding practices	Who feeds the infant or child?
	What are the cultural rules or norms about breast feeding, mealtime, self-feeding, eating certain foods?
	When is independence in feeding expected?
Sleeping patterns	Do children sleep with parents?
	How do parents respond to the infant during the night?
	What are appropriate responses to crying?
Discipline	Is disobedience tolerated?
	How strict are the rules governing behavior?
	Who disciplines the child?
	How do the parents discipline their child?
Perception of disability	Do the parents believe that a disability can improve?
	Do they feel responsible for the disability?
	Do family members feel that they can make a difference in improving the disability?
	Are spiritual forms of healing valued?
Help seeking	From whom does the family seek help?
	Does the family actively seek help or do the family members expect help to come to them?
Communication and interaction	Does the family use a direct or indirect style of communication?
	Do family members share emotional feelings?
	Is most communication direct or indirect?
	Does the family value socializing?

Adapted from Wayman, K.I., Lynch, E.W., & Hanson, M.J. (1990). Home-based early childhood services: Cultural sensitivity in a family systems approach. *Topics in Early Childhood Special Education 10*, 65–66.

narrative reasoning, asking, "What story am I in?" The home environment and the family members' interactions help to reveal their cultural values. When therapists ask open-ended questions, they can elicit information about the family's routines, rituals, and traditions to provide an understanding of the cultural context. The culturally competent therapist demonstrates an interest in understanding the family's culture, an acceptance of diversity, and a willingness to participate in traditions or cultural patterns of the family. In home-based services, cultural competence may mean removing shoes on entrance, accepting foods when offered, scheduling therapy sessions around holidays, and accommodating language differences. In center-based services, cultural sensitivity remains important, although a family's cultural values may be more difficult to ascertain outside the home. A culturally competent therapist inquires about family routines, cultural practices, traditions, and priorities; demonstrates a willingness to accommodate to these cultural values; and integrates her or his intervention recommendations into the family's cultural practices.

Assistive Technologies and Universal Access

Assistive technologies have significantly improved the quality of life for persons with disabilities. Computers, power mobility, augmentative communication devices, and environmental control units have greatly enhanced functional performance, making it possible for children to participate in roles previously closed to them. IDEA and other laws encourage states to provide assistive technology to students. These laws have increased the momentum for using assistive devices with children; however, the IDEA mandate is not funded, meaning that local school districts and other sources need to provide the funding for assistive technology.

Use of Assistive Technology in the Child's Daily Routine

A broad array of technology has become available, particularly in the area of mobility and communication. As the availability of a range of assistive technology increases, decision making about the optimal technology to improve a child's function has become more difficult. At times, the technology that seems to offer the most functionality to the child is not the best choice because it is too complicated and time intensive for the teacher to implement in the classroom with 20 other children. Assistive technology must match the child's abilities and performance limitations and enable the child to perform age- and developmentally appropriate activities. The adults in the child's environment must support the technology by dedicating the time needed to help the child

to use it in functional ways. For example, an Alphasmart, which is a lightweight transportable word processor, matches the needs of fourth and fifth graders whose handwriting is illegible. The technology is a practical solution because it is relatively simple to operate and students quickly become independent in its use, alleviating the need for the teacher's time to set up the device and check on its use. Voice-recognition word processing software is available for children with more significant motor skills limitation, yet it has not been as successfully implemented in classrooms. At this time, voice-recognition programs continue to require an extensive learning process in which the computer learns the student's speech and the student learns how to use his or her voice to operate the program. Voice-recognition software (e.g., Dragon Naturally Speaking) is also challenging to implement in a noisy classroom, and in most situations it is not appropriate for one student to talk out loud in the classroom.

Although a therapist can extensively train a student to use power mobility, an augmentative communication device, or an adapted computer, the child's skills with the technology will not generalize into everyday routines unless parents, teachers, and aides are sufficiently comfortable with and knowledgeable about the technology. The importance of those closest to the child being able to implement the technology and troubleshoot when necessary implies that the occupational therapist educate them extensively about how to apply the technology and remain available to problem-solve the issues that inevitably arise. Sometimes the solutions that work best are low-technology devices, because the personnel working with the child do not have the time and expertise to implement high technology devices.

One trend observed in school systems is that the occupational therapist serves as an assistive technology consultant or becomes a member of a district-wide assistive technology team. The teams have been formed given the increased prevalence of technology use in public schools and the need for experts who can dedicate time to learning about emerging technology. An assistive technology team makes recommendations to administrators on equipment to order, trains students to use computers and devices, troubleshoots technology failures, determines technology needs, and provides ongoing education to staff and families. One role of a school or district assistive technology team is to promote universal access.

Universal Access

The concept of universal access is now widespread, and it refers to the movement to develop devices and design environments that are accessible to everyone. When schools invest in universal access for their learning technology, all students can access any or most of the school's computers, and adaptations for visual, hearing, motor, or cognitive impairment can be made on all or most of the school's computers. Universal access means that the system platforms can support the software with accessibility options and that a range of keyboards, mice, and switches are available for alternative access. Universal access also refers to physical access. At present, children in power or manual wheelchairs should be able to access all environments, including recreational facilities, sports arenas, swimming pools, playgrounds, and community centers. Schools are now designed to accommodate additional computers in classrooms. Desks are designed for laptop computers, and some desks are accessible to wheelchairs.

With the accessibility options available on Windows and the Macintosh operating system, computer programs can be easily adapted. For example, the cursor can be enlarged, and most computer applications and word processing programs offer multiple methods of augmented visual and auditory feedback (see Chapter 18).

Hammel and Niehaus (1998) outlined the involvement of occupational therapists in general technology to ensure accessibility for students with disabilities. School-based occupational therapists should demonstrate the following competencies:

- Operate major computing systems used in public schools and troubleshoot system problems.
- Make major operating systems accessible to people with disabilities.
- Operate general application programs (e.g., word processing, databases, graphics), teacher utility tools, and computer-based instruction.

The continued advancement of assistive technology suggests that assistive technology specialists are needed. Occupational therapists can pursue certification by the Rehabilitation Engineering Society of North America (RESNA) or attend continuing education classes on assistive technology. Occupational therapists with expertise in assistive technology become valuable members of technology teams in school districts or those in assistive technology clinics of hospitals and rehabilitation centers.

Evidence-Based Practice

With the goal of providing the best services possible, occupational therapists and other health care professionals are seeking and using practices and approaches that have research evidence of effectiveness. In **evidence-based practice**, occupational therapists emphasize integrating research findings into their practice and using research evidence in clinical reasoning. The use of databases on evidence-based medicine has become essential to clinical decision making. Sackett, Rosenberg, Muir Gray, Haynes, and Richardson (1996) defined evidence-based medicine as "the conscientious, explicit, and judi-

cious use of current best evidence in making decisions about the care of individual patients" (p. 71). Therefore, evidence-based practice does not mean that intervention becomes based solely on research findings. It does mean that occupational therapists consider the research evidence, along with their own experiences and family priorities when making intervention decisions (Law & Baum, 1998; Sackett et al., 1996).

The body of research literature supporting occupational therapy with children remains limited when compared to other disciplines (e.g., psychology); however, often research studies and clinical trials in other disciplines have relevance to occupational therapy practice. Research evidence is readily available and accessible through Internet sources. A list of links to health care research databases can be found in Appendix 1-A. The steps in applying evidence-based practice are listed in Box 1-2.

In searching for research to inform a clinical decision, the occupational therapist weighs the strength or importance of each study. Studies that provide the most important research evidence are meta-analyses or reviews of clinical trials. The findings of these studies generally have good applicability to practice because they combine the findings of studies that have met a rigorous standard established by the authors. Findings from a rigorous randomized clinical trial also provide strong evidence for practice, followed by results from studies using quasi-experimental designs. Pre-experimental studies and descriptive designs can provide information relevant to clinical decision making; however, their findings are not as strong and should be applied with caution. Outcome research can assist practitioners in establishing benchmarks or standards for performance and client programs;

BOX 1-2   **Steps in Evidence-Based Practice**

STEP 1
- Convert the need for information (about intervention effects, prognosis, therapy methods) into an answerable question.

STEP 2
- Search the research databases using the terms in the research question.
- Track down the best evidence to answer that question.

STEP 3
- Critically appraise the evidence for its
  - validity (truthfulness)
  - impact (level of effect)

STEP 4
- Critically appraise the evidence for its applicability (usefulness in your practice) priorities

STEP 5
- Implement the practice or apply the information. Evaluate the process.

however, descriptive outcome studies do not provide strong evidence for the effectiveness of a specific intervention.

The conceptual and practice models listed in Box 1-3 are important to occupational therapy for children and have been investigated using experimental designs. Summaries of the efficacy research in each of the areas are presented in this section.

Neurodevelopmental Treatment

Outcomes of neurodevelopmental treatment (NDT) with children who have cerebral palsy or delayed motor function were investigated primarily in the 1970s through early 1990s. Results of these studies are inconclusive. Three quasi-experimental studies of NDT found significant improvement in the sample receiving intervention using NDT (Carlsen, 1975; Mayo, 1991; Scherzer, Mike, & Ilson, 1976). Palmer et al. (1988) completed a randomized clinical trial examining the effect of physical therapy using a neurodevelopment treatment versus infant stimulation. The participants were infants, 12 to 19 months of age, with mild to severe spastic diplegia. The Bayley Scales of Infant Development (Bayley, 1993) were administered preintervention and postintervention. The group that received infant stimulation demonstrated greater increases in motor scale scores than the group that received neurodevelopmental physical therapy. The authors concluded that their findings did not support neurodevelopment physical therapy with infants with spastic diplegia. Limitations of the study were lack of fidelity checks of intervention implementation and use of an instrument (i.e., the Bayley) that is not sensitive to changes in motor performance. Two more recent studies also found no differences in the performance of children who received NDT and those who received no treatment or an alternate treatment (Law et al., 1991; Law et al., 1997).

The most recent study by Law and others (1997) found that functional performance in children who received intensive NDT and casting was no different than the performance of children who received regular occupational therapy that emphasized functional activities.

The children in this study were between 18 months and 4 years from eight children's rehabilitation centers in Ontario, Canada. All of the participants had cerebral palsy with upper extremity involvement. A crossover design was used where children received intensive NDT with casting or regular occupational therapy for 4 months, no treatment for 2 months (wash-out period), and then 4 months of the alternate intervention. The Peabody Developmental Motor Scales (PDMS) and the QUEST (which rates the quality of arm movement patterns) were the primary outcome measures. The children in both groups improved significantly in both measures. Those who wore their casts longer (more than 20 hours per week) improved more on the PDMS.

Together, the studies of NDT indicate weak support for this interventional method. By clinical report, it is effective for certain children, primarily those with cerebral palsy, in developing specific motor skills (Howle, 2002). These studies suggest that an NDT approach should be selectively applied to achieve specific outcomes. The inconclusive evidence also suggests that the performance areas targeted when using NDT should be specifically and routinely measured to determine whether progress toward expected outcomes is satisfactory.

Sensory Integration

The original studies that compared sensory integration with no treatment (e.g., Ayres, 1972, 1977) demonstrated significant positive effects. These studies used samples of children with learning disabilities and compared sensory integration to no treatment. Although the effect sizes for Ayres' original studies were high, the sample sizes were low.

Recent studies have found that the effects of intervention using a sensory integration approach are equivalent to the effects of alternative treatment approaches. Polatajko, Kaplan, and Wilson (1992) analyzed seven randomized clinical trials of sensory integration treatment that used two or more groups and included a comparison or control group. All studies were of children with learning disabilities between the ages 4.8 and 13 years. The outcome variables included academic performance, visual-motor, sensory-motor, and language performance. The seven clinical trials did not provide any statistical evidence that sensory integration treatment improved academic performance. Several of the studies found that sensory and motor performance improved with sensory integration intervention. Most of the results with sensory integration intervention were similar to the results with perceptual motor intervention. A limitation cited by Polatajko et al. (1992) was that sensory integration treatment in a research context is quite different from sensory integration treatment in a clinic where therapists can individualize each session to the needs of the child.

The meta-analysis of sensory integration treatment by Vargas and Camilli (1999) showed small treatment effects, substantiating the earlier findings of Polatajko et al. (1992). Using a criterion-based selection process, Vergas and Camilli found 14 studies of sensory integration compared to no treatment and 11 of sensory integration compared to an alternative treatment (usually perceptual motor activities). Effect sizes were calculated and weighted for sample size. For comparisons of sensory integration to no treatment, the average effect size was .29, which is a low effect size. When sensory integration is compared to an alternative treatment, the effect size was .09, which means that the effects of sensory integration were not significantly different from those of other treatments. The authors reported that the average effect size for earlier studies (before 1982) was higher (.60) than the average effect size for studies after 1982 (.03). The skill areas that improved were psycho-educational and motor performance areas. Although the effects of sensory integration appear to be small, findings of significant improvement in motor performance following sensory integration treatment are consistent.

Sensory Modalities

Application of sensory modalities has also been studied, generally in small samples and with positive results. These studies investigate the application of a specific sensory modality to achieve specific behavioral/performance outcomes in a group of children with the same diagnosis or similar problems. The efficacy of using touch pressure to gain behavioral changes in children with autism or attention deficit hyperactivity disorder (ADHD) has been researched (Edelson, Goldberg, Edelson, Ken & Grandin, 1999; Fertel-Daly et al., 2001; VandenBerg, 2001). Edelson et al. investigated the efficacy of the Hug Machine, which is a device that provides touch pressure through the sides of the body. Using a sample of children with autism, participants who received the Hug Machine treatment twice a week were compared to a control group. The participants who used the Hug Machine exhibited a significant reduction in tension and a slight change in anxiety. Physiological measures were not significantly different between groups.

Two recent studies examined the effect of pressure through wearing a weighted vest. Fertel-Daly and colleagues (2001) examined the effects of a weighted vest on five preschool children with pervasive developmental disorders. Using an ABA single-subject design, vests were worn for 2 hours per day, 3 days a week, for 5 weeks, with baseline (wearing no vest) data collected before and after the intervention. Attention, number of distractions, and duration of self-stimulation behavior were measured. All participants demonstrated increased attention and decreased distractibility, and four of five showed decreased self-stimulation behaviors. VandenBerg (2001) also examined the effects of a weighted vest on four children diagnosed with ADHD. The children demonstrated greater on-task behaviors when wearing the vests. The summary of the studies using small samples found that touch pressure and deep pressure, applied intermittently, can decrease tension and anxiety, improve attention, and increase on-task behavior.

Another study of sensory modalities (Schilling et al., 2003) examined the effects from children sitting on therapy balls on in-seat behavior and legible word productivity. Occupational therapists sometimes recommend that students sit on therapy balls in the classroom to give them additional vestibular and proprioceptive input while sitting. The children can bounce to stay attentive and alert and receive additional vestibular/proprioceptive feedback when they shift their weight through the ball's movement. Using a multiple baseline single subject design, all participants (n = 3) improved in in-seat behavior and legible word productivity (Schilling et al., 2003). The balls seemed to help in sensory modulation with the participants, and they represent a nonintrusive method to provide enhanced sensory input during the school day. The outcome measures, staying in one's seat and legible word productivity, are important academic-related outcomes. All of these sensory modalities studies used small samples, so larger group studies are needed. Each demonstrated that interventions focused on physiological impairments (sensory modulation) using specific sensory modalities produced performance outcomes that enhanced the child's ability to participate in home and school environments.

Collaborative Consultation

The types of service delivery have been the focus of outcome studies. In occupational therapy, the application of consultation has been examined, comparing it with one-on-one models of intervention. These studies have shown that collaborative consultation is as effective as or more effective than direct services. In a study with preschool children that extended 7 months, direct individual services (n = 8) were compared to group consultation services (n = 8) (Davies & Gavin, 1994). The progress of the children's motor skills was similar in the two samples, indicating that positive outcomes could be achieved when group interventions with consultation were used. In a pilot study of 14 kindergarten children, the levels of achievement of individualized education program (IEP) goals were compared with the achievement levels of children who received direct intervention or consultation. Children achieved nearly three fourths of their IEP goals whether they received consultation or direct services (Dunn, 1990). Teachers expressed more positive feedback toward the occupational therapy services when the therapist provided consultation. Kemmis and Dunn (1996) examined the effectiveness of weekly occupational therapy consultation with teachers. During each week of the school year, teachers and occupational therapists dedicated 60 minutes to plan intervention. Students who were the focus of these weekly meetings achieved a success rate of 63% on their intervention goals.

Using a quasi-experimental design, Dreiling and Bundy (2003) compared a consultative model to direct (and indirect) intervention. Eleven children were in the consultation group, and 11 were in the direct-indirect intervention group. In the consultation group, the therapists were in the classrooms one day a week and met with the teaching staff twice a month. Following a year of intervention, the number of goals achieved was not significantly different between the two groups (56% of goals were achieved by the consultation group and 50% by the direct intervention group). This effect size was low, indicating that the same benefits were achieved by each intervention method. Although these studies of consultation used small sample sizes, together they suggest that consultation that facilitates achievement of the child's goals, has at least the same effects as direct intervention models, and has positive benefits in developing relationships between occupational therapists and other professionals who are working with the child.

Occupation as an Intervention Means

Occupation as a means for improving performance has been well researched. Occupations that are effectively used as means to intervention outcomes must have purpose and meaning (Trombly, 1995). The purpose is the goal of the intervention activity, and the meaning is the value of the activity. As discussed in the first part of this chapter, through clinical reasoning the therapist learns what the child values and what has meaning. When possible, the goal should be the same as that of the child's, although the goal is often established by external demands (e.g., children are expected to learn keyboarding in fifth-grade curriculum). Perhaps most important, the meaning or theme of an activity should reflect the child's values and interests.

Although most studies of the effectiveness of meaningful occupation or purposeful activity use adults as subjects, the results have important implications for occupational therapy with children. These studies support the use of occupation as a means for improving client performance and suggest that occupational therapists continue to refine their occupation-based models of intervention. Examples of studies of the effects of occupational context on performance are replete in the occupational therapy literature. A few examples are described in this section. Lin, Wu, Tickle-Degnen, & Coster (1997) completed a meta-analysis of studies of occupation as means. They concluded that intervention providing purposeful activity produces better-quality client performance (e.g., improved motor function) than a therapist and client focus on movement in isolation. To evaluate the effect of having a concrete goal, Van der Weel, Van der Meer, and Lee (1991) compared children's range of motion in supination when moving a drumstick to moving to an abstract command. The movement range was significantly greater with the concrete task. Sietsema, Nelson, Mulder, Mervau-Scheidel, & White (1993) also investigated the difference in shoulder range of motion when participants with brain injury reached to play a computer game versus when they reached for an abstract target. Range of motion was significantly greater when playing the game.

Nelson and colleagues extensively investigated the effect of enhanced context or enhanced meaning on client performance during an activity. In these studies (e.g., Bloch, Smith, & Nelson, 1989; Lang, Nelson, & Bush, 1992; Miller & Nelson, 1987; Riccio, Nelson, & Bush, 1990), the clients were given either a rote exercise or a meaningful activity with enhanced context with a purposeful goal. Their studies and others (e.g., Murphy, Trombly, Tickle-Degnen, & Jacobs, 1999) demonstrated that when the meaning of an activity was enhanced by producing an end product, playing a game, or providing a specific context, the clients performed longer, with greater effort, and with higher quality (e.g., greater range of motion, smoother and more organized movement). These outcomes suggest that meaningfulness in intervention activities motivates children to perform at optimal levels. By extension, it is probable that meaningful intervention activities are practiced in and generalized to other contexts, because the child values them. The effectiveness of occupation as an intervention means and consultation as the primary model of service delivery are important concepts in practice with children. The evidence supports the effectiveness of these concepts and validates the model presented in this chapter that included these concepts as essential elements of occupational therapy intervention.

Family-Centered Care

Family-centered care is a model advocated in the literature and the legislation for individuals with disabilities. Although it is well described in the literature, efficacy studies investigating the outcomes of family-centered care are few. Rosenbaum, King, Law, King, & Evans (1998) reviewed clinical trials of family-centered health care. They identified five clinical trials, published from 1983 to 1995, most of which used a parent education model as part of intervention for chronically ill children.

The positive outcomes of the family-centered interventions when compared to child-focused models included improved child skills, increased parent satisfaction with care, and enhanced child psychological adjustment.

Although clinical trials of family-centered care by occupational therapists have not been published, a number of occupational therapy scholars have examined the outcomes of elements of family-centered care. VanLeit and Crowe (2002) investigated the effects of a program designed to help mothers of children with disabilities improve their use of time and the quality of their occupations through an occupational therapy-led support group. Following their participation in the group, the mothers (n = 19) reported improved performance and satisfaction using the Canadian Occupational Performance Measure when compared to a control group (n = 19). Measures of time use and time perception were no different between the two groups. Investigating the effects of a similar program, qualitative data from the participating mothers were analyzed (Helitzer, Cunningham-Sabo, VanLeit, & Crowe, 2002). This support group program was designed to help mothers cope with difficulties in daily routines with a child with disabilities. The mothers who participated in six weekly small group sessions perceived that their self-image had changed and their coping strategies had increased. This series of studies (Helitzer et al., 2002; VanLeit, & Crowe, 2002) demonstrated the positive effects of implementing support groups designed to help mothers improve their ability to cope with the daily care of a child with special needs. Elements of the intervention that seemed effective were use of small groups of mothers who could support each other, acknowledgement of the stress and challenges inherent in raising a child with special needs, using mothers' accounting of their own routines and activity demands to make recommendations, and allowing mothers to think through their routines and their challenges to develop their own solutions. Family-centered care involves basic and simple elements of good communication and caring, such as listening, demonstrating respect, and providing honest, informative answers to questions; yet these simple elements seem to have important effects on child and family outcomes.

Evidence-based practice means that occupational therapists access research to guide their practice and implement approaches that have known efficacy. Although occupational therapy experimental design research remains limited, the body of research useful to practice is substantial. Occupational therapists must learn to access, analyze, and apply clinical research to offer the most effective services.

SUMMARY

This chapter introduces the book by defining basic concepts in occupational therapy evaluation and intervention. It also describes evolving concepts that support best practices with children. It concludes by defining the commitment of occupational therapists to using evidence-based outcomes research in clinical problem solving. Through this commitment, occupational therapists make decisions about intervention using their experience and training, the child's and family's priorities, and research evidence.

Occupational therapy practice with children has matured in the past two decades from a profession that relied on basic theory to drive decision making to one that recognizes the complexities and multiple dimensions of clinical reasoning. A primary goal of this book is to define and illustrate the application of research evidence in clinical reasoning. The remaining chapters of the book expand on the basic concepts presented in this chapter by exploring the breadth of occupational therapy for children, explaining theories that guide clinical reasoning in each practice domain, illustrating practice models in educational and medical systems, and describing intervention strategies with evidence of efficacy.

STUDY QUESTIONS

1   For each aspect of clinical reasoning, identify a clinical problem and describe how an occupational therapist would use that aspect of clinical reasoning to make a decision.

2   What are the characteristics of scales or assessments to evaluate (a) participation, (b) performance and performance limitations, and (c) client factors and impairments in a 5-year-old child with severe cerebral palsy? (See Chapters 7 and 8.)

3   Define narrative reasoning. Why is this type of reasoning important to all levels of evaluation? List important sources that the therapist uses to develop the "child's story."

4   IDEA states that infant services should be provided in natural environments and school-aged children should receive services in the least restrictive environment. How are these requirements the same, and how are they different? (Access IDEA online at www.IDEApractices.org.) Compare the rules and etiquette when providing services in the home versus services in the classroom.

5   Consider a second-grade student who uses high technology (e.g., power mobility, augmentative communication device, adapted computer) to function in the classroom. Define methods that help integrate his or her assistive technology into classroom routine. Describe how the occupational therapist can include the teacher, teacher's aide, and student's peers in this goal.

REFERENCES

Americans with Disabilities Act. (1990). Public Law 101-336, 104.

Amundson, S. (1996). *Evaluation Tool of Children's Handwriting.* Homer, AK: OK Kids.

Ayres, A.J. (1972). Improving academic scores through sensory integration. *Journal of Learning Disabilities, 5,* 339-343.

Ayres, A.J. (1977). Effect of sensory integrative therapy on the coordination of children with choreoathetoid movements. *American Journal of Occupational Therapy, 31,* 291-293.

Bayley, N. (1993). *Bayley Scales of Infant Development* (2nd ed.). San Antonio, TX: Psychological Corporation.

Bloch, M.W., Smith, D.A., & Nelson, D.L. (1989). Heart rate, activity, duration, and effect in added-purpose versus single-purpose jumping activities. *American Journal of Occupational Therapy, 43,* 25-30.

Bundy, A. (1997). Play and playfulness: What to look for. In D. Parham & L. Fazio (Eds.), *Play and occupational therapy for children* (pp. 52-66). St. Louis: Mosby.

Bundy, A.C. (2002). Play theory and sensory integration. In A.C. Bundy, S. Lane, & E. Murray (Eds.), *Sensory integration: Theory and practice* (2nd ed.). Philadelphia: Lippincott Williams & Wilkins.

Bundy, A., & Koomar, J.A. (2002). Orchestrating intervention: The art of practice. In A. Bundy, S.J., Lane, & E.A. Murray (Eds.), *Sensory integration: Theory and practice* (2nd ed., pp. 242-260). Philadelphia: Lippincott, Williams & Wilkins.

Butler, C. (1986). Effects of powered mobility on self-initiated behaviors of very young children with locomotor disability. *Developmental Medicine and Child Neurology, 28,* 325-332.

Butler, C. (1988). High tech tots: Technology for mobility, manipulation, communication, and learning in early childhood. *Infants and Young Children, 2,* 55-73.

Campos, J.J., & Bertenthal, B.I. (1987). Locomotion and psychological development in infancy. In K.M. Jaffe (Ed.), *Childhood powered mobility: Developmental, technical, and clinical perspectives. In proceedings of the RESNA First Northwest Regional Conference* (pp. 11-42). Washington, DC: RESNA Press.

Carlsen, P.N. (1975). Comparison of two occupational therapy approaches for treating the young cerebral-palsied child. *American Journal of Occupational Therapy, 29,* 267-272.

Case-Smith, J. (1998). Thinking out of the box. In J. Case-Smith (Ed.), *Occupational therapy: Making a difference in school based practice.* Bethesda: AOTA.

Chan, S.Q. (1990). Early intervention with culturally diverse families of infants and toddlers with disabilities. *Infants and Young Children, 3* (2), 78-87.

Children's Defense Fund. (2003). Leave no child behind. Retrieved on March 31, 2004, at www.childrensdefense.org/earlychildhood.

Cripe, J.W., & Venn, M.L. (1997). Family-guided routines for early intervention services. *Young Exceptional Children, 2,* 18-26.

Davies, P.L., & Gavin, W.J. (1994). Comparison of individual and group/consultation treatment methods for preschool children with developmental delays. *American Journal of Occupational Therapy, 48,* 155-161.

Deater-Deckard, K., Dodge, K.A., Bates, J.E., & Petit, G.S. (1996). Physical discipline among African American and European American mothers: Links to children's externalizing behaviors. *Developmental Psychology, 6,* 1065-1072.

Deboer, A. (1986). *The art of consulting.* Chicago: Arcturus Books.

Dreiling, D.S., & Bundy, A.C. (2003). A comparison of consultative model and direct-indirect intervention with preschoolers. *American Journal of Occupational Therapy, 57,* 566-569.

Dunn, W. (1990). A comparison of service-provision models in school-based occupational therapy services: A pilot study. *Occupational Therapy Journal of Research, 10* (5), 300-320.

Edelson, S.M., Goldberg, M., Edelson, M.G., Kerr, D.C., & Grandin, T. (1999). Behavioral and physiological effects of deep pressure on children with autism: A pilot study evaluating the efficacy of Grandin's Hug Machine. *American Journal of Occupational Therapy, 53,* 145-152.

Fertel-Daly, D., Bedell, G., & Hinojosa, J. (2001). Effects of a weighted vest on attention to task and self-stimulatory behaviors in preschoolers with pervasive developmental disorders. *American Journal of Occupational Therapy, 55,* 629-640.

Fidler, G.S., & Fidler, J.W. (1978). Doing and becoming: Purposeful action and self-actualization. *American Journal of Occupational Therapy, 32,* 305-310.

Fleming, M. (1994). Procedural reasoning: Addressing functional limitations. In C. Mattingly & M.H. Fleming, *Clinical reasoning: Forms of inquiry in a therapeutic practice* (pp. 137-177). Philadelphia: F.A. Davis.

Folio, R., & Fewell, R. (2000). *Peabody developmental motor scales* (2nd ed.). Austin, TX: Pro Ed.

Garcia Coll, C., & Magnuson, K. (2000). Cultural differences as sources of developmental vulnerabilities and resources. In S.J. Meisels & J.P. Shonkoff (Eds.), *Handbook of early childhood intervention* (2nd ed., pp. 94-114). Cambridge: Cambridge University Press.

Haack, I., & Haldy, M. (1998). Adaptations and accommodations for sensory processing problems. In J. Case-Smith (Ed.), *Occupational therapy: Making a difference in school system practice.* Bethesda: American Occupational Therapy Association.

Hammel, J., & Niehues, A. (1998). Integrating general and assistive technology into school-based practice: Process and information resources. In J. Case-Smith (Ed.), *Occupational therapy: Making a difference in school system practice.* Bethesda: American Occupational Therapy Association.

Hammill, D.D., Pearson, B.N.A., & Voress, J.K. (1993). *Developmental Test of Visual Perception* (2nd ed.). Austin, TX: Pro Ed.

Hanft, B., & Place, P.A. (1996). *The consulting therapist.* San Antonio, TX: Therapy Skill Builders.

Helitzer, D.L., Cunningham-Sabo, L.D., Vanleit, B., & Crowe, T.K. (2002). Perceived changes in self-image and coping strategies of mothers of children with disabilities. *Occupational Therapy Journal of Research, 22,* 25-33.

Holm, M., Rogers, J.C., & James, A.B. (2003). Treatment of activities of daily living. In M.E. Neistadt & E.B. Crepeau (Eds.), *Willard & Spackman's occupational therapy* (pp. 323-363). Philadelphia: Lippincott Williams & Wilkins.

Howle, J. (2002). *Neuro-developmental treatment approach: Theoretical foundations and principles of clinical practice.* Laguna Beach, CA: The North American Neuro-Developmental Treatment Association.

Humphry, R. (2002). Young children's occupations. *American Journal of Occupational Therapy, 56,* 171-179.

Individuals with Disabilities Education Act. Amendments of 1997 (P.L. 105-17). 20 U.S.C. 1400 et seq.

Jarrett, R. (1996). African American family and parenting strategies in impoverished neighborhoods. *Qualitative Sociology, 20,* 275-288.

Kemmis, B.L., & Dunn, W. (1996). Collaborative consultation: The efficacy of remedial and compensatory interventions in school contexts. *American Journal of Occupational Therapy, 50,* 709-717.

Kimball, J. (1999). Sensory integration frame of reference: Postulates regarding change and application to practice. In P. Kramer & J. Hinojosa, *Frames of reference of pediatric occupational therapy* (2nd ed.). Philadelphia: Lippincott Williams & Wilkins.

Koomar, J., & Bundy, A. (2002). Creating direct intervention from theory. In A.C. Bundy, S.J. Lane, & E.A. Murray (Eds.), *Sensory integration: Theory and practice* (2nd ed., pp. 261-307). Philadelphia: F.A. Davis.

Kramer, P., & Hinojosa, J. (1999). *Frames of reference for pediatric occupational therapy* (2nd ed.). Philadelphia: Lippincott Williams & Wilkins.

Lang, E.M., Nelson, D.L., & Bush, M.A. (1992). Comparison of performance in materials-based occupation, imagery-based occupation, and rote exercise in nursing home residents. *American Journal of Occupational Therapy, 46,* 607-611.

Law, M., & Baum, C. (1998). Evidence-based occupational therapy. *Canadian Journal of Occupational Therapy, 65* (3), 131-135.

Law, M., Cadman, D., Rosenbaum, P., Walter, S., Russell, D., & DeMatteo, C. (1991). Neurodevelopmental therapy and upper-extremity inhibitive casting for children with cerebral palsy. *Developmental Medicine and Child Neurology, 33,* 379-387.

Law, M., Russell, D., Pollock, N., Rosenbaum, P., Walter, S., & King, G. (1997). A comparison of intensive neurodevelopmental therapy plus casting and a regular occupational therapy program for children with cerebral palsy. *Developmental Medicine and Child Neurology, 39,* 664-670.

Lin, K.-C., Wu, C.-Y., Tickle-Degnen, L., & Coster, W. (1997). Enhancing occupational performance through occupationally embedded exercise: A meta-analytic review. *Occupational Therapy Journal of Research, 17,* 25-47.

Lynch, E., & Hanson, M. (1997). *Developing cross-cultural competence* (2nd ed.). Baltimore: Brookes.

Lynch, E., & Hanson, M. (1993). Changing demographics: Implications for training in early intervention. *Infants and Young Children, 6* (1), 50-55.

Mattingly, C. (1994). The narrative nature of clinical reasoning. In C. Mattingly & M.H. Fleming (Eds.), *Clinical reasoning: Forms of inquiry in a therapeutic practice* (pp. 239-269). Philadelphia: F.A. Davis.

Mattingly, C., & Fleming, M.H. (1994). *Clinical reasoning: Forms of inquiry in a therapeutic practice.* Philadelphia: F.A. Davis.

Mayo, N.E. (1991). The effects of physical therapy for children with motor delay and cerebral palsy. *American Journal of Physical Medicine and Rehabilitation, 70,* 258-267.

McCollum, J.A. (2002). Influencing the development of young children with disabilities: Current themes in early intervention. *Child and Adolescent Mental Health, 7* (1), 4-9

McCollum, J.A., & Hemmeter, M.L. (1997). The effects of intervention on parent-child interaction when young children have disabilities. In M.J. Guralnick (Ed.), *The effectiveness of early intervention: Second generation research* (pp. 549-576). Baltimore: Brookes.

Miller, H., & Heaphy, T. (1998). Sensory processing in preschool children. In J. Case-Smith (Ed.), *Occupational therapy: Making a difference in school system practice,* Bethesda: American Occupational Therapy Association.

Miller, L., & Nelson, D. (1987). Dual-purpose activity versus single-purpose activity in terms of duration on task, exertion level, and affect. *Occupational Therapy in Mental Health, 7,* 55-67.

Miller, L.J., Reisman, J.E., McIntosh, D.N., & Simon, J. (2001). An ecological model of sensory modulation: Performance of children with Fragile X Syndrome, Autism, Attention-Deficit/Hyperactivity Disorder, and Sensory Modulation Dysfunction. In S.S. Roley, E.I. Blanche, & R.C. Schaaf (Eds.), *Understanding the nature of sensory integration with diverse populations* (pp. 57-88). San Antonio, TX: Therapy Skill Builders.

Murphy, S., Trombly, C., Tickle-Degnen, L., & Jacobs, K. (1999). The effect of keeping an end-product on intrinsic motivation. *American Journal of Occupational Therapy, 53,* 153-157.

Nelson, D.L., Konosky, D., Fleharry, K., Webb, R., Newere, K., Hazboun, V.P., Fontane, C., & Licht, B.C. (1996). Effects of an occupationally embedded exercise on bilaterally assisted supination in persons with hemiplegia. *American Journal of Occupational Therapy, 50,* 639-646.

Palmer, F.B., Shapiro, B.K., Wachtel, R.C., Allen, M.C., Hiller, J.E., Harryman, S.E., Mosher, B.S., Meinert, C.L., & Capute, A.J. (1988). The effects of physical therapy on cerebral palsy. *New England Journal of Medicine, 318,* 803-808.

Polatajko, H.J., Kaplan, B., & Wilson, B. (1992). Sensory integration treatment for children with learning disabilities: Its status 20 years later. *Occupational Therapy Journal of Research, 36,* 571-578.

Riccio, C.M., Nelson, D.L., & Bush, M.A. (1990). Adding purpose to the repetitive exercise of elderly women through imagery. *American Journal of Occupational Therapy, 44,* 714-719.

Richardson, P. (2003, March). From roots to wings: Social participation for children with physical disabilities. *Developmental Disabilities Special Interest Section Quarterly, 26,* 1-4.

Rogoff, B. (2003). *The cultural nature of human development.* New York: Oxford University Press.

Rogoff, B., & Morelli, G. (1989). Perspectives on children's development for cultural psychology. *American Psychologist, 44,* 343-348.

Rorie, J.L., Paine, L.L., & Barger, M.K. (1996). Primary care for women—Cultural competence in primary care services. *Journal of Nurse-Midwifery, 41* (2), 92-100.

Rosenbaum, P., King, S., Law, M., King, G., & Evans, J. (1998). Family-centred service: A conceptual framework and research review. *Physical & Occupational Therapy in Pediatrics, 18,* 1-20.

Rubin, K., Fein, G.G., & Vandenberg, B. (1983). Play. In P.H. Mussen (Ed.), *Handbook of child psychology: Vol. 4* (4th ed., pp. 693-774). New York: Wiley & Sons.

Sackett, D.L., Rosenberg, W.M.C., Muir Gray, J.A., Haynes, R.B., & Richardson, W.S. (1996). Evidence-based medicine: What it is and what it isn't. *British Medical Journal, 312,* 71-72.

Schell, B (2003). Clinical reasoning: The basis of practice. In E.B. Crepeau, E.S. Cohn, & B.A.B. Schell, *Williard & Spackman's occupational therapy* (10th ed., p. 135). Philadelphia: Lippincott Williams & Wilkins.

Scherzer, A.L., Mike, V., & Ilson, J. (1976). Physical therapy as a determinant of change in the cerebral palsied infant. *Pediatrics, 53,* 47-52.

Schilling, D.L., Washington, K., Billingsley, F.F., & Deitz, J. (2003). Classroom seating for children with attention deficit hyperactivity disorder. *American Journal of Occupational Therapy, 57,* 534-541.

Schopler, E. (1994). A statewide program for the treatment and education of autistic and related communication handicapped children (TEACCH). *Psychoses and Pervasive Developmental Disorders, 3,* 91-103.

Schopler, E., Mesibov, G.B., & Hearsey, K. (1995). Structured teaching in the TEACCH systems. In E. Schoper & G.B. Mesibov (Eds.), *Learning and cognition in autism* (pp. 243-268). New York: Plenum Press.

Sharifzadeh, V.S. (1997). Families with Middle Eastern roots. In E. W. Lynch & M. Hanson (Eds.), *Developing cross-cultural competence* (2nd ed., pp. 441-482). Baltimore: Brookes.

Sietsema, J.M., Nelson, D.L., Mulder, R.M., Mervau-Scheidel, D., & White, B.E. (1993). The use of a game to promote arm reach in persons with traumatic brain injury. *American Journal of Occupational Therapy, 47,* 19-24.

Tickle-Degnen, L. (1998). Using research evidence in planning treatment for the individual client. *Canadian Journal of Occupational Therapy, 65* (3), 152-159.

Tickle-Degnen, L., & Coster, W. (1995). Therapeutic interaction and the management of challenge during the beginning minutes of sensory integration treatment. *Occupational Therapy Journal of Research, 15,* 122-141.

Trombly, C.A. (1995). Occupation: Purposefulness and meaningfulness as therapeutic mechanisms. *American Journal of Occupational Therapy, 49,* 960-972.

U.S. Census Bureau (2002). 2002 American Community Survey Profiles. Retrieved on March 31, 2004, at www.census.gov/acs.

VandenBerg, N.L. (2001). The use of a weighted vest to increase on-task behavior in children with attention difficulties. *American Journal of Occupational Therapy, 55,* 621-628.

Van der Weel, F.R., Van der Meer, A.L.H., & Lee, D.N. (1991). Effect of task on movement control in cerebral palsy: Implications for assessment and therapy. *Developmental Medicine and Child Neurology, 33,* 419-426.

VanLeit, B., & Crowe, T.K. (2002). Outcomes of an occupational therapy program for mothers of children with disabilities: Impact on satisfaction with time use and occupational performance. *American Journal of Occupational Therapy, 56,* 402-410.

Vargas, S., & Camilli, G. (1999). A meta-analysis of research on sensory integration treatment. *American Journal of Occupational Therapy, 53,* 189-198.

Vygotsky, L. (1978). *Mind in society.* Cambridge: Harvard University Press.

Willis, W. (1997). Families with African American roots. In E. W. Lynch & M. Hanson (Eds.), *Developing cross-cultural competence* (2nd ed., pp. 165-208). Baltimore: Brookes.

Wolfberg, P.J. (2003). *Peer play and the autism spectrum: The art of guiding children's socialization and imagination.* Shawnee Mission, KS: Autism Asperger Publishing Company.

World Health Organization. (2001). *ICF: International classification of functioning, health, disability and participation.* Geneva, Switzerland: WHO.

Zuniga, M.E. (1997). Families with Latino roots. In E.W. Lynch & M. Hanson (Eds.), *Developing cross-cultural competence* (2nd ed., pp. 209-250). Baltimore: Brookes.

1-A Evidence-Based Occupational Therapy Links

OCCUPATIONAL THERAPY SYSTEMATIC EVALUATION OF EVIDENCE: OTSEEKER

www.otseeker.com

OTseeker is a database that contains abstracts of systematic reviews and randomized controlled trials relevant to occupational therapy. Trials have been critically appraised and rated to assist in evaluating their validity and interpretability. These ratings assist therapists in judging the quality and usefulness of trials for informing clinical intervention. OTseeker links to trials through a wide range of sources. Included on the site is a search function, a tutorial on evidence-based practice, systematic reviews, randomized controlled trials, and critical appraisal. Links to other sites on evidence-based practice are provided.

OCCUPATIONAL THERAPY EVIDENCE-BASED PRACTICE RESEARCH GROUP

www.fhs.mcmaster.ca/rehab/ebp

The McMaster Occupational Therapy Evidence-Based Practice group focuses on research to critically review evidence regarding the effectiveness of occupational therapy interventions and to develop tools for evaluation of occupational therapy programs. This site is only partially developed.

CENTRE FOR EVIDENCE-BASED MEDICINE

www.cebm.utoronto.ca

Includes critical appraisal sheets, resources for teaching evidence-based medicine, calculators for interpreting effect sizes, numbers to treat, and other statistics. Teaching resources are available for different medical disciplines. The site provides examples of clients, important clinical questions, and an analysis of the literature to predict the likelihood of specific outcome. The information in the site follows and supports the original work of Sackett, Straus, Richardson, Rosenberg, and Haynes.

TREATMENT OUTCOMES COMMITTEE OF THE AMERICAN ACADEMY FOR CEREBRAL PALSY AND DEVELOPMENTAL MEDICINE

www.aacpdm.org/home.html

The Treatment Outcomes Committee of the American Academy for Cerebral Palsy and Developmental Medicine (AACPDM) aims to critically appraise research relevant to developmental disability. It then presents the results in summarized evidence tables. Discussions debate the issue of "levels of evidence." The site classifies levels of evidence, giving detailed recognition of evidence for single subject designs.

PEDro-PHYSIOTHERAPY EVIDENCE DATABASE

http://ptww.cchs.usyd.edu.au/pedro

PEDro refers to the Physiotherapy Evidence Database and is an initiative of the Centre for Evidence-Based Physiotherapy (CEBP) in Sydney, Australia. PEDro aims to give physiotherapists and others rapid access to bibliographic details and abstracts of randomized controlled trials and systematic reviews in physiotherapy. All randomized controlled trials included in the database have been rated on the PEDro rating scale for quality (from 0-10) to discriminate between trials that are likely to be valid and interpretable and those that are not. PEDro contains many trials of relevance to occupational therapy.

REHAB TRIALS

www.rehabtrials.org

Rehab Trials is a registry of randomized controlled trials related to rehabilitation. Populations include people with spinal cord injury, stroke, traumatic brain injury, amputations, and studies with both adults and children. Intervention studies include technology and equipment, pressure garments, cushions, and constraint-induced movement therapy.

COCHRANE LIBRARY

www.update-software.com/cochrane

The Cochrane Library consists of a regularly updated collection of evidence-based medicine databases, including The Cochrane Database of Systematic Reviews, which provides high-quality information to people providing and receiving care and those responsible for research, teaching, funding, and administration at all levels.

Cochrane Reviews (the principal output of the Collaboration) are published electronically in successive issues of *The Cochrane Database of Systematic Reviews*. Preparation and maintenance of Cochrane Reviews is the responsibility of international collaborative review groups. At the beginning of 2001, the existing review groups covered all of the important areas of health care. The members of these groups—researchers, health care professionals, consumers, and others—share an interest in generating reliable, up-to-date evidence relevant to the prevention, treatment, and rehabilitation of particular health problems or groups of problems.

DATABASE OF ABSTRACTS OF REVIEWS OF EFFECTIVENESS (DARE)

http://agatha.york.ac.uk/darehp.htm

DARE (the Database of Abstracts of Reviews of Effects) contains summaries of systematic reviews that have met strict quality criteria. Each summary also provides a critical commentary on the quality of the review. DARE covers a broad range of health care related topics and can be used for answering questions about the effects of health care interventions, as well as for developing clinical guidelines and policy making. DARE is available free of charge on the Internet (http://nhscrd.york.ac.uk) and as part of the Cochrane Library.

NATIONAL GUIDELINE CLEARINGHOUSE

www.guidelines.gov/index.asp

National Guideline Clearinghouse (NGC) is a public resource for evidence-based clinical practice guidelines. NGC is sponsored by the U.S. Agency for Healthcare Research and Quality (formerly the U.S. Agency for Health Care Policy and Research), www.ahrq.gov, in partnership with the American Medical Association, www.ama-assn.org, and the American Association of Health Plans, www.aahp.org.

EVIDENCE-BASED MEDICINE TOOLKIT

www.med.ualberta.ca/ebm/ebm.htm

This is a collection of tools for identifying, assessing, and applying relevant evidence for better health care decision making. The appraisal tools are adapted from the Users' Guides series prepared by the Evidence-Based Medicine Working Group and originally published in the *Journal of the American Medical Association (JAMA)*.

SEARCHING FOR EVIDENCE

www.med.usf.edu/CLASS/Gene/web.htm

This site provides a compilation of useful resources of medical evidence that can be found on the Internet.

PUBMED CLINICAL QUERIES

www.ncbi.nlm.nih.gov/entrez/query/static/clinical.html

This site identifies only clinical queries. Four study categories are provided, and the emphasis may be more sensitive (i.e., most relevant articles but probably some less relevant ones) or more specific (i.e., mostly relevant articles but probably omitting a few). As a result, only experimental design studies with their abstracts are listed; therefore, only high-validity studies are provided.

NETTING THE EVIDENCE

www.shef.ac.uk/~scharr/ir/netting

This site provides an extensive listing of web sites related to evidence-based practice. It contains many useful links to important evidence-based practice sites. It has a library of resources describing evidence-based practice and critical appraisal and using outcomes in practice.

2 Teaming

Jane Case-Smith

KEY TERMS

Multidisciplinary professional teams
Collaboration
Model of team dynamics
Team interaction models
Team process

CHAPTER OBJECTIVES

1 Describe professionals in other disciplines who provide services to children with disabilities and to their families.
2 Describe the dynamics of team function.
3 Compare team function in medical, educational, and early intervention systems.
4 Describe the elements of the team process, including communication, decision making, consensus building, and conflict resolution.
5 Discuss issues in the team process that affect team effectiveness.

A child with disabilities benefits most from holistic intervention. Therefore the collaborative efforts of a multidisciplinary team of professionals are needed to design and provide the intervention program. In the medical, educational, and community-based settings in which children are served, individualized plans of intervention are developed, and child outcomes become the responsibility of teams of professionals. Often the child's individualized plan calls for the involvement of specialized professionals, who then make up the team for the child; that is, certain services become responsible for implementing the plan. The makeup of the team is determined by the type of setting in which services are received, the child's age, the type and severity of the child's disabilities, and community resources. For example, a child with a high-level spinal cord injury will benefit from the services of an occupational therapist, a physical therapist, a nurse, a social worker, a rehabilitation engineer, and others, depending on the individual situation. A young child with Down syndrome often receives services from an occupational therapist, a speech-language pathologist, a physical therapist, a special educator, a nurse, a social worker, an optometrist, and a physician. Teams in rural areas often have fewer members, because specialists are not available.

The professionals involved with the child and family change over time, and new professionals participate in the child's care during medical crises and hospital admissions, during periods of vocational training, and with transitions from early intervention to preschool and from preschool to school. Because a team of professionals from multiple disciplines defines the context for almost all pediatric occupational therapy practice, it is essential that therapists develop skills in collaboration. Effective teaming skills can be as important as the technical and professional skills that define the therapists' professions.

This chapter describes the professionals of other disciplines who work with occupational therapists. A model of team dynamics is explained and then exemplified for medical, educational, and early intervention teams. Finally, effective team processes are identified and discussed.

SERVICE PROVIDERS WHO WORK WITH OCCUPATIONAL THERAPISTS

Physicians

The primary physician for children is often a pediatrician or family practitioner. Physicians in pediatric specialty areas may also provide medical care (e.g., pediatric neurology, surgery, orthopedics, and ophthalmology). Physicians who provide medical care to children have completed internships and residencies in pediatrics and related specialty areas and have successfully completed board certification examinations. Standards of pediatric practice mandate the identification of developmental delays as part of the routine care of the well child. Because most children obtain health care on an ongoing basis from birth, pediatricians and family practitioners are in an ideal position to identify, evaluate, treat, and refer children with developmental delays.

The responsibilities of the pediatrician or family practitioner include identifying children for referral to early intervention and providing families with information about early intervention (Wachtel & Compart, 1996). The family often needs a physician's referral to become eligible for early intervention services and specific prescriptions for physical and occupational therapy services. In a recent survey of pediatricians, screening and referral practices were identified. Most pediatricians (90%) primarily use an informal process and nonstandardized screening techniques to identify children with developmental disabilities (American Academy of Pediatrics, Division of Child Health Research, 2003). Physicians report that they feel competent in identifying motor disabilities and do not feel as competent in identifying learning disabilities. When pediatricians have patients who have developmental disabilities, approximately half report participating in the interdisciplinary team assessments. Most of their participation is consultative, involving phone calls and submission of the medical record.

In addition to identifying children at risk and making appropriate referrals, the physician manages diagnostic workup examinations to determine the causes of disabilities. Often it is important to research the medical cause of a disability to determine its course and prognosis, and in the case of a genetic disorder, it is essential to identify the likelihood of recurrence of the disability in the family. Some conditions (e.g., autism, attention deficit disorder) benefit from pharmaceutical treatment, which must be initiated and managed by a physician.

Children with disabilities generally have more medical problems than other children. For example, children with spina bifida are vulnerable to orthopedic, respiratory, and circulatory problems. Children with cerebral palsy require ongoing medical management related to orthopedic, neurologic, and respiratory concerns. All children with chronic medical problems require ongoing monitoring by their pediatricians and other medical specialists. The role of the physician on the team varies from consultant to leader, depending on the system in which the team is functioning and the medical stability of the child. In the hospital and other medical systems, the physician provides team leadership (discussed later in the section on medically based teams).

Nurses

Registered nurses (RNs) make up the largest segment of the health care work force. To become an RN or professional nurse, candidates must graduate from a state-approved school of nursing. There are two types of degree programs: a 2-year associate degree program, usually offered at community colleges, and a 4-year baccalaureate degree program from a college or university. In recent years hospital-based diploma programs have shown decreased enrollment; in 2000 they represented 30% of the RN population. In the same year, 40% of nurses were trained in associate degree programs and 29% received basic nursing education in baccalaureate programs (American Nurses Association, 2001).

Generic nursing education includes courses in the biologic, behavioral, and social sciences. Basic courses include biology, anatomy and physiology, pharmacology, pathophysiology, nutrition, growth and development, system theory, and interpersonal relationship. Nurses prepared at the bachelor's degree level receive education in community health, including principles of interdisciplinary and interagency service coordination or care management and nursing research (Cox, 1996).

All RNs must pass licensure examinations after completing their accredited generalist educational program. Each state defines the scope of nursing practice and standards for licensure in a Nurse Practice Act, and many states have developed continuing education requirements for nurses as a prerequisite for maintaining licensure (American Nurses' Association, 2004).

In March 2000, approximately 60% of employed RNs worked in hospitals, almost 18% worked in community or public health settings, and 9% worked in ambulatory care settings, most often physicians' offices (American Nurses' Association, 2001). Today, nurses who work with children are employed in diagnostic clinics, child development centers, outpatient and health department clinics, and home health services. Nurses who work in schools provide medical care by administering medicines, implementing routine medical procedures (e.g., asthma treatment or catheterization), and performing health screenings.

The role of a nurse in early intervention includes (1) diagnosing and treating health problems in children and families; (2) screening and assessing the psychologic, physiologic, and developmental characteristics of the child and family for early identification, referral, and intervention; (3) planning and coordinating with the family and interdisciplinary team; (4) providing intervention to the family to improve the child's and family's health and developmental status; and (5) evaluating the effectiveness of the nursing care provided (American Nurses' Association Consensus Early Intervention Committee, 1993).

Nurses often serve as case managers in early intervention (Collins, 1995; Hansen, Holaday, & Miles, 1990) Their case management activities may include locating community activities, helping family members gain understanding of the child's individual education plan, making periodic telephone calls to assess the child's and family's status, providing information about parent groups, and helping parents contact families with similar problems.

Today, more than 20% of RNs seek education beyond their basic nursing training and have postgraduate degrees and specialist credentials. The *clinical nurse specialist* has an advanced nursing degree and can implement certain procedures traditionally performed by a physician or can perform these procedures under the direct supervision of a physician. These nurses can establish their own practices in a community, but generally they establish a close working relationship with a specific physician or group of physicians. The roles of the clinical nurse specialist include (1) assessing health status, (2) diagnosing human responses to actual or potential health problems, (3) planning and implementing specific therapeutic intervention, and (4) evaluating client outcomes (American Association of Colleges of Nursing, 2004).

Nurse practitioners hold an advanced degree in a specialty area of nursing practice. These nurses can practice independently; that is, without direct physician supervision. The major activities of nurse practitioners include screening, completing health histories, performing physical and psychologic examinations, managing care during wellness and illness, teaching, consulting and collaborating, conducting client follow-up examinations and referrals, promoting positive health, and managing personnel and administration (Cox, 1996). A nurse practitioner can diagnose illness and can manage many illnesses in the chronic stage; nurse practitioners, therefore, provide some of the care previously provided only by physicians. Nurse practitioners focus on health maintenance, disease prevention, counseling, and patient education (American College of Nurse Practitioners, 2004).

Pediatric nurse practitioners work with pediatricians and health care teams in clinics, offices, schools, public health departments, and hospitals. The activities of pediatric nurse practitioners include providing health maintenance care for children, performing screening and well child examinations, diagnosing and treating common childhood illnesses, performing immunizations, and providing anticipatory guidance regarding common health problems (National Association of Pediatric Nurse Practitioners [NAPNAP], 2004).

Licensed practical nurses (LPNs) complete 12- to 16-month training programs, usually after high school, and take examinations in the state in which they will practice. These training programs do not necessarily result in a degree. LPNs provide bedside care and work under the supervision of RNs. *Nurse's aides* are trained at the associate degree level in vocational or on-the-job programs in medical facilities.

Physical Therapists

Physical therapy and occupational therapy are known together as the *rehabilitation therapies* (or related services in the schools), and therapists in these two professions work closely in a variety of settings. Physical therapists and occupational therapists share similar or common goals for their clients and offer complementary approaches to intervention. For example, both therapies address activities of daily living (ADLs), but they approach these outcomes using different techniques and theories, and complementary recommendations then are made to the family.

Physical therapists assess joint motion, muscle strength and endurance, the function of the heart and lungs, and the performance of activities required in daily living, among other responsibilities. Treatment includes therapeutic exercise, cardiovascular endurance training, and training in ADLs (American Physical Therapy Association [APTA], 1999).

The minimum educational requirement to become a physical therapist is a post-baccalaureate degree (e.g., master's or doctoral degree in physical therapy) from an accredited program. A growing number of institutions now offer the doctor of physical therapy (DPT) degree; there were 81 such programs in the United States in 2003. Approximately 200 U.S. colleges and universities offer professional education programs in physical therapy. At all entry levels of physical therapy education, the graduates must pass a state-administered licensure examination, which allows the candidate to practice in that state.

Physical therapy professional educational programs prepare students to be generalists, capable of entering general settings, such as hospitals or rehabilitation centers. The entry level curriculum provides basic information about working with children and families; however, pediatric content is not a primary emphasis of the course work. Physical therapists provide intervention to children with neuromuscular, musculoskeletal, or cardiopulmonary impairments. Approximately 5% of all physical therapists work in schools, and a higher percentage provide pediatric services in hospitals, rehabilitation centers, clinics, and homes.

In the regulations for Part C of the Individuals with Disabilities Education Act, the legal definition of physical therapy services is given as those activities that promote "sensorimotor function through enhancement of musculoskeletal status, neurobehavioral organization, perceptual and motor development, cardiopulmonary status, and effective environmental adaptation" (Individuals with Disabilities Education Act [IDEA], 1997, Sec. 303.12). Specific services of physical therapists, as defined in IDEA, are to:

- Provide treatment to increase joint function, muscle strength, mobility, and endurance
- Address gross motor skills that rely on the large muscles of the body involved in physical movement and range of motion
- Help improve the student's posture, gait, and body awareness
- Monitor the function, fit, and proper use of mobility aids and devices (Federal Regulations, Sec. 300.24 [b] [8]; National Dissemination Center for Children with Disabilities, 1999)

The services provided by pediatric physical therapists are listed in Table 2-1.

TABLE 2-1 Services for Children Provided by Physical Therapists

Developmental Activities
Strengthening
Movement and mobility
Tone management
Motor learning
Balance and coordination
Recreation, play, and leisure
Adaptation of daily care activities and routines
Equipment design, fabrication, and fitting
Orthotics and prosthetics
Burn and wound care
Cardiopulmonary endurance
Safety and prevention programs
Use of assistive technology

From American Physical Therapy Association, Section on Pediatrics (2003) *The A, B, C's of pediatric physical therapy.* Retrieved March 25, 2004, from www.pediatricapta.org/graphics/Gen%20Ped%20PT.pdf.

A physical therapist assistant works under the supervision of the physical therapist. These individuals assist the physical therapist in implementing treatment programs, training children in exercises and ADLs, and conducting treatment, and they report the child's responses to the physical therapist. A physical therapist assistant must complete a 2-year educational program, typically offered through a community or junior college. The program consists of 1 year of general education and 1 year of technical courses on physical therapy procedures that includes clinical experience.

Speech-Language Pathologists

Occupational therapists work closely with speech-language pathologists, particularly when children have feeding and oral motor problems, augmentative communication needs, or global neuromotor and developmental delays. Occupational therapists share knowledge and philosophy with speech therapists. Speech-language pathologists hold a master's or doctoral degree. Approximately 242 colleges and universities provide graduate programs in speech-language pathology. To practice, graduates must receive the Certificate of Clinical Competence of the American Speech-Language-Hearing Association (ASHA), and in most states speech-language pathologists can practice only with a license (American Speech-Language-Hearing Association [ASHA], 2002). To earn the certificate, a speech-language pathologist must have a graduate degree and almost 400 hours of supervised clinical experience, must complete a clinical fellowship, and must pass a written examination. Almost 60% of speech therapists work in schools or preschools. Others work in clinics, hospitals, speech and language centers, and home health agencies.

According to the ASHA (2002), speech pathologists work to prevent speech, voice, language, communica-tion, swallowing, and related disabilities. They screen, identify, assess, diagnose, refer, and provide treatment and intervention, including consultation and follow-up services, to children at risk for speech, voice, language, communication, swallowing, and related disabilities. Speech-language pathologists select, prescribe, dispense, and provide services that support the effective use of augmentative and alternative communication devices and other communication prostheses and assistive devices (Box 2-1). They also work with children who have oral motor problems that cause eating and swallowing disorders. Part C of IDEA defines speech-language pathology as services that include identification, referral, and intervention for "children with communicative or oropharyngeal disorders and delays in development of communication skills" (IDEA, 1997, Sec. 303.12).

In recognition of the importance of social behaviors and cognition in addition to language, the practice of speech pathology with young children has shifted its focus from language to the broad area of communication (Lorsardo, 1996). Speech therapists or communication specialists also appreciate the relationship between communication and other domains of development (e.g., motor performance, social-emotional function, and adaptive behaviors).

School Psychologists

A school psychologist is a professional psychologist who has completed a field placement program in school psychology. This individual has specialized training in both psychology and education. All psychologists have a master's or doctoral degree and have satisfactorily completed at least 1 year of supervised experience. For certification in school psychology, most states require a 2- or 3-year specialist level or post-master's degree in school psychology.

School psychologists function as independent practitioners. They conduct a multifaceted psychologic and psychoeducational assessment of children and adolescents (National Association of School Psychologists [NASP], 2004). Their primary roles in assessment are to identify an educational diagnosis and to assist in determining the level of inclusion that would most benefit the student.

Psychologic and psychoeducational assessment includes the following areas:
- Academic skills
- Learning aptitudes
- Personality and emotional development
- Social skills

Although most occupational therapists associate school psychologists with assessment and diagnosis, their roles are more comprehensive. The goals of school psychologic services are to promote mental health and facilitate student learning. To meet these goals, school psychologists consult and collaborate with parents, school

BOX 2-1 Scope of Practice of Speech-Language Pathologists

1 Providing prevention, screening, consultation, assessment and diagnosis, treatment, intervention, management, counseling, and follow-up services for disorders of the following:
  - Speech
  - Language, including comprehension and expression in oral, written, graphic, and manual modalities; language processing, preliteracy and language-based literacy skills, including phonologic awareness
  - Swallowing or other upper aerodigestive functions, such as infant feeding and aeromechanical events
  - Cognitive aspects of communication
  - Sensory awareness related to communication, swallowing, or other upper aerodigestive functions
2 Establishing augmentative and alternative communication techniques and strategies, including developing, selecting, and prescribing such systems and devices.
3 Providing services to individuals with hearing loss and their families/caregivers.
4 Screening the hearing of individuals for the purpose of referral for further evaluation and management.
5 Using instrumentation to observe, collect data, and measure parameters of communication and swallowing.
6 Selecting, fitting, and establishing effective use of prosthetic/adaptive devices for communication, swallowing, or other upper aerodigestive functions.
7 Collaborating in the assessment of central auditory processing disorders.
8 Educating and counseling individuals, families, co-workers, educators, and other persons in the community regarding acceptance, adaptation, and decision making about communication, swallowing, or other upper aerodigestive concerns.
9 Advocating for individuals through community awareness, education, and training programs to promote and facilitate access to full participation in communication, including the elimination of societal barriers.
10 Collaborating with and providing referrals and information to audiologists, educators, and health professionals as individual needs dictate.
11 Addressing behaviors and environments that affect communication, swallowing, or other upper aerodigestive functions.
12 Providing services to modify or enhance communication performance.
13 Recognizing the need to provide and appropriately accommodate diagnostic and treatment services to individuals from diverse cultural backgrounds and adjust treatment and assessment services accordingly.

Modified from American Speech-Language-Hearing Association (ASHA). (2002). *Scope of practice in speech-language pathology.* Retrieved March 14, 2004, from www.asha.org.

officials, and outside personnel regarding mental health, behavioral, and educational concerns. These services often entail counseling or family dialog. Most often school psychologists intervene when behavioral and mental health issues affect a student's performance. When student behavioral problems are identified, school psychologists often determine the appropriate referrals for mental health services (NASP, 2000).

School psychologists also provide direct services to individual students and groups to enhance mental health, behavior, social competency, and academic status. Using consultation and monitoring models, school psychologists work with teachers and related service providers who interact with students on a daily basis. School psychologists also provide prevention services to identify potential learning difficulties, design programs for children at risk for failure, help parents and teachers develop skills for coping with disruptive behavior, and develop school-wide initiatives to make schools safer and more effective (NASP, 2000).

Social Workers

Professional social workers are the nation's largest group of providers of mental health services. The primary focus of the social work profession is to help people participate in their social environments. Social workers help children and families link to community agencies, obtain financial assistance, and find resources when mental health is at risk. They also provide counseling and coordination of interagency services for their clients.

A professional social worker has earned a bachelor's or a master's degree in social work and meets state certification or licensure requirements. Most states that certify clinical social workers require a master's degree in social work, at least 2 years' experience, and an examination. Social workers practice in many settings, including family service and child welfare agencies, community mental health centers, schools, and hospitals. The social worker with a bachelor's degree can work in a variety of settings, primarily performing case management activities. Social work case managers help link clients to community resources and help coordinate services for clients who need comprehensive care (National Association of Social Workers [NASW], 2002).

Social workers in clinical and school settings provide counseling and consulting services. The roles of social workers in schools include social assessment and counseling; outreach and liaison among school, home, and community agencies; case management; advocacy; and education and training of staff (e.g., related to social emotional and risk issues of students).

The legal definition of social work in Part C of IDEA includes the following:
  - Making home visits to evaluate a child's living conditions and patterns of parent-child interaction
  - Conducting an emotional-developmental assessment of the child within the family context
  - Providing individual and family-group counseling with parents and other family members, and appropriate social skill–building activities with the child and parents
  - Working with those problems in a child's and family's living situation (home, community, and

any center where early intervention services are provided) that affect the child's maximum utilization of early intervention services; and

- Identifying, mobilizing, and coordinating community resources to enable the child and family to receive maximum benefit from early intervention services (National Dissemination Center for Children with Disabilities, 1999)

Teachers and Special Educators

Teachers, in collaboration with special educators, design and provide instruction to students with disabilities. Because students with disabilities are routinely included in general education classrooms in their neighborhood schools, special education teachers often work in teams with general education teachers. Occupational therapists and certified occupational therapy assistants work closely with teachers, often directly in the classroom. Therapists consult with teachers and provide other types of support (e.g., teaching, modifying the curriculum for students with disabilities, setting up assistive technology for classroom use).

Teachers and special educators are certified or licensed in specialty areas of instruction that define the grades and types of student they are qualified to teach (e.g., early childhood, learning disability). All teachers and all early intervention specialists (sometimes called *early childhood specialists*) have at least a bachelor's degree. With a bachelor's or master's degree in special education and successful completion of a teaching internship, the individual earns a teaching certificate in one of the student diagnostic categories. To maintain their license or certification, teachers are required by most states to complete graduate courses. Many states require teachers to work toward and achieve a master's degree within a specified period after employment.

Educators work with other team members in child assessment, program planning, and implementation. They administer cognitive and academic tests and collect evaluation data on the students. Often they coordinate comprehensive assessments of students to ensure that all relevant areas are evaluated and the process is completed in a timely manner.

The special educator frequently coordinates the planning process by calling together team members to develop the Individualized Education Program (IEP) or the Individualized Family Service Plan (IFSP). With an individualized program in place, the educator selects, adapts, and implements instructional strategies that address the developmental and educational needs of the child. These professionals select, manage, and present the curriculum and learning materials, and they manage the classroom environment, creating surroundings conducive to learning. In the case of home schooling or home-based services, the special educator helps families establish home environments that promote development and learning. Teachers often ask for consultation from related service personnel (e.g., occupational therapists) to help solve problems when specific issues arise or when students fail to meet expectations.

Most classrooms have teaching assistants or aides who are trained to assist the professional teacher in the classroom. Aides help with the logistics of student function, (e.g., getting dressed for recess, monitoring hallways, assisting in feeding, setting up learning areas). Aides often work directly with children with disabilities, assisting them in classroom activities. A teaching assistant usually has an associate of arts degree and a teaching associate's certificate. Teaching assistants have a minimum of a high school diploma, whereas aides do not have any minimal degree requirement.

Summary

A number of trends in education, certification, and qualifications can be observed in the related professions that work with occupational therapists and certified occupational therapy assistants. Most of these related professions require a master's degree to practice with children and families, and most of these professionals are licensed or certified according to state law. Such individuals, therefore, have legal definitions and scopes of practice. Most professionals who work with children have multiple levels of education and credentialing that define levels of authority and independence in practice. With support personnel to assist in teaching and implementing intervention, collaborative teams of supervisors and associates (e.g., occupational therapists and occupational therapy assistants) work together to provide comprehensive and cost-effective services.

The national organizations for the professions discussed in this section have established standards of practice that define the roles and values of each profession. The national organizations publish ethical statements with their standards of practice that confirm the profession's ethical values and assure the public that its professionals are fair, truthful, competent, and respectful of consumers' confidentiality and individual rights.

This section described only a few of the professionals who work with occupational therapists and certified occupational therapy assistants (see the list of services in Table 2-2). Each profession has its own scope of practice and makes unique contributions to the medical, school-based, or early intervention team. Learning about the educational background and scope of practice of other professionals on the team is the first step in collaborative teamwork. This knowledge allows appropriate referrals to be made, and each professional's expertise can be used in team decisions. An understanding of the discipline-specific roles of each team member promotes

TABLE 2-2   Disciplines Listed in the Individuals with Disabilities Education Act (IDEA)

Part B: School Programs	Part C: Early Intervention
FAPE offers services that meet state standards; they are provided under public supervision by qualified personnel. FAPE includes the following: ■ Special education (specially designed instruction) that meets the unique educational needs of the child, including classroom, physical education, home, hospital, and institution instruction, and vocational education if specially designed ■ Related services needed by the child to benefit from special education are the following: 1 Speech and hearing therapy 2 Psychologic sessions 3 Physical and occupational therapy 4 Recreation 5 Social work 6 Counseling 7 Medical diagnosis and evaluation 8 Parent training and counseling 9 Assistive technology devices and instruction 10 Rehabilitation counseling 11 School health program	Early intervention is designed to 1 Meet developmental needs of the child and family relative to the child's development; and 2 Meet state standards, providing services under public supervision by qualified personnel. Early intervention includes the following services: 1 Family training, counseling, home visits 2 Special instruction 3 Speech therapy 4 Hearing therapy 5 Occupational therapy 6 Physical therapy 7 Psychologic sessions 8 Service coordination 9 Medical diagnosis or evaluation 10 Early identification, screening, and assessment 11 Health program 12 Social work 13 Vision 14 Nursing 15 Nutrition 16 Assistive technology devices and instructions 17 Transportation and financial counseling

FAPE, Free appropriate public education.

team communication and the team process, as described in the next sections.

MODEL OF TEAM DYNAMICS

The team of professionals who provide services to children tends to be fluid and dynamic, with roles and membership shifting in response to the client's needs and system changes. Team interaction is one of the most rewarding and potentially challenging aspects of pediatric occupational therapy. Becoming an effective team member requires a unique set of competencies. Interpersonal communication, conflict resolution, decision making, consultation, and leadership are among the skills that are essential for an effective team member.

This section describes a model of team dynamics based on interacting components that determine a team's effectiveness and productivity (Figure 2-1). The model's components are the team's (1) mission and purpose, (2) composition and structure, and (3) interaction model. These elements determine the manner in which the team functions and are nested in a system or practice context. The primary contexts for children's services are hospitals or medical systems, schools, and community early intervention programs. The context or organizational system often determines the team's mission, structure, and interaction model, which can vary, even within a system (e.g., teams in the public school system may use multidisciplinary or

SYSTEM-PRACTICE CONTEXT

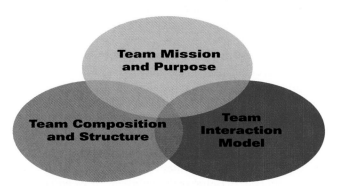

FIGURE 2-1   Model of team dynamics.

interdisciplinary models). This section applies the model of team dynamics to medical, educational, and early intervention systems.

MEDICAL SYSTEMS

Team Mission

Children's hospitals and hospitals with pediatric units provide medical, surgical, and psychiatric testing and treatment. Their clients include newborns with medical problems and children who are ill or who have been injured. The aim of a hospital-based team is to restore or promote health (Figure 2-2). As part of the

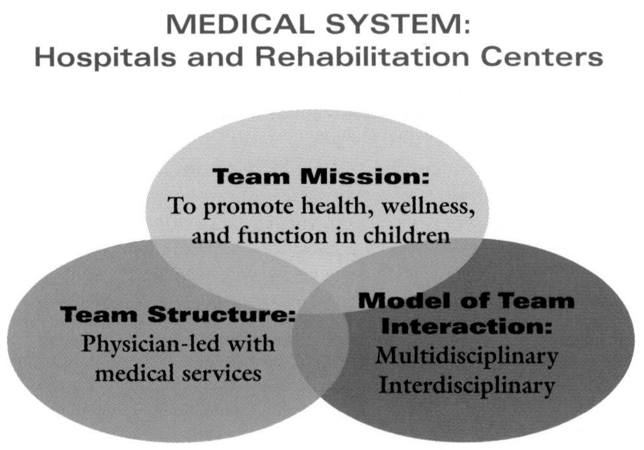

MEDICAL SYSTEM:
Hospitals and Rehabilitation Centers

Team Mission:
To promote health, wellness, and function in children

Team Structure:
Physician-led with medical services

Model of Team Interaction:
Multidisciplinary
Interdisciplinary

FIGURE 2-2 Example of team dynamics in the medical system.

individual's health, medical systems also promote *function*, generally defined in medical settings as independence in ADLs. Various health care professionals provide care under the direction of a physician. From the first day of admission, the desired outcome for the child is discharge from the hospital in a medically stable and healthy condition. Therefore the goal on entrance into the system is that the child leave the system as quickly and as medically well as possible. A secondary goal of the hospital team is placement of the child in appropriate services that meet the individual's developmental, functional, and educational needs.

When the child has a specific diagnosis or health problem, care plans and critical pathways are developed to guide the medical intervention. A *critical pathway* is a standard protocol used to guide a child's treatment and to assess whether the most efficacious treatments are being used. Critical pathways also provide a method for evaluating outcomes. *Care plans* determine when specific services are initiated and then provide broad guidelines for what should be provided. They are one tool that helps hospital personnel make efficient use of resources, shorten the hospital stay, and lower readmission rates. They reflect the expanding focus of hospitals on cost-effective measures, examination of outcomes, and management of resources.

Team Composition and Structure

Hospitals traditionally have used a physician-led team model. A child is admitted to the physician's care, and the physician determines the tests, procedures, and treatments the child receives. The physician refers the child to other health professionals when another professional's scope of practice matches the treatment interventions the child needs. Sometimes the team is made up of a physician and a nurse. Other clients require the services of a nurse, social worker, occupational therapist, physical

therapist, and speech-language pathologist. The child's medical problem determines the composition of the team and the unit to which he or she is admitted. Teams may form quickly and temporarily around a single case (e.g., the physical therapist or occupational therapist who can take a new referral is on the team). Hospitals also may have long-standing core teams with an established membership; these teams often serve children with chronic health problems (e.g., a multidisciplinary feeding team, an human immunodeficiency virus [HIV] clinic team, or a myelomeningocele team).

The roles of the medical team members are usually inequitable, with the physician as the designated leader. The physician-led team is essential to the operation of intensive care, surgical, or acute care units. The leadership position of the physician is not as established in rehabilitation or chronic care teams. When care is long term and less medically critical, a nurse or rehabilitation therapist may share in the leadership roles. A hierarchy of power and linear relationships among team members may not be as apparent. On these chronic care or rehabilitation teams, the physician may function as a consultant, and members may have more equality. In other clinical practices managed by health maintenance organizations (HMOs), nurse practitioners may provide numerous medical services and are considered leaders of the medical team.

Team Interaction Model:
Multidisciplinary and Interdisciplinary

Although the lines of authority may vary in certain medical teams, most use the multidisciplinary team model. This model evolves when the membership of the team frequently changes, generally in response to the child's medical problem. In multidisciplinary teams, members function relatively autonomously. Each is respected for his or her expertise in a defined practice area. Members have a good understanding of other professionals' scopes of practice and rely on these team members to fulfill their roles. For example, in a neonatal intensive care unit (NICU), all team members acknowledge that the dietitian provides new mothers with information on infant feeding formulas before discharge. This team also relies on the physical therapist to provide positioning recommendations to parents at the time of the newborn's discharge. Teams that are more established and are assigned to units with children who have comprehensive rehabilitation needs may use interdisciplinary models.

In a multidisciplinary model, professionals complete separate assessments and make individual treatment plans. Intervention is generally carried out in separate one-on-one sessions. Communication is informal and tends to be triggered by a patient's immediate needs rather than an established team meeting time (e.g., a quick call from the nurse to the occupational therapist to inform him or her that an infant appears alert and ready for an oral feeding). The medical chart is a primary form of communication. Communication tends to focus on essential elements of the child's care and tasks that need to be accomplished to restore health or meet the functional goals that will lead to discharge. Communication often results in actions and leads to other immediate communications, reflecting the rapid pace of the medical system. The medical goals are held as priorities and usually supersede social and behavioral goals.

A multidisciplinary, hospital-based team functions well when the membership is stable and when team members perceive that they have equal status with one another. Teams are most likely to achieve equality of member status when goals for the client expand beyond the child's medical needs to social, developmental, and functional needs. Hospitals and medical systems have long-standing teams on special units (e.g., NICU, rehabilitation units) or in specialty clinics (e.g., cerebral palsy clinic). These teams, which establish developmental and functional goals for the client, in addition to health goals, use the interdisciplinary models (Miller et al., 2001).

In contrast to the multidisciplinary team, the interdisciplinary team requires group synthesis (Box 2-2). The professionals have substantial knowledge of the other disciplines, and this awareness enables each professional to speak and understand the language of the others. Roles on an interdisciplinary team are more flexible and more equitable. Inpatient rehabilitation programs (see Chapter 25) generally have interdisciplinary teams. A well-defined program often prescribes the team roles. The Commission for Accreditation of Rehabilitation Facilities (CARF) requires that programs define admission and discharge criteria, services, and protocols for certain conditions, as well as methods for evaluating programs.

Miller et al. (2001) described an interdisciplinary feeding team in which a range of medical professions (e.g., occupational therapy, nutrition, speech-language pathology, psychology, gastroenterology) provided integrated, well-coordinated services. Because children with complex feeding problems frequently have weight loss, nutritional deficiencies, and physiologic and behavioral issues, care by an integrated team with members who understand all the issues is essential. As an example, establishing a diet for a child requires that team members collaborate to accommodate the child's current medications, sensory and nutritional needs, and behavioral issues around food preferences, as well as the family's cultural preferences.

On rehabilitation units, comprehensive plans involving multiple services are developed for individual children. The team members work together toward mutually agreed-upon functional outcomes. Co-treatments are common; therapists meet with the child's family to

BOX 2-2 Hospital-Based Interdisciplinary Team

After suffering severe head trauma, Phil was a patient for 2 months at Children's Hospital on its rehabilitation unit. An interdisciplinary team, which included a nurse, social worker, occupational therapist, certified occupational therapy assistant, physical therapist, and speech-language pathologist, cared for Phil during his stay. A school psychologist, dietician, and clinical psychologist consulted with the team. In the first weeks the team evaluated and monitored Phil as he transitioned from a comatose state to a conscious condition. The occupational therapy assistant implemented a sensory stimulation program, and the physical therapist initiated upright posture and performed passive range-of-motion exercises.

Phil became alert and responsive 2 weeks after his injury. At that time, both therapists completed a separate evaluation related to each professional domain of concern. At the beginning of the third week, all team members met with the family to review their assessment results and recommendations. After an hour's discussion the team developed a plan that reflected the parents' concerns and priorities, the medical concerns, and the therapists' recommendations.

Initially, emphasis was placed on mobility and activities of daily living (ADLs), and the physical and occupational therapists took leadership roles in determining Phil's daily regimen of activities. During the fourth week, the team met and decided to prioritize speech goals for the following 2 weeks and to evaluate and order assistive technology, including a wheelchair and laptop computer. Both would be needed for Phil's return to school. ADLs remained an emphasis with these expanded goals.

At the end of the sixth week, the hospital team met with the school-based team to determine revised priorities, based on the expectations of the school environment. Written and oral communication and school functions were emphasized.

In the last 2 weeks of Phil's hospital stay, team members frequently met to discuss his technology needs for home and school and to plan a home program. They discussed which scenarios were optimum for follow-up, and it was determined that the school therapists could carry out most of Phil's program, with limited outpatient follow-up by the hospital team.

This example of an interdisciplinary medical team illustrates the need for frequent meetings at critical points to make program changes, to address technology needs, to develop recommendations, and to complete discharge planning. Although the roles are delineated, team members understand the benefit of frequent communication, and the goals reflect the input of several members, including the family. Flexible models of intervention are used, including co-treatments, consultations with other professionals, and transference of leadership among various team members.

address issues such as selection of mobility and augmentative communication devices or strategies for managing posttraumatic brain injury aggression. Although assessment may be carried out in one-on-one sessions, members participate together in program and discharge planning. A case manager, usually a nurse or sometimes a social worker, coordinates the individualized care plan. Not only is the case manager knowledgeable about the rehabilitation unit's services and the team's therapists, he or she is also familiar with the services the child and family will need as they transition into the community.

Parents' roles on the hospital team are usually limited and prescribed. Family members defer to the physician and other health care personnel because of their expertise and professional prestige (Gilkerson, 1990). Although parents are the experts about their child, they admit that they are not the authority on health conditions. In particular, parents of a child with a newly diagnosed illness or disability may find it difficult to understand or accept their child's condition. Therefore they are not prepared to participate as members of a hospital-based team. Parents' participation is also affected by the stress induced by the child's illness and hospitalization, external demands on their lives that continue despite the trauma (e.g., other children in the family), and the simple logistics of scheduling team and parent meetings. Often parents form individual relationships with the professionals of the team and recognize that limited participation on the team may be adequate, particularly when their individual communication is shared with other team members.

Summary

Medical teams generally are led by physicians and often are managed by nurses. Composition of the team may change according to the patient's medical issues and needs for medical expertise. Hospital-based teams often form quickly, work efficiently, and disband when the patient's health problems have been resolved. Rehabilitation teams and specialist teams for children with chronic health problems tend to have routine interactions over time and to function using an interdisciplinary model. In an interdisciplinary model, team members collaborate at different points in the continuum of patient care. Although interdisciplinary team members most often administer evaluations and provide intervention independently; they plan together, collaborate to write the patient's goals, and regularly communicate about the patient's progress.

EDUCATIONAL SYSTEM

Team Mission

The mission of a school-based team is to provide children with the knowledge and skills to live productive lives in society (Figure 2-3). Public schools are primarily (i.e., approximately 80%) funded by their local communities and are therefore responsible to those communities. Teams in schools design and plan the curriculum, implement instruction and intervention, and evaluate student outcomes. In recent years, schools have become responsible not only for designing and providing age-appropriate curricula with individual plans for children in

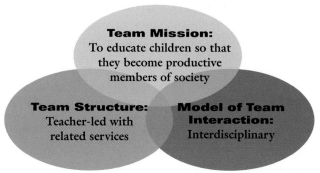

EDUCATION SYSTEM:
Public Schools and Alternative Schools

FIGURE 2-3 Example of team dynamics in the educational system.

special education, but also for demonstrating student outcomes, including students who receive special education services (IDEA Practices, 2004).

Team Composition and Structure

The members of the school-based team are defined by, and related services are listed in, IDEA (see Table 2-2). In addition to the services of the regular and special educators, a student is entitled to related services that enable him or her to benefit from special education (IDEA, 1997). Although some educational teams (e.g., diagnostic teams) have stable membership, more often the membership of an educational team fluctuates according to the needs of the student.

A child's IEP defines which service providers participate in the child's educational program, and it determines the level of service to be provided. Therefore an IEP defines how a team organizes and structures the levels of participation around an individual child. If services are defined as "consultation," interaction and communication between therapists (the consultants) and teacher (the consultee) become the predominant method of service delivery. If the team decides that occupational therapy direct services are needed, a combination of service delivery models is implemented, which may include (1) one-on-one intervention inside or outside the classroom, (2) consultation with the teacher and other related service providers, and (3) group sessions with children. After direct interventions and consultation, a student may receive monitoring services to determine whether the higher levels of performance achieved during intervention are maintained. Team structure and roles are governed by decisions made at the beginning of the year, and they reflect the parents' priorities, assessment results, educational priorities, and educational outcomes as defined by the school system.

The teacher or special educator is often the leader of the team, coordinating the related services listed on the

IEP and ensuring that certain educational priorities are achieved. The teacher's role as leader is a natural one, because he or she spends the most time with the students in the classroom. The teacher is most knowledgeable about the student's curriculum and expected learning outcomes and often has greater access to the parents for ongoing communication. Because team members have equal status, roles and responsibilities are shared, all members contribute to problem solving, and decisions about a student's program are made collaboratively.

Some therapy services are obtained under contract from other agencies; therefore the related service personnel are not actual employees of the school system. This structure can be challenging for the team, particularly when the contract therapist is considered an outsider or is consistently unavailable for team meetings. When members are not full participants, the team is fractured, and the result may be duplication of services or missed opportunities for the student. Teams involving contracted agencies can create challenges for the team leader, and extra steps must be taken to maintain the flow of communication among all members.

The 1997 IDEA amendments specify that teams must write integrated student goals focused on academic or functional competencies. Teams determine which academic goals have priority and need the support of related services. Occupational therapists are listed as a service to be provided to help the child meet specific academic or functional goals. For example, the occupational therapist may provide services to help a child learn to use a computer or an augmentative communication device to achieve specific communication goals. The writing of integrated goals that best serve the child requires collaboration and frequent communication among team and family members.

Team Interaction Model: Interdisciplinary

As described under medical system teams, members of school-based interdisciplinary models value the contribution of each discipline and work to ensure regular and systematic communication. Team members recognize that their knowledge, skills, roles, and responsibilities overlap and therefore routinely meet to discuss and clarify their roles regarding a specific student. The support of the school's administration is essential to the success of an interdisciplinary educational team. Research confirms the need for this support and for an organizational structure that recognizes the importance of team collaboration (Giangreco, 1995; Giangreco, Edelman, & Nelson, 1998).

The creation of collaborative cultures among educators and related services requires promotion of collegiality and meaningful connections (Louis & Kruse, 1996). A congenial school is one with strong interpersonal relationships among team members, energetic dialogs among team members about practices with students, tolerance of disagreement, and a deep sense of commitment (Gossen & Anderson, 1995). Creation of a congenial school requires that educators and related service practitioners spend time together, have frequent opportunities for communication, and learn together.

Five characteristics mark the interrelationships of a successful school-based interdisciplinary team:

1 Goals are developed and decisions are made by consensus.
2 Collaborative strategies are used.
3 Team members work in proximity to each other when possible.
4 Team members meet both formally and informally.
5 Team members demonstrate flexibility in the roles they assume.

Decision Making by Consensus

Consensus in decision making is important to the function of interdisciplinary teams. "By reaching mutually valued agreements, team members strengthen and extend the development of their shared framework, have opportunities to learn from and support each other, and establish clearly communicated expectations designed to facilitate effective service provision" (Giangreco, 1995, p. 60-61). When members agree, goals and plans can be supported and implemented. Consensus is signified by all team members, including the family, signing the Individualized Education Program. When team members do not achieve consensus, relationships tend to erode, and conflicts develop. Conflicts can be destructive to the implementation of a child's program. Conflict resolution involves objectively examining the issues and then reexamining the goals for the child. Generally, focusing on the child's goals helps resolve conflict concerning discipline-specific strategies. (Consensus building and conflict resolution are discussed in the final section of this chapter.)

Developing Collaborative Strategies

Interdisciplinary teams understand the importance of collaboration in planning goals and strategies. Most children benefit from interventions that are applied consistently across team members; therefore it becomes imperative that team members keep each other informed as to what strategies are attempted, which work well, and which do not. For example, the preschool teacher and occupational therapist may decide to implement a sensorimotor activity with 5-year-olds after their writing and spelling lesson. Each child takes turns on the balls, scooter boards, trampoline, and swings in games led by the teacher and occupational therapist. These activities emphasize various themes, including body scheme, numbers and counting, seasons, and holidays. Through discussion about how these activities fit into the day's routines, the teacher and therapist decide to implement the sensorimotor program before writing and spelling to promote the children's optimal arousal for the sedentary tasks that follow.

Barnes and Turner (2001) found that occupational therapists and teachers collaborated frequently, generally to review the child's progress toward his or her current goals and to make adjustments to the child's program. Teachers felt that the occupational therapists' contribution was greater when the collaboration was higher (more frequent). Student achievement of goals did not increase with greater collaboration, possibly because with collaboration comes greater accountability and more scrutiny of the child's achievement. Also, often the children who require the greatest degree of collaboration may be the most challenging, may have more significant disabilities, and may be less likely to progress.

Working in Proximity to Each Other

Collaboration is easiest to achieve when members work in proximity to each other. Providing occupational therapy services in a classroom, rather than in a separate clinic or area, helps promote interdisciplinary teaming. When in the classroom, the therapist can model for the teacher, can learn from the teacher, and can best address educational outcomes that relate to the classroom curriculum (Rainforth & York-Barr, 1997). Informal communication between the teacher and therapist while in the classroom contributes to an understanding of each other's discipline roles.

Block scheduling, a method particularly suited to preschool classrooms, refers to a block of time in the morning or afternoon during which a therapist is in one classroom. In some settings, the block of time is shared with other therapists (e.g., both speech and occupational therapists are in the kindergarten room on Wednesday afternoons). During this time, the therapist may work with several different children, may lead one or two small group activities, and may participate in general classroom instruction. Often most of the children in the room receive direct input from the therapist during the block of time. Block scheduling allows (1) support activities to be scheduled at the same time, (2) time for teachers and practitioners to work intensively with small groups of students, (3) minimal disruption of instruction, and (4) time for teachers and therapists to hold team meetings (Snell, Lowman, & Canady, 1996).

Meeting Formally and Informally

The school administration must recognize the importance of formal and informal meetings and allow time for both when determining scheduling and staffing. Administrators who do not recognize the value of team meetings may write contracts for occupational therapy services that cover only the treatment times specified on the IEP. As result, therapists are not paid and cannot afford to schedule time for meetings or for communications. This lack of administrative support is detrimental to the team.

In a study of school-based collaborative practices between teachers and occupational therapists, Barnes and Turner (2001) found that most collaboration between occupational therapists and teachers occurred informally, such as in the classroom, offices, and hallways. Formal meetings were rare; only 15% of the respondents indicated that they met regularly in a formal format.

Demonstrating Flexibility

Interdisciplinary teams must be flexible. Team leadership is shared by all team members and shifts from member to member, depending on the issue or task. The leadership qualities of team members are recognized and promoted. Flexibility regarding discipline roles (Box 2-3) allows

---

BOX 2-3 Flexible Discipline Roles

Patricia is a 9-year-old student with spastic hemiparesis and severe communication delays. The team developed an Individualized Education Program (IEP) that identified mobility, keyboarding, and communication goals. Initially, emphasis was placed on ambulation using a hemiwalker, and the physical therapist had precedence in the child's schedule. The occupational therapist and teacher helped emphasize this primary goal.

Halfway through the year, the family and team decided that powered mobility was optimum during the school day, and a powered wheelchair was obtained. The team met to revise Patricia's IEP. Independent ambulation became a secondary goal, and concerns about her difficulty with oral and written communication were given priority in the team's discussion. With new goals in speech and written communication, the level of direct services provided by the speech-language pathologist and occupational therapist increased. Keyboarding and use of an augmentative communication device became the emphasis of the occupational therapy intervention. The occupational and speech-language therapists scheduled in-class time together to help Patricia learn to use her new device in her classroom. They used in-class time to determine how, when, and where Patricia could best use the device.

By the end of the year, Patricia's homeroom teacher supported the use of her device in the classroom. The occupational therapist switched to working with Patricia during her computer laboratory time using "Intellitool" programs, and the speech-language therapist assumed a leadership role in developing an appropriate vocabulary that related to the curriculum of her classroom on her augmentative communication device.

This example emphasizes the level of flexibility needed by team members to accommodate the evolving needs of the student.

professionals to focus on the priority needs of the child rather than rigid adherence to their scope of practice.

Summary

When interdisciplinary teams in the school succeed, it is always the student who benefits. The time that team members dedicate to team function can be as valuable as the time for direct services with the child. The challenge comes in learning how to support the teacher. The occupational therapist may have to sacrifice scheduled time with a student to listen to a teacher's concerns, express an interest in what the class is learning, or solve a problem that has become a troubling issue for the teacher. Support of the teacher and his or her role and responsibilities is essential to the development of a climate in which the team can flourish. This collaboration is often returned in the form of support for the goals that are the occupational therapist's responsibility. Time with the teacher supports the communication that is critical to an understanding both of the student's progress in the curriculum and of his or her needs that may interfere with progress.

In summary, team relationships require nurturing. Time together, positive interactions, trust, and respect are essential foundations on which team collaboration is built. Trust and respect develop when a therapist contributes to the classroom routine and supports the teacher and other team members by listening and acting on promises. The occupational therapist asks for the opinions of team members and welcomes feedback regarding recommendations she or he has made. To build congenial communities, therapists and teachers must place priority on collegiality, positive attitudes, supportiveness, and openness.

EARLY INTERVENTION SYSTEM

Team Mission

The early intervention system is designed to provide multidisciplinary, interagency services to infants and toddlers with disabilities and their families (Figure 2-4). A major role of early intervention systems is the identification of infants at risk for disability and those who will benefit from these services. Once an infant enters the early intervention system, optimizing his or her developmental function becomes the focus. Professionals recognize the importance of intervention during this early period of neuroplasticity and rapid development of function. In addition, professionals embrace the concept that the family is the constant in the infant's life, and services must include support of the family's ability to promote the child's development. An emphasis on family involvement has become a universal characteristic of early

EARLY INTERVENTION SYSTEM:
Community agencies, homes, childcare centers

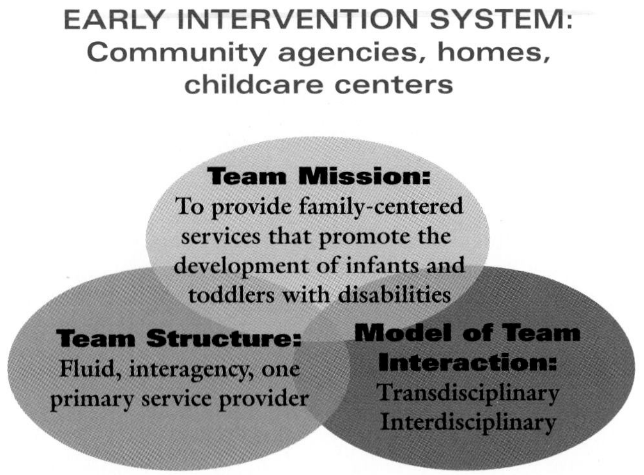

FIGURE 2-4   Example of team dynamics in early intervention systems.

intervention programs. In family-centered services, professionals form partnerships with parents to develop a mutually agreed-upon program for the infant. This program may include direct services to the infant or direct services to the parents or both. Parents participate in early intervention services to the extent that they are willing and comfortable. At times, parents may be the leader of the team; in other instances, parents may primarily be the recipients of services.

Some unique aspects make early intervention systems different from medical or educational systems. First, early intervention systems were built on a range of services established for families and children that existed in each state before the implementation of early intervention legislation. Today, as a result, multiple agencies participate in the provision of services, and interagency agreements characterize every intervention system. Teams in this system are not only multidisciplinary in nature, they are also interagency in structure. Because members of the team are employed in different agencies, the need to coordinate the services is great. The role of service coordinator is highlighted in the early intervention legislation and is an important function in early intervention teams. This individual coordinates the IFSP process to ensure that it is consistent and comprehensive and that it helps link the family with other community agencies.

Second, with the family as the center of the team, members acknowledge the need to assume roles with flexibility. When supported by other team members, professionals act in roles that are outside their discipline's scope of practice; they also teach parts of their roles to other members of the team. According to IDEA, services must be provided in the child's natural environment, which is often the home or childcare center. The IFSP is viewed as a dynamic or fluid document, and families can add or revise goals as intervention progresses without reconvening a full team meeting.

Team Composition and Structure

The early intervention services available to families, as defined by IDEA, are listed in Table 2-2. In addition to this list of professional services, the law clearly places the parents in an essential role as members of the early intervention team. The IFSP lists both infant and family goals, as well as the needed supports related to the concerns and priorities the family has for the infant. The structure of the early intervention team is circular, with members sharing equal status. Leadership roles are shared, and service delivery is flexible so that services accommodate family priorities. Community-based teams tend to have stable and enduring membership, which can strengthen the team's cohesiveness. Because a high level of flexibility is required and the family is the center of services, transdisciplinary models of teamwork are developed.

Team Interaction Model: Transdisciplinary and Interdisciplinary

A transdisciplinary approach is based on the assumption that coherence is promoted when the family primarily interacts with one professional (McGonigel & Garland, 1988). Team members work together to evaluate the infant and to design a program that is implemented by one team member. The family's entrance into therapy and intervention programs becomes easier because the family primarily relates only to one individual. This individual consults with other professionals on the team to answer the family's questions and design appropriate intervention strategies. The occupational therapist frequently provides consultation, explaining to the primary service provider strategies to promote the child's development and achievement of the outcomes identified by the team. When the occupational therapist is the primary service provider, she or he becomes the recipient of consultation for professionals in other disciplines.

In this model, assessment is planned, implemented, and summarized by the team as a whole. All team members assess the child, often in an arena assessment (see Chapter 21). In the arena model, one team member interacts with the child while other members observe the child and interact with the parents, asking them to help interpret the child's behaviors. Throughout the process, team members explain the assessment model to the parents and encourage them to ask questions. After observing the child, the team assembles to interpret their observations (Linder, 1993).

All team members (including the parents) come together with assessment results and their interpretations to develop the IFSP. Planning begins by asking the family to communicate their concerns and priorities. The team helps the family members articulate what they would like the early intervention team to address in the form of outcomes. Each outcome has prescribed services (e.g.,

occupational therapy, nutrition, social work), and those professionals take responsibility for achieving it. The service delivery setting (e.g., home, clinic) is also defined, based on the family's preferences. Services in the infant's natural environment are emphasized. The *natural environment* includes home and community settings in which children without disabilities participate.

In the transdisciplinary model (sometimes called a *coaching model*), all team members commit to teaching, learning, and working across disciplinary boundaries (Bruder & Bologna, 1993). Team members share information based on their disciplinary knowledge that contributes to the child's intervention program. After the IFSP meeting, one or two members assume responsibility for carrying out the recommendations and strategies. The primary interventionist and the parents learn to recognize when the expertise of the occupational therapist or another therapist is needed. Because responsibility for the plan rests primarily with one individual, team members must be well versed in the skills and resources of the other professionals on the team. This model works only when team members frequently call on their colleagues to solve problems and for consultation. It is particularly appropriate for infants who are medically fragile and do not tolerate multiple sources of stimulation.

An occupational therapist is most effective in coaching other team members to implement a technique or strategy when she or he (1) has experience in implementing the strategy, (2) feels that the team member has the skills and underlying knowledge to implement the strategy correctly, (3) recommends a strategy that is relatively easy to master and fits well into the child's and family's everyday routines, and (4) recommends a strategy that has very little chance of causing harm. Highly specialized techniques should not be transferred to other professionals, particularly when incorrect application could be detrimental to the infant.

The advantage of a transdisciplinary model is that unnecessary duplication and fragmentation are avoided. The team adopts the family's goals; as a result, goals tend to be functional and holistic and in the context of the child's natural environment. The transdisciplinary model enables professionals to learn from each other and expand their professional knowledge into related disciplines. "At its best, the transdisciplinary approach can limit the intrusiveness in and disruption of family lives that occur when teams require families to work separately with each discipline" (Garland, 1994, p. 99).

A transdisciplinary approach requires that professionals willingly share discipline-related information. Coaching a team member to implement strategies typically implemented by occupational therapists initially may be perceived as a threat. However, because this model involves sharing of knowledge and frequent collaborative decision making, all team members have the potential to grow beyond their disciplinary boundaries in a process generally perceived to be enriching. To successfully coach another team member, the occupational therapist must assess the team member's preferred learning style and provide information according to that learning style. Successful coaching requires the occupational therapist to consider how much information to provide, the format for that information, the timing for teaching, a means for checking on progress, and the types of reinforcement needed.

Summary

Early intervention teams create equality of roles across disciplines and agencies. Nontraditional team members may be involved because of the expanded focus on child and family. Team members share strategies designed to help the family and child attain the outcomes they seek, with one team member consistently interacting with the family. Transdisciplinary teams can provide consistent, holistic services to young families when team members achieve a high level of collaboration and communication.

TEAM PROCESS

Qualities of Effective Teams

An effective team has specific characteristics and qualities. Its members' discipline skills and expertise are important; however, technical skills are not sufficient to make teaming work. In teams that function well, members also have positive interpersonal skills, strong problem-solving ability, openness, and supportiveness (LaFasto & Larson, 2001). Teams work best when they are composed of good problem solvers who are active and constructive in team discussions. During problem solving, members should maintain a focus on the key issues and family priorities.

An important aspect of a strong team is that its members share a purpose or goal. The clarity of this purpose defines the focus of the team and affects how well their efforts coalesce. A shared purpose can help ground the team and provide a point of reference when decisions are made for an individual child. This shared purpose tends to be broad and inclusive, reflecting the service delivery system. An example of a shared purpose for a medical-based team is to promote maximal health, wellness, and function in the child. A shared purpose for an educational-based team may be to promote the child's full participation in the school and community or to maximize a child's ability to participate in and contribute to society.

Teams work best when team members assume a variety of roles in addition to their professional roles. Two types of roles critical to team function are task-oriented and interaction-oriented roles. To help the team stay on task, make decisions, and develop a work plan, certain team members should assume task-oriented roles, such as (1) seeking information, (2) summarizing, (3) recording, (4) asking questions, and (5) providing information (Rainforth & York-Barr, 1997). These roles move the team forward, help them stay on course, and provide the energy to accomplish the work.

For teams that function together over time, it is important that certain team members take on interaction-oriented roles. In these roles the occupational therapist may encourage, use humor to diffuse tension, offer support, or be a harmonizer, compromiser, or active listener (Rainforth & York-Barr, 1997). The harmonizers and compromisers on the team provide the glue that helps team relationships grow. Relationship-oriented members improve cohesion and help the members enjoy each other and the team process. Task-oriented and interaction-oriented roles are as important to the team's outcomes as discipline expertise.

Although certain team members may excel at interaction, it is important that all members have open communication. Openness means that members are straightforward in responding to one another, that they are honest about their perceptions, and that they are open to creative solutions. When members are open to solutions that reflect different disciplinary perspectives, interventions are likely to be more holistic and comprehensive. Although sometimes professionals are sensitive to what they think parents can assimilate, they should never mislead them or purposely omit information. When information is difficult to deliver, such as an explanation of a new diagnosis, professionals should convey the information honestly, with empathy, and in a heartfelt manner.

Supportiveness among team members means that each member pitches in when needed, maintains a positive outlook, and is willing to take responsibility. Supportive team members are easy to work with, listen to others' ideas, and are sensitive to others' feelings (LaFasto & Larson, 2001). Rainforth and York-Barr (1997) defined the types of supports that team members can provide to one another:

- Resource support (e.g., materials, funding information, community resources and agencies)
- Moral support (e.g., listening and encouraging)
- Technical support (e.g., specific and individualized strategies, instructional methods, and adaptations of those methods)

Combinations of these three types of support are also generally used with teachers, other professionals, and parents.

Resources that occupational therapists bring to the team may include materials for classroom or home use, such as adapted equipment, handouts, or written instruction. Encouraging feedback from teachers about the strategies they are implementing or the progress noted in a child exemplifies moral support. Moral support also can mean that an occupational therapist slips out of a discipline-specific role and provides what is needed at the moment, such as comforting a child while the nurse gives an injection; helping a teacher calm a child having a tantrum; and co-leading a song with the music teacher for a group of preschool children. Technical support involves providing expertise to enhance a child's ability to participate in play and school activities, ADLs, or community life. Support involves not only the range of assistive technology, but also specialized techniques that promote a child's function.

Structures that Promote Collaboration

Models of service delivery can promote teaming and partnerships. Block scheduling, explained earlier, allows team members to schedule their therapy times together in the classroom, increasing opportunities for collaboration and communication. Another service delivery model that supports teaming and can promote the child's functional performance is co-teaching. In co-teaching, the occupational therapist and teacher plan an instructional session that they implement together. Occupational therapists frequently have co-taught handwriting to elementary-age students. They also co-lead sensorimotor sessions or circle time activities with preschool children. Teachers reported feeling energized by co-teaching and indicated that they perceived a greater sense of community by sharing their teaching role (Murata, 2002).

Another structure that can enable strong teamwork is the establishment of a core team and an extended team (Giangreco, 2000). The core team has substantial regular involvement with the student, and the extended team is composed of professionals whose involvement is less frequent or more focused. The core team is often made up of the teachers, assistants, and parents, whereas the extended team often comprises the therapists and consulting professionals. The identification of two team levels allows services to be provided more efficiently. Not everyone needs to attend meetings, although all members need to be informed about the child's progress. Giangreco (1995, 2000), who recommends the use of core teams, reported that children with multiple disabilities have an average of 11 members on their teams. This model allows the family to interact with a smaller number of professionals, giving them more opportunity to develop close relationships.

A critically important organizational structure that supports an effective team process is scheduled meeting times. When communication occurs only by chance or when members meet informally, opportunities for team decision making and consensus building are lost. Team meetings allow for planning and provide time for the development and expansion of programs and services.

Scholars and experts on teamwork (Katzenbach & Smith, 1993; LaFasto & Larson, 2001; Rainforth & York-Barr, 1997) have provided guidelines for implementing effective team meetings. According to their research, team meetings are effective when:

1 Meeting times are honored by participants.
2 The team leader develops an agenda, which members are welcome to amend, and which then is followed in the meeting.
3 Members actively listen to each other.
4 The discussion focuses on the agenda and the clients.
5 Members freely share their perceptions, including their perceptions of group process at the end of the meeting.

Establishing a structure in which teams can flourish is essential. Administrative support of teaming is vital; this allows the team quality time to meet, to encourage communication, to build a sense of community, and to ensure that children's services are planned through team-based decisions. System supports are the foundation of effective teamwork, but they are not sufficient in themselves to achieve it; the interactions and interpersonal skills of team members also determine effectiveness.

Communication

The goal of team communication is that professionals and family members develop *shared meaning* about their concerns and priorities for the child and about the system (Case-Smith & Wavrek, 1998). Because the language used by health care professionals is often technical and medically related, families can easily misunderstand its meaning. Occupational therapists and other team members must make a concerted effort to use lay terminology to describe function, rather than neurophysiologic components, and to work with families to develop shared meaning about the child and the system. Descriptive *everyday language* adds to the comfort level and understanding of fellow team members. Even when professionals use simple, direct language, the message can be misunderstood. The family's ability to assimilate information may also be limited in times of stress, such as when the child is hospitalized. As a general rule, professionals should use simple messages and repeat information when it is essential that parents understand.

Parents usually reinforce intervention goals when team members explain recommendations in sufficient depth, reinforce each other's suggestions, welcome parental feedback, and incorporate the parents' ideas into a suggested activity. Such collaboration requires time and willingness to develop a shared meaning of what is best for the child.

When team members have developed effective communication systems, collaboration and integrated service delivery becomes possible. Teams use three methods for reaching decisions: problem solving, decision making by consensus, and conflict resolution. Each method is based on open lines of communication, a willingness and initiative to share information, and a commitment to team collaboration.

Team Problem Solving

In the first step of team problem solving, it is often important to identify who needs to be involved in discussing the problem. Not all team members must participate, but access to those with relevant expertise is critical to the process. In team problem solving, the members use a five-step process to ensure that all solutions are considered and to encourage all members to contribute (Box 2-4).

Team problem solving offers the following advantages:

1 More diverse knowledge and perspectives are brought to bear on the problem.

2 Great interest in the problem is stimulated because of the attention of numerous individuals.

3 The resulting solution is greater than the sum of the individual contributions.

4 Inappropriate solutions are rejected.

Teams can have difficulty at any point in the process. Frequently teams do not take the time to state the problem clearly and gather the necessary information. Often members settle for a strategy before alternatives have been thoroughly discussed (Johnson & Johnson, 1994). Successful problem solving requires that teams agree on the problem and remain open to solutions without judging their value too quickly.

An educational team, in particular, engages in a problem-solving process when the student's performance does not match the expectations of the curriculum or when anticipated progress is not achieved. In problem-solving meetings in the schools, teams search for the least intrusive solutions that can be implemented in the regular classroom and those that are consistent with the IEP in place. School teams work to develop creative solutions that use in-place resources, because resources are often limited.

Decision Making by Consensus

Only in very rare situations are decisions in medical, educational, and early intervention systems made unilaterally. Although each professional may assess the child, these interpretations and recommendations must always be given to the team so that the recommendations can be prioritized and integrated with other similar interpretations of team members. Decision making, therefore, is never reductionistic; the team and family make all important decisions. Although this process requires time and resources, it eliminates duplication, and the team is able to focus on the most important goals and services for the child and family.

Innovative and effective plans that the team and family can commit to implementing, therefore, require the "buy in" of all members. When all members agree to implement an intervention plan, the participation of each member increases, and the plan is more likely to succeed. To reach team consensus, members must actively participate and negotiate, with the voice of each member equally important. Decisions by consensus take more time and require more adaptability and flexibility by team members than other decision-making models. However, consensus building around an individual child is summative and, over time, enhances team cohesiveness.

In team planning meetings that include parents (e.g., IFSP and IEP meetings), the parent has the deciding voice. To assume the role of decision maker, a parent must be informed about how the team operates, how he or she can participate in the process, and how an intervention plan is developed. Given clear and specific

---

BOX 2-4   Steps in Team Problem Solving

STEP 1: DEFINE THE PROBLEM OR ISSUE.
- The problem is defined clearly and objectively.
- The team develops a comprehensive description of the problem, including individual and environmental factors that influence the issue.
- Team members make a commitment to solving the problem.

STEP 2: GATHER INFORMATION ABOUT THE PROBLEM.
- Team members work to understand the problem thoroughly.
- Barriers and supports/resources are identified.

STEP 3: GENERATE AND CONSIDER ALTERNATIVE STRATEGIES.
- Alternative strategies are formulated.
- Creative and divergent thinking is helpful.
- Team members identify as many strategies as possible to reduce barriers and increase supports.

STEP 4: DECIDE ON AND IMPLEMENT A STRATEGY.
- Each alternative is discussed, with team members identifying the resources needed and assessing the probability of success.
- Consensus decision making is used.
- Once a decision has been made, a plan is developed for achieving the solution.
- The plan identifies specific action, the team members responsible, and a timeline for implementation.

STEP 5: EVALUATE THE SUCCESS OF THE PLAN.
- The team determines whether the strategies were correctly implemented and, if they were, the outcome of each strategy.
- If the outcome does not meet the goals, the barriers are analyzed, new approaches are generated, an alternative strategy is selected, and a new plan is developed.

Modified from Johnson, D.W., & Johnson, F.P. (1994). *Joining together: Group theory and group skills* (5th ed.). Englewood Cliffs, NJ: Prentice-Hall; and Rainforth & York-Barr (1997).

information about the team's assessment and planning process and the type of intervention the program offers, the parents can take leadership roles in building consensus for their important concerns regarding their child. Bailey (1991) made the following suggestions for practices that can increase the family's role in reaching team consensus.

1 At the beginning of the meeting, the team leader states the purpose of the meeting and its desired outcome. All participants describe their roles as they relate to the child.

2 Members explain the format of the meeting to the parents; that is, what they can expect to happen during the meeting.

3 Families are invited to speak first. They should be asked to share their perspectives and describe their observations of the child.

4 Any medical, technical, or discipline-specific terms are immediately explained in lay language.

5 Members readily admit when they do not know the answer to a question. Honesty is most important. Misinformation can have severely negative effects on relationships and trust building.

6 Families should never be placed in the middle of a professional disagreement. When professionals disagree, they should be open about their opinions but should make every attempt not to confuse the family or break their trust in the team.

7 Consensus on goals for the child and intervention strategies results when professionals communicate openly and clearly and when they consider the child's and family's needs above their professional identities and personal interests. (Additional discussion of communication strategies for consensus building is found in Chapter 5.)

Conflict Resolution

When disagreement arises regarding the intervention plan or service implementation, negotiation strategies should be used to resolve the conflict in a positive and constructive way. *Negotiation* is a process by which people who want to come to an agreement, but who disagree about the nature of the agreement, establish a plan accepted by all. Negotiation requires clear communication of the options and possible solutions. Team members should present clear rationales for the goals or solutions that they propose. The proposed goals should relate directly to the entire team's concerns and priorities and particularly to those of the family.

The first step in negotiation among team members is to identify the overall goal. When the team members disagree on specific objectives or activities, a global goal (e.g., promotion of the child's optimal health and development) on which all members agree becomes the starting point for compromise. Common interests related to the general goal can be established by first reconfirming the common purpose. With overall goals in mind, compatible intervention strategies can be identified. Conflicting interests need to be made explicit (Brandt, 1993).

Successful negotiation and problem resolution are more likely to be achieved when (1) members are separated from the problem, (2) mutual interests and gains are accentuated, and (3) objective criteria are used to evaluate the solutions generated (Fisher & Ury, 1981). The problem therefore needs to be *depersonalized*, or viewed as separate from the individuals involved and their interpersonal interactions. All common interests and concerns should be identified, and they should relate to the child or to the concerns of family members. The solutions generated should be specific and concrete. They may need to be prioritized so that the team has an initial emphasis. Finally, criteria should be established to evaluate progress toward resolution of the conflict. Short-term objectives with explicit criteria allow the family and team to measure immediate progress and adjust to the plan, which prevents negative feelings and conflict. These problem-solving strategies help the team to reach agreement on intervention goals and to support each other and the family in reaching those goals.

When disagreements cannot be resolved by team members, it is helpful for the team to obtain data regarding the problem and potential solutions. Data about the student during a trial of an intervention can promote objective decision making. For example, if the team cannot decide whether a student should be using power or manual mobility, data about the child's function during trials of each mobility type would enable the team to come to consensus on the most appropriate device. When objective data can be obtained prior to decision making, the team is likely to reach consensus and make good decisions (Rainforth & York-Barr, 1997).

Summary

An occupational therapist's teaming skills are as important to effective intervention as discipline-specific techniques. Contributing to a team, collaborating with its members, and negotiating opinions are competencies that require effort and team experience to develop. Garland (1994) summarized how professionals can become contributing, collaborative team members:

1 Strive for consistency between one's discipline-specific goals and philosophy and those of the team.

2 Ask for clarification regarding one's role and the roles of other team members.

3 Promote openness and clarity of communication.

4 Offer one's knowledge and skills and express a willingness to use the resources of the other team members.

5   Develop decision-making and problem-solving skills.

6   Communicate a willingness to accept responsibility for the work of the team.

7   Develop skills in managing and using conflict productively.

8   Seek and use performance feedback from team colleagues.

As described in the model of team dynamics, the environment must be conducive to the growth and development of a collaborative team. Administrative and organizational supports are essential to team function, and these supports influence the type of team interaction that evolves.

STUDY QUESTIONS

1   Describe the roles of the physician and nurse in the hospital, school, and early intervention systems. What are the implications for the team when the role of medical professionals shifts from team leaders to consultants?

2   Identify areas of overlap in the scope of practice of physical therapy and occupational therapy with children. What are advantages and disadvantages of the overlap in scope of practice?

3   What is the role of the teacher in the hospital? Given a child with head trauma who has spent 2 months on a rehabilitation unit, describe how the hospital-based teacher may optimally function during the child's transition from hospital to his former classroom.

4   Compare the advantages and disadvantages of primary communication with other professionals on your team through (1) written reports, (2) files and charts, (3) electronic mail, (4) telephone contact, (5) face-to-face meetings, and (6) informal conversations in the lunchroom.

5   Identify the variables that promote the effectiveness of a team, including system and individual characteristics important to the development of a cohesive team.

REFERENCES

American Academy of Pediatrics, Division of Child Health Research. (2003). *Screening for developmental disabilities.* Retrieved March 15, 2004, from www.aap.org/research/periodicsurvey/ps13exm.htm

American Association of Colleges of Nursing. (2004). *Your career: A look at the facts.* Retrieved June 12, 2004 from *www.nursing.about.com.*

American College of Nurse Practitioners. (2004). *What is a nurse practitioner?* Retrieved March 15, 2004, from www.nurse.org/acnp/facts

American Nurses Association. (2001). *Analysis of the American Nurses Association staffing survey.* Retrieved April 14, 2004 from *www.nursingworld.org.*

American Nurses Association. (2004). *Planning a nursing career.* Retrieved June 12, 2004 from www.nursingworld.org.

American Nurses Association. (2004). *Nursing facts: Today's registered nurse—numbers and demographics.* Retrieved March 15, 2004, from www.nursingworld.org.

American Nurses' Association, Early Intervention Consensus Committee. (1993). *National standards of nursing practice for early intervention services.* Lexington: University of Kentucky College of Nursing.

American Physical Therapy Association (APTA). (1999). APTA Background Sheet 1999, Retrieved on March 25, 2004 at www.apta.org.

American Speech-Language-Hearing Association (ASHA). (2002). *Scope of practice in speech-language pathology.* Retrieved March 23, 2004, from www.asha.org.

Bailey, D.B. (1991). Building positive relationships between professionals and families. In M.J. McGonigel, R.K. Kaufmann, & B.H. Johnson (Eds.), *Guidelines and recommended practices for the Individualized Family Services Plan* (pp. 29-38). Bethesda, MD: Association for the Care of Children's Health.

Barnes, K.J., & Turner, K.D. (2001). Team collaborative practices between teachers and occupational therapists. *American Journal of Occupational Therapy, 55,* 83-89.

Brandt, P. (1993). Negotiation and problem-solving strategies: Collaboration between families and professionals. *Infants and Young Children, 5* (4), 787-884.

Bruder, M.B., & Bologna, T. (1993). Collaboration and service coordination for effective early intervention. In W. Brown, S.K. Thurman, & L.F. Pearl (Eds.), *Family-centered early intervention with infants and toddlers: Innovative cross-disciplinary approaches* (pp. 103-127). Baltimore: Brookes.

Case-Smith, J., & Wavrek, B. (1998). Models of service delivery and team interaction. In J. Case-Smith (Ed.), *Pediatric occupational therapy and early intervention* (pp. 83-109). Boston: Butterworth-Heinemann.

Collins, R.M. (1995). Nurses in early intervention. *Pediatric Nursing, 21* (6), 529-531.

Cox, A.W. (1996). Preparing nurses. In D. Bricker & A. Widerstrom (Eds.), *Preparing personnel to work with infants and young children and their families: A team approach* (pp. 161-180). Baltimore: Brookes.

Fisher, R., & Ury, W. (1981). *Getting to yes: Negotiation agreement without giving in.* New York: Viking Press.

Garland, C.W. (1994). World of practice: Early intervention programs. In H. Garner & F. Orelove (Eds.), *Teamwork in human services: Models and applications across the life span* (pp. 89-116). Boston: Butterworth-Heinemann.

Giangreco, M.F. (1995). Related services decision making: A foundational component of effective education for students with disabilities. *Occupational and Physical Therapy in Educational Environments, 15* (2), 47-67.

Giangreco, M.F. (2000). Related services research for students with low-incidence disabilities: Implications for speech-language pathologist in inclusive classrooms. *Language, Speech, and Hearing Services in Schools, 31,* 230-239.

Giangreco, M.F., Edelman, S.W., & Nelson, C. (1998). Impact of planning for support services on students who are deaf-blind. *Journal of Visual Impairment and Blindness, 92,* 18-29.

Gilkerson, L. (1990). Understanding institutional functioning style: A resource for hospital and early intervention collaboration. *Infants and Young Children, 2,* 22-30.

Gossen, D., & Anderson, J. (1995). *Creating the conditions: Leadership for quality schools.* Chapel Hill, NC: New View.

Hansen, S., Holaday, B., & Miles, M.S. (1990). The role of pediatric nurses in a federal program for infants and young children with handicaps. *Journal of Pediatric Nursing, 5* (4), 246-251.

IDEA Practices. (2004). IDEA: *The Law,* Retrieved March 24, 2004, from www.ideapractices.org.

Individuals with Disabilities Education Act (IDEA), Amendments of 1997 (P.L. 105-17). U.S.C. 1400 (et seq.).

Johnson, D.W., & Johnson, F.P. (1994). *Joining together: Group theory and group skills* (5th ed.). Englewood Cliffs, NJ: Prentice-Hall.

Katzenbach, J.R., & Smith, D.K. (1993). *The wisdom of teams: Creating the high-performance organization.* Boston: Harvard Business School Press.

LaFasto, F., & Larson, C. (2001). *When teams work best.* Thousand Oaks, CA: Sage Publications.

Linder, T. (1993). *Transdisciplinary play-based assessment.* Baltimore: Brookes.

Lorsardo, A. (1996). Preparing communication specialists. In D. Bricker & A. Widerstrom (Eds.), *Preparing personnel to work with infants and young children and their families: A team approach* (pp. 91-114). Baltimore: Brookes.

Louis, K.S., & Kruse, S. (1996). *Professionalism and community: Perspectives on reforming urban schools.* Thousand Oaks, CA: Corwin Press.

McGonigel, M.T., & Garland, C.W. (1988). The individualized family service plan and the early intervention team: Team and family issues and recommended practices. *Infants and Young Children, 1,* 10-21.

Miller, C.K., Burklow, K.A., Santoro, K., Kirby, E., Mason, D., & Rudolph, C.D. (2001). An interdisciplinary team approach to the management of pediatric feeding and swallowing disorder. *Children's Health Care, 30* (3), 201-218.

Murata, R. (2002). What does team teaching mean? A case study of interdisciplinary teaming. *The Journal of Educational Research, 96* (2), 67-77.

National Association of Pediatric Nurse Practitioners (NAPNAP). (2004). *Scope and standards of practice for pediatric nurse practitioners,* Retrieved June 15, 2004, from www.napnap.org/.

National Association of School Psychologists (NASP). (2000). *Standards for training and field placement programs in School Psychology.* Retrieved June 12, 2004, from www.nasponline.org.

National Association of School Psychologists (NASP). (2004). *What is a school psychologist?* Retrieved March 23, 2004, from www.nasponline.org/about_nasp

National Association of Social Workers (NASW). (2002). *The power of social work.* Retrieved March 23, 2004, from www.socialworkers.org.

National Dissemination Center for Children with Disabilities (1999). *Related services.* Retrieved March 24, 2004, from www.nichcy.org.

Rainforth, B., & York-Barr, J. (1997). *Collaborative teams for students with severe disabilities: Integrating therapy and education services (2nd Ed.)* Baltimore: Brookes.

Snell, M.E., Lowman, D.K., & Canady, R.L. (1996). Parallel block scheduling: Accommodating students' diverse needs in elementary schools. *Journal of Early Intervention, 20* (3), 265-278.

Wachtel, R.C., & Compart, P.J. (1996). Preparing pediatricians. In D. Bricker & A. Widerstrom (Eds.), *Preparing personnel to work with infants and young children and their families: A team approach* (pp. 181-198). Baltimore: Brookes.

SUGGESTED READINGS

American Academy of Pediatrics. (2001). *Role of the pediatrician in family-centered early intervention services.* Retrieved September 1, 2003, from www.aap.orga/policy/re0037.html.

American Physical Therapy Association, Section on Pediatrics. (2003). *The ABCs of pediatric physical therapy.* Retrieved March 24, 2004, from www.pediatricapta.org.

Cochrane, C.G., Farley, B.G., & Wilhelm, I.J. (1990). Preparation of physical therapist to work with handicapped infants and their families: Current status and training needs. *Physical Therapy, 70,* 372-380.

Council for Exceptional Children. (2004). *CEC Code of Ethics and Standards of Practice.* Retrieved March 14, 2004, from www.cec.sped.org.

Fullan, M. (1993). *Change forces: Probing the depths of educational reform.* New York: Falmer Press.

Giangreco, M.F., Dennis, R., Edelman, S., & Cloninger, C. (1994). Dressing your IEPs for the educational climate: Analysis of IEP goals and objectives for students with multiple disabilities. *Remedial and Special Education, 15* (5), 288-296.

Giangreco, M.F., Edelman, S., & Dennis, R. (1991). Common professional practices that interfere with the integrated delivery of related services. *Remedial and Special Education, 12* (2), 16-24.

Giangreco, M.F., Edelman, S.W., Luiselli, R.E., & MacFarland, S.Z. (1996). Support service decision-making for students with multiple service needs: Evaluation data. *The Journal of the Association for Persons with Severe Handicaps, 221,* 135-144.

Soderberg, G.L. (1993). The twenty-seventh Mary McMillan lecture: On passing from ignorance to knowledge. *Physical Therapy, 73,* 797-808.

U.S. Department of Labor, Bureau of Labor Statistics. (2004). Licensed practical and licensed vocational nurses. Retrieved February 24, 2002, from www.bls.gov/oco/ocos102.htm.

WEB SITES

American Academy of Pediatrics
www.aap.orga/policy
American Academy of Pediatrics, Division of Child Health Research
www.aap.org/research.html
American College of Nurse Practitioners
www.nurse.org/acnp

American Nurses' Association
www.nursingworld.org
American Physical Therapy Association, Section on Pediatrics
www.pediatricapta.org
American Speech-Language-Hearing Association (ASHA)
www.asha.org
Council for Exceptional Children
www.cec.sped.org
IDEAPractices
www.ideapractices.org

National Association of Pediatric Nurse Practitioners (NAPNAP) www.napnap.org
National Association of School Psychologists
www.nasponline.org
National Association of Social Workers
www.socialworkers.org
National Dissemination Center for Children with Disabilities
www.nichcy.org
U.S. Department of Labor, Bureau of Labor Statistics
www.bls.gov

Foundations for Occupational Therapy Practice with Children

Mary Law ■ Cheryl Missiuna ■ Nancy Pollock ■ Debra Stewart

CHAPTER OBJECTIVES

1 Explain the history and evolution of theories pertaining to child development.
2 Define the term *occupation* and describe the study of occupation with emphasis placed on the occupations of children.
3 Explain what is meant by person-environment congruence.
4 Articulate the concepts and principles that define family-centered services.
5 Explain the developmental and learning theories of the early and middle 1900s, which provided the foundation for occupational therapy theories.
6 Explain and apply cognitive models of practice.
7 Use a dynamic systems approach to explain how children develop motor skills.
8 Explain how the person-environment-occupation model is used with other specific models of practice in occupational therapy intervention with children.
9 Describe and apply acquisitional theories and approaches.
10 Define and explain the appropriate use of neurodevelopmental and sensory integration therapy approaches.
11 Describe strategies that exemplify each practice model using the client examples provided.
12 Compare and contrast intervention activities derived from different theoretical approaches and practice models.

INTRODUCTION

Chapter 3 discusses the current conceptual and theoretical foundations of occupational therapy practice with children. This chapter is organized into four sections, beginning in section 1 with a brief overview of the historical and current perspectives on the theories that underlie current service provision: development, occupation, and environment. Section 2 focuses on foundational theories for occupational therapy practice. In section 3, an overall framework for occupational therapy practice with children is discussed, based on a person-environment-occupation (PEO) perspective. This discussion is followed by overviews of current models of practice, ranging from an occupation-based approach to a neuromaturation-based approach. Section 4 of this chapter illustrates the application of these models of practice to specific practice scenarios, demonstrating the connection of theories, models of practice and assessment, and intervention strategies.

Occupational therapists have developed and used theory as the basis for professional practice for many years. Early developers of occupational therapy focused on the theories of occupation and the use of time (Meyer, 1922; Slagle, 1922). Theories of development, which influenced theories of occupation, came into use in the 1920s and 1930s. Theories and models of practice related to neurointegrative and environmental approaches were not developed until the 1940s (McColl et al., 2003). In the past three decades, a reemergence of the theories of occupation has occurred, and several models of practice have been developed using these concepts.

SECTION 1: OCCUPATIONAL THERAPY PRACTICE WITH CHILDREN

When most people recall their childhood, summer is remembered as a time when friends spent the entire day playing outside. Children moved from activity to activity as a group, enjoying one another's company and participating in a variety of play activities. Most adults have fond memories of these days. At the time, however, the children did not think about the reasons they engaged in play activities or why particular activities were enjoyable. It was just fun! Occupational therapists, however, have a different perspective on play.

Play is considered one of the primary occupations of childhood. Occupational therapists understand that play is essential for development, and they study the concepts and assumptions that underlie the theories of play. Occupational therapists realize that multiple, interrelated factors within the child, family, and environment influence a child's ability to engage in play. All therapists, either implicitly or explicitly, base their practice on a theoretical rationale: play is the primary occupation of childhood. Through the use of theory, assessment, and clinical reasoning, occupational therapists hypothesize and then develop interventions to improve the occupational performance of children.

A *theory* is defined as a set of facts, concepts, and assumptions that together are used to describe, explain, or predict phenomena. Theories help organize selected aspects of the world in a systematic manner. Using theory, occupational therapists organize knowledge, understand observations, and explain or predict occupational function and dysfunction. Theories, therefore, provide a guide or rationale for occupational therapy intervention. Theories form the foundation for *models of practice,* or frames of reference, that guide the day-to-day delivery of occupational therapy services. A model of practice (also called a frame of reference) is the practical expression of theory and provides therapists with specific methods and guidelines for occupational therapy intervention. Models of practice draw from one or more theories and use concepts and assumptions to delineate the specific details of an occupational therapy practice, including who receives intervention, what intervention strategies are used, and when and where intervention is provided. The expected results from the delivery of an occupational therapy service are also based on the model of practice and the results expected in each practice situation.

Concepts Influencing Occupational Therapy Practice with Children
Development

Perspectives on development and occupation have changed over the past century with changes in our knowledge about children, the factors affecting their development, and their basic need for engagement in purposeful tasks and activities. *Developmental theories* focus on explaining the processes by which infants mature and gain skills to become fully functioning adults. At the core of developmental theories is an explanation of the relationship between human biologic capacity and maturation and the influence of the environment on the behavioral experiences of the individual. In fact, developmental theories tend to be distinguished from each other by the specific weighing of these two factors, nature or nurture, or by the emphasis on a particular aspect of human biologic function or environment. For example, behavioral theories focus more on the influence of the environment on human development, whereas *psychoanalytic theories* focus on biologic determinants of behavior.

Although the emphases can differ, developmental theorists generally agree that human development is both the process and the product of biologic maturation and environmental experiences. *Development* may be defined as the sequential changes in function that occur with maturation of the individual or species. These sequential changes should be differentiated from the concept of *growth,* which refers to maturational changes that are physically measurable. In the past, different dimensions of development have been emphasized. For example, *longitudinal development* focuses on the stages of development, whereas *hierarchical development* focuses on the prerequisite skills needed for higher level skills. Evolving views and theories of development place less emphasis on the stages and components of development and more on the person as a whole and his or her development in relation to environment, roles, and occupations (Humphry, 2002). The emerging theories of person-environment relations and complex systems have influenced these changes.

Occupation

Theories of occupation have changed since the early 1900s. The ideals of moral treatment were prominent in the early part of the twentieth century, particularly the concept that daily routines and occupations improve a person's health. Although the profession of occupational therapy had not yet developed, physicians and others in health care began to focus on the use of a "work cure." The following excerpt from the *Journal of the American Medical Association* is an excellent example of the value placed on occupation at the time:

> How does occupation affect a cure? One thing is certain, that the coated tongue, the obstinate constipation, the diminished secretions, the sallow complexion and the other symptoms of ill health that very stubbornly resist other methods of treatment gradually disappear when patients are engaged in suitable occupation, and we can nearly always look forward with confidence for a marked

improvement in mental condition (Moher, 1907, p. 1666).

The decade after this article was published saw the beginning of a new profession called occupational therapy. Throughout the 1920s and into the 1930s, the focus of occupational therapy was the development of the idea of occupation as cure, which also defined the occupations best used for specific medical problems. Occupational therapists used the principles of graded, purposeful activity and a balance of work, rest, and play as the basis for treatment methods (McColl et al., 2003; Slagle, 1922).

In the 1940s, changes in the medical arena, particularly with the discovery of antibiotics and the advancement of specific medical and surgical techniques, had a tremendous influence on the way in which occupational therapists used occupation in treatment. The development of specific techniques increased, and more focus was placed on programs of activities of daily living. Occupational therapy treatment focused on the prescription of activities with specific aims (Hyatt, 1946). For example, the flexion, extension, pronation, supination (FEPS) loom was developed to ensure that targeted ranges of movement were achieved. As a result of these changes, treatment became "medicalized." In other words, the focus of occupational therapy became a series of technical activities rather than purposeful occupation. The influence of the medical model on the profession dominated for three decades and remains a predominant influence today.

As the 1960s ended, occupational therapists were increasingly uncomfortable with the technical focus of their profession. There was a call for more emphasis on the development of theory and a renewed interest in the roots of the profession: occupation (Yerxa, 1967). During this time, Reilly (1966, 1974a) described a theory of occupational behavior in which the individual strives to develop skills and competencies directed toward mastery and achievement. Work and play were viewed as the contexts in which these developments occur. Fidler and Fidler (1978) focused on the importance of purposeful activity, or *doing*, in the development of self and the prevention of dysfunction. Kielhofner and Burke (1980), building on Reilly's work, described a model of human occupation that incorporated a systems theoretical view of the nature of occupation. This model expanded the understanding of life roles and the powerful influence they have on experience and health.

In the past 15 years, a specific academic discipline called *occupational science* became a basis of occupational therapy (Yerxa et al., 1989). Study of the human as an occupational being is essential to an understanding of the complexity of engagement in occupation and the relationship between occupation and human health. Wilcock described the human need to use time in a purposeful way. "This need is innate and related to health and survival because it enables individuals to utilize their biologic capacities and potential and thereby flourish" (Wilcock, 1993, p. 23).

As the study of occupation has developed, occupational therapy scholars have proposed definitions of occupation. Clark and colleagues defined occupations as "chunks of daily activity that can be named in the lexicon of the culture" (Clark et al., 1991, p. 301). Christiansen and co-workers defined occupation as the "ordinary and familiar things that people do every day" (Christiansen, Clark, Kielhofner, & Rogers, 1995, p. 1015). The definition adopted by the Canadian Association of Occupational Therapists (CAOT) states that "occupation refers to a group of activities and tasks of everyday life, named, organized, and given value and meaning by individuals and a culture" (CAOT, 1997, p. 34).

Each definition refers to daily activities or "chunks" of activity. Because of this daily activity concept, occupation is often thought of as simple; that is, activities that people perform each day to look after themselves, to be productive, and to enjoy life. The definition of occupation becomes more complex with the inclusion of its meaning or purpose. The meaning of an occupation for an individual or the value of an occupation determined by a culture begins to show the many layers of occupation and the central relationship of occupation to the human experience.

Occupation is a basic human need (CAOT, 1997). Dunton (1919) expressed his belief that occupation is as necessary to life as food and drink. Occupation also is an important determinant of health. Health can be strongly influenced by a person's engagement in meaningful occupations, and conversely, the absence of meaningful occupation can have dire health consequences (Wilcock, 1998). Occupation serves as a means of organizing time, space, and materials. Patterns, habits, and roles evolve through the organization of occupation (Kielhofner, 1997). Occupations change over the life span (as do patterns of time use), representing occupational development.

Play is a key area of occupational focus in practice with children. Play is often described as a primary occupation of childhood (Knox, 1997). Most of the focus in the occupational therapy literature has been on play as a therapeutic medium and as a reflection of development (Stewart et al., 1996). Parham (1996) referred to this description as the *functional view of play;* that is, play serves other functions, such as the development of motor or cognitive skills. A recent survey confirms that pediatric occupational therapists most often use play in therapy as a medium for developing both the skills underlying function (e.g., understanding cause-and-effect relationships, exploring an object by manipulating it) and an understanding of the rules that guide behavior (e.g., taking turns) (Couch, Deitz, & Kanny, 1998). Occupational therapists often observe children's play and play with them when trying to determine their level of development in performance areas and performance components (Linder, 1994). Less often, but probably more important, therapists view play as the outcome of interest, the end rather than the means. Parham suggested that therapists must understand that "play is important for its own sake, not only because it subserves other important functions" (Parham, 1996, p. 78).

Occupation plays a dual role in the occupational therapy profession, as both the focus of intervention and the medium through which occupational therapists often intervene. For example, a child may be struggling at school to successfully fulfill his or her role as a student because of an attention deficit disorder. The student's academic occupations are negatively affected, as is his or her social occupation of maintaining positive peer relationships. The occupational therapist analyzes the daily occupations in which the child is expected to participate, determines the personal and environmental factors that are influencing the child's performance, and uses some of these occupations (e.g., entering a play group, independently completing desk work) to facilitate the child's performance.

Occupational analysis is frequently used to gain an understanding of the roles, tasks, activities, and skills required by the individual to perform meaningful occupations successfully in specific contexts (Watson, 1997). The recent development of occupation-focused assessment tools, such as the School Function Assessment (Coster, Deeny, Haltiwanger, & Haley, 1998), indicates that the profession is moving forward in applying increased theoretical knowledge about occupation to the practice of occupational therapy.

When occupational therapists use an occupation-based model of practice, the desired outcome is the achievement of optimal occupational performance for a child. What do the professionals know about the occupational performance of children with special needs? According to the National Health Interview Survey of 1992 to 1994, 6.5% of children in the United States with disabilities are limited to some degree in their participation in daily activities (Newacheck & Halfon, 1998). They reported that children with physical disabilities are "two to three times more likely to be unable to perform their usual activities than children with other conditions (e.g., asthma)" (Newacheck & Halfon, 1998, p. 612). Children with special needs also have lower rates of participation in ordinary daily activities (Brown & Gordon, 1987; Pless, Cripps, Davies, & Wadsworth, 1989; Sloper, Turner, Knussen, & Cunningham, 1990; Law, Seep et al., 1999). This pattern of restricted occupation appears to start in early childhood and is ingrained by the adolescent years. Children with special needs also experience social isolation (Anderson & Clarke, 1982; Cadman, Boyle, & Szatmari & Offord, 1987; LaGreca, 1990; Blum, Resnick, Nelson, & St. Germaine, 1991; Law & Dunn, 1993). Clearly, encouraging participation in the typical activities of childhood needs to be the major focus of pediatric occupational therapy.

Environment

Human ecology is the study of human beings and their relationships with their environments. *Environments* are the contexts and situations that occur outside individuals and elicit responses from them, including personal, social, institutional, and physical factors. Environmental factors can facilitate or limit engagement in occupation (Law, 1991). A concept prevalent in the human development literature and more recently in health care is person-environment congruence, or *environmental fit*, which is described as the congruence between individuals and their environments (Stewart & Law, 2003).

How has environment historically been viewed in occupational therapy? Early in the development of occupational therapy, little was written about the influence of the environment. The few references to the environment in early occupational therapy literature focused on how the physical environment influenced the recovery of the client (McColl et al., 2003). In the 1930s, environmental theories had not yet been developed, but the literature introduced general ideas about the ways in which occupational therapy could provide an environment conducive both to recovery and to the development of skills. Modification of the environment to influence client behaviors was first suggested in the 1940s. During the 1950s and 1960s, the literature continued to describe both the role of the environment in occupational therapy as an influence on behavior and the ways in which enrichment of the environment, or the creation of *prosthetic environments*, could minimize disability.

Over the past two decades, occupational therapists have stressed the importance of the interaction between individual and environment. Specific models of practice have been developed with a focus on environment (Dunn, Brown, & McGuigan, 1994; Law et al., 1996). Systems theory, emphasizing the interdependent relationship between individual and environment, formed the basis for concepts that define occupational therapy and models of practice. Primary models of practice address the environment in terms of its cultural, social, institutional, and physical dimensions and the transactional relationship between people and the environments in which they live, work, and play (Rigby & Letts, 2003; Yerxa et al., 1989).

Two theories from environment-behavior studies and theories related to risk and resilience are presented in these pages, because these theories are most applicable to occupational therapy practice in pediatrics. (The reader is directed to Law et al. [1996, 1997] for information on other environment-behavior theories and models.)

Bronfenbrenner (1977), with a background in developmental psychology, focused his study on the *social* development of the individual. He believed that an interdependent relationship existed between a person and social settings. A person is viewed as a social agent who interacts with all levels of the environment to develop and bring meaning to his or her life. The environment is described in terms of the social and cultural settings around a person. Levels of the environment are defined by their proximity to the individual; that is, family is most important, then friends and extended family, and then the community and society. Changes at any level of the environment influence a person's behavior. Throughout his or her life, a person constantly adapts to changes in the environment.

According to Bronfenbrenner's theories of social development, occupational therapists are part of a person's social environment. These theories help the therapist understand life span changes in clients in the context of their social settings. The interdependence between a person and the social environment helps therapists to expand intervention strategies to include families and communities.

Ecologic psychologists E. Gibson and J. Gibson considered the interdependence of a person with his or her environment to be an explanation of *perceptual* development. E. Gibson (1988) described the motivation of a person to perform meaningful tasks and to learn about the various aspects of the environment that enable the individual to reach his or her goals. J. Gibson (1977, 1979) described the importance of the environment as constraining or enhancing the performance of tasks, a relationship he labeled *affordance*. Successful adaptation to the environment occurs when a person matches his or her activities to the affordances of the environment or when the person modifies the environment to ensure successful completion of an activity.

The Gibsons' theories emphasize the importance of understanding a child's development in the context of daily surroundings and activities. Occupational therapists are encouraged to provide opportunities in which a child can explore and learn about the environment in a manner suitable to achieving his or her goals.

Risk and Resilience

Several theories and research programs have been developed to explain the ways the environment influences the developmental outcomes of children and adolescents. Most of this work focuses on the participation of children and youth in everyday activities and on factors that either place children and adolescents at risk for poor outcomes or help them achieve optimal outcomes. For example, psychologist Emi Werner studied the people of Kauai for more than 40 years. Her research indicated that participation in extracurricular activities plays an important role in the lives of resilient adolescents, especially when they participate in activities that are cooperative in nature (Werner, 1989).

The risk and resilience literature attempts to explain why some children have better outcomes than others who were raised in similar circumstances. Researchers such as Rutter (1990) and Garmezy (1985) have identified protective factors related to the child, the family milieu, and the social environment. For example, attributes of the child that influence positive outcomes include strong self-esteem and positive communication skills (Garmezy, 1985; Werner, 1989, 1994). Attributes of the family that influence positive outcomes include family cohesion and harmony (Garmezy, 1985). Attributes of the social environment that promote resilience include extended social support and availability of external resources (Garmezy, 1985). Environmental factors, such as family-centered service delivery, acceptance of community attitudes, supportive home environments, and mentoring relationships with adults, have been shown to have a positive influence on child development (Richmond & Beardslee, 1988; Wallander & Varni, 1989; Werner, 1994). Emerging evidence indicates that it is the total number of risk factors to which a child is exposed and the resources available to promote resilience for that child that ultimately are predictive of the child's vulnerability to future adverse events and developmental outcomes (Engle, Castle, & Meno, 1996; Sandler, 2001).

Family-Centered Service

During the past 20 years, families of children with disabilities have increased their role in determining and implementing services for their children. Families have been leaders in promoting family-centered service, a philosophy of service provision that emphasizes the central role of families in making decisions about the care their children receive. Although client-centered and family-centered practice first originated in the 1940s, after Carl Rogers published a book on clinical intervention for the problem child (Rogers, 1939), only recently has implementation of the principles of family-centered service become a standard of practice. Challenged by the changes in the health services field and an increased demand by consumers for involvement in the services they receive, health care providers have made great strides in implementing family-centered service.

The term *family-centered service* arose from early intervention programs. The three important concepts that define family-centered service are (1) parents know their children best and want the best for their children; (2) families are different and unique; and (3) optimal child functioning occurs in a supportive family and community context.

In family-centered service, the family's right to make autonomous decisions is honored. The relationship between the family and professionals is a partnership in which the family defines the priorities for intervention and, with the service provider, helps direct the intervention process (Dunst, Trivette, & Deal, 1988). In working with families, service providers emphasize education to enable parents to make informed choices about the therapeutic needs of their child (Bazyk, 1989). Intervention is based on the family's visions and values; service providers recognize their own values and do not impose them on the family. The family's roles and interests, the environments in which the family members live, and the family's culture make up the context for service provision (Law, 1991). Individualization of both the assessment and intervention processes is essential to family centeredness. Intervention is viewed as a dynamic process in which clients and parents work together as partners to define the therapeutic needs of the child with a disability. Services are designed to fit the needs of the family, rather than forcing the family to fit the needs of the service providers or the intervention policies already in place.

Increasing evidence in the literature indicates that interdisciplinary, family-centered service for children with disabilities leads to increased family satisfaction and may lead to greater functional improvement in children with disabilities (Mahoney & Bella, 1998; Mahoney & O'Sullivan, 1990). Research has demonstrated that parents feel greater control when service providers are positive and proactive and promote parental participation and competency. In contrast, a lack of control is associated with behaviors that are unresponsive to the family's needs, are paternalistic, and that fail to recognize or accept family decisions (Dunst, Trivette, Davis, & Cornwall, 1988).

Moxley-Haegert and Serbin (1983) found that teaching parents to recognize developmental gains in their delayed infants increases parents' participation and enhances developmental gains for the child. In a randomized, controlled trial involving 219 families, Stein and Jessop (1984, 1991) demonstrated that an integrated, community-based program that focused on the whole family and its needs led to greater parental satisfaction with care and better psychologic adjustment of the child.

The findings of a recent survey completed by 494 parents, 324 service providers, and 15 chief executive officers from 16 organizations delivering children's rehabilitation services indicate that parental satisfaction with service is primarily determined by the family-centered culture at the organization and by parental perceptions of family-centered service (Law et al., in press). Occupational therapists who work with children enhance the effectiveness of their services when they practice from a family-centered perspective.

World Health Organization International Classification of Functioning, Disability, and Health

It is useful for occupational therapists to have a knowledge of the World Health Organization (WHO) International Classification system, which is used in the broad rehabilitation and disability arena. The *International Classification of Impairments, Disabilities, and Handicaps* (ICIDH) was first developed and published in 1980 (WHO, 1980). The development of software that categorizes and selects outcome measures (Law, King et al., 1999) is an example of a way that occupational therapists have used this classification.

The revised classification system is titled the *International Classification of Functioning, Disability, and Health,* or ICF (WHO, 2001). The ICF views functioning at three levels: the body (structure and function), the person (activities), and society (participation). It also includes the domain of environmental factors, which can have a significant influence on a person's functioning and health. The ICF model of functioning, disability, and health depicts the dynamic interaction between a person and his or her environment at all levels of functioning. As the ICF becomes globally adopted as a classification system and model of functioning and health, occupational therapists are encouraged to apply it to research, education, and clinical practice. The American Occupational Therapy Association (AOTA) has acknowledged the strong connection between concepts of occupation in the field of occupational therapy and participation in the ICF by establishing "engagement in occupation to support participation" as the profession's targeted outcome (AOTA, 2002).

SECTION 2: FOUNDATIONAL THEORIES

Foundational theories form the basis of occupational therapy intervention approaches. These theories come from many fields of study, ranging from the biologic sciences to social sciences to humanities. Occupational therapists draw from a wide range of foundational theories to explain occupational performance. Most theories used by occupational therapists who work in pediatrics are concerned with change. Such theoretical perspectives complement the therapist's view of human development as changes that occur in the function of an individual or a species. Considering the complex nature of the PEO perspective and the transactions involved in occupational performance, a number of foundational theories are relevant. This section reviews the theories most commonly used by occupational therapists who work with children and adolescents with disabilities.

Developmental Theories

Developmental theories explain and describe the different components of a person as they relate to occupational performance. Different theorists have focused on particular components of the individual in an effort to explain developmental function and dysfunction. The most common theories used by occupational therapists are presented.

Freud and Psychosexual Stages

Discussion of the theory proposed by Sigmund Freud (1966) focuses on personality development. Freud (1856-1939) proposed that personality arises from the biologic, instinctual energy of the individual and that this energy is differentiated through typical environmental experiences at different ages (Table 3-1). He believed that personality forms during the first few years of life, as children pass through a series of psychosexual stages of development. Each stage of development focuses on distinct pleasure-sensitive areas of the body, called *erogenous zones.*

Freud's model of personality includes three main concepts: id, ego, and superego. The *id* is the initial, motivating part of a person's personality and is present at birth. It represents the psychic energy, the impetus for all behavior. The id contains both the life and death instincts of the individual. The id operates for pleasure, whereas the *ego* operates in reality. As the ego develops, a child learns to cope with the real world. The ego also protects itself against anxiety with defense mechanisms that reduce or redirect anxiety in various ways. Beginning around age 4 or 5, Freud believed that the *superego* emerged, which is the voice of conscience.

Freud is best known for his systematic study and organization of concepts related to the unconscious. The *unconscious* is the region of the mind where thoughts, feelings, and memories, of which the person mostly is unaware, are stored. Dreams were viewed as an expression of a person's unconscious wishes.

Although many of Freud's theories have been questioned over the years, his concepts of the unconscious and the psychosexual aspects of personality development have contributed significantly to our understanding of human nature (Myers, 2001). Many developmental models, including those in occupational therapy and psychoanalysis, incorporate some of Freud's concepts. For example, pediatric therapists often refer to the oral-anal stages of infant development. Also, some therapists still use projective tests and techniques to address personality characteristics such as unconscious wishes and conflicts.

TABLE 3-1 Contrasted Sequences of Selected Stage Theories

Age	Freud: Psychosexual Development	Erikson: Ego Adaptation	Piaget: Cognitive Development	Kohlberg: Moral Development
6 mo	Pregenital period	Basic trust vs mistrust	Sensorimotor period	Preconventional morality: Punishment and obedience
1 yr	Oral stage ↓			
18 mo	Anal stage	Autonomy vs doubt and shame		
2 yr			Preoperational period: preconceptual phase ↓	
3 yr	Phallic stage	Initiative vs guilt	Initiative thought phase	
4 yr		↓		
5 yr		Industry vs inferiority		
6 yr	Latency period			Instrumental relativism
7 yr			Concrete operational period	
8 yr				
9 yr				Conventional morality; Social conformity
10 yr				
11 yr	Genital stage		Formal operational period	Law and order
12 yr		Self-identity vs role diffusion		
13 yr				
14 yr				
15 yr				
16 yr				Postconventional morality: Social contracts
17 yr				
18 yr	↓	Intimacy and solidarity vs isolation ↓	↓	Universal ethics ↓

Erikson and Psychosocial Development

Eric Erikson (1964) was a student of Freud's, and his theory of development reflects that affiliation. Erikson is viewed as the father of ego psychology. His work demonstrates a more optimistic view of human nature and focuses on the functions of the ego in response to the environment. He believed that personality is based on more than instinct, and he gave priority to the adaptive response of the ego in the development of the individual.

Erikson conducted extensive studies of children, including cross-cultural comparisons. He believed that play afforded the best opportunity for observation of adaptive and maladaptive responses of the ego. His theories emphasize environmental influences and are applicable across cultures, which make them especially useful for occupational therapists.

Erikson divided the life span into eight stages of psychosocial development. Each stage is represented by a personal-social crisis that gives impetus to growth of the ego. His model begins with exploration and leads to mastery. The concepts of mastery and achievement characterize development throughout childhood and adolescence (see Table 3-1). Each stage results in the acquisition of an abstract personality quality, such as hope or wisdom (Hall & Lindzey, 1978). This text briefly describes the first five stages, through adolescence.

Basic Trust versus Mistrust.   The infant, from birth to about 18 months, develops *psychologic trust,* the eagerness to approach new experiences without fear. Trust develops through the caregiving attentions of the parents. The initial sense of trust comes from the infant's realization that survival needs will be met and that he or she can exist in a state of comfort. The most difficult task for the infant is to maintain this trust in the absence of his or her parents. Erikson believed that parents must gradually provide opportunities for separation, although they should be experiences that do not provoke excessive anxiety. Infants who successfully resolve this stage acquire *hope.*

Autonomy versus Doubt and Shame.   The 2- to 4-year-old toddler experiences autonomy rather than doubt and shame. This stage is characterized by holding on and letting go and is exemplified by the crisis that occurs through the toilet-training process. Erikson specified the relationship of autonomy to the child's increasing control over his or her body. This stage brings independent movement away from the parents, enabling the child to explore the environment. Parents must provide opportunities for the child to make choices and develop a sense of self-controlled *will.*

Initiative versus Guilt.   The newly autonomous preschool-age child has mastered basic motor skills and must now build a repertoire of social skills to deal with the outer world. Central to this development is the achievement of gender role identity. Children primarily learn gender roles through imitation of parents and possibly teachers. Through imitation, children learn to assume responsibility for themselves in familiar and comfortable environments. Evident in their complex play scenarios and newly achieved self-care skills is a sense of *purpose.*

Industry versus Inferiority.   The elementary school child experiences a period of slow, steady growth. The need for security is transferred from the family to the peer group, as the child attempts to master the activities appropriate for his or her age. The peer group is used as a standard of performance against which the child can measure his or her own skills. Through sports, games, and school achievements, the child gains a sense of *competence.*

Self-Identity versus Role Diffusion.   Erikson studied the period of adolescence in detail. The masterful school-age child is suddenly shaken by the physiologic changes of puberty and must struggle to regain control over his or her body, identity, and future. During adolescence, prolonged childhood ends and society asks the adolescent to make choices about adult roles. The adolescent experiments with patterns of identity until a sense of continuity and control over the ego is regained and a perspective of the future is acquired. Despite the often-turbulent conflicts between adolescents and their elders, Erikson believed the actions of both are directed to the same end: helping adolescents clarify their roles as members of society. Through resolution of the identity crisis, the individual gains continuity of the past with the future—a sense of *fidelity.*

Piaget and Cognitive Development

Jean Piaget (1971) was concerned with the developmental adaptation of the individual in response to ongoing environmental experiences. He defined *adaptation* as the child's ability to adjust to change to fit into his or her environment, and he examined adaptation through the child's relationships with human and nonhuman objects and through time and space. Piaget (1952) introduced the idea that children are intrinsically motivated to learn from their surroundings and that they act on, rather than simply react to, their environment (Krantz, 1994). Piaget used the terms *cognitive structures,* or *schema,* to describe the way in which children represent objects, events, and relationships in their minds. Piaget viewed every interaction as an opportunity either to assimilate new knowledge into existing structures or to adapt existing structures to accommodate new information. *Accommodation* is new learning, and it is believed to be the way that the cognitive progress is made. Piaget's developmental stages have been the focus of research and critique; however, his descriptions of the gradual accumulation of knowledge in specific content areas remain valid concepts in child development.

Piaget believed the child organizes his experiences into mental schemes (concepts) through mental operations. Operations may be defined as the cognitive methods used by the child to organize his or her schemes and experiences to direct his or her actions. The totality of operational schemes available to the child at any given time constitutes the adapted intelligence, or *cognitive competence,* of the child.

Piaget believed that an invariant, hierarchical development of cognition proceeded from the simple to the complex, from the concrete to the abstract, and from personal to worldly concerns. He specified four maturational levels or periods of cognitive function: sensorimotor, preoperational, concrete operational, and formal operational (see Table 3-1) (Flavell, 1985). He believed that this sequence of development leads to the cognitive maturity of adulthood. The culmination of these levels is a person with values, goals, and plans and an understanding of his or her purpose in society.

A knowledge of Piaget's theory is important to occupational therapists who plan programs for children. Regardless of the therapeutic approach used in treatment, the therapist interacts with a thinking child. It is essential that the selection and structure of an activity be in accordance with the operational skills and concepts of the child.

The primary focus of Piaget's concept is an explanation of cognitive learning, but Schmidt (1988) developed the idea further in the area of motor learning. He proposed that motor schemas are formed as combinations of (1) the initial conditions of the movement, (2) the specific parameters used to create it, (3) the knowledge of the results in the environment, and (4) the sensory consequences of the movement. Through repeated experiences, the child abstracts relationships among these four features and is considered to have learned a new movement.

Kohlberg and Moral Development

Lawrence Kohlberg (1978) was interested in the relationship between the concepts of cognitive development and the acquisition of moral value schemes. He designed a series of fascinating experiments that presented moral dilemmas to children and young adults of different ages. Like Maslow, whose theories are described in the next section, Kohlberg did not judge the correctness of children's choices; instead, he collected data about the concepts used by the children to make moral decisions. He found these concepts to be patterned, sequential, and somewhat linked to age. His model of moral development describes three discrete levels: preconventional morality, conventional morality, and postconventional morality. Each of these levels has two complementary stages (see Table 3-1).

It is interesting to note that Kohlberg's stages are chronologically behind those of Piaget, indicating that levels of cognition must be mature before an individual can use the higher level operative methods to examine abstract issues of morality. By adulthood, the individual develops a mature sense of morality and uses moral thinking in dealing with everyday situations.

Maslow and the Hierarchy of Basic Needs

Abraham Maslow is generally considered the father of humanistic psychology in the United States (Hall & Lindzey, 1978). He outlined a hierarchy of basic human needs that is believed to follow a longitudinal sequence (Maslow, 1968, 1970, 1971). At the base of his hierarchy are *physiologic needs,* such as food, water, rest, air, and warmth, which are necessary to basic survival. The next level is characterized by the *need for safety,* broadly defined as the need for both physical and physiologic security. The *need for love and belonging* promotes the individual's search for affection, emotional support, and group affiliation. The *need for a sense of self-esteem,* which is defined as the ability to regard the self as competent and of value to society, is evidenced as an individual grows. The *need for self-actualization,* which represents the highest level, is attained through achievement of personal goals.

Maslow proposed that each of these needs serves as a motivator to achieve a higher level of human potential. A progression of development takes place that begins with the satisfaction of biologic and egocentric needs. It proceeds through the needs for social group affiliation and culminates in the use of intellectual capacities to affect the broader community of the individual. If the lower level needs are not met, the individual is not able to direct his or her energies toward higher levels. For example, a child that comes to school hungry finds it difficult to concentrate on the classroom learning activities. Recognition of a child's needs and the hierarchy of development of these basic needs is important for occupational therapists who strive to help children achieve personal goals.

Rogers and the Development of Self

Carl Rogers (1969) believed that people have an inborn need for self-actualization. The central idea of Rogers' theory is the individual's inner experiencing; that is, how the individual perceives himself or herself and his or her relationships and environment. Rogers acknowledged the instrumental influence of the environment in the development of self, but he believed that the individual has the capacity to choose responses to the environment that allow him or her to maintain a sense of personal control.

Rogers is best known for his formulation of client-centered therapy. Like Erikson, Rogers believed that each individual has, and must find within himself or herself, the resources for growth, adaptation, and self-actualization. Client-centered therapy is designed to elicit these resources; the therapist takes a nondirective role that encourages the client to express his or her own desires and interests and to act on these. Occupational therapists have embraced a client-centered approach to practice for many years, because it fits with the philosophy that a client should be actively engaged in the therapy process.

Learning and Systems Theories

Most important to occupational therapy are theories that integrate concepts about people, their environments, and their occupations. A discussion of these learning and systems theories follows.

Learning Theories

Development has been defined as an "evolution of predictable sequences of interactions between a child and the objects in his or her environment" (Lyons, 1984, p. 446). Developmental theories, which provide stages or markers of progress against which a child can be compared, were emphasized in the previous section in this chapter. Traditional views of development emphasize the dominant role of the maturation of the central nervous system (CNS). More recently, occupational therapists have begun to understand that cognitive and motor progress is possible through a dynamic process in which the CNS develops as the child attempts to solve cognitive and movement problems. This process is called *learning;* that is, the acquisition of knowledge through experience in a way that leads to a permanent change in behavior. In occupational therapy theory, it is helpful to examine theories of motor learning, cognitive progress, and motivation for change. In all three domains, learning occurs when children find solutions to problems and thereby acquire functional skills.

Before the ways children learn are examined, it is important to review the different dimensions in which tasks may vary, because each of these dimensions is relevant to the way in which tasks are learned.

1 *Simple-complex.* Simple tasks, such as reaching for an object, require a decision followed by a sequenced response. Complex tasks, such as handwriting, require the integration of information from a variety of sources and the application of underlying rules that guide performance (Colley & Beech, 1989).

2 *Open loop–closed loop.* In an open-loop task, a motor program is put into place before the action begins and is not modified during the performance of a task. An example of an open-loop task is throwing a ball. In a closed-loop task, the child continues to monitor and respond to feedback that he or she receives intrinsically from the body and extrinsically from the environment. An example of a closed-loop task is cutting out a shape using scissors (Adams, 1971).

3 *Environment changing–environment stationary.* The difficulty of learning a task is tremendously influenced by the extent to which the task is predictable. When the environment is changeable or variable, the child has to learn the movement and learn to monitor the environment to adapt to change. Running on rough terrain or playing soccer are examples of tasks in which the environment is constantly changing. This concept is not to be confused with the open- and closed-loop features of the task previously described. Brushing the teeth and playing the piano are tasks in which the child must monitor sensory feedback during the performance of the tasks (closed loop), but the environment remains stationary (Sugden & Sugden, 1990).

4 *Novel-acquired.* During the first performances of a task, the child combines what he or she knows about the task with information from the environment. The child then makes a workable procedure that is controlled, slow, and full of effort. With repeated performance of the task, however, multiple procedures are collapsed and run more automatically. With practice, the speed of performance increases and the effort decreases (Anderson, 1982).

5 *Task modality.* The ease or difficulty of learning a task depends on the match between the way the task is presented and the preferred learning style of the child. Some children learn best through auditory or visual methods; others prefer movement and touch. The modality of the task (e.g., visual, oral, physical, figural) is another factor that influences learning.

Skinner and Behaviorism.   The past 50 years have witnessed tremendous progress in the field of learning theories. Early learning theorists, such as Thorndike, emphasized the association between a behavior and the resulting reward or punishment as a simple explanation of behavioral change. Skinner (1953) described perhaps the best known learning theory from this era. Skinner believed that the environment shapes all human behaviors and that behaviors may be randomly emitted in response to an environmental stimulus. In other words, a person tries a behavior that worked in a previous situation, or an involuntary, reflexive response is elicited by an environmental stimulus. The behavior is then reinforced by the environmental consequences that follow. This sequence—stimulus situation, behavioral response, and environmental consequence—constitutes a *contingency of behavior,* the mechanism by which the environment shapes behavior.

Skinner (1976) stated that through natural occurrences in the environment, a child's adaptive behaviors are reinforced, and behaviors that are not adaptive are ignored or punished. The child usually associates positive reinforcement (reward) with a pleasant experience. Behavior is strengthened and maintained as long as it is generally effective in obtaining positive reinforcement. If reinforcement is absent (i.e., not given) and therefore negative, positive behavior may be extinguished.

Skinner believed that all behavior is a result of the environmental control of the individual, culture, and species. He specified that humans, species, and culture are all part of the environment, therefore they control as much as they are controlled. Problems arise when an environment changes and becomes inconsistent with prior contingency patterns. For example, children use one set of behaviors with their families and another set with friends. Behaviors that are reinforced by friends may bring complaints from or may be ignored by parents.

Extensive research has confirmed that when particular behaviors result in specific, consistent consequences, these behaviors can be modified. Skinner (1953) believed that a process called *shaping* creates new behaviors. Shaping involves breaking down a complex behavior into components and reinforcing each behavior individually and systematically until it approximates the desired behavior. Critics of this theory cite its failure to explain personality traits (e.g., motivation) and cognitive abilities (e.g., imagination and creativity) and its tendency to generalize across age and gender spectrums with no recognition of developmental differences.

Social Cognitive Theories.
The initial acquisition of highly complex and abstract behaviors was difficult for learning theorists to explain until the advent of the social cognitive theory proposed by Bandura (1977, 1982, 1989). This theory introduced the idea that children can learn by observing the behavior of others. Bandura's theory has two important concepts: acquisition and performance. During *acquisition* a child observes the behavior of others and determines the consequences, and these observations are stored in memory for later use. *Performance* refers to the idea that the child may decide to perform the behavior, depending on the child's perception of the situation and the consequences. Bandura believed that critical factors in the child influence the learning process, including the child's perception of his or her competencies, a topic that is addressed later in this section. Bandura's introduction of the importance of the social context to the child's ability to learn and his recognition that a child's thoughts and beliefs also influence his or her learning ability are important to occupational therapists.

Vygotsky (1978) also recognized that learning is developed in a social context, and he believed that cognitive development occurs through the gradual internalization of concepts and relationships encountered through social interactions. Although he agreed with Piaget that children develop as a result of engagement in activity, he believed that learning also requires interaction with others who are more cognitively competent. He suggested that children first experience activities (e.g., problem solving) in situations in which a child, an activity, and a significant other are components. The adult initially does most of the cognitive work, but gradually the adult's speech is internalized by the child and, with experience and application, becomes part of the child's cognitive repertoire (Missiuna, Malloy-Miller, & Mandich, 1998).

Vygotsky introduced the critical concept of a *zone of proximal development,* which he conceptualized as "the distance between the actual developmental level as determined by independent problem-solving and the level of potential development as determined through problem-solving under adult guidance or in collaboration with more capable peers" (Vygotsky, 1962, p. 86).

Vygotsky believed that the zone of proximal development reflects the learning potential of the child at a moment in time. When an adult and a child experience an activity together, they interpret the objects and events differently. Vygotsky suggested that the adult use language to help the child redefine the situation so that adult and child have a shared definition. When a learning opportunity is created that provides an optimal balance between the child's existing skills and the challenge of the task, the adult can model language and behavior that will help the child progress.

Vygotsky's emphasis on the interaction involving children's learning, their environment, the type of instruction provided, and their culture was a precursor to many of the dynamic systems models that influence learning theory today.

Information Processing.
The computer has served as a source of inspiration for learning theories that study the manner in which children learn, attend, remember, and solve problems. These theories are called *information processing theories,* and they all focus on the system by which children extract information from the environment, interpret the information, and organize a behavioral response. The theories of many widely recognized researchers (e.g., Case, 1985; Shiffrin & Atkinson, 1969; Siegler, 1983) fit this framework. Although the learning theories differ slightly, similarities exist in the basic beliefs about learning.

Information processing theories are usually portrayed as flowcharts that represent the source of the sensory *input,* the method of accessing memories and solving problems (called *throughput* or *elaboration*), and the *output,* which is the result or solution. Some theorists add a *feedback loop* to explain the acquisition of knowledge and the use of the results of actions (e.g., Sternberg, 1984). Like social cognitive theory, information processing theory emphasizes change as a continuous process of learning and explains age differences as improvement in children's problem-solving abilities with experience (Krantz, 1994). Information processing theories have been developed for and applied to both the cognitive and motor domains.

Factors that Influence Learning.   A discussion of learning theories cannot be completed without briefly considering the factors in the child that are believed to influence learning, such as motivation, attitude, and self-perception. The relationship between learning and other affective components is complex. It is widely accepted that children's motivation to perform occupations is influenced by their perceptions of their efficacy, regardless of whether these perceptions are correct (Bandura, 1993). If children experience success in learning situations, it is assumed that they increase their perceived competence and internal control, gain support from significant others, and show pleasure at mastering the task. The assumption is made that children are more likely to seek out optimal challenges if they have experienced success. The corollary of this theory is that children who experience repeated failure begin to avoid challenges and are less likely to seek out new learning situations (Harter, 1978).

Therapists need to be aware of the importance of providing successful learning opportunities and optimal challenge situations. It is also important to note, however, that when children are young, they may not have the metacognitive awareness required to compare their own performance accurately to that of others. This lack of awareness may actually have an adaptive purpose in childhood. The fact that young children do not evaluate their own performance increases the likelihood that they will put energy and effort into practicing skills in a wide variety of environments with little concern about their actual competency (Bjorklund & Green, 1992). As children develop, however, their expectation of competence becomes more specific to the type of task and is influenced by their prior experiences with that task, their observations of typically developing peers performing it, and the evaluative feedback provided by credible adults (Bandura, 1997).

Another consideration for the occupational therapist relates to what happens to the learning once the skill is acquired. Children do not always automatically transfer the skills they have learned; they often require instruction and guidance to transfer the knowledge and skills from one task to another and to generalize these skills to different environments. Some researchers propose that generalization be shown as much attention and emphasis as that given to initial skill acquisition (Gresham, 1981). As the research on the ways children learn is reviewed, the ability of theory to explain learning and performance in a functional context and in a variety of settings requires reflection.

Dynamic Systems Theory

Emerging theoretical ideas from systems theory influence today's thinking in many areas of development in children, and these ideas are beginning to lead to the creation of alternative models of practice for therapy intervention. In contrast to a hierarchical model of neural organization, systems theory (also called *dynamic systems theory*) proposes a flexible model of neural organization in which the functions of control and coordination are distributed among many elements of the system rather than vested in a single hierarchical level (VanSant, 1991). Work that led to the development of dynamic systems theory includes research by Bernstein (1967), who used concepts from physics related to movement and applied these ideas to motor development. Bernstein proposed that the CNS controls groups of muscles (not individual muscles) and that these groups can change motor behavior on their own without CNS control. These ideas challenge the traditional view that the brain controls all motor behavior.

Systems theorists do not believe in the formation of schema, patterns, or representations of learning; rather, they suggest, the parameters of the actual situation influence the learning that takes place at that point in time (Eliasmith, 1998). Systems theory has its roots in geometric concepts, and at the most basic level, a dynamic system is simply something that changes over time. Dynamic systems theorists emphasize that learning does not occur just in the brain "since the nervous system, the body, and environment are all constantly changing and simultaneously influencing each other" (Van Gelder, 1995, p. 373). In this approach, the therapist looks for periods of stability in learning and watches for signs that a child is ready to shift to a qualitatively different type of behavior. Identification of the system variables that drive the transition from one level to another facilitates learning (Burton & Miller, 1998). These variables can be related to the child, the task, or the environment. Thelen (1995) suggested that variables such as physical growth and biomechanics may be more important for motor learning in infancy, whereas factors such as experience, practice, and motivation may be more influential in the learning of motor activities in an older child.

In this theoretical approach, instead of viewing behavior (e.g., motor skills) as predetermined in the CNS, systems theory views motor behavior as emerging from the dynamic cooperation of the many subsystems in a task-specific context. The CNS is seen as only one of the components underlying movement changes. Other elements include the infant's biomechanical, psychologic, and social environments and the task itself (Heriza, 1991).

The dynamic systems approach is developed from a functional rather than a structural framework. It implies that all factors contributing to the motor behavior are important and exert an influence on the outcome. It represents an ecologic approach in that a child's functional performance depends on the interactions of the child's inherent and emerging skills, the characteristics of the desired task or activity, and the environment in which the activity is performed. Dynamic systems theory has many similarities to the emerging occupational therapy theories that focus on person, environment, and occupation relationships (see Chapter 4).

Research in dynamic systems theory has focused on explaining the ways new skills are learned (Evans, 2002; Mitchell, 1995; Thelen, Schoner, Scheier, & Smith, 2001; Thelen & Spencer, 1998). The learning of new movements or ways of completing an activity requires that previously stable movements be broken down or become unstable. New movements and skills emerge when a critical change occurs in any of the components that contribute to motor behavior. These periods of change are called *transitions*. Motor change in young children is envisioned as a series of events during which destabilization and stabilization of movement take place before the transitional phase movement becomes stable and functional (Piper & Darrah, 1994).

The period of instability that occurs in a transitional phase is seen as the optimal time to effect changes in movement behavior. Three characteristic situations mark the transitional stage:

1 Variability in motor performance increases.
2 When changes in movement occur, return to a stable pattern takes longer.
3 Children display more interest in trying a new motor task. For example, when changing to a walk from a crawl, children interrupt the normal efficient crawl by standing up from time to time. They start to take steps when holding onto someone's hand. Children like to be upright and begin to spend less time in crawling. Ultimately they take their first independent steps.

In children with impairments such as cerebral palsy (CP), constraints hinder the emergence of motor functions. *Constraints* in the child are limitations imposed on motor behaviors by the child's physical, social, cognitive, and neurologic characteristics. The constraint that traditionally has received most attention is the integrity of the CNS; less frequently, other biomechanical constraints are considered, such as biomechanical forces, muscle strength, or a disproportionate trunk-to-limb ratio. *Environmental constraints* include physical, social, and cultural factors not related to a specific task. One example of a physical constraint is the surface on which the child acts (e.g., the incline or texture of the surface); a social constraint could be a parent's lack of reinforcement of the acquisition of motor behaviors. *Task constraints* are restrictions on motor behavior imposed by the nature of the task. Established motor behaviors may be altered by specific task requirements. For example, when faced with the task of crawling on rough terrain, infants may alter motor behavior by extending their knees and "bear walking." When a child reaches for a ball, the ball's size influences the shape of the child's hand and the approach taken (e.g., one hand versus two). The unique features of these tasks have shaped the child's motor behavior.

SECTION 3: MODELS OF PRACTICE USED BY OCCUPATIONAL THERAPISTS

This section of the chapter focuses on models of practice developed specifically for occupational therapy assessment and intervention with children. Section 3 begins by providing an example of a theoretical framework that focuses on occupation and occupational performance. The authors believe that occupational therapy assessment and intervention should always reflect an occupation-based theoretical perspective. Discussion of this overall framework is followed by overviews of specific models of practice used with children and youth. These models of practice are used in conjunction with an overall focus on occupation and occupational performance.

As discussed earlier in this chapter, several theoretical models primarily address the concepts of occupation and occupational performance. These theoretical models provide a means by which occupational therapists can understand the PEO relationship and use it in clinical practice. Examples of current and emerging models that provide this perspective include the following:

- Person-environment-performance (Christiansen & Baum, 1991, 1997)
- Ecology of human performance (Dunn, Brown, & McGuigan, 1994)
- Model of human occupation (Kielhofner, 1995)
- Person-environment-occupation (PEO) model (Law et al., 1996)
- Occupational adaptation (Schkade & Schultz, 1992)
- Contemporary task-oriented approach (Mathiowetz & Bass Haugen, 1994)

All these models support an occupation-based approach to occupational therapy practice. In each, the influence of the environment occupational performance is discussed. Differences between these models include their relative emphasis on specific concepts, such as roles, and the distinction between occupation and occupational performance. In most of these models, the focus of primary intervention is on the person, with relatively less emphasis on changing environments. In contrast, the ecology of human performance and PEO models focus equally on facilitating change in the person, occupation, and/or environment. The model of human occupation is the model that has been most studied and validated. The other models are newer, and research about their use is emerging. The choice of the most appropriate model for a specific area of practice depends on the therapist's knowledge and experience and the context of practice.

To illustrate in more detail the use of a theoretical model to ensure that occupational performance is the focus of clinical practice, the PEO model is described below.

The PEO model was developed using theoretical foundations from the *Canadian Guidelines for Occupational Therapy,* environmental-behavioral theory, and work by Csikszentmihalyi & Csikszentmihalyi (1988) on the theory of optimal experience. The PEO model outlines the concepts of person, environment, and occupation as follows:

- *Person:* A unique being who, across time and space, participates in a variety of roles important to him or her.
- *Environment:* Cultural, socioeconomic, institutional, physical, and social factors outside a person that affect his or her experiences.
- *Occupation:* Groups of self-directed, functional tasks and activities in which a person engages over the life span (Law et al., 1996).

The PEO model suggests that occupational performance is the result of the dynamic, transactive relationship involving person, environment, and occupation (Figure 3-1). Across the life span and in different environments, the three major components—person, environment, and occupation—interact continually to determine occupational performance. Increased congruence, or fit, among these components represents more optimal occupational performance (Figure 3-2).

The PEO model is used as an analytic tool to identify factors in the person, environment, or occupation that facilitate or hinder the performance of occupations chosen by the person. Occupational therapy intervention can then focus on facilitating change in any of these three dimensions to improve occupational performance. Specific models of practice, as outlined in the next section of this chapter, can be used in conjunction with the PEO model to address specific performance components or environmental conditions that impede occupational performance.

Specific Models of Practice

The models of practice or frames of reference currently used in occupational therapy with children and youth can be classified into two types: occupation-based models and neuromaturation-based models. Occupation-based models of practice were more recently developed and are based primarily on contemporary theoretical approaches such as systems theory and integrative models of development. Neuromaturation-based models of practice have been used in practice longer and are based on a hierarchical approach to development; they emphasize both performance components and aspects of occupational performance as desired outcomes.

Occupation-Based Models of Practice

Cognitive Approaches

Cognitive approaches are "top down" or occupation-based approaches because the emphasis in therapy is on assisting the child to identify, develop, and use cognitive strategies to perform daily occupations effectively. The following distinct approaches are classified as cognitive models of practice:

- Cognitive behavior modification (Kendall, 1993; Meichenbaum, 1977)
- Cognitive strategy training (McCormick, Miller, & Pressley, 1989)
- Verbal self guidance (Martini & Polatajko, 1998)
- Cognitive orientation to daily occupational performance (Polatajko et al., 2001)
- Passport to learning (Leew, 2001)

All cognitive approaches emphasize increasing a child's repertoire of cognitive strategies and improving the child's ability to select, monitor, and evaluate his or her usage of these strategies during the performance of a task. The inherent assumption is that improved performance results from the dynamic interaction of the

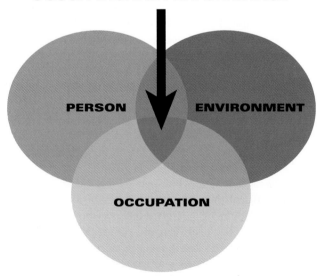

OCCUPATIONAL PERFORMANCE

PERSON   **ENVIRONMENT**

OCCUPATION

FIGURE   3-1 Person-environment-occupation model. (From Law, M., Cooper, B., Strong, S., Stewart, D., Rigby, P., & Letts, L. [1996]. The person-environment-occupation model: A transactive approach to occupational performance. *Canadian Journal of Occupational Therapy, 63* [1], 9-23.)

MAXIMIZES FIT
and therefore maximizes occupational performance

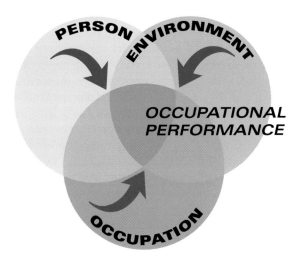

MINIMIZES FIT
and therefore minimizes occupational performance

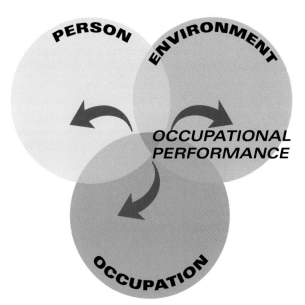

FIGURE 3-2   Person-environment-occupation analysis. (From Law, M., Cooper, B., Strong, S., Stewart, D., Rigby, P., & Letts, L. [1996]. The person-environment-occupation model: A transactive approach to occupational performance. *Canadian Journal of Occupational Therapy, 63* [1], 9-23.)

child's movement skills with the parameters of the task in the context in which it needs to be performed. Therefore cognitive strategies are discovered, applied, and evaluated during task performance in the child's typical environments (Missiuna, Mandich, Polatajko, & Malloy-Miller, 2001).

The cognitive model of practice requires that the therapist identify and use a global problem-solving strategy, which provides a consistent framework within which the child discovers specific strategies applicable to tasks that he or she either needs or wants to perform. This global strategy is based on the five-stage problem-solving structure first outlined by Luria (1961). Using occupational therapy terminology, these steps include (1) task analysis, (2) anticipation of the child's difficulties, (3) exploration and selection of task-specific strategies, (4) application of a strategy to the task, and (5) evaluation of the strategy's effectiveness (Missiuna, Malloy-Miller, & Mandich, 1998). The task-specific strategies a child discovers are unique to him or her. However, they may help the child become more aware of his or her personal biomechanics (e.g., "You need to reach out with both hands to catch a big ball."); motor learning (e.g., "Watch someone else first, then try it."); or implicit sensory feedback (e.g., "You need to hold the pen more firmly."); as well as the aspects of the task (e.g., "The cookie dough is easier to knead than stir."). The strategies that the therapist helps the child discover initially may seem to be compensatory, but once they are internalized, the child's

cognitive skills develop, and he or she becomes able to approach, learn, and perform tasks more effectively. The atmosphere in the therapy session is one of acceptance and support for taking risks. Although the child guides the selection of activities, the therapist is always aware of the generalization and task-specific strategies that the child needs to learn and creates opportunities for the discovery of these to occur (Missiuna et al., 2001; Polatajko, Mandich, & Missiuna et al., 2001).

Because the selection of tasks is critical to the approach, a client-centered tool must be used that allows the child to identify goals for intervention. An appropriate goal-setting instrument for use with children older than 9 years of age is the Canadian Occupational Performance Measure (COPM) (Law et al., 1998); for children 5 to 9 years of age, the Perceived Efficacy and Goal Setting (PEGS) system can be used (Missiuna & Pollock, 2000). The cognitive approach is probably not a suitable model of practice for children under 5 years of age because of its emphasis on the development of metacognitive skill and knowledge.

One of the key features of a cognitive model of practice is the way in which the therapist helps the child explore strategies, make decisions, apply strategies, and evaluate their use. The therapist does not give instruction. Rather, he or she uses questions to help children (1) discover the relevant aspects of the task, (2) examine how they are currently performing the task, (3) identify where they are getting "stuck," (4) creatively think about alternative solutions, and (5) try out these solutions and evaluate them in a supportive environment. Once a strategy is found to be helpful, the therapist uses questions to help the child "bridge" or generalize the strategy, eliciting from the child other times and situations in which that strategy may apply (Polatajko, Mandich, & Missiuna et al., 2001).

In recent years a particular cognitive approach, the cognitive orientation to daily occupational performance (CO-OP) (Polatajko, Mandich, & Miller et al., 2001), has been researched systematically to determine whether it is an effective model to use with children with developmental coordination disorder. Evidence is accumulating that CO-OP is effective at enabling skill acquisition and that it also results in generalization and transfer of learned skills (Polatajko, Mandich, & Missiuna et al., 2001). A randomized clinical trial comparing CO-OP with an equivalent number of sessions of direct skill training showed that, although children in both groups improved and achieved motor goals, the gains in the CO-OP group were greater; long-term maintenance both of the motor goals and of the cognitive strategies was significantly stronger in the CO-OP group, which led parents to report greater satisfaction with this treatment approach (Miller et al., Mandich, & Macnab, 2001).

Through research such as this, a variety of cognitive strategies have been identified that seem to be helpful to many different children experiencing occupational performance difficulties. Videotape analysis has been used to systematically identify and describe some of these strategies (Mandich, Polatajko, Missiuna, & Miller, 2001). It appears that children need to be able to state and apply a global executive strategy, such as "Goal, Plan, Do, Check" (Meichenbaum, 1977) to guide their problem solving. In addition, specific strategies seem to be useful for improving their performance, including verbal self-guidance (child talks himself or herself through the motor sequence); feeling the movement (drawing attention to an aspect of the sensation of movement as it is performed); motor mnemonic (labeling a body position or motor sequence); body position (verbalizing or directing attention to the body position or body parts relative to the task); and task specification (discussing specific parts of the task or actions to change the task) (Mandich, 1997; Mandich et al., 2001). Research is underway to examine whether children who have more significant cognitive or affective limitations need to learn the same types of strategies or whether additional strategies are required.

In summary, occupational therapists who use a cognitive model of practice (1) focus on the occupations a child wishes to perform rather than on foundational skill building; (2) use a general problem-solving framework that guides the child to discover, select, apply, and evaluate the use of specific cognitive strategies; (3) use process questions to increase the child's awareness of the use of strategy during the performance of daily tasks; and (4) plan for transfer and generalization of the strategies that the child has learned (Missiuna et al., 1998; Polatajko, Mandich, & Missiuna et al., 2001).

Compensatory and Environmental Approaches.

Occupational performance is successful when the demands of the task, the skills of the child, and the features of the environment are congruent. When the skills of the person do not meet the demands of the task in the environment, occupational performance decreases. Most of the models of practice in occupational therapy, particularly with children who are still developing, focus on increasing the child's skills. The compensatory model of practice operates from the assumption that the emphasis should be on adapting the demands of the task or modifying the environment in a way that "compensates" for the limitations of the person. Performance of the occupation increases because of the compensation; however, the task is often performed in a manner that is not described as typical. Teaching clients to use compensatory techniques has an immediate and direct link to improved performance of everyday occupations.

The compensatory approach has two major concepts: *compensation*, which involves making children aware of their difficulties and teaching them strategies for coping with these problems; and *adaptation*, which involves changing the task or the environment to accommodate the difficulties (Kielhofner, 1997). In compensatory strategy, the child is trained to compensate for motor patterns or cognitive functions that are ineffective by using intact behaviors or abilities that can be substituted for behaviors that are impaired (Neistadt, 1990). In the motor domain, the child with limited use of intrinsic hand muscles can learn to manipulate objects on a table rather than in the hand. In the cognitive domain, therapists may teach children to use *cognitive prostheses*, such as memory notebooks or lists of the sequence of steps in an activity, with the expectation that, over time, the child may internalize the content supported by these external cues. When skills are still insufficient to enable performance, task adaptation is used to modify the demands of a task to bring it to the competence level of the child. Task demands are analyzed and functional limitations are identified, and difficulties then are creatively circumvented. For example, a child with a learning disability may be able to complete a page of arithmetic problems when the font is enlarged and the paper has a color tint.

With children, the compensatory approach often complements other approaches that focus on skill building. Methods for adapting tasks are selected not only so that the child succeeds at a particular task, but also to promote skills in similar tasks and in other environments. For example, a boy with poor drawing skills can create a picture using peel-off stickers of animals. Although this adaptation allows the boy to create a picture more easily than drawing with markers, peeling off and placing the stickers provide practice of fine motor skills, specifically bilateral coordination, isolated finger movements, spatial relations, and use of force. Practice in these skills may generalize to other art activities, and the easy success the child achieves when using colorful animal stickers may encourage him to attempt other art activities.

Psychosocial Approaches. Occupational therapists use a variety of psychosocial approaches when working with children and adolescents experiencing problems in occupational performance because of social, emotional, or behavioral issues or difficulties with relationships. Several of these approaches, such as a cognitive approach or the compensatory and environmental approach, are discussed elsewhere in this chapter. These approaches are grounded in theories that focus on the development of self, on family and peer relationships, and on the aspects of the social and cultural environment that influence each of these. Although the number of occupational therapists who work with children with chronic mental health issues is relatively small, all occupational therapists who work in pediatrics use the concepts of psychologic and social development implicitly, because developing the ability to maintain relationships with peers and significant others is an essential part of the occupational performance of childhood and adolescence.

Models of practice that focus on social behavior and the development of self place fairly equal emphasis on the person and the social environment. Personal attributes, such as temperament, self-esteem and self-efficacy, problem-solving ability, and social skills, are considered important determinants of healthy functioning. Environmental influences on behavior and social development suggest the need to consider the expectations and social elements of the home, school, and community environments and to recognize the importance of friends in a young person's life. For the occupational therapist, the critical consideration is the impact of the person's attributes and environmental influences on the child's ability to participate in daily occupations.

Given the complex nature of behavior and social relationships, occupational therapists often draw on a number of intervention approaches in this model of practice. The therapist's knowledge of normal behavior, vulnerabilities associated with particular disabilities, attachment, coping skills, and compatibility of temperaments may guide intervention with a parent-child dyad. Cognitive behavioral strategies may be used by occupational therapists to help young people who are depressed or socially withdrawn develop strategies that encourage participation in social situations.

Coping Model. The coping model (Williamson & Szczepanski, 1999; Zeitlin & Williamson, 1994) addresses psychosocial function, uses cognitive behav-

ioral strategies, and is congruent with the PEO model. Therapists who use this model emphasize the use of coping resources that enable the child to meet challenges posed by the environment. The goal is to improve the child's ability to cope with stress in personal, social, and other occupational performance areas. When children are successful in coping with their own personal needs and the demands of the environment, they feel good about themselves and their place in the world. Coping strategies are learned, and children build on previous successful experiences in coping with environmental expectations (Zeitlin & Williamson, 1994).

All children experience stress when faced with physical, cognitive, and emotional challenges. When these challenges are successfully met by the child's inner resources and caregiving supports, the result is a sense of motivation, learning, and mastery. Stress can evoke negative feelings when the child's resources are poorly matched to the environment's demands (e.g., the child becomes upset when picked up quickly from the floor because he or she cannot tolerate the intensity of the stimulation, and parent holding and protection are not available). Both internal and external resources assist in the process of coping. Internal coping resources include coping style, beliefs and values, physical and affective states, and developmental skills. External coping resources include human supports and materials and environmental supports.

INTERNAL AND EXTERNAL COPING RESOURCES. Children have unique patterns of sensorimotor organization, reactivity, and self-initiation (Zeitlin, Williamson, & Szczepanski, 1988). Children exhibit different levels of *sensory reactivity,* which determines arousal and activity levels and is basic to all interactions. *Coping style* comprises the way the child reacts to social interactions and responds to environmental events. Intrinsically motivated and self-initiated behaviors are part of a child's coping style. Examples of these behaviors are the child's exploration of objects and space, initiation of interaction, and persistence in activities. Self-initiated behaviors are particularly important to occupational therapists, because many children with disabilities show limited spontaneous behaviors when exploring the environment, initiating play, and persisting in activity.

The terms *beliefs* and *values* describe the way the child views himself or herself and the world. Beliefs are reflected in the child's self-esteem and can be inferred from behavior. Values reflect a child's desires and preferences and are demonstrated in activity preferences and task mastery. A child's beliefs and values are strongly influenced by the family's beliefs and cultural background.

Physical and affective states influence the child's ability to cope with environmental stress. Energy, endurance, moods, and emotions define the child's ability to respond to, engage in, and persist in activity.

Chronic illness, emotional instability, and depression influence the child's ability to handle the demands of the environment effectively.

Developmental skills and competence are the internal resources a child brings to a task. As the child matures, he or she is able to handle increasingly complex demands. Often a child with disabilities is placed in situations that match the chronologic age (e.g., a preschooler play group) but not necessarily the developmental age. When expected behaviors do not match developmental skills (e.g., to sit quietly and attend), children experience stress and generally seek external coping supports.

Human supports are people in the child's environment who support the child's coping efforts. Parents and other primary caregivers are the most significant external resources for coping in the child's early years (Williamson & Szczpanski, 1999). Parents buffer the child's exposure to stress, make demands, model coping behaviors, encourage and assist the child in coping efforts, and give contingent feedback.

The family provides material supports and resources, including food, clothing, shelter, and medical services, as well as toys and activities. Environmental supports are the spaces and materials available to the child. Coping skills are influenced by the organization of materials, light intensity, noise level, and temperature. Environmental resources may include adapted equipment and technology associated with comfort and functional support.

EFFECTIVE COPING. The child successfully copes with new challenges when (1) he or she has underlying resources that enable a successful response to an environmental demand or new situation; (2) human supports are provided to facilitate his or her performance (e.g., the therapist gives the child a visual or verbal cue); and (3) environmental supports are provided that enable the child to feel safe and comfortable, be attentive and engaged, and feel calm and organized (e.g., a classroom that is quiet and well-organized and that has a comfortable lighting level and temperature). The therapist continually evaluates whether the child's skills (internal resources) and environmental supports (external resources) are adequate to meet the demands of the activity. When the child exhibits ineffective coping strategies, the therapist adjusts the task demands and provides more human or environmental support to enable the child to succeed in his or her coping efforts. Failure in an activity is not always avoided because feedback from inadequate performance can help the child learn to evaluate his or her coping efforts and adapt or modify his or her response.

To facilitate effective coping, Williamson and Szczepanski defined three postulates:

1 The occupational therapist can grade the environmental demands to ensure that they are congruent with the child's adaptive capabilities. For example, the environment of a child with attention deficit hyperactivity disorder (ADHD) can be adapted by reorganizing materials to reduce visual demands and enhance visual attention. To enhance the social skills of children with behavioral disorders, a shortage of materials for an art activity can be placed on the table to encourage sharing among the children.

2 The therapist can design intervention activities to enhance the child's internal and external coping resources. Intervention focuses on the child's resources, including coping style, beliefs and values, physical and affective states, developmental skills, human supports, and material and environmental supports. Coping is supported when beliefs and values contribute to a positive sense of self. The therapist can foster a positive sense of self and can involve the child in activities that promote self-efficacy. For older children, the therapist can facilitate group discussions of personal goals and plans for reaching these goals. Personal social skills may be emphasized by practice of social skills in the context of games with peers. Activities that emphasize group skills, such as problem solving, sharing, and communication, can help older children develop improved personal social skills that can be generalized to school and extracurricular activities.

3 The therapist can provide appropriate, contingent responses to the child's coping efforts. Timely, positive, and explicit feedback to the child's coping efforts helps the child experience a sense of mastery. Feedback that effectively enhances coping efforts emphasizes self-directed, purposeful behaviors. Therefore the therapist supports child-initiated activity and provides feedback that encourages the extension and elaboration of emerging skills. Because research suggests that children with disabilities tend to assume passive, dependent roles, highly structured and therapist-directed activities should be replaced with child-initiated activities that are specifically and appropriately reinforced and then generalized to other situations (Williamson & Szczepanski, 1999).

Social Skills Development. Intervention that develops positive coping strategies in children and adolescents with psychosocial dysfunctions can be essential for promoting the ability to participate in meaningful daily activities and relationships. Occupational therapists working with older children and adolescents with mental health problems often use social skills groups to promote coping effectiveness and occupational performance. A group milieu allows young people to master developing skills in a safe and supportive environment.

Current approaches may also target the broader environment as the focus of intervention, by means of the following:

- Family education and counseling
- Consultation to caregivers and service providers in schools and community programs

- Peer support and activity groups
- Development of strong social networks

Social networks have been shown to help a person establish positive attitudes and role behavior, maintain and improve self-esteem, and develop moral and social values (Hansen, Watson-Perczel, & Christopher, 1989; Christopher, Nangle, & Hansen, 1993). Other studies have identified the interactive, protective factors in child, family, and social environment that enable a child to be resilient to the effects of disability (Garmezy, 1985; Rutter, 1990).

Research on psychosocial approaches is difficult to review because of its scope and because of the variety of types of practice and their implementation across different disciplines. Evidence in the literature supporting the use of specific approaches is minimal. Reinecke, Ryan, and DuBois (1998) completed a meta-analysis of cognitive behavioral approaches for adolescents with symptoms of depression. Six clinical trials were reviewed, and this type of approach was shown to be effective in alleviating depression, with moderate maintenance of the effect over time. Studies on the effectiveness of social skills training have been conducted with adolescents with conduct disorders (Tisdelle & St. Lawrence, 1988), with depression (Fine, Forth, Gilbert, & Haley, 1991; Plienis et al., 1987; Reed, 1994), with schizophrenia (Hayes, Halford, & Varghese, 1991), and with autism (Plienis et al., 1987). Although many of these studies have methodologic limitations, the results seem to offer support for social skills interventions in improving self-esteem, positive affect, problem-solving, and social behaviors.

Systems Approaches. Systems theory concepts are applied primarily in occupational therapy intervention in areas of motor development and play. Application of these concepts is challenging, because using this approach broadens the focus of intervention to include all factors (environmental, family, child, occupation) that influence the performance of a specific task. From the literature that discusses the application of systems theory or dynamic systems theory to occupational therapy intervention, the following principles emerge:

- Assessment and intervention strategies must recognize the inherent complexity of task performance. The most useful assessment strategy is to develop a "picture" or "profile" of the ways performance components and environmental and task factors affect performance of the tasks the child wants to accomplish. Assessment of only one or a few components (e.g., balance, mood, tone) is not likely to lead to the most effective identification of constraints (Darrah & Barlett, 1995).
- The focus of assessment and intervention is on the interaction of the person, the environment, and the occupation. Therapy begins and ends with a focus on the occupational performance tasks a child or youth wants to, needs to, or is expected to perform. When

a child shows readiness and motivation to attempt a task or activity, the focus of intervention on that particular activity can effect changes in his or her performance (Law et al., 1998).

- The therapy process focuses on identification and change of child, task, or environmental constraints that prevent the achievement of the desired activity. Some of these factors may be manipulated to enhance the functional motor task or goal; others may be managed by providing the missing component during the execution of the task. Parts of activities can be changed (e.g., different toy sizes). Activities should be practiced in a variety of environments that can facilitate completion of the task and promote the flexibility of movement patterns. Activities incorporated into the child's daily routine provide more opportunities for finding solutions for functional motor challenges.
- With intervention through the systems approach, the focus on changing environments and occupations is equal to or greater than the focus on changing the inherent skills of the child or adolescent. Intervention is best accomplished in natural, realistic environments. The accomplishment of whole occupations, not parts of them, is emphasized. The goal in therapy is to enable a child to accomplish an identified activity, rather than promote change in a developmental sequence or improve the quality of the movement.
- Children must practice a newly found skill. Practice and repetition of activities are also the rule for children without disabilities who are developing any new skill.

Models of practice for therapy assessment and intervention, based on dynamic systems theory, are beginning to emerge, although challenges to implementation remain (Darrah & Barlett, 1995; Case-Smith, 1996). Common among these models is the focus on successful achievement of the functional goal rather than on the development of typical patterns of movement (Burton & Davis, 1996; Darrah, Law & Pollock, 2001; Ketelaar et al., 2001). Burton and Davis developed an ecologic task assessment tool to ensure that the task and environment are compatible with the abilities of the child (Burton & Davis, 1996). Ketelaar et al. (2001), in a study of 55 children receiving either functional therapy based on dynamic systems theory or therapy aimed at developing "typical" movement patterns, found that children in the functional therapy group demonstrated significantly more functional skills (mobility and self-care) as measured by the Pediatric Evaluation of Disability Inventory (Haley, Coster, Ludlow, Haltiwanger, & Andrellos, 1992).

Law et al. (1998) used the systems theory to develop a family-centered, functional approach to intervention. In their approach, the focus of assessment is the child's ability to achieve functional tasks and the identification of factors in the child, task, or environment that enable or constrain performance. The COPM, an individualized, family-centered measure, has been used with parents to enable them to identify tasks and activities that their child is beginning to do, trying to do differently, or showing an interest in doing (Law et al., 1998). The actual behavior of the child is the most important determinant of these activities. Therapists and parents then work together to observe these activities and ensure that the child attempts and remains interested in a new task. Once it has been determined that a child is trying to accomplish a new task or trying to accomplish an already achieved task in a new way, the therapist and parents together identify the constraints (child, environmental, task) preventing successful completion of the task.

Intervention focuses on changing constraining factors to facilitate performance. Intervention is provided only when it has been identified that a child is ready to accomplish a task and when constraints have been identified for which intervention or compensation can be provided. In three single case studies of this approach, intervention was designed to change only the environmental or task constraints. In this study, children also achieved significant changes in function (Lammi & Law, 2003). Intervention emphasizes practice of tasks in context and does not focus either on the achievement of performance within a hierarchical developmental framework or on the achievement of improved quality of movement. Intervention focuses on changing a broad range of constraints in the child, task, and environment to facilitate performance.

Mary Reilly and other occupational therapists have focused on play behavior using a systems approach. Reilly (1962, 1974b) originally developed a theory of occupational behavior to conceptualize the roles of being a child, a student, a worker, and an adult. She focused on the importance of play in the development of occupational behavior. She saw play as the occupation of the child, having an organizational effect on behavior. She believed that play forms the basis for adult competence and that play gives meaning to the daily life of a child.

Reilly described two major theoretical orientations: (1) an appreciative system of learning and (2) play progression. The appreciative system of learning states that learning takes place as the individual tries to relate external facts to internal values. The learning process is based on personal values, and through these values a person derives meaning from the external world. The individual's imagination is critical to learning. Play progresses through three hierarchical levels: (1) exploration, (2) competence, and (3) achievement. Through play the child learns different rules, which can then be used in future interactions. Play serves as the foundation for adult competency.

Play competence is complex, because it involves the child's interaction with different environments (physical, social, cultural) and includes both action and attitude (Ferland, 1997). A child's attitude toward play is called *playfulness*. These concepts form the basis of new approaches to occupational therapy assessment and intervention in the area of play (Bundy, 1991, 1993; Ferland, 1997; Parham & Primeau, 1997).

Motor Learning. Motor learning as a model of practice focuses on helping the child achieve goal-directed functional actions. It may initially appear to be a skill-building approach, because the focus is on the acquisition of skills involved in movement and balance. However, motor learning is actually an occupation-based approach, because it is directed toward the search for a motor solution that emerges from an interaction of the child with the task and the environment.

When a child is learning a new functional task, a general movement structure is brought into place that takes into consideration the relationship involving the child's movement capabilities, the environmental conditions, and the action goal. When the task is performed repeatedly, these correspondences become more refined, and the goal is achieved more successfully. Specific processes, such as muscle contraction patterns, stabilization and positioning of joints, and response to gravity and other forces, are only crudely organized at first. However, with continued practice, these become more organized and finely tuned (Gentile, 1998). These patterns are called *movement synergies,* or *coordinative structures,* and they represent the child's preferred strategy for solving a task in the most energy-efficient way (Thelen, 1995). Children with motor programming and motor control deficits often have difficulty establishing the timing and sequencing of synergies of movement. When using a motor learning model of practice, the therapist evaluates and then facilitates the development of the postural control and movement synergies necessary for achievement of a functional goal (Blanche, 1998). In addition to knowledge about movement, the major concepts that therapists need to understand are the importance of feedback, both intrinsic and extrinsic, and of the variables that affect the practice of a specific task.

Different types of feedback contribute to the motor learning process. Feedback is *intrinsic* when it is produced by the child's sensory systems and is inherent in a task. An example of intrinsic feedback is information that is available to the child through vision, proprioception, sensation, or kinesthesia. *Extrinsic* feedback is provided to the child by an external source, such as the therapist, or by observation of the results of one's actions (Nicholson, 1996). *Knowledge of results* is a type of extrinsic feedback in which the therapist provides information to the child about the relationship between the actions and the goal, but only after the fact. For example, a child who is throwing a basketball toward the hoop may be told that the ball is not going high enough and therefore is missing the hoop. *Knowledge of performance* is a type of extrinsic feedback that emphasizes the pattern of movement and its relationship to achievement of the task. In the same example, the child may be told that he is not extending his arms far enough before releasing the ball. In both cases, the therapist's feedback focuses on the outcome of the action, not on the child's effort.

Research on the scheduling, frequency, and amount of feedback that best promote learning has been published (e.g., see Lee, Swinnen, & Serrien, 1994). Studies have shown that immediate extrinsic feedback may prevent the learner from paying attention to the intrinsic sources of feedback that are always available, such as vision and proprioception. This lack of attention to intrinsic feedback may make the learner dependent on information from the person providing instruction (Schmidt, 1988).

Very little research has focused on the effect of different types of feedback on task performance with children experiencing occupational performance difficulties. However, research investigating motor learning principles with children with movement difficulties has suggested that these children may not solve movement problems in a typical way. The research suggests that extrinsic sources of feedback that focus a child's attention on specific aspects of the task and on important sensory cues may be important (Lefebvre & Reid, 1998).

Another important concept in motor learning is the influence of different types of practice on learning and performance. There is no question that practice of a task is beneficial to learning. The difficulty confronting most therapists is the dilemma of whether to practice the *whole* task or only *parts* or components of the task. Study results indicate that the benefits of practicing either the whole task or parts of the task depend on the inherent goals of the task (Shumway-Cook & Woollacott, 1995). If the task is one in which the coordination or timing of the parts is important to the task, then whole-task practice is more effective for learning. Examples of these continuous types of tasks are walking, swinging at a ball, and bicycling. If a task contains distinct parts that can be performed in a serial manner, these can be practiced as parts of the task. A child learning soccer can be taught how to kick the ball as a discrete task. Most occupations involving movement are actually a combination of continuous and discrete tasks. Consequently, application of the whole task must follow teaching of the parts. Learning to ride a tricycle, for example, does not have the same requirement for integrating balance as bicycling. Therefore the child can focus on learning to pedal separately from steering, but he or she must then combine them.

Another important consideration in planning practice sessions is the use of random versus blocked practice. During random practice, the environmental conditions vary slightly each time; blocked practice involves drilling the task over and over in the same way. Random practice produces better learning, because the variable practice allows the child to solve a slightly different movement "problem" every time (Lee et al., 1994). In this way the child defines more quickly the parameters relevant to the particular plan of action (Gentile, 1998).

Some of the key techniques that therapists use in this model of practice are giving verbal instructions and demonstrating movement strategies. Verbal instructions focus on the relationship between the child and the objects in the environment and emphasize key movement features directly related to achievement of the functional goal (Gentile, 1998). The extent to which a therapist should use physical handling to guide or demonstrate movement has been a subject of some debate (Nicholson, 1996). Some suggest that providing manual guidance can be helpful during the initial teaching of a movement because it may clarify the goal, guide selective attention, and help the child organize and plan the movement. Others stress that guidance or facilitation of movement should not be used or should be removed as soon as possible, arguing that the therapist rapidly becomes part of the environment, which alters the performance context and the intrinsic feedback available to the child (Gentile, 1998).

Finally, as discussed earlier in this chapter with regard to children's learning, a distinction must be drawn between the performance of a skill that may take place while the child is in a therapy session and the actual learning of that skill. Modern perspectives of motor learning recognize that learning takes place only when there is evidence of a relatively permanent change in the child's ability to respond to a movement problem or to achieve a movement goal (Missiuna & Mandich, 2002). The learning of a new motor skill needs to be evaluated through tests of retention and transfer, not just immediate changes in performance (Ma, Trombly, & Robinson-Podolski, 1999). Therefore, although therapists who use a motor learning model of practice may be pleased that a child has demonstrated acquisition of the original action goal, they also must create opportunities for the child to demonstrate that learning during a subsequent therapy session (retention), on a closely related task (transfer), or in a different setting (generalization).

To summarize, a therapist using a motor learning model of practice:

1 Analyzes the movement synergies the child uses to achieve the functional action goal
2 Considers the child's stage of learning and determines how best to facilitate the provision of both extrinsic and intrinsic feedback to improve the efficiency of the movement
3 Provides opportunities for optimal practice of the goal
4 Promotes independent performance and decision making as soon as possible and evaluates whether the motor learning has been acquired, transferred, and generalized

Approaches to Learning and Behavior. Occupational therapists and other professionals use theories about learning and behavior to promote development in areas of function that involve learning complex skills and behaviors. Traditionally, this was known as an acquisitional approach, because it emphasized the notion of developing or acquiring new skills. It is similar to the *teaching-learning approach* described in occupational therapy literature. Self-care and handwriting are examples of areas of occupational performance to which occupational therapists have applied an acquisitional approach.

The underlying assumptions and concepts of an acquisitional or teaching-learning approach originated from the field of behavior studies and have evolved as understanding of learning theory has advanced. Some of these assumptions and concepts are:

1   Skills can be improved through practice, repetition, feedback, and reinforcement.
2   The focus of intervention is on the skill itself (e.g., handwriting) and not on the specific components (e.g., fine motor control, in-hand manipulation, grasp). Intervention involves direct training of the skill.
3   Brief, frequent (e.g., daily) treatment sessions are considered most effective for learning a skill.
4   The skill may be divided into subskills, which may be taught as components of the targeted skill. However, as each new subskill or component is acquired, the new learning is combined with the components already mastered to reinforce learning. It is understood that remediation of performance components alone does not necessarily effect change in higher level skills.
5   For learning to occur, the intervention must be matched to the individual needs of the child and should be meaningful to the child.

Handwriting is an area of occupational performance in which an acquisitional approach has been advocated (see Chapter 17). Although few studies of the effectiveness of the acquisitional approach to handwriting have been published, many remedial handwriting programs are commercially available. A few published studies have demonstrated that the use of acquisitional principles by therapists and educators in a positive, interesting, and dynamic learning environment promotes the development of handwriting (Barchers, 1994; Milone & Waslyk, 1981). Some handwriting studies provide therapists and educators with strategies for remediation that use some of the concepts previously listed (Bergman & McLaughlin, 1988; Graham & Miller, 1980). Further research is needed to determine the effectiveness of this approach with different populations of children across a broad range of skills and areas of occupational performance.

Sensory Processing Approach. Sensory processing is an emerging occupational therapy approach that has developed from sensory integration theory (see the next section). The focus of sensory processing is on the modulation of sensory input by the nervous system and how it affects task performance. Miller and Lane (2000) described sensory processing as "reception, modulation, integration and organization of sensory stimuli, including behavioral responses to sensory input" (p. 2). It is hypothesized that children can be underresponsive to sensory input, overresponsive, or a combination of the two. This inability to modulate sensory input results in problems such as hypersensitivity or gravitational insecurity and is hypothesized to affect sensorimotor and cognitive development, behavior, social interactions, and daily occupational performance.

Children with a sensory processing disorder may show poor registration of sensation, may be hypersensitive to stimuli, may avoid certain sensations, or may seek particular inputs (Dunn, 1997). These disorders may be present in children with a variety of developmental disorders, and they are often described in children with pervasive developmental disorders or autism (Baranek, Foster, & Berkson, 1997; Keintz & Dunn, 1997; Watling, Deitz, & White, 2001; Yack, Sutton, & Aquilla, 1998). Dunn and colleagues (Dunn, 1994, 1999; Dunn & Brown, 1997; Ermer & Dunn, 1997) have developed evaluation tools for identifying sensory processing problems in children and adults. A number of authors have proposed treatment programs to address sensory processing disorders (Miller, Wilbarger, Stackhouse, & Trunnell, 2002; Reisman & Hanschu, 1992; Wilbarger, 1995; Williams & Shellenberger, 1994).

Preliminary evidence drawn from case studies and single-subject design research has shown some positive outcomes using sensory integration therapy with children with autism and pervasive developmental disorders (Case-Smith & Bryan, 1999; Linderman & Stewart, 1999; Stagnitti, Raison, & Ryan, 1999); however, the literature lacks any large controlled trials that evaluate the efficacy of these treatment approaches. Although there is significant intuitive appeal for sensory processing disorders as explanatory models for children's observed behaviors, more research is required to validate these theories and to investigate appropriate interventions.

Neuromaturation Approaches

Neuromaturation approaches in occupational therapy refer to approaches based primarily on a hierarchical, staged development of the nervous system. These methods focus largely on changing performance components during therapy intervention. The assumption is that functional improvement results from changes in performance components. Neuromaturation approaches are supported primarily by developmental theories.

Neurodevelopmental Theory. Historically, the primary concept underpinning a neurodevelopmental therapy (NDT) approach to practice was that normal postural reactions are necessary for normal movement and that these postural reactions are for the most part automatic (Bobath, 1980). Although this intervention approach continues to focus on problems in postural control and motor coordination, as seen in cerebral palsy, the principles underlying the treatment approach have expanded to include motor learning and dynamic systems theories. In addition, NDT principles have shifted to recognize the importance of the environment and to place more emphasis on activities that are clearly functional and meaningful to the child (Howle, 2002).

When evaluating a child using this approach, the therapist analyzes the child's movements to identify missing or atypical muscular-skeletal elements that create functional limitations. These missing elements become one focus of intervention and are used to select the developmental level of therapeutic activities. Therapeutic handling is integral to the NDT approach and is used to facilitate postural control and movement synergies and to inhibit or constrain motor patterns that, if practiced, would lead to secondary deformities and dysfunction (Howle, 2002). A therapist applying NDT strategies focuses on changing movement patterns to achieve the best energy-efficient performance for the individual in the context of age-appropriate tasks.

As the therapist manually guides and handles the child in the context of an activity, these elements are always combined with the child's active participation. With the therapist's guidance, the child practices sequences of movements in slightly different ways to reinforce learning of the task. This practice is important for making a movement strategy functional and automatic. Therapists emphasize quality of movement (e.g., accuracy, quickness, adaptability, and fluency). Although, therapeutic handling remains an integral part of NDT, practitioners use many treatment methods, "manipulating the individual task or the environment in order to positively influence function" (Howle, 2002, p. 63).

Acknowledging that NDT principles have changed over the years to incorporate theories of motor learning and dynamic systems theory, clinical evaluation studies of the neurodevelopmental therapy approach (many of which were completed more than 10 years ago) have raised questions about its efficacy. Eight comparison studies of this approach for children with cerebral palsy have been conducted over the past 20 years. In these studies, the NDT approach has been compared with no therapy (Wright & Nicholson, 1973), with functional therapy (Carlsen, 1975; Scherzer, Mike, & Ilson, 1976;

Sommerfeld, Fraser, Hensinger, & Beresford, 1981), with infant stimulation (Palmer et al., 1988), with Vojta therapy (D'Avignon, 1981) and with differing intensities of therapy (Law et al., 1991; Mayo, 1991). The results of these trials were mixed, with three demonstrating no difference (Law et al., 1991; Sommerfeld et al., 1981; Wright & Nicholson, 1973), three supporting neurodevelopmental therapy (Carlson, 1975; Mayo, 1991; Scherzer et al., 1976), and two supporting alternate treatments (D'Avignon, 1981; Palmer et al., 1988). The more rigorous randomized clinical trials have generally produced results that do not support the efficacy of the neurodevelopmental approach (Piper, 1990). A recent systematic review of neurodevelopmental therapy concluded that "the preponderance of results. . . . do not confer any advantage to NDT over alternatives to which it was compared" (Butler & Darrah, 2001, p. 789). The only consistent effect of NDT that was statistically significant was an immediate effect on range of motion. Despite lack of evidence on efficacy, NDT remains an important and widely used approach with children who have cerebral palsy and CNS dysfunction affecting motor performance. Because the conceptual basis of NDT has evolved over the past decade, a first step in additional research on its efficacy would be to operationalize the new concepts into treatment protocols that can be measured and replicated for research purposes.

Sensory Integration. The theory of sensory integration, together with the treatment approach derived from that theory, grew from the work of Jean Ayres (1969, 1972a, 1972b). Ayres developed her theory in an effort to explain behaviors observed in children with learning difficulties based on neural functioning. Specifically, she hypothesized that some children with learning difficulties experience problems in "organizing sensory information for use" (Ayres, 1972a). She named this neural process *sensory integration*. Since Ayres' original work, she and many others have conducted research aimed at evaluating the process of sensory integration, defining subtypes of sensory integrative dysfunction, and determining the efficacy of sensory integration therapy (SIT).

SIT is based on assumptions drawn from neuromaturation theory and systems theory (Fisher & Murray, 1991). Neuromaturation concepts, such as hierarchical organization of cortical and subcortical areas, developmental sequence of learning and skill acquisition, and neural plasticity, are crucial to an understanding of the mechanisms of sensory integration. Systems theory also underlies sensory integration, because the focus is on the child seeking sensory input and using adaptive behavior as an organizer of the input. Based on these assumptions, the SIT approach seeks to provide the child with enhanced opportunities for controlled sensory input, with a particular emphasis on vestibular, proprioceptive, and tactile input, in the context of meaningful activity. In intervention the therapist facilitates an adaptive response, which requires the child to integrate the sensory information. Sensory integration is hypothesized to improve through this process. More recent literature has integrated occupation-based perspectives and emerging theories of motor development in the reconceptualization of sensory integration, but the methods used in SIT remain essentially unchanged (Bundy & Murray, 2002).

Much of Ayres' work, and that of her colleagues, was devoted to the development of evaluation tools that could clearly identify individuals with sensory integrative dysfunction. The Southern California Sensory Integration Tests (Ayres, 1972c, 1980) and the more recent Sensory Integration and Praxis Tests (Ayres, 1989) are the result of this work. Included in this area of identification and evaluation are a number of studies aimed at describing different subtypes of sensory integrative dysfunction (Ayres, 1965, 1972d, 1977, 1989; Ayres, Mailloux, & Wendler, 1987). These identified dysfunction subtypes include somatodyspraxia, bilateral integration and sequencing, postural ocular movements, and sensory modulation. Some of these results have been called into question based on the validity of the methods used to determine the subtypes (Cummins, 1991). In a large confirmatory factor analysis study, Mulligan (1998) described a four-factor model comprising visual-perceptual deficits, somatosensory deficits, bilateral integration and sequencing deficits, and dyspraxia.

Another area of intense research effort has been evaluation of the efficacy of SIT for children with learning problems. Early work by Ayres (1972b, 1978) and others (Ottenbacher, Short, & Watson, 1979; Ayres & Mailloux, 1981) had reported positive changes resulting from SIT in such outcomes as motor, academic, and language performance. Reviews of more recent studies, however, called their results into question, citing substantial methodologic flaws in the research methods (Hoehn & Baumeister, 1994). Studies in the late 1980s and the 1990s evaluated the efficacy of SIT using more rigorous methods, including randomized controlled trials. In a systematic review of these studies, Polatajko and colleagues concluded that "the review has failed to find any statistical evidence that SIT improves the academic performance of learning disabled children more than a placebo. With respect to sensory or motor performance, the results are not consistent, but do suggest that, statistically, overall SIT may be similar to perceptual motor training" (Polatajko, Kaplan, & Wilson, 1992, p. 337). Using meta-analysis techniques, Vargas and Camilli (1999) concurred with these conclusions. They found that early efficacy studies of sensory integration produced large positive effects, but studies conducted after 1982 did not yield significant positive effects. The more recent

studies of SIT demonstrated effects equal to those of alternative treatments in the participants' psychoeducational and motor performance areas, with no improvement noted in sensory perceptual areas (Vargas & Camilli, 1999).

Despite the negative findings related to sensory integration research, SIT is widely practiced in the field of occupational therapy and remains a powerful force in clinical reasoning in the field of pediatrics. In a survey of occupational therapists working with children with autism, fully 99% of the therapists reported using sensory integration techniques with their clients (Watling, Deitz, Kanny, & McLaughlin, 1999). Kaplan, Polatajko, Wilson, and Faris (1993) suggested the following possible explanations for this continued support:

1 An intense bond is formed between child and therapist during SIT that has multiple positive influences.
2 The child is perceived to improve even though SIT may not be the cause of the improvement.
3 Sensory integration theory is useful for reframing the thinking about what underlies a child's behavior, leading to a more positive view of the child.

Recent research has also included parents' perceptions of change in their children and in themselves as a result of occupational therapy that used SIT (Cohn, Miller, & Tickle-Degnen, 2000; Cohn, 2001). Parents reported positive changes in their children's social participation, perceived competence, and self-regulation. The parents valued the new understanding of the child's behavior and used this perspective to support and advocate for the child more effectively. Ayres' work has had a significant impact on occupational therapy practice with children, and its controversial nature has led to an increased sophistication and rigor in the scholarly work accomplished in the field of occupational therapy.

Developmental Approaches. During the 1960s and 1970s, occupational therapists working with children had a strong developmental perspective. Several experts in the field developed approaches for their work with children that were based on earlier developmental theories from other disciplines. These theories attempted to explain the functioning and growth of children and adolescents from an occupational therapy perspective. Perhaps the best known occupational therapy theorist of this time was Lela Llorens (1969, 1976, 1991). She identified a developmental frame of reference that focused on the physical, social, and psychologic aspects of life tasks and relationships. Llorens viewed the role of the occupational therapist to be one of facilitating development and assisting in the mastery of life tasks and the ability to cope with life expectations. Occupational therapists in pediatrics still refer to models of average skill development for different age groups when they assess children (Case-Smith, 2001).

A spatiotemporal adaptation model of practice that views development as a spiraling process, moving from simple to complex, was proposed by Gilfoyle, Grady, and Moore (1990). Adaptation is viewed as a continuous process of interaction involving the individual, time, and space. Many of the concepts of the spatiotemporal adaptation model of practice are drawn from an understanding of the central nervous system and from theoretical material produced by Piaget (1971) and other developmental theorists.

The adaptation process has four components: assimilation, accommodation, association, and differentiation. *Assimilation* is the reception of sensory stimuli from internal and external environments. *Accommodation* is the motor response to these stimuli. *Association* is the organized process of relating current sensory information with the current motor response and then relating this relationship to past responses. *Differentiation* is the process of identifying the specific elements in a child's situation that are useful and relevant to another situation to refine the responsive pattern. Based on prior experience, the child develops a sense of what is useful and what is not useful to motor activity in the current situation. In this view of development, the child is continually modifying older, more primitive behaviors for effective motor responses, rather than continually acquiring new skills.

Recent theories and models of development in the occupational therapy literature incorporate new concepts of PEO relationships, dynamic systems theories, and life span changes. Instead of focusing on different components of functioning, such as motor, social, or cognitive development, occupational therapy theorists are addressing the development of occupation across the life span (Davis & Polatajko, 2004; Humphry, 2002).

Two emerging occupational perspectives on development remain in the conceptual and exploratory stages of theory development and require further research and validation. In one of these proposals, Humphry suggests a dynamic system perspective in a model of developmental processes. The complex, reciprocal, and nonlinear relationships of a child's innate characteristics and the environmental factors in the development of occupation form a key concept in this model (Humphry, 2002). Other key constructs include experience, self-organization, and emergent behaviors that have no predetermined patterns. This perspective acknowledges the complexity of learning to do and refining occupation over the life span.

In the other new proposal, Davis and Polatajko (2004) offer an occupational perspective on development constructed from the developmental literature. They take an interactionist perspective on development, viewing individuals and their environments in a reciprocal relationship that delineates human development across the life span (Davis & Polatajko, 2004).

Three principles that govern this dynamic relationship are provided in a model of occupational development. The first principle, continuity, recognizes that occupational development is a continuous, lifelong process. The second principle, multiple determinicity, holds that no single factor determines development, but rather that multiple personal and environmental determinants exist. The third principle, multiple variations and changing mastery, characterizes the patterns of occupational development and proficiency across the life span (Davis & Polatajko, 2004).

SECTION 4: CLINICAL APPLICATION EXAMPLES

In this section, three case examples are used to outline the different assessment and intervention strategies and expected outcomes for the models of practice discussed in the preceding section. The examples include a young child with CP, a school-age child with developmental coordination disorder, and an adolescent with sensory modulation and behavioral problems. For each example, the most commonly used approaches are selected for the clinical situation. These choices do not mean that other approaches cannot be used, but they are applied less often.

Case Example 1

Stacey is a 3-year-old girl who has CP with moderate quadriplegia. She is able to walk short distances using a walker. Her parents have set current goals for Stacey that include household mobility, participation in dressing tasks, and improvement of participation with peers in play in her preschool. In this example, the discussion focuses on the goal of participation in play with peers (Table 3-2).

Case Example 2

Brian is a 9-year-old boy with developmental coordination disorder. He is isolated from his peers at school, is clumsy, has difficulty performing any tasks requiring handwriting, is poorly organized, and has trouble staying on task (Table 3-3). A COPM was completed with Brian, and he identified the following occupational performance issues:
1 Messy desk
2 Disorganized written work; illegible handwriting
3 Difficulty getting out for recess on time

Case Example 3

Chris is a 15-year-old high school student who is currently struggling to complete grade 10. He has dropped one subject in the current year and has been labeled an underachiever. He has difficulty taking notes in class and reorganizing his work. He has been referred to a community psychiatric service because of problems with low mood, lack of motivation in his academic and social life, poor social adjustment, and disturbed family relations.

His parents complain that Chris regularly lies to them about petty thefts from the home and that hours of confrontation and badgering by them are required to get the truth. They report various other instances of misbehavior. Chris has had trials of medication for ADHD and depression with limited success, and on one occasion he took a dangerous overdose of medication.

He presents himself as a somewhat disheveled youth who denies any knowledge or insight into his difficulties. His parents are firm in their conviction that he requires intensive intervention (Table 3-4).

TABLE 3-2 Case Study 1: Stacey

Practice Model	Assessment Strategy	Clinical Reasoning Used to Explain Client Problem	Clinical Reasoning Used to Guide Intervention and Predict Outcome	Expected Outcome
Dynamic systems	Stacey's spontaneous posture and movement during functional activities are observed. Physical assessment of muscle tone, postural alignment, balance, coordination, and potential for change is completed. The Gross Motor Function Measure is used to assess gross motor skills.	Postural and movement impairments are restricting Stacey's ability to perform functional activities and to move efficiently throughout her environment.	Within the context of functional activities, the therapist uses handling techniques to facilitate or inhibit posture and movement to increase Stacey's ability to perform. Emphasis is placed on preparation, sensory input, weight bearing, initiation of movement, stability, and alignment. Repetition and practice reinforce the new learning.	Stacey will move more easily, efficiently, and independently and engage in play with her peers.
Motor learning	Observe the motor requirements of various play situations in the preschool. Observe Stacey's current ability to perform each of these (e.g., ambulation to play area, ability to sit in a stable position and use both hands in play).	Stacey will participate in play situations more easily if she is able to move to and from the play areas and to use her hands for play while in a seated position.	Therapist will identify movement positions or transitions necessary for play. Therapist will set up the environment so as to facilitate practice of these. During practice, therapist will use verbal instruction or physical guidance to improve performance.	Through varied practice in situations that are motivating for her, Stacey will learn to use intrinsic and extrinsic feedback more effectively to guide movement. Over time, the movement positions or transitions will become more functional, and she will be able to engage in play situations more easily.
Neurodevelopment	Observe Stacey moving in the environment, in particular movement transitions; perform a physical assessment of tone, ROM, strength, reflex development, righting reactions, and equilibrium responses; use the Gross Motor Function Measure to assess gross motor skills.	Atypical tone and movement patterns are inhibiting the development of more normal patterns and limiting Stacey's mobility.	Therapy is provided to decrease the influence of tone and to promote the development of normal movement patterns. The sensorimotor experience of normal movement will reinforce new movement strategies. Handling and facilitation techniques are used to accomplish these goals.	Stacey will experience less influence of abnormal tone on movement and more normal movement patterns. Increased functional movement will allow her to engage in play with peers. Her risk for contractures and deformities will be decreased.

ROM, Range of motion.

TABLE 3-3 Case Study 2: Brian

Practice Model	Assessment Strategy	Clinical Reasoning Used to Explain Client Problem	Clinical Reasoning Used to Guide Intervention and Predict Outcome	Expected Outcome
Cognitive Approaches	Use observations, interview, and the Sensory Profile to examine Brian, performing each of the tasks identified by the COPM. Identify the specific strategies he uses or does not use and note the points at which he appears to get "stuck."	Brian does not know the strategies he needs to complete each task effectively and efficiently and/or he is unable to select appropriate strategies to achieve his goal.	Using guided discovery and mediation, it is possible to teach Brian generalizable organizational strategies that will help him organize his desk, his written work, and the sequence in which he dons his outdoor clothing for recess.	Brian will be able to implement task-specific and global strategies that will help him organize any task that has multiple parts or that requires a sequence of actions. Brian will be able to generalize these strategies to other settings and transfer them to other tasks.
Compensatory/task	Observe the classroom materials and procedures that are in place for each task. Discuss options with the teacher for making each task easier for Brian.	Brian currently does not have the skills needed to cope with the demands of the tasks. Each task needs to be adapted to ensure his success in the classroom.	Brian will be provided with modified materials that will help him organize his desk (e.g., color-coded notebooks to match textbooks; colored schedule on the wall), his written output (e.g., raised lined paper), and his locker (e.g., sequence of instructions posted on locker door).	With modifications in place, Brian will become more successful at performing these tasks. This will ultimately improve his ability to complete tasks efficiently and to participate with his peers. Over time, other interventions can be used to improve his skills.
Sensory integration	Assess Brian using tools such at the Sensory Integration and Praxis Tests (SIPT), Clinical Observation of Motor and Postural Skills (COMPS), as well as observation in classroom, playground, home, interview Brian, his teacher and his parents.	Brian is not integrating sensory input from different sensory systems effectively leading to maladaptive responses, limiting the development of new skills and the ability to respond effectively to environmental demands.	Provide controlled sensory input, in particular tactile, vestibular and proprioceptive to Brian with a demand for an adaptive response through goal directed, meaningful play activities. This will facilitate sensory integration.	Brian will interact more effectively in his environment; should generalize to all environments as he progresses. Outcome would be a closer relationship between environmental expectations and Brian's performance or response.
Sensory processing	Use observation and interview, checklists e.g., Sensory Profile to look at Brian's behavior and history in different environments, look for patterns of behaviors potentially indicating underlying difficulties processing or modulating sensory input	Brian's behavior and functioning is a reflection of sensory processing/ modulation abilities. He is seeking to modulate input to the CNS through various sensory systems	Modify task and environmental factors to alter sensory experience for Brian, work towards him taking responsibility to do this himself. Increase his awareness of what he needs and how to get it in a functional activity and/or socially acceptable manner, some believe in use of specific sensory input e.g., deep pressure to change the child's CNS state, but minimal evidence to support this at present	Improved modulation of sensory input will prepare Brian for learning and help him to benefit from teaching in class, and participation in school activities.

COPM, Canadian Occupational Performance Measure.

TABLE 3-4 Case Study 3: Chris

Practice Model	Assessment Strategy	Clinical Reasoning Used to Explain Client Problem	Clinical Reasoning Used to Guide Intervention and Predict Outcome	Expected Outcome
Learning/behavior models	Assessment of school-based "skills" (areas of occupational performance), including handwriting, organization skills	Chris's acquisitional skills (handwriting, organization) appear to have significant gaps that would benefit from a behavior/learning approach.	Chris's handwriting and organizational skills could improve with an intensive, repetitive program that focuses on the acquisition or learning of these skills.	If Chris identified a need to improve his handwriting and organization and he was motivated to work on acquiring these skills, a regular program could be successful in improving his occupational performance in these two areas.
Sensory processing	Assessment of Chris's ability to process sensory information (e.g., tactile, vestibular, visual, auditory, proprioceptive)	Chris has difficulty modulating sensory stimuli when there is input from more than one source (i.e., visual and auditory combined). Handwriting skills are affected by poor proprioceptive feedback and low tone in the upper extremities.	If Chris and his teachers develop an awareness of his sensory processing challenges, he will be able to develop cognitive strategies for coping with multiple sensory input. A multisensory handwriting program may improve his speed and legibility.	Chris and his teachers will develop strategies for modulating sensory stimuli at school that will enable him to focus more on the tasks of schoolwork. Handwriting speed and legibility may improve somewhat to enable Chris to keep up with the written demands at school.
Compensatory/environmental	Assessment of Chris's current environment and the fit of environmental demands with his skill level	The demands of the school environment are not matched to Chris's skills, resulting in anxiety and behavioral problems. The family is concerned but confused about Chris's behavior.	If Chris becomes more aware of his difficulties in the school environment, he can use compensatory strategies to cope with the demands. Environmental adaptation of difficult tasks and people's expectations is needed to create a more supportive environment for Chris.	With the development of compensatory strategies and environmental adaptations, the P-E fit will improve, and Chris will experience increased satisfaction with his school performance. Family and teacher education will help his parents understand his difficulties and will increase supportive strategies.

P-E, Person-environment.

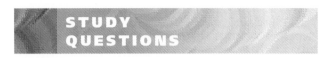

STUDY QUESTIONS

1 As the occupational therapist, you recently initiated services with a 10-year-old girl with spina bifida. Her lesion is at the T1 level, and she uses a motorized wheelchair. She has difficulty with lower extremity dressing and the dressing involved in catheterization. Using the dynamic systems model, identify variables that would likely affect dressing goals.

2 You work with a 4-year-old boy with autism who has severe communication problems, stereotypic movement, and hypersensitivities. This boy has particular problems in making transitions from the classroom to the playground, cafeteria, and bus. Describe two strategies derived from a compensatory approach that you might use to help him make transitions without causing a temper

tantrum. Describe one strategy using a sensory processing approach that should be considered to help him make transitions out of the classroom.

3 In therapy with a child with dyspraxia, you are working on cutting with scissors. At present the child alternates hands, holds the scissors with the forearm pronated and wrist flexed, and makes only snips when attempting to cut paper. Use a motor learning approach to design an intervention activity to promote scissors cutting. Explain the types of feedback that you would give the child to reinforce learning.

4 An 8-year-old girl with sensory processing problems is referred to the school-based occupational therapist. She appears to be sensory seeking and is very active in the classroom. She hits and bites other children and does not seem aware that these behaviors are socially inappropriate. She focuses most effectively when given deep pressure, but her attention span remains limited to 10 minutes. Apply the coping model to design three intervention strategies that can help this girl cope and develop peer relations in the second grade classroom.

REFERENCES

Adams, J.A. (1971). A closed-loop theory of motor learning. *Journal of Motor Behavior, 3*, 111-149.

American Occupational Therapy Association. (2002). Occupational therapy practice framework: Domain and process. *American Journal of Occupational Therapy, 56*, 609-639.

Anderson, E.M., & Clarke, L. (Eds.). (1982). *Disability and adolescence*. New York: Methuen.

Anderson, J.R. (1982). Acquisition of cognitive skill. *Psychological Review, 89*, 369-406.

Ayres, A.J. (1965). Patterns of perceptual motor dysfunction in children: A factor analytic study. *Perceptual and Motor Skills, 20*, 335-368.

Ayres, A.J. (1969). Deficits in sensory integration in educationally handicapped children. *Journal of Learning Disabilities, 2*, 160-168.

Ayres, A.J. (1972a). *Sensory integration and learning disorders*. Los Angeles: Western Psychological Services.

Ayres, A.J. (1972b). Improving academic scores through sensory integration. *Journal of Learning Disabilities, 5*, 338-343.

Ayres, A.J. (1972c). *Southern California sensory integration tests manual*. Los Angeles: Western Psychological Services.

Ayres, A.J. (1972d). Types of sensory integrative dysfunction among disabled learners. *American Journal of Occupational Therapy, 26*, 13-18.

Ayres, A.J. (1977). Cluster analyses of measures of sensory integration. *American Journal of Occupational Therapy, 31*, 362-366.

Ayres, A.J. (1978). Learning disabilities and the vestibular system. *Journal of Learning Disabilities, 11*, 18-29.

Ayres, A.J. (1980). *Southern California sensory integration tests manual: Revised*. Los Angeles: Western Psychological Services.

Ayres, A.J. (1989). *Sensory integration and praxis tests*. Los Angeles: Western Psychological Services.

Ayres, A.J., & Mailloux, Z.K. (1981). Influence of sensory integrative procedures on language development. *American Journal of Occupational Therapy, 35*, 383-390.

Ayres, A.J., Mailloux, Z.K., & Wendler, C.L.W. (1987). Developmental dyspraxia: Is it a unitary function? *Occupational Therapy Journal of Research, 7*, 93-110.

Bandura, A. (1977). Self-efficacy: toward a unifying theory of behavior change. *Psychological Review, 84*, 191-215.

Bandura, A. (1982). Self-efficacy mechanism in human agency. *American Psychologist, 37*, 122-147.

Bandura, A. (1989). Human agency in social cognitive theory. *American Psychologist, 44*, 1175-1184.

Bandura, A. (1993). Perceived self-efficacy in cognitive development and functioning. *Educational Psychologist, 28*, 117-148.

Bandura, A. (1997). *Self-efficacy: The exercise of control*. New York: Freeman.

Baranek, G.T., Foster, L.G., & Berkson, G. (1997). Sensory defensiveness in persons with developmental disabilities. *Journal of Autism and Developmental Disorders, 29*, 213-224.

Barchers, S.I. (1994). *Teaching language arts: An integrated approach*. Minneapolis: West Publishing.

Bazyk, S. (1989). Changes in attitudes and beliefs regarding parent participation and home programs: An update. *American Journal of Occupational Therapy, 43*, 723-728.

Bergman, K.E., & McLaughlin, T.F. (1988). Remediating handwriting difficulties with learning disabled students: A review. *Journal of Special Education, 12*, 101-120.

Bernstein N. (1967). *Coordination and regulation of movements*. New York: John Wiley & Sons.

Bjorklund, D.F., & Green, B.L. (1992). The adaptive nature of cognitive immaturity. *American Psychologist, 47*, 46-54.

Blanche, E.I. (1998). Intervention for motor control and movement organization disorders. In J. Case-Smith (Ed.), *Pediatric occupational therapy and early intervention* (2nd ed.). (pp. 255-276). Boston: Butterworth-Heinemann.

Blum, R.W., Resnick, M.D., Nelson, R., & St. Germaine, A. (1991). Family and peer issues among adolescents with spina bifida and cerebral palsy. *Pediatrics, 88* (22), 280-285.

Bobath, K. (1980). *A neurophysiological basis for the treatment of cerebral palsy*. London: Heinemann Books.

Bronfenbrenner, U. (1977). Toward an experimental ecology of human development. *American Psychologist, 32*, 513-531.

Brown, M., & Gordon, W. (1987). Impact of impairment on activity patterns of children. *Archives of Physical Medicine and Rehabilitation, 68*, 828-832.

Bundy, A.C. (1991). Play theory and sensory integration. In A.G. Fisher, E.A. Murray, & A.C. Bundy (Eds.), *Sensory integration: Theory and practice* (pp. 46-68). Philadelphia: F.A. Davis.

Bundy, A.C. (1993). Assessment of play and leisure: Delineation of the problem. *American Journal of Occupational Therapy, 47*, 217-222.

Bundy, A., & Murray, E. (2002). Sensory integration: A. Jean Ayres' theory revisited. In A. Bundy, S. Lane, & E. Murray

(Eds.), *Sensory integration theory and practice* (2nd ed.). (pp. 3-34). Philadelphia: F.A. Davis.

Burton, A.W., & Davis, W.E. (1996). Ecological task analysis: utilizing intrinsic measures in research and practice. *Human Movement Science, 15,* 285-314.

Burton, A.W., & Miller, D.E. (1998). *Movement skill assessment.* Champaign, IL: Human Kinetics.

Butler, C., & Darrah, J. (2001). Effects of neurodevelopmental treatment (NDT) for cerebral palsy: an AACPDM evidence report. *Developmental Medicine and Child Neurology, 43(11),* 778-90.

Cadman, D., Boyle, M., Szatmari, P., & Offord, D.R. (1987). Chronic illness, disability, and mental and social well-being: Findings of the Ontario child health study. *Pediatrics, 79,* 805-813.

Canadian Association of Occupational Therapists (CAOT). (1997). *Enabling occupation: An occupational therapy perspective.* Ottawa, ON: Canadian Association of Occupational Therapists (CAOT).

Carlsen, P.N. (1975). Comparison of two occupational therapy approaches for treating the young cerebral-palsied child. *American Journal of Occupational Therapy, 29,* 267-272.

Case, R. (1985). *Intellectual development: Birth to adulthood.* Orlando, FL: Academic Press.

Case-Smith, J. (1996). Analysis of current motor development theory and recently published infant motor assessments. *Infants and Young Children, 9* (1), 29-41.

Case-Smith, J. (2001). Development of childhood occupations. In J. Case-Smith (Ed.), *Occupational therapy for children.* (4th ed.). (pp. 71-94). St. Louis: Mosby.

Case-Smith, J., & Bryan, T. (1999). The effects of occupational therapy with sensory integration emphasis on preschool age children with autism. *American Journal of Occupational Therapy, 53,* 489-497.

Christiansen, C., & Baum, C. (1991). *Occupational therapy: Overcoming human performance deficits.* Thorofare, NJ: Slack.

Christiansen, C., & Baum, C. (1997). *Occupational therapy: Enabling function and well-being.* Thorofare, NJ: Slack.

Christiansen, C.H., Clark, F., Kielhofner, G., & Rogers, J. (1995). Position Paper: Occupation. *American Journal of Occupational Therapy, 49,* 1015-1018.

Christopher, J.S., Nangle, D.W., & Hansen, D.J. (1993). Social skills interventions with adolescents. *Behavior Modification, 17,* 314-338.

Clark, F.A., Parham, D., Carlson, M.E., Frank, G., Jackson, J., Pierce, D., et al. (1991). Occupational science: Academic innovation in the service of occupational therapy's future. *American Journal of Occupational Therapy, 45,* 300-310.

Cohn, E.S. (2001). Parent perspectives of occupational therapy using a sensory integration approach. *American Journal of Occupational Therapy, 55,* 285-294.

Cohn, E., Miller, L.J., & Tickle-Degnen, L. (2000). Parental hopes for therapy outcomes: Children with sensory modulation disorders. *American Journal of Occupational Therapy, 54,* 36-43.

Colley, A.M., & Beech, J.R. (1989). *Acquisition and performance of cognitive skills.* New York: John Wiley & Sons.

Coster, W., Deeny, T., Haltiwanger, J., & Haley, S. (1998). *School function assessment.* San Antonio: Psychological Corporation.

Couch, K.J., Deitz, J.C., & Kanny, E.M. (1998). The role of play in pediatric occupational therapy. *American Journal of Occupational Therapy, 52,* 111-117.

Csikszentmihalyi, M., & Csikszentmihalyi, I.S. (1988). *Optimal experience: Psychological studies in flow in consciousness.* Cambridge: Cambridge University Press.

Cummins, R.A. (1991). Sensory integration and learning disabilities: Ayres' factor analysis reappraised. *Journal of Learning Disabilities, 24,* 160-168.

Darrah, J., & Barlett, D. (1995). Dynamic systems theory and management of children with cerebral palsy: unresolved issues. *Infants and Young Children, 8,* 52-9.

Darrah, J., Law, M., & Pollock, N. (2001). Innovations in practice: Family-centered functional therapy—a choice for children with motor dysfunction. *Infants and Young Children, 13* (4), 79-87.

D'Avignon, M. (1981). Early physiotherapy ad modum Vojta or Bobath in infants with suspected neuromotor disturbance. *Neuropediatrics, 12,* 232-241.

Davis, J., & Polatajko, H. (2004). Occupational development. In C.H. Christiansen & E.A. Townsend (Eds.), *Introduction to occupation: The art and science of living* (pp. 91-120). Upper Saddle River, NJ: Prentice-Hall.

Developmental Coordination Disorder (DCD) Research Group. (1995). *CO-OP: Cognitive orientation to daily occupational performance.* Unpublished manuscript. London, ON: University of Western Ontario.

Dunn, W. (1999) *The sensory profile user's manual.* San Antonio: Psychological Corporation.

Dunn, W. (1994). Performance of typical children on the sensory profile: an item analysis. *American Journal of Occupational Therapy, 48,* 967-974.

Dunn, W. (1997). The impact of sensory processing abilities on the daily lives of young children and their families: A conceptual model. *Infants and Young Children, 9,* 23-35.

Dunn, W., & Brown, C. (1997). Factor analysis on the sensory profile from a national sample of children without disabilities. *American Journal of Occupational Therapy, 51,* 490-495.

Dunn, W., Brown, C., & McGuigan, A. (1994). The ecology of human performance: A framework for considering the effect of context. *American Journal of Occupational Therapy, 48,* 595-607.

Dunst, C., Trivette, C., & Deal, A. (1988). *Enabling and empowering families: principles and guidelines for practice.* Cambridge, MA: Brookline Books.

Dunst, C.J., Trivette, C.M., Davis, M., & Cornwall, J. (1988). Enabling and empowering families of children with health impairments. *Child Health Care, 17,* 71-81.

Dunton, W.R. (1919). *Reconstruction therapy.* Philadelphia: W.B. Saunders.

Eliasmith, C. (1998). The third contender: A critical examination of the dynamicist theory of cognition. In P. Thagard (Ed.), *Mind readings: Introductory selections on cognitive science* (pp. 303-333). Cambridge, MA: MIT Press.

Engle, P.L., Castle, S., & Meno, P. (1996). Child development: vulnerability and resilience. *Social Science and Medicine, 43* (5), 621-635.

Erikson, E.H. (1964). *Childhood and society* (2nd ed.). New York: W.W. Norton.

Ermer, J., & Dunn, W. (1997). The sensory profile: A discriminant analysis of children with and without disabilities. *American Journal of Occupational Therapy, 51,* 283-290.

Evans, J.L. (2002). Variability in comprehension strategy use in children with SLI: a dynamical systems account. *International Journal of Language and Communication Disorders, 37* (2), 95-116.

Ferland, F. (1997). *Play, children with physical disabilities and occupational therapy: The Ludic model.* Ottawa, ON: University of Ottawa Press.

Fidler, G.S., & Fidler, J.W. (1978). Doing and becoming: purposeful action and self-actualization. *American Journal of Occupational Therapy, 32,* 305-310.

Fine, S., Forth, A., Gilbert, M., & Haley, G. (1991). Group therapy for adolescent depressive disorder: A comparison of social skills and therapeutic support. *Journal of the American Academy of Child and Adolescent Psychiatry, 30,* 79-85.

Fisher, A.G., & Murray, E.A. (1991). Introduction to sensory integration theory. In A.G. Fisher, E.A. Murray, & A.C. Bundy (Eds.), *Sensory integration: Theory and practice* (pp. 3-26). Philadelphia: F.A. Davis.

Flavell, J. (1985). *Cognitive development.* Englewood Cliffs, NJ: Prentice-Hall.

Freud, S. (1966). *Psychopathology of everyday life. [Ed. Alan Tyson, Trans. James Strachey.].* Oxford: W. W. Norton & Co.

Garmezy, N. (1985). Stress-resistant children: The search for protective factors. In J.E. Stevenson (Ed.), Recent research in developmental psychopathology. *Journal of Child Psychology and Psychiatry Book* (Suppl. No. 4, pp. 213-233). Oxford: Pergamon Press.

Gentile, A.M. (1998). Implicit and explicit processes during acquisition of functional skills. *Scandinavian Journal of Occupational Therapy, 5,* 7-16.

Gibson, E. (1988). Exploratory behavior in the development of perceiving, acting and acquiring of knowledge. *Annual Review of Psychology, 39,* 1-41.

Gibson, J. (1977). The theory of affordances. In R. Shaw & J. Bransford (Eds.), *Perceiving, acting and knowing* (pp. 67-82). Hillsdale, NJ: Erlbaum.

Gibson, J. (1979). *The ecological approach to visual perception.* Boston: Houghton-Mifflin.

Gilfoyle, E.M., Grady, A.P., & Moore, J.C. (1990). *Children adapt* (2nd ed.). Thorofare, NJ: Slack.

Graham, S., & Miller, L. (1980). Handwriting research and practice: a unified approach. *Focus of Exceptional Children, 13,* 1-16.

Gresham, F. (1981). Social skills training with handicapped children: A review. *Reviews in Educational Research, 51,* 139-176.

Haley, S.M., Coster, W.J., Ludlow, L.H., Haltiwanger, J., & Andrellos, P. (1992). *Administrative manual for the Pediatric Evaluation of Disability Inventory.* San Antonio: Psychological Corporation.

Hall, C.S., & Lindzey, G. (1978). *Theories of personality* (3rd ed.). New York: John Wiley & Sons.

Hansen, D.J., Watson-Perczel, M., & Christopher, J.S. (1989). Clinical issues in social skills training with adolescents. *Clinical Psychology Review, 9,* 365-391.

Harter, S. (1978). Effectance motivation reconsidered: Toward a developmental model. *Human Development, 21,* 34-64.

Hayes, R.L., Halford, W.K., & Varghese, F.N. (1991). Generalization of the effects of activity therapy and social skills training on the social behavior of low functioning schizophrenic patients. *Occupational Therapy in Mental Health, 11,* 3-20.

Heriza, C.B. (1991). Motor development: traditional and contemporary theories. In M. Lister (Ed.), *Contemporary management of motor control problems: Proceedings of the II-step conference.* Alexandria, VA: Foundation for Physical Therapy.

Hoehn, T.P., & Baumeister, A.A. (1994). A critique of the application of sensory integration therapy for children with learning disabilities. *Journal of Learning Disabilities, 27,* 338-350.

Howle, J.M. (2002). *Neurodevelopmental treatment approach: Theoretical foundations and principles of clinical practice.* Laguna Beach, CA: Neuro-Developmental Treatment Association.

Humphry, R. (2002). Young children's occupations: Explicating the dynamics of developmental processes. *American Journal of Occupational Therapy, 56,* 171-179.

Hyatt, G.B. (1946). Occupational therapy: Can doses be exact? *Occupational Therapy and Rehabilitation, 25,* 57-61.

Kaplan, B.J., Polatajko, H.J., Wilson, B.N., & Faris, P.D. (1993). Reexamination of sensory integration treatment: A combination of two efficacy studies. *Journal of Learning Disabilities, 26,* 342-347.

Keintz, M.A., & Dunn, W. (1997). A comparison of the performance of children with and without autism on the Sensory Profile. *American Journal of Occupational Therapy, 51,* 530-537.

Kendall, P.C. (1993). Cognitive-behavioral therapist with youth: Guiding theory, current status and emerging developments. *Journal of Consulting and Clinical Psychology, 61,* 235-247.

Ketelaar, M., Vermeer, A., Hart, H., van Petegem-van Beek, E., & Helders, P. (2001). Effects of a functional therapy program on motor abilities of children with cerebral palsy. *Physical Therapy, 81,* 1534-45.

Kielhofner, G. (1995). *A model of human occupation: Theory and application* (2nd ed.). Baltimore: Williams and Wilkins.

Kielhofner, G. (1997). *Conceptual foundations of occupational therapy.* (2nd ed). Philadelphia: F.A. Davis.

Kielhofner, G., & Burke, J. (1980). A model of human occupation. Part 1. Conceptual framework and content. *American Journal of Occupational Therapy, 34,* 572-581.

Knox, S. (1997). Development and current use of the Knox Preschool Play Scale. In L.D. Parham & L.S. Fazio (Eds.), *Play in occupational therapy for children.* St. Louis: Mosby.

Kohlberg, L. (1978). Revisions in the theory and practice of moral development. *New Directions in Child Development, 2,* 83-87.

Krantz, M. (1994). *Child development: Risk and opportunity.* Belmont, CA: Wadsworth.

LaGreca, A.M. (1990). Social consequences of pediatric conditions: Fertile area for future investigation and intervention? *Journal of Pediatric Psychology, 15,* 285-307.

Lammi, B., & Law, M. (2003). Family-centred functional therapy: A single subject study of the effects of addressing the task and the environment in preschool aged children with CP. *Canadian Journal of Occupational Therapy, 70* (5), 285-297.

Law, M. (1991). The environment: A focus for occupational therapy. *Canadian Journal of Occupational Therapy, 58,* 171-179.

Law, M., & Dunn, W. (1993). Perspectives on understanding and changing the environments of children with disabilities. *Physical and Occupational Therapy in Pediatrics, 13* (3), 1-17.

Law, M., Baptiste, S., Carswell, A., McColl, M., Polatajko, H., & Pollock, N. (1998). *Canadian occupational performance measure* (3rd ed.). Ottawa, ON: Canadian Association of Occupational Therapists (CAOT).

Law, M., Cadman, D., Rosenbaum, P., DeMatteo, C., Walter, S., & Russell, D. (1991). Neurodevelopmental therapy and upper extremity casting: Results of a clinical trial. *Developmental Medicine and Child Neurology, 33,* 334-340.

Law, M., Cooper, B., Strong, S., Stewart, D., Rigby, P., & Letts, L. (1996). The person-environment-occupation model: A transactive approach to occupational performance. *Canadian Journal of Occupational Therapy, 63* (1), 9-23.

Law, M., Cooper, B., Strong, S., Stewart, D., Rigby, P., & Letts, L. (1997). Theoretical contexts for the practice of occupational therapy. In C. Christiansen & C. Baum (Eds.), *Occupational therapy: Enabling function and well-being.* Thorofare, NJ: Slack.

Law, M., Haight, M., Milroy, B., Willms, D., Stewart, D., & Rosenbaum, P. (1999). Environmental factors affecting the occupations of children with physical disabilities. *Journal of Occupational Science, 6* (3), 102-110.

Law, M., Hanna, S., King, G., Hurley, P., King, S., Kertoy, M., & Rosenbaum, P. (in press). Factors affecting family-centred service delivery for children with disabilities. *Child: Care, Health and Development.*

Law, M., King, G., MacKinnon, E., Russell, D., Murphy, C., & Hurley, P. (1999). *All about outcomes.* (CD-ROM). Thorofare, NJ: Slack.

Lee, T.D., Swinnen, S.P., & Serrien, D.J. (1994). Cognitive effort and motor learning. *Quest, 46,* 328-344.

Leew, J. (2001). Passport to learning: A cognitive intervention for children with organizational difficulties. *Physical and Occupational Therapy in Pediatrics, 20* (2/3), 145-160.

Lefebvre, C., & Reid, G. (1998). Prediction in ball catching by children with and without a developmental coordination disorder. *Adapted Physical Activity Quarterly, 15,* 299-315.

Linder, T.W. (1994). *Transdisciplinary play-based assessment.* Baltimore: Brookes.

Linderman, T., & Stewart, D. (1999). Sensory integrative-based occupational therapy and functional outcomes in young children with pervasive developmental disorders: A single subject study. *American Journal of Occupational Therapy, 53,* 145-152.

Llorens, L.A. (1969). Facilitating growth and development: The promise of occupational therapy. *American Journal of Occupational Therapy, 24,* 93-101.

Llorens, L.A. (1976). *Application of developmental theory for health and rehabilitation.* Rockville, MD: American Occupational Therapy Association.

Llorens, L.A. (1991). Performance tasks and roles throughout the life span. In C. Christiansen & C. Baum (Eds.), *Occupational therapy: Overcoming human performance deficits* (pp. 45-68). Thorofare, NJ: Slack.

Luria, A. (1961). *The role of speech in the regulation of normal and abnormal behaviors.* New York: Liveright.

Lyons, B.G. (1984). Defining a child's zone of proximal development: Evaluation process for treatment planning. *American Journal of Occupational Therapy, 38,* 446-451.

Ma, H., Trombly, C. A., & Robinson-Podolski, C. (1999). The effect of context on skill acquisition and transfer. *American Journal of Occupational Therapy, 53,* 138-144.

Mahoney, G., & Bella, J. (1998). An examination of the effects of family-centered early intervention on child and family outcomes. *Topics in Early Childhood Special Education, 18* (2), 83-94.

Mahoney, G., & O'Sullivan, P. (1990). Early intervention practices with families of children with handicaps. *Mental Retardation, 28,* 169-176.

Mandich, A., Polatajko, H., Missiuna, C., & Miller, L. (2001). Cognitive strategies and motor performance in children with developmental coordination disorder. *Physical and Occupational Therapy in Pediatrics, 20* (2/3), 125-143.

Martini, R., & Polatajko, H. (1998). Verbal self-guidance as a treatment approach for children with developmental coordination disorder: A systematic replication study. *Occupational Therapy Journal of Research, 18,* 157-181.

Maslow, A.H. (1968). *Toward a psychology of being.* Princeton, NJ: Van Nostrand.

Maslow, A.H. (1970). *Motivation and personality.* New York: Harper & Row.

Maslow, A.H. (1971). *The farther reaches of human nature.* New York: Viking Press.

Mathiowetz, V., & Haugen, J.B. (1994) Motor behavior research: Implications for therapeutic approaches to central nervous system dysfunction. *American Journal of Occupational Therapy, 48* (8), 733-745.

Mayo, N.E. (1991). The effect of physical therapy for children with motor delay and cerebral palsy. *American Journal of Physical Medicine and Rehabilitation, 70,* 258-267.

McColl, M., Law, M., Stewart, D., Doubt, L., Pollock, N., & Krupa, T. (2003). *Theoretical basis of occupational therapy* (2nd ed.). Thorofare, NJ: Slack.

McCormick, C.B., Miller, G., & Pressley, M. (1989). *Cognitive strategy research: From basic research to educational applications.* New York: Springer-Verlag.

Meichenbaum, D. (1977). *Cognitive-behavior modification: An integrative approach.* New York: Plenum Press.

Meyer, A. (1922). The philosophy of occupational therapy. *Archives of Occupational Therapy, 1,* 1-10.

Miller, L.J., & Lane, S. J. (2000). Towards a consensus in terminology in sensory integration theory and practice. Part 1. Taxonomy of neurophysiological processes. *Sensory Integration Special Interest Section, 23,* 1-4.

Miller, L.J., Wilbarger, J., Stackhouse, T., & Trunnell, S. (2002). Clinical reasoning in occupational therapy: The STEP-SI model of intervention of sensory modulation dysfunction. In A. Bundy, S. Lane, & E. Murray (Eds.), *Sensory integration therapy and practice* (2nd ed.). (pp. 435-451). Philadelphia: F.A. Davis.

Miller, L., Polatajko, H., Missiuna, C., Mandich, A., Macnab, J., & Malloy-Miller, T. (2001). A pilot trial of a cognitive treatment for children with developmental coordination disorder. *Human Movement Science, 20,* 183-210.

Milone, M.N. Jr., & Waslyk, T.M. (1981). Handwriting in special education. *Teaching Exceptional Children, 14,* 58-61.

Missiuna, C., & Mandich, A. (2002). Integrating motor learning theories into practice. In S. Cermak & D. Larkin (Eds.), *Developmental coordination disorder* (pp. 221-233). Albany, NY: Delmar.

Missiuna, C., & Pollock, N. (2000). Perceived efficacy and goal setting in young children. *Canadian Journal of Occupational Therapy, 67,* 101-109.

Missiuna, C., Malloy-Miller, T., & Mandich, A. (1998). Mediational techniques: Origins and application to occupational therapy in pediatrics. *Canadian Journal of Occupational Therapy, 65,* 202-209.

Missiuna, C., Mandich, A., Polatajko, P., & Malloy-Miller, T. (2001). Cognitive orientation to daily occupational performance (CO-OP). Part 1. Theoretical foundations. *Physical and Occupational Therapy in Pediatrics, 20* (2/3), 69-81.

Mitchell, P.R. (1995). A dynamic interactive developmental view of early speech and language production: Application to clinical practice in motor speech disorders. *Seminars in Speech & Language, 16,* 100-109.

Moher, T.J. (1907). Occupation in the treatment of the insane. *Journal of the American Medical Association, 158,* 1664-1666.

Moxley-Haegert, L., & Serbin, L.A. (1983). Developmental education for parents of delayed infants: Effects on parental motivation and children's development. *Child Development, 54,* 1324-1331.

Mulligan, S. (1998). Patterns of sensory integration dysfunction: A confirmatory factor analysis. *American Journal of Occupational Therapy, 52,* 819-828.

Myers, D.G. (2001) *Psychology (6th ed.).* New York: Worth Publishers.

Neistadt, M.E. (1990). A critical analysis of occupational therapy approaches for perceptual deficits in adults with brain injury. *American Journal of Occupational Therapy, 44,* 299-304.

Newacheck, P., & Halfon, N. (1998). Prevalence and impact of disabling chronic conditions in childhood. *American Journal of Public Health, 88* (4), pp. 610-617.

Nicholson, D.E. (1996). Motor learning. In C.M. Fredericks & L.K. Saladin (Eds.), *Pathophysiology of the motor systems: Principles and clinical presentations* (pp. 238-254). Philadelphia: F.A. Davis.

Ottenbacher, K., Short, M.A., & Watson, P.J. (1979). Nystagmus duration changes in learning disabled children during sensory integrative therapy. *Perceptual and Motor Skills, 48,* 1159-1164.

Palmer, F.B., Shapiro, B.K., Wachtal, R.C., Allen, M.C., Hiller, J.E., Harryman, S.E., et al. (1988). The effects of physical therapy on cerebral palsy: A controlled trial in infants with spastic diplegia. *New England Journal of Medicine, 318,* 903-908.

Parham, L.D. (1996). Perspectives on play. In R. Zemke & F. Clark (Eds.), *Occupational science: The evolving discipline.* Philadelphia: F.A. Davis.

Parham, L.D., & Primeau, L. (1997). Play and occupational therapy. In L.D. Parham & L.S. Fazio (Eds.), *Play in occupational therapy for children.* St. Louis: Mosby.

Piaget, J. (1952). *The origins of intelligence in children.* New York: International Universities.

Piaget, J. (1971). *Psychology and epistemology: towards a theory of knowledge.* New York: Viking Press.

Piper, M.C. (1990). Efficacy of physical therapy: Rate of motor development in children with cerebral palsy. *Pediatric Physical Therapy, 2,* 126-130.

Piper, M.C., & Darrah, J. (1994). Motor assessment of the developing infant. Philadelphia: W.B. Saunders.

Pless, I.B., Cripps, H.A., Davies, J.M.C., & Wadsworth, M.E.J. (1989). Chronic physical illness in childhood: Psychological and social effects in adolescence and adult life. *Developmental Medicine and Child Neurology, 31,* 746-755.

Plienis, A.J., Hansen, D.J., Ford, F., Smith, S., Stark, L., & Kelly, J. (1987). Behavioral small group training to improve the social skills of emotionally-disordered adolescents. *Behavior Therapy, 18,* 17-32.

Polatajko, H.P., Kaplan, B.J., Wilson, B.N. (1992). Sensory integration treatment for children with learning disabilities: Its status 20 years later. *Occupational Therapy Journal of Research, 12,* 323-341.

Polatajko, H.J., Mandich, A.D., Miller, L.T., & Macnab, J.J. (2001). Cognitive orientation to daily occupational performance (CO-OP). Part 2. The evidence. *Physical and Occupational Therapy in Pediatrics, 20* (2/3), 83-106.

Polatajko, H.J., Mandich, A.D., Missiuna, C., Miller, L.T., Macnab, J., Malloy-Miller, T. (2001). Cognitive orientation to daily occupational performance (CO-OP). Part 3. The protocol in brief. *Physical and Occupational Therapy in Pediatrics, 20* (2/3), 107-123.

Reed, M.K. (1994). Social skills training to reduce depression in adolescents. *Adolescence, 29,* 293-302.

Reilly, M. (1962). Occupational therapy can be one of the great ideas of 20th century medicine. *American Journal of Occupational Therapy, 16,* 87-105.

Reilly, M. (1966). A psychiatric occupational therapy program as a teaching model. *American Journal of Occupational Therapy, 20,* 61-67.

Reilly, M. (1974a). Occupational behavior: A perspective on work and play. *American Journal of Occupational Therapy, 25,* 291-296.

Reilly, M. (1974b). *Play as exploratory behavior.* Beverly Hills, CA: Sage Publications.

Reinecke, M.A., Ryan, N.E., & DuBois, D.L. (1998). Cognitive-behavioral treatment of depression and depressive symptoms during adolescence: A review and meta-analysis. *Journal of the American Academy of Child and Adolescent Psychiatry, 37,* 26-34.

Reisman, J., & Hanschu, B. (1992). *Sensory integration inventory: Revised for individuals with developmental disabilities.* Hugo, MN: PDP Press.

Richmond, J.B., & Beardslee, W.R. (1988). Resiliency: Research and practical implications for pediatricians. *Journal of Developmental and Behavioral Pediatrics, 9,* 157-163.

Rigby, P., & Letts, L. (2003). Environment and occupational performance: Theoretical considerations. In L. Letts, P. Rigby, & D. Stewart (Eds.), *Using environments to enable occupational performance.* (pp. 17-32). Thorofare, NJ: Slack.

Rogers, C.R. (1939). *The clinical treatment of the problem child.* Boston: Houghton-Mifflin.

Rogers, C.R. (1969). *Freedom to learn.* Columbus, OH: Merrill.

Rutter, M. (1990). Psychosocial resilience and protective mechanisms. In J. Rolf, A.S. Masten, D. Cicchetti, K. Nuechterlein, & S. Weintraub (Eds.), *Risk and protective factors in the development of psychopathology* (pp. 181-214). Cambridge: Cambridge University Press.

Sandler, I. (2001). Quality and ecology of adversity as common mechanisms of risk and resilience. *American Journal of Community Psychology, 29* (1), 19-61.

Scherzer, A.L., Mike, V., & Ilson, J. (1976). Physical therapy as a determinant of change in the cerebral palsied infant. *Pediatrics, 53,* 47-52.

Schkade, J.K., & Schultz, S. (1992). Occupational adaptation: Toward a holistic approach for contemporary practice, Part 1. *American Journal of Occupational Therapy, 46,* 829-837.

Schmidt, R.A. (1988). *Motor control and learning: A behavioral emphasis.* Champaign, IL: Human Kinetics.

Shiffrin, R.M., & Atkinson, R.C. (1969). Storage and retrieval processes in long-term memory. *Psychological Review, 76,* 179-193.

Shumway-Cook, A., & Woollacott, M.H. (1995). *Motor control: Theory and practical applications.* Baltimore: Williams & Wilkins.

Siegler, R.S. (1983). Five generalizations about cognitive development. *American Psychologist, 38,* 263-277.

Skinner, B.F. (1953). *Science and human behavior.* New York: Free Press.

Skinner, B.F. (1976). *Walden two.* New York, New York: Macmillan.

Slagle, E.C. (1922). Training aides for mental patients. *Archives of Occupational Therapy, 1,* 11-17.

Sloper, P., Turner, S., Knussen, C., & Cunningham, C. (1990). Social life of school children with Down's syndrome. *Child: Care, Health and Development, 16* (4), 235-251.

Sommerfeld, D., Fraser, B.A., Hensinger, R.N., & Beresford, C.V. (1981). Evaluation of physical therapy service for severely mentally impaired students with cerebral palsy. *Physical Therapy, 61,* 338-344.

Stagnitti, K., Raison, P., & Ryan, P. (1999). Sensory defensiveness syndrome: A paediatric perspective and case study. *Australian Occupational Therapy Journal, 46,* 175-187.

Stein, R.E.K., & Jessop, D.J. (1984). Does pediatric home care make a difference for children with chronic illness? Findings from the pediatric ambulatory care treatment study. *Pediatrics, 73,* 845-853.

Stein, R.E.K., & Jessop, D.J. (1991). Long-term mental health effects of a pediatric home care program. *Pediatrics, 88,* 490-496.

Sternberg, R.J. (1984). Mechanisms of cognitive development. *American Psychologist, 38,* 263-277.

Stewart, D., & Law, M. (2003). The environment: Paradigms and practice in health, occupational therapy and inquiry. In L. Letts, P. Rigby, & D. Stewart (Eds.), *Using environments to enable occupational performance* (pp. 3-15). Thorofare, NJ: Slack.

Stewart, D., Pollock, N., Law, M., Ferland, F., Rigby, P., Toal, C., et al. (1996). Occupational therapy and children's play. Practice paper. *Canadian Journal of Occupational Therapy, 63,* insert.

Sugden, D.A., & Sugden, L. (1990). *The assessment and management of movement skill problems.* Leeds: School of Education.

Thelen, E. (1995) *Motor development: A new synthesis.* American Psychologist, *50* (2) 79-95.

Thelen, E., Schoner, G., Scheier, C., Smith, L. (2001). The dynamics of embodiment: A field theory of infant preservative reaching. *Behavioral and Brain Sciences, 24,* 1-86.

Thelen, E., Spencer, J.P. (1998). Postural control during reaching in young infants: A dynamic systems approach. *Neuroscience and Behavioral Reviews, 22,* 507-14.

Tisdelle, D.A., & St. Lawrence, J.S. (1988). Adolescent interpersonal problem-solving skill training: Social validation and generalization. *Behavior Therapy, 19,* 171-182.

Van Gelder, T. (1995). What might cognition be, if not computation? *Journal of Philosophy, 91,* 345-381.

VanSant, A.F. (1991). Neurodevelopmental treatment and pediatric physical therapy: A commentary. *Pediatric Physical Therapy, 3,* 137-141.

Vargas, S., & Camilli, G. (1999). A meta-analysis of research on sensory integration treatment. *American Journal of Occupational Therapy, 53,* 180-198.

Vygotsky, L.S. (1962). *Thought and language.* Cambridge, MA: MIT Press. (Original work published in 1934)

Vygotsky, L.S. (1978). Mind in society: The development of higher mental processes. In M. Cole, V. John-Streiner, S. Scribner, & E. Souberman (Eds.), *Mind in society.* Cambridge, MA: Harvard University Press.

Wallander, J., & Varni, J. (1989). Social support and adjustment in chronically ill and handicapped children. *American Journal of Community Psychology, 17* (2), 185-201.

Watling, R., Deitz, J., & White, O. (2001). Comparison of sensory profile scores of young children with and without autism spectrum disorders. *American Journal of Occupational Therapy, 55,* 416-423.

Watling, R., Deitz, J., Kanny, E.M., & McLaughlin, J.F. (1999). Current practice of occupational therapy for children with autism. *American Journal of Occupational Therapy, 53,* 498-505.

Watson, D.E. (1997). *Task analysis: An occupational performance approach.* Bethesda, MD: American Occupational Therapy Association (AOTA).

Werner, E.E. (1989). High-risk children in young adulthood: A longitudinal study from birth to 32 years. *American Journal of Orthopsychiatry, 59,* 72-81.

Werner, E.E. (1994). Overcoming the odds. *Developmental and Behavioral Pediatrics, 15,* 131-136.

Wilbarger, P. (1995). The sensory diet: Activity programs based on sensory processing theory. *Sensory Integration Special Interest Section Newsletter, 18,* 1-4.

Wilcock, A. (1993). A theory of human need for occupation. *Occupational Science: Australia, 1,* 17-24.

Wilcock, A. (1998). Reflections on doing, being, becoming. *Canadian Journal of Occupational Therapy, 65,* 248-256.

Williams, M.S., & Shellenberger, S. (1994). *How does your engine run? A leader's guide to the alert program for self-regulation.* Albuquerque, NM: Therapy Works.

Williamson, G., & Szczepanski, M. (1999). Coping frame of reference. In P. Kramer & J. Hinojosa (Eds.), *Frames of reference in pediatric occupational therapy.* Baltimore: Williams & Wilkins.

World Health Organization. (1980). *International classification of impairments, disability and handicap.* Geneva: World Health Organization.

World Health Organization. (2001). *International classification of disability, functioning and health.* Geneva: World Health Organization.

Wright, T., & Nicholson, J. (1973). Physiotherapy for the spastic child: An evaluation. *Developmental Medicine and Child Neurology, 15,* 146-163.

Yack, E., Sutton, S., & Aquilla, P. (1998). *Building bridges through sensory integration.* Weston, ON: Authors.

Yerxa, E.J. (1967). Authentic occupational therapy. *American Journal of Occupational Therapy, 21,* 1-9.

Yerxa, E.J., Clark, F., Frank, G., Jackson, J., Parham, D., Pierce, D., et al. (1989). Occupational science: The foundation for new models of practice. *Occupational Therapy in Health Care, 6,* 1-17.

Zeitlin, S., & Williamson, G.G. (1994). *Coping in young children: Early intervention practices to enhance adaptive behavior and resilience.* Baltimore: Brookes.

Zeitlin, S., Williamson, G.G., & Szczepanski, M. (1988). *Early coping inventory.* Bensenville, IL: Scholastic Testing Service.

Development of Childhood Occupations

Jane Case-Smith

Neuromaturational theory
Dynamic systems theory
Perceptual-action coupling
Functional synergies
Cultural practices
Occupations within cultural, social, and physical
  contexts
Play development

1 Explain historical and current theories of child development.
2 Explain the development of functional performance using current psychologic theories.
3 Analyze how occupations develop through cultural practices.
4 Explain how individual biologic systems and cultural, social, and physical contexts contribute to a child's occupational performance in the first 10 years of life.
5 Describe the development of play in children.

An understanding of child development is foundational knowledge for pediatric occupational therapists. Researchers from many disciplines, including medicine, psychology, education, sociology, and occupational therapy, have contributed to the literature on human development, and the different perspectives they provide should be woven into a holistic and comprehensive understanding of how children become adults.

Occupational therapists want to know *what* developmental changes occur in children and *how* children develop their unique personhood. The answers to these questions provide essential knowledge for evaluating children and for determining the appropriate materials, activities, and environments to support children's skill development and participation in their communities.

This chapter focuses on child development theories, with emphasis on concepts that have emerged in the past 2 decades. The first section discusses emerging concepts that explain how children develop and what variables and interactions influence developmental outcomes. In the second part of the chapter, a model for the development of childhood occupations is applied to children's development of play in the first 10 years of life.

DEVELOPMENTAL THEORIES AND CONCEPTS

Researchers of the 1930s and 1940s were concerned with identifying the sequence of skill maturation that defined normal development. Gesell (Gesell et al., 1940; Gesell, 1945; Gesell & Amatruda, 1947) and McGraw (1945) assumed that normal development was revealed through a specific skill sequence that reflected maturation of the central nervous system (CNS). They believed that the sequence of motor, cognitive, socioemotional, and language skill development was relatively unaffected by the infant's experiences. The work of these neuromaturational theorists in documenting this developmental sequence has been well respected and has allowed the creation of developmental assessment tools. The sequence of normal development has been particularly important in identifying children with disabilities. Gesell believed that variations in the normal sequence of development indicate CNS dysfunction. Identifying children with developmental deficits or significant delays remains an important function of physicians, nurses, occupational therapists, and others who provide early intervention services.

Neuromaturation

Neuromaturational theory frequently has been used to explain motor development (e.g., Ellison, 1994; Milani-Comparetti & Gidoni, 1967). According to neuromaturational theory, brain stem structures develop first, as evidenced by the reflexive responses of the newborn (e.g., automatic grasp, asymmetric tonic neck reflex), which are controlled by neural pathways originating in the brain stem. Cortical structures appear to develop later, as evidenced by the coordinated and planned actions of the child. The infant's increasing control of action and movement indicates not only development and myelination of the midbrain and cortical structures, but also simultaneous inhibition of brain stem control of movement. The three primary principles of neuromaturational theory are:

1 Movement progresses from primitive reflex patterns to voluntary, controlled movement. In newborn and young infants, motor reflexes provide the first methods of interaction with the environment (e.g., reflexive grasp) and are essential to life (e.g., sucking and swallowing reflex). Because early reflexive movements serve functional needs, the newborn appears surprisingly competent. These reflex patterns subside as balance, postural reactions, and voluntary motor control emerge (i.e., when the infant learns to roll, sit, creep, stand, and walk).

2 The sequence and rate of motor development are consistent among infants and children. The developmental scales of Gesell and Amatruda (1947), Illingworth (1966, 1984), Bayley (1993), and others are based on a typical rate and sequence of development. By assuming that the sequence of milestones (i.e., major motor accomplishments) is constant and predictable, the normative developmental sequence can be used to diagnose neurologic impairment and disability.

3 Low-level skills are prerequisites for certain high-level skills. For example, infants develop motor control in a cephalocaudal direction, with head control maturing first, followed by trunk control sufficient for independent sitting, and finally pelvic control sufficient for standing and walking.

In assuming a hierarchy of CNS function, the neuromaturational theory limited the thinking on how a child learns to act in the environment. Using current research models (e.g., Gibson, 1995; Gottlieb, 1997; Thelen, 1995; Thelen, Corbetta, & Kamm, et al., 1993), it has become apparent that multiple variables at different levels influence the child's skill development. The child learns occupations through interaction with his or her environment rather than through the emergence of a predetermined scenario reflecting neuromaturational principles.

Development in Social and Physical Contexts

Piaget (1952) expanded our understanding of a child's maturation by emphasizing that development is an interplay between the environment and the child's innate abilities (see Chapter 3). Piaget emphasized the maturation of cognitive structures that enable the child to understand the environment, language, and social action.

Infants develop an understanding of the world by interacting with the environment. The impact of environment on the child's development changes as the child becomes increasingly able to assimilate the complexities of physical and social events. Piaget documented the child's acquisition of symbolic thought and formal cognitive operations, because these reflect genetic endowment and are reinforced by experiences in an environment that responds in predictable ways. For example, Piaget documented the early development of tool use. He observed that children at 8 to 10 months manipulate two objects and can move an obstacle to get an interesting object. By 12 months, infants can relate an object to other objects, in addition to relating the objects to themselves. At this stage, infants use a stick to rake in an object out of reach. By 18 months, infants begin to use trial and error to solve problems. At 24 months of age, they no longer exclusively need physical manipulation to solve problems and begin to demonstrate use of mental manipulation (Piaget, 1952; McCarty, Clifton, & Collard, 2001).

Recent research studies have shown that cognitive structures develop at earlier ages than Piaget assumed. Infants as young as 1 month demonstrate the ability to associate learning from one sensory system with another sensory system. For example, they recognize objects with their eyes that they previously felt in their mouths (Mandler, 1990). In addition, at 9 months, infants can remember an event 1 week after it happened (Metzoff & Moore, 1992).

McCarty et al. (2001) found that children can manipulate and use tools at ages younger than Piaget documented. Their research demonstrated how children 9 to 19 months solved problems in how to approach the grasp and use of a spoon. A spoon loaded with food was presented to the child in different orientations. Children 9 to 14 months of age picked up the spoon using an awkward grasp and then attempted to adjust the spoon's orientation to get the food into their mouths. Children 19 months old planned how to grasp and orient the spoon to get the food before acting, avoiding the use of awkward grasps that required adjusting. This study showed that children as early as 19 months can solve problems without physical manipulation and trial and error to handle a tool accurately.

Another developmental theorist, Vygotsky (1978), believed that children learn in social interactions. He demonstrated that children learn through *scaffolding*, or support, provided by caregivers and teachers. A *just right* challenge in the child's zone of proximal development enables the child to take the next step in skill development. The *zone of proximal development* is the distance between the child's current developmental level (skills the child performs independently) and the potential (next) developmental level (skills the child performs when guided by an adult). Parents and other family members intuitively provide environmental challenges that encourage the infant to exhibit a higher skill level and then support the infant's efforts to reach that level. Parents and siblings naturally promote the infant's development by modeling actions, assisting the infant's first attempts to perform an action, and reinforcing his or her efforts with praise and expressions of delight.

Piaget, Vygotsky, and the many subsequent developmental theorists have examined how human development transpires through a dynamic interplay involving the child and the child's cultural, social, and physical environments. Researchers of child development have documented differences in the rate of development in socioeconomic groups, regions, and individuals. For example, rates of development appear different in rural versus urban areas (Touwen, 1979; von Hofsten, 1993). Children's rate of development also differs among cultural groups and generations, in part because of differences in nutrition and childcare practices. In human development research, the emphasis currently is on the variations expressed by individual infants and on what human systems and environmental constraints contribute to these variations.

Studies that analyze the uniqueness of individual performance often use longitudinal and qualitative approaches to analyze the performance of children over time and in natural contexts. Because these longitudinal studies document the patterns of development over time, they uncover how individual systems are constructed and assembled. Longitudinal approaches make it possible to relate transitions of subsystems to each other and to other dynamic growth parameters (von Hofsten, 1993). Understanding *how* children acquire qualitative differences in functional performance and *how* they become unique individuals can begin by focusing on the variables that influence a child's developmental course. The following sections examine current theories of development that explain the interplay and relationships among a child's biologic functions, occupations, and social, physical, and cultural contexts.

DYNAMIC SYSTEMS THEORY

Dynamic systems theory refers to performance or action patterns that emerge from the interaction and cooperation of many systems, both internal and external to the child (Thelen, 2002). In the context of child development, performance patterns emerge from the interaction of an individual's systems and performance contexts as the child strives to achieve a functional goal (Mathiowetz & Haugen, 1994, 1995). The dynamic systems theory is most useful in describing how specific motor and process skills develop.

In this model, a child's behaviors and actions are initially highly variable, with many degrees of freedom. The first actions of the infant have been described as random and uncontrolled. Development of skill proceeds by means of constraint of these degrees of freedom as the child gains control of his or her actions. Behavior, therefore, is not prescribed by a hierarchical arrangement of the CNS, but rather emerges from external and internal constraints. These constraints provide information to the brain and body systems that set the boundaries or limits for the child's behavior (Clark, 1997).

Humans are complex biologic systems comprising many subsystems (e.g., motor sensory, perceptual, skeletal, and psychologic subsystems). These subsystems are in constant flux, interacting according to the task at hand and conditions in the environment. The child's actions during the performance of a task, therefore, are the result of the subsystems' interaction with each other and with the environment. These individual systems come together and self-organize in a coordinated way to achieve the child's goal. For example, initially a child is interested in exploring the sensory characteristics of a toy. As he or she reaches for the toy, grasps it, brings it to midline in hand-to-hand play, and finally to the mouth, the child's attention and cognitive focus are not on planning each of these actions. Instead, they are on assimilating the toy's actions and perceptual features.

Longitudinal studies reveal that children demonstrate unique trajectories of development and that variations in functional performance among children persist into adulthood. Thelen and her colleagues demonstrated the uniqueness of motor development in a study of reaching in 4- and 5-month-old infants (Thelen et al., 1993). Each 5-month-old infant was able to reach toward an object, but the patterns demonstrated were quite unique. Some infants demonstrated a slow, cautious first approach to the object, whereas others made ballistic arm movements in an attempt to reach it. Although all first reaches tended to be circuitous, the amount of correction made to obtain the object, the speed at which the attempt was made, and the angle at which arms were held toward the object were different.

In a similar way, between 8 and 10 months, most infants acquire the motivation to be independently mobile. The need to self-initiate movement from place to place emerges as an important task, or goal, to accomplish. This goal reflects the infant's curiosity about the environment, a desire to explore space, and a determination to reach a specific play object. Although mobility becomes a common goal of an infant toward the end of the first year, the method used to achieve that mobility varies greatly. Some infants roll to another space in the room, whereas others scoot on their buttocks in a sitting position. Some infants push backward while lying in a prone position, and others creep forward to explore their environment. How the infant achieves mobility is influenced by many contributing body systems (e.g., strength, coordination, and sense of balance and movement). Conditions in the environment also influence infant mobility (e.g., the surfaces on which the child plays, the encouragement provided by caregivers, and the way in which the task is presented).

Perceptual Action Reciprocity

Perception and action are interdependent and inextricably linked. An individual's perception of the environment informs action, and the individual's actions provide feedback about movement, performance, and consequences in the environment. Initially, many of the child's actions are exploratory in nature; that is, the child moves fingers over the surfaces of objects to learn their shape, texture, and consistency. The child waves an object in the air to hear the sounds it makes and to feel its weight. These actions help the child perceive sensory and perceptual features (affordances) of objects. *Affordance* is the fit between the child and his or her environment (Gibson, 1979, 1997). The environment and objects in it offer the child opportunities to explore and act. This action is based on what the environment affords, as well as the child's perceptual capability to recognize affordances in that environment. For example, colorful, noise-making toys afford manipulation because they have movable parts and rounded surfaces and easily fit into an infant's hand. Learning about affordances entails exploratory activities. Individual finger movements, thumb opposition, hand-to-hand transfer, and eye-hand coordination are facilitated by the physical characteristics of the toy.

Manipulation is guided by visual, tactile, and kinesthetic input (Rochat, 1989; Ruff, 1989). Exploration of objects begins with visual exploration and mouthing (Rochat & Gibson, 1985). By 6 months, infants prefer exploring with their eyes and hands (Rochat, 1989). Fingering and manipulation skills increase substantially between 6 and 12 months, enabling infants to gather more precise information about objects. By 12 months, infants detect object properties with increasing specificity and learn to adjust their exploratory action (Adolph, Eppler, & Gibson, 1993). For example, to perceive the consistency of a soft, squishy object, a child squeezes it, and to perceive the texture or velvet or corduroy, he or she runs the fingers back and forth over it.

Through object manipulation, the child develops haptic perception (i.e., an understanding of objects' shape, texture, and mass). Bushnell and Boudreau (1993) propose that specific motor skills are required to develop haptic perception. They note that infants learn to identify an object's sensory qualities (e.g., texture, consistency, temperature, contour) only when they develop the motor skills to explore each different sensory quality. For example, an infant does not accurately discriminate texture until he or she can explore texture by moving the fingers back and forth (at about 6 months).

The child also cannot discriminate hardness until 6 months, when he or she can tighten and lessen the grip while holding an object (Bushnell & Boudreau, 1993). Because configural shape requires that two hands be involved in exploring an object's surfaces, children typical cannot accurately perceive shape until 12 months. These examples demonstrate that haptic perception develops in association with the child's development of manipulation skills. Once the child learns to discern the perceptual qualities of the object being handled, he or she begins to master the use of tools and objects in communication and cognitive tasks.

Functional Performance: Flexible Synergies

As mentioned, the infant begins life with few constraints on performance, which permits the greatest variability in the system for the generation of spontaneous movements. This variability permits flexibility for exploration of the environment and rapid perceptual and cognitive learning. The infant quickly selects functional synergistic movement patterns. For example, from birth the infant demonstrates a pattern of hand-to-mouth movement (e.g., to calm himself or herself by sucking on a fist). Only minimal adaptive changes are made in this synergistic pattern (shoulder rotation and horizontal adduction, elbow flexion and forearm pronation, followed by supination and neutral wrist position) as the child learns to feed himself or herself with various utensils.

Because synergies that enable tool use are softly assembled around the goal of the task at hand, they are stable but flexible units. Synergies have specific consistent characteristics, such as the sequence of movements and the ratio of joint movement, which can be adjusted to accommodate each new situation. This *adaptable stability* is a hallmark of normal movement (Cioni et al., 1997).

The functional synergies that characterize a child's development of occupations are highly adaptable and highly reliable. The child self-organizes these synergies around goals, and his or her first goals are embedded in and organized around play (as described in the second part of this chapter).

Development of Performance Skills

How does a child learn new performance skills? How does competence develop during childhood? Children generally transition through three stages of learning to acquire a new skill (Gibson, 1997; Piper & Darrah, 1994). The first stage involves exploratory activity. The first year of life is primarily a period of sensorimotor exploration. Exploration occurs naturally in all human beings, generally when an individual is presented with a new object or task. Through exploration, a child learns about self and the environment. In this stage the child experiments with objects and activities using different systems, new combinations of perception and movement, and new sequences of action. In this exploratory stage or when challenged by a new and difficult task, a child tends to demonstrate primitive movement. New challenges tend to elicit lower levels of skills, because these can be accessed more easily than the child's highest level skills, which demand more energy and effort (Granott, 2002). By using lower level skills to address new problems, the child can focus on perceptual learning about the task before beginning to use higher level skills, which ultimately allow more success in performing the task. Gilfoyle, Grady, and Moore (1990) noted that when children are first challenged with a new and difficult task (e.g., a first step), they use primitive movement patterns (e.g., balance by stiffening the legs and trunk) before progressing to integrated skill.

In the second stage of learning, perceptual learning, the child begins to use the feedback and reinforcement received from his or her exploration. In this transitional stage, the child begins to exhibit consistency in the movement patterns used to accomplish tasks. Because this second stage is a phase of perceptual learning, and certain actions that were tried initially are discarded as ineffective. Interest in the activity remains high as perceptual learning continues and is inherently motivating and meaningful to the child. In this stage, the child appears focused on learning and attempts activities multiple times. The child may fluctuate between higher and lower levels of skill. Connolly and Dalgleish (1993) found considerable variability when toddlers attempted to use a spoon. Greer and Lockman (1998) found similar variability when 3-year-olds attempted to use a writing tool. At times the children grasped the tool using an adult gripping pattern, and at other times they used a primitive, full hand grasp. Mature patterns are selected more often as children enter the third stage of skill learning.

In the third stage of learning, skill achievement, the child selects the action pattern that works best for achieving a goal. The pattern selected is comfortable and efficient for the child. Selection of a single pattern indicates both perceptual learning and increased self-organization. During this end stage of learning, the child demonstrates flexible consistency in performance. He or she uses the same pattern and approach to the task but easily adapts the pattern according to task requirements. High adaptability is always characteristic of a well-learned task. Another attribute of learned performance is the use of action patterns that are orderly and economical. Children continue to practice performance when given opportunities in the environment. The third stage of learning leads to exploration of new and different activities, therefore a child's learning continues into new performance arenas, expanding his or her occupations.

DEVELOPMENT OF HUMAN OCCUPATIONS

To understand the development of human occupations, the occupational therapist must have a complete understanding of the ways in which cultural, social, and physical contexts contribute to a child's development. Human development occurs in a family and a community with specific cultural, social, and physical characteristics (Figure 4-1). A child performs and masters activities according to his or her inherent facility and genetic endowment and the supports and constraints in the environment. Therefore, to understand a child's performance, one must examine the interactions of occupations and activities, individual process and motor skills, and context.

Occupations, Activities, and Skills

Children tend to accomplish certain occupations and their corresponding tasks in a sequence that is common to typically developing children. However, the way these tasks are accomplished is unique for each child. A child learns new occupations based on the facility that she or he brings to the activity. Motor, cognitive, sensory or perceptual, communicative, and socioemotional systems contribute to occupational performance. The strengths and constraints of each system determine the quality and developmental level of performance. These systems are interdependent; that is, they work together in such a way that the strengths of one system (e.g., visual) can support limitations in others (e.g., kinesthetic). Which systems are recruited for a task varies according to the novelty of the activity and the degree to which the task has become automatic. For example, research has shown that handwriting involves visual, perceptual, kinesthetic, visual-motor, cognitive, and language systems (Cornhill & Case-Smith, 1996; Tseng & Murray, 1994). Initially handwriting is guided by the visual system, but after it has been practiced and learned, it is guided primarily by the kinesthetic system. Occupations such as feeding may involve somatosensory skills more than visual skills. Feeding behaviors are reflexive at birth and continue to involve primarily automatic responses as the infant becomes a child.

Contexts for Development

Children develop occupations through participation in family activities and cultural practices. As a child participates in the family's cultural practices, he or she learns occupations and performance skills that enable him or her to become a full participant in the community. Rogoff explains that, "People develop as participants in cultural communities. Their development can be understood only in light of the cultural practices and

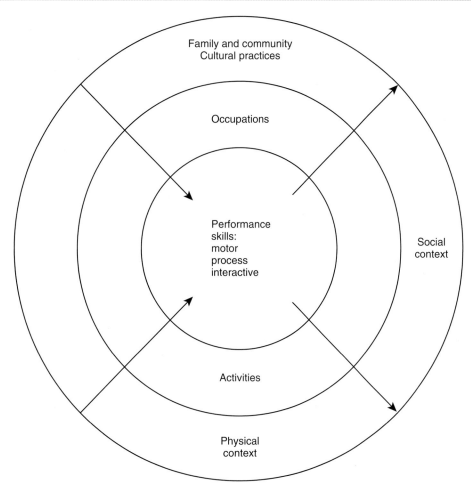

FIGURE 4-1 Model of the development of child occupations.

circumstances of their communities" (Rogoff, 2003, pp. 3-4). Variations in the child's play activities (e.g., how he or she builds with wooden blocks, draws a picture of himself or herself, or sings a song) reflect the child's biologic abilities and the influence of cultural, social, and physical contexts.

A child's cultural, social, and physical contexts change through the course of development and tend to expand as the child matures. The environment surrounds and supports the child's action; it also forces the child to adapt and assists or accommodates that adaptation. As a child perceives the affordances of the environment, he or she learns to act on those affordances, expanding a repertoire of actions. At the same time, the child's understanding of how the world responds to his or her actions increases. Rogoff (2003) argued that culture affects every aspect of the child's development, which cannot be understood outside this context. The child is nested in his or her family, culture, and community, which have influenced the child's genetic makeup and continue to provide his or her learning environment. By recognizing this influence, occupational therapists always view the child in his or her cultural context and work as change agents within that context.

Figure 4-1 illustrates how the child's skills and occupations are embedded in his or her family's and community's cultural practices. Cultural practices are the routine activities common to a people of a culture and may reflect religion, traditions, economic survival, community organization, and regional ideology. The child learns motor and process skills through his or her participation in these cultural practices. Reciprocally, a child's motor and process skills enable him or her to participate in the occupations and cultural practices of the child's family and community. The arrows represent these reciprocal influences.

Cultural Contexts

To fully understand how children develop through participation in cultural practices, Rogoff and her colleagues have studied child development in various cultures, including the European American culture. Their findings, as well as the findings of occupational therapists (e.g., Bazyk, Stalnaker, Llerena, Ekelman, & Bazyk, 2003), have expanded our understanding of how children develop and have broadened the definition of typical child development.

Cultures vary in many aspects, such as the roles of women and children, values and beliefs about family and religion, family traditions, and the importance of health care and education. The continuum of interdependence versus autonomy of individuals varies in cultural groups and is a significant determinant of childhood occupations. The value a people or community places on interdependence among its members versus individual autonomy creates differences in child-rearing practices and different experiences for developing children.

Most middle-class European Americans value independence as a primary important goal for their children. U.S. parents encourage individuality, self-expression, and independence in their children's actions and thoughts. To foster early independence in children, U.S. parents do not sleep with their infants. Generally at the earliest age, infants sleep in their own crib and room. Yet this practice is unusual compared with other societies in the world, such as Asia, Africa, and South America, where infants sleep in their parents' bed or room (Morelli, Rogoff, Oppenheim, & Goldsmith, 1992). For example, Japanese parents report that co-sleeping facilitates infants' transformation from separate individuals to persons able to engage in interdependent relationships. Japanese parents are interested in promoting continued reciprocity with their children, encouraging the primacy of family relationships (Rogoff, 2003).

One consequence of the early separation of infants from their parents for sleeping is that middle-class U.S. parents often engage in elaborate and time-consuming bedtime routines. In contrast, Mayan parents reported that they do not use bedtime routines (e.g., stories or lullabies) to coax babies to sleep (Rogoff, Mosier, Mistry, & Goncu, 1993). To encourage interdependence, Mayan parents hold their infants continuously, and they often hold them so that they can orient to the group (i.e., facing other members of the group rather than their mothers). By observing others more than watching the mother, infants become aware of their adult community. In the Latino culture, which also encourages interdependence, parents are permissive and indulgent with young children. Latino parents do not push developmental skills, in part because they value interdependence with the family as opposed to autonomy of the individual (Zuniga, 1998).

In general, cultures that value independence over interdependence also value competition over cooperation. Korean American children have been found to be more cooperative in play than European American children. Mexican children also are more likely to cooperate than European American children (Rogoff, 2003). These examples briefly illustrate how cultural beliefs influence the ways parents raise their children and communities support and challenge children.

Social Contexts

Culture influences the social relationships that envelop the child, yet certain aspects of the child's social context appear to be independent of cultural influences and are consistent across cultures. This section defines elements of the social context particularly important to a child's development. The most important relationships formed during infancy are those with parents and/or primary caregivers. When caregivers are sensitive and responsive to the infant, healthy socioemotional development results (Easterbrooks & Biringer, 2000). Infants' interactions with parents serve to enhance the infants' basic physiologic and regulatory systems. When parents attune to the infant's sensory modulation and arousal needs and support these needs, the infant develops secure attachment. Mothers who modulate their behaviors to match their infants' needs for stimulation and comfort also promote the infants' abilities to self-regulate. The child's interaction with a caregiver gives him or her essential information about how self and other are related, which becomes important to engaging in future relationships. Attachment patterns seem to influence the child's style of interaction and engagement in later years. A study of toddlers' problem solving showed that securely attached toddlers display more enthusiasm and task enjoyment (Matas, Arend, & Sroufe, 1978). Sensitive responding consolidates the infant's sense of efficacy and provides a foundation of security for confident exploration of the environment (Easterbrooks & Biringer, 2000).

Csikszentmihalyi and Rathunde (1998) described parenting as a dance between supporting and challenging the child. Supporting the child enables him or her to assimilate or explore the environment; that is, to play. Parental challenge requires a child to accommodate and conform. Parenting provides a combination of these supports and challenges. Rogoff (1990) defines the support-challenge combination of guided participation as adults challenging, constraining, and supporting children in solving problems. All parents use some measure of support to bolster children's attempts to master skills and some degree of challenge to move children toward higher levels of mastery. These elements are subtly provided by parents in the ways they present tasks and in when and how they instruct or intervene. Effective guidance relies on careful observation of the child's cues. Sensitivity and responsivity to the child's needs appear to be among the most important variables in the promotion of child development (Lerner, Anderson, Balsano, Dowling, & Bobek, 2003). The concept of guided participation is similar to Vygotsky's notion of the zone of proximal development. In guided participation, emphasis is placed on parents' sensitivity to the child's skills to determine the level of support or challenge needed.

In typical situations, infants receive care from multiple care providers, including childcare providers, grandparents, and other adults. The infant may or may not attach to caregivers other than the parents or primary caregivers; however, these social relationships are important to the infant's emotional development and provide him or her with opportunities to develop social skills. According to a study by the National Institute of Child Health and Human Development (NICHHD), 84% of 12-month-old infants were in nonparent childcare for part of the day (NICHHD, 2000). The study revealed that positive caregiving occurred when children were in smaller groups, child-adult ratios were low, caregivers did not use an authoritarian style, and the physical environment was safe, clean, and stimulating. Family factors predicted child outcomes even for children who spent many hours in childcare. The family environment appears to have a significantly greater effect on a child's development than the childcare environment (Fitzgerald, Munn, Cabrera, & Wong, 2003).

Physical Contexts

The physical environment surrounds and supports the child's action; it forces the child to adapt his or her actions to meet the demands and constraints of the physical surroundings. As a child perceives the affordances of the environment, he or she learns to act on those affordances, thus expanding a repertoire of actions. At the same time, the child's understanding of how the world responds to his or her actions increases. Gibson (1995) explained how a child's exploration of physical surfaces and objects allows him or her to develop and practice mobility and manipulation skills. Examples of the interactions of a child and his or her physical environments and the developmental consequences are presented in the second part of the chapter.

EXPLANATORY THEORIES OF CHILD DEVELOPMENT OUTCOMES

Humans have the capacity to change across the life span. Although the degree of change is not limitless and is constrained by biologic and contextual factors, human development is believed to have relative *plasticity* (Lerner, Anderson, Balsano, Dowling, & Bobek et al., 2003). This concept has obvious importance to occupational therapists, who provide intervention services designed to change and promote children's performance. Gottlieb (1992) defines plasticity as a fusion of the organism (the child) and the environment (including its cultural, physical, and socioeconomic characteristics). Individual development involves the emergence of new structural (e.g., cellular) and functional components (e.g., body systems). The child's experiences produce new neurologic connections (i.e., new associations) and structural changes (e.g., physical growth), and it is the relationships among components, not the components themselves,

that are most important to development. Acknowledgement of the system's *plasticity* places the focus on the child's potential for change and on the contextual features that promote or limit the child's performance.

The congruence, or *goodness of fit*, between the child and his or her social and physical context determines the quality of development, influencing which occupations are reinforced and which are hindered. *Positive goodness of fit*, meaning that the social and physical environment support the child's skill development, can increase the child's developmental trajectory. Lack of goodness of fit can create disruption of psychologic development and may put the child at risk for behavioral or academic problems.

Chess and Thomas (1984, 1999) asserted that if a child's characteristics provide a good fit (or match) with the demands of a particular setting, adaptive outcomes result. The child's *temperament* is an important determinant in how well a child matches the caregiving environment (Lerner et al., 2003). *Temperament* is an important attribute in the child's social interaction. According to Thomas and Chess (1977), *temperament* refers to the child's behavioral style, and it is believed to be innate and learned. Nine areas of temperament have been identified: (1) activity level, (2) approach or withdrawal, (3) distractibility, (4) intensity of response, (5) attention span and persistence, (6) quality of mood, (7) rhythmicity, (8) threshold of response, and (9) adaptability. Each of these areas contributes uniquely to the child's ability to form social relationships and to respond to the social environment (Thomas & Chess, 1977).

Each of these areas of temperament forms a continuum: extreme temperament levels are associated with problematic behaviors, and moderate levels are related to easy and appropriate behaviors. Children who exhibit extreme temperament characteristics (e.g., those who are highly active, moody, or irritable) have been identified as *difficult*. The difficult child may not fit with the expectations and schedules of caregivers. Others with happy moods and moderate intensity of response are considered *easy*. A child with an easy temperament may be rhythmic and have positive moods and may have a better fit with caregivers. A match of parent and infant temperament can facilitate strong attachment, just as a mismatch can create difficulties in attachment.

To illustrate how temperament affects goodness of fit, children with arrhythmic, poorly regulated sleep/wake cycles were reported to be difficult to manage by European American families in which the parents worked and needed a consistent routine of sleeping patterns. Puerto Rican parents did not have difficulty accommodating children with poorly regulated sleep/wake cycles because they molded their schedules around them and allowed their children to sleep when they wanted. In the Puerto Rican families, the incidence of child behavior problems was very low, particularly before school age when a school schedule was imposed (Lerner et al., 2003). These studies and many others (Chess & Thomas, 1999) suggest that the child's temperament and behavior affect goodness of fit between the caregiver and the child, which in turn influences developmental outcomes.

Developmental outcomes have also been attributed primarily to the child's personality. Research has shown that certain children attain positive developmental outcomes despite a poor caregiving environment. *Resiliency* refers to a child's internal characteristics that enable him or her to thrive and develop despite high-risk factors in the environment. The concept of resiliency emerged from studies of child development in which the context included risk factors known to have negative effects (e.g., child abuse, parental mental illness or substance abuse, socioeconomic hardship) (Werner, 2000). A resilient child has protective factors that enable him or her to develop positive interpersonal skills and general competence despite stressful or traumatic experiences or social environments known to limit developmental potential (e.g., an adolescent, single parent). Resilient infants are characterized as active, affectionate, good natured, and easygoing. *Protective factors* include alertness, the ability to be easily soothed, and social responsiveness (Werner, 2000). Resilient toddlers display many of these characteristics, and in one study were reported to be alert, cheerful, responsive, self-confident, and independent (Werner & Smith, 1992).

A child's *resiliency versus vulnerability* also seems to relate to basic physiologic characteristics. Children with low cardiovascular reactivity and high immune competence cope better with stressful situations and are less vulnerable to illness when stressed (Werner, 2000). In middle childhood, well-developed problem solving and communication skills are important to a child's ability to deal with stress. Resilient boys and girls tend to be reflective rather than impulsive, demonstrate an internal locus of control, and use flexible coping strategies in overcoming adversity (Werner, 2000).

These concepts suggest that in the interpretation of the influence of environmental factors on a child's development, variables internal to the child can overcome negative contextual variables, including those believed to have a profound influence (e.g., poor caregiving). A resilient child does not necessarily have the highest levels of motor and cognitive competence, but this child does have essential social, interaction, and communication skills that enable him or her to engage in positive experiences with others.

Taken together, the theories that explain how children grow and develop into competent adults and full participants in the community suggest that a child's development of occupations must always be understood as a fusion of the child's biologic being and his or her cultural, social, and physical contexts, or as an interaction of these elements.

CHILDREN'S SKILLS, OCCUPATIONS, AND CULTURAL, SOCIAL, AND PHYSICAL CONTEXTS

The following section describes the child's development of motor and process skills through play occupations as defined by his or her cultural, physical, and social contexts. For three age groups—infancy, early childhood, and middle childhood—typical play occupations and activities are described. The individual abilities and contexts that contribute to the development of play occupations are then identified. Although children's occupations are similar within a particular age level, the contexts, individual abilities, and activities are varied and diverse, resulting in a unique occupational performance for each child. The uniqueness of a child's development and how these components relate in individuals are the keys to analysis of the development of occupational performance.

This section of the chapter describes the development of play occupations, acknowledging that it is influenced by cultural, physical, and social contexts. Although the child learns occupations other than play (e.g., those related to school function), occupational therapists most often use play activities to engage the child in the therapeutic process. Play activities serve as the means to improve performance because they are self-motivating and offer goals around which the child can self-organize (Parham & Primeau, 1997). Children put effort and energy into play activities, because they are inherently interesting and fun. (A more detailed description of play as a goal and modality of therapy can be found in Chapter 16.) Descriptions of a child's development of feeding, self-care, and school function are presented in other chapters (Chapters 15 and 22). The contribution of communication abilities is also important to the development of play and other childhood occupations, but it is not discussed in this chapter because language and communication are not primary concerns for occupational therapists.

Infants: Birth to 2 Years
Play Occupations

The play occupations of infants in the first 12 months are exploratory and social; that is, they are related to bonding with caregivers (Boxes 4-1 and 4-2). As in every stage, these occupations overlap (i.e., bonding occurs during exploratory play with the parent's hair and face, and the parent's holding supports the infant's play with objects). Much of the infant's awake and alert time is

BOX 4-1 Development of Play Occupations: Infants— Birth to 6 Months

PLAY OCCUPATIONS
Exploratory Play
Sensorimotor play predominates.

Social Play
Focused on attachment and bonding

PERFORMANCE SKILLS
Fine Motor/Manipulation
Develops accurate reach to object
Uses variety of palmar grasping patterns
Secures object with hand and brings to mouth
Transfers objects hand to hand
Examines objects carefully with eyes
Plays with hands at midline

Gross Motor/Mobility
Lifts head (3 to 4 months) raises trunk when prone (4 to 6 months)
Sits propping on hands
Plays (bounces) when standing with support from parents
Rolls from place to place

Process: Cognitive
Repeats actions for pleasurable experiences
Integrates information from multiple sensory systems

Social/Interaction
Coos, then squeals
Smiles, laughs out loud
Expresses discomfort by crying
Communicates simple emotions through facial expressions

BOX 4-2 Development of Play Occupations: Infants— 6 to 12 Months

PLAY OCCUPATIONS
Exploratory Play
Sensorimotor play evolves into functional play.

Functional Play
Begins to use toys according to their functional purpose

Social Play
Attachment, relating to parents or caregivers

PERFORMANCE SKILLS
Fine Motor/Manipulation
Mouths toys
Uses accurate and direct reach for toys
Plays with toys at midline; transfers hand to hand
Bangs objects together to make sounds
Waves toys in the air
Releases toys into container
Rolls ball to adult
Grasps small objects in fingertips
Points to toys with index finger, uses index finger to explore toys
Crudely uses tool

Gross Motor/Mobility
Sits independently
Rolls from place to place
Independently gets into sitting
Pivots in sitting position
Stands, holding on for support
Plays in standing when leaning on support
Crawls on belly initially, then crawls on all fours (10 months)
Walks with hand held (12 months)

Process: Cognitive
Responds to own name
Recognizes words and family members' names
Responds with appropriate gestures
Listens selectively
Imitates simple gestures
Looks at picture book
Begins to generalize from past experiences
Acts with intention on toys

Social/Interaction
Shows special dependence on mother
Plays contently when parents are in room
Interacts briefly with other infants
Plays give and take

spent in exploratory play, often play that occurs in the caregiver's arms or with the caregiver nearby.

Exploratory play is also called *sensorimotor play*. Rubin (1984) defined *exploratory play* as an activity performed simply for the enjoyment of the physical sensation it creates. It includes repetitive movements to create actions in toys for the sensory experiences of hearing, seeing, and feeling. The infant places toys in his or her mouth, waves them in the air, and explores their surfaces with his or her hands. These actions allow for intense perceptual learning and bring delight to the infant (without any more complex purpose).

In the second year of life, the infant engages in *functional*, or *relational*, *play*; that is, an object's function is understood, and that function determines the action (Boxes 4-3 and 4-4). Initially, children use objects on themselves (e.g., pretending to drink from a cup or to comb the hair). These self-directed actions signal the beginning of *pretend play* (Piaget, 1952). The child knows cause and effect and repeatedly makes the toy telephone ring or the battery-powered doll squeal to enjoy the effect of the initial action.

By the end of the second year, play has expanded in two important ways. First, the child begins to combine actions into play sequences (e.g., he or she relates objects

to each other by stacking one on the other or by lining up toys beside each other). These combined actions show a play purpose that matches the function of the toy. Second, 2-year-old children now direct actions away from themselves. The objects used in play generally resemble real-life objects (Linder, 1993). The child places the doll in a toy bed and then covers it. The child pretends to feed a stuffed animal or drives toy cars through a toy garage. At 2 years of age, play remains a very central occupation of the child, who now has an increased attention span and the ability to combine

BOX 4-3   Development of Play Occupations: Infants— 12 to 18 Months

PLAY OCCUPATIONS
Relational and Functional Play
Engages in simple pretend play directed toward self (pretend eating, sleeping)
Links two or three schemes in simple combinations
Demonstrates imitative play from an immediate model

Gross Motor Play
Explores all spaces in the room
Rolls and crawls in play close to the ground

Social Play
Begins peer interactions
Parallel play

PERFORMANCE SKILLS
Fine Motor/Manipulation
Holds crayon and makes marks; scribbles
Holds two toys in hand and toys in both hands
Releases toys inside containers, even small containers
Stacks blocks and fits toys into form space (places pieces in board)
Attempts puzzles
Opens and shuts toy boxes or containers
Points to pictures with index finger
Uses two hands in play, one to hold or stabilize and one to manipulate

Gross Motor/Mobility
Sits in small chair
Plays in standing
Walks well, squats, picks up toys from the floor
Climbs into adult chair
Flings ball
Pulls toys when walking
Begins to run
Walks upstairs with one hand held
Pushes and pulls large toys or boxes on floor

Process: Cognition
Acts on object using variety of schema
Imitates model
Understands how objects work
Understands function of objects
Uses trial-and-error in problem solving
Recognizes names of various body parts

Social/Interaction
Moves away from parent
Shares toys with parent
Responds to facial expressions of others

BOX 4-4   Development of Play Occupations: Toddlers— 18 to 24 Months

PLAY OCCUPATIONS
Functional Play
Multischeme combinations
Performs multiple related actions together

Pretend or Symbolic Play
Makes inanimate objects perform actions (dolls dancing, eating, hugging)
Pretends that objects are real or symbolize another objects

Social Play
Participates in parallel play
Imitates parents and peers in play
Participates in groups of children
Watches other children
Begins to take turns

Gross Motor Play
Enjoys sensory input of gross motor play

PERFORMANCE SKILLS
Fine Motor/Manipulation
Completes four- to five-piece puzzle
Builds towers (e.g., four blocks)
Holds crayon in fingertips and draws simple figures (straight stroke or circular stroke)
Strings beads
Begins to use simple tools (e.g., play hammer)
Participates in multipart tasks
Turns pages of book

Gross Motor/Mobility
Runs; squats; climbs on furniture
Climbs on jungle gym and slides
Moves on ride-on toy without pedals (kiddy car)
Kicks ball forward
Throws ball at large target
Jumps with both feet (in place)
Walks up and down stairs

Process: Cognitive
Links multiple steps together
Has inanimate object perform action
Begins to use nonrealistic objects in pretend play
Continues to use objects according to functional purpose
Object permanence is completely developed.

Social/Interaction
Expresses affection
Shows wide variety of emotions: fear, anger, sympathy, joy
Can feel frustrated
Enjoys solitary play, such as coloring, building
Laughs when someone does something silly

multiple actions in play. The emergence of *symbolic*, or *imaginary, play* with toys and objects offers the first opportunities for the child to practice the skills of living.

The child also engages in gross motor play throughout the day. As he or she becomes mobile, exploration of space, surfaces, and large action toys becomes a primary occupation. Movement is also enjoyed simply as movement; the child delights in swinging and running or attempting to run and moving in water or sand. Deep proprioceptive pressure and touch are craved and requested. As in exploratory play, the child's exploration of space involves simple, repeated actions in which the goal appears to be sensation. Often extremes in sensation seem to be enjoyed and are frequently requested. Repetition of these full-body kinesthetic, vestibular, and tactile experiences appears to be organizing to the CNS.

In addition, this repetition is important to the child's development of balance, coordination, and motor planning. Hence, the occupational goal of movement and exploration becomes the means for development of multiple performance areas.

In the first year, the goal of an infant's *social play* is attachment, or bonding, to the parent. As described by Greenspan (1990), this is a period in which the infant falls in love with his or her parents and learns to trust the environment because of the care and attention provided by the parents or caregivers. These occupations are critical foundations to later occupations that involve social relating and demonstration of emotions. At 1 year of age, infants play social games with parents and others to elicit responses. Although infants at this age engage readily with individuals other than family, they require their parents' presence as an emotional base and return to them for occasional emotional refueling before returning to play.

By the second year, children exhibit social play in which they imitate adults and peers. Imitation of others is a first way to interact and socially relate (Papalia & Olds, 1995). Both immediate and deferred imitation of others is important to social play as children enter preschool environments and begin to relate to their peers.

Performance Skills

Sensorimotor Skills

The newborn's motor responses contribute to perceptual development and organization. Gross motor activity begins prenatally in response to vestibular and tactile input inside the womb. The first movements of newborns appear to be reflexive; however, on closer examination, they reveal the ability to process and integrate sensory information. The newborn demonstrates orientation and attention to visual, auditory, and tactile stimuli. An important fact is that the newborn also exhibits *habituation*, or the ability to extinguish incoming sensory information (e.g., ability to sleep by blocking out sound in a noisy nursery).

In the first month of life, the infant moves the head side to side when in a prone position and rights the head when supported in sitting. By 4 months, the prone infant lifts the head to visualize activities in the room. This ability to lift and sustain an erect-head position appears to relate to the infant's interest in watching the activities of others, as well as improved trunk strength and stability. As the infant reaches 6 months, he or she demonstrates increased ability to maintain upright posture when in a prone position. The infant can also move side to side on the forearms, then the hands, and can lift an arm to grasp a toy. Over the next 6 months, this dynamic, postural stability prepares the infant to become mobile.

Rolling is normally the infant's first method of becoming mobile and exploring the environment. Initially, rolling is an automatic reaction of body righting; usually the infant first rolls from the stomach to the side and then from the stomach to the back. By 6 months the infant rolls sequentially to progress across the room. Heavy or large babies may initiate rolling several months later, and infants with hypersensitivity of the vestibular system (i.e., overreactivity to rotary movement) may avoid rolling entirely.

Most infants enjoy supported sitting at a very early age. As their vision improves in the first 4 months, they become more eager to view their environment from a supported sitting position. The newborn sits with a rounded back and a head that is erect only momentarily. Head control emerges quickly. By 4 months, the infant can hold the head upright with control for long periods, moving it side to side with ease. Most 6-month-old infants sit alone by propping forward on the arms, using a wide base of support with the legs flexed. However, this position is precarious, and the infant easily topples when tilted. Many 7-month-old infants sit independently. Often their hands are freed for play with toys, but they struggle to reach beyond arm's length.

By 8 to 9 months, the infant sits erect and unsupported for several minutes. At that time, or within the next couple months, the infant may rise from a prone posture by rotating (from a side-lying position) into a sitting position. This important skill gives the infant the ability to progress by creeping to a toy; and then, after arriving at the toy, to sit and play. By 12 months, the infant can rise to sitting from a supine position, rotate and pivot when sitting, and easily move in between positions of sitting and creeping.

After experimenting with pivoting and backward crawling in a prone position, the 7-month-old infant crawls forward. He or she may first attempt belly crawling using both sides of the body together. However, reciprocal arm and leg movements quickly emerge as the most successful method of forward progression. Crawling in a hands-and-knees posture (sometimes called *creeping*) requires more strength and coordination than belly crawling. The two sides of the body move reciprocally. In addition, shoulder and pelvic stability are needed for the infant to hold his or her body weight over the hands and knees. Mature, reciprocal hands-and-knees crawling also requires slight trunk rotation (Figure 4-2). Through the practice of crawling in the second 6 months of life, the child develops trunk flexibility and rotation. Most 10- to 12-month-old infants crawl rapidly across the room, over various surfaces, and even up and down inclines.

Infants at 5 and 6 months delight in standing, and they gleefully bounce up and down while supported by their parents' arms. The strong vestibular input and practice of patterns of hip and knee flexion and extension are important to the development of full upright posture after 1 year. The young infant also prepares for a full

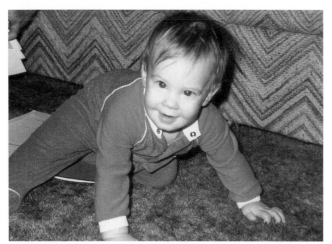

FIGURE 4-2 Crawling allows the child to develop trunk rotation and transitional movements.

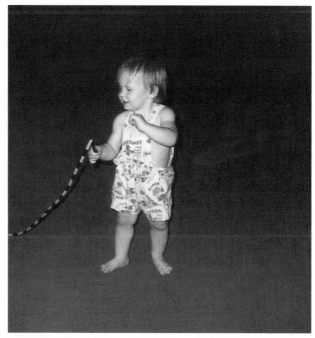

FIGURE 4-3 Infant's first stance is characterized by a wide base and high guard arm position.

upright posture by standing against furniture or the parent's lap. A 10-month-old infant practices rising and lowering in upright postures while holding onto the furniture. By pulling up on furniture to standing, the infant can reach objects previously unavailable. This new level of exploration and increase in potential play objects motivates infants to practice standing and motivates parents to place breakable objects on higher shelves. At 12 months the infant learns to shift the body weight onto one leg and to step to the side with the other leg. The infant soon takes small steps forward while holding onto furniture or the parent's finger.

The infant's first efforts toward unsupported forward movement through walking are often seen in short, erratic steps, a wide-based gait, and arms held in high guard (Figure 4-3). All these postural and mobility skills contribute to the infant's ability to explore space and to obtain desired play objects. By 18 months, the infant prefers walking to other forms of mobility, but balance remains immature, and the infant falls frequently. He or she continues to use a wide-based gait and has difficulty with stopping and turning. Infants remain highly motivated to practice this new skill, however, because walking brings new avenues of exploration and a sense of autonomy, and the parent must now protect the infant from objects that could not previously be reached and from spaces that could not previously be explored.

The newborn moves his or her arms in wide ranges, mostly to the side of the body. In the first 3 months, the infant contacts objects with the eyes more than with the hands. However, the infant soon learns to swipe at objects placed at his or her side. This first pattern of reaching is inaccurate, but by 5 months, the accuracy of reaching toward objects greatly increases. The infant struggles to combine grasp with reach and may make several efforts to grasp an object held at a distance. As postural stability increases, the infant also learns to

control arm and hand movements as a means of exploring objects and materials in the environment. By 6 months, direct unilateral and bilateral reaches are observed, and the infant smoothly and accurately extends his or her arm toward a desired object (von Hofsten, 1993).

Grasp changes dramatically in the first 6 months (Figure 4-4). Initially, grasping occurs automatically (when anything is placed in the hand) and involves mass flexion of the fingers as a unit. The object is held in the palm rather than distally in the fingers or fingertips. Three- to 4-month-old infants, therefore, squeeze objects within their hands, and the thumb does not appear to be involved in this grasp. At 4 to 5 months, the infant exhibits a palmar grasp in which flexed fingers and an adducted thumb press the object against the palm. At 6 months, the infant uses a radial palmar grasping pattern in which the first two fingers hold the object against the thumb. The infant secures small objects using a raking motion of the fingers, with the forearm stabilized on the surface.

Grasp continues to change rapidly between 7 and 12 months (Corbetta & Mounoud, 1990). A radial digital grasp emerges in which the thumb opposes the index and middle finger pads. At approximately 9 months, wrist stability in extension increases, and the infant is better able to use the fingertips in grasping (e.g., the infant can use fingertips to grasp a small object, such as a cube or cracker). A pincer grasp, with which the infant holds small objects between the thumb and finger pads, develops by 10 to 11 months. The 12-month-old infant uses

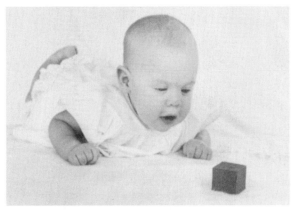

3 months
Looks at cube

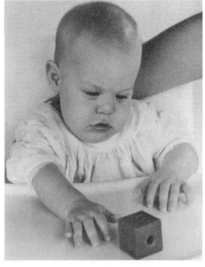

5 months
Looks and approaches

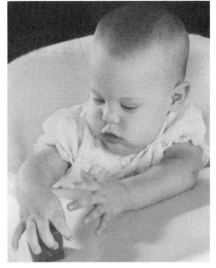

6 months
Looks and crudely grasps with whole hand

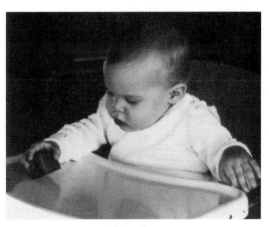

9 months
Looks and deftly grasps with fingers

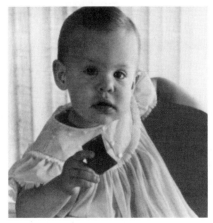

12 months
Looks, grasps with forefinger and thumb,
and deftly releases

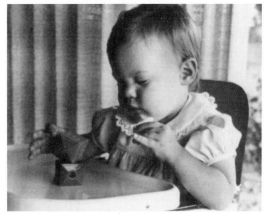

15 months
Looks, grasps, and releases, to build a tower
of two blocks

FIGURE 4-4 Developmental progression of prehensile behavior. (From Ingalls, A.J., & Salerno, M.C. [1983]. *Maternal and child health nursing* [3rd ed.]. St. Louis: Mosby.)

a variety of grasping patterns, often holding an object in the radial fingers and thumb. The infant may also grasp a raisin or piece of cereal with a mature pincer grasp (i.e., one in which the thumb opposes the index finger).

In the second year of life, grasping patterns continue to be refined. The child holds objects distally in the fingers, where holding is more dynamic. By the end of the second year, a tripod grasp on utensils and other tools may be observed. Other grasping patterns may also be used, depending on the size, shape, and weight of the object held. For example, tools are first held in the hand using a palmar grasp and then a digital grasp. Blended grasping patterns develop toward the end of the second year, allowing the child to hold a tool securely in the ulnar digits while the radial digits guide its use.

Voluntary release of objects develops at about 8 months. The first release is awkward and is characterized by full extension of all fingers. The infant becomes interested in dropping objects and practices release by flinging them from the high chair. By 10 months, objects are purposefully released into a container, one of the first ways the infant relates separate objects. As the infant combines objects in play, release becomes important for stacking and accurate placement. For example, the play of 1-year-old children includes placing objects in containers, dumping them out, and then beginning the activity again.

Between 15 and 18 months, the infant demonstrates release of a raisin into a small bottle and the ability to stack two cubes. Stacking blocks is part of play, because the infant now has the needed control of the arm in space, precision grasp without support, controlled release, spatial relations, and depth perception. The infant can also place large, simple puzzle pieces and pegs in the proper areas. At the same time, the infant acquires the ability to discriminate simple forms and shapes. Therefore the infant's learning of perceptual skills is supported by his or her improved manipulative abilities, and increased perceptual discrimination promotes the infant's practice of manipulation (Pehoski, 1995).

The complementary use of both hands to perform a desired task develops between 12 months and 2 years. During this time one hand is used to hold the object while the other hand manipulates or moves the object. In general, the 1-year-old child switches which hand is the "doing" hand and which is the "holding" hand. It is not until the third year that children consistently demonstrate use of two hands in simultaneous, coordinated actions (e.g., using both hands to string beads or button a shirt) (Fagaard, 1990).

Process and Cognition.   In the first 6 months, the infant learns about the body and the effects of its actions. Interests are focused on the actions of objects and the sensory input these actions provide. The infant's learning occurs through the primary senses: looking, tasting, touching, smelling, hearing, and moving. The infant

enjoys repeating actions for their own sake, and play is focused on the action that can be performed with an object (e.g., mouthing, banging, shaking), rather than the object itself (Linder, 1993). By 8 to 9 months, the infant understands object permanence; that is, he knows that an object continues to exist even though it is hidden and cannot be seen (Cohen & Cashon, 2003)

By 12 months, the infant's understanding of the functional purpose of objects increases. Play behaviors are increasingly determined by the purpose of the toy, and toys are used according to their function. The infant also demonstrates more goal-directed behaviors, performing a particular action with the intent of obtaining a specific result or goal. Tools become important at this time, because the infant uses play tools (e.g., hammers, spoons, shovels) to gain further understanding of how objects work.

In the second year, the child can put together a sequence of several actions, such as placing small people in a toy bus and pushing it across the floor. The sequencing of actions indicates increasing memory and attention span. Some of the first sequential behaviors illustrate the child's imitation of adult or sibling actions, therefore increased ability to imitate and increased play sequences appear to develop concurrently (Figure 4-5 A & B).

Interaction and Social Relations.   The infant's emotional transition from the protective, warm womb to the moment of birth is a dramatic change. The primary purpose of the newborn's system is to maintain body functions (i.e., the cardiovascular, respiratory, and gastrointestinal systems). However, as the infant matures, the focus shifts to increasing competence in interaction with the environment. The sense of basic trust or mistrust becomes a main theme in the infant's affective development and is highly dependent on the relationship with the primary caregivers. According to Erikson (1963), the first demonstration of an infant's social trust is observed in the ease with which he or she feeds and sleeps.

The basic trust relationship has varying degrees of involvement. Parent-infant bonding is not endowed but is developed from experiences shared between parent and child over time. These feelings are seen in the progression of physical contact between parent and infant. Klaus and Kennell (1976) discussed the importance of the face-to-face position and eye-to-eye contact between parents and infant as part of the attachment process.

In the second year of life, the parents (or caregivers) remain the most important people in the child's life. Toddlers practice their autonomy around parents, but they have no intention of giving up reliance on them and may become upset or frightened when the parents leave. Two-year-old children are interested in other children, but they tend to watch them rather than verbally or physically interact with them. In a room of open spaces, these children are likely to play next to each other. Their

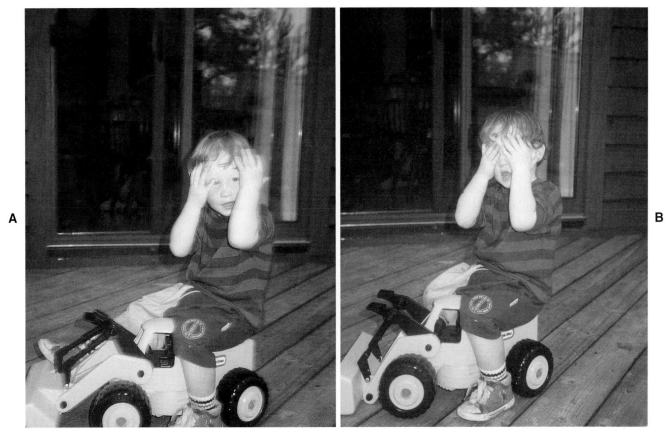

FIGURE 4-5 This 2-year-old boy engages in social play, imitating an adult, sequencing action, taking turns, and demonstrating understanding of object permanence on self (e.g., hiding his eyes).

side-by-side play often involves imitation, with few oral acknowledgments of each other.

Contexts of Infancy

Cultural Contexts

The family's cultural beliefs and values influence caregiving practices and determine many of the child's earliest experiences. The following two examples illustrate specific ways cultural beliefs and values influence an infant's development by influencing feeding and co-sleeping practices. Breast feeding and bottle feeding practices vary in different cultures and ethnic groups. Although practices vary in the United States, European American mothers tend to breast-feed the first 6 months. Mothers often establish a feeding schedule, separating feedings by longer intervals as the infant matures. African American families transition to table food quickly, and infants generally eat only table food by 1 year (Willis, 1998). In contrast, Chinese and Filipino infants are often breast-fed on demand until 2 to $2\frac{1}{2}$ years of age (Chan, 1998a, 1998b). These parents tend to be indulgent, carrying and holding their infants throughout the day, even during naps. When the infants are not held, they are kept nearby and picked up immediately if they cry (Chan,

1998b). In many countries, children are fed certain foods as medicine; that is, to improve health or prevent illness. For example, in the Middle East, infants are given tea and herbal mixtures to prevent or cure illness, and a dietary balance of hot and cold foods is believed to be essential to good health (Sharifzadeh, 1998).

Children around the world are encouraged to self-feed at different ages using different utensils and methods. In India, toddlers learn to use only the right hand to eat. The left hand is dirty and is used only to clean oneself after defecation. As children learn to self-feed, parents often restrain the left hand (Rogoff, 2003). As a result, the right hand develops early advanced skills to manipulate and prehend food without the assistance of the left. These self-feeding practices can contribute to children's rapid maturation of right hand dexterity. Studies of Japanese child have shown higher level fine motor skills compared with American children. The greater fine motor skills of Chinese children have been attributed, in part, to their early use of chopsticks as feeding utensils (Wong, Chan, Wong, & Wong, 2002).

In most U.S. homes, children sleep separated from their parents. For the earliest ages, children are placed in a separate crib and generally a separate room. Middle-class parents believe that infants and toddlers need to learn to sleep independently and to become independent in self-care skills as soon as is possible. In most societies outside the United States, infants sleep with their mothers (Rogoff, 2003). Mayan infants and toddlers sleep in the same room with their parents, often in the mother's bed (Morelli, Rogoff, Oppenheim, & Goldsmith, 1992). Asian and Middle Eastern parents tend to sleep with their infants, because they believe that these sleeping arrangements are important to nurturing and bonding. In some African American and Appalachian families, parents sleep with their infants. Close physical contact at night and then into the day can foster interdependence within families, in contrast to the independence that most U.S. parents often foster in their children.

Physical Contexts. Although many infants have a supplemental play area in a childcare center, the home provides the infant's first play environment. The crib is often a play environment, providing a place for comforting toys (e.g., music boxes and colorful mobiles). Other early play spaces include the playpen, infant seat, or swing. The infant also spends time playing on the floor's carpeted surface or on a blanket. Because the infant is not yet mobile, safety is not as much of a concern as it will be in the next 2 years of life. Early play also occurs in the parent's or caregiver's arms. Exploratory play and attachment occupations are pursued on the parents' laps, and the infant is fascinated by the parents' faces and clothing. At the same time, the infant feels safe and comforted by the parent's presence.

In the second 6 months, the infant requires less support to play, and a major role of the parent becomes one of protector from harm. As the infant becomes more mobile, spaces are closed and objects now within reach are removed. Exploration of all accessible spaces becomes an infant's primary goal.

In the second year of life, the child's environment may expand to the yard, to the neighbors' homes and yards, and to previously unexplored spaces in the home. Most children have opportunities for play in their home's yard or in the fenced-in areas of their childcare centers. Although the child's increasing interest in visiting outdoor spaces provides important opportunities for sensory exploration, it also creates certain safety concerns. Parents therefore invest in gates and other methods of restricting the child's mobility to safe areas.

Early Childhood: Ages 2 to 5 Years
Play Occupations

The three types of play that predominate in early childhood are (1) *dramatic,* or *symbolic, play,* (2) *constructive play,* and (3) *rough-and-tumble,* or *physical, play* (Boxes 4-5 and 4-6). Similar changes are observed in each type of play. First, the child's play becomes more elaborate; that is, the child now combines multiple steps and

---

BOX 4-5 Development of Play Occupations: Preschoolers— 24 to 36 Months

PLAY OCCUPATIONS
Symbolic Play
Links multiple scheme combinations into meaningful sequences of pretend play
Uses objects for multiple pretend ideas
Uses toys to represent animals or people
Plays out drama with stuffed animals or imaginary friends

Constructive Play
Participates in drawing and puzzles
Imitates adults using toys

Gross Motor Play
Likes jumping, rough-and-tumble play
Makes messes

Social Play
Associative, parallel play predominates

PERFORMANCE SKILLS
Fine Motor/Manipulation
Snips with scissors
Traces form, such as a cross
Colors in large forms
Draws circles accurately
Builds towers and lines up objects
Holds crayon with dexterity
Completes puzzles of four to five pieces
Plays with toys with moving parts

Gross Motor/Mobility
Rides tricycle
Catches large ball against chest
Jumps from step or small height
Begins to hop on one foot

Process: Cognitive
Combines actions into entire play scenario (e.g., feeding doll, then dressing in nightwear, then putting to bed)
Shows interest in wearing costumes; creates entire scripts of imaginative play

Social/Interaction
Cooperative play, takes turns at times
Shows interest in peers, enjoys having companions
Begins cooperative play and play in small groups
Shy with strangers, especially adults
Engages in dialog of few words

---

multiple schema. Short play sequences become long scripts involving several characters or actors in a story (Linder, 1993; Knox, 1997). Second, play becomes more social. The preschool-age child orients play toward peers, involving one or two peers in the story and taking turns playing various roles. When preschool-age children play with peers, the interaction appears to be as important as the activity's goal. As the child approaches 5 years of age, all play becomes increasingly social, generally involving a small group of peers (Papalia & Olds, 1995).

Beginning at 2 years of age and continuing through the early childhood years, the child's play is symbolic and

BOX 4-6 Development of Play Occupations: Preschoolers— 3 to 4 Years

PLAY OCCUPATIONS
Complex Imaginary Play
Creates script for play in which pretend objects have actions that reflect roles in real or imaginary life

Construction Play
Creates art product with adult assistance
Works puzzles and blocks

Rough-and-Tumble Play
Enjoys physical play, swinging, sliding at playground, jumping, running

Social Play
Participates in circle time, games, drawing and art time at preschool
Engages in singing and dancing in groups
Associative play: plays with other children, sharing and talking about play goal

PERFORMANCE SKILLS
Fine Motor/Manipulation
Uses precision (tripod) grasp on pencil or crayon
Colors within lines
Copies simple shapes; begins to copy letters
Uses scissors to cut; cuts simple shapes
Constructs three-dimensional design (e.g., three-block bridge)

Gross Motor/Mobility
Jumps, climbs, runs
Begins to skip and to hop
Rides tricycle
Stands briefly on one foot
Alternates feet walking upstairs
Jumps from step with two feet

Process: Cognitive
Uses imaginary objects in play
Has dolls and little men carry out roles and interact with other toys
Categorizes and sorts objects

Social/Interaction
Attempts challenging activities
Prefers play with other children; group play replaces parallel play
Follows turn-taking in discourse and is aware of social aspects of conversation
Shows interest in being a friend
Prefers same sex playmates

imaginative. The child pretends that dolls, figurines, and stuffed animals are real. He or she may also imitate the actions of parents, teachers, and peers. At ages 3 and 4, pretend play becomes more abstract, and objects, such as a block, can be used to represent something else. Pretend play now involves many steps that relate to each other. Children develop scripts as a basis for their play (e.g., one child is the father and one is the mother). They base these scripts on real-life events and play their roles with enthusiasm and imagination, creating their own stories and enjoying the power of their imaginary roles. Their dramatic play is quite complex at this time. However, when they are in small groups, their interaction with their peers seems to be more important than the play goal, and they can easily turn to new activities suggested by one of the group. By 5 years of age, this imaginary play is predominantly social, as small groups of two and three join in cooperative play. About one third of the time, a 5-year-old child engages in pretend play (Rubin, Maioni, & Hornung, 1976). However, this pretend play is based on imitation of real life and dressing up to play certain roles (e.g., firefighter, police officer, ballerina). Although children of this age demonstrate some understanding of adult roles, they erroneously assume that roles are one dimensional (e.g., a firefighter has one role, that of putting out fires). Through pretending, children develop creativity, problem solving, and an understanding of another person's point of view (Singer & Singer, 1990) (Boxes 4-7 and 4-8).

Play that involves building and construction also teaches the child a variety of skills during early childhood. At first these skills are demonstrated in the completion of puzzles and toys with fit-together pieces. However, with mastery of simple pegs and puzzles, the child becomes more creative in construction. For example, the 4-year-old child can develop a plan to build a structure with blocks and then carry out the steps to complete the project. With instructions and a model, the 5-year-old child can make a simple art project or create a three-dimensional design. A 5-year-old child can also put together a 10-piece puzzle. The final product has become more important, and the child is motivated to complete it and show others the final result. The planning and designing involved in building and construction play helps the child acquire an understanding of spatial perception and object relationships. This activity also appears to be foundational to academic performance in school.

Children from 2 to 5 years of age are extremely active and almost always readily engage in rough-and-tumble play. They continue to delight in movement experiences that provide strong sensory input. Activities such as running, hopping, skipping, and tumbling are performed as play without any particular goal. Although rough-and-tumble play generally involves other children, it is generally noncompetitive and rarely organized. Children enjoy this activity for the simple, simultaneous pleasure of movement as they play together.

In associative physical play, children are generally more interested in being with other children than in the goal of the activity. However, it is important to note that some children enjoy primarily social play, whereas others enjoy solitary play. These differences do not relate to ability as much as they relate to preferences and temperament (Papalia & Olds, 1995).

BOX 4-7   Development of Play Occupations: Preschoolers— 4 to 5 Years

PLAY OCCUPATIONS
Games with Rules
Begins group games with simple rules
Engages in organized play with prescribed roles
Participates in an organized gross motor game such as kick ball, "duck, duck, goose"

Construction Play
Takes pride in products
Shows interest in the goal of the art activity
Constructs complex structures

Social Play; Dramatic Play
Participates in role play with other children
Participates in dress up
Tells stories
Continues with pretend play that involves scripts with imaginary characters

PERFORMANCE SKILLS
Fine Motor/Manipulative
Draws using a dynamic tripod grasp
Copies simple shapes
Completes puzzles of up to 10 pieces
Uses scissors to cut out squares and other simple shapes
Colors within the lines
Uses two hands together well, one stabilizing paper or object and other manipulating object
Draws stick figure or may begin to draw trunk and arms
Copies own name
Strings 1/4-inch beads

Gross Motor/Mobility
Jumps down from high step; jumps forward
Throws ball
Hops for long sequences (four to six steps)
Climbs on playground equipment, swinging from arms or legs
Throws ball and hits target
Skips for a long distance
Walks up and down stairs reciprocally

Process: Cognitive
Understands rules to a game
Remembers rules with a few reminders
Makes up stories that involve role playing with other children
Participates in goal-oriented, cooperative play with two or three other children
Participates in planning a play activity
Begins abstract problem solving

Social/Interaction
Enjoys clowning
Sings whole songs
Role plays based on parents' roles

BOX 4-8   Development of Play Occupation: Kindergartners— 5 to 6 Years

PLAY OCCUPATIONS
Games with Rules
Board games
Computer games with rules
Competitive and cooperative games

Dramatic Play
Elaborate imaginary play
Role plays stories and themes related to seasons or occupations
Emphasis is on reality
Reconstructs real world in play

Sports
Participates in ball play

Social Play
Participates in group activities
Organized play in groups
Goal of play (winning) may compete with social interaction at times

PERFORMANCE SKILLS
Fine Motor/Manipulation
Cuts with scissors
Prints name from copy
Copies triangle; traces diamond
Completes puzzles of up to 20 pieces
Traces letters, begins to copy letters
Manipulates tiny objects in fingertips without dropping
Uses two hands together in complementary movements

Gross Motor/Mobility
Hops well for long distances
Skips with good balance
Catches ball with two hands
Kicks with accuracy
Stands on one foot for 8 to 10 seconds

Process: Cognitive
Reasons through simple problems
Bases play more on real life than imaginary world
Participates in organized games
Uses complex scripts in play
Demonstrates deferred imitation

Social/Interaction
Participates in groups of two to four that play in organized, complex games
Has friends (same sex)
Enjoys singing and dancing; reflects meaning of words and music
Demonstrates understanding of others' feelings

Performance Skills

Sensorimotor Skills

Young children are amazingly competent individuals, and their repertoire of motor function leaps forward during the preschool years (see Performance Skills in Boxes 4-6, 4-7, and 4-8). By age 2, the child walks with an increased length of stride and an efficient, well-coordinated, and well-balanced gait. Children do not exhibit true running (characterized by trunk rotation and arm swing) until 3 to 4 years of age, because running requires greater strength and balance than walking. The 4-year-old child demonstrates a walking pattern similar to that of an adult. By 5 to 6 years of age the mature running pattern has developed, and children test their speed by challenging each other to races.

As mobility develops, children gain access to spaces previously unavailable to them. By 2 years of age, a child walks stairs without holding onto a parent's hand, and at $2\frac{1}{2}$ years the child can walk downstairs without support. The $3\frac{1}{2}$-year-old child walks up and down stairs by alternating the feet and without needing to hold onto a rail.

Running and stair climbing become possible, in part, because the child's balance increases. Emerging balance can be observed as the 2-year-old child briefly stands on one foot. By 5 years of age, the child can balance on one foot for several seconds and walk on a curb without falling (Folio & Fewell, 2000). Between 3 and 5 years, the child may successfully attempt to use skates or roller blades (Figure 4-6).

Jumping is first observed in the 2-year-old child. This skill requires strength, coordination, and balance. By 3 years of age the child can jump easily from a step. Hopping requires greater strength and balance than jumping and is first observed at $3\frac{1}{2}$ years. Skipping is the most difficult gross motor pattern, because it requires sequencing of a rhythmic pattern that includes a step and a hop. A coordinated skipping pattern is not observed until 5 years of age (Knobloch & Pasamanick, 1974).

Two-year-old children begin to pedal tricycles and move small riding toys. By 3 years of age they can pedal a tricycle but may run into objects. The 4-year-old child can steer and maneuver the tricycle around obstacles.

By $2\frac{1}{2}$ years most children can catch a 10-inch ball. This pattern of maturity enables the 4-year-old child to catch a much smaller ball successfully, such as a tennis ball (Folio & Fewell, 2000). The first pattern of throwing involves a pushing motion, with the elbow providing the force for the throw. The 4-year-old child demonstrates more forward weight shift with throwing, thereby increasing the force of the ball and the distance thrown. Kicking emerges in the 2- to 3-year-old child, with accurate kicking to a target exhibited by 6 years of age. Ball skills become increasingly important as the child begins participating in organized sports during the primary grades.

Early childhood is a time of rapid improvement in fine motor and manipulation performance. By 4 years of age children learn to move small objects efficiently within one hand (i.e., in-hand manipulation). By 4 years of age a child can hold several small objects in the palm of the hand while moving individual pieces with the radial fingers (Pehoski, 1995). In-hand manipulation indicates that isolated finger movement is well controlled and that the thumb easily moves into opposition for pad-to-pad prehension. These skills also indicate that the child can modulate force and that he or she has an accurate perception of the gentle force needed to handle small objects with the fingertips (Case-Smith & Berry, 1998; Pehoski, 1995).

With efficient in-hand manipulation, the preschool child also learns the functional use of drawing and cutting tools. The preschool child grasps a pencil using a tripod or quadripod grasp (i.e., with the pencil resting between the thumb and first two fingers or between the thumb and first three fingers). At first the child holds the pencil with a static tripod grasp and uses forearm and wrist movement to draw. However, the 5-year-old child develops a mature, dynamic tripod. In this grasp pattern the pencil is held in the tips of the radial fingers and is moved using finger movement. By controlling the pencil using individual finger movements, the child can make letters and small forms.

Drawing skills progress from drawing circles to lines that intersect and cross in a diagonal (e.g., an X). The 5-year-old child can draw a person with multiple and recognizable parts. Drawing is often a strong interest at this age and therefore contributes to the child's imaginative play. He or she can also draw detailed figures created in the imagination (i.e., monsters, fairies, and other fanciful creatures).

The development of scissors skills follows the development of controlled pencil use. The first cutting skill, observed at 3 years, is snipping with alternating full-finger extension and flexion. Between 4 and 6 years, bilateral hand coordination, dexterity, and eye-hand coordination improve, enabling the child to cut out simple shapes. Mature use of scissors is not achieved until 5 to 6 years, because it requires isolated finger

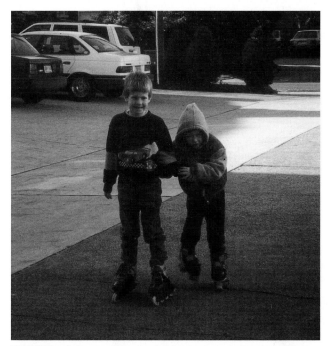

FIGURE 4-6 Preschool children demonstrate sufficient equilibrium for roller skating.

movements, simultaneous hand control, and well-developed eye-hand coordination for cutting accuracy (Folio & Fewell, 2000).

Other fine motor skills acquired during the preschool years are important to the child's constructive and dramatic play. Activities such as putting puzzles together, building towers, stringing small beads, using keys, and cutting out complex designs usually require dexterity, bilateral coordination, and motor planning.

Process and Cognition.   Preschool-age children create symbolic representations of real life objects and events during play. In addition, they begin to plan pretend scenarios in advance, organizing who and what are needed to complete the activity. Play becomes an elaborate sequence of events that is remembered, acted out, and later described for others. For example, the child may act out the role of an adult, imitating action remembered from an earlier experience. This form of role play demonstrates the child's understanding of how roles relate to actions and how actions relate to each other (e.g., the child may role play a grocery store clerk, displaying items for sale, taking money from the customer, and placing the money in a toy cash register).

Abstract thinking begins in the preschool years as the child pretends that an object is something else. For example, the child may pretend a block is a doll bed; later the same block may become a telephone receiver or a train car.

The motor skills noted in early childhood also reflect cognitive skills. To construct a three-dimensional building, the child must have the ability to discriminate size and shape. Building in three dimensions also requires spatial understanding and problem-solving skills. When building from a set of blocks, the child usually must first categorize and organize the blocks. Next, the child must solve the problem of how to fit them together to replicate a model or create the imagined structure.

In a similar way, the emergence of drawing skills reflects both cognitive abilities and fine motor skills. The 3-year-old child makes crude attempts to represent people and objects in drawings. By 4 years of age a child can draw a recognizable person, demonstrating the ability to select salient features and represent them on a two-dimensional surface. The 4-year-old child not only identifies the parts of a person but also relates them correctly, although the size of the parts is rarely proportional to real life. At 5 years the child's drawing is more refined, more realistic, and better proportioned. By this age, pictures begin to tell stories and reflect the child's emotions (Linder, 1993).

Interaction and Social Relations.   In early childhood, interaction and play with peers take on increasing importance. Children become social beings and identify themselves as individuals (i.e., separate from parents). Erikson (1963) defined the first psychosocial phase of early childhood as *autonomy versus shame and doubt.*

Autonomy dominates the psychosocial development from 2 to 4 years. The child is adamant about making personal decisions. The development of trust in the environment and improvements in language bring forth control over self, strengthening the child's autonomous nature.

The discovery of the body and how to control it promotes independence in self-care. Success in acting independently instills a sense of confidence and self-control. However, the negative side of autonomy is a sense of shame or doubt. This feeling comes when the child acts independently and is told that he or she has done something wrong (i.e., misbehaved). The child needs to learn which independent actions meet the approval of adults.

Erikson described the latter part of early childhood as a period of *initiative versus guilt.* Children need to achieve a balance between initiative to act independently and the responsibility they feel for their own actions. Children 4 to 5 years old explore beyond the environment, discovering new activities. They seek new experiences for the pleasure of learning about the environment and for the opportunities they offer for exploration. If the child's learning experiences are successful and effective and his or her actions meet parental approval, a sense of initiative is developed. Through these activities the child learns to question, reason, and find solutions to problems.

Adult-child relationships and early home experiences also influence later peer relations. According to research, children whose attachments to their mothers are rated as secure tend to be more responsive to other children in childcare settings. They are also more curious and competent (Jacobson & Wille, 1986; Youngblade & Belsky, 1992). Peer play becomes an important avenue for the child's development of social and cognitive abilities.

The development of autonomy provides a foundation for the child's imagination. Now the young child explores the world not only through the use of his or her senses but also by thinking and reasoning. Although play can be reality based, it usually includes fantasy, wishes, and role play. Words, rhymes, and songs also complement this type of play (Figure 4-7).

Contexts

Cultural and Social Contexts

The social roles of young children vary across cultures. In the United States, the importance of interaction with peers is stressed at young ages. Most American children begin to interact with their peers (same age group) at about 3 years of age. Same-age peers become increasingly important through elementary school and dominate the social life of a teenager. In the United States and much of the world, children are grouped exclusively by age. These age groupings may provide more

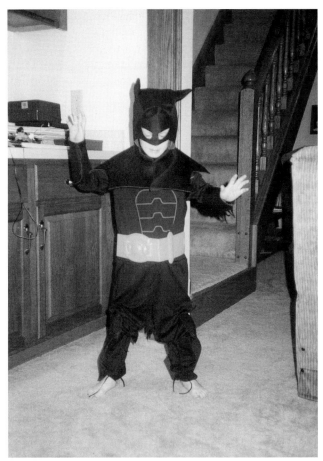

FIGURE 4-7 Three- and 4-year-old children love dressing in costumes and spending hours in the character suggested by those costumes.

opportunities for play, but they also diminish opportunities for older children to teach and nurture younger children. Younger children have fewer opportunities to imitate older children. Children in other parts of the world play and socialize with people of different ages. For example, in Mayan communities, children spend almost all of their time with siblings and other young relatives of a wide range of ages (Bazyk et al., 2003). In Polynesia, children remain with family members, including extended family. They socially participate in mixed age groups, playing "on the edge" and watching intently until they can join in the play. In Mexican families, toddlers play with children of various ages. Often they play with older siblings. This "enduring social network" remains in place over time to care for, teach, and discipline children to adulthood (Rogoff, 2003).

When children spend days with a variety of ages, they have many opportunities to imitate and learn from older children and adults. Caring friendships are developed with family and friends of various ages and of varying relationships. Interaction with children of varying ages

provides children the opportunity to practice teaching and nurturance with young children and to imitate older children (Whiting & Edwards, 1988). In contrast, the age-based groupings used in U.S. childcare centers and preschools reduce children's opportunities to learn from engaging with younger (and older) children.

At very young ages, Mayan children play within their parents' work activities (Bazyk et al., 2003). For example, children engage in play activities while helping their mothers wash clothes. The children's play in the Mayan culture was tolerated during daily work activities but was not specifically encouraged (Bazyk et al., 2003). These researchers found that children's work was playful, blurring the European American distinction between work and play. When children play in work activities, they are learning skills that will serve them well in adulthood. These natural occurrences in Mayan communities stand in contrast to U.S. customs, in which imitation and pretend playing of adult roles is orchestrated in groups of preschoolers in childcare centers. American parents specifically design and encourage their children's play, at times becoming playmates with children. Most parents in the United States believe that play is important to their children's development, therefore they create opportunities for play time and encourage play skills (Rogoff, 2003).

Physical Contexts. By the age of 5, a child's outdoor environment has expanded beyond the areas around the home and childcare center. A variety of outdoor environments offer space for rough-and-tumble play, and expanded social and physical environments give the child new opportunities for learning (and generalizing) the skills he or she has achieved. Although adult supervision remains essential, the entire neighborhood may become the child's playground.

The availability of new indoor environments is also to be expected. Preschool classrooms usually have centers for different types of activities (e.g., creating art, listening to stories, playing games). In addition, community groups often sponsor a variety of indoor activities (e.g., preschool gymnastics, organized play programs) in which the child can take part.

Expanded environments offer children the opportunity to adapt play skills learned at home to the constraints of new spaces. For example, the child who climbs and slides down the stairs at home learns to climb a 6-foot ladder and slide down the slide in the neighborhood park. Parks and playgrounds also provide the child with new surfaces that challenge balance and equipment that offers intense vestibular experiences.

Cultural and socioeconomic differences can influence a child's physical environment. Inner city parents frequently confine their children to the immediate household and forbid them to go outside after school, particularly to play. These protective strategies limit children's exposure to dangerous neighborhood influences,

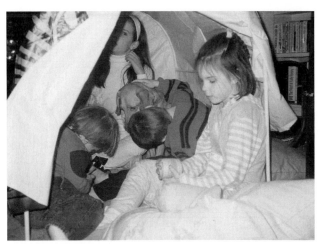

FIGURE 4-8 Pup tents become a haven for quiet play.

but they also severely restrict the physical context available for play (Garcia Coll & Magnuson, 2000).

Most preschool-age children also enjoy spending time in quiet spaces. Children, especially those who demonstrate overreactivity to sensory input, may feel drawn to quiet, enclosed spaces (e.g., a space behind the couch, the safe haven of their bedrooms, a small tent in the corner of the playroom) (Figure 4-8). Quiet spaces can be organizing and calming after a day in a childcare center. Other children who may have underreacting sensory systems may seek stimulating environments that are full of activity, or they may create their own high activity in an otherwise quiet space.

When placed in new environments, children often respond by instinctively exploring the new spaces (e.g., hallways, cupboards, corners, furniture). Exploring the features of an environment can help orient children to the spaces that surround them, can promote perceptual learning, and can provide an understanding of the play possibilities in that environment.

Middle Childhood: Ages 6 to 10 Years
Play Occupations

Although 6-year-old children continue to enjoy imaginative play, they begin increasingly to structure and organize their play. By 7 and 8 years of age, structured games and organized play predominate (Box 4-9). *Games with rules* are the primary mode for physical and social play. Groups of children organize themselves, assign roles, and explain (or create) rules to guide the game they plan to play. The goal of the game now competes with the reward of interacting with peers, and children become fascinated with the rules that govern the games they play.

At 7 and 8 years of age, children do not understand that rules apply equally to everyone involved in the game, and they are often unable to place the rules of the

---

BOX 4-9 Development of Play Occupations: Middle Childhood—6 to 10 Years

PLAY OCCUPATIONS
Games with Rules
Computer games, card games that require problems solving and abstract thinking

Crafts and Hobbies
Has collections
May have hobbies

Organized Sports
Cooperative and competitive play in groups/teams of children
Winning and skills are emphasized.

Social Play
Play includes talking and joking
Peer play predominates at school and home.

PERFORMANCE SKILLS
Fine Motor/Manipulation
Good dexterity for crafts and construction with small objects
Bilateral coordination for building complex structure
Precision and motor planning evident in drawing
Motor planning evident in completion of complex puzzles

Gross Motor/Mobility
Runs with speed and endurance
Jumps, hops, skips
Throws ball well at long distances
Catches ball with accuracy

Process: Cognitive
Abstract reasoning
Performs mental operations without need to physically try
Demonstrates flexible problem solving
Solves complex problems

Social/Interaction
Cooperative, less egocentric
Tries to please others
Has best friend
Is part of cliques
Is less impulsive, able to regulate behavior
Has competitive relationships

---

game above the personal need to win (Florey & Greene, 1997). However, breaking the rules may incur the criticism of peers, who also acknowledge the importance of rules at this time. By 9 and 10 years of age, children are more conscientious about obeying rules.

By 8 and 9 years, children become interested in sports, and parents are generally supportive of sports activities. Although a form of play, organized sports can assume a serious nature (i.e., intrinsic motivation and the internal sense of control are overridden by the external demands of practice and serious competition with peers).

Interest in creating craft and art projects continues in middle childhood. During this time, the child shows an increased ability to organize, to solve problems, and to create from abstract materials. However, the completion of craft and art projects continues to require the support of adults to organize materials and identify steps. The final product, which is relatively unimportant to younger children, is now valued.

In middle childhood, children play in cooperative groups and value interaction with their peers. When friends come together, almost all activity is play and fun. Simply talking and joking become playful and entertaining. Children spend more than 40% of their waking hours with peers (Cole & Cole, 1989). In these peer groups, children learn to cooperate but also to compete (Florey & Greene, 1997). They are now interested in *achievement* through play; they recognize and accept an outside standard for success or failure and criteria for winning or losing. With competition in play comes risk taking and strategic thinking. Children who compete in sports and other activities exhibit courage to perform against an outside standard (Reilly, 1974).

Performance Skills

Sensorimotor Skills

During the elementary school years, motor development continues to focus on the refining of previously acquired skills. With this refinement, hours of repetition of activities to attain mastery of common interests are observed. Children ride bicycles, scale fences, swim, skate, and jump rope (Knobloch & Pasamanick, 1974; Stone & Church, 1973) (Figure 4-9). Although motor capabilities are highly varied for this age group, balance and coordination improve throughout the middle childhood years, providing children with the agility to dance and play sports with proficiency. Research indicates that children who master physical skills tend to exhibit high self-esteem (Short-DeGraff, 1988). Not only does self-esteem improve as children master physical skills, but peer acceptance improves as well.

Performance of fine motor skills in middle childhood includes efficient tool use (e.g., scissors, tweezers) and precise drawing skills. Children handle and manipulate materials (fold, sort, adhere, cut) with competency. The drawing skills of 8- and 9-year-old children demonstrate appropriate proportions and accuracy, and handwriting skills improve in speed and accuracy as children learn manuscript and then cursive writing. These improvements provide evidence of increased dexterity and coordination. Construction skills, manipulation, and abilities to use tools continue to generalize across performance areas with increases in speed, strength, and precision.

Process and Cognition. In middle childhood, concepts and relationships in the physical world are understood and applied. The child relates past events to future plans and comprehends how situations change over time. Thinking has become more flexible and abstract. The child has become a reasoning individual who can solve problems by understanding variables and weighing pertinent factors before making decisions.

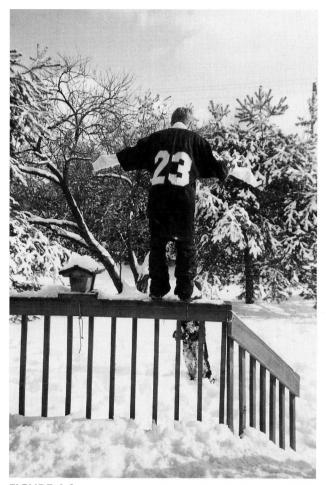

FIGURE 4-9 Balance is excellent in 9- and 10-year-old children, who skillfully conquer icy railings.

In the past, children could apply only one solution, and they often were stuck when the solution of choice did not work. By 8 and 9 years of age, however, they recognize that different solutions can be tried, and they arrive at answers through abstract reasoning rather than through concrete trial and error. At this age, children can also pay attention to more than one physical characteristic at a time and can systematically put elements together (Papalia & Olds, 1995).

In play, children order objects by size or shape, demonstrating the ability to discriminate perceptual aspects of objects and to order them accurately. They also understand the relationship of the whole to the parts, and they imagine pieces as parts of a whole. Children at 9 and 10 years of age can give instructions to others and tell stories in detail.

By middle childhood, children learn to combine tasks and routines into complex games and competitive sports. Because a number of rules are needed to play sports, such as baseball or hockey, the child understands the need to combine the rules into a complete game. To participate in the activity successfully, he or she also understands when rules apply and how they relate to each other.

Interaction and Social Relations. Children in middle childhood focus on meeting challenges in themselves as well as challenges presented by others. Children appreciate the recognition that comes with successful completion of assignments or projects. Comparison with peers is increasingly important during this time. If a child's schoolwork is compared with the work of a more successful student, a negative evaluation can reduce his or her sense of mastery and may produce feelings of inferiority.

School-age children seek independence of identity. They are not as egocentric as young children and demonstrate a more objective view of themselves. Children at this age have a definite subculture, or clique, that includes only certain friends (Papalia & Olds, 1995). At this age, children are quick to criticize those who do not conform to the group esthetic. Therefore rejection by the child's peers may result from a lack of conformity in dress or physical appearance. Children who are rarely praised by their peers, who have difficulty communicating, or who do not know how to initiate relationships are less likely to have close friendships.

During middle childhood, children become disinterested in adults, including their parents. The values of peers become significantly more important than those of adults. Data indicate that children between 7 and 10 years of age are highly compliant with and easily shift in the direction of their peers (Costanzo & Shaw, 1966).

The child's progression from games with some structure and flexible rules to highly competitive games demonstrates progression in moral development. Early in the child's thinking (before 7 years of age), rules are viewed as absolute, sacred, and unchangeable. Children 7 to 10 years old recognize that rules come from someone in authority, and they accept what this authority says. However, late in the elementary school years, children cast aside their beliefs in the absolute infallibility of rules, because they have gained the knowledge that people are the creators of rules. Questioning of the rules and the authority who makes them begins at this age (Florey & Greene, 1997).

Contexts

Cultural Contexts

European American young children rarely participate in work roles. Chores are rarely given to children under 8 or 9 years of age. Many American families do not expect children to take responsibility for chores until the age of 10 or 11. In contrast, Polynesian children develop household skills by 3 or 4 years, at which time they gather wood, sweep, or run errands to the store. In West Africa, children have duties and run errands when they are 3 years old. In Kenya, 8-year-old girls perform most of the housework (Rogoff, 2003). In countries other than the United States and Europe, the typical age for children to assume work responsibilities is 5 to 7 years. In a study of 50 communities, children at 5 to 7 years are given responsibility for caring for younger children, for tending animals, and for carrying out household chores (Rogoff et al., 1975).

Mayan children are continuously at their parents' side during work days. At early ages, they participate in work tasks, such as running errands and helping with cleanup. Bazyk et al. (2003) found that although Mayan children began work activities at a very early age, they embedded play in these chores. Children in Central Africa acquire work experience from toddler age, and by age 12 they can kill game, make medicines, trap animals, and garden (Rogoff, 2003). Ogunnaike and Houser (2002) examined the effects of participation in work activities and errands on cognitive performance in young Yoruban children. In Yoruba, young children are taught to be helpful, responsible, and respectful. Before age 5, Yoruban girls are taught how to perform household chores, such as washing, sweeping, cooking, and caring for younger siblings. By middle childhood, the girls take full responsibility for these work roles. The number of errands a child was required to run and cognitive performance were significantly related, and the results of this study seemed to indicate that having children run errands and participate in work tasks at an early age enhances cognitive competence (Ogunnaike & Houser, 2002).

In the United States, most children and youth have very few opportunities to work with adults. Rogoff (2003) believes that American children are missing valuable opportunities for learning and gaining self-satisfaction. Compared with practices in societies outside the United States, the lack of work opportunities for American children limits their practice of skills important to their future and may delay their entry into adult work roles.

Physical Contexts

In middle childhood the child's play environment is now large and complex; more activities take place in the neighborhood and at school. The school's playground supports both social and physical play of small groups (or pairs) of children. Play occurs on ball fields and in community centers, amusement parks, and sports arenas. Organized activities often are sponsored by churches or by groups such as the Young Men's Christian Association (YMCA). By middle childhood, children have the mobility skills to maneuver through all environments (e.g., rough terrain, busy city streets). The society of school-age children dominates neighborhood streets and backyards, with bicycle races and spontaneous street hockey games. These children explore the woods and go on adventures in nearby parks to find areas unexplored by others. Although supervision by adults is still needed at times, intermittent supervision usually suffices.

SUMMARY

A child's development of occupational performance is influenced by many systems and variables in the individual and in the environment. The individual patterns observed in children provide insight into how and why a child follows a certain developmental trajectory. Sensorimotor, cognitive, and social interaction skills support the child's performance in play occupations. At the same time, a child's activities are highly influenced by his or her cultural, social, and physical contexts. As an essential occupation of childhood, play provides a means of understanding and appreciating a child's performance. A child's play reveals the complexities of individual, activity, and environmental interaction. This interaction is the essence of a child's development of occupations.

STUDY QUESTIONS

1 Apply the stages of learning to a child's development of the pencil grasp for writing.
2 Describe the development of social play for a child from age 2 to 6 years. Explain how an occupational therapist would use this information when designing an intervention plan.
3 Compare a sensorimotor play activity appropriate for 2-year-old to one appropriate for a 5-year-old. How do these activities differ?
4 Two 4-year-old children are playing house; one is the father and one is the mother. They have decided to have a play dinner that they will make in their play kitchen. At this time, they are setting the table using play silverware and plates from the small kitchen's cupboard. Analyze this play activity by identifying the motor, sensory, cognitive, and interactive abilities needed to set the table for a play dinner. List cultural, social, and physical variables that may affect the children's performance of this activity.

REFERENCES

Adolf, K.E., Eppler, M.A., & Gibson, E.J. (1993). Development of perception of affordances. In C. Rovee-Collier & L.P. Lipsitt (Eds.), *Advances in infancy research* (Vol. 8, pp. 51-98). Norwood, NJ: Ablex.

Bayley, N. (1993). *Bayley Scales of Infant Development* (rev. ed.). San Antonio: Psychological Corporation.

Bazyk, S., Stalnaker, D., Llerena, M., Ekelman, B., & Bazyk, J. (2003). Play in Mayan children. *American Journal of Occupational Therapy, 57,* 273-283.

Bushnell & Boudreau. (1993). Motor development and the mind: the potential role of motor abilities as a determinant of aspects of perceptual development. *Child Development 64(4):* 1005–1021.

Case-Smith, J., & Berry, J. (1998). Preschool hand skills. In J. Case-Smith (Ed.), *Making a difference in school based practice* (pp. 1-45). Bethesda, MD: American Occupational Therapy Association (AOTA).

Chan, S. (1998a). Families with Asian roots. In E.W. Lynch & M.J. Hanson (Eds.), *Developing cross-cultural competence* (2nd ed., pp. 251-354). Baltimore: Brookes.

Chan, S. (1998b). Families with Filipino roots. In E.W. Lynch & M.J. Hanson (Eds.), *Developing cross-cultural competence* (2nd ed., pp. 355-408). Baltimore: Brookes.

Chess, S., & Thomas, A. (1984). *The origins and evolution of behavior disorders: Infancy to early adult life.* New York: Brunner/Mazel.

Chess, S., & Thomas, A. (1999). *Goodness of fit: Clinical applications from infancy through adult life.* New York: Brunner/Mazel.

Cioni, G., Ferrari, F., Einspieler, C., Paolicelli, P., Barbiani, T., & Prechtl, H.F. (1997). Comparison between the observation of spontaneous movements and neurologic examination in preterm infants. *Journal of Pediatrics, 130,* 704-711.

Clark, J. (1997). A dynamical systems perspective on the development of complex adaptive skill. In C. Dent-Read & P. Zukow-Goldring (Eds.), *Evolving explanations of development: Ecological approaches to organisms-environment systems.* Washington, DC: American Psychological Association.

Cohen, L.B., & Cashon, C.H. (2003). Infant perception and cognition. In R.M. Lerner, M.A. Easterbrooks, & J. Mistry (Eds.), *Handbook of psychology: Vol. 6. Developmental psychology* (pp. 65-90). New York: John Wiley & Sons.

Cole, M., & Cole, S. (1989). *The development of children.* New York: Scientific American Books.

Connolly, K.J., & Dalgleish, M. (1993). Individual patterns of tool use by infants. In A.F. Kalverboer, B. Hopkins, & R. Geuze (Eds.), *Motor development in early and later childhood: Longitudinal approaches* (pp. 174-204). Cambridge: Cambridge University Press.

Corbetta, D., & Mounoud, P. (1990). Early development of grasping and manipulation. In C. Bard, M. Fleury, & L. Hay (Eds.), *Development of eye-hand coordination across the life span.* Columbia: University of South Carolina Press.

Cornhill, H., & Case-Smith, J. (1996). Factors that relate to good and poor handwriting. *American Journal of Occupational Therapy, 50,* 732-739.

Costanzo, P.R., & Shaw, M.E. (1966). Conformity as a function of age level. *Child Development, 37,* 967-975.

Csikszentmihalyi, M., & Rathunde, K. (1998). The development of the person: An experiential perspective on the ontogenesis of psychological complexity. In W. Damon (Series Ed.) & R.M. Lerner (Vol. Ed.), *Handbook of child psychology: Vol 1. Theoretical models of human development* (5th ed., pp. 635-684). New York: John Wiley & Sons.

Easterbrooks, M.A., & Biringen, Z. (2000). Mapping the terrain of emotional availability and attachment. *Attachment and Human Development, 2,* 123-129.

Ellison, P.H. (1994). *The INFANIB: A reliable method for the neuromotor assessment of infants.* Tucson: Therapy Skill Builders.

Erikson, E.H. (1963). *Childhood and society* (2nd ed.). New York: W.W. Norton.

Fagaard, J. (1990). The development of bimanual coordination. In C. Bard, M. Fleury, & L. Hay (Eds.), *Development of eye-hand coordination across the life span*. Columbia: University of South Carolina Press.

Fitzgerald, H., Munn, T., Cabrera, N., & Wong, M.M. (2003). Diversity in caregiving contexts. In R.M. Lerner, M.A. Easterbrooks, & J. Mistry (Eds), *Handbook of psychology: Vol 6. Developmental psychology* (pp. 135-169). New York: John Wiley & Sons.

Florey, L.L., & Greene, S. (1997). Play in middle childhood: A focus on children with behavior and emotional disorders. In L.D. Parham & L. Primeau (Eds.), *Play in occupational therapy for children* (pp. 26-143). St. Louis: Mosby.

Folio, M.R., & Fewell, R.R. (2000). *Peabody Developmental Motor Scales* (rev. ed.). Austin: Pro-Ed.

Garcia Coll, C., & Magnuson, K. (2000). Cultural differences as sources of developmental vulnerabilities and resources. In J.P. Shonkoff & S.J. Meisels (Eds.), *Handbook of early childhood intervention* (2nd ed., pp. 94-114). Cambridge: Cambridge University Press.

Gesell, A. (1945). *The embryology of behavior: The beginnings of the human mind*. New York: Harper & Brothers.

Gesell, A., & Amatruda, G. (1947). *Developmental diagnosis* (2nd ed.). New York: Harper & Row.

Gesell, A., Halverson, H.M., Thompson, H., Ilg, F.L., Castner, B.M., Ames, L.B., et al. (1940). *The first five years of life*. New York: Harper & Row.

Gibson, E.J. (1997). An ecological psychologist's prolegomena for perceptual development: A functional approach. In C. Dent-Read & P. Zukow-Goldring (Eds.), *Evolving explanations of development: Ecological approaches to organisms-environment systems*. Washington, DC: American Psychological Association.

Gibson, J.J. (1979). *The ecological approach to visual perception*. Boston: Houghton-Mifflin.

Gibson, J.J. (1995). Exploratory behavior in the development of perceiving, acting, and the acquiring of knowledge. In L.P. Lipsitt & C. Rovee-Collier (Eds), *Advances in infancy* (pp. xxi-lxi). Norwood, NJ: Ablex.

Gilfolye, E., Grady, A., & Moore, J. (1990). *Children adapt* (2nd ed.). Thorofare, NJ: Slack.

Gottlieb, G. (1997). *Synthesizing nature-nurture: Prenatal roots of instinctive behavior*. Hillsdale, NJ: Erlbaum.

Granott, N. (2002). How microdevelopment creates macrodevelopment: Reiterated sequences, backward transitions, and the zone of current development. In N. Granott & J. Parziale (Eds.), *Microdevelopment: Transition processes in development and learning* (pp. 213-242). Cambridge: Cambridge University Press.

Greenspan, G. (1990). *Infancy and early childhood: The practice of clinical assessment and intervention with emotional and developmental challenges*. New York: International Universities Press.

Greer, T., & Lockman, J.J. (1998). Using writing instruments: Invariances in young children and adults. *Child Development, 69*, 888-902.

Illingworth, R.S. (1966). The diagnosis of cerebral palsy in the first year of life. *Developmental Medicine and Child Neurology, 8*, 178-194.

Illingworth, R.S. (1984). *The development of the infant and young child*. Edinburgh: Churchill Livingstone.

Jacobson, S.L., & Wille, D.E. (1986). The influence of attachment pattern on developmental changes in peer interaction from the child to the preschool period. *Child Development, 57*, 338-347.

Klaus, M.H., & Kennell, J.H. (1976). *Maternal-infant bonding*. St. Louis: Mosby.

Knobloch, H., & Pasamanick, B. (1974). *Gesell & Amatruda's developmental diagnosis* (3rd ed.). New York: Harper & Row.

Knox, S. (1997). Development and current use of the Knox Preschool Play Scale. In L.D. Parham & L. Primeau (Eds.), *Play in occupational therapy for children* (pp. 35-51). St. Louis: Mosby.

Lerner, R.M., Anderson, P.M., Balsano, A.B., Dowling, E.M., & Bobek, D.L. (2003). In R.M. Lerner, M.A. Easterbrooks, & J. Mistry (Eds.), *Handbook of psychology: Vol. 6. Developmental psychology* (pp. 535-558). New York: John Wiley & Sons.

Linder, T. (1993). *Transdisciplinary play-based assessment* (rev. ed.). Baltimore: Brookes.

Mandler, J.M. (1990). A new perspective on cognitive development in infancy. *American Scientist, 78*, 236-243.

Matas, L., Arend, R.A., & Sroufe, L.A. (1978). Continuity and adaptation in the second year: The relationship between quality of attachment and later competence. *Child Development, 49*, 547-556.

Mathiowetz, V., & Haugen, J. (1994). Motor behavior research: Implications for therapeutic approaches to central nervous system dysfunction. *American Journal of Occupational Therapy, 48*, 733-745.

Mathiowetz, V., & Haugen, J. (1995). Evaluation of motor behavior: Traditional and contemporary views. In C.A. Trombly (Ed.), *Occupational therapy for physical dysfunction* (4th ed., pp. 157-186). Baltimore: Williams & Wilkins.

McCarty, M.E., Clifton, R.K., & Collard, R.R. (2001). The beginnings of tool use by infants and toddlers. *Infancy, 2* (2), 233-256.

McGraw, M. (1945). *The neuromuscular maturation of the human infant*. New York: Macmillan.

Metzoff, A.N., & Moore, M.K. (1992). Early imitation within a functional framework: The importance of person identity, movement, and development. *Infant Behavior and Development, 15*, 470-505.

Milani-Comparetti, A., & Gidoni, E.A. (1967). Pattern analysis of motor development and its disorders. *Developmental Medicine and Child Neurology, 9*, 625-630.

Morelli, G.A., Rogoff, B., Oppenheim, D., & Goldsmith, D. (1992). Cultural variation in infants' sleeping arrangements: Questions of independence. *Developmental Psychology, 28*, 604-613.

National Institute of Child Health and Human Development (NICHHD), Early Child Care Research Network. (2000). Characteristics and quality of child care for toddlers and preschoolers. *Applied Development Science, 4* (3), 116-135.

Ogunnaike, O.A., & Houser, R.F. (2002). Yoruba toddlers' engagement in errands and cognitive performance on the Yoruba Mental Subscale. *International Journal of Behavioral Development, 26* (2), 145-153.

Papalia, D.E., & Olds, S.W. (1995). Human development (6th ed.). New York: McGraw-Hill.

Parham, L.D., & Primeau, L. (1997). Play and occupational therapy. In L.D. Parham & L. Fazio (Eds.), *Play in occupational therapy for children* (pp. 2-22). St. Louis: Mosby.

Pehoski, C. (1995). Object manipulation in infants and children. In A. Henderson & C. Pehoski (Eds.), *Hand function in the child* (pp. 136-153). St. Louis: Mosby.

Piaget, J. (1952). *The origins of intelligence in children* (M. Cook, Trans.) New York: International Universities Press.

Piper, M.C., & Darrah, J. (1994). *Motor assessment of the developing infant.* Philadelphia: W.B. Saunders.

Reilly, M. (Ed.). (1974). *Play as exploratory learning.* Beverly Hills, CA: Sage Publications.

Rochat, P. (1989). Object manipulation and exploration in 2- to 5-month-old infants. *Developmental Psychology, 25,* 871-884.

Rochat, P., & Gibson, E.J. (1985). Early mouthing and grasping: Development and cross-modal responsiveness to soft and rigid objects in young infants. *Canadian Psychology, 26* (2), 452.

Rogoff, B. (2003). *The cultural nature of human development.* New York: Oxford University Press.

Rogoff, B., Mosier, C., Mistry, J., & Goncu, A. (1993). Guided participation in cultural activity by toddlers and caregivers. *Monographs of the Society for Research in Child Development, 58* (8), 1-179.

Rogoff, B., Selless, M.J., Pinotta, S., Fox, N., & White, S.H. (1975). Age of assignment of roles and responsibilities to children: A cross-cultural survey. *Human Development, 18,* 353-369.

Rubin, K. (1984). *The Play Observation Scale.* Ontario, Canada: University of Waterloo.

Rubin, K., Maioni, T.L., & Hornung, M. (1976). Free play behaviors in middle-class and lower-class children: Parten and Piaget revisited. *Child Development, 47,* 414-419.

Ruff, H.A. (1989). The infant's use of visual and haptic information in the perception and recognition of objects. *Canadian Journal of Psychology, 43,* 302-319.

Sharifzadeh, V.S. (1998). Families with Middle Eastern roots. In. E.W. Lynch & M.J. Hanson (Eds.), *Developing cross-cultural competence* (2nd ed., pp. 409-440.). Baltimore: Brookes.

Short-DeGraff, M. (1988). *Human development for occupational and physical therapists.* Baltimore: Williams & Wilkins.

Singer, D.G., & Singer, J.L. (1990). *The house of make-believe: Play and the developing imagination.* Cambridge, MA: Harvard University Press.

Stone, J.L., & Church, J. (1973). *Childhood and adolescence: A psychology of the growing person* (3rd ed.). New York: Random House.

Thelen, E. (1995). Motor development: A new synthesis. *American Psychologist, 50,* 79-95.

Thelen, E. (2002). Self-organization in developmental processes: Can systems approaches work? In M. Johnson & Y. Munakata (Eds.), *Brain development and cognition: A reader* (2nd ed., pp. 544-557). Malden, MA: Blackwell Publishers.

Thelen, E., Corbetta, D., Kamm, K., Spencer, J., Schneider, K., & Zernicke, R.F. (1993). The transition to reaching: Mapping intention and intrinsic dynamics. *Child Development, 64,* 1058-1098.

Thomas, A., & Chess, S. (1977). *Temperament and development.* New York: Brunner/Mazel.

Touwen, B.C.L. (1979). *Examination of the child with minor neurological dysfunction: Clinics in development medicine 71.* London: Heinemann.

Tseng, M., & Murray, E. (1994). Differences in perceptual-motor measures in children with good and poor handwriting. *Occupational Therapy Journal of Research, 14* (1), 19-36.

von Hofsten, C. (1993). Studying the development of goal-directed behaviour. In A.F. Kalverboer, B. Hopkins, & R. Geuze (Eds.), *Motor development in early and later childhood: Longitudinal approaches.* New York: Cambridge Press.

Vygotsky, L.S. (1978). *Mind in society: The development of higher psychological processes.* Cambridge, MA: Harvard University Press.

Werner, E.E. (2000). Protective factors and individual resilience. In J.P. Shonkoff & S.J. Meisels (Eds.), *Handbook of early childhood intervention* (pp. 115-134). Cambridge: Cambridge University Press.

Werner, E.E., & Smith, R.S. (1992). *Overcoming the odds: High risk children from birth to adulthood.* Ithaca, NY: Cornell University Press.

Whiting, B., & Edwards, C.P. (1988). A cross-cultural analysis of sex differences in the behavior of children aged 3 through 11. In G. Handel (Ed.), *Childhood socialization* (pp. 281-297). Cambridge, MA: Harvard University Press.

Willis, W. (1998). Families with African American roots. In E.W. Lynch & M.J. Hanson (Eds.), *Developing cross-cultural competence* (2nd ed., pp. 165-208). Baltimore: Brookes.

Wong, S., Chan, K., Wong, V., & Wong, W. (2002). Use of chopsticks in Chinese children. *Child: Care, Health, and Development, 28,* 157-163.

Youngblade, L.M., & Belsky, J. (1992). Parent-child antecedents of 5-year-olds' close friendships: A longitudinal analysis. *Development Psychology, 28* (4), 700-713.

Zuniga, M.E. (1998). Families with Latino roots. In E.W. Lynch & M.J. Hanson (Eds.), *Developing cross-cultural competence* (2nd ed., pp. 209-250). Baltimore: Brookes.

SUGGESTED READINGS

Emde, R.N. & Robinson, J. (2000). Guiding principles for a theory of early intervention: A developmental-psychoanalytic perspective. In J. Shonkoff & S. Meisels (Eds.), *Handbook of early intervention* (2nd ed., pp. 169-178). Cambridge: Cambridge University Press.

Furono, S., O'Reilly, K.A., Hosaka, C.M., Inatsuka, T.T., Zeisloft-Falbey, B., & Allman, T. (1984). *Hawaii early learning profile.* Palo Alto, CA: VORT.

Goldfield, E.C., Kay, B.A., & Warren, W.H. (1993). Infant bouncing: The assembly and tuning of action systems. *Child Development, 64,* 1128-1142.

Lerner, R.M. (1998). Theories of human development: Contemporary perspectives. In W. Damon (Series Ed.) & R.M. Lerner (Vol. Ed.), *Handbook of child psychology: Vol. 1. Theoretical models of human development* (pp. 1-24). New York: John Wiley & Sons.

Newell, K.M. (1986). Constraints on development of coordination. In M.G. Wade & H.T.A. Whiting (Eds.),

Motor development in children: Aspects of coordination and control (pp. 341-360). Dordrecht, Netherlands: Martinus Nijhoff.

Piek, J. P. (2002). The role of variability in early motor development. *Infant Behavior & Development 25* (4), 452-465.

Rubin, K.H., Fein, G.G., & Vandenberg, B. (1983). Play. In E.M. Hetherington (Ed.), *Handbook of child psychology: Socialization, personality and social development* (pp. 693-774). New York: John Wiley & Sons.

von Hofsten, C. (1982). Eye-hand coordination in the newborn. *Developmental Psychology, 18* (3), 450-461.

Working with Families

Ruth Humphry ■ Jane Case-Smith

Family as a dynamic system
Family occupations: routines, traditions and celebrations
Functions of a family
Family adaptation and resilience

Family diversity
Family-centered services
Parent-professional collaboration
Families facing multiple challenges

CHAPTER OBJECTIVES

1 Describe the occupations and functions of families using the family systems theory.
2 Appreciate the diversity of families and define methods to learn about a family's culture and background.
3 Explore the implications of having a child with special needs with regard to the co-occupations of family members.
4 Analyze the implications of having a child with special needs with regard to family function.
5 Synthesize information about the family life cycle and transitions to identify times of potential stress for families of children with special needs.
6 Specify the roles of the occupational therapist in collaboration with families.
7 Understand how to establish and maintain collaborative relationships with a family.
8 Enact alternative methods of communication that promote family-therapist partnerships.
9 Describe ways families can participate in intervention services.
10 Explain strategies for supporting the strengths of families facing multiple challenges.

This chapter introduces a range of issues related to families, particularly families of children who have special developmental or health care needs. It considers how family members fulfill the functions of a family by collectively engaging in daily or weekly activities and by sharing special events. The chapter explores a range of factors that contribute to the variety of families with which therapists may work in providing occupational therapy for children. Having presented this background in the occupations of families and family diversity, the chapter then turns to the ways the special needs of children bring opportunities and challenges to families. This discussion includes the ways that having a child with disabilities can influence how family members organize their time, engage in activities, and interact with one another. Throughout the chapter the importance of a family-centered philosophy and evidence from the literature are discussed.

REASONS TO STUDY ABOUT FAMILIES

The development of children's occupations cannot be understood without insight into what shapes their daily activities. In the family context, young children first learn about activities, how to perform them, what activities mean, and what to expect as the outcomes of their efforts (Humphry, 2002). Although children's activities vary from one culture to the next, universally their families play a major role in guiding children in how to spend their time, what to do, and why the things they do are important (Larson & Verma, 1999; Rogoff, 2003). For example, Ogunnaike and Houser (2002) reported that in an African community, 2-year-old children watch their older siblings contributing to the household economy, and the younger ones then also want to help. Toddlers are taught to run errands for their mothers by going to neighbors' houses to borrow things. These children experience their activities as important, a way of showing that they are responsible and can contribute to the family. Furthermore the researchers reported that the toddlers given responsibilities, rather than allowed to entertain themselves through play, performed better on standardized tests of mental abilities than those not included in household tasks. In contrast, in the United States, 2-year-olds are not expected to run errands or contribute. Instead, they are closely supervised, and play is encouraged as a way to spend their time and help them learn (Rogoff, 2003). The better occupational therapists understand the influences on the way families operate in their daily routines and their goals for the ways children spend their time, the better prepared the therapists will be to support each family in helping the child engage in activities the family values.

Another reason to study families explicitly is to circumvent the inclination to reference one's own family experiences as a template for the way families operate. Walsh (2002) points out that when people speak of "the family," they suggest a socially constructed image of a "normal" family, giving the impression that an ideal family exists in which optimal development occurs. In reality, many different types of families are successfully raising children. In this chapter, two or more people who share an enduring emotional bond and commitment to pool resources can be seen as a family. Families may comprise people who are blood relatives or whose relationship may be legally defined, but increasingly, people are coming together and defining themselves as a family (Fine, Demo, & Allen, 2000; Laird, 2003; Walsh, 2003). This chapter focuses on families raising children. One or more parents, grandparents, and stepparents, as well as adoptive or foster parents, can successfully bring up children. Unless germane to the discussion of family diversity, the authors refer to the caregiving adult relationship as "the parent" of the child.

A third reason to study families is that the involvement of family members is central to the best practice of occupational therapy. In addition to organizing and enabling daily activities, the family provides the child's most enduring set of relationships throughout childhood, into early adulthood, and possibly beyond. During the course of his or her lifetime, a person with a disability may receive services from people working through health services, educational programs, and social agencies. These relationships exist because professionals bring expertise required by the special needs of the young person. Over time, the type of skills needed changes, and new professionals enter the young person's life. The family represents a source of continuity across this changing pattern of professional involvement. The family forms a unique emotional attachment to their child, and their continuous involvement gives them special insight into the child's needs, abilities, and occupational interests. In light of the family's expertise, occupational therapists strive to collaborate with family members, following their lead and supporting their efforts in promoting the well-being and development of the child with special developmental or health care needs (Lawlor & Mattingly, 1998).

Finally, including families in the process of providing services for children is not just best practice; it is the law. In recognizing the power of families, federal legislation requires service providers and educators to seek the input and permission of a parent or guardian on any assessment, intervention plan, or placement decision. The importance of the family in the early part of the child's life (from birth to 3 years old) is reflected by the emphasis on family-centered services in Part C of the Individuals with Disabilities Education Act (IDEA) (IDEA, 1997). It requires providers to talk with parents and develop an Individualized Family Service Plan (IFSP) regarding the resources the family needs to promote the child's optimal development. Later, in the school system, parents are involved in developing the Individualized Educational Program (IEP), which guides special education and related services (see Chapter 22).

THE FAMILY: A GROUP OF OCCUPATIONAL BEINGS

Family members, individually or together, engage in a variety of different activities that are part of home management, caregiving, employed work, education, play, and leisure domains and that help them feel connected to each other. A father fulfills one of his family roles by picking up groceries on his way home from work or a child studies for a test because his parents expect good grades. Family occupations occur when daily activities and special events are shared by family members. A parent helping her son study for the test, the whole family going to a movie, or brothers shooting baskets together are examples of family occupations. By engaging in occupations together families with children fulfill the functions of a family expected of them by members of their community. Societies first anticipate that families provide children with a cultural foundation for their development as occupational beings. Family members share and transmit a *cultural model*, a habitual framework for thinking about events, for determining which activities should be done and when, and for deciding on how to interact (Gallimore & Lopez, 2002). By providing a cultural foundation, families ensure that children learn how to approach, perform, and experience activities in a manner consistent with their cultural group. This cultural learning process enables children to acquire the occupations that will make their participation in a variety of contexts possible (Box 5-1).

Occupations have meaning because they convey a sense of self, connect us to other people and link us to place (Hasselkus, 2002). Routine family occupations and special events also form the basis for repeated interpersonal experiences that give family members a sense of support, identity, and emotional well-being. The importance of family occupations is reflected by the fact that families create special activities for the specific purpose of spending time together (Schultz-Krohn, 2004).

Families are also expected to help their children develop fundamental routines and life style habits that contribute to their physical health and well-being. It is in the context of receiving care and sharing in family activities that children acquire skills that lead to their independence in activities of daily living (ADLs) and that

BOX 5-1 Outcomes of Family Occupations

Family occupations contribute to the following outcomes for children
1 Establish a cultural foundation for learning occupations that enables children to participate in a variety of contexts.
2 Help shape children's basic sense of identity and emotional well-being.
3 Help children learn to master routines and habits that support physical health and well being.
4 Foster readiness to learn and to participate in educational programs.

they learn habits that will influence their health across the life span. For example, in the context of sharing in family dinners and leisure activities after dinner, children establish habits that can reduce or increase future problems with obesity.

A final function of a family is to prepare children for formal or informal educational activities and whatever other practices the community uses to prepare young people to become productive adults (Rogoff, 2003). Parents, in the context of their daily routines, give children experiences that influence how they approach learning.

Family resources are properties within families that family members use to engage in a balanced pattern of needed and desired activities in a way that enables them to fulfill the family functions described above. Some family members engage in productive activities that enable them to bring in *financial resources* so that the family can acquire material things such as a place to live, food, and clothing. The financial resources also determine what types of community activities are available for family members. *Human resources* comprise the knowledge and skills family members bring to activities. For example, a teenager who learns to use the Internet at school brings these skills home and can help her parent learn how to pay bills on line. *Time* is a third resource families invest to engage in activities that enable them to fulfill family functions. Finally, experiencing close interpersonal relationships during shared activities draws on family members' *emotional energy*, another family resource that is invested in some activities but not others (J.M. Patterson, 2002; Walsh, 2002).

Guided by their cultural models, special circumstances, and community opportunities for activities, families use their resources in different ways. For example, one family may choose to pay (using financial resources) to have the yard work done so that time (another asset) on Saturday afternoons can be used for having a picnic together. Another family invests interpersonal energies (an emotional resource) to get everyone to help with the yard work on Saturday afternoon so that money will be available to pay for music lessons. Financial, human, and

emotional resources, as well as time, are not limitless, and in healthy families, members negotiate a give and take of their assets. For example, mothers of children with attention deficit hyperactivity disorder (ADHD) set aside extra time to help with their children's activities and rely on hired help or assistance from other family members to get household tasks done (Segal, 2000). Typically families with children have a hierarchical organization in which one or more family members (e.g., a parent) take major responsibility for determining how the resources are distributed, enabling the family to engage in activities that enable it to fulfill family functions.

SYSTEM PERSPECTIVE OF FAMILY OCCUPATIONS

A metaphor that helps in understanding families and their occupations is to think of a family as a dynamic system in which its members, as parts of the system, engage in occupations together to fulfill the functions of a family. As a complex social system, family members have to coordinate what they do and when they do things to share in family routines, traditions and celebrations (Box 5-2). As with any system, *interdependent influences* exist among the different parts; that is, the activity of one person can influence the activities of other members. For example, a sixth grader may ask to stay after school with his friend, which means he is not available to watch his sister that afternoon while his mother shops. Consequently, the mother brings her daughter to the grocery store. Shopping with the preschool daughter takes the mother longer than shopping alone. As a result, they do not get home as quickly, and dinner is started late. The interdependent nature of family members' activities is illustrated by the fact that the boy's choice of what he wanted to do in the afternoon altered the activities of his mother and sister and indirectly affected the family's mealtime routine that evening. Recognizing that a family functions as a whole, a therapist that suggests an after-school horseback riding class for a child with cerebral palsy can appreciate that the recommendation must

BOX 5-2 Key Concepts of a Family System Model

1 A family system is composed of individuals who are interdependent and have reciprocal influences on each other's occupations.
2 Within the family, subsystems are defined with their own patterns of interaction and shared occupations.
3 A family must be understood as a whole, and it is more than the sum of the abilities of each member.
4 The family system works to sustain predictable patterns in family occupations and to be part of a larger community.
5 Change and evolution are inherent in a family.
6 A family, as an open system, is influenced by its environment.

be weighed in light of the family resources and the implications of that activity for the entire family system.

Not all members share in all activities that contribute to family functions; at times, certain family members form a special interactive relationship, or *subsystem,* to engage in shared activities. For example, during caregiving, a parent and child (adult-child subsystem) engage in co-occupations, such as dressing and feeding, in which the child learns more independence in doing ADLs (Zemke & Clark, 1996). Other subsystems include a couple planning the family vacation or brothers and sisters (sibling subsystem) playing softball together. During family occupations, the performance of one family member is part of the social context of the other family members' performance and subjective experience of the activity. Therefore shared activities hold special meaning and motivation for certain family members that may not be shared with other family members. In working with children, the occupational therapist frequently interacts with the mother and child (Lawlor & Mattingly, 1998). However, if therapists recognize that not all family functions are accomplished by the parent-child subsystem, they can find ways to involve other family members, such as siblings, in developing activities (e.g., play routines) with children who have special needs.

With all the activities a family does and the different members who can carry out these tasks, it would become confusing and draw on family resources if everyone had to negotiate daily who was going to do what, when, and in which way. An effective family system organizes itself into *predictable patterns* of daily and weekly activities and familiar ways with special events. Guided by their cultural models, families settle into *daily routines* for various household activities. These daily routines include interactive rituals that take on symbolic meaning and seem so matter of course that people do not think of doing them any other way, and they resist changing them (Gallimore & Lopez, 2002). Bedtime routines for a child, for example, can have a set sequence of taking a bath, brushing teeth and the parent reading a book. If routines are interrupted, even by a welcomed event, such as a grandparent coming to visit, family members invest extra family resources reconfiguring their daily routines under the changed circumstances. For example, time is spent making up a bed on the sofa rather than giving the daughter a bath, and emotional energy is expended to help the daughter fall asleep in the living room so that the grandparent can sleep in her bedroom. Families may experience the disruption of their daily routines as unsettling and taxing, and it is not uncommon to hear family members sigh in relief when they can return to predictable patterns; that is, when "things get back to normal."

In addition to routines for daily or weekly activities (Figure 5-1), families also establish predictable patterns

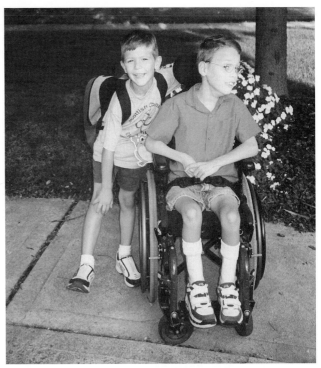

FIGURE 5-1 Michael and his brother wait for the school bus. (Courtesy Jill and Mark McQuaid, Dublin, Ohio.)

for what they do during special events. *Family traditions,* such as cooking special food for birthday celebrations or sharing leisure activities on Sunday afternoons, help families develop a sense of group cohesion and emotional well-being for family members (Figure 5-2). Families may decide to maintain their traditions, because these customary activities fulfill family functions, rather than address an individual member's needs. For example, a family that traditionally vacations with grandparents for several weeks in the summer may value the way special occupations together reinforce their sense of being a family. Conflict with the occupational therapist could arise if the therapist assumes that the family will shorten the traditional vacation to attend some therapy sessions during the summer. When the occupational therapist offers a range of options and asks the family to set priorities, family members can consider all their routines and traditions and determine how they want occupational therapy services to fit into their lives.

Celebrations are predictable patterns of doing activities, such as religious rituals, that are shared with members of the community. Therefore what is done during family celebrations is common to what other families that share a similar background do for the same celebration. This link to others gives family members a sense of meaning associated with their special events that connects them to a community of families. Therapists may be asked for assistance so that children can participate in celebrations. For example, a parent may want positioning suggestions so that her daughter with cerebral palsy

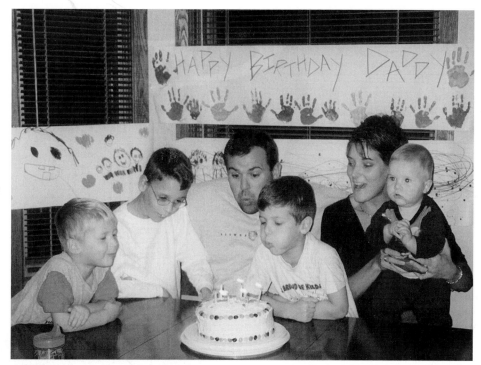

FIGURE 5-2 Michael's family celebrates Dad's birthday. (Courtesy Jill and Mark McQuaid, Dublin, Ohio.)

will be comfortable during Christmas Eve services. The family of a boy with sensory processing problems may need ideas for coping that they can use while attending a Fourth of July fireworks display with the neighbors. By enabling the children's occupational engagement, the entire family participates in community celebrations and confirms their identity as a family like every other family raising children.

Among the researchers who have investigated family routines and practices, Fiese and colleagues (Fiese & Tomcho, 2001; Markson & Fiese, 2000) have examined the meaning of routines and related ritual interactions of families' daily activities and religious celebrations. Their studies showed that families that reported finding more meaning and commitment to their routines and special activities experienced better health of family members and stronger interpersonal relationships.

FAMILY ADAPTATION, AND RESILIENCE

As a dynamic system that exists over time, change and evolution are inherent in being a family. Thus, despite the inclination of families to organize their activities into predictable patterns in the form of their routines, traditions, and celebrations, internal or external forces press for family adaptation or changes what they do and how they interact. J.M. Patterson (2002) described a variety of pressures that can alter family activities. These might include daily hassles, such as multiple demands on a

parent's time or unpredictable transportation, as well as positive life transitions, such as the birth of a baby or an older son leaving home to take a job, which alter household routines. Other events requiring family adaptation in their routines and traditions may be unexpected, such as job loss, illness, or an event that affects the community (e.g., a tornado). To accommodate these pressures and change their activity patterns, families reorganize family resources and negotiate new ways of doing things. When the disruption of daily routines exceeds a family's resources, the family may need to eliminate some valued routines, and if the demands of the situation continue to exceed resources, the family becomes unable to fulfill its functions.

The process of *adaptation* starts when a family recognizes the state of affairs, an interruption in their activities or a loss of emotional well-being (Grant, Ramcharan, & Goward, 2003; J.M. Patterson, 2002). Gathering information and talking among themselves about their different perspectives of a disruptive event enables family members to construct a shared meaning of the demands of the situation and to evaluate their options for meeting the challenge. Families use a variety of strategies to make sense of what is happening (Walsh, 2002). For example, they can tell stories about a similar instance or another generation that experienced a comparable event. They can redefine what seems like a catastrophic event by making a comparison with another family in which something they see as more devastating has occurred. For example, finding spiritual meaning in an adverse event is a way of changing how it is experienced. Regardless of the strategy used, by co-constructing their own definitions of events, families diminish the feeling of being out of control, and based on how they define the state of affairs, they can allocate resources to manage the situation.

The family members' ability to communicate with each other is important to co-construction of meaning and adaptation of daily routines. Families engage in affective and instrumental communication. In *affective communication,* family members express their care for and support of each other. In *instrumental communication,* members give each other role assignments, establish schedules, make decisions, and resolve conflicts. Clear, effective communication is important for establishing meaning for an event or problem and for planning resolution of the crisis. As Patterson put it, "A family's belief in their inherent ability to discover solutions and new resources to manage challenges may be the cornerstone of building protective mechanisms and thereby being resilient" (J.M. Patterson, 2002, p. 243).

Families demonstrate resilience when they draw on resources to reconstruct their routines or create new ones that enable them to continue to fulfill family functions. For example, McCubbin, Balling, Possin, Frierdich, & Bryne (2002) identified factors that contributed to families' resilience and ability to manage when children were diagnosed with cancer. Based on their interviews of 42 parents, they found *resiliency factors* that made it easier for the family to construct new routines to deal with the situation. These families drew on their own resources, such as religious beliefs and the emotional support of each other, and then reset their definition of how they would live or operate as a family. The parents rearranged their routines so that one parent could be with the child receiving inpatient medical treatment while the other stayed at home with the siblings. Parents reported that they also drew on resources in their community. For example, when neither of them had time to cook, members from their church brought in meals so the family could share meals together.

Occupational therapists who recognize the power of daily routines and family traditions are sensitive to disruption of a family's pattern of activities and can assist parents in reestablishing or creating meaningful family routines. For example, the occupational therapist may suggest strategies that enable a child with a gastrostomy tube to participate in the family mealtime (e.g., explaining to the parents what foods the child can safely "taste" at the dinner table). The therapist can also help families find ways to make important traditions possible. If a child with autism has difficulty in a new environment, the therapist can recommend ways to help the child adjust by suggesting that he carry a CD player with his favorite music when trying to leave home for the traditional family vacation.

IMPORTANCE OF FAMILY ECOLOGY

As with any other open system, the social and physical features surrounding the family influence it. Cultural models are partly shaped by values, beliefs, and ways of thinking shared with others who have similar backgrounds (Gallimore & Lopez, 2002). In addition, the occupations of families do not take place just within the home. Many of the resources for family activities that enable families to function effectively are available in the neighborhood and the larger community. Proximity to places of worship, stores, and friends is part of the family's ecology and influences how family members spend their time. At a slightly more removed level, family functions are supported when social institutions make services available (e.g., a health department that runs an immunization clinic, the volunteer group that helps parents choose the best childcare centers, businesses that raise money for a school system).

The advantage of an ecologic perspective is that it raises awareness of the ways things distant from the family and beyond its control influence how the family fulfills its functions. Forces that change the family ecology can be remote and the influence indirect. For example, a large corporation that decides to cut its work force causes job loss in the neighborhood and forces people to leave the area to find employment. Suddenly the parents no longer have a baby-sitter and have to change leisure time activities. On an even more distant level, shifts in public attitudes during a particular period of time influence the environment and resources for families. For example, families can be affected by the attitudes of voters who determine public policies about the rights of people with disabilities, universal health care coverage, welfare reform, and the rights of undocumented immigrants (Fine, Demo, & Allen, 2000).

For therapists working with children with special needs and their families, it is especially important to take an ecologic perspective and to investigate whether families can access a range of community activities that will enable them to fulfill their functions. For example, in a survey of family-centered services in Ontario, King et al. (2003) found that communities vary in how they support the inclusion of families raising children with disabilities. Limited access to recreational resources and lack of social support for parents reduce the participation of children with special needs in leisure activities. Therapists who strive to enable children's occupations that lead to participation in community contexts are no longer focused on the occupation of individual children. Turnbull, Turbiville, and Turnbull (2002) propose a collaborative empowerment model in which families draw on their knowledge of their children's abilities and receive support from other families and professionals to make changes at the community level. By joining with families in advocating for children's rights, occupational therapists contribute to a synergistic force that increases the family's access to resources outside their homes and helps them function as a family.

SOURCES OF DIVERSITY IN FAMILIES

Families with children who need occupational therapy services come from many different backgrounds and in a variety of forms, and therapists working with these children have the rewarding opportunity to learn from their families. Therapists must find a balance between focusing on the similarities and appreciating the differences among families (Allen, Fine, & Demo, 2000). Because individuals are inclined to view the world through their own cultural model and to use personal experiences as a point of reference, it takes professional commitment to becoming skilled at working with a variety of different families. A qualitative study of mothers who had immigrated to the United States from Asian countries illustrates how the cultural model of a service provider dominated the suggestions she gave a Korean family whose son had suffered a traumatic brain injury. The mother commented, "You know that Oriental men are not used to doing household chores. My social worker would tell my husband about all the work that I have to do and ask him what work he would be willing to take over to give me relief. She laid the foundation for my husband to begin to help me, but it is hard for him to know what to do" (Raghavan, 1998, p. 62).

Families differ from one another in a number of ways. Three sources of family diversity discussed below are the family's ethnic background, family structure, and socioeconomic status. A fourth section considers differences in parenting styles and practices.

Currently family researchers and service providers have focused on understanding how a family's culture and traditions affect child-rearing practices and how these might be adaptive, strengthening a family or bringing about positive developmental outcomes (Koramoa, Lynch, & Kinnair, 2002). Families have patterns of different characteristics (e.g., family structure, family income, having a family member with a disability), and the ecology in which families function varies (e.g., religious opportunity, crime rate in the neighborhood, period in history). Therefore generalizations of research findings about diverse family groups are rarely accurate, and sensitivity to the unique differences of each family is always needed.

Ethnic Background

Ethnicity is a term used to group families that share a common nationality or language. It tends to be a broad concept, and heterogeneity among families within

groups described as Latino, African American, Anglo-American, or Asian should be anticipated. Furthermore, people may identify themselves as belonging to more than one ethnic group, making it harder to use the concept to guide the way one works with families. Coll and Pachter (2002) offer two reasons for retaining ethnicity as an important variable when working with families raising children. First, families that are not part of the dominant ethnic group experience a discontinuity between their cultural models and the majority culture that shapes the social institutions. Thus a cultural gap may exist between health systems and educational programs and the families of minority ethnic groups. In addition, as the proportion of ethnic groups grows in the United States, the sons and daughters of these groups make up a larger proportion of the overall population of children in this country. Occupational therapists who serve children with special needs can anticipate working with an ever-growing, ethnically diverse group of families. In the following discussion, the influence of ethnic background on the ways a family fulfills its functions and raises its children is considered first. The special issues of recent immigrants then are considered.

Ethnic groups share cultural practices that can determine who has the authority to allocate family resources and a value system that sets priorities for family routines and special events. Families in an ethnic group may have similar daily activities, ways of interacting, and ways of thinking about events and may find similar meaning in their routines, traditions, and celebrations. Differences among ethnic groups are expressed in gender role expectations, child-rearing practices, and expectations at certain ages, as well as in definitions of health and views of disability. Cultural practices are not static traits; rather, they change when members of the group adapt to new situations (Harwood, Leyendecker, Carlson, Asencio, & Miller, 2002). Therapists encounter families with cultural models that reflect not only their culture of origin but also the group's history, the factors that caused the group to relocate, their economic concerns, and experiences with racism and other forms of prejudice that influence how or where families live.

Although every family wants their children to be successful members of the community, their vision of how they will participate in different contexts varies among different ethnic groups and influences how children spend their time and what is expected of them (Larson & Verma, 1999). The influence of ethnic background on how children are raised is illustrated in a study conducted by Carlson and Harwood (2003), who investigated how much structure and control Anglo-American and Puerto Rican mothers asserted over their infants during ADLs. The Anglo-American parents appeared to value individuality, responding to and supporting child-initiated activities rather than dominating them. Puerto Rican parents, on the other hand, encouraged more cooperation. The researchers observed mothers in their daily routines and found that Puerto Rican mothers controlled their infants' behaviors more than the Anglo-American mothers, who tolerated more off-task behaviors. Carlson and Harwood pointed out that Puerto Rican parents are guided by the anticipation that their children will join a Puerto Rican community that values respectful co-operation. The Anglo-American willingness to follow the child's lead is compatible with valuing individual autonomy. Without insight into ethnic differences, a therapist watching parent-child interaction may mistakenly interpret a Puerto Rican mother's physical control and effort to divert a child's attention to the needs of others as intrusive and insensitive to the toddler's sense of identity and self-efficacy. Therapists avoid this type of error by understanding what a parent hopes to achieve before formulating an opinion about the appropriateness of a family's interactive routines.

The influx of recent immigrants expands the diversity within ethnic groups that therapists will encounter. Within a community, one family may have members who have been in a country for generations, and the family next door may have recently relocated to the country. Migration affects the family and how it functions at multiple levels (Falicov, 2003). First, relocation to another country frequently includes a series of separations and reunions of children from immediate family members. Suarez-Orozco, Todorova, and Louie (2002) found that 85% of the 385 youths in their sample of recent immigrants had been separated from a parent and nearly half had lived apart from both of their parents during the process of family migration. Although the length of separation varied, it was not unusual for a child to have been apart from the father for 2 years or longer. In some families the tradition of having a child live with a grandparent or other relative may buffer the initial separation and help reduce the stress. Yet when the children are brought into the United States to join their immigrant parents, they must leave behind a caregiver and familiar community. Researchers found that reunification could be protracted, because families may not have been able to pay for travel or housing for all family members, meaning people arrived in stages months or years apart. In addition, when both parents immigrated ahead of their children, it was not unusual for the children subsequently brought into the country to have to adjust to living not only with their parents again but also possibly with younger siblings born in the new country. Therapists working with immigrant families need to be sensitive to the possibility of family friction, depression, and a sense of uncertainty among family members.

For each immigrant family, the process of *acculturation* varies; this is the process of selectively blending their traditions in how things are done, what activities are important, and interactive styles with the cultural practices of the majority group (Falicov, 2003). Parenting practices might insulate children from exposure to the language, ways, and values of the majority culture until the children go to school. For example, enrolling children in childcare programs may seem the equivalent of child abandonment in some cultures, and families may bring a grandparent with them as part of the immigration process so that both parents can find paid employment. This may mean that children entering school have had few experiences beyond their home environment. In school, surrounded by new peers, the children's acculturation process is influenced, creating conflict among family members (Coll & Pachter, 2002). Unfortunately, feeling disconnected from home or discriminated against at school leads some youths to drop out of school as a way to ease the tension (Harwood et al., 2002).

Family Structure

Family features, such as the presence of children in the household, marital status, sexual orientation, and age/generation, are factors described as the *family structure* (Allen et al., 2000). Family structure in combination with its cultural model influences how the family organizes itself to fulfill essential roles, such as caregiving of dependent family members or allocation of family resources. For example, in multigenerational families, a grandmother may act as the head of the household and the primary caregiver to the grandchildren while her adult child is employed outside the home. As discussed earlier, the idea that there is a best family structure in which children are raised is a myth (Walsh, 2002). For example, single-parent families have been portrayed as dysfunctional and as leaving children more vulnerable to having problems (Amato, 2000). However, Larson (2001) sampled the activities and emotions during activities of employed mothers in two-parent or single-parent homes of adolescents and found that this stereotype of the single-parent home was not necessarily the rule. Single mothers in his study experienced less stressed, more flexible routines after a day at work and friendlier relationships with their teenagers than did their counterparts in two-parent homes. Mothers with a husband reported more hassles trying to make and serve dinner by a designated dinnertime and experienced housework as more unpleasant. Larson speculates that the negotiation of responsibilities and trying to live up to expectations of being a "wife" in a two-parent home contributed to these differences. Clearly, every family structure has advantages and risk factors (Larson, 2001).

During their childhood many children experience changes in the family structure. Unwed mothers may marry, or parents in a family may divorce and later one or both may remarry. A child may transition from a two- to a three-generation family when an aging grandparent moves into the home. Therapists should talk with family members in an inclusive manner that does not suggest an assumed family structure. Asking a parent or child, "Can you tell me about your family?" does not suggest any expectations about who is in a family and helps family members openly express their definition of who is in their family.

Gay, lesbian, and bisexual families reflect one variation of family structure that therapists encounter. Children may be the products of a parent's previous heterosexual relationship or may be born or adopted into families headed by adults who are gay, lesbian, or bisexual (C.J. Patterson, 2002). Because parents do not want to expose their children to the prejudice of homophobia, many are reluctant to be identified, and estimates of the number of parents who are not heterosexual range from 1% to 12% of families (Stacey & Biblarz, 2001). Many of the issues and needs of all parents are expressed by gay, lesbian, and bisexual parents (Park, 1998).

Because sexual orientation has been the basis for judicial decisions that have denied people parenting rights, recent studies have investigated the issue of whether the sexual orientation of the parent affects the child's behaviors or influences the child's sexual orientation. Studies comparing the psychological adjustment and school performance of children being raised by lesbian or gay parents to those of children with heterosexual parents have generally found no differences (C.J. Patterson, 2002). Further illustrating the importance of an ecologic perspective, Stacey and Biblarz (2001) noted that researchers of child development need to examine not only a family's structure, but also how the family fits into its community. When parents who are gay or lesbian reside in a community accepting of different orientations, the parents may be more likely to engage in open discussion about sexual preferences. Not being part of such a community can be considered a risk factor. For example, Oswald and Culton (2003) interviewed gay, lesbian, bisexual, and transgender people living in a rural Midwest area. Many of these individuals reported a sense of being disconnected from the community, and their network of social support was fragmented. A family living under these circumstances may be less open to social support offered by people outside the family at times of crisis and thus not as resilient as one living in a cosmopolitan community that was accepting of a parent's life style.

Marital status is another source of differences in family structure. A multitude of factors influence the decision to have or not to have children and whether the mother is married to or living with the father (Musick, 2002). A third of the births in the United States are to unmarried women (National Center for Health Statistics, 2000). Although the majority of single-parent households are headed by women, the number of fathers who are single parents has increased (U.S. Bureau of the Census, 2000).

Although it is possible for a single parent to raise competent, well-adjusted children (Amato, 2000; Murray,

Bynum, Brody, Willert, & Stephens, 2001), as Entwisle and Alexander (2000) summarize in their longitudinal study of more than 700 first graders over the first 5 years of school, single-parent homes, when no other adults were in the home, were associated with children's poorer school performance. First, a single adult is less likely to have financial resources than two-adult families. In addition, the younger the person was at the time of transition into parenthood, the less likely he or she is to have completed higher education which will also impact financial resources. Time is another family resource that can be in short supply in single-parent families, especially when there are a number of young children who need physical assistance throughout their daily activities.

A final source of stress, divorce, the way many single-parent families are formed, can be a source of disruption that alters household routines, traditions, and celebrations. Factors that contribute to positive developmental outcomes for children after couples break up include the parents' psychological well-being, economic resources, whether the family is part of a larger kinship network, and how parents navigate the separation and dissolution process. For example, Greene, Anderson, Hetherington, Forgatch, & DeGarmo (2003) reported contradictory findings regarding how well children adjust after their parents' divorce. Initially parenting practices were erratic, and the parent-child relationship, especially between custodial mothers and young sons, could be stormy. Yet, 2 years after a divorce, many of the problems had diminished; therefore some of the consequences of divorce depend on where in the adjustment process researchers conduct their study. Anderson (2003) argued that the best way to strengthen single-parent families was to empower parents by recognizing their strengths and encouraging them to reestablish routines. The therapist can be supportive by acknowledging that these parents face considerable challenges in raising children alone and by aiding the parent in identifying resources such as friends, extended family, religious groups, and other single parents.

When birth parents are unable or unavailable to care for children, *kinship care* is a way to preserve family ties that might be lost if children are placed in foster homes (Kelley, Whitley, Sipe, & Yorker, 2000). Households in which grandparents are raising their grandchildren are examples of kinship care and are a growing source of differences between families. These families, primarily headed by middle-aged or older women and disproportionately by women of color, are often formed after adverse events, such as child neglect or abandonment, maternal substance abuse, or incarceration or death of the parents (Joslin, 2000; Kelley et al., 2000). Much of the research on grandparents raising their children's children explores the issue of caregiver stress. Evidence from both qualitative and quantitative studies suggests that grandparents caring for their grandchildren (or great-grandchildren) find it both rewarding and challenging (Baird, John, & Hayslip, 2000; Kelley et al., 2000). Grandparents reported satisfaction in being able to "be there" for the child or children and reported that they have had to learn new parenting skills in response to the new generation. However, they also experienced parenting stress, which was exacerbated when they lacked social support, had limited financial resources, or were in poor health. When a child is reported to have behavioral or health problems, the caregiving demands increase the grandparents' sense of emotional distress (Hayslip, Emick, Henderson, & Elias, 2002).

Socioeconomic Status

The influence of the family's socioeconomic status (SES) on children occupations and development is complex (Hoff, Laursen, & Tardif, 2002). First, SES is difficult to discuss because many people, despite a growing gap between families with and without resources (Rank, 2000), are uncomfortable acknowledging that they live in a stratified society. Another reason that SES is difficult to study as it relates to development is because SES reflects a composite of different factors, including the social prestige of family members, the educational attainment of the parents, and the family income. These factors influence each other and have varying implications for how a family fulfills its functions through their daily routines and special events. For example, a parent's educational background not only affects potential employment, it also influences parenting practices. Education affects how an adult incorporates new ideas about a healthy life style and child development. Low household income contributes to a family's SES and limits another family resource, finances. Finally any one of these factors, if positive, can help mediate the effect of the others. For example, a child of a low income family in which the caregiving grandmother is a highly respected member of her church might find that the neighbors monitor his activities.

Another issue is that financial resources fluctuate for many families changing according to the employment status of different family members (Rank, 2000). Factors that influence employment, such as a below-average education, inability to speak English, or disability of a family member, leaves families more vulnerable as job opportunities come or go. When employment is found, the job may not pay enough to meet the family's needs, leaving the family with no resources if unexpected events occur. Falling into poverty has implications for how the family is able to support the health of its members (Rank, 2000). A poor diet, impoverished living conditions, reduced utilization of preventive health care services, and inability to control environmental factors can lead to health problems such as asthma or mental illness (e.g., depression). Researchers have demonstrated that low

income or limited education is associated with differences in the amount and content of parents' interaction with their children (Bradley, Corwyn, McAdoo, & Coll, 2001; Hoff et al., 2002; Rogoff, 2003). In these circumstances parents may not be as responsive, addressing the child less often, providing fewer learning opportunities, and not engaging in an interactive teaching process.

Nonetheless, it is necessary to look beyond simple associations between poverty and parenting, because some parents do better than others despite a low SES (Murray et al., 2001). Occupational therapists need to understand how some parents living in poverty adapt and raise children successfully. For example, single parents who have strict disciplinary standards may seem harsh. However, their parenting practices may be grounded in an anticipation that their children will grow into a world where obedience to people in authority is important for keeping a job. Other parents who restrict their children's community activities may be effective in monitoring who they are with, minimizing the negative influences of poor neighborhoods. When a therapist is sensitive to and deeply understands a family with a low SES, she or he can make recommendations that help the child with special needs while supporting the family in their precarious position.

Parenting Style and Practices

The parenting and raising of a well-adapted child are complex issues that have attracted the interest of many researchers (Bornstein, 2002). The individual interactive style and parenting practices of an adult raising a child are additional factors that must be considered in gaining an understanding of the diversity of families. Steinberg and Silk (2002) distinguish between *parenting style,* the emotional climate between parent and child, and *parenting practices,* goal-directed activities parents do in raising their children. For example, two parents may believe that if they want their children to do well in school, it is their responsibility to spend time with the children reviewing their homework (a parenting practice). However, the interpersonal interactions while they engage in this shared activity (parenting style) can be distinctly different. One parent may discuss the work and help the child find solutions to problems, whereas the other parent may feel he has the emotional energy only to point out errors. What leads to individual differences in how people parent? An ecologic and transactional perspective of development and parenting encourages therapists to consider family resources and the adult's psychological background, personal history, and personality, which are in constant interaction with characteristics of the child being parented (Kotchick & Forehand, 2002; Sameroff & Fiese, 2000).

Regardless of ethnic background, poverty status, and parenting practices, a parenting style that is warm, responsive, and positive and that provides structure and learning opportunities is associated with children who rank higher on many measures of social and cognitive development (Bradley et al., 2001; Steinberg & Silk, 2002). For example, in a study of low-income, rural African American families. Brody, Dorsey, Forehand, and Armistead (2002) found that children whose school behavior was reported to be good had mothers who combined a supportive relationship with watchful monitoring of their children's behavior and activities.

Dialog between parents and therapists does not always go smoothly, and the collaborative nature of the relationship is sometimes lost if the parent and therapist hold different ideas about parenting style or parenting practices. This tension increases if the parent worries about the therapist's disapproval (Lawlor & Mattingly, 2001). The professional cannot assume greater knowledge than the parent about what the child needs to be able to do or about the interactive style that best accompanies shared activities. At the same time, therapists can be supportive and can empower parents by working with them so that family resources such as time and emotional energy are available when shared activities occur.

Therapists' Professional Responsibility in Light of Family Diversity

As discussed in the previous sections, family diversity is a social construct (Fine et al., 2000) defined in the eyes of the beholder; that is, families that appear atypical may be defined as "just an average family" in another era or culture. At the same time, Walker (2002) argued that it is not sufficient to strive to treat all families the same, because each family has different needs and expectations for how professionals can support them. Each family deserves to be seen in light of what makes it unique and how very similar it is to all other families raising children. An initial step toward recognizing differences among families is to reflect on one's own cultural model and associated beliefs and critically analyze how knowledge about families is constructed (Allen et al., 2000; Rogoff, 2003). Finding other people who can share an insider perspective because they have been part of a similar family and reading the literature are helpful ways to gain an understanding of families with different backgrounds. Occupational therapists who acknowledge that every family has unique features and needs initiate conversations that solicit the parent's explanation about family membership, the family's cultural model, and the activities valued for and by the child. Talking with parents about how they do things together during their daily and weekly routines and the meanings they give these shared activities is a place to start. With these understandings, the therapist can design interventions that fit into daily routines and are compatible with family traditions.

IMPACT ON THE FAMILY OF A CHILD WITH A HEALTH OR DEVELOPMENTAL PROBLEM

When families experience new demands and stresses, they continue to function by creating meaning about the stressful event and by working as a system to adapt and continue their daily activities. A child with exceptional health or developmental needs creates new demands on a family system, and families with sufficient resources and flexibility respond by adapting their daily routines and special events so that they can fulfill their family functions. Bernheimer and Keogh illustrated the importance of family resilience in the conclusion of their longitudinal study of families of children with special needs: "The majority of our families are doing quite well. Like the children in our study, they share common characteristics but are strikingly unique in many ways. They are adapting and adjusting within their physical and cultural environments, and are making decisions about the organization of their lives and about their children, consistent with their values and beliefs and with what they think is important" (Bernheimer & Keogh, 1995, p. 429).

Three research issues limit discussion of how having a child with special needs influences the ways families engage in daily and weekly activities and special events to fulfill their functions. First, in many studies examining family experiences with a child with special needs, the research participants were two-parent, Anglo-American families. Thus what we know about families who are raising children with disabilities is not well generalized to families with other ethnic backgrounds or family structures. Second, psychologists and family researchers have conducted much of the research on the consequences of having a child with special needs. Therefore the literature offers a better developed picture of how family members feel and relate to each other than of how they spend their time together and find meaning in their activities. Finally, because the family is seen as a whole social system, it is very difficult to generalize across families raising children with different diagnoses. With some developmental disabilities, such as autism and learning disabilities, the family may not have a diagnosis for several years and may have evolved coping strategies to deal with the behavioral or learning issues without understanding the basis for the problems and without resources and interventions to help (Rolland, 2003). In other families, the children's problems may be chronic or their health or rate of development may gradually decline, or the family may experience a series of crises and remissions. These differences alter the pattern of time use, the parenting style, and the activities that make up each family's daily routines.

FAMILY RESOURCES AND A CHILD WITH SPECIAL NEEDS

Having a child with special needs does not eliminate any of the functions of a family. That is, through their activities, families continue to provide a cultural and psychosocial foundation and to guide their children's experiences in activities that will lead to optimal health and participation in the larger community. Understanding how families make choices in light of finite resources and their vision of children's futures puts some of these decisions families make about daily activities and what they want to work on in a different light (Kellegrew, 2000). For a period, especially when a problem is recently diagnosed or when medical treatment is needed, family resources (e.g., time, money, and emotional energy) may be directed primarily to the needs of the child (Melamed, 2002). For example, a mother who has a full-time job to help pay medical and therapy bills and spends 4 hours a day feeding her medically fragile child has limited time and emotional energy to devote to helping another child with homework or to sharing in recreational activities. Yet, over time, this allocation of resources may have negative implications for family members, and if the feeding problems are chronic, other choices may need to be made.

Financial Resources

Having a child with special needs has implications for family economics. Parents with children who have disabilities have many hidden and ongoing expenses When children are hospitalized, many expenses (e.g., days out of work, childcare for siblings, transportation, meals, motel rooms) are incurred in addition to costs not covered by insurance. Mothers on welfare reported that they face multiple barriers (LeRoy, 2004). Though they wanted to become self-sufficient, employment seemed like a distant dream as they struggled with transportation and finding childcare, particularly for older children.

Although financial problems create added stress, therapists are often reluctant to discuss finances, especially costs associated with their own services. In a sample of mothers of children with cerebral palsy, Nastro found that insurance coverage was inadequate to meet the families' needs. As one mother reported, "Each piece of equipment has a big price tag. Even the smallest piece has a couple hundred dollar price tag. Most insurance companies do not cover it. Medicaid does not cover everything" (Nastro, 1992, p. 52). Also, many insurance plans have caps on the number of therapy visits allowed per year. Therefore parents must cut back on services or pay for sessions by finding a way to save somewhere else.

Children who require extensive medical treatment can bring economic devastation to a family, especially when insurance coverage is inadequate (Kirk, 1998).

Another challenge to financial resources occurs when a parent decides to remain unemployed so that he or she has time to provide extra caregiving. In a study of how parents spend their time, mothers of children with Down syndrome worked significantly fewer paid hours than mothers of children without disabilities. As a result, the mothers of children with Down syndrome had reduced earning capacity (Barnett & Boyce, 1995). Financial strain is increased in single-parent homes. Mothers of preschoolers with special needs were less likely to work outside the home than single mothers of typically developing young children (Porterfield, 2002). With one spouse unable to take on paid employment, these households are at higher risk for problems associated with low income. Case-Smith (2004) found that mothers of children with medical conditions left employment due to the frequency of their children's illness. These children needed specialized medical care (i.e., nursing care) that prohibited their attending community childcare centers. The need to stay home with a child who has multiple medical needs and frequent illness and lack of community childcare for such a child may become a particularly difficult situation for a single parent to manage.

Human Resources

The human resources important to a family in raising children are education, practical knowledge, and problem-solving ability. An understanding of the basis of the child's problems and of possible adaptations is a powerful resource in helping families establish effective patterns of daily activities. As a parent, Marci Greene (1999) observed that a comprehensive parent-professional partnership should include ongoing parent education. Initially parents want additional information about their children's conditions and about accessing services (Knox, Parmenter, Atkinson, & Yezbeck, 2000). However, parents appreciate dialog with professionals beyond informational topics such as the development of feeding skills or behavioral management. Parents want professionals to share conceptual knowledge as well (Greene, 1999).

Families who are coping with stress have reported that "the ability to build on personal experience and expertise" is an essential coping strategy (Grant & Whittell, 2000, p. 261). Parents may develop this knowledge through parent to parent groups in which families can share strategies with other families who have similar types of issues (Fox, Vaughn, Wyatte, & Dunlap, 2002). For therapists, listening to parents and individualizing the information, as well as connecting family members to other resources, helps build the parents' personal resources.

Time Resources

Daily and weekly activities, by their very definition, require time investment, and every family at one time or another experiences stress because there are too many things to be done and not enough time. Children with disabilities often depend on caregivers longer than typically developing children, and the extra daily care or supervision needed may extend for many years (Fox et al., 2002). The amount of time spent in shared activities around caregiving can be wearing and frustrating and can reduce the family's time for recreation and social gatherings. In a study of more than 200 families of children with Down syndrome, mothers spent three times as much time in childcare as mothers of typically developing children (Barnett & Boyce, 1995). The fathers of children with Down syndrome spent twice as much time in childcare as fathers of typically developing children. One commonly used coping strategy of family caregivers is to organize the day into well-established routines (Grant & Whittell, 2000). Helitzer, Cunningham-Sabo, VanLeit, and Crowe found that mothers of children with disabilities reported that they used "structure, routine, and organized time management as a way to maintain a sense of control" (Helitzer et al., 2002, p. 28). However, their busy, structured lives often were disrupted by crises, such as trips to the hospital or urgent care department, and as a result, the mothers felt they were "living on the edge" and that every disruption in their routines was experienced as a crisis.

Service providers can be a source of threat to the family's time and emotional resources. Greene described how her family "experienced the burden of home programming" as occupational, physical, and speech therapists made separate recommendations that would require an hour and a half a day (Greene, 1999, p. 150). These home assignments became a source of guilt and marital difficulty as the family struggled to meet the needs both of their daughter and of her typically developing sibling.

Crowe (1993) found that mothers of children with multiple disabilities spent significantly more time in childcare activities and less time in socialization than mothers of typical children. In a qualitative study of parents of children with chronic medical conditions and disabilities, parents reported that they had round-the-clock responsibilities in administering medical procedures and performing caregiving tasks (Case-Smith, 2004). They described the challenges of "always being there" to care for their child's extraordinary medical needs and to engage their very dependent child in developmentally appropriate activities. These parents, whose children were often ill and even hospitalized, were always "on call" and often had to cancel activities outside the home when the child was ill.

Emotional Energy

Families of children with disabilities may experience special forms of stress, social isolation and less psychologic well-being than families with typically developing children (DeGrace, 2004; Dyson, 1993; McGuire, Crowe, Law, & VanLeit, 2004). Some researchers report that parents of children with disabilities experience recurrent grief. This sorrow characterizes the initial diagnosis and can recur at developmental milestones or transitions. Fox et al. (2002) conducted a qualitative investigation to understand how children with developmental delays and behavioral problems influenced the family's life style. Their parents suggested that dealing with the child's needs required a lot of emotional energy from the different family members. One theme, "it's a 24-hour, 7-day-a-week involvement," was supported by stories of frustration from responding to challenging behaviors and applying parenting practices that would meet the needs of their children. Parents reported that individuals who offered "a shoulder to lean on" and professional assistance, encouragement, and information were particularly helpful.

The literature reports that parents of children with disabilities may experience anxiety and depression (Olsson & Hwang, 2001). Mothers appear more vulnerable than fathers. In a study of 216 families of children with autism and mental retardation and 214 families of children without disabilities, Olsson and Hwang (2001) found that mothers of children with autism were more depressed than mothers of children with mental retardation and that both groups were more depressed than mothers of children without disabilities. The fathers in these families did not exhibit more depression than fathers of typical children. Mothers' self-competence may be more related to the parenting role than that of fathers, and mothers may be more vulnerable when stressful difficulties arise in the parenting domain (Olsson & Hwang, 2001). Hastings (2003) investigated levels of stress, depression, and anxiety in a cohort of 18 couples with children with autism. Mothers and fathers felt similar levels of stress; however, mothers were more anxious. Mothers may feel more responsibility for the child (Hastings, 2003) and may take on a larger part of the extra care that a child with disabilities requires (Olsson & Hwang, 2001).

When children have chronic medical problems that require round-the-clock use of technology, parents often find themselves exhausted and sleep deprived. Some of the consequences for parents whose children require routine medical procedures are anxiety and depression due to the risks inherent in the administration of the medical procedures (Kirk, 1998). When parents must administer medical procedures beyond the typical parent-child activities of nurturance, caregiving, and play, they appear to experience stress and anxiety. In addition, they often do not have the time and resources to access energizing and relaxing activities, such as socializing and recreation (Kirk, 1998).

SUPPORTING PARTICIPATION IN FAMILY LIFE

Development of Independence in Self-Care and Health-Maintenance Routines

Occupational therapists who understand the nature of family occupations can help parents manage and adapt daily living tasks with their children. The therapist asks first about daily routines and tasks that seem the most difficult. Then the therapist asks the parent where help is needed. After observing the parent feeding or dressing the child, the occupational therapist engages the parent in a discussion of alternative strategies that help the child perform daily living activities with greater skill and independence (Figure 5-3). With knowledge of the biomechanics of lifting and moving, the therapist considers whether the task is performed in a way that conserves energy and avoids injury. This consideration is especially important when a physical impairment significantly limits mobility. Strategies to help a 5-year-old bathe, dress, and use the toilet may no longer be safe for the parent's back when the child becomes an adolescent.

Routines that lead to more independence in self-care provide opportunities to enrich the child's learning.

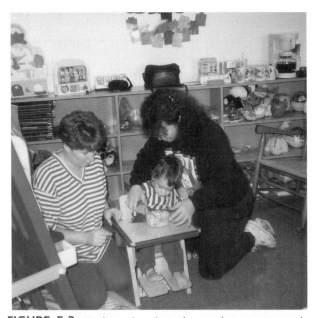

FIGURE 5-3 A therapist gives the mother recommendations for increasing the child's skills in self-feeding. Supportive positioning equipment and adapted feeding utensils make the task easier for the child and the mother.

During dressing, the child can improve strength by pulling up pants and increase language by naming colors found on the clothing. Therapists can suggest how to turn tasks into learning situations. As with all suggestions, the parent weighs the costs and benefits. Often, the occupational therapist hears, "That just won't work for us." When this happens, a number of different strategies are needed to reach the same goal.

Becoming independent in self-care occupations frequently requires repeated practice until performance becomes a habit. Occupational therapists who understand principles of behavior management can help parents reinforce a child's efforts at independence. Continuity in frequently repeated self-care occupations, such as using the toilet and eating with utensils, is increased through communication between among the occupational therapist, teacher, parents, and others. A notebook that the child carries between school and home may serve this purpose.

Any extra time that the therapist asks the parent to spend teaching new steps in self-care should be in response to a parent's identified need. In addition, the effort should be justified by evidence that the altered routine has a good chance of bringing an immediate change. Alternative suggestions should be made quickly when an adapted technique does not work. The goal of occupational therapy recommendations should be to benefit the entire family by increasing the child's independence at minimal cost in time and energy to the parents. As stated by Bernheimer and Keogh (1995), "successful interventions are the ones that can be woven back into the daily routine; they are the threads that provide professionals with the means to reinforce, rather than fray, the fabric of everyday life" (p. 430) (Figure 5-4).

Participation in Recreation and Leisure Activities

King et al. (2003) propose that the family's ability to engage family members in recreational and leisure activities is the result of a multidimensional process that includes the community, the family, and the child with a disability (Figure 5-5). Their conceptual framework draws on literature in leisure studies and work with families of children with special needs. Some factors can directly influence participation, such as an inclusive program wherein which peers and activity leaders support and believe in the child's ability to participate (Figure 5-6). Other factors, like such as the extent to which the parents perceive acceptance from friends and neighbors and how parents view being active, indirectly shape whether families choose to participate in recreational activities in the community. Parents of children with developmental delays and behavioral problems will sometimes stop taking their child out in response as a

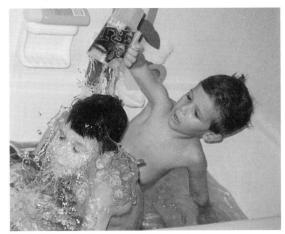

FIGURE 5-4 Michael's bath time routine allows him to practice a range of skills, including play and social interaction. (Courtesy Jill and Mark McQuaid, Dublin, Ohio.)

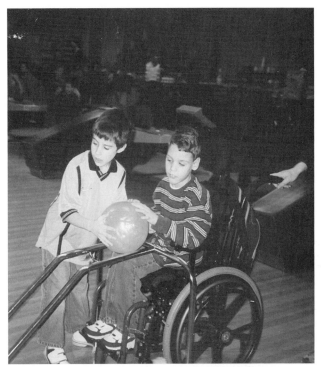

FIGURE 5-6 Michael bowls with a friend. (Courtesy Jill and Mark McQuaid, Dublin, Ohio.)

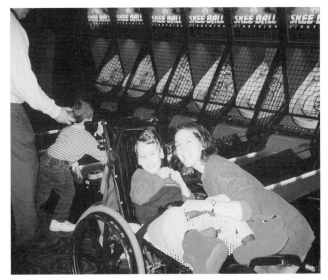

FIGURE 5-5 Recreational opportunities in the community provide an important family occupation.

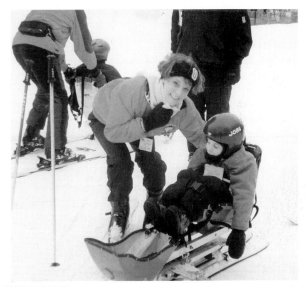

FIGURE 5-7 Most skiing facilities have equipment for children unable to stand independently.

result of negative reactions of other people to their child's noises or tantrums (Fox et al., 2002). Resources, such as money to purchase equipment and time to transport children, influence the extent to which a family can participate in recreational activities (Figure 5-7).

Occupational therapists can communicate that they respect the value of recreation and leisure by including it in assessment and intervention plans. Therapists can suggest adapted equipment the child can use to make recreational activities possible. With the passage of the Americans with Disabilities Act (1990), more recreational opportunities became available to individuals with disabilities. Information about community recreational activities is often available in local newsletters (Figure 5-8). Therapists can note which activities are accessible and appropriate for children with disabilities.

They can also suggest strategies for making the family's outings more successful, such as providing headphones for a child with auditory sensitivity. Practitioners can also help parents accomplish caregiving tasks efficiently to make more time available for recreation. Scheduling therapy and education programs to enable families to engage in recreational activities can also support family function.

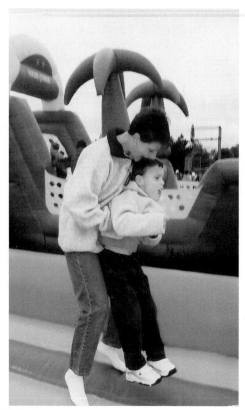

FIGURE 5-8 Activity centers with soft mats, bolsters, balls, and tunnels for tumbling offer safe and accessible environments for children with physical disabilities.

Socialization and Participation in Social Activities

Socialization is not only needed for health, it is an important mechanism for preparing family members to enter their cultural group and participate in community activities. Most families of children with disabilities, particularly those with problem behaviors, report that far too few opportunities exist for participation in the community. Families perceive that they are the only socialization agent for their children, because community social activities simply do not accommodate their children (Turnbull & Ruef, 1997). In addition, children with disabilities may interact more frequently with adults than with peers, particularly if they have classroom aides. Constant interaction with adults to the exclusion of peers may exacerbate feelings of incompetence in interactions with peers.

Children with disabilities, particularly problem behaviors, face a "glaring void of friendships" (Turnbull & Ruef, 1997, p. 224). Educational and intervention programs should focus more attention on helping friendships to develop and flourish. Although professionals have created more activities and environments that include children with disabilities, they have not necessarily encouraged mutual and reciprocal friendships to develop. Turnbull and Ruef urge professionals to focus on understanding the components of friendship and the connections that form into mutual friendships.

The presence of disability in the child may also create barriers to the parents' opportunities to socialize. Families of children with special needs often feel that they have less time to spend participating in social activities. Because childcare is typically difficult to arrange and must be set up in advance, taking advantage of spontaneous social opportunities is rarely possible (Patterson & Blum, 1996). Children who act out or demonstrate disruptive behaviors may be particularly difficult to manage in social situations.

Parents often find it helpful to develop friendships with other parents experiencing similar circumstances. A number of studies have found that increased social supports are associated with healthier family functioning and lower levels of stress (Gavidia-Payne & Stoneman, 1997; VanLeit & Crowe, 2002). Helitzer et al. (2002) implemented a program for mothers of children with disabilities to address their concerns and difficulties in daily routines and coping. The mothers were encouraged to provide emotional support to one another and to assist each other in resolving specific dilemmas in daily routines. These mothers perceived that they had changed their self-image and coping strategies through participation in the group sessions. They placed great value on having "a supportive opportunity to discuss their feelings and thoughts in a setting that was nonjudgmental and comfortable" (VanLeit & Crowe, 2002, p. 408). Schultz and Schultz (as cited in VanLeit & Crowe) implemented a similar program and found that parents perceived positive emotional outcomes. These programs can offer mothers social supports, strategies to help in coping, and practical ideas that make everyday life easier. Social supports appear to help parents adapt to stress and have a more positive attitude toward their children. These social supports appear to be of equal or greater importance to families than professional services (Britner, Morog, Pianta, & Marvin, 2003).

Fostering Readiness for Community Living

Families of children with disabilities express concerns about the future of their children with disabilities, particularly once they have left school, worrying that they do; they worry that these children will not have the life skills needed to live independently (Knox et al., 2000). As children become adolescents and then young adults, parents need information on possible living arrangements in the community. Often young adults are capable of leaving home but need support persons and arrangements for short- or long-term supervision and monitoring. These young adults do not have many options, and the options either may be overly restrictive (in order to secure funding) or may not provide sufficient supervision. Parents of young adults with disabilities emphasize the need for information on housing, particularly innovative supported living arrangements. For these young adults to succeed in living in the community with support, families need assistance in finding roommates, other support persons, funding, and arrangements for supervision and monitoring (Turnbull & Ruef, 1997).

Young adults with disabilities face many challenges in finding and maintaining employment (Turnbull & Ruef, 1997). Families and professionals need to work together to advocate for changes in the community to create opportunities for young adults to become employed and productive members of society (see Chapter 26).

FAMILY LIFE CYCLE

As discussed earlier, family systems undergo metamorphosis and adapt as family members change. Some transitions can be anticipated with developing children and seem to be tied to age more than ability. For example, *normative events* in children that require adjustments in families include the birth of a child, starting kindergarten, transitions between schools, leaving high school, and living outside the home. Other changes in the family are not anticipated. *Non-normative events* may include a grandparent coming to live with the family or a parent accepting a different job in another city. Families that are cohesive and adaptable adjust interactive routines, reorganize daily activities, and return to a sense of "normal" family life. If interactive routines and role designation are too rigidly set, the family may not be able to operate effectively through periods of transition. This is especially true if the family experiences unanticipated, threatening events, such as a job loss or a medical crisis. All families use coping strategies to accommodate periods of transition. Lawlor and Mattingly (1998) found that families express frustration that therapists do not engage them in anticipatory planning. Parents want to understand that they have reason to expect their disabled child will have a place in society and an opportunity to engage in socially valued occupations throughout adulthood.

Occupational therapists must also understand that all families are unique. Although life-cycle models consist of predictable events, the individuality of each family is acknowledged. The characteristics and issues at each life stage are highly variable, and each family moves through the stages at different rates. For example, family members may experience and resolve their feelings when they first learn about their child's diagnosis. However, the family also experiences cycles of sadness and acceptance later, within and between life stages. Issues that the family seemed to resolve when the child was an infant may occur again when the child reaches school age and an "educational diagnosis" is made or a learning problem is identified. Other life stage—related events, such as the child's ability to develop friendships when first entering grade school, may become an issue again, such as when the child enters high school (Turnbull & Turnbull, 1997).

Finally, the nature of the family structure can result in different members of the family being at different stages at the same time. Therefore characteristics of the family members and the child's phase of development must be considered. For example, in a skipped-generation family, grandparents frequently have to deal with changes associated with old age at the same time they are parenting their grandchildren. In other families, parents may be taking care of their elderly parents in addition to caring for a child with special needs. Similarly, a young couple may have more energy and resources to cope with the birth of a child with special needs than does an older couple with four other children participating in school activities.

Early Childhood

Identifying a child as being at risk for health or developmental problems is not always a simple process. Unless the child is born with medical problems, or with congenital problems in a body structure, or has features that suggest a syndrome, many children are not diagnosed until months, and sometimes years later. Families that describe their experiences in raising a child with a disability frequently recall their journey by looking back to a period when "something was not right" (Fox et al., 2002). Families of children with pervasive developmental delays recall a sense that they had to search for a diagnosis with repeated testing and visits to several clinics or evaluation centers. After receiving a diagnosis and ending a period of uncertainty, families hope for a period of stability.

Parents whose first child has special needs do not have the same experiences to draw on as families with older children (Grant & Whittell, 2000). Parents of young children may ask questions such as: "Do you think he can go into a regular classroom?" and "Do you think she will be able to live on her own some day?" Thoughtful responses to these questions recognize the parents' need for optimism and hope. However, the responses must be honest and realistic. Even therapists with years of experience and extensive knowledge about disability and development cannot make definitive statements about the future. Long-range predictions about when the child will achieve a certain milestone or level of independence are always speculative. However, parents experience frustration and feel frustrated when they are told that the future cannot be predicted. Therapists can help parents understand the range of possibilities by telling them about the continuum of services for older children and young adults in the community. Talking with parents of older children with a similar condition or hearing the therapist's story of a child with the same characteristics provides some insight into the future. Even without knowing the child's developmental course, parents start to develop an understanding that services are in place, and they begin to create new stories about their child's future.

Armed with information about the system, their rights, and the resources available to them in their communities, parents can solve problems and independently access needed services. The caregiving routines of parents whose young child has a disability are not particularly different from those of all parents of young children. At this time in the child's life, the parent's work consists of managing the child's play environment and introducing new, developmentally appropriate objects and materials. The parent ensures safety and may adjust or arrange the play environment so that the infant can access objects of interest. Feeding, diapering, bathing, and daily care are also natural parenting activities at this time. Only when infants and young children have serious medical conditions or behavioral problems are daily occupations significantly altered.

When children are medically unstable but still at home, a family may have home-based nursing for extended periods (i.e., months to several years). Murphy (1997) described the stress created by the constant presence of nurses and professional care providers constantly present in the home. Role ambiguity often results when parents feel that they must take on unpaid nursing work and nurses take on parenting roles. Parents also report stress from a lack of privacy and the continual feeling that they are "on duty." Parents of medically fragile children must make tremendous accommodations and should elicit high levels of sensitivity and responsiveness from professionals. For example, when parents have a medically unstable infant and around-the-clock, in-home nursing care, services such as respite become a priority.

School Age

When a child enters school, the family is excited about the new opportunities for learning and the child's new demonstration of independence. However, school entry is not always a positive event for families of children with disabilities. Families that experienced early intervention services may be disappointed to find fewer family services and less family support offered by the school. Typically, parents are not encouraged to attend classes or school-based therapy sessions. Many parents view the transition to school as an opportunity to be less involved and a sign of their child's maturation. To ease the transition from home to school, the parents of special-

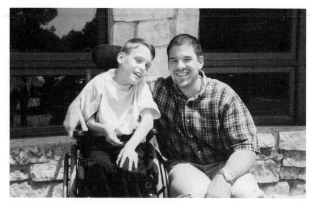

FIGURE 5-9 Michael has an aide at school who supports his participation in both academic and nonacademic activities. (Courtesy Jill and Mark McQuaid, Dublin, Ohio.)

needs children should learn about the school's programs, schedules, rules, and policies (Figure 5-9).

For children with mild learning disabilities, entry into school may be the first time that the gap between a child's performance and teachers' expectations for him or her performance is identified. Therefore this may also be the first time that parents receive information that their child has special needs. When this is the case, parents can experience surprise, disbelief, or relief.

To the school-age child, making friends and maintaining friendships become critically important. Some parents report concern if their children appear lonely, isolated, and friendless. Turnbull and Ruef (1997) found that children with behavioral problems have no friends, leaving the parents with the additional responsibility of creating and supervising play opportunities with other children. Teachers and therapists can use different strategies to promote friendships in inclusive environments. Typically developing peers can take turns being a child's "special buddy," and they can offer assistance with projects or tutoring. In situations in which social stigma is an issue, peer relations can be promoted by explaining the disability to the other children and by designing classroom activities that promote cooperation and positive interaction.

Adolescence

Adolescence is a challenging and potentially stressful time for all families. Several issues emerge in the lives of children with disabilities when they reach adolescence. Parents may need to prepare the young person to handle his or her growing sexual needs. In certain cases parents face decisions about their child's use of birth control and protection from sexually transmitted diseases. With adolescence, new concerns about a son's or daughter's vulnerability increase.

Although the child usually is well-accepted by family members, the social stigma incurred from peers and others may increase during adolescence. As one mother said, "The community accepts our children much more easily when they are small and cute. Babyish mannerisms are no longer acceptable. . . . [Our son] has had real problems with his social relationships. He simply does not know how to initiate a friendship. He has difficulty maintaining a sensible conversation with his peers. He doesn't handle teasing well, so he is teased unmercifully" (Anderson, 1983, p. 90).

The cute child with unusual behaviors may become a not-so-cute adolescent with socially unacceptable behaviors. As one parent explained why her son was not invited to a Christmas party, "Everyone in the family was invited except Billy. I thought it must be an oversight, but the friend later explained apologetically, 'I thought Billy's presence might make the other guests uncomfortable.' This kind of attitude is difficult to accept, particularly when he had been included very successfully in a similar party. I find myself crying at the unfairness" (Schulz, 1985, p. 16).

Other parents have reported difficulty in caring for their child's growing physical needs. As the child reaches adulthood, parents who are reaching middle age may feel their strength and energy declining.

> The sapping of energy occurs gradually. The isolation it imposes does, too. As I work professionally with young mothers, I see them coping energetically with the demands of everyday life. They are good parents, caring ones, doing everything possible to help their child [with a disability] reach full potential, sometimes doing more than they have to; and if they have other children, they are doing the same for them. Most of these mothers even get out, see friends, attend meetings, volunteer in the community, and do all the things their friends and families expect them to do. All this is at least possible when one's child is little, though it demands enormous energy. But to look at the mothers of children who have turned into teenagers is to see the beginnings of the ravages. Their life style is changing. They go out less, see fewer people, do less for their children. They are stripping their living to the essentials (Morton, 1985, p. 144).

FAMILY SYSTEMS

Parents

Regardless of the type of family structure (e.g., traditional, nontraditional, blended, or three-generation households), caregiving adults sharing parental duties need to coordinate their efforts. These adults form the *parent subsystem* of the family, which can be a positive force and can contribute to the child's ability to face developmental challenges. Researchers have found a number of different solutions in how parents distribute childcare, realizing that the different forms may all be

adaptive if they enable the system to operate and meet family functions (Hombeck et al., 1997; Weiss, Marvin, & Pianta, 1997). Studies have found that additional time in caregiving co-occupations is required in the mother-child subsystems (Crowe, 1993). The type of disability the child has and its severity affect the amount of time required; for example, Crowe (1993) found that mothers of children with multiple disabilities spent at least 1 hour more a day on child-related activities compared with mothers of children with Down syndrome. Disabilities that seem to create more stress and caregiving effort for the family include autism, severe and multiple disabilities, behavior disorders, and medical problems that require frequent hospitalization and in-home medical care.*

Researchers have reported that mothers experience stress from the increased workload of caring for a child with disabilities (Hastings, 2003; Olsson & Hwang, 2001; Willoughby & Glidden, 1995). In addition, mothers may experience more stress than their husbands because they are typically the primary parent working with the intervention team, and, as a result, face great demands on their time and communication skills (Lawlor & Mattingly, 1998). Mothers often become the conduit for communication, responsible for transferring information and expectations between clinic and family. Therefore mothers must be sensitive to the perspectives of both the professionals and family members.

Some researchers have found that fathers can be more at risk for stress than mothers because they feel isolated and helpless compared to the mother, who is more involved. Young and Roopnarine (1994) found that fathers spend about one third the time caring for their children that mothers do. Also, fathers may lack social supports compared with their spouses. Scholars have come to recognize the multidimensional process influencing what fathers do and why they do it (Parke, 2002) They also have noted that fathers are more sensitive than mothers to the influence of the ecology of the family and the attitude of others.

Other studies have found that mothers and fathers report similar levels of stress related to a child with disabilities (King et al., 1996; Nagy & Ungere, 1990). Although stress levels were similar (King et al.), mothers attended 80% of the child's intervention sessions compared with fathers, who attended 33%. The problem that arises from fathers' inability to attend therapy is that information is often conveyed via the mother. Therapists should identify and use more direct methods of communicating with the father to ensure that information is

---

* Turnbull & Turnbull, 1997; Olsson & Hwang, 2001; VanLeit & Crowe, 2002; Hastings, 2003; Rivers & Stoneman, 2003; and Case-Smith, 2004.

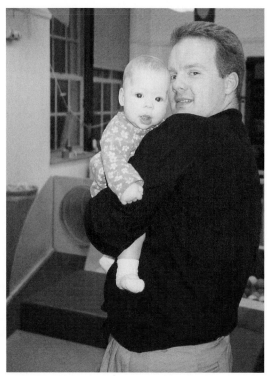

FIGURE 5-10 Father enjoys holding his child while attending an early intervention program in the evening with his family.

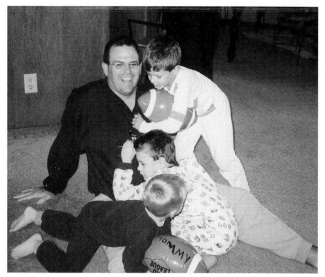

FIGURE 5-11 Playtime with Dad before bed.

transmitted accurately and to unburden the mother of the responsibility of transmitting information.

Ninio and Rinott (1988) recommended a number of strategies for encouraging the father's participation. Programs that seem to best support the father's involvement actively attempt to involve the father in planning meetings, offer convenient scheduling for therapy and meetings, such as evenings or weekends (King et al., 1996), focus on providing information about the disability and community resources, and provide opportunities for the father to enjoy activities with his child (Figures 5-10, 5-11). When the father is the family's primary decision maker, it is critical that he receive complete information about the decisions that need to be made, including the purchase of assistive technology and accessing resources for the child.

A child with disabilities can also affect the relationship between husband and wife. Although there is evidence that a child with disabilities can stress the marital relationship and decrease marital satisfaction, some parents have reported that their marriage was strengthened (Rivers & Stoneman, 2003). Differences in marital satisfaction between families of children with disabilities and those of typically developing children tend to be minimal (e.g., Britner, Morog, Pianta, & Marvin, 2003). Stress in dealing with the child may bring parents together for problem solving, and they may rely on each other for emotional support and coping. A strong relationship between husband and wife seems to buffer parenting stress. Britner et al. found that mothers who reported high levels of marital satisfaction also reported less parental distress and found their supports and interventions to be more helpful.

Siblings

As was suggested in the discussion of the system perspective, family members reciprocally influence one another in a dynamic way. Having a brother or sister with special needs changes the experiences of other children growing up in that family (Figure 5-12).

Williams et al. (2002) have investigated the question of how having a sibling with special needs influences the

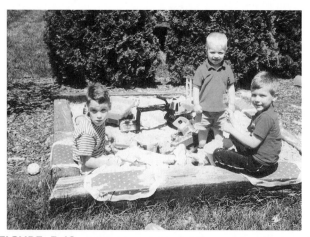

FIGURE 5-12 Michael and his brothers enjoy backyard play. A sandbox is a fail-proof medium that provides equal opportunity for multiple levels of play. (Courtesy Jill and Mark McQuaid, Dublin, Ohio.)

typically developing brother or sister. Using a method that allowed them to track direct and indirect effects (structural equation model), they investigated factors that might influence behavioral problems or the self-esteem of children who had a sibling that had either a chronic illness (e.g., cancer, diabetes, or cystic fibrosis) or a developmental disability (e.g., autism, cerebral palsy). They considered factors that might influence the typical child's experiences, such as how much the child understood about the disease, the sibling and his or her attitude and social support. They also asked the mother about the mood and emotional closeness of the family (family cohesion). The researchers reported that the family's SES, family cohesion, and the siblings' understanding of the disease were related to whether or not the typically developing sibling had behavioral problems. They also found that when the siblings felt supported, their behavior, mood, and self-esteem were more positive than when they felt unsupported.

Siblings are an important source of support to each other throughout life. In general, the relationships between children with disabilities and their siblings are strong and positive (Stoneman, 2001) (Figure 5-13). However, the research findings are varied across types of disabilities and sibling place in the family (older or younger). Research reports have shown that when the child with a disability has more severe disabilities, the quality of sibling interaction decreases (Stoneman, 2001).

Siblings without disability generally select play activities in which the child with a disability can participate, such as rough-and-tumble play rather than symbolic play. Conflict among siblings may be higher when a child has a disability such as hyperactivity or behavioral problems. Conflict tends to be lower when a child has Down syndrome or mental retardation. Often the roles of siblings are asymmetric, with the typically developing child dominating the child with a disability. Siblings may be asked to take on caregiving roles, and assuming caregiving roles can have both positive and negative effects (Stoneman, 2001). Siblings learn to relate and interact in the context of a family. Positive and solid marital systems seem to promote more positive sibling relationships, and marital stress has a deleterious effect on sibling relationships. Rivers and Stoneman (2003) studied the effects of marital stress and coping on sibling relationships when one child had autism. Using multiple self-report measures of siblings and parents, they found that when marital stress is greater, the sibling relationship is more negative. This study confirmed the importance of examining sibling relationships in the context of the family, recognizing that all family subsystems affect each other.

As occupational therapists promote engagement in a full range of activities as a way of helping the child participate in family life, the inclusion of siblings, not just as helpers but as members of the family, is an important step in occupation-centered practice. The therapist can collaborate with family members regarding ways to structure activities and choose the location and timing for activities to help families manage or minimize aggressive or annoying behaviors of the child with special needs. Peer support groups for the typically developing siblings can also be occupation-centered (Parker, 2003). Therapists can develop a recreational program for brothers and sisters of children with whom they work so that the siblings can meet one another and realize that their family is not the only one that faces challenging behaviors. These groups generally have open-ended discussions about what it means to have siblings with disabilities. When possible, siblings should be involved in occupational therapy sessions. They are likely to be the best playmates and can often elicit maximum effort from their brother or sister. In addition, sibling involvement gives the therapeutic activity additional meaning (play), and siblings can act as models for teaching new skills and providing needed support in a natural context (e.g., they can help the child with special needs learn a puzzle or game).

Extended Family

In the extended family, the experience of having a child with special needs depends on the meaning family members bring to their relationship with the child. For some grandparents, grandchildren represent a link to the future and an opportunity for vicarious achievement. Researchers find that when children have disabilities, grandparents express both positive and negative feelings and go through a series of adjustments similar to those

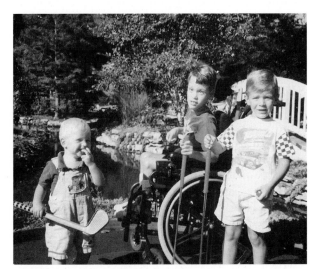

FIGURE 5-13 Although Michael is the oldest of four boys, his younger brothers already take the initiative to help him participate. A round of miniature golf requires his brothers' assistance, which does not detract from the fun. (Courtesy Jill and Mark McQuaid, Dublin, Ohio.)

of the parents (Schimoeller & Baranowski, 1998). Many of the negative feelings, such as anger and confusion, appear to decrease with time. However, some never completely disappear. Positive feelings, such as acceptance and a sense of usefulness, increase over time. A grandparent's educational level and sense of closeness to the child are positively associated with greater involvement with the child. Factors, such as the grandparent's age and health and the distance the grandparent lives from the child, do not appear to influence involvement (Figure 5-14). Grandparents learn information about their grandchild's condition primarily through the child's parents. However, some seek information from other sources, such as support groups for grandparents of special-needs children.

Patterson, Garwick, Bennett, and Blum (1997) interviewed parents of children with chronic conditions about the behavior of extended family members. Family members, such as grandparents, uncles, and aunts of the child, were especially important to fathers and mothers for emotional and practical assistance. When extended family members were not supportive, parents expressed frustration and hurt by over their lack of contact. In addition, parents recalled examples of times family members made insensitive comments about the child, ignored the child, or did not want to talk about the child's disability. Parents of children with behavioral problems reported that extended family members tended to blame the child's actions on the parents' inability to discipline correctly (Turnbull & Ruef, 1997). Families may be reluctant to ask relatives for assistance, wishing instead that they might volunteer (Grant & Whittell, 2000). With the consent of the parents, occupational therapists can encourage extended family members to become more involved by offering to share information with them and inviting them to therapy sessions. In this way, therapists can help families build on important social and emotional resources.

FAMILY RESILIENCE AND GETTING ON WITH LIFE

An important philosophic shift has occurred over the past few decades in the way families of children with special needs are viewed by professionals. The original assumption, that the presence of a disabled member led to family dysfunction and a life of recurring sorrow, has been replaced by more neutral descriptions of the adjustment process (Helff & Glidden, 1998). Parents of children with special needs say that their children bring growth-producing challenges, and a sense of pride, fulfillment, and joy to their families (Stallings & Cook, 1997; Turnbull, Blue-Banning, Turbiville, & Park, 1999). The strength and resilience of many families in meeting life events and achieving a level of happiness and life satisfaction can be a source of inspiration to occupational therapists.

The fact that most families successfully adjust to children's disabilities should not lead occupational therapists to ignore the initial and ongoing challenges that families face. Times of coping and adaptation vary according to whether a family must adjust to an acute traumatic event leading to a disability or the family gains a gradual, unfolding understanding of the child's developmental differences. After the diagnostic period, when the child's problems are identified, the family goes about the process of living. During this period the demands for adaptation and coping vary. The following sections describe how occupational therapists can offer support, intervention services, and education to families.

COLLABORATING WITH FAMILIES

Parent-professional collaboration grows from an appreciation that by working in partnership both the occupational therapist and parent have important expertise and knowledge that will make a difference in a child's life. The sustained involvement and special insights families bring has been discussed earlier; this section goes into more specificity regarding the different ways occupational therapists work with families.

Family-centered services are described by professionals in early intervention programs in a variety of different ways (Unger, Jones, Park, & Tressell, 2001). Definitions vary from acting as service coordinators, to addressing the needs of the family for financial and social

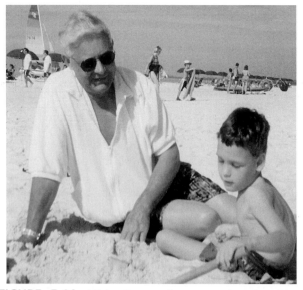

FIGURE 5-14 Michael's grandparents enjoy their time with him and offer important support to his parents. (Courtesy Jill and Mark McQuaid, Dublin, Ohio.)

resources as part of an intervention program, to involving family members as part of a team that makes decisions relative to a child's program. Three complementary models for family-centered services are (1) family support, (2) therapist and teacher services, and (3) parent education.

Family support is designed to bolster a network of social support to enhance the family's natural strengths and family functions. DeGrace (2004) recommended not being so focused on the child's issues that a therapist does not recognize how the disability impacts family occupations. Social support, such as being able to talk with other parents, decreases the family members' feelings of isolation and stress, which detract from their potential to optimize the developmental outcome of the child with special needs (McGuire, Crowe, Law, & VanLeit, 2004). Promoting a family's well-being through emotional support and practical suggestions allows families to engage in responsive interaction with their children (Dunst, 2000). The occupational therapist's role in providing family support is to help the family secure needed resources and to capitalize on its existing competencies and strengths.

Direct services are provided when the therapist engages a child in an activity with the goal of promoting the child's skill acquisition and minimizing the consequences of a disability. Other family members may be present and participating in the therapeutic activity, but the occupational therapist's attention is on promoting the child's engagement in the activity.

Parent education has a number of purposes and should be individualized to the parents' interests, learning styles, and knowledge levels. In parent-mediated therapy, the caregiver is taught how to engage the child in an activity designed to achieve a parent-identified goal or outcome (Mahoney et al., 1999). Strong evidence indicates that the more adults who are raising a child know about development, the more responsive and supportive they are in interacting with that child and the better prepared they are to foster optimal development (Shonkoff & Phillips, 2000; Wacharasin, Barnard, & Spieker, 2003). Parents of children with delays are not looking for developmental milestones; their efforts to engage their children in daily activities are not informed by hearing that typically children feed themselves with spoons between 15 and 24 months or don simple clothing between 2 and 3 years. Parents want to hear how children with special needs learn things that other typically developing children seem to teach themselves. Kaiser and Hancock (2003) reported on an effective, systematic approach to teaching parents new skills. First, the parents identified the outcome or skills they wanted to foster, and the interventionists then guided them in what to do and how to implement child instruction within the natural flow of everyday activities.

Parent education is likely to be effective when the child demonstrates interest in doing the activities the team has targeted. At that point the therapist becomes a "coach" who facilitates an exchange of ideas that helps the parent discover ways of helping the child learn the activity (Rush, Shelden, & Hanft, 2003). This dialog includes periods of observation and reflection. Coaches bring both didactic and pragmatic understanding of the intervention strategy and serve as a resource (Kaiser & Hancock, 2003). Unlike in direct therapy, the parent is the focus of the therapist's attention, and the parent is the one interacting with the child. The concept of coaching avoids an approach that can give the impression that therapists have more expertise in how to raise children than parents do. Parent education requires a range of skills, including an understanding of development and a well-grounded expertise in how to implement an intervention that has proved effective (Kaiser & Hancock, 2003). Therapists who understand the principles of adult learning, who have a clear idea of what they want to teach, and who are skillful observers are likely to be effective parent educators.

Establishing a Partnership

The first interactions of the therapist with a family open the door to the establishment of a partnership. In a family-centered approach, the therapist demonstrates a family orientation that establishes trust and builds rapport. The practitioner conveys to the family "a willingness to orient services to the whole family, rather than just the child" (McWilliam, Tocci, & Harbin, 1998, p. 212). The therapist's initial interview reflects an interest not only in the child's behaviors but also in the family's concerns with managing those behaviors. These first interactions demonstrate that an equal partnership is desired and encourage a give-and-take of information. At the same time, parents begin to understand that professionals are there to help them and to provide information and resources that support the child's development.

Trust building is not easily defined, and it is associated with nonverbal language and words. Thinking the best of families is important to the development of this partnership. This may not always be easy, particularly when the family's life style contradicts that of the professional. Being positive and maintaining a nonjudgmental position with a family can be challenging, but it is essential to establish trust and build on a trusting relationship.

In a qualitative study in which 137 families were interviewed about their partnerships with service providers (Blue-Banning, Summers, Frankland, Nelson, & Beegle, 2004), families emphasized that partnerships were built on equality and reciprocity. A sense of equality was created when professionals acknowledged the validity of the parents' point of view, and partnerships flourish when there are opportunities for each member to contribute. Turnbull et al. (1999) advocated expanding the definition of parent education to one in which a collaborative exchange of information occurs among parents, professionals, and people in the community. If parent education focuses on helping the parent minimize the child's disability and optimize developmental gains, the focus is too narrow. Furthermore, if teaching is always a one-way process, it does not necessarily strengthen the family by recognizing their expertise. Rather, Turnbull et al. (1999) suggest that programs involve parents who are knowledgeable about community organizations and activities designed for children with special needs. Then parents can become the educators. By bringing together a collaborative team that includes people in community agencies and organizations, parents can contribute their expertise on how to work with children who have special needs.

Providing Helpful Information

Parents of children with disabilities report that information is a primary need from service providers (Grant & Whittell, 2000; Greene, 1999). In a study of family-centered early intervention programs, mothers reported the frequency of specific family services. The services provided, in order of frequency, were (1) child information, (2) educational activities, (3) systems engagement, (4) personal-family services, and (5) resource assistance (Mahoney & Bella, 1998). The information that therapists provide to families about the intervention system prepares the families to work with existing systems, to use resources available, and to understand their rights as consumers. This information also enables the family members to become informed decision makers and to choose their level of participation in the intervention program.

Child-related information that may be of benefit to parents includes information about the child's development, the disability, the child's health, and assessment results. To provide up-to-date information, therapists must continually engage in reading and other professional development activities. Naturally, families want the most accurate and complete information, which places a responsibility on professionals to obtain current information and to continually update their skills. The families in one qualitative study "admired providers who were willing to learn and keep up to date with the technology of their field. . . . a competent professional is someone who is not afraid to admit when he or she does not know something, but is willing to find out" (Blue-Banning et al., 2004, p. 178).

Although parents express that they want information about their child and about the diagnosis, it must be given in a supportive manner. Service providers who focused on the negative aspects of the child's condition or compared the child to typically developing peers were viewed as not supportive (Patterson et al., 1997). Once a deficit has been identified and the child qualifies for services, hearing the child's developing abilities expressed as delays or deficits can be hurtful for the parents. Describing what the child has accomplished using a criterion-referenced instrument, such as using the Pediatric Evaluation of Disability Inventory (Haley, Coster, Ludlow, Haltiwanger, & Andrellos, 1992), helps parents remain positive and encouraged. Using an occupation-centered approach, the therapist asks what self-care activities the child is attempting or what play skills are emerging. Articulating a therapeutic goal linked to an emerging skill that the parents have identified reduces professional jargon and helps parents understand how the intervention plan relates to their child. Typically, parents hope to receive recommendations for activities that help the child play, for toys that match the child's abilities, and for strategies that lead to independence in self-care. They also look to the therapist for help in managing motor impairments or differences in sensory processing that limit occupational performance.

Respecting and Accepting Family Diversity

Respect for and acceptance of family diversity is demonstrated when professionals acknowledge that all families have strengths and resources. The positive aspects of families are recognized and used as the foundation for the intervention program. Parent participants in focus groups defined respect as simple courtesies from professionals, such as being on time to meetings (Blue-Banning et al., 2004). The professionals who were interviewed linked respect to being nonjudgmental and accepting of families. When professionals are disrespectful to families, parents may become reluctant to access services or may lose their sense of empowerment. Demonstrating respect for families becomes particularly important when they are of different racial, ethnic, cultural, and socioeconomic status.

Families from different cultures often have different perspectives on child rearing, health care, and disabilities. Table 5-1 lists cultural characteristics, examples, and the possible consequences for intervention programs.

Therapists need to be sensitive to the implications of these subtle differences in child rearing. For example, in one family, all of the children slept in the parents' bed for their first 12 years. This tradition made it difficult to increase the independence and self-sufficiency of a 10-year-old boy with myelomeningocele. Although the therapist was concerned about the child's dependence on bedtime routines, the parents were not. If the therapist gave the family recommendations for increasing inde-

TABLE 5-1 Cultural Considerations in Intervention Services

Cultural Considerations	Examples	May Determine
Meaning of the disability	Disability in a family may be viewed as shameful and disgraceful or as a positive contribution to the family.	Level of acceptance of the disability and the need for services
Attitudes about professionals	Professionals may be viewed as persons of authority or as equals.	Level of family members' participation; may be only minimal if the partnership is based only on respect or fear
Attitudes about children	Children may be highly valued.	Willingness of the family to make many sacrifices on behalf of the child
Attitudes about seeking and receiving help	Problems in the family may be viewed as strictly a family affair or may be easily shared with others.	Level of denial; may work against acknowledging and talking about the problem
Family roles	Roles may be gender specific and traditional or flexible. Age and gender hierarchies of authority may exist.	Family preference; may exist for the family member who takes the leadership role in the family-professional partnership
Family interactions	Boundaries between family subsystems may be strong and inflexible or relaxed and fluid.	Level of problem sharing/solving in families; family members may keep to themselves and deal with problems in isolation or may problem solve as a unit.
Time orientation	Family may be present or future oriented.	Family's willingness to consider future goals and future planning
Role of the extended family	Extended family members may be close or distant, physically and emotionally.	Who is involved in the family-professional partnership
Support networks	Family may rely solely on nuclear family members, on extended family members, or on unrelated persons. Importance of godparents	Who can be called on in time of need
Attitude toward achievement	Family may have a relaxed attitude or high expectations for achievement.	Goals and expectations of the family for the member with the disability
Religion	Religion and the religious community may be strong or neutral factors in some aspects of family life.	Family's values, beliefs, and traditions as sources of comfort
Language	Family may be non-English speaking, bilingual, or English speaking.	Need for translators
Number of generations removed from country of origin	Family may have just emigrated or may be several generations removed from the country of origin.	Strength and importance of cultural ties
Reasons for leaving country of origin	Family may be immigrants from countries at war.	Family's readiness for involvement with external world

From Turnbull, A.P., & Turnbull, H.R. (1990). *Families, professions and exceptionality: A special partnership* (pp. 156-157). Columbus, OH: Merrill.

pendence that included having the child sleep in his own bed, the parents' responses may have been negative. Choosing to change a family routine is entirely a parental decision. The parents may indicate that they prefer that the occupational therapist focus on activities other than those that challenge the family's values.

Providing Flexible, Accessible, and Responsive Services

Because each family is different and has individualized needs, services must be flexible and adaptable. The occupational therapist should continually adapt the intervention activities as the family's interests and priorities change. Responsiveness entails "doing whatever needs to be done" as a clear demonstration of commitment to the child and family (McWilliam, Tocci, & Harbin, 1998).

Families value the commitment of professionals to their work and feel that it is important that professionals view them as "more than a case" (Blue-Banning et al., 2004). Parents expressed appreciation when professionals exhibited "above and beyond" commitment by meeting with them outside the workday, remembering their child's birthday, or bringing them materials to use.

Although therapists are often flexible and responsive to the child's immediate needs and the parent's concerns, the range of possible services is sometimes limited by the structure of the system. When a parent desires additional services, a change in location (e.g., home-based versus center-based care), or services to be provided at a different time, the therapist may or may not be able to accommodate the request because of the therapist's schedule. Often the agency or school system enforces policies regarding the therapist's caseloads and scope of services. Practitioners are caught in the middle, between the system's structure and individualized family needs. A ready solution does not always exist for the therapist who is constrained by time limitations and the demands of a large caseload.

Much of the time the therapist recognizes that he or she cannot change the structure of the system and must work as efficiently as possible within the system. At the same time, the therapist should inform the family of the program's rules and policies so that they are aware of the constraints of the system. The occupational therapist can also take the initiative to work toward changing the system to allow more flexibility in meeting family needs. Some suggestions for therapists from parents on providing flexible and responsive services include the following (Turnbull & Turnbull, 1990):

1 Listen with empathy to understand family concerns and needs.
2 Verbally acknowledge family priorities.
3 Make adaptations to services based on "parents" input.
4 Explain the constraints of the system when the parents' requests cannot be met.
5 Suggest alternative resources to parents when their requests cannot be met within the system.
6 Discuss parents' suggestions and requests with administrators to increase the possibilities that policies and agency structure can change to benefit families.

Respecting Family Roles in Decision Making

Parents should be the primary decision makers in intervention for their child. Although professionals tend to acknowledge readily the role of the parents as decision makers, they do not always give parents choices or explain options in ways that enable parents to make good decisions. Too often, plans that should be family-centered are written in professional jargon and do not always address family concerns (Boone, McBride, Swann, Moore, & Drew, 1998). Parents are involved in decision making about their child in the following ways:

1 Parents can defer decision making to the therapist. Deferring to the therapist may reflect confidence in the therapist's judgment and may be an easy way for parents to make a decision about an issue that they do not completely understand.
2 Parents have veto power. It is important that parents know that they have the power to veto any decision made or goal chosen by the team. Awareness of the legitimacy of this role gives parents assurance that they have an important voice on the team and can make changes, should they desire them. This role appears to be quite satisfying to parents (McBride et al., 1993).
3 Parents share in decision making. As described in the previous section, when parent-professional partner-

ships have been established, the parents fully participate in team discussions that lead to decisions about the intervention plan. Service options and alternatives are made clear, and parents have the information needed to make final decisions. Requests of parents are honored (within the limitations of the program). In a qualitative study in which families were interviewed, McBride and others (1993) found that although family members assumed limited roles in decision making and were provided few meaningful choices, most families reported satisfaction with these practices. Families cannot always be given a wide range of choices about who will provide services and when and where these services will be provided. However, their role in decision making should still be emphasized. Families who are empowered to make decisions early in the intervention process will be are better prepared for that role throughout the course of the child's development. In most cases, assessment of choices and good decision making are skills that parents promote in their children as they approach adulthood.

COMMUNICATION STRATEGIES

As previously discussed, a priority of parents is to receive information regarding child development in general and what to expect for their own child's development. They also desire information about the diagnosis or disability, therapeutic activities to enhance the child's skills, and methods to cope with the disability within the family's routine. Therapists have tremendous amounts of information to impart to parents. Effective helping is most likely to occur when the information given is requested or sought by the parent (Dunst et al., 1994). Effective communication is built on trust and respect; it requires honesty and sensitivity to what the parent needs to know at the moment.

Occupational therapists communicate with parents using a variety of methods: formal and informal, written, verbal, and nonverbal. The following section describes communication strategies consistent with the principles described earlier. The strategies are based primarily on feedback from parents regarding what they have found to be effective help from occupational therapists (Case-Smith & Nastro, 1993; Hinojosa, Sproat, Mankhetwit, & Anderson, 2002).

Formal Team Meeting with the Family

Sometimes the therapist's first meeting with a family is a formal team meeting to develop an IFSP or IEP or a rehabilitation plan. To increase the parents' participation and comfort level in such a planning meeting, it is important to provide them with specific information about the purpose, structure, and logistics of the meeting. Information about parental rights must be explained to parents before and during the meeting. Professionals may need to decipher legal terms so that parents have practical knowledge regarding IDEA safeguards. Prior to an IFSP or IEP meeting, parents should be informed of the questions that the team members may ask (e.g., "What are your visions for your child?"), so that they can formulate thoughtful responses. Parents should receive assessment results before the meeting. As a result, parents have an opportunity to think about the assessment and to be prepared to discuss their goals for the child in the team meeting. A telephone call before the meeting also gives the therapist an opportunity to ask about the parents' concerns and to prepare options for meeting those concerns in the child's educational program or intervention plan.

In a parent-professional conference, family members need to feel comfortable and connected to the other team members. The conference should begin with the introduction of all members and a discussion of the purpose of the meeting. Professionals should encourage parents to ask questions, express opinions, or take notes. After the introductions, family members should be encouraged to share information, using open-ended questions. For example, the therapist might begin, "What are your primary concerns about Jim and school right now?" All team members should respectfully attend to what the parents say, ask for clarification when needed, and indicate understanding by paraphrasing or summarizing the information.

When professionals share information, they should use jargon-free language, avoiding technical terms. When technical terms are used, they must be explained in ways that everyone can understand. Professionals should begin with positive points and then explain problems and deficits. In describing the problems, anecdotes or real examples of the child's performance should be given. Parents appreciate it when occupational therapists are sensitive to the parents' responses to new information and provide opportunities for questions. When information is provided in writing, parents have an opportunity to read it later, without the presence of a group of professionals (Turnbull & Turnbull, 1997).

After plans and decisions about goals have been made, they should be summarized. Plans should be specific and should include dates, tasks, and the names of those who are responsible for the plans. The meeting should end on a positive note, with plans made for another meeting or the next mode of communication. Again, parents find it helpful when verbalized plans are provided to them later in writing.

Informal Meetings

Many parents prefer informal, individual meetings with the occupational therapist to structured, more formal meetings. Meetings during or after the child's therapy, although convenient, are not always ideal. The therapist

needs to be organized and prepared for parent encounters. Often the answer to a casual question, such as, "How is Sherry doing in occupational therapy?" holds great importance for the parent. Casual or general responses are not adequate. The therapist should give specific examples of recent performance or should state when reevaluation will occur and how those results will be reported.

When unplanned meetings occur, the therapist needs to listen to and acknowledge the parent's concerns. When the parent asks for specific information about intervention or intervention goals, the therapist should indicate that he or she prefers to respond after reviewing daily notes and charts on the child. The therapist can later make a telephone call to the parent with the child's chart in hand to avoid giving the parent erroneous or misleading information.

Written and Electronic Communication

In many intervention settings, particularly in the schools, parents are not physically present, and regular communication with family members relies on written strategies. Because written communication does not require the sender and recipient to be in the same place at the same time, it is a practical and important way to maintain communication with parents.

Notebooks

Notebooks shared between therapists and parents seem to be a highly valued and successful way for parents to keep important information and to have a regular, reliable method for expressing concerns. In the notebook, team members may describe a new skill the child demonstrated that day, an action by the child that delighted the class, an upcoming school event, or materials requested from the parent. It may also include snack information or the current strategy for working on self-feeding. The parents can share their perceptions of the child's feelings, new accomplishments at home, or new concerns. Regardless of whether the therapist and parent have face-to-face contact, notebooks are important. Home-based therapists may initiate a notebook for the parent to record significant child behaviors and for the therapist to make weekly suggestions for activities. In the neonatal intensive care unit, notebooks are sometimes kept at the infant's bedside. These notebooks provide a method for the parents and therapists to communicate with the nursing staff on successful strategies for feeding and handling the infant.

Handouts

When judiciously used and appropriate to the child, handouts can be helpful and valued by the parents.

Handouts should be individualized and applicable to the family's daily routine. Handouts copied from books and manuals are appropriate if they are individualized. Many parents prefer pictures and diagrams. One mother expressed her appreciation of handouts, saying, "The home-based therapist who came out would not only show me and do things, she would watch me handle Martin and correct me if I did it wrong. She brought me pictures and diagrams and explained what each meant. . . . I still go back to them at times" (Nastro, 1992, p. 70).

Other mothers have said that photographs are also helpful. In the hospital, occupational therapists often take photographs of the child in a good position for feeding or other caregiving tasks to serve as a reminder to parents and staff on ways to improve postural alignment.

Electronic Mail and Other Methods of Communication

Electronic mail has become an easy way to stay in touch with parents. As an end- of- the- day activity, it offers the therapist a method for noting any particular daily occurrences that would be of interest to the parents. Regardless of whether the family has access to electronic communication, a regular progress report is important to parents and is required in most school systems. A simple report covering a few areas of performance may be more meaningful to the parents than a lengthy, complicated report. Child quotes and reports of specific performance send the message that the child is receiving individualized attention.

Telephone calls and simple notes sent home are good ways to maintain communication regarding issues on which the parents and therapist have a common understanding. However, informal communication methods are not appropriate when the therapist has concerns or issues about the child. If the therapist expects a lengthy discussion, the telephone is not the method of choice, although a call may be used to set up a meeting.

Some therapists use videotapes to convey information about handling, feeding, and positioning methods. When selecting videotaping as a method of conveying information, the therapist should keep in mind that parents must invest time in watching the tape; short clips of direct relevance to current goals are most efficient.

HOME PROGRAMS

Throughout this text, recommendations have been given for ways to integrate therapeutic strategies into the daily occupations of children, with the clear recognition that learning occurs best in the child's natural environment. Skills demonstrated in therapy translate into meaningful functional change only when the child can generalize the skill to other settings and demonstrate the skill in his or her daily routine. Therapists often recommend home activities for parents to implement with their child, so that he or she can apply new skills at home.

Before making recommendations the therapist should ask the parents about daily routines and the typical flow of family activities during the week. Understanding which routines and traditions hold special meaning for the family will help therapists focus. The therapist and parents discuss family occupations during the day and identify naturally occurring opportunities to teach the child new skills by understanding what needs to occur and deciding when it will work for them. The result of this close examination of the typical week enables the therapist and parents to embed goals and activities in interactive routines where the therapeutic process does not diminish the value and pleasure.

Hinojosa (1990) and Case-Smith and Nastro (1993) examined the ways mothers use home programs and the characteristics of home programs that parents value and implement. Hinojosa completed a qualitative study in which eight mothers of preschool children with CP were interviewed. Most of the mothers did not carry out the suggested home programs. Mothers reported that they did not have the time, energy, or confidence to follow the programs effectively. Hinojosa suggested that it is inappropriate to expect mothers to follow a strict home program. Instead, therapists should assist mothers in adaptive ways to meet their children's needs with minimal disruption to their lives. He described the resultant home intervention as "mother directed," meaning that the mother made the decision as to how therapy might be implemented at home (Hinojosa, 1990).

Case-Smith and Nastro (1993) replicated Hinojosa's study using a sample of mothers from Ohio who had young children with CP. Each had accessed private and publicly funded therapies. Initially, when their children were infants, these mothers had participated extensively in home programs. They indicated that these efforts were self-motivated and did not feel that the specific home programs were "an imposed expectation" on the part of the therapists. As the children reached preschool age, the mothers no longer implemented home programs with their children. Reasons for discontinuing home programs included lack of time and increased resistance on the part of their children. Lyon (1989) expressed a mother's perspective on implementing the implementation of therapy at home:

"I've come to terms with being 'only human.'" If I could ensure that Zak could go through the day always moving in appropriate ways, flexing when he should flex, straightening when he should straighten, and play and learn and experience and appreciate . . . I would; but, that is not possible. I do have a responsibility to help

Zachary develop his motor skills, but I also have a responsibility to help him learn about life. So on those days when we have so much fun together or are so busy that bedtime comes before therapy time, I finally feel comfortable that I have given him something just as vital to his development, a real mom" (Lyon, 1989, p. 4).

Although mothers tend not to implement specific prescribed strategies, they report appreciating the therapists' suggestions and ideas about home activities that promote child development or make caregiving easier. Case-Smith and Nastro (1993) found that the mothers in their sample frequently used the handouts with specific activities and recommendations long after they had been given to them. Summers et al. (1990), explained that parents found written materials and videotapes helpful because they were "not always ready to hear, understand, or accept some information, but that it could be available for later use" (p. 91). At the same time, it is important to realize that written material may be a less-effective form of communication for families in which reading is not an already established way to learn about child development.

Positive relationships with families seem to develop when open and honest communication is established, and when parents are encouraged to participate in their child's program to the extent that they desire. When asked to give advice to therapists, parents stated that they appreciated (1) specific objective information; (2) flexibility in service delivery; (3) sensitivity and responsiveness to their concerns (McWilliam et al., 1998); (4) positive, optimistic attitudes (Case-Smith & Nastro, 1993); and (5) technical expertise and skills (Blue-Banning et al., 2004). One mother expressed that hope and optimism are always best. "Given a choice, I would want my therapist to be an optimist and perhaps to strive for goals that might be a bit too optimistic, keeping in mind that we might not come to that" (Nastro, 1992, p. 64). McWilliam et al. describe this positive attitude as "a belief in parents' abilities, a nonjudgmental mind-set and optimistic view of children's development, and an enthusiasm for working with families" (p. 213).

WORKING WITH FAMILIES FACING MULTIPLE CHALLENGES

Features that contribute to diversity in families are characteristics that occupational therapists welcome and accommodate in providing individualized services. For example, parents dealing with their own chronic physical illnesses may need help dealing with energy or emotional support as they experience social stigma associated with an illness such as HIV/AIDS (Opaccich & Savage, 2004). The principles presented in this text remain critically important, but they are more difficult for therapists to implement when they are working with families facing multiple challenges. Challenges to a family's ability to fulfill its functions (e.g., living in poverty, acute onset of a disability in the parent) increase the vulnerability of children with special needs and add unique challenges to family functions. By identifying protective factors that bolster the child's resilience, the therapist can approach issues from a positive perspective to support strengths, capitalize on family assets, and work to make maximum use of community resources.

The occupational therapist grounded in family systems perspective and committed to empowering families will work effectively with a whole family system in a family-centered manner, regardless of the type of disability of one or more family members (Brown, Humphry, & Taylor, 1997). Understanding and valuing how the family system orchestrates members' occupations to fulfill family function allows the occupational therapist to take a holistic view of the family's needs and priorities. Although parents advocate a positive view, it is important to recognize when an unusual parental behavior reflects family dysfunction (e.g., child abuse, child neglect). Issues in child abuse and child neglect are discussed in Chapter 13. When family dysfunction is pervasive, most occupational therapists need input from colleagues with expertise in counseling and family systems. Services for the child with special needs continue, but the therapist considers ecological and family systems factors in collaborating with the team to set priorities and provide services.

Families in Chronic Poverty

Chronic poverty has a pervasive effect on family and child experiences. The majority of families receiving public assistance are children and mothers with poor educational backgrounds, an inconsistent work history, and low-wage jobs. Welfare recipients are often stereotyped as lazy and unmotivated, and as having children just to make money off the system (Seccombe, James, & Walters, 1998). The process of "qualifying" for services can be frustrating, depersonalizing, and degrading. Once the family qualifies for help, resources are not always enough for it to make ends meet. In interviews with hundreds of single mothers living on welfare or working in low-paying jobs, Edin and Lein (1996) found that both groups had to engage in a variety of survival strategies to access enough resources to meet their families' needs. Both groups reported sharing apartments and working on the side or having a second job. In addition, both groups relied on financial assistance from their social network, such as the child's father or family and friends.

Seccombe and colleagues (1998) conducted an ethnographic study of women receiving welfare and asked about their reasons for needing assistance. Although the participants realized that the United States culture tends to emphasize individual responsibility for rising above poverty, many of the women believed that bad luck was a primary reason their families needed assistance. Single parents are particularly vulnerable (Edin & Lein, 1996); without family members to help, these mothers lack control over the events in their lives. Unexpected events, such as a car breaking down or special meetings at school about a child, can cause the parent to miss hours at a job and can increase financial strain. Some women have reported that they returned to welfare and Medicaid "for the child" (Seccombe et al., 1998). Poverty represents a multidimensional issue, and therapists cannot make assumptions about the reasons a family lives in poverty.

Poverty is a burden born by a disproportionate number of children. In 2001 it was estimated that 16.3% of all children lived in poverty while only 10.1 percent of the population 18 to 64 years old were living in poverty (U.S. Bureau of the Census, 2002). Furthermore, poverty occurs at a higher rate among some minority families, where 31% of the African American young people under 18 live below the poverty line and 28% of the Hispanic children do. Because children in families with poor housing and low limited access to basic services are more likely to experience health problems, occupational therapists must consider issues related to poverty in making their interventions appropriate to the family SES. Recognizing that poverty creates a unique cultural worldview enables therapists to consider what it means to provide family-centered services (Humphry, 1995). For example, a different worldview of time, with the emphasis on the here and now, makes it harder to schedule or keep appointments. Families of low SES are rarely able to follow through with their plans. Therefore, planning for the future has little meaning, and participating in the setting of annual goals at IFSP or IEP meetings may not be considered important.

Further, increasing the vulnerability of children with special needs who live in poverty are the multiple challenges that put their parents at greater risk for poor parenting. In one study almost one half (45%) of the mothers struggled with depression, and fewer than one half reported that they had a family member who could help baby-sit (Schteingart, Molnar, Klein, Lowe, & Hartmann, 1995). Even with incentives such as diapers, toys, and food, low-income mothers got their children to an early intervention program only 40% to 50% of the time, compared with the 75% of the time for middle-income mothers (Brinker, 1992). Therapists who are aware that poverty creates special conditions strive to individualize intervention plans and consider how formal support can replicate the positive effects of social support to promote better parenting (Brinker, 1992; Dunst, Trivette, & Jodry, 1997). The following case study describes intervention that reinforces family strengths and addresses important environmental issues that influence this child's development.

Case Study

Jason and his mother, Ms. Thorp, lived in a government-subsidized, one-bedroom apartment, and they received food stamps and welfare assistance. Because it was a dangerous neighborhood, Ms. Thorp tried to keep Jason inside as much as possible. At his 4-year-old annual physical, the physician noticed that Jason was not completely toilet trained. His mother stated that he did not use a spoon, and that he demonstrated limited expressive vocabulary. An interdisciplinary assessment at the Developmental Evaluation Center revealed a short attention span, a below-average self-care standard score on the Pediatric Evaluation of Disabilities Inventory, and 20% delay in expressive language. The occupational therapist also noted that Jason demonstrated poor fine motor skills (i.e., he did not complete puzzles, color with a crayon or cut along a line). On the fine motor scales of the Peabody Developmental Motor Scales, Jason was below the 10th percentile. Because Jason had not been exposed to a varied learning environment, the team recommended that he enroll in a childcare program with children his own age. They also recommended that the speech-language pathologist and occupational therapist consult with his teacher.

In developing an IEP, his mother, with input from the social worker, had selected a childcare program. Because it was near her home, she could walk Jason to school, saving him an hour-long van ride to the Head Start program on the other side of town. The teachers welcomed him and thought that they could work on toilet training, but they insisted that Jason needed to be able to feed himself lunch before he entered the program.

The therapist discussed Jason's use of a spoon with Ms. Thorp, but she did not instruct her to force Jason to use utensils. The therapist recalled hearing that children living in poverty were less likely to have meals in a particular location or at regular times, and she realized that strategies at different levels would be needed to achieve spoon feeding.

The therapist decided that she could be supportive and effective in changing mealtime routines by providing services in the home, rather than at the clinic. Therefore she visited Jason's home later that week. At the beginning of the home visit, the therapist realized that the family had no kitchen table. In talking about their daily schedule, Ms. Thorp reported that they did not awaken at any specific time. However, Jason was usually up by 11:30 AM to watch his favorite television show. She reported that watching television together was an activity she enjoyed with her son.

Ms. Thorp gave Jason a cheese sandwich sometime in the late morning. She selected cheese sandwiches because the nutritionist said they were good, and Jason did not make a mess when he walked around with them. Ms. Thorp reported that she was not a "morning person," so she frequently did not have breakfast or lunch. Instead, she snacked during the day. For dinner, she frequently made chicken or hamburgers, which she and Jason ate in the living room. The plate was placed on the coffee table, and Jason stood near it and finger fed himself. If she made something like pinto beans, Ms. Thorp fed Jason so that he would not make a mess. She explained, "When we moved in, there were bugs everywhere. I fought hard to kill them because I know they are dirty. I know if he makes a mess with food, the bugs will be right back!"

The therapist brought a cup of pudding as a treat for Jason, and she asked him to spoon it himself. They sat Jason in the corner of the sofa. When he was handed the spoon, he dipped it into the pudding, inverted the spoon as he brought it to his mouth, and sucked the pudding from the spoon. Ms. Thorp became upset when pudding dropped from his spoon onto his shirt. She took the spoon away and fed him the rest of the pudding.

The therapist wanted to understand Jason's weekly routine. She learned that Jason spent every Tuesday night with his father, who would take him out for an ice cream cone. His maternal grandmother occasionally watched Jason on weekends when Ms. Thorp supplemented their income by filling in as a cook's assistant in a coffee shop. The therapist interpreted the family's strengths as the following:

1 Ms. Thorp is a devoted mother who wants her son to be healthy and wants a clean apartment.
2 Ms. Thorp listens to and follows the advice of the nutritionist.
3 The Thorps share an interactive routine around a television show in the morning, which helps create temporal organization.
4 Jason's family includes extended family, who see him regularly.

Her concerns about Jason learning to spoon feed include the following:

1 Jason does not have a place for meals, and he rarely sees another person using a spoon.
2 Meals are typically foods that can be eaten with the fingers.
3 Jason does not use tools well, and Ms. Thorp does not want him to be messy.
4 Ms. Thorp is easily overwhelmed by details, and she does not seem to solve problems easily.

The next time she visited, the therapist brought a stool from the physical therapy equipment library. They adjusted the height so that it could be pulled up to the coffee table, creating a place for Jason to sit and eat. She also purchased two place mats with his favorite cartoon hero on them. The therapist brought a can of macaroni and cheese for Jason to eat. Jason loved his "chair" and

table. When given the spoon to eat macaroni from a bowl, he scooped but inverted the spoon on the way to his mouth. He looked surprised and then finger fed himself the noodles. Together the therapist and Ms. Thorp planned that Jason would have "noodles" as lunch, and they agreed that lunch would occur immediately before Jason's favorite TV show.

On her third home visit, the therapist arranged to come in the evening when Jason's father came to take him for ice cream. When she arrived, Ms. Thorp returned the stool because her mother had a stool Jason could use. The therapist explained to Jason's father that his son needed more practice using a spoon. He agreed to get cups of ice cream instead of ice cream cones and to eat with Jason.

Within 4 weeks of the therapist's third visit, Ms. Thorp reported that Jason was successfully using a spoon. The team arranged for Jason to begin preschool the next week.

Parents with Special Needs

Parents themselves may have special needs that require an emphasis on supportive services. Parents who face physical or sensory challenges may need help in solving problems, such as monitoring the activity of an active child or being alerted to the cry of an infant (Meadow-Orlans, 1995). Occupational therapists, who work from the perspective that parenting reflects a process of co-occupation, can assist the parent in the modification of tasks. For example, adapting the location of routines, such as diaper changing and infant bathing, can enable parents with physical limitations to participate in caregiving and simple routines that build affection between the parent and child. Therapists can explore the use of adaptive equipment, such as motion detectors or sound-activated alarm systems, to compensate for the parents' sensory deficits and ensure responsiveness to their child's cues. Most parents who have had long-term experiences with a physical limitation independently develop creative solutions for providing care for their children, and they only occasionally seek a therapist's assistance in determining how to perform specific caregiving tasks.

Parents who struggle with drug addiction or mental illness (MI) may worry whether they are up to caregiving responsibilities (McKay, 2004). They often require counseling, mental health services, and opportunities to participate in support groups. When parents have special needs that strongly influence their caregiving ability, their needs often become the first emphasis of intervention.

Parents with mental retardation (MR), MI, or drug addiction are at risk for having children with developmental disabilities. Professionals have questioned the competency of parents with MR. However, with support systems in place, these parents can be surprisingly successful. Parents at risk because of MR or MI appear to be most successful in caring for young children when they are married, have few children, have adequate financial support, and have multiple sources of support (Tymchuk, Andron, & Unger, 1987).

In providing support to parents with MR, Espe-Sherwindt and Kerlin (1990) recommended that professionals focus on the parents' internal and external control, self-esteem, social skills, and problem-solving skills. Therapists can help empower parents to make their own decisions, thereby increasing their sense of self-control. Often individuals with MR or drug addiction have low self-esteem and lack confidence in their ability to make decisions. Because self-esteem is important in interactions with children, this aspect of interaction should be considered.

Professionals should also focus on helping parents with MR and MI build problem-solving skills. Everyday care for children requires constant problem solving. Many times professionals give advice or recommendations without encouraging the parents to solve the problem or independently to try their own actions first. When others direct parents, they become more dependent. However, when parents successfully solve a problem, they become empowered to act independently in daily decision making. Problem solving can be taught and modeled. Espe-Sherwindt and Kerlin (1990) suggested that teaching problem-solving skills in daily caregiving could be critical to parents' development of caregiving competence.

When occupational therapists work with parents with MR or MI, it becomes essential to know the parents' learning styles and abilities. Many times instructions need to be repeated and reinforced. Therapists must use good judgment in what techniques are taught to these parents, with emphasis on safe and simple methods. The occupational therapist should also recognize the need for additional supports to help parents with MR access those needed services. Regular visits in the home by aides, nurses, or teaching assistants can meet the level of support needed. If the occupational therapist communicates his or her goals and strategies to the visiting aide, therapy activities are more likely to be implemented by the parents and other professionals working with the family.

Working with parents with MR or MI can be frustrating when appointments are missed or requests are not followed. Therefore an understanding of the parents' needs is essential. The development of simple, repetitive routines and systems that the parents can learn and follow enables them to become competent caregivers. With support, they can offer a child a positive and loving environment that fosters both health and development.

Professionals use a variety of strategies to deal with challenging families. When families have continual stress and problems, it is important for therapists to begin to build trust slowly, to share observations and concerns, and to accept parents' choices (DeGangi, Wietlesbach, Poisson, Stein, & Royeen, 1994). When parents do not seem to understand the intervention process, professionals can attempt to establish rapport by using concrete, simple terms; by providing both written and oral information; and by providing ideas that would immediately help the child. Professionals also report that parents can better articulate their concerns when services were are home based, when lay terminology is used, and when services are presented in a slow, nonjudgmental way (DeGangi et al., 1994). Focusing on the child's strengths and developing trust and responsiveness are also important when parents are coping with their own challenges.

SUMMARY

Working with families is one of the most challenging and rewarding aspects of pediatric occupational therapy. The family's participation in intervention is of critical importance in determining how much the child can benefit. Therapy goals and activities that reflect the family's priorities often result in meaningful outcomes.

This chapter described families as systems with unique structures and interactive patterns. The potential effects of a child with a disability on a family's occupations were related to implications for the occupational therapist's role. Issues that arise during different stages of the family's life cycle were described. In the final section, principles and strategies for working with families were discussed. The strategies included communication methods to inform and involve parents in the intervention program. It is critically important that the occupational therapist show sensitivity to the family's values and interests, respect the family's values and interests, maintain a positive attitude, continually update skills, obtain current information to give parents, and offer consistent, positive support of family members.

STUDY QUESTIONS

1 Randomly select 10 friends (include at least five people of different ages). Ask them to write down the names of everyone in their family and to include anyone they want. Write a definition of "the family" that would include all the characteristics of the families described by your subjects. (Idea adapted from Levin and Trost, 1992.)

2 Use Table 5-1 to identify your own cultural characteristics. Of which characteristics would you want an occupational therapist to be aware

of if he or she were giving services to your family?

3 The priorities of parents change over the life cycle. Describe two priorities of the parents of a low-functioning infant with severe and multiple disabilities. Describe the priorities of the same parents during the child's early school years and adolescence. Describe the role of the occupational therapist in meeting each priority need.

4 List three strategies that the occupational therapist might use in working with a family with an income below the poverty level in which the father is of normal intelligence and the mother has moderate MR. Neither parent works outside the home, and they have a 2-year-old daughter with moderate delays in language and fine-motor skills.

REFERENCES

Allen, KR., Fine, M.A., & Demo, D.H. (2000). An overview of family diversity: Controversies, questions and values. In D.H. Demo, K.R. Allen, & M. A. Fine (Eds.), *Handbook of family diversity* (pp. 1-14). New York: Oxford University Press.

Amato, P.R. (2000). Diversity within single-parent families. In D.H. Demo, K.R. Allen, & M. A. Fine (Eds.), *Handbook of family diversity* (pp. 149-172). New York,: Oxford University Press.

Americans with Disabilities Act (1990) (PL101-336) 42, U.S.C.A 12134 et seq.

Anderson, C. (2003). The diversity, strengths and challenges of single-parent households. In F. Walsh (Ed.), *Normal family processes: Growing diversity and complexity.* (3rd ed., pp. 121-152). New York: Guilford Press

Anderson, D. (1983). He's not "cute" anymore. In T. Dougan, L. Isbell, & P. Vyas (Eds.), *We have been there* (pp. 90-91). Nashville, TN: Abington Press.

Baird, A., John, R., & Hayslip, B. (2000). Custodial grandparenting among African Americans: A focus group perspective. In B. Hayslip & R.G. Glen (Eds.), *Grandparents raising grandchildren: Theoretical, empirical, and clinical perspectives* (pp. 1250-144). New York: Springer Publishing.

Barnett, S., & Boyce, G.C. (1995). Effects of children with Down syndrome on parents' activities. *American Journal of Mental Retardation, 100* (2), 115-127.

Bernheimer, L.P., & Keogh, B.K. (1995). Weaving interventions into the fabric of everyday life: An approach to family assessment. *Topics in Early Childhood Special Education, 15,* 415-433.

Blue-Banning, M., Summers, J.A., Frankland, H.C., Nelson, L.L., & Beegle, G. (2004). Dimensions of family and professional partnerships: Constructive guidelines for collaboration. *Exceptional Children, 70* (2), 167-184.

Boone, H.A., McBride, S.L., Swann, D., Moore, S., & Drew, B.S. (1998). IFSP practices in two states: Implications for practice. *Infants and Young Children, 10* (4), 36-45.

Bornstein, M.H. (2002). *Handbook of parenting* (2nd edition, vols. 1-5). Mahwah, NJ: Lawrence Erlbaum.

Bradley, R.H., Corwyn, R.F., Burchinal, M., McAdoo, H.P., & Coll, C.G. (2001). The home environments of children in the United States: Part 2. Relations with behavioral development through age thirteen. *Child Development, 72,* 1868-1886.

Bradley, R.H., Corwyn, R.F., McAdoo, H.P., & Coll, C.G. (2001). The home environments of children in the United States: Part 1. Variations by age, ethnicity, and poverty status. *Child Development, 72,* 1844-1867.

Brinker, R.P. (1992). Family involvement in early intervention: Accepting the unchangeable, changing the changeable, and knowing the difference. *Topics in Early Childhood Special Education, 12* (3), 307-332.

Britner, P.A., Morog, M.C., Pianta, R.C., & Marvin, R.S. (2003). Stress and coping: A comparison of self-report measures of functioning in families of young children with cerebral palsy or no medical diagnosis. *Journal of Child and Family Studies, 12,* 335-348.

Brody, G.H., Dorsey, S., Forehand, R., & Armistead, L. (2002). Unique and protective contributions of parenting and classroom processes to the adjustment of African American children living in single parent families. *Child Development, 73,* 274-286.

Brown, S.M., Humphry, R., & Taylor, E. (1997). A model of the nature of family-therapist relationships: Implications for education. *American Journal of Occupational Therapy, 51,* 597-603.

Carlson & Harwood. (2003). Attachment, culture, and the caregiving system: The cultural patterning of everyday experiences among Anglo and Puerto Rican mother-infant pairs. *Infant-Mental-Health-Journal, 24,* 53-73.

Case-Smith, J. (2004). Parenting a child with a chronic medical condition. *American Journal of Occupational Therapy, 58.*

Case-Smith, J., & Nastro, M. (1993). The effect of occupational therapy intervention on mothers of children with cerebral palsy. *American Journal of Occupational Therapy, 46,* 811-817.

Coll, C.G., & Pachter, L.M. (2002). Ethnic and minority parenting. In M.H. Bornstein (Ed.), *Handbook of parenting* (2nd edition., vol 4) (pp. 1-20). Mahwah, NJ: Lawrence Erlbaum.

Crowe, T.K. (1993). Time use of mothers with young children: The impact of a child's disability. *Developmental Medicine and Child Neurology, 35,* 612-630.

DeGangi, G.A., Wietlesbach, S., Poisson, S., Stein, E., & Royeen, C. (1994). The impact of culture and socioeconomic status on family-professional collaboration: Challenges and solutions. *Topics in Early Childhood Special Education, 14* (4), 503-520.

DeGrace, B.W. (2004). The everyday occupation of families with children with autism. *American Journal of Occupational Therapy, 58.*

Dunst, C.J. (2000). Revisiting "rethinking early intervention." *Topics in Early Childhood Special Education, 20,* 95-104.

Dunst C.J., Trivette, C.M., & Deal, A. (1994). *Supporting and strengthening families: Methods, strategies and practices.* Cambridge, MA: Brookline Books.

Dunst, C.J., Trivette, C.M., & Jodry, W. (1997). Influences of social support on children with disabilities and their families.

In M.J. Guralnick (Ed.), *The effectiveness of early intervention* (pp. 499-522). Baltimore: Paul H. Brookes.

Edin, K., & Lein, L. (1996). Work, welfare, and single mothers' economic survival strategies. *American Sociological Review, 61,* 253-266.

Entwisle, D.R., & Alexander, K.L. (2000). Diversity in family structure: Effects on schooling. In D.H. Demo, K.R. Allen, & M.A. Fine (Eds.), *Handbook of family diversity* (pp. 316-337). New York: Oxford University Press.

Espe-Sherwindt, M., & Kerlin, S.L. (1990). Early intervention with parents with mental retardation: Do we empower or impair? *Infants and Young Children, 2,* (4), 21-28.

Falicov, C.J. (2003). Immigrant family processes In F. Walsh (Ed.), *Normal family processes: Growing diversity and complexity* (3rd ed., pp. 280-300). New York: Guilford Press.

Fiese, B.H., & Tomcho, T.J. (2001). Finding meaning in religious practices: The relation between religious holiday ritual and marital satisfaction. *Journal of Family Psychology, 15,* 597-609.

Fine, M.A., Demo, D.H., & Allen, K.R. (2000). Family diversity in the 21st century: Implications for research, theory and practice. In D.H. Demo, K.R. Allen, & M.A. Fine (Eds.), *Handbook of family diversity* (pp. 440-448). New York: Oxford University Press.

Fox, L., Vaughn, B.J., Wyatte, M.I., & Dunlap, G. (2002). "We can't expect other people to understand": Family perspectives on problem behaviors. *Exceptional Children, 68,* 437-450.

Gallimore, R., & Lopez, E.M. (2002). Everyday routines, human agency and ecocultural context: Construction and maintenance of individual habits. *Occupational Therapy Journal of Research, 22,* 70-77.

Gavidia-Payne, S., & Stoneman, Z. (1997). Family predictors of maternal and paternal involvement in programs for young children with disabilities. *Child Development, 68,* 701-717.

Grant, G., Ramcharan, P., & Goward, P. (2003). Resilience, family care and people with intellectual disabilities. *International Review of Research in Mental Retardation, 26,* 135-173.

Grant, G., & Whittell, B. (2000). Differentiated coping strategies in families with children or adults with intellectual disabilities: The relevance of gender, family composition and the life span. *Journal of Applied Research in Intellectual Disabilities, 13,* 256-275.

Grant, G., Ramcharan, P., & Goward, P. (2003). Resilience, family care and people with intellectual disabilities. *International Review of Research in Mental Retardation, 26,* 135-173.

Greene, M. (1999). A parent's perspective. *Topics in Early Childhood Special Education, 19,* 147.

Greene, S.M., Anderson, E.R., Hetherington, E.M., Forgatch, M.S., & DeGarmo, D.S. (2003). Risk and resilience after divorce. In F. Walsh (Ed.), *Normal family processes: Growing diversity and complexity* (3rd ed., pp. 96-120). New York: Guilford Press.

Haley, S.M., Coster, W.J., Ludlow, L.H., Haltiwanger, J.T., & Andrellos, P.J. (1992). *Pediatric Evaluation of Disability Inventory.* San Antonio: Psychological Corporation.

Harwood, R.L., Leyendecker, B., Carlson, V.J., Asencio, M., & Miller, A.M. (2002). Parenting among Latino families in the U.S. In M.H. Bornstein (Ed.), *Handbook of parenting: Social conditions and applied parenting* (2nd ed.). Mahwah, NJ: Erlbaum.

Hasselkus, B.R. (2002). The meaning of everyday occupation. Thorofare, NJ: Slack.

Hastings, R.P. (2003). Child behavior problems and partner mental health as correlates of stress in mothers and fathers of children with autism. *Journal of Intellectual Disability Research, 47,* 231-237.

Hayslip, B., Emick, M.A., Henderson, C.E., & Elias, K. (2002). Temporal variations in the experience of custodial grand parenting: A short-term longitudinal study. *Journal of Applied Gerontology, 21,* 139-156.

Helff, C.M., & Glidden, L.M. (1998). More positive or less negative? Trends in research on adjustment of families rearing children with developmental disabilities. *Mental Retardation, 36,* 457-464.

Helitzer, D.L., Cunningham-Sabo, L.D., VanLeit, B., & Crowe, T.K. (2002). Perceived changes in self-image and coping strategies of mothers of children with disabilities. *Occupational Therapy Journal of Research, 22* (1), 25-33.

Hinojosa, J. (1990). How mothers of preschool children with cerebral palsy perceive occupational and physical therapists and their influence on family life. *Occupational Therapy Journal of Research, 10,* (3), 144-162.

Hinojosa, J., Sproat, C.T., Mankhetwit, S., & Anderson, J. (2002). Shifts in parent-therapist partnerships: Twelve years of change. *American Journal of Occupational Therapy, 56,* 556-563.

Hoff, E., Laursen, B., & Tardif, T. (2002). Socioeconomic status and parenting. In M.H. Bornstein (Ed.), *Handbook of parenting* (2nd ed., vol 2, pp. 231-252). Mahwah, NJ: Erlbaum.

Hombeck, G.N., Gorey-Ferguson, L., Hudson, T., Seefeldt, T., Shapera, W., Turner, T., & Uhler, J., et al. (1997). Maternal, paternal, and marital functioning in families of preadolescents with spina bifida. *Journal of Pediatric Psychology, 22,* 167-181.

Humphry, R. (2002). Young children's occupations: Explicating the dynamics of developmental processes. *American Journal of Occupational Therapy, 56,* 171-179.

Humphry, R. (1995). Families living in poverty: Meeting the challenge of family-centered services. *American Journal of Occupational Therapy, 49,* 687-693.

Humphry, R. (2002). Young children's occupations: Explicating the dynamics of developmental processes. *American Journal of Occupational Therapy, 56,* 171-179.

Individuals with Disabilities Education Act of 1997 (IDEA). (P.L. 105-117).

Joslin, D. (2000). Emotional well-being among grandparents raising children affected and orphaned by HIV disease. In B. Hayslip, & R.G. Glen (Eds.), *Grandparents raising grandchildren: Theoretical, empirical, and clinical perspectives* (pp. 87-105). New York: Springer Publishing Company.

Kaiser, A.P., & Hancock, T.B. (2003). Teaching parents new skills to support their young children's development. *Infants and Young Children, 16,* 9-22.

Kellegrew, D. (2000). Constructing daily routines: a qualitative examination of mothers with young children with disabilities. *American Journal of Occupational Therapy, 54,* 252-259.

Kelley, S.J., Whitley, D., Sipe, T.A., & Yorker, B.C. (2000). Psychological distress in grandmother kinship care providers: The role of resources, social support and physical health. *Child Abuse and Neglect, 24,* 311-321.

King, G.A., King, S.M., & Rosenbaum, P.L. (1996). How mothers and fathers view professional caregiving for children with disabilities. *Developmental Medicine and Child Neurology, 38,* 397-407.

King, G., Law, M., King, S., Rosenbaum, P., Kertoy, M.K., & Young, N.L. (2003). A conceptual model of factors affecting the recreation and leisure participation of children with disabilities. *Physical and Occupational Therapy in Pediatrics, 23,* 63-89.

Kirk, S. (1998). Families' experiences of caring at home for a technology-dependent child: A review of the literature. *Child: Care, Health and Development, 24* (2), 101-114.

Knox, M., Parmenter, T.R., Atkinson, N., & Yezbeck, M. (2000). Family control: The views of families who have a child with an intellectual disability. *Journal of Applied Research in Intellectual Disabilities, 13,* 17-28.

Koramoa, J., Lynch, M.A., & Kinnair, D. (2002). A continuum of child-rearing: Responding to traditional practices. *Child Abuse Review, 11,* 415-421.

Kotchick, B.A., & Forehand, R. (2002). Putting parenting in perspective: A discussion of the contextual factors that shape parenting practices. *Journal of Child and Family Studies, 11,* 255-269.

Laird, J. (2003). Lesbian and gay families. In F. Walsh (Ed.), *Normal family processes: Growing diversity and complexity (3rd Ed).* New York: Guilford Press.

Larson, R. (2001). Mothers' time in two-parent and one-parent families: The daily organization of work, time for oneself, and parenting of adolescents. *Minding the Time in Family Experiences: Emerging Perspectives and Issues* (vol. 3, pp. 85-109). New York: Elsevier Science.

Larson, R.W., & Verma, S. (1999). How children and adolescents spend time across the world: Work, play, and developmental opportunities. *Psychological Bulletin, 125,* 701-736.

Lawlor, M.C., & Mattingly, C.F. (1998). The complexities embedded in family-centered care. *American Journal of Occupational Therapy, 52,* 259-267.

Lawlor, M.C., & Mattingly, C.F. (2001). Beyond the unobtrusive observer: Reflections on researcher-informant relationships in urban ethnography. *American Journal of Occupational Therapy, 55* (2), 147-154.

LeRoy, B.W. (2004). Mothering children with disabilities in the context of welfare reform. In S.A. Escaile, & J.A. Olson (Eds.), *Mothering occupations: Challenge, agency, and participation* (pp. 372-390). Philadelphia: F.A. Davis.

Levin, I., & Trost, J. (1992). Understanding the concept of family. *Family Relations, 41,* 348-351.

Lyon, J. (1989). I want to be Zak's mom, not his therapist. *Developmental Disabilities Special Interest Section Newsletter, 12* (1), 4.

Mahoney, G., & Bella, J. (1998). An examination of the effects of family-centered early intervention on child and family outcomes. *Topics in Early Childhood and Special Education, 18* (2), 83-94.

Mahoney, G., Kaiser, A., Birolametto, L., MacDonald, J., Robinson, C., Safford, P., & Spiker, D., et al. (1999). Parent education in early intervention: A call for a renewed focus. *Topics in Early Childhood Special Education, 19,* 131-140.

Markson, S., & Fiese, B.H. (2000). Family rituals as a protective factor for children with asthma. *Journal of Pediatric Psychology, 25,* 471-479.

McBride, S.L., Brotherson, M.J., Joanning, H., Whiddon, D., & Dermitt, A. (1993). Implementation of family-centered services: Perceptions of families and professionals. *Journal of Early Intervention, 17,* 414-430.

McCubbin, M., Balling, K., Possin, P., Frierdich, S., & Bryne, B. (2002). Family resilience in childhood cancer. *Family Relations, 51,* 103-111.

McGuire, B.K., Crowe, T.K., Law, M., & VanLeit, B. (2004). Mothers of children with disabilities: Occupational concerns and solutions. *OTJR: Occupation, Participation and Health, 24,* 54-63.

McKay, E.A. (2004). Mothers with mental illness: An occupation interrupted. In S.A. Escaile, & J.A. Olson (Eds.), *Mothering occupations: Challenge, agency, and participation* (pp. 238-258). Philadelphia: F.A. Davis.

McWilliam, R.A., Tocci, L., & Harbin, G.L. (1998). Family-centered services: Service providers' discourse and behavior. *Topics in Early Childhood and Special Education, 18* (4), 206-221.

Meadow-Orlans, K.P. (1995). Sources of stress for mothers and fathers of deaf and hard of hearing infants. *American Annals of the Deaf, 140* (4), 352-357.

Melamed, B.G. (2002). Parenting the ill child. In M.H. Bornstein (Ed.), *Handbook of parenting* (2nd ed., vol 5, pp. 329-348). Mahwah, NJ: Lawrence Erlbaum.

Morton, K. (1985). Identifying the enemy: A parent's complaint. In H.R. Turnbull & A. Turnbull (Eds.), *Parents speak out: Now and then* (pp. 143-148). Columbus, OH: Merrill.

Murphy, K.E. (1997). Parenting a technology assisted infant: Coping with occupational stress. *Social Work in Health Care, 24* (3/4), 113-126.

Murray, V.M., Bynum, M.S., Brody, G.H., Willert, A., & Stephens, K. (2001). African American single mothers and children in context: A review of studies on risk and resilience. *Clinical Child and Family Psychology Review, 4,* 133-155.

Musick, K. (2002). Planned and unplanned childbearing among unmarried women. *Journal of Marriage and Family, 64,* 915-929.

Nagy, S., & Ungerer, J. (1990). The adaptation of mothers and fathers to children with cystic fibrosis: A comparison. *Children's Health Care, 19* (3), 147-154.

Nastro, M. (1992). An ethnographic study of mothers of children with cerebral palsy and the effect of occupational therapy intervention on their lives. (Unpublished master's thesis, Ohio State University, Columbus).

National Center for Health Statistics. (2000). Unmarried Childbearing retrieved July 2003 from www.cdcgov/nchs/fastats/unmarry.htm.

Ninio, A., & Rinott, N. (1988). Fathers' involvement in the care of their infants, and their attributions of cognitive competence to infants. *Child Development, 59,* 652-663.

Ogunnaike, O.A., & Houser, R.F. (2002). Yoruba toddlers' engagement in errands and cognitive performance on the Yoruba Mental Subscale. *International Journal of Behavioral Development, 26,* 145-153.

Opacich, K., & Savage, T.A. (2004). Mothers with chronic illness: Reconstructing occupation. In S.A. Escaile, & J.A. Olson (Eds.), *Mothering occupations: Challenge, agency, and participation* (pp. 217-237). Philadelphia: F.A. Davis.

Olsson, M.B., & Hwang, C.P. (2001). Depression in mothers and fathers of children with intellectual disability. *Journal of Intellectual Disability Research, 45,* 535-543.

Oswald, R.F., & Culton, L.S. (2003). Under the rainbow: Rural gay life and its relevance for family providers. *Family Relations, 52,* 72-81.

Parke, R.D. (2002). Fathers and families. In M.H. Bornstein (Ed.), *Handbook of parenting* (2nd edition, vol 3, pp. 27-74). Mahwah, NJ: Lawrence Erlbaum.

Park, C.A. (1998). Lesbian parenthood: A review of the literature. *American Journal of Orthopsychiatry, 68,* 376-389.

Parker, K. (2003). Determined spirits: Opportunities to be and do (Unpublished masters project, University of North Carolina, Chapel Hill, NC).

Patterson, C.J. (2002). Lesbian and gay parenthood. In M.H. Bornstein (Ed.), *Handbook of parenting* (2nd Edition) (ed., pp. 317-338). Mahwah, NJ: Lawrence Erlbaum Associates.

Patterson, J.M. (2002). Integrating family resilience and family stress theory. *Journal of Marriage and Family, 64,* 349-360.

Patterson, J.M., & Blum, R.W. (1996). Risk and resilience among children and youth with disabilities. *Archives of Pediatric Adolescent Medicine, 1150,* 692-698.

Patterson, J.M., Garwick, A.W., Bennett, F.C., & Blum, R.W. (1997). Social support in families of children with chronic conditions: Supportive and nonsupportive behaviors. *Developmental and Behavioral Pediatrics, 18,* 383-391.

Porterfield, S.L. (2002). Work choices of mothers in families with children with disabilities. *Journal of Marriage and Family, 64,* 972-981.

Raghavan, B. (1998). An ethnographic study of Asian mothers of children with disabilities: Implications of cultural influences for health care professionals. (Unpublished master's thesis, Ohio State University, Columbus).

Rainforth, B., & Salisbury, C. (1988). Functional home programs: A model for therapists. *Topics in Early Childhood Special Education, 7* (4), 33-45.

Rank, M.R. (2000). Poverty and economic hardship in families. In D.H. Demo, K.R. Allen, & M.A. Fine (Eds.), *Handbook of family diversity* (pp. 293-315). New York: Oxford University Press.

Rivers, J.W., & Stoneman, Z. (2003). Sibling relationships when a child has autism: Marital stress and support coping. *Journal of Autism and Developmental Disorders, 33* (4), 383-394.

Rogoff, B. (2003). *The cultural nature of human development.* New York: Oxford University Press.

Rolland, J.S. (2003). Mastering family challenges in serious illness and disability. In F. Walsh (Ed.), *Normal family processes: Growing diversity and complexity.* (3rd ed., pp. 460-489). New York: Guilford Press.

Rush, D.D., Shelden, M.L., & Hanft, B.E. (2003). Coaching families and colleagues: A process for collaboration in natural settings. *Infants and Young Children, 16,* 33-477.

Sameroff, A.J., & Fiese, B.H. (2000). Transactional regulation: The developmental ecology of early intervention. In J.P. Shonkoff & S.J. Meisels (Eds.), *Handbook of early childhood intervention* (2nd ed., pp. 135-159). New York: Cambridge Press.

Schimoeller, G.L., & Baranowski, M.D. (1998). Intergenerational support in families with disabilities: Grandparents' perspective. *Families in Society: The Journal of Contemporary Human Services, 79,* 465-476.

Schteingart, J.S., Molnar, J., Klein, T.P., Lowe, C.B., & Hartmann, A.H. (1995). Homelessness and child functioning in the context of risk and protective factors moderating child outcomes. *Journal of Clinical Child Psychology, 24,* 320-331.

Schultz-Krohn, W. (2004). Meaningful family routines in a homeless shelter. *American Journal of Occupational Therapy, 58.*

Schulz, J.B. (1985). The parent-professional conflict. In H.R. Turnbull, & A.P. Turnbull (Eds.), *Parents speak out: Then and now* (2nd ed., pp. 3-22). Columbus, OH: Merrill.

Seccombe, K., James, D., & Walters, K.B. (1998). "They think you ain't much of nothing": The social construction of the welfare mother. *Journal of Marriage and the Family, 60,* 849-865.

Segal, R. (2000). Adaptive strategies of mothers with children with ADHD: Enfolding and unfolding occupations. *American Journal of Occupational Therapy, 54,* 300-306.

Shonkoff, J.P., & Phillips, D.A. (2000). From neurons to neighborhoods: The science of early childhood development. Washington, DC: National Academy Press.

Stacey, J., & Biblarz, T.J. (2001). How does the sexual orientation of parents matter? *American Sociological Review, 66,* 159-183.

Stallings, G., & Cook, S. (1997). *Another season: A coach's story of raising an exceptional son.* Boston: Little, Brown.

Steinberg, L., & Silk, J.S. (2002). Parenting adolescents. In M.H. Bornstein (Ed.), *Handbook of parenting* (2nd edition., vol 1) (pp. 103-133). Mahwah, NJ: Lawrence Erlbaum.

Stoneman, Z. (2001). Supporting positive sibling relationships during childhood. *Mental Retardation and Developmental Disabilities Research Reviews, 7,* 134-142.

Suarez-Orozco, C., Todorova, I.L.G., & Louie, J. (2002). Making up for lost time: The experiences of separation and reunification among immigrant families. *Family Process, 41,* 625-643.

Summers, J.A., Dell'Oliver, C., Turnbull, A.P., Benson, H., Santelli, E., Campbell, M., & Siegel-Causey, E. (1990). Examining the individualized family service plan process: What are family and practitioner preferences? *Topics in Early Childhood Special Education, 10,* (2), 78-99.

Turnbull, A.P., Blue-Banning, M., Turbiville, V., & Park, J. (1999). From parent education to partnership education: A call for a transformed focus. *Topics in Early Childhood Education, 19,* 164-172.

Turnbull, A.P., & Ruef, M. (1997). Family perspectives on inclusive lifestyle issues for people with problem behavior. *Exceptional Children, 63,* 211-227.

Turnbull, A.P., & Turnbull, H.R. (1990). *Families, professions and exceptionality: A special partnership* (pp. 156-157). Columbus, OH: Merrill.

Turnbull, A.P., & Turnbull, H.R. (1997). *Families, professionals, and exceptionality: A special partnership* (3rd ed.). Columbus, OH: Merrill.

Turnbull, A.P., Turbiville, V., & Turnbull, H.R. (2002). Evolution of family-professional partnerships: Collective empowerment as the model for the early twenty-first century. In J.P. Shonkoff & S.J. Meisels (Eds.), *Handbook of early childhood intervention* (2nd ed., pp. 630-650). New York: Cambridge University Press.

Tymchuk, A.J., Andron, L., & Unger, O. (1987). Parents with mental handicaps and adequate child care: A review. *Mental Handicap, 15,* 49-54.

Unger, D.G., Jones, C.W., Park, E., & Tressell, P.A. (2001). Promoting involvement between low-income single caregivers and urban early intervention programs. *Topics in Early Childhood Special Education, 21,* 197-212.

United States Bureau of the Census. (2002). America's families and living arrangements: Population Characteristics retrieved August 2003 from www.census.gov U.S Department of Commerce Economics and Statistics Administration.

VanLeit, B., & Crowe, T.K. (2002). Outcomes of an occupational therapy program for mothers of children with disabilities: Impact on satisfaction with time use and occupational performance. *American Journal of Occupational Therapy, 56,* 402-410.

Wacharasin, C., Barnard, K.E., & Spieker, S.J. (2003). Factors affecting toddler cognitive development in low-income families: implications for practitioners. *Infants and Young Children, 16,* 175-187.

Walker, S. (2002). Culturally competent protection of children's mental health. *Child Abuse Review, 11,* 380-393.

Walsh, F. (2002). A family resilience framework: Innovative practice applications. *Family Relations, 51,* 130-137.

Walsh, F. (Ed.) (2003). *Normal family processes: Growing diversity and complexity* (3rd ed.). New York: Guilford Press.

Weiss, K.L., Marvin, R.S., & Pianta, R.C. (1997). Ethnographic detection and description of family strategies for child care: Application to the study of cerebral palsy. *Journal of Pediatric Psychology, 22,* 263-278.

Williams, P.D., Williams, A.R., Graff, J.C., Hanson, S., Stanton, A., Hafeman, C., Liebergen, A., Leuenberg, K., Setter, R.K., Ridder, L., Curry, H., Barnard, M., Sanders, S., et al. (2002). Interrelationships among variables affecting well siblings and mothers in families of children with chronic illness or disability. *Journal of Behavioral Medicine, 25,* 411-424.

Willoughby, J.C., & Glidden, L.M. (1995). Fathers helping out: Shared child care and marital satisfaction of parents of children with disabilities. *American Journal of Mental Retardation, 99,* 399-406.

Young, D.M., & Roopnarine, J.L. (1994). Fathers' childcare involvement with children with and without disabilities. *Topics in Early Childhood Special Education, 14*(4), 488-502.

Zemke, R., & Clark, F. (1996). Co-occupations of mothers and children: Introduction. In R. Zemke, & F. Clark (Eds.), *Occupational science: The evolving discipline.* Philadelphia: F.A. Davis.

WEB SITES

Family Village: www.familyvillage.wisc.edu/
This site integrates information, resources, and communication opportunities on the Internet for individuals with cognitive and other disabilities, for their families, and for service providers. This site includes informational resources on specific diagnoses, communication connections, adaptive products and technology, adaptive recreational activities, education, worship, and health issues, as well as disability-related media and literature.

Support for Families of Children with Disabilities (SFCD): www.supportforfamilies.org/aboutus.html
SFCD is a parent-run, San Francisco–based, nonprofit organization founded in 1982. This site provides information, resources, and support to families of children with disabilities so that they can make informed choices for their children.

U.S. Department of Health and Human Services, Administration for Children and Families (ACF): www.acf.dhhs.gov/
The ACF is a federal agency that funds state, territory, local, and tribal organizations to provide family assistance (welfare), child support, child care, Head Start programs, child welfare, and other programs relating to children and families.

FAMILIES OF LESBIANS, GAYS, AND BISEXUAL OR TRANSGENDER INDIVIDUALS

Parents Families and Friends of Lesbians and Gays (PFLAG): www.pflag.org

COLAGE (Children of Lesbians and Gays Everywhere (COLAGE): www.colage.org

National Clearinghouse on Child Abuse and Neglect Information: http://nccanch.acf.hhs.gov/index.cfm
This organization is a service of the Children's Bureau of the U.S. Department of Health and Human Services' Administration for Children and Families. It collects, organizes, and disseminates information on all aspects of child maltreatment. The mission of the Clearinghouse is to connect professionals and concerned citizens to timely and well-balanced information on programs, research, legislation, and statistics regarding the safety, permanency, and well-being of children and families.

RESOURCES FOR FAMILIES AND CHILDREN WITH DISABILITIES

http://naic.acf.hhs.gov/pubs/r_disa.cfm
This web site lists organizations for families with children with specific disorders. Each organization is linked to its web site.

5-A A Parent's Perspective

Beth Ball

When I was first asked to contribute to this chapter, I reflected on the myriad experiences and feelings that have emerged as a result of having children with disabilities. This seemed too vast a topic to be captured in a few typed pages. The following is a brief glimpse into my thoughts and feelings about life with my three disabled children. There is much more than facts or history about our lives. There is, of course, emotion—deep and undeniable—and there is poetry. There is the first shed tear of realization that my child will have a life that is more difficult than most. There is the happy smile of childhood shared with supportive therapists and teachers. There is the frustrated panic of adolescence, when social situations are hard and troublesome and when the phone does not ring on Saturday night.

Initial Response

Learning about the disabilities of each of my children came at different times in their lives. The impact varied because of the timing of the news and the disability of each child. Benjamin was born on a warm June day in 1971. On the delivery table, the nurse turned the mirror away, and I didn't understand why I couldn't see the baby. Everything seemed to happen in slow motion. The physician held him up and announced that he was a boy, but there was a small problem. His right arm tapered from the elbow to a thumblike digit for a right hand, and his left arm ended in a modified claw hand, having a center cleft halfway into his palm and syndactyl webbing between the outside fingers.

The nurse placed him on my tummy, and he peed a fountain all over the sterile drapes. She said, "That works," which was comforting, but scary, because I had not considered that other things could be wrong.

It was not until that night when I had him all to myself in the privacy of my own room that I felt the bifid femur of his right leg; the block at his knee that refused to let it extend; the very thin lower leg, which turned out to be missing the tibia; and the clubfoot. I discovered all of these problems one at a time. The sick feeling in my stomach was guilt. There must have been something that I had done wrong that had caused this. Even though I had followed all the doctor's instructions, I must have missed something. What would everyone think? I must not be good enough to have a child.

Mick, my husband, and I were lucky to have a wonderful pediatrician whose first advice was exactly what we needed to hear. He told us not to withdraw from our family and friends (alluding to the feelings of shame and guilt that we had not overtly expressed). He told us to allow them to give us support, that they would only want to help. The unspoken message that they would not judge us was very important.

And so we started on our journey of new experiences with orthopedic surgeons, prosthetists, genetic counselors, neurologists, urologists, internists, and pediatricians. Later came occupational therapists, physical therapists, ENT (ear, nose, and throat) specialists, vision therapists, special education teachers, and psychologists. We searched for answers to "Why?" We searched for options to deal with the issues of discrepancies in leg length and hand function. We searched for resolution to our own feelings. But we were fortunate because, as husband and wife, we never blamed each other.

Mick and I started the journey together, and we have always turned to each other for support. Sometimes it was an "us against the world" attitude and a fierce, protective response that got us through the hard times. When joyous times came, they did so with the realization that it had taken all our efforts to get there. The reason that we have been able to deal with the problems and come out on top is that we have a commitment to each other and a deep faith in God. This statement is much too simplistic for the deep feelings of need, grace, and oneness that we have. This oneness has allowed us to go forward to meet challenges as they have come.

Another reason we have been able to go forward is that we see each of our children as a gift. They are grace without gracefulness. They are charm without all the social skills. They are fun with a sometimes struggling sense of humor. They are individuals who have enriched our lives and given us humility, wonder, and awe at their commitment to living, loving, and succeeding.

Accessing Services and Resources

Gaining services and resources for our children has not come without pain, questioning, depression, and anger. It has been a constant struggle. We faced the first barrier when we attempted to find the money to cover the costs of prosthetics and medical care for our son. When we were told that it would be better to amputate Benj's leg above the knee than to try to keep it and work through the lack of joints and musculature, we were also told about the costs of prosthetics. One of the first things our orthopedic surgeon told us was that we needed to find a source of funding, because prosthetics would cost more than a small house by the time Benj was 16.

I will not go into all the details, but I will give you a few insights into what parents must face when they do not know where to turn to find funds. The doctors have a few ideas, but they are not the source of information in this area. Agencies and hospitals may have more information, but getting connected to the right person to gain the information is not an easy task. A major stumbling block to searching for and finding help is a set of feelings that include shame for begging and not being good enough to support the needs of your child yourself.

In the search for money to cover the costs of prosthetics, we approached a well-known agency because we knew that they worked with individuals who had physical disabilities. They had fund-raising campaigns that were earmarked for this purpose. After being told that providing prosthetics was not among their services, and because this was the third or fourth rejection that we had encountered, Mick broke down and joined me in some tears. We were then informed that we had better pull ourselves together. This was our child and our responsibility, and we had better "face it." Shame turned to anger as we left. I felt judged, and included in the anger was the fear that we would not be able to provide for Benj. How could this man judge us? Why didn't this administrator of an agency that provides services to children with disabilities and parents have more empathy for our situation? If he didn't help, then to whom could we turn?

This experience made us more leery of asking for assistance. Luckily, the Shriners accepted our application, and they provided most of the funds for Benj's prosthetics until he turned 18. I do not want to think of what might have happened if we had not had their help. Dealing with financial issues created a new level of trauma that was added to our earlier pain.

However, what we discovered from this process were the necessary and valuable aspects of networking. It was through work, friends, and family that we made contact with the Shriners. It was through people at school that we were put in touch with the local Special Education Regional Resource Center and became a part of the Parent Advisory Council. It was through many of the parents that we met in these places that we learned about the Ohio Coalition for the Education of Children with Disabilities. It has always been invaluable to us to be able to share with other parents who have similar feelings, frustrations, and breakthroughs. If it had not been for these people and these agencies, we would not have received valuable personal, educational, and emotional support that we needed.

Whose Grief, Whose Struggle?

Many people have tried to describe the feelings that occur when a child with a disability comes into a family. The grief cycle (the same cycle that we go through when a loved one dies) is sometimes used to explain how families deal with the news that their child is disabled. When my children were small, the path of feelings about their disabilities could be set aside for the new dream of having the brightest, cutest, most wonderful child with special needs. I dreamed of the well-spoken poster child. These dreams might have also been called denial and led others to believe that I was unaware of the true impact of my children's problems. In truth, that may have been so.

The feelings do not come from the big picture of the disability. They come from all the little incidents. For example, when Benj was 12 or 13 months old, I took him out of a nice, warm tub of sudsy water and stood his chubby, slippery little nude body next to the tub so that he could hold on while I toweled him dry. He stood straight and tall on his left leg, but as I watched, he tried to bear weight on his useless, dangling right leg. He bent his left leg so that his right toes touched the floor, and then he leaned forward to see why he could not reach the floor with his right foot. It was a moment of revelation for me. Until that moment, I think that all the focus had been on me: my inadequacy, my problem, my pain. This was harder; it was too deep even for tears. This was Benj's life, *his* surgeries, *his* pain, and *his* inability to run swiftly through life. My role was to help and support him. Of course, every now and then, I have my own private pity party. However, it is not my pain that is the issue; it is theirs. Somehow, for me, there is a deeper pain in watching someone I love struggle than the pain I feel when struggling myself.

In our minds, Jessica, our second child, had no disabilities through her first 5 years of life. She did have four eye surgeries by age 5 (due to crossed eyes, muscle imbalance, and rotary nystagmus). During her preschool years, she attended a church-related preschool. At parent conference times, when the teacher would indicate problems or ask pointed questions about behaviors at home, I would justify Jessica's performance by telling myself, or Mick, that every surgery sets a child back about 3 months.

When Jessica was old enough to go to kindergarten, we were called into a special conference in which we were carefully told that she was not ready to do so. I did not hear anything else that day. The impact of that statement and the carefully worded explanation were like an icy shower. It was almost as if I had awakened from a dream with a clear vision of how disabled and delayed my daughter really was. I felt guilty and ashamed. I am an occupational therapist, and I know developmental milestones. I had let my doctor and others calm my fears about delays in walking, ataxia, and fine motor challenges because I did not want to believe that this second child of mine could have more than visual impairments. I was in denial for 5 years, helped by well-meaning people who did not want to hurt me. Jessica's diagnoses from her new physicians included mild cerebral palsy, amblyopia, monocular vision, strabismus, and minimal peripheral vision.

It's OK to Be This Way

One night after Jessica's conference, I received an answer to my prayer of "Where do I go from here?" I attended a presentation by Ken Moses, a psychologist and counselor who writes and speaks about parenting children with disabilities. I then experienced a new step on my journey. He spoke about the grief cycle and how we are grieving, not for a lost child, but for a lost dream. His discussion supported what I had been feeling and experiencing. The most important factor to me was the permission he gave me to feel the way I did. He emphasized how important denial is in helping us to deal with life-affecting decisions. He pointed out that denial buys us the time to gather our resources so that we can deal head on with problems.

Ken Moses also spoke about the importance of recognizing that anger gives us the energy to take action. Many times our children's disabilities required so many appointments, surgeries, exercises, prescriptions, Individualized Education Program (IEP) meetings, and other details that I was left with only enough energy to put one foot in front of the other. I ignored or put on hold things or decisions that I should have taken care of immediately. Often it was anger that got me off my duff and sparked my determination to get things done. I learned that unless anger is turned inward or unleashed on others, it can actually help. I came away from this talk with a sense of relief. To have these feelings was normal, and I was not a bad person, mom, or therapist. It continues to bother me when professionals criticize parents for being in denial. My position is that these parents don't yet have the resources they need to deal with their child's disability. So give them some!

Where Do We Go from Here?

Decisions are forced on parents. There are medical decisions, therapy decisions, educational decisions, second opinion decisions, and decisions made in the middle of the night and in the emergency room. Some decisions are avoided until the last possible moment. Decision making starts immediately with a diagnosis or with the search for a diagnosis. What doctor should we use? What hospital? What about insurance? How much intervention do we need? How much do we want? What will they think if we say no to this thing that they think is important for our family? Is it important?

When Jessica was in elementary school, we would wait for the bus together. Each morning while sitting on our staircase landing, Jessica and I spent 20 minutes practicing eye exercises. Some days it was easy; other days Jessica would complain, resist, and attempt to divert my attention from the task. One day, when she was 7 or 8 years old, we were doing her exercises and discussing her braces, her eye surgery, and her occupational therapy session scheduled for that afternoon. She wanted to know for the thousandth time why we had to do these things. I explained that we were trying to fix things so she would have an easier time of it. She suddenly looked up at me and asked, "Is there anything about me that you don't have to fix?" I quickly named all of her gifts and attributes that I treasured. Later, as Jessica's bus turned the corner, I was left sitting on the steps with feelings of emptiness and guilt. I also had a new insight into the impact of countless therapy sessions, surgeries, and home programs.

This incident also made me face another aspect of denial. There is an unavoidable fact that there are some aspects of disabilities that cannot be fixed. I became an occupational therapist so that I could help people and make things better for them. I truly believed (and believe) that I could help eliminate some problems, that I could help heal hurts, and that I could provide training so that people could be more independent. Once I saw Jessica's problems, I was off and running. I wanted to make up for lost time. Fear drove me to leave no stone unturned if I thought that it would help Jessica get better.

There have been several types of denial that I have experienced. I denied that there was a problem. I denied my feelings about the problem. I denied that the problem may still exist, even after a lot of intervention. In the school setting, I denied that there were some areas that did not need to be addressed, and I pushed for intervention where it sometimes was not needed. Recently, I have recognized another form of denial: that helping our children with their schoolwork might create a dependency on others for that help. Mick and I always helped our children with their homework and school projects. I rationalized that their success with their schoolwork would help them achieve in life. Their work ethic for school was high. Unfortunately, because we provided continual support in completing their homework, they never had the opportunity to fail. It is now very clear to me that children have to learn responsibility for themselves and that failure is a vital part of the learning process. I wanted to cushion my children's self-esteem by ensuring that they were successful in school. However, with the complex pattern of learning and growth, there is no clear path for children who have more challenges than most. Children with disabilities do need more help with schoolwork, but how much is too much? Lessons learned later are just as valuable, but they are more challenging because there is more at stake.

School

Other than their child's medical issues, qualifying for special education is one of the greatest traumas parents of a special needs child will encounter. It is obvious that Benj has an orthopedic handicap. However, to qualify for special education, we had to go through an intake process. Benj had to be tested, and we waited with baited breath. He did qualify, and Benj attended kindergarten through third grade in a school that had an orthopedic handicap program. He was in a self-contained classroom for disabled children until third grade.

When attention turned to education instead of surgeries and therapies, we found that physical disabilities are more apparent than learning disabilities. Soon our priorities switched to cognition and classroom skill building. During that time Benj was retained in first grade because the teachers had decided that he had a learning disability. This evaluation provided another chance for the ever-present grief cycle to jump up and bite us. Acceptance of the physical part of the disability was almost in place. However, this new evaluation crushed my new dream of having the brightest, most socially adept physically disabled child. I went through an equally bitter (if not more so) period of blame and self-pity. Once again, I also feared for his success.

When Jessica was tested, we requested the testing because the preschool had prepared us for the possibility that she would have trouble learning. The school said that it was too early to find a discrepancy, but we pursued it, and one was found. She qualified for the learning-disabled program. For each of the next 5 years, Jessica's resource room moved from one school to another. This meant that each year, she had to adjust to a new building, new teachers, and new classmates. When Jessica was in fourth grade, we were told to take her to counseling because she was withdrawn and had no friends on the playground. Guess why. When she was in sixth grade, we moved to another district because it had neighborhood schools with special education resources in each building. There, too, the resource room for her particular grade level was not in the neighborhood school. We couldn't win!

When Benj was in third grade, Mick and I decided that he would benefit from being in the regular classroom for most of his instruction. We were a little ahead of the curve regarding inclusion, and our request received quite a response! In 1980 Benj was a pioneer. That year was difficult for us because we decided to change priorities to allow the learning-disabled program

to meet his needs. One of the most intimidating places in the world is a room full of educators, including heads of programs, psychologists, teachers, occupational therapists, and physical therapists. The only ones that believe that you are doing the right thing for your child seem to be you and your husband. Allowing the school's learning disability (LD) program to meet our son's needs turned out to be the right decision, but I still get stomach cramps when it is time for an IEP meeting (even an IEP meeting in which I am the occupational therapist).

When we find ourselves making judgments about families, a red flag needs to go up. As was pointed out earlier in this chapter, each family has a different structure and different values. Decision making in each family is complicated and sacred. I know many people thought we were crazy when we decided to have a third child. Some were even brave enough to tell us so to our faces. Service providers held their breath, and educators looked for another Ball child in their classrooms. Having another child was a decision about which Mick and I prayed. This time in our lives was like a pause in a heartbeat, filled with hope and fear but also with the knowledge that we were in it together.

Alexander was born on a cold day in February of 1981. He had no physical problems, but he was just as colicky as the other two children. He walked at 9 months and never stopped after that. He was very busy. In preschool meetings, I was the one to point out discrepancies in Alexander's progress. The teacher complimented me on being accepting, and I carefully informed her that I had been through this twice before and had not been as accepting then. I told her that that was okay, too. My children had not fallen off the face of the earth because it took time for me to face their delays. They were doing just fine, and parents need to be allowed to feel the way they do. However, that did not mean that professionals should not be honest with them!

Receiving sympathetic and respectful honesty is the only way to know that I know I have all the facts before I make a decision. Honesty is a gift that you, as a therapist, give parents. It does not mean that parents will hear you, that they will follow your suggestions, or even that you are always right. But your honest appraisal of the situation gives parents a piece of the picture and the truth that they need to help their child succeed. It helps if you take the time to listen to the parents' dreams or if you help them put words to those dreams. Many times I could not even express my dreams because they were caught under the lump of fear deep in my soul. There were, and still are, weeks that I cannot deal with the long term. I can only take it one crisis at a time. There are days when I do not even know that I have a dream for my children. But there are other days when I clearly see the life that my children may achieve, and that is where I like to be.

Alexander has turned out to be borderline gifted and learning disabled, with attention deficit disorder and dyslexia. His disabilities were identified between kindergarten and first grade, again at our insistence. Alexander continues to reverse letters as he reads and writes. He often reads the end of words first. At age 9, he wrote out, in bold letters on a T-shirt, a commitment to avoid drugs: "Lust say on." Classic notes left for me on the kitchen counter often told me that his "homework is bone" or the "bog has ben out."

Alexander's disability has also been difficult on me and my husband. The feelings of loss and sadness that accompanied identification and the knowledge that we had somehow failed resurfaced. Again I had to fight for services. I also had to watch him struggle through years of extra tutoring, vision therapy, and occupational therapy just to begin to decode words. Alexander has borne the burden of being the articulate, social child. He has struggled with feelings of guilt that his disabilities are not as great as those of his siblings. He has received counseling to help him deal with these feelings as well as feelings of his own inadequacy.

However, part of Alexander's disability was a gift for me. He always needed books read to him for school. When he could not get a particular book on tape or he needed to complete one in a hurry, I spent time reading with him. We have shared insights on comparisons of religions, how Native Americans smoke peace pipes, and how to save yourself if you become lost in the middle of a forest. It has been cherished time that would not have occurred if he had the ability to read on his own.

Gifts and Dreams

Recently I heard that old saying, "I'm playing the hand I've been dealt." I think that applies to all of us. It seems to me that everyone has many sources of grief in their lives. We, as the parents of children with disabilities, can focus on the delays and the fears. We should be allowed to feel the feelings that are associated with this situation. However, I think that you'll find that most of us are proud of our children's accomplishments: learning to put on a prosthesis alone, learning to turn a somersault by herself, or hitting the right key on the keyboard to match the screen.

There are some things our children will never be able to do, activities they choose not to attempt. Jessica has chosen not to pursue bike riding. Benj has chosen not to alternate his feet on the stairs. Alexander has chosen not to read piano music. All of these things would be next to impossible for them, but I never told them they couldn't do them. Parents are always in the position of encouraging the impossible. Because they are more objective, help givers and professionals think that parents are denying reality. However, the reality is that it is the child who will ultimately determine what he or she can or cannot do. We have made and will make many mistakes parenting our children with disabilities, but we refuse to let their disabilities limit the possibilities.

I remember crying over *The Velveteen Rabbit* when I read it to the kids. It seemed that the problems of my children kept them from being "real" too. I knew that all the love I was showering on them could not change their physical makeup; however, I also knew that the love I was showering on them might help them cope with their "realness." Benj has told me that he will run in heaven, and I believe that. I also know that all three of them run in their hearts everyday here, and that others seeing them are challenged to be more themselves.

As part of my job, I was asked to evaluate a student who had hands similar to Benj's "claw" hand. He had a hearing impairment, and the special education team met to determine how best to serve him in the school setting. When we sat down in the meeting, one of my colleagues made a comment about his hands. She said she couldn't understand why his parents didn't have his hands "fixed." They looked so strange. I sucked in a breath and my heart pounded. I could not respond. I felt immobilized in my chair, without a voice. How did my colleague have the right to judge that the boy's hands needed fixing? My pounding heart was accompanied by the resounding thought, "He has a right to those hands, his hands. He has a right to be different." In part I had these feelings because I had evaluated his hand skills and knew that despite how different his hands appeared, he was able to use them skillfully. Only after the meeting was I able to express what I thought and felt. I realized that this person had made the comment because she thought that "fixing" his hands would take away the staring and teasing that always accompany looking different.

To express my feelings, I wrote my colleague a letter. In it I explained that my husband and I had made the decision to partly increase function in Benj's left hand when he was 7 months old, wishing it would look more like everyone else's. It was hard to admit that I had those feelings. I told her that Benj's right arm, which we affectionately call "Super Pinky," will never look like everyone else's. I told her about the scars on his hand and the scars on his wrist from the site where the graft skin was taken. I talked about Benj's surgery allowing for a little stronger grasp but not full extension or flexion. I told her that the young man about whom she had commented had an adapted grasp for scissors and functional cutting skills.

My letter also explained that this is a bigger issue than hands; it is about attitudes. I see our roles as professionals who work with children who are different as teaching not only the children, but also everyone else. The message about our kids needs to be that different is not worse, just different. I know that people have the capacity to be open to difference. If we lived in a perfect world, all differences would be OK, and we would not feel that we have to fix them. However, we live in the ever-present face-lift, nose fix, and "Extreme Makeover" society. People are judged on their appearance. Part of our role as professionals is to learn to accept differences, particularly in appearance, and not to try to fix everything. Our job is to help others understand that different is not wrong. This is a very simplistic view of a complex problem.

When I told Benj about the incident, he said, "That person is not cold. She just doesn't know all the facts. If God wanted everyone to look like everyone else, He wouldn't have made handicapped people. There have been times when I wanted to look like everyone else. True people are the ones who remember you for more than your physical side, and that's what really matters. True people are able to look at you and not think you are different, but that you are unique."

Benj is now 31 and has married a young lady with spina bifida. He has a new diagnosis of spinal muscle atrophy. He is gradually losing function in his remaining leg. He and I are in denial about this, but we know that we have always taken one day at a time. He and his wife are working toward independence in all areas of their lives. Jessica is working in a grocery and has had several poems published. Alexander is a carpentry apprentice, married to a wonderful young lady, and has just had a beautiful daughter. As parents of children with disabilities, we continue to be very involved in our children's lives beyond the usual time. My dreams for them remain the same as when they were small: that they will be happy, that they will be as independent as they can be, and that they will always have someone who loves them. As the kids have grown into adults, we have had to practice involvement and support without control. We have also had to deal with our emotions, because the disabilities our children have are for life.

In all stages and at all ages, families of people with disabilities value support and resources. If you take the time to hear a parent's dream, you may hear the sound of laughter and tears. You may hear the strong heartbeat of anger or the resistance to a life that is less than it can be. As a therapist, you are a gift to parents whose lives you touch. You have a solution to some of their frustrations. You have the opportunity to be as honest as you can be and to provide them with the information they need to make decisions. You are the answer to some parent's question.

Thank you.

Beth Ball is the mother of three children with disabilities. She is also an occupational therapist and has worked in the school system a number of years.

Common Conditions that Influence Children's Participation

Sandra L. Rogers

Burn injury
Cardiopulmonary
  dysfunctions
Developmental
  disabilities
Infectious conditions
Musculoskeletal
  disorders
Neoplastic disorders

Neuromuscular
  disorders
Pervasive
  developmental
  disorders (PDDs)
Toxic agents
Traumatic brain injuries
  (TBIs)

CHAPTER OBJECTIVES

1 Describe the incidence, signs and symptoms, causes, and pathologic conditions of common medical diagnoses in children.
2 Describe the primary medical conditions associated with major developmental disabilities.
3 Explain how functional performance is affected by various medical, pathologic, and developmental conditions.
4 Explain precautions and special considerations for working with children who have specific medical conditions and/or developmental disabilities.

This chapter is intended to familiarize the occupational therapist with some of the major medical conditions, diseases, and disabilities of children who receive occupational therapy services. Pediatric conditions can be differentiated in several ways: congenital or acquired, acute or chronic, stable or aggressive, discrete or pervasive, occurring at different stages of development, or according to body systems affected. None of these alone is totally satisfactory; however, the body systems approach is the simplest and most useful for educational and reference purposes.

The chapter therefore is organized in a body systems format; it includes sections on traumatic brain injury, burn injury, and pervasive developmental disorders. The chapter provides information on the incidence and prevalence, signs and symptoms, causes, pathologic abnormalities, general medical treatment, and prognosis of the conditions described. Functional performance and treatment issues are also introduced. Pediatric psychiatric conditions are reviewed in Chapter 13, and neonatal medical conditions are described in Chapter 20. No single chapter can provide complete information about all conditions that may affect children. Many of the other chapters detail the appropriate occupational therapy evaluation, planning, treatment, and follow-up guidelines. A list of more comprehensive medical texts is provided at the end of the chapter.

CARDIOPULMONARY DYSFUNCTIONS

Cardiopulmonary dysfunctions are conditions that affect the cardiac and respiratory systems of the infant and child; they include congenital and acquired conditions that affect the child's health and ability to participate fully in life's occupations and roles.

Congenital Heart Disease

Most cardiac problems in children are congenital in nature or occur secondary to other conditions. These disorders are serious, frightening, and sometimes life-threatening. This section discusses several of the major common anomalies found in the heart and major vessels.

Congenital heart disease is the major cause of death in the first year (other than prematurity) and occurs in approximately 8.6 children per 1,000 births (Centers for Disease Control and Prevention, 2002). According to the Centers for Disease Control and Prevention (CDC), an average of 4,423 babies are born in the United States each year with heart malformations (CDC). Heart defects are also common components of syndromes and have a higher prevalence in chromosomal disorders. The cause of most congenital heart defects is unknown, but numerous studies have linked congenital heart disease to specific chromosomal abnormalities, and several diseases have been linked to specific gene defects.

Three major cardiovascular changes must take place at birth. The foramen ovale, the hole between the right and left atria, must close. In addition, the ductus arteriosus and ductus venosus must close to allow blood to flow to the lungs and to the liver, respectively. Many complications can arise if these changes do not occur. Another cardiovascular complication that may occur during the perinatal period is *intracranial hemorrhage.* This condition may occur prenatally, during the birth process, or postnatally. The site and the extent of the bleeding affect the prognosis. For example, extracranial bleeding, or *cephalohematoma,* is considered minor and usually does not cause permanent damage. Conversely, subdural, subarachnoid, and intraventricular hemorrhages are more serious and, depending on the extent of damage, may cause seizures, brain damage, cerebral palsy, and death (Bernstein, 2004).

Heart defects are classified according to the hemodynamic characteristics of blood flow deficits; that is, deficits that result in (1) increased pulmonary blood flow, (2) decreased pulmonary blood flow, (3) obstructed blood flow, and (4) mixed blood flow (Wong & Hockenberry-Eaton, 2001). Deficits that increase the amount of pulmonary blood flow include one of the most common conditions found in premature newborns, *patent ductus arteriosus (PDA).* In this condition the ductus arteriosus does not constrict, which can lead to heart failure and inadequate oxygenation of the brain. Treatment includes administration of the drug indomethacin, which often triggers closure of the arterial wall. Surgery follows if the drug is not an effective treatment (Bernstein, 2004; Curry, 2002). The other major congenital malformations that result in an increase in pulmonary blood flow are *atrial septal defects (ASDs),* and *ventricular septal defects (VSDs).* An ASD is an opening in the septum between the right and left atrial chambers (Figure 6-1). It can be any size and can occur anywhere along the septum. Because of the opening, when the left atrium contracts, blood is sent into the right atrium; this is called a *left-to-right shunt.* Left-to-right shunts cause more blood than normal to be sent to the lungs, resulting in *wet lungs,* a condition that makes the lungs more susceptible to upper respiratory infection. A left-to-right shunt also causes the right atrium, and especially the right ventricle, to work much harder and eventually can cause heart failure in the older child. Symptoms include poor exercise tolerance and small size for age. Information for diagnosis is gathered from the

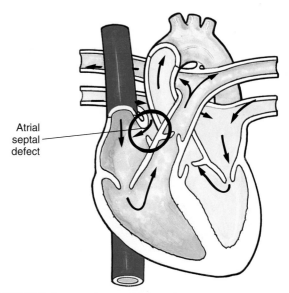

Atrial septal defect

FIGURE 6-1 Atrial septal defect. (From Wong, D.L. [1999]. *Whaley and Wong's nursing care of infants and children* [6th ed.]. St. Louis: Mosby.)

physical examination (i.e., detection of the characteristic heart murmur), evaluation of chest x-ray films and electrocardiograms, and the use of echocardiography or heart catheterization (Bernstein, 2004).

Surgical procedures are implemented if the child is in distress. The surgery may be performed early, or it may be postponed until the child is 4 or 5 years of age. Until that time the child is closely watched for complications, especially for signs of heart failure (Bernstein, 2004; Curry, 2002). VSDs are the most common type of congenital cardiac malformation and are often more serious than ASDs. A VSD consists of a hole or opening in the muscular or membranous portions of the ventricular septum (Figure 6-2).

In a VSD the blood flows from the left ventricle to the right ventricle (a left-to-right shunt), and as in an ASD, an increased amount of blood is pumped to the lungs. The defect is considered less serious if the opening is in the membranous section of the septum and more serious if multiple muscular holes are present (Wong & Hockenberry-Eaton, 2001).

Symptoms associated with VSDs include feeding problems, shortness of breath, increased perspiration, fatigue during physical activity, increased incidences of respiratory infections, and delayed growth. Causative factors are often idiopathic, but congenital infections, various teratogenic agents, and genetic predisposition may contribute to the cause (Park & George, 2002).

As with an ASD, the diagnosis of VSD is based on the murmur and on the findings of chest x-ray films, electrocardiograms, echocardiograms, and heart catheterization. Improvement often occurs after 6 months of age, and more than 50% of cases correct themselves by 5 years

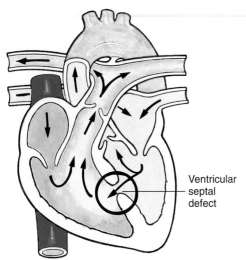

FIGURE 6-2   Ventricular septal defect. (From Wong, D.L. [1999]. *Whaley and Wong's nursing care of infants and children* [6th ed.]. St. Louis: Mosby.)

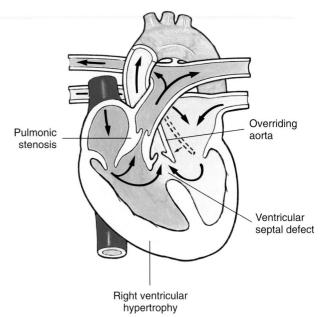

FIGURE 6-3   Tetralogy of Fallot. (From Wong, D.L. [1999]. *Whaley and Wong's nursing care of infants and children* [6th ed.]. St. Louis: Mosby.)

of age (Park & George, 2002). However, if the extent of damage is great or if the hole does not repair itself, surgical procedures to close the defect may be needed early in the child's life.

Children with a VSD must be carefully monitored to avoid the life-threatening condition known as *Eisenmenger's complex,* in which pulmonary vascular obstruction can occur as a result of prolonged exposure to increased blood flow and high pressure. Eventually the heart is no longer capable of pumping against the increased pulmonary pressure, the child goes into congestive heart failure, and blood pools in the right ventricle. This development is a medical emergency that requires immediate surgical intervention.

The prognosis for infants with VSDs continues to improve with advances in surgical techniques and the management of heart failure. These children are at risk for several serious complications, including cardiovascular accident (CVA), embolism, brain abscess, growth retardation, seizures, and death (Park & George, 2002).

Tetralogy of Fallot (*TOF*) is a defect of decreased pulmonary blood flow. As its name implies, TOF is associated with four different problems: (1) pulmonary valve or artery stenosis with (2) a VSD present prenatally, causing (3) right ventricular hypertrophy and (4) override of the ventricular septum by the aorta (Figure 6-3). Physiologically, the unoxygenated returning blood cannot easily exit to the lungs because of the pulmonary stenosis. Instead, it takes two paths of least resistance: the defect, creating a right-to-left shunt, and the aorta (Bernstein, 2004).

Symptoms of TOF include central cyanosis, coagulation defects, clubbing of the fingers and toes, feeding difficulties, failure to thrive, and dyspnea (Wong &

Hockenberry-Eaton, 2001). The cause of TOF is probably similar to that of VSD. The insult to the developing fetus is believed to occur in the early weeks of fetal development, when the right ventricle is at a critical stage (Park & George, 2002). The diagnosis of TOF is usually based on the presence of cyanosis; analysis of the heart murmur; electrocardiographic demonstration of right ventricular hypertrophy and right axis deviation; chest x-ray films that show the characteristic boot-shaped heart, and echocardiographic demonstration of the overriding aorta (Bernstein, 2004; Park & George).

TOF initially is managed with medication, and surgery is delayed as long as possible. In severe cases a temporary shunt may be inserted to bypass the stenosis. Usually the Blalock-Taussig surgical procedure is used until complete corrective surgery can be performed, in which the pulmonary outflow obstruction is removed, the VSD is closed, and the aorta may be enlarged. As with VSDs, the prognosis is improving as techniques and maintenance improve. The operative mortality rate has been reduced from 10% to 5%, but the surgery is still a dangerous and complicated procedure (Wong & Hockenberry-Eaton, 2001).

A common congenital heart defect that affects mixed pulmonary flow is *transposition of the great vessels (TGV),* also known as *transposition of the great arteries (TGA).* In this condition, the pulmonary artery leaves the left ventricle and the aorta exits the right ventricle with no communication between the systemic and pulmonary circulations. The severity of the condition depends on the amount of circulatory mixing that occurs between the two sides. Circulatory mixing occurs as a result of co-existing congenital cardiac defects (e.g., a VSD or pulmonary stenosis) or congenital transposition of the ventricles, called *corrected transposition* (Park & George, 2002). The severity of the symptoms varies, but cyanosis, congestive heart failure, and respiratory distress are common.

The diagnosis of TVG is made through heart catheterization and through echocardiography; both procedures can identify the transposition. The condition is treated surgically. One technique involves enlargement of the foramen ovale. To accomplish this, a catheter with a balloon tip is inserted through the foramen ovale into the left atrium and then pulled back through the opening, enlarging it and thereby increasing the flow of oxygenated blood to the right atrium (Bernstein, 2004). Another procedure involves excision of the atrial septum and insertion of a patch that redirects the blood flow. In a third, more recently developed technique, the great vessels are severed at their bases and reattached to the proper ventricles. The main pulmonary artery is anastomosed to the proximal aorta, and the ascending aorta is anastomosed to the proximal pulmonary artery (Bernstein, 2004; Park & George, 2002).

The operative mortality rate for TGV is 5% to 10%, regardless of the surgical procedure used. In later life these children have been known to develop arrhythmias and ventricular dysfunctions.

A child with congenital cardiac defects that have not yet been repaired can be expected to have reduced endurance for exertion but may be normal in other ways. This child may want to participate in a range of self-care and play activities. Pacing and the selection of appropriate activities may be essential to the child's health and ability to participate in family and peer activities. After surgery and throughout life, general health maintenance is essential in these individuals, including a well-balanced diet, aerobic exercise, and avoidance of smoke inhalation (Bernstein, 2004).

The occupational therapist may deal directly or indirectly with the consequences of congenital cardiac defects. For example, these defects are often secondary diagnoses in children with genetic syndromes. Children with Down syndrome or other types of mental retardation (MR) may have histories of congenital heart problems. In these cases, occupational therapists must be aware of associated signs and symptoms, treatment procedures, complications of medications, and the effect of the condition on the child's functioning.

Dysrhythmias

Irregular cardiac rhythms, or *dysrhythmias,* are not as common in children as in adults. However, the incidence of these problems is increasing, possibly because more children with congenital heart defects are surviving

surgery, which may leave them with a residual dysrhythmia. The three classes of dysrhythmia are bradydysrhythmia, tachydysrhythmia, and conduction disturbances. The diagnosis of dysrhythmia is based primarily on standard and 24-hour electrocardiographic monitoring (Brook, 1998).

Bradydysrhythmia is an abnormally slow heart rate. The most common type is a complete heart block, or *atrioventricular (AV) block.* This condition is common after surgery or myocardial infarction and occasionally may require a pacemaker. Sinus bradycardia can be caused by anoxia or autonomic nervous system disorder. In this condition the child's heart rate may be reduced to less than 60 beats per minute (bpm), and extra beats and slow nodal rhythms also may be present (Park & George, 2002).

Tachydysrhythmia is an abnormally fast heart rate. Sinus tachycardia can be a symptom of several other conditions, including fever, anxiety, anemia, and pain. *Supraventricular tachycardia (SVT)* is a heart rate of 200 to 300 bpm and is among the most common disturbances in children. SVT is a serious condition that can lead to congestive heart failure. The child with SVT is irritable, eats poorly, and is pale. In some cases a vagal maneuver, such as the Valsalva maneuver, can reverse the SVT, but in other cases the child may require hospitalization, esophageal overdrive pacing, or synchronized cardioversion (Wong & Hockenberry-Eaton, 2001).

Conduction disturbances are common after surgery and may be temporary. Premature contractions may be atrial, ventricular, or junctional. These sometimes can be handled with interim or permanent pacing, depending on the nature and severity of the disturbance (Bernstein, 2004).

Neonatal Respiratory Problems

Respiratory problems are common in newborns and can be dangerous. Some of these problems are acute, and others are considered chronic lung diseases. Respiratory distress problems may be caused by prematurity, aspiration of amniotic fluid or meconium, malformation or tumors of the respiratory organs, neurologic disease, central nervous system (CNS) damage, drugs, air trapped in the chest or pericardium (the sac surrounding the heart), and pulmonary hemorrhages (Haddad & Fontan, 2004).

An acute respiratory problem often found in newborns, especially preterm infants, is *respiratory distress syndrome.* This disease is caused by a deficiency of *surfactant,* the chemical that prevents the alveoli from collapsing during expiration. Because surfactant is not produced until about the thirty-fourth to the thirty-sixth week of gestation, many premature infants are born with this deficiency. As the air sacs collapse, oxygen absorption and carbon dioxide elimination are hindered.

Treatment includes administration of surfactant and supplemental oxygen, and ventilator support may be needed. Most infants begin to recover after 3 to 4 days of treatment, as the baby's body begins to produce surfactant. In some newborns, respiratory distress syndrome results in chronic lung problems (Stoll & Kliegman, 2004a).

Chronic lung disease implies a long-term need for supplemental oxygen. The chronic lung disease often seen in neonatal centers is *bronchopulmonary dysplasia (BPD)*. These newborns have had some type of acute respiratory problem that required prolonged use of mechanical ventilation and other types of necessary but perhaps traumatic intervention. In BPD the airways thicken, excess mucous forms, and alveolar growth is retarded. As a result, these children often are susceptible to respiratory infections and other respiratory problems. Problems such as BPD that are associated with the techniques used to save newborns' lives are called *iatrogenic disorders*.

The artificial respirators currently used are sophisticated machines that allow careful control of oxygen mixtures. They are designed to maintain a constant pressure on the alveoli, thus keeping them open in the absence of surfactant. This is known as *positive end-expiratory pressure (PEEP)*, which has significantly lowered the rate of fetal death and the overall risk of severe developmental delays (Stoll & Kliegman, 2004a). Currently, many newborns with respiratory distress are given surfactant at birth, which allows them to breathe independently despite lung immaturity. Early administration of surfactant has greatly reduced the incidence of BPD and has improved the mortality rate in very premature infants.

Asthma

Asthma is a chronic inflammatory disorder characterized by bronchial smooth muscle hyperreactivity that causes airway constriction in the lower respiratory tract, difficulty breathing, and bouts of wheezing. It is one of the most common long-term respiratory disorders of childhood. In most children with asthma, the first symptoms appear in early childhood, before 5 years of age (Emond, Camargo, & Nowak, 1998; Rabinovitch & Gelfand, 1998). Asthma appears to be an inherited trait and is often associated with familial patterns of allergy.

Exposure to an allergen, smoking, cold air, exercise, inhaled irritants, and viral infection may trigger asthma attacks (Wong & Hockenberry-Eaton, 2001). The attacks are characterized by smooth muscle spasm of the bronchi and bronchioles and inflammation and edema of the mucous membranes with accumulation of mucous secretions. The child has difficulty breathing, particularly in expiration; the forceful expiration through the narrowed bronchial lumen creates the characteristic wheezing. The child also has a hacking, nonproductive cough.

This experience can be frightening for the child, and the symptoms may worsen in response to the panic. The effort of breathing may also result in sore ribs and exhaustion. *Status asthmaticus* is a serious asthmatic condition in which medications typically prescribed do not improve the condition and emergency medical intervention is needed (Haddad & Fontan, 2004; National Institutes of Health [NIH], 1997).

Treatment for asthma may include environmental control measures, skin testing, immunotherapy for allergies, emotional support, and a combination of pharmacologic agents, usually beta-adrenergic agonists and methylxanthine (Emond et al., 1998; Wong & Hockenberry-Eaton, 2001). These drugs may be related to school performance problems and in some cases can cause dependencies. Monitoring of the child's schoolwork and teaching him or her about the use and abuse of the medications should minimize difficulties in this area. The goal of nonpharmacologic therapy is prevention, and occupational therapists can help prevent or reduce the child's exposure to airborne allergens and irritants in a therapy setting. The goal of pharmacologic therapy is to prevent or control asthma symptoms, reduce the frequency and severity of asthma exacerbations, and reverse airflow obstruction. Occupational therapists, therefore, should be knowledgeable about the use of asthma medications, including metered-dose inhalers (Emond et al.).

Children with asthma may be fearful of overexertion and may be concerned about contact with triggering allergens. This may result in a self-limited life style. Teaching the child to manage the condition, respond calmly to stress, and pace activities can be essential to maintaining a normal childhood pattern. Structured peer group activities can also be useful in preventing social isolation. Breathing exercises, stretching, and controlled breathing can assist in management of the attacks (Emond et al., 1998).

Cystic Fibrosis

The most common serious pulmonary and gastrointestinal problem of childhood is *cystic fibrosis (CF)*. This inherited autosomal recessive disorder is related to a gene located on chromosome 7. In the United States, the incidence of CF is 1 in 3,500 births among white children and 1 in 17,000 births among African American children (Boat, 2004). CF is a multisystem disease that appears to be related to an impermeability of epithelial cells to chloride; as a result, the exocrine (mucus-producing) glands malfunction, producing secretions that are thick, viscous, and lacking in water (Boat). The thick secretions block the pancreatic ducts, bronchial tree, and digestive tract.

One of the earliest signs of CF, *meconium ileus,* occurs in the newborn. A thick, puttylike substance that cannot be eliminated blocks the small intestine (Wong & Hockenberry-Eaton, 2001). The abdomen becomes distended, and the child is unable to pass stools; if the condition goes untreated, vomiting and dehydration occur (Boat, 2004).

Chronic pulmonary disease is the most serious complication of CF. A chronic cough, wheezing, lower respiratory infections, abscesses and cysts, hemoptysis, and recurrent pneumothorax are examples of the serious pulmonary complications that develop in CF. Other complications often result from hypoxemia, nasal polyps, and enlargement of the right side of the heart (right ventricular hypertrophy), which eventually may cause heart failure (Wong & Hockenberry-Eaton, 2001).

In addition, CF typically affects sodium absorption–inhibiting factor, and as a result excessive amounts of sodium chloride are secreted from the sweat glands onto the skin. Mothers may detect a salty taste when they kiss their children. This may alert the physician, who can perform a simple diagnostic procedure known as the *sweat test*. For this test, an electrode is placed on the skin, causing the child to sweat at the contact site, and a sample of the sweat is taken. Detection of an excessive level of sodium chloride establishes the diagnosis (Boat, 2004).

Pancreatic insufficiency causes characteristic foul-smelling, greasy stools. Associated problems include malabsorption; clinical diabetes; deficiencies of vitamins A, E, and K; and gastrointestinal obstruction. In the liver, bile ducts also become blocked, resulting in destruction of cells behind the blocked ducts. Although this is a serious problem, a positive point is that children's livers are often capable of regeneration.

Medical management of CF generally consists of vigorous pulmonary therapy, inhalation therapy, chest physical therapy, antibiotic therapy, bronchodilator therapy, anti-inflammatory treatment, endoscopy and lavage, and nutritional therapy (Boat, 2004). Efforts are made to keep the lungs as free as possible; these may involve physical or respiratory therapy techniques such as mist tent therapy, intermittent positive pressure breathing, aerosol therapy, and postural drainage techniques (Wong & Hockenberry-Eaton, 2001).

A child with CF frequently spends time in and out of hospitals with various complications and for various treatments. These children may have a series of crises alternating with periods of comparative health, although a general degeneration occurs. Children whose primary symptoms are gastric inflammation have a better prognosis than those whose initial problems are related to respiratory functioning. All require a careful balance of nutrition, fluid intake, and exercise. Boys generally have a longer life span than girls, but degeneration of body functions and death occur for many in their teens and early twenties (Wong & Hockenberry-Eaton, 2001). Early detection and treatment have been shown to prolong life. The child and family may need assistance in dealing with grief and impending death.

Medical, nursing, dietary, and respiratory therapy are central to the treatment of a child with CF. Respiratory therapists may play a key role by providing postural drainage, chest clapping, and chest expansion exercises. The occupational therapist may be concerned with energy conservation (activities that promote efficient breathing) and prevocational, recreational, and psychosocial support groups. Social, psychologic, and pastoral staff may provide essential family support.

HEMATOLOGIC DISORDERS

Several hematologic disorders affect child development and function. This section addresses some of the disorders most commonly seen by occupational therapists as primary or secondary diagnoses.

Sickle Cell Anemia

Sickle cell anemia comprises a group of diseases, called *hemoglobinopathies,* in which adult hemoglobin A (HbA) is partly or completely replaced by abnormal sickle hemoglobin (Wong & Hockenberry-Eaton, 2001). *Homozygous sickle cell disease* (i.e., *sickle cell anemia [SCA]*) is a hereditary, chronic form of anemia characterized by the presence of abnormal sickle (crescent shaped) erythrocytes that contain an abnormal type of hemoglobin called *hemoglobin S (HbS)* (Figure 6-4). The inheritance pattern is that of an *autosomal recessive disorder;* that is, if both parents have sickle cell trait (persons with both normal HbA and abnormal HbS), there is a 25% chance that they will produce a child with SCA. In the United States most cases of SCA occur in African American infants (the incidence is about 8% among these infants). SCA is rare in white infants but can be found in people of Hispanic, Middle Eastern, and Mediterranean ancestry (Wong & Hockenberry-Eaton). The condition now can be detected in newborns. A few states require sickle cell screening for all newborns, and more states are considering this course of action.

The clinical course for children with SCA is marked by episodes of severe worsening, called *sickle cell crises,* which can be grouped into four types (Steinberg, 1996). *Aplastic* and *hyperhemolytic crises* are characterized by imbalances in the production of red blood cells and by their premature destruction. This may cause the hemoglobin level to decrease by 50%, necessitating immediate transfusions. *Sequestration crises* are marked by sudden, rapid enlargement of the spleen. This type of SCA traps much of the blood volume and can cause shock or death. *Painful,* or *vaso-occlusive, crises* are characterized by pain in the hands, feet, toes, and abdomen.

SCA affects other organs as well. Lungs may become infected, and hypoxemia is common; liver and kidney

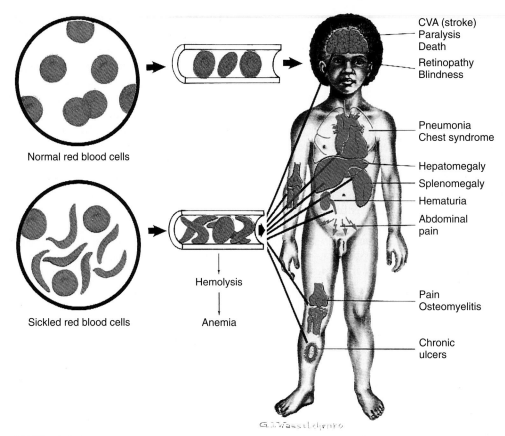

Normal red blood cells

Sickled red blood cells

CVA (stroke)
Paralysis
Death

Retinopathy
Blindness

Pneumonia
Chest syndrome

Hepatomegaly

Splenomegaly

Hematuria

Abdominal
pain

Hemolysis

Anemia

Pain
Osteomyelitis

Chronic
ulcers

FIGURE 6-4 Differences between normal and sickled blood cells. (From Wong, D.L. [1999]. *Whaley and Wong's nursing care of infants and children* [6th ed.]. St. Louis: Mosby.)

involvement causes urine problems and hematuria; CVAs may occur; the legs may develop ulcers; and spleen damage can leave the child defenseless against major infections (Steinberg, 1996). In addition, children with SCA experience chronic anemia, delayed growth, and delayed sexual maturation, and they have an increased risk of septic infection.

Sickle cell symptoms do not usually appear until the fourth month of life. However, screening can be done on the newborn with a blood test, the *Sickledex*. This test is followed by hemoglobin electrophoresis, which can provide a definitive diagnosis and allows for early identification and treatment (Steinberg, 1996). Early diagnosis (prior to 3 months of age) allows initiation of appropriate treatment and thereby minimizes complications. There is no cure for sickle cell disease. Treatment focuses on reducing the sickling phenomenon and treating the medical emergencies and their sequelae. Medical management includes bed rest, hydration, electrolyte replacement, oxygen therapy, analgesics, antibiotics, periodic exchange transfusions, and sometimes splenectomy (Wong & Hockenberry-Eaton, 2001). Current research is focusing on the possible use of hydroxyurea and erythropoietin to increase the concentration of fetal hemoglobin and reduce complications. Bone marrow transplantation has been performed in some cases and

holds promise for a cure, but its use currently is limited by a lack of suitable donors, the high mortality rates, and proper patient selection.

Even with medical treatment, children with SCA may experience anoxia, CVAs, seizures, and cardiac failure. Disability and death are common (Steinberg, 1996). Many children have no symptoms and participate in typical occupations. Physical and sexual development is delayed in adolescents. Rehabilitation and school-based professionals may provide treatment for the functional deficits created by these serious complications (Wong & Hockenberry-Eaton, 2001). Supportive counseling, activity adaptation, family support, and monitoring of the child's day-to-day functions are also important roles for occupational therapists.

Hemophilia

The *hemophilias* are a group of conditions characterized by prolonged clotting (coagulation) times and abnormal and excessive bleeding. This bleeding occurs any place in the body, either spontaneously or after serious or minor trauma. There are two major types of hemophilia. *Hemophilia A*, or *classic hemophilia*, is caused by a plasma deficiency of factor VIII, which is necessary for blood coagulation. This factor, also called *antihemophilic globulin (AHF)*, is produced by the liver and is essential for the formation of thromboplastin in phase I of blood coagulation. *Hemophilia B (Christmas disease)* results from a deficiency of clotting factor IX. The hemophilias are sex-linked recessive hereditary disorders and occur almost exclusively in boys (Wong & Hockenberry-Eaton, 2001). The incidence is 1 in 5,000 in males. Among those who have the disease, about 85% have a factor VIII deficiency, and about 15% have a factor IX deficiency. The incidence is equally represented in all ethnic groups. The severity of the disease depends on the amount of clotting factor; the less clotting factor present, the more severe the disease (Montgomery & Scott, 2004).

Symptoms are not usually noticeable or bothersome until near the end of the first year of life, when a child begins to crawl and walk and soft tissue hemorrhages (i.e., easy bruising, intramuscular hematomas, hemarthroses) begin to occur. Soft tissue hemorrhages and hemarthroses are treated at home by replacing the missing factor to a level that again controls the bleeding (Montgomery & Scott, 2004). This is called *replacement therapy,* and most children can be trained to administer their own infusions.

Bleeding into joints *(hemarthrosis),* a hallmark of hemophilia, can cause severe musculoskeletal problems that can lead to joint deterioration if left untreated. Consequently, the child may have increasing difficulty with ambulation and functional activities. A number of procedures can be used to protect the joints. Blood can be drained from a joint, chemical agents can be injected into the joint, and specific preventive range-of-motion (ROM) activities can be initiated. Chronic arthropathy is the major long-term disability of hemophilia. Surgical procedures, such as joint replacements or synovectomies, carry some element of risk for hemophiliac clients (Montgomery & Scott, 2004). Recreational activities must be carefully chosen to avoid trauma, and this can be frustrating to the child and may limit social interaction. Children with hemarthrosis may frequently miss school during crisis periods.

The prognosis for children with hemophilia depends on management of the condition and the avoidance of *bleeds* in critical organs. Intracranial hemorrhage is one of the most dreaded and serious complications of hemophilia. The treatment of hemophilia has improved sufficiently over the past 20 years to make a normal life expectancy possible (Montgomery & Scott, 2004; Wong & Hockenberry-Eaton, 2001).

MUSCULOSKELETAL DISORDERS

Bone tissue is one of the few body tissues that actively regenerate themselves. The skeletal system is malleable; it deposits or reabsorbs bone based on the stresses it receives. Elements of the skeletal system include the bones, joints, cartilage, and ligaments. The muscular system includes the muscle fibers and their covering of fascia; it is activated by the nerves and moves the bones to create functional motion. Tendons connect the muscular and skeletal systems at the origins and insertions of the muscles (Morrissy & Weinstein, 2001).

Bone is mesenchymal tissue. As the child develops, the bone is first laid down as either membranous or cartilaginous tissue and gradually becomes ossified through a calcium deposition process called *endochondral ossification*. The bones initially are formed early in fetal development. The growth and ossification processes in long bones occur at the epiphyseal plates; these structures, which are located at the ends of the bones and are covered in articular cartilage, form the associated joints. Growth and ossification continue until 25 years of age, at which time the epiphyses fuse (Morrissy & Weinstein, 2001). Bones without physeal plates (i.e., the pelvis, scapulae, carpals, and tarsals), grow by appositional bone growth from their surrounding perichondrium and periosteum. The bones of the spine, metacarpals, metatarsals, and phalanges grow by a combination of appositional and endochondral ossification (Thompson, 2004).

The musculoskeletal system can be affected by genetic and congenital disorders, trauma, infection, and metabolic, endocrine, circulatory, and neurologic disorders (Morrissy & Weinstein, 2001). This section addresses some of the major musculoskeletal disorders.

Congenital Anomalies and Disorders

A relatively large number of the conditions that affect the musculoskeletal system have a genetic or congenital cause. These conditions often affect the child throughout life, causing disability, deformity, and sometimes death.

Osteogenesis imperfecta (OI), also called *brittle bones,* is a disorder characterized by decreased bone deposition due to an inability to form type 1 collagen. In most cases OI is transmitted by an autosomal dominant gene. However, the most severe fetal type has an autosomal recessive inheritance pattern (Leet, Dormans, & Tosi, 2002). This condition can run several different courses, from mild to severe, with most individuals having a milder form of the disease. OI has an incidence of 1 in 20,000 births.

In all cases the bones are unusually fragile, and even minor trauma can cause a fracture. The severity of the disorder varies greatly, depending on the time of onset (Table 6-1). Multiple fractures or repeated fracture of the same bone may cause a limb to become misshapen and eventually muscularly underdeveloped because of the long periods of immobilization and disuse. Prevention must be attempted at least with padded arm and leg protectors and orthoses. Surgical insertion of metal rods and segmental osteotomies may be helpful for providing

TABLE 6-1 Effects of Onset of Osteogenesis Imperfecta

Type	Severity	Effect
Fetal	Most severe	Fractures occur in utero and during birth; mortality is high.
Infantile	Moderately severe	Many fractures occur in early childhood; severe limb deformities and growth disturbances also occur.
Juvenile	Least severe	Fractures begin in late childhood; by puberty, bones often begin to harden, and fewer fractures occur. Dental problems may be present.

internal support and correcting deformities that may develop. As the child grows, the rods must be replaced to accommodate the growth.

Over time, children with OI can be expected to develop progressive deformities. In addition, their activity patterns are affected by caution and time spent in casts. With the fetal and infantile forms of the disorder, maternal education in handling and positioning is essential to prevent fractures during childcare activities. Children with OI need to be involved in monitored movement activity so that muscle strength and the postural effects of weight bearing and exercise can be achieved (Wong & Hockenberry-Eaton, 2001). Children with less severe forms of OI may participate in many normal activities, including some sports. Novel treatments for OI are being tested. They include medications that stop bone resorption (and thereby increase bone density), bone marrow transplantation, and gene therapy to replace the incorrect message in collagen metabolism (Leet et al., 2002).

Marfan's syndrome, or *arachnodactyly,* is an autosomal dominant trait marked by excessive growth at the epiphyseal plates (i.e., tall stature), arachnodactyly (the fingers are long, slender, and curved, resembling a spider's legs), skull asymmetry, and alterations in the joints, eyes, heart, and aorta. The incidence is 1 to 2 per 100,000 population. The joints are lax and hypermobile, and striated muscles are poorly developed. Visual problems are often present because of the dislocation of the lens (Morrissy & Weinstein, 2001). Symptoms include increased height and decreased weight for age, excessively long extremities, scoliosis, coxa vara, depressed sternum, stooped shoulders, elastic skin, and fragility of the blood vessels. A child with Marfan's syndrome may begin walking later than usual because of decreased postural stability, but the child will not necessarily have developmental delays. Longevity is diminished because of cardiac complications. Treatment is symptomatic and addresses any skeletal deformities, such as scoliosis, that interfere with function (Robinson, 2004).

Achondroplasia, or *chondrodystrophia,* is the most common cause of dwarfism. Dwarfism is caused by stunting of epiphyseal plate growth and cartilage formation. Achondroplasia is an autosomal dominant trait, and frequent spontaneous mutations are known to occur. The limb bones continue to grow to appropriate widths but are abnormally short. Individuals with achondroplasia rarely grow to more than 4 feet in height. Although skull size is normal, face size may be small, with a prominent forehead and jaw and a small nose. Trunk growth is near normal. Skeletal abnormalities include lumbar lordosis, coxa vara, and cubitus varus. There is no cure for achondroplasia. Adults may experience back pain and occasionally paralysis caused by spinal stenosis. Surgical treatment occasionally may be necessary to relieve neurologic complications, improve functional movement, or correct extreme deformities (Morrissy & Weinstein, 2001).

Arthrogryposis multiplex congenita is characterized by incomplete fibrous ankylosis, or contracture of many or all of the child's joints at birth. With amyoplasia, the primary form of arthrogryposis, both the upper and lower extremities are involved. The cause is unknown, but these children have few anterior horn cells in the spinal cord, which may indicate a neuropathic cause. The child has stiff, spindly, and deformed joints and may also have clubfoot, hip dislocation, or characteristic posturing. The knee and elbow joints may appear thickened, and muscles may be absent or incompletely formed. The anterior horn cells of the spinal cord may be absent, in which case the child may also experience paralysis. Treatment focuses on maintaining and increasing functional ROM and strength. Splints, serial casts, surgery, and daily stretching may be included in this regimen (Morrissy & Weinstein, 2001; Thompson, 2004). Adapted equipment and training for activities of daily living (ADLs), school, play, and work performance may assist the child in optimal functioning.

A common abnormality of the foot is *congenital clubfoot,* or *talipes equinovarus.* The incidence of congenital clubfoot is high (1 to 2 per 1,000) and much higher when a sibling has clubfoot (1 in 35). In 1999 more than 3,200 infants were born with clubfoot, and boys were affected twice as frequently as girls (CDC, 2002; Morrissy & Weinstein, 2001). The pattern of presentation suggests inheritance through a single autosomal dominant gene. The condition may be unilateral or bilateral, and the major clinical features are forefoot adduction and supination, heel varus, equinus of the ankle, and medial deviation of the foot (Figure 6-5). Some of the bones involved may be malformed, and the muscles of the lower leg are often underdeveloped. In a small number of cases, paralysis and permanent deformity may be present.

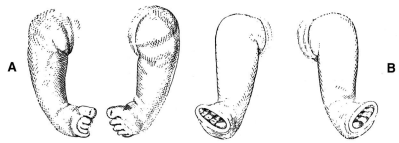

FIGURE 6-5 Bilateral congenital talipes equinovarus. **A,** Before correction. **B,** Undergoing correction in plaster casts. (From Brashear, H.R., & Raney, R.B. [1986]. *Handbook of orthopedic surgery* [10th ed., p. 39]. St. Louis: Mosby.)

In some cases clubfoot is associated with other congenital problems and conditions, but the exact cause or causes of clubfoot are unclear. During fetal development, development of the muscles on the medial and posterior aspects of the legs is adversely affected, and as a result, these muscles are shorter than normal (Morrissy & Weinstein, 2001). These contractions, in turn, lead to the bone and joint problems. The clubfoot deformity can be corrected with taping, the use of malleable splints, serial casting, or orthopedic surgery. The soft tissue surgeries may be combined with bony operations, such as arthrodesis of joints, osteotomies, and insertion of a bone wedge on the medial side of the calcaneus, to correct the line of weight bearing (Morrissy & Weinstein). This treatment reduces foot mobility but increases function and stability. The prognosis is good for children who are treated early.

The analogous condition in the upper extremity, *congenital clubhand,* is far less common and is associated with partial or full absence of the radius and bowing of the ulnar shaft. The radial musculature, nerves, and arteries may be absent or underdeveloped. Often the hand remains functional. Treatment includes progressive casting and ROM exercises, static or dynamic splinting, or surgery; however, these procedures provide more cosmetic than functional benefit. The child with congenital clubhand may occasionally require some training or adaptations for school or ADLs (Morrissy & Weinstein, 2001).

Developmental dysplasia of the hip (congenital hip dislocation) is almost as common as clubfoot, having an incidence of 1.5 per 1,000 live births (CDC, 2002). The condition is often bilateral and occurs nine times more often in girls than in boys (Thompson, 2004). The causes of congenital hip dislocation (head out of the socket) and subluxations (head partly out of the socket) are both genetic and environmental. Hip laxity may be genetically inherited or may be a result of a hormonal secretion of the uterus. Environmental factors related to hip dislocation include birth complications from uterine pressure and poor presenting positions. Dislocation or subluxation of the unstable hip also may be caused by sudden, passive extension or by positioning that keeps the legs extended and adducted (Salter, 1999).

Early diagnosis of congenital dislocation of the hip is critical because delay can cause serious and permanent disabilities. Three clinical observations that may be used in diagnosing this condition in infants are Ortolani's sign, Galeazzi's sign, and Barlow's test. The result of the Barlow test (the most critical test for newborns) is considered positive if the unstable hip clicks out of the acetabulum when the leg is abducted and pressure is placed on the medial thigh (Morrissy & Weinstein, 2001). Ortolani's sign is a maneuver to reduce a recently dislocated hip. For this maneuver the infant's knees and hips are flexed, and the femur is alternately adducted and pressed downward and then abducted and lifted. If the hip is unstable, it dislocates when adducted but returns to the socket when abducted. The evaluator feels and often hears a click as this happens. With Galeazzi's sign, one knee is lower than the other when the child is placed in the supine position on a table with the knees flexed to 90 degrees. This results from the dislocated femur lying posterior to the acetabulum (Thompson, 2004).

In the older child with congenital hip dislocation, Trendelenburg's sign is seen. With this sign, the hip drops to the opposite side of the dislocation and the trunk shifts toward the dislocated hip when the child is asked to stand on the foot of the affected side (Morrissy & Weinstein, 2001).

If treatment is begun within the first few weeks of life, normal development of the hip nearly always can be ensured. The longer the dislocation goes unresolved, the poorer the prognosis. Specific treatment techniques vary according to the age of the client when treatment is initiated, but generally the techniques involve stabilizing the hip in an abducted and flexed position to facilitate femoral and acetabular development. This stabilization may be accomplished with splints, traction, the hip spica plaster cast, or the pillow splint (Morrissy & Weinstein, 2001; Salter, 1999). If these methods do not correct the disorder, several surgical procedures may be performed to correct bony and soft tissue problems. In severe cases, arthrodesis or total replacement arthroplasty may be performed. Again, every infant should be examined for this deformity in the first weeks of life to prevent the complications this defect can cause.

Hypoplasia or *aplasia* is the underdevelopment of an organ because of a decrease in the number of cells, whereas *aplasia* is the failure of an organ to develop at all. These are relatively rare conditions that occur in the fibula, tibia, and femur (limiting gait and stability) or in the clavicles and radius. Other congenital defects occasionally seen are *Sprengel's deformity* (congenital high scapula), recurvatum of the knee, and alignment deformities (Salter, 1999; Thompson, 2004).

Limb Deficiencies

Limb deficiencies in children are most commonly attributable to congenital malformations. A small number occur because of accidents or as the result of surgery to prevent the spread of cancer, such as Ewing's sarcoma. Congenital limb deficiencies occur more frequently in the upper extremities. Limb deficiencies and malformations may be familial or may result from early fetal insult or, rarely, from congenital constricting bands. With congenital constricting bands, the soft tissue and overlying skin on a small body part fail to grow in circumference. If the constriction is severe enough, the band stops distal limb circulation, causing gangrene and intrauterine amputation (Morrissy & Weinstein, 2001). Traumatic amputations are becoming less common because of better emergency care and the improved ability of surgeons to reattach a traumatically removed body part. Congenital malformations of the hands or feet, usually in the fingers and toes, occur in 1 per 600 live births (Morrissy & Weinstein). According to the CDC, more than 3,200 babies are born with polydactyly, syndactyly, or adactyly each year (CDC, 2000).

Polydactyly is an excess of fingers or toes. This is a relatively common condition that may involve one or more extra complete digits or duplication of only part of a digit. Bony changes may be present or just extra soft tissue. In most cases surgical amputation or reconstruction is performed early in childhood, particularly if the hand is involved. *Syndactyly,* or webbing between the fingers or toes, occurs frequently. It is most common in the upper extremity and in boys. It sometimes co-exists with polydactyly, which makes repair more complicated. In simple cases the fingers are surgically separated in early childhood (Morrissy & Weinstein, 2001; Trumble, 2000). Extensive hand therapy is usually unnecessary, although splinting and scar reduction may be helpful in some cases. *Bradydactyly* and *microdactyly* are overly large or small digits, respectively. Plastic surgery may be performed if the digits are unsightly or impair function (Trumble).

Congenital limb deficiencies include amelia, phocomelia, paraxial deficiency, and transverse hemimelia (Figure 6-6). *Amelia* is the absence of a limb or the distal

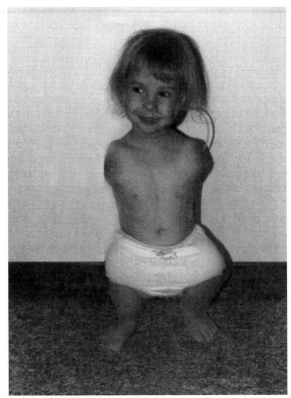

FIGURE 6-6   Child with multiple congenital limb deficiencies, including bilateral transverse upper arm deficiency and bilateral proximal femoral focal deficiency. (From Stanger, M. [1994]. Limb deficiencies and amputations. In S. Campbell [Ed.], *Physical therapy for children.* New York: W.B. Saunders.)

segments of a limb. With *phocomelia* the child may have a fully or partly formed distal extremity but is missing one or more proximal segments of the limb. With *paraxial deficiencies* the proximal part of the limb is correctly developed, but either the medial or lateral side of the rest of the limb may be missing. *Transverse hemimelia* is the amputation of a limb segment across the central area. It is common for a child with malformation of one body part to have bilateral or hemilateral problems (Trumble, 2000).

Children with congenital limb deficiencies may require surgery for removal of skin flaps or "nuisance" parts if these interfere with function. It is common for children to have some shoulder, trunk, and rib asymmetries as well. These children are fitted with prostheses as early as 2 months but usually by 6 months of age. Hybrid and myoelectric prosthesis have developed significantly in the past 5 years, eliminating some of the prior limitations of prosthetic use (i.e., lack of combination of both force and manipulation in one device), making the use of a prosthesis more realistic and appropriate (Morrissy & Weinstein, 2001). Early and appropriate matching of the child to the prosthetic device allows the child to incorporate the prosthesis into his or her body image; it promotes balance, prevents scoliosis, facilitates bilateral function, and reduces dependence on the residual limb for tactile input. A multidisciplinary prosthetic team often follows the child's development into adolescence and his or her family (Trumble, 2000).

Hybrid and myoelectric devices should be considered as the initial prostheses. When these devices are applied early in development, the child develops a more intuitive use of the available muscle groups to power the prosthesis. Infants with upper extremity amputations are often given a passive mitt, or a terminal device (TD) without cabling. This allows the child to hold objects that are placed in the hand and to develop early eye-hand skills. Active TD use is instituted between 15 and 24 months of age; elbow operation, if necessary, is not introduced until the child is developmentally able to operate the mechanism. As the child grows and matures, new prostheses are fabricated that reflect the child's increased size and skills. As expected, this process is more complex for upper extremity amputees than for lower extremity amputees and for children with multiple amputations (Morrissy & Weinstein, 2001).

Acquired limb deficiencies are treated much like those of adults, except that tasks must be developmentally structured and sequenced. Bimanual activities for play, school, and self-care are emphasized. Learning to independently apply, remove, and care for the prosthesis is also part of the treatment process for school-age children. The child must be taught ADL skills, with and without the prosthesis, and may require assistance and adaptations for some school, work, and play tasks. Occasionally children experience overgrowth of the long bones, resulting in pain and possibly skin penetration and infection. Conservative skin stretching and surgical revision may be necessary (Morrissy & Weinstein, 2001). Psychosocial, self-concept, and social play experiences may assist these children, particularly as they approach puberty.

Juvenile Rheumatoid Arthritis

Juvenile rheumatoid arthritis (JRA) is a major cause of physical disability in children younger than 16 years of age. It has an overall prevalence of 113 per 100,000 children, and approximately 260,000 children in the United States have the disease (Trumble, 2000). JRA usually begins between 2 and 4 years of age and is more common in girls (Morrissy & Weinstein, 2001). It is the most common form of arthritis in children. There is no single test to diagnose the disease; the diagnosis is made on the basis of persistent arthritis in one or more joints for at least 6 weeks after other possible illnesses have been ruled out. Sometimes a variety of tests may be needed to arrive at a firm diagnosis.

Arthritis is best described by four major changes that may occur in the joints. The most common features of JRA are joint inflammation, joint contracture (stiff, bent joint), joint damage, and/or alteration or change in growth. Other symptoms include joint stiffness after rest or decreased activity (also referred to as *morning stiffness* or *gelling*) and weakness in muscles and other soft tissues around involved joints. Children vary in the degree to which they are affected by any particular symptom (Wong & Hockenberry-Eaton, 2001).

Rheumatoid arthritis is a systemic disease that affects every aspect of an individual's life. It is characterized primarily by inflammatory changes in and destruction of the synovial joints (Figure 6-7). The exact cause of JRA is unknown, but factors believed to play undefined roles in its cause include genetics, emotional trauma, histocompatibility antigens, viruses, and antigen-antibody immune complexes (Morrissy & Weinstein, 2001).

JRA is usually described as having three different forms: (1) pauciarticular, (2) polyarticular, and (3) systemic. The pauciarticular form usually affects fewer than five joints. Involvement is often asymmetric, and there are few or no systemic manifestations. The joints most

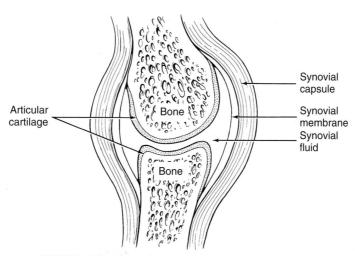

FIGURE 6-7 Components of a typical synovial joint.

often affected are the knees, hips, ankles, and elbows. Overgrowth of the long bones surrounding the inflamed joint often causes gait problems and flexion contractures. Many children who have pauciarticular JRA develop iridocyclitis, an inflamed condition of the iris and ciliary body of the eye that can lead to blindness if not treated.

With polyarticular JRA the onset is often abrupt and painful, with symmetric involvement of the wrists, hands, feet, knees, ankles, and sometimes the cervical area of the spine. This resembles adult rheumatoid arthritis, and rheumatoid nodules on extensor surfaces indicate a more severe course. Five or more joints are affected, and as many as 20 to 40 separate joints may be involved; other symptoms include a low-grade fever, malaise, anorexia, listlessness, and irritability (Miller & Cassidy, 2004).

Systemic JRA, or *Still's disease,* consists of polyarticular symptoms plus involvement of other organs, such as the spleen and lymph nodes (Morrissy & Weinstein, 2001). Signs and symptoms include high fever, rash, anorexia, enlargement of the liver and spleen, and an elevated white blood cell count. Epiphyseal plates adjacent to an affected joint may initially show an acceleration of growth but later may be destroyed, causing local growth delay.

Medical management primarily centers on the use of therapeutic drugs, such as nonsteroidal anti-inflammatory analgesics. Corticosteroids are used to manage overwhelming inflammatory or systemic illness or as a bridge therapy in children who are not yet responsive to other medications. Surgical repair and reconstruction are seldom recommended for children. Other forms of treatment may include splinting, active and passive ROM exercises, and monitoring of joint motion to maintain maximal function and prevent deformity.

The prognosis for JRA varies, depending on a number of factors, but it is important to remember that the largest percentage of children (with the pauciarticular type of JRA) recover completely within 1 to 2 years. Only about 15% of all children with JRA have permanent disabilities (Miller & Cassidy, 2004).

Children with JRA may have pain at times, may show signs of fatigue, and may have reduced ROM in one or more joints. As a result, they may have difficulty performing ADLs and certain school tasks. Adaptive equipment such as pen and pencil grips, dressing aids, and built-up handles on utensils or other adaptations to feeding equipment often improve functioning and reduce fatigue and stress on joints. Seating needs must be monitored to help reduce fatigue and prevent harmful pressure on joints (Trumble, 2000).

Play and recreational activities may be adapted to allow full participation and to maintain strength and ROM. Children with severe deficits may require prevocational evaluation and treatment. Child and parent education in joint protection and energy conservation techniques is essential for children with JRA at all ages and stages (Trombly & Radomski, 2002).

Soft Tissue Injury

Children, being active and busy, are frequently subject to traumatic injury, particularly soft tissue injury. *Contusions* are injuries and tears of the soft tissue, skin, muscles, and subcutaneous tissue. When they occur, an inflammatory response results and the child experiences pain, swelling, and hemorrhagic responses. Contusions are not usually serious in the typically developing child but can be difficult for children with a disordered response to trauma (e.g., hemophilia). *Crush injuries* are common in children (e.g., fingers caught in doors), can also involve bone and nails, and may swell and be painful (Morrissy & Weinstein, 2001).

A *dislocation* occurs when forces on a joint pull or push it out of its socket. This injury creates obvious problems in alignment, as well as deformity and immobility. Dislocations should be reduced as soon as possible so that inflammation does not increase the pain and difficulty of this procedure. After reduction the child's extremity is usually immobilized for some time to allow healing. If the forces exerted on the ligaments are strong enough to tear them, the injury is called a *sprain*. These forces also may damage muscles, nerves, tendons, and blood vessels in the area. Several "special" tests of joint laxity can be used for sprain evaluation. Pain may or may not be severe, but swelling and favoring of the extremity usually are seen. Sprains must be positioned and immobilized for an extended period and in severe cases may be casted or splinted for 3 to 6 weeks (Morrissy & Weinstein, 2001).

Fractures

Fractures are extremely common in children. They can occur prenatally and perinatally in children with other pathologic conditions but are uncommon in typically developing infants. As children grow older and their independence and activity level increases, they may be injured in automobile, skateboard, and bicycle accidents, in falls, and while participating in sports. Childhood fractures can also be caused by child abuse. An unusually high number of fractures may trigger an investigation into the possibility that abuse has occurred.

Fractures may be classified in many ways. An *open,* or *compound, fracture* is an open wound or penetration caused by an object outside the body or caused by extrusion of bone from within the body. A *closed fracture* is one in which no penetration has occurred. Open fractures present added difficulties because the wound must be closed in addition to treatment of the fracture. The risks of infection and soft tissue and nerve damage are higher with open fractures, and complications are more common (Salter, 1999; Thompson, 2004).

Displacement and malalignment of bones often complicate traumatic fractures. Figure 6-8 shows some of the most common types of malalignment caused by serious fractures. Children's fracture patterns are not identical to those of adults. Their bones may buckle or bend rather than break because their bones are thinner and less solid. *Greenstick fractures* occur when the bone is not completely separated on one side, much as a twig breaks when bent. Sometimes the bone breaks completely, but the periosteal covering remains intact, holding the fragments together. This *periosteal hinge* may assist or complicate fracture reduction. *Comminuted fractures* occur when multiple fragments are created by the injury (Salter, 1999).

Children's ligaments are often stronger than their epiphyseal plates. Therefore when stress is applied, it is more common to find a fracture than a dislocation or sprain. Fractures involving the epiphyseal growth plate, which account for 15% of childhood fractures, are of particular concern because they may affect the growth and alignment of the bone and the integrity of the joint in later life. The type of problem and its severity depend on the location and extent of the injury in relation to the growth plate. Figure 6-9 presents the Salter-Harris classification system (Salter, 1999). Under this system, more severe injuries are given higher numbers. Fractures that cross the joint surface generally are the most serious because they may result in uneven growth on the joint surface and thereby impair the normal slide, glide, and alignment of the joint in adolescence and adulthood.

Treatment of fractures requires open or closed reduction, or realignment, of the bony fragments and immobilization until the bone heals. Open surgical reduction

is rare in children but may be performed for injuries to the growth plate and serious compound or comminuted fractures (Salter, 1999). Fractures in children heal more quickly than those in adults. Young children and infants may heal in 2 to 4 weeks and school-age children in 6 weeks. Adolescents require immobilization for the same 8 to 10 weeks required by adults with similar injuries (Morrissy & Weinstein, 2001; Salter).

Immobilization is usually achieved through use of a cast, although in severe cases pins, traction, and external fixation may be used. The advent of synthetic, fiberglass, and polyurethane resin casting materials has been an advantage for children because these materials are waterproof and come in bright colors. Children with casts should be checked to ensure that circulation and skin integrity are maintained under the cast and that the cast is not breaking down from active use. A child in traction may need adapted devices and activities to maintain independence while he or she is immobilized. Prevention of skin breakdown is also a concern for any individual for whom bed rest is prescribed (Salter, 1999).

Torsion Deformities

Particularly in children, prolonged twisting forces may cause changes in epiphyseal plate growth, causing the long bones to twist in the direction of the abnormal force. These are known as *internal, external,* or *combinational torsional deformities* (Salter, 1999). For example, "toeing out," which is characterized by externally rotated feet and knees and limited internal rotation of the femur, is common in young children. This deformity is often seen in infants who habitually sleep in the prone position with their legs externally rotated, causing external femoral torsion. Conversely, children who spend

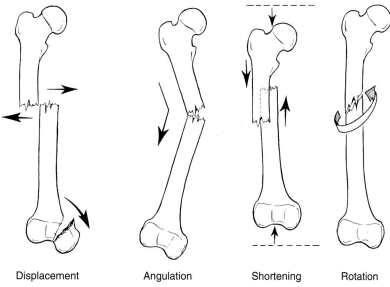

Displacement   Angulation   Shortening   Rotation

FIGURE 6-8   Types of malalignment caused by fractures.

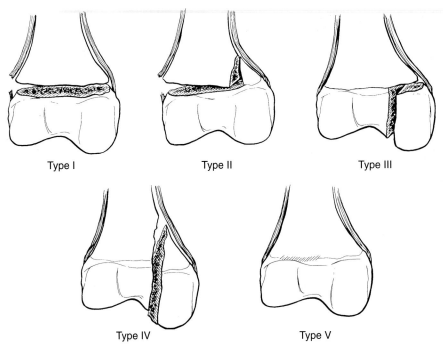

FIGURE 6-9 Salter-Harris classifications of epiphyseal plate injuries.

a great deal of time sitting on the floor with knees in front, feet out to the side, and femurs internally rotated (the "television position," or "W-sitting"), may begin to "toe in" as a result of the internal femoral tension.

Bowlegs, or genu varum, are an example of a deformity caused by combinational torsional forces (i.e., prolonged internal torsion to the tibia and external torsion to the femur). This deformity is often present at birth because of prenatal posturing, but it usually corrects itself unless compounded by specific neuromuscular problems or unusual sleeping and sitting postures that continue to apply the abnormal torsions (Salter, 1999).

Curvature of the Spine

Lordosis, kyphosis, and scoliosis are the three major deformities of the spine. These conditions may occur functionally, posturally, and structurally; they may occur secondary to muscle imbalance, bony deformities, or other pathologic conditions such as cerebral palsy; or they may occur idiopathically. They may be congenital or acquired. In most cases the cause of these disorders is unknown, although some familial patterns exist (Salter, 1999) (Figure 6-10). *Lordosis* is an anteroposterior curvature in which the concavity is directed posteriorly. Also called *hollow back*, this condition often occurs secondary to other spinal deformities or to an anterior pelvic tilt. It usually is predominantly in the lumbar area of the back and occasionally is painful. It can also occur secondary to extreme obesity, hip flexion contractures, or conditions such as muscular dystrophy. Lordosis may occur during the adolescent growth spurt experienced by many

girls. Treatment focuses on correcting the underlying conditions, stretching tight hip flexors, and strengthening the abdominal musculature. Postural training and occasionally, in severe cases, back bracing are included.

The opposite anteroposterior curvature, with the convexity posterior, is called *kyphosis*. With this condition, also called *round back* and, in adolescents, *Scheuermann's disease,* the curvature is usually primarily in the upper back. The deformity is common in children and adolescents and usually is the result of faulty posture. This is particularly true as the teenage girl's skeletal growth outpaces her muscular growth. The deformity can occur in children with spina bifida cystica or arthritis. Treatment depends on the cause and severity of the problem. In mild cases postural training and strengthening activities such as weight training, swimming, and dance are often useful. Thoracic kyphosis requires the use of a Milwaukee brace. In severe cases, a combination of anterior spinal release and fusion and posterior spinal fusion and instrumentation may be used to guide and support the spine (Morrissy & Weinstein, 2001; Thompson, 2004).

Scoliosis is the most common and serious of the spinal curvature disorders, usually involving lateral curvature, spinal rotation, and thoracic hypokyphosis. Treatment is considered when a lateral curvature of more than 10 degrees is present. Lateral curvature of the spine is often accompanied by rotation of the vertebral bodies. Functional scoliosis is flexible and can be caused by poor posture, leg length discrepancy, poor postural tone, hip contractures, or pain. Congenital scoliosis is usually structural in nature, caused by abnormal spinal or spinal cord structure. Diseases of the nervous system or spine

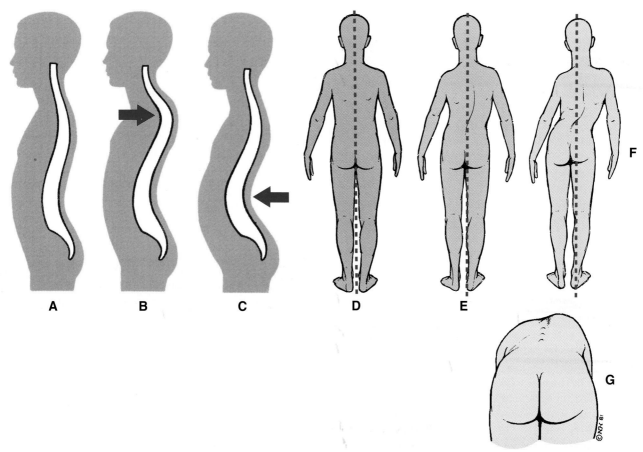

FIGURE 6-10 Defects of the spinal column. **A,** Normal spine. **B,** Kyphosis. **C,** Lordosis. **D,** Normal spine in balance. **E,** Mild scoliosis in balance. **F,** Severe scoliosis not in balance. **G,** Rib hump and flank asymmetry seen in flexion caused by rotary component. (Redrawn from Hilt, N.E., & Schmitt, E.W. [1975]. Pediatric orthopaedic nursing. In Wong, D. (Ed.), *Pediatric nursing*. St. Louis: Mosby.)

also may result in scoliosis. However, most cases of scoliosis have no known cause.

Scoliosis is rarely painful. The diagnosis is based on careful examination and history taking. If preliminary evaluation and palpation suggest the condition, radiographic analysis is also used. Structural scoliosis often progresses over time; the vertebral bodies may become wedge shaped and rotate toward the convex part of the curve, and the intervertebral disk may shift and deform (Salter, 1999). Curves of less than 20 degrees are considered mild. Those of more than 40 degrees may result in permanent deformity, and those of 65 to 80 degrees may result in reduced cardiopulmonary function. Skin breakdown between the ribs and pelvis may also develop in some cases.

Treatment includes orthotic intervention and surgical spinal fusion. The two most common types of bracing are the Boston brace, created from prefabricated plastic shells, and a thoracolumbosacral orthotic (TLSO). Exercise alone is rarely effective for managing scoliosis but may be helpful in strengthening spinal and abdominal muscles during treatment. If surgery is indicated, postoperative therapy and adapted ADLs are sometimes needed; in general, children and adolescents progress well after surgery and maintain a normal life style into adulthood (Salter, 1999; Thompson, 2004).

NEUROMUSCULAR DISORDERS

Children with neuromuscular disorders constitute a large percentage of the clients of occupational therapy practice. Several conditions involve impairment of the neurologic system, resulting in interference with the child's ability to interact effectively with the environment. The site of damage may be the brain, spinal cord, peripheral nerves, neuromuscular junction, or the muscle itself. The disorder may interfere with the reception and processing of sensory input or the ability to act effectively on the environment, or a combination of these may result. Neuromuscular deficits may occur before, at, or after birth. This section addresses several of the major conditions in this category.

Cerebral Palsy

Cerebral palsy (CP) is characterized by nonprogressive abnormalities in the developing brain that create a cascade of neurologic, motor, and postural deficits in the developing child. The incidence of CP is estimated to be 1.4 to 2.4 per 1,000 live births, and although this rate has remained constant over a 30-year period, the causes have changed. Because of a rise in the survival rate of very premature infants in both the very low birth weight and extremely low birth weight categories, a rise in the incidence of CP with spastic diplegia, often associated with prematurity and low birth weight, has been noted. On the other hand, athetoid CP, often attributed to fetal asphyxia and hyperbilirubinemia, has decreased in developed countries (Pellegrino, 2002). It is estimated that 5,000 infants and 1,200 to 1,500 preschool children are diagnosed with CP each year.

Although a pattern of motor and postural deficits is a defining feature of CP, many secondary disorders typically co-exist with this diagnosis. Cognitive, sensory, and psychosocial deficits often compound motor impairments and subsequent functioning (Pellegrino, 2002). Although CP is usually the result of injury or disease at or before birth (congenital CP), children injured in early childhood display similar symptoms and are sometimes classified as having CP (acquired CP). CP is expressed through variable impairments in motor and postural control, coordination of muscle action, and sensation that typically are classified according to the type and distribution of motor impairment (Stanley, Blair, & Alberman, 2000).

The various causes of congenital CP can be grouped according to premature birth or term birth. Prematurity now accounts for the majority of known causes for CP. This increased rate may be associated with the central nervous system's vulnerability to insult (i.e., increased sensitivity to bleeding near the lateral ventricles, which has a cascading effect on further CNS development) during gestational weeks 26 to 32.

Cerebrovascular accident (CVA), developmental brain abnormalities, placental abruption, fetomaternal hemorrhage, placental infarction, and maternal exposure to environmental toxins have also been associated with CP. In addition, maternal infections such as cytomegalovirus, syphilis, varicella virus, and toxoplasmosis can be secondary causes of CP. Causes of acquired CP include trauma, intracranial hemorrhage, CNS infections, near drowning, hypoxia, and metabolic disorders.

Early diagnosis of CP is important to elicit the services that the child and family may need to optimize the child's potential for development and to prevent secondary disabilities. To develop a definitive diagnosis, a team of developmental specialists conducts thorough physical and developmental evaluations. These evaluations usually take place over a period of months in early development. The team may include a pediatrician, an occupational and a physical therapist, a developmental nurse, and a speech-language pathologist. Retention of primitive reflexes and automatic reactions, variable tone, hyperresponsive tendon reflexes, asymmetry in the use of extremities, clonus, poor sucking or tongue control, and involuntary movements may indicate the presence of CP. Motor delays coupled with delays in other developmental areas or with a discrepancy in cognitive development are also strong indicators. Infants who weigh less than 1,500 g at birth are particularly vulnerable and must be monitored closely (Johnston, 2004a; Pellegrino, 2002). Each child with CP has a unique set of problems. Comprehensive ongoing medical assessment is necessary in children diagnosed with CP to treat medical sequelae associated with the condition.

Characteristically, the child with CP shows impaired ability to maintain normal postures because of a lack of muscle co-activation and the development of abnormal movement compensations. These compensatory patterns develop in certain muscle groups to maintain upright postures and to effect movement against gravity. For example, the child's poor head control, resulting from poor co-activation of cervical flexors and extensors, causes the center of gravity to move anteriorly; this results in compensatory reactions in the thoracic and lumbar spine as the child attempts to stay upright. Likewise, hyperreactive responses to tactile, visual, or auditory stimuli may result in fluctuations of muscle tone that often adversely affect postural control and further diminish coordinated responses in everyday activities.

Classification of Cerebral Palsy

The locale of the lesion affects the development and quality of movement patterns present in the child with CP. For example, CP with spasticity indicates a lesion in the motor cortex. Lesions in the basal ganglia typically cause fluctuations in muscle tone that are described as *diakinesis, dystonia,* or *athetosis.* Cerebellar damage tends to produce the unstable movements characteristic of the ataxic child.

The variability of the movement and postural disorder may be classified according to which limbs are affected. Involvement of the upper and lower extremities on one side is *hemiplegia,* involvement of all limbs is *tetraplegia* or *quadriplegia* and *diplegia* when the child demonstrates quadriplegia with mild upper extremity involvement and significant impairment of function in lower extremities.

Several classifications of CP have been developed according to the quality of tone, disorder distribution, and locale of brain lesions. These classifications are featured in Table 6-2. Characteristics are described according to quality and distribution of muscle tone, ROM, quality of movement, presence of reflexes and reactions,

TABLE 6-2 Cerebral Palsy Classifications

	Severe Spasticity	Moderate Spasticity	Mild Spasticity	Pure Athetosis	Athetosis with Spasticity	Athetosis with Tonic Spasms	Choreoathetosis	Flaccid	Ataxia
Quality of tone	Severely increased tone; flexor and extensor co-contraction are constant; tone is high at rest, during sleep, or when awake; tone pattern is more proximal than distal	Moderately increased tone; near normal at rest but increases with excitement, movement attempts, effort, emotion, speech, sudden stretch; agonists and distal muscles more spastic	Mildly increased or normal tone at rest but increases with effort or attempts to move or attempts at quicker movements	Fluctuation of tone from low to normal; no or little spasticity; no co-activation of flexors and extensors	Fluctuates from normal to high; some ability to stabilize proximally; moderate proximal spasticity and distal athetosis	Unpredictable tone changes from low to very high; either all flexion or extension of extremities	Constant fluctuations from low to high with no co-contraction; jerky involuntary movements more proximal than distal	Fluctuating, markedly low muscle tone; seen at birth, or toddler initially classified as flaccid, later classified as spastic, athetoid, or ataxic	Ranges from near normal to normal; increased tone, when present, usually involves lower extremity flexion
Distribution of tone	Quadriplegia, but may also manifest as diplegia or paraplegia	Same as in severe spasticity	Same as in severe spasticity, but diplegia and hemiplegia more common	Quadriplegia with occasional hemiplegia	Same as in athetosis	Quadriplegia, hemiplegia, or monoplegia	Quadriplegia	Quadriplegia	Quadriplegia
Range of motion	Abnormal patterns can lead to scoliosis, kyphosis, hip/knee/finger deformity; forearm pronation contracture, hip subluxation, heel cord subluxation with equinovarus or equinovalgus; decreased trunk, shoulder, and	More available movement and more flexor/extensor imbalance can lead to kyphosis, lordosis, hip subluxations or dislocations, hip and knee flexion contractures; tight hip internal rotators and adductors; heel cord shortening; foot rotation	Limitations more distal than proximal; minimal deformities	Transient subluxation of joints such as shoulders and fingers; may have valgus on feet or knees; rarely any deformities	Incidence of scoliosis; some flexion deformities at hips, elbows, and knees; usually full range of motion proximally and hypermobile distally	More pronounced scoliosis; more dislocation of arm because of flailing spasm; possible kyphoscoliosis, hip dislocation on skull side, flexion contracture on hips/knees, subluxation of hips, fingers, or lower jaw	Many involuntary movements with extreme ranges but no control at midrange; deformities rare, but tendency for shoulder and finger subluxation	Hypermobile joints that tend to sublux; flat chest; later, range limitations due to limited movement	Range usually not a problem; decreased range, when present, usually in flexion

Continued

TABLE 6-2 Cerebral Palsy Classifications—cont'd

	Severe Spasticity	Moderate Spasticity	Mild Spasticity	Pure Athetosis	Athetosis with Spasticity	Athetosis with Tonic Spasms	Choreoathetosis	Flaccid	Ataxia
	pelvic girdle mobility; limited midrange control where co-contraction is least balanced.								Lacks point of stability, therefore co-activation is difficult; uses primitive rather than abnormal patterns, hence gross, total patterns; incoordination, thus dysmetria disdiadochokinesia, tremors at rest, symmetric problems
Quality of movement	Decreased midrange, voluntary, and involuntary movements; slow and labored stereotypical movements	May be able to walk; stereotypical, asymmetric, more associated reactions; total movement synergies	Often able to walk; seems driven to move; has increased variety of other movements, some stereotypical	Writhing involuntary movements, more distal than proximal; no change with intention to move; many fixation attempts caused by decreased ability to stabilize	Decreased ability to grade movements; decreased midline control and selective movement; proximal stability and distal choreoathetosis; varies with case	Extreme tonic spasm without voluntary control; some involuntary movement, distal more than proximal	Wide movement ranges with no gradation; jerky movements more proximal than distal; no selective movement or fixation of movement; weak hands and fingers	Ungraded movements; slow movements difficult; many static postures, as if hanging on to anatomic structures instead of active control	
Reflexes and reactions	Obligatory primitive reflexes (positive support, ATNR, STNR, neck righting); protective, righting, and equilibrium reactions are often absent.	Strong primitive reflexes—Moro, startle, TNR, TLR, positive support prominent; decreased neck righting; associated reactions strong; righting may be present, but equilibrium reaction develops to sitting and kneeling	Primitive reflexes used for functional purposes and not obligatory; righting, protective, and equilibrium reactions delayed but established; may not develop higher level reactions	Primitive reflexes not usually obligatory or evoked; protective and equilibrium reactions usually present but involuntary movements affect grading	TNR/TLR strong but intermittent and modified by involuntary movements; equilibrium reactions, when present, unreliable and may or may not be used	Strong ATNR, STNR, TLR; protective and equilibrium reactions absent during spasm, otherwise present, unreliable, or absent	Intermittent TNR; righting and equilibrium reactions present to some extent, but abnormal coordination; abnormal upper extremity protective extension possible, but often absent	Usually less reactive because of decreased tone; righting is delayed; delayed protective extension more available than equilibrium reaction	May develop righting reactions, but these are uncoordinated, exaggerated, and poorly used; equilibrium reactions, when developed, are not coordinated; needs wide base of support because of poor weight shifting

	1	2	3	4	5	6	7	8	9
Oral motor	Immobile, rigid chest; shallow respiration and forced expiration; lip retraction with decreased lip closure and tongue thrust; communication through forced expiration	Not as involved as in severe spasticity	Increased mobility, thus more respiratory function for phonation; shortness of breath limits sentence length; better ability to dissociate mouth parts, but poor lip closure causes drooling	Fluctuations adversely affect gross and fine motor performance; volume of speech may go up or down with breath; feeding may be decreased due to instability and tongue/jaw/swallow incoordination	Difficulty with head control, thus decreased oral motor; decreased coordination of suck/swallow, resulting in decreased feeding and speech	Feeding may be difficult because aspiration is unpredictable; severe language and speech impairment caused by decreased control	Facial grimaces, dysarthria, irregular breathing, difficulty sustaining phonation, poor intraoral and extraoral surfaces	Quiet, soft voice because of decreased respiration; delayed speech; increased drooling; often expressionless face	Speech is monotone, very slow; uses teeth to stabilize tongue or hold cup to mouth when drinking; decreased articulation
Associated problems	Seizures, cortical blindness, deafness, MR, malnutrition, prone to URTI	Seizures, MR, perceptual motor problems, imbalance of eye musculature	Seizures, less MR, perceptual problems	Hearing loss, less MR		Same as in athetosis	Same as in athetosis	Obesity, sensory impairment, URTI	Nystagmus, MR, sensory problems; uses vision for righting and as reference point for movement
Personality characteristics	Passive, dependent; resistant and adapts poorly to change; anxious and fearful of being moved; generally less frustrated than athetoid individuals	Lesser degree of traits seen in severe spasticity	More frustrated and critical about self because of awareness of better performance; more patient than children of same age	Emotional lability; less fearful of movement; more outgoing, but tends to be frustrated		Same as in athetosis	Same as in athetosis	Visually attentive, cannot move, therefore is a "good" baby; decreased motivation	Does not like to move

Modified from Bobath, B. (1978). *Classification of types of cerebral palsy based on the quality of postural tone.* London: The Bobath Centre.

ATNR, Asymmetric tonic neck reflex; *STNR,* symmetric tonic neck reflex; *TNR,* tonic neck reflex; *TLR,* tonic labyrinthine; *MR,* mental retardation; *URTI,* upper respiratory tract infection.

oral motor problems, associated problems, and personality characteristics.

Although CP is considered nonprogressive, abnormal movement patterns, muscle tone, and sensory function, combined with the effects of gravity and normal growth, may cause the child to develop contractures and deformities over time. Function may become more limited as the child grows to adulthood. Furthermore, the effects of normal aging may result in decreased function, physical discomfort, and arthritic responses over time (Nelson, 2001).

Language and intellectual deficits often co-exist with CP. Delays in cognitive development and below-average intelligence have been seen in 50% to 75% of children with CP. This impairment may range from mild to profound (Pellegrino, 2002). Speech disturbances occur in approximately 30% of these children. Articulation problems may be associated with impairment of tongue and lip movements. Speech and language problems may be receptive or expressive, relating to central processing impairment. Limitations in communication tend to isolate the child, may create stress and frustration for the child and parent, and can negatively affect the development of psychosocial skills. Use of augmentative communication equipment can prevent some of these consequences of speech impairment and is critical for increasing the communication abilities of children with severe CP (Nelson, 2001).

Seizure disorders occur in approximately 50% of children with CP, and the incidence appears to be higher among children with spastic disorders (Johnston, 2004a). In children with severe seizures, some degeneration may continue after birth. Anticonvulsant drugs are commonly used to control seizure activity. These drugs must be carefully monitored and may affect the state of the child's digestion and gums, requiring feeding adjustments and good dental care.

Feeding problems are associated with the abnormal oral movements, tone, and sensation. The child may be hypersensitive or hyposensitive to touch around and in the mouth, and sucking, chewing, and swallowing may be difficult to initiate or control (Pellegrino, 2002). The child's diet may need to be adjusted, and special feeding techniques may be required. These children also may require medication to maintain regularity of elimination. Positioning helps improve postural stability for feeding and toileting (Nelson, 2001).

Several sensory deficits may be present. Problems with the visual system may include impaired vision, blindness, limitations in eye movements and eye tracking, squinting, strabismus, eye muscle weaknesses, and eye incoordination. In addition, children with CP may have visual perception problems that can interfere with school progress. It is estimated that 40% to 50% of children with CP have visual defects of some type and require glasses or low vision and visual-perceptual training. Auditory disturbances include hearing problems (acuity), which can range from slight hearing loss to total deafness. Auditory perceptual problems and agnosia are also common. An estimated 25% of children with CP have some type of auditory disturbance and may require hearing aids (Stanley et al., 2000).

Children with CP must be monitored for signs of behavioral problems and psychosocial delays that can become serious if not found and corrected early. Evaluation of these areas, emotional support, normalization of social experiences, and behavior management programs should be integral parts of the total assessment and treatment regimen for these special children (Pellegrino, 2002).

Antispasticity oral medications (e.g., diazepam, baclofen, and dantrolene) have shown limited effectiveness in improving muscle tone in children with spasticity. The medications can reduce spasticity or rigidity and improve comfort in older children for short periods. These medications work on the neurotransmitter acetylcholine (ACh) and are fast acting. Significant side effects occur with many children, including drowsiness, excessive drooling, and physical dependency, all of which tend to outweigh the potential benefit of the medication (Pellegrino, 2002).

Several injectable agents are now available that can target localized areas of spasticity more effectively. Implanted medication pumps are being used with children who have severe spasticity. The pump is inserted into the skin of the abdomen, and the catheter is routed to the lumbar spine, where it is placed in the intrathecal space. This placement allows delivery of antispasticity medication (primarily baclofen) into the spinal cord, where it can directly inhibit motor nerve conduction. The major advantages of the pump include lower and more controlled doses of medication and decreased spasticity (Pellegrino, 2002; Stanley et al., 2000). Mechanical failures, infection, and the need for intensive medical intervention may rule out some children as candidates for this treatment. In addition, the long-term effects of such treatment for children remain unclear (Johnston, 2004a).

When spasticity is severe, neural blocks may be used to disrupt the reflex arc (Pellegrino, 2002). Recently, injectable botulinum toxin has been used to block the nerve-muscle junction effectively. Botulinum toxin is deadly in the general circulation, but when injected intramuscularly in minute quantities, it blocks the neuromuscular junction effectively for 3 to 6 months. This allows the child to use the muscle without the interference of spasticity. The long-term benefits of treatment have yet to be well researched, but no serious side effects have been documented.

Orthopedic surgery traditionally has been used to correct joint deformities, to balance uneven muscular action, and to reduce contractures that have resulted from abnormal and asymmetric tone. The most frequently performed surgeries include tendon release (permanent lengthening of a muscle) and tendon transfer (moving the point of attachment of a tendon on bone). Both procedures require the use of a cast for 6 to 8 weeks after surgery, and because overall muscle tone is not changed, the procedures may need to be repeated (Menkes, 2001).

Other possible surgeries include correction of hip deformities or dislocations and scoliosis. A new surgical technique, called the *Lucque procedure,* is currently recommended for aggressive treatment of scoliosis (Pellegrino, 2002). Orthotic management in support of surgery or to reduce tone, prevent contractures, or stabilize or position often improves and increases functional activity. Tone-reducing or inhibitive casts made for the lower extremity can gently strengthen and lengthen spastic muscles. Often a series of casts is applied to increase ROM gradually. When ROM within normal limits has been achieved, the cast is worn intermittently to maintain the increased muscle length. Active and passive ROM activities, positioning and handling to enhance postural tone, and orthotics may be used alone or in combination to improve the child's functional independence (Nelson, 2001).

Neurosurgical intervention for spasticity has been aimed at the brain, spinal cord, and peripheral nerves. For example, cerebellar or dorsal column stimulators have been implanted, but the results have been disappointing. Currently, selective posterior rhizotomy (SPR) is the most widely used neurosurgical procedure. In SPR 50% of the dorsal rootlets at L2-S2 are severed to muscles determined to be spastic, as tested by electromyography (EMG) during surgery. Good candidates for SPR include those with a diagnosis of spastic diplegia, normal cognitive status, no fixed deformities, and good underlying muscle strength in the spastic muscles (Park & Owen, 1992).

The initial studies for SPR provide encouraging data for functional changes, although others have indicated that long-term risks must be balanced with the potential for sustained functional improvements. Reported changes include improved motor control, gait, upper extremity functioning, sitting balance, and responsiveness to other treatment strategies (Loewen, Steinbok, Holsti, & MacKay, 1998; Steinbok, Reiner, & Kestle, 1997). However, some studies have indicated that serious side effects and long-term complications may result from SPR, including persistent back pain, neurogenic bowel and bladder, spondylolisthesis, spondylolysis, severe lumbar lordosis, and sensory changes (McLaughlin et al., 1998).

Although the prognosis varies for each type of CP, children with CP typically live to adulthood, but their life expectancy may be less than that of the normal population. The reason for the shorter life expectancy is not known. Some speculate that it is related to persistent alterations in physiologic and immunologic functioning, the implications of which are not fully understood (Rogers, Coe, & Karaszewski, 1998). The functional prognosis varies greatly from type to type, with hemiplegia and spastic diplegia having a better prognosis than the more severe, rigid types. Depending on their ability to attain independence or modified independence with assistive devices and technology, children with CP may experience the full range of life events (Pellegrino, 2002), although they may have limitations in all areas of human occupation to some degree. Although there is no evidence that specific treatment approaches in physical or occupational therapy can prevent or correct CP, there is evidence that therapy that seeks to optimize development is important (Butler & Darrah, 2001). Functional performance in self-care and independent living, school and work performance, play, and recreation all may need to be addressed at some point in the child's life. Parents may require support and respite, as well as education, to care for the child with CP and to meet the needs of the family as a whole (Nelson, 2001).

Seizure Disorders and Epilepsy

Epilepsy is a chronic neurologic condition of recurrent seizures that occur with or without the presence of other brain abnormalities. A *seizure* may be defined as a temporary, involuntary change of consciousness, behavior, motor activity, sensation, or automatic functioning (Weinstein, 2002). Provoked seizures occur frequently in children as a result of fever, acute illness, or CNS infection or after traumatic brain injury (Menkes, 2001).

A *seizure* starts with an excessive rate and hypersynchrony of discharges from a group of cerebral neurons that spreads to the adjoining cells, called the *epileptogenic focus* (Weinstein, 2002). Some seizures may be directly attributed to the factor or factors that trigger the seizure. For example, acute factors often described are hypoglycemia, fever, trauma, hemorrhages, tumors, infections, and anoxia. Other seizures may be attributed to previous scarring and structural damage or to hormonal changes. Many seizures, especially in children, have no discernible underlying disease and therefore are idiopathic in nature (Menkes, 2001).

Seizures are classified by their clinical signs or symptoms and electroencephalographic (EEG) characteristics. The two major types of seizure according to this form of categorization are (1) *generalized seizures,* which involve the entire cerebral cortex, and (2) *partial seizures,* which begin in a single location and remain limited or spread to become more generalized. Generalized seizures can be further divided into tonic-clonic, absence, atypical absence, myoclonic, and atonic forms. Partial seizures can be either simple or complex and are the most common type of seizure disorder found in childhood;

approximately 60% of cases are partial seizures. An individual may experience both generalized and partial seizures, which is called a *mixed seizure disorder* (Wong & Hockenberry-Eaton, 2001).

Of the generalized seizures, the tonic-clonic type occurs most frequently. A child having a *tonic-clonic seizure* may have an aura, or sensation, that the seizure is about to begin. This nonspecific seizure can occur at any age and involves excessive neuronal firing from both hemispheres in a symmetric pattern. This is usually followed by a loss of consciousness, during which the body becomes rigid, or tonic, and then rhythmic clonic contractions of all the extremities occur. Incontinence is common. The seizure may last 5 minutes and is followed by a postictal period that may last 1 to 2 hours, during which the child is drowsy or in a deep sleep (Weinstein, 2002).

A second type of generalized seizure, *absence seizure,* is characterized by a momentary loss of awareness and the absence of motor activity except eye blinking or rolling. There is no aura, the seizure usually lasts less than 30 seconds, and there is no postictal period. The onset of these seizures occurs in the first decade of life. Abrupt interruption of an activity, a glazed look, stares, and unawareness of surroundings characterize a child having an absence seizure. This may be mistaken for daydreaming. Absence seizures are uncommon in children and early adolescents, accounting for only 5% of all seizures (Weinstein, 2002).

Two other mild forms of generalized seizure are (1) *myoclonic seizures,* which consist of contractions by single or small groups of muscles, and (2) *akinetic seizures,* in which the primary problem is a loss of muscle tone. Children rarely have serious seizures for an extended period (30 minutes or longer). This condition is called *status epilepticus* and requires medical management to maintain body functions and hydration. Intravenous anticonvulsant medication is also indicated to treat this condition.

In *complex partial seizures,* which usually originate in the temporal lobe, children may show automatic reactions such as lip smacking, chewing, and buttoning and unbuttoning of clothing. These seizures are focal, and the characteristics are similar to those of absence seizures. In addition, the individual may appear to be confused and disorganized and may have sensory experiences, such as smelling and tasting items not in the environment and hearing sounds of various types.

Simple partial seizures usually involve the motor cortex and result in clonic activity of the face or extremities. Psychic symptoms include visual hallucinations, illusions, auditory hallucinations, or olfactory sensations. The typical seizure includes nighttime awakenings and twitching of facial muscles; this twitching interferes with speech and spreads to the hands (Weinstein, 2002).

Infantile spasms pose a serious threat to development. They typically begin at 6 months and disappear by 24 months. During this time, development appears to stop and skills may be lost. Early treatment with adrenocorticotropic hormone can inhibit the seizure activity; however, the effects on development are almost inevitable. More than 90% of children with known causes for their seizures have mental retardation (MR) (Weinstein, 2002).

The incidence and prevalence of seizures are difficult to estimate. The incidence of generalized seizures, including tonic-clonic, absence, and myoclonic seizures, has been reported to be approximately 2.5 per 1,000 children. The incidence of partial seizures has been reported to be 1.7 to 3.6 per 1,000 children, and unclassified and mixed seizures account for 2 per 1,000 (Menkes, 2001). Many of these unclassified and mixed seizures may occur infrequently and cease as the child matures.

A child who has a seizure must undergo a thorough evaluation to determine the factors that caused the seizure. A family history, medical history, and developmental history must be completed, as well as an EEG to help determine the type of seizure.

Anticonvulsive medications are administered in an attempt to control the seizures. In theory these medications increase the intensity required to trigger the seizure or eliminate the recruitment of surrounding cells. Weinstein (2002) has described some of the common side effects of these anticonvulsive medications, including cataracts, weight gain, high blood pressure, pathologic fractures, drowsiness, hair loss or gain, nausea, liver damage, vomiting, gum enlargement, hyperactivity, anorexia, and lymphoma-like syndrome. Commonly prescribed medications include valproic acid (Depakene), phenytoin (Dilantin), phenobarbital, ethosuximide (Zarontin), and carbamazepine (Tegretol).

Balancing the dosage of anticonvulsant medications can be a difficult process and is often repeated at various times as the child grows and matures. Antiepileptic medication is often withdrawn or reduced if the child has been seizure-free with a normal EEG for at least 2 years. Withdrawal is done slowly and with caution, and health care workers are often asked to monitor the child closely during this period (Menkes, 2001; Weinstein, 2002).

A number of antiepileptic therapies based on old treatments are regaining favor as a result of new research. One example is the ketogenic diet, which consists of a carefully monitored intake of fats, sugars, and carbohydrates that forces the body to use fat rather than carbohydrates for energy and alters neurotransmitters (Hemingway, Freeman, Pillas, & Pyzik, 2001). The urine must be monitored to ensure adequate spillage of ketones. Short-term side effects include metabolic acidosis and electrolyte disturbances, uric acid kidney stones, and diarrhea and vomiting. When the child has been seizure free for a period of 9 months the diet can be terminated.

Surgical intervention is used if adequate control of the seizures cannot be achieved with medication. Surgical interventions that seek to cure epilepsy have been shown to be effective by reducing the seizure focus of the brain, particularly in complex partial seizures arising from the mesial temporal lobe. *Hemispherectomy,* involving removal of most of one side of the brain, is used for seizures that arise from multiple foci in one side of the brain and for progressive unilateral disorders. Palliative surgical interventions include corpus callosotomy and electrical stimulation of the vagus nerve or the thalamus for intractable mixed seizures that have an onset that cannot be localized to one area or that arise from both hemispheres. The timing for surgery is determined by the effectiveness of medication, seizure severity, and the impact of epilepsy on the child's functioning (Menkes, 2001).

Even with optimal care, only about 50% to 75% of children can be controlled completely with medication. Having a seizure can be frightening to the child and those around him or her. When a child has a seizure, staff members must remain calm, move spectators away, and protect the child. Box 6-1 presents an outline of the emergency treatment procedures for seizures. Most children with seizure disorders have normal intelligence scores, are controlled by a single antiepilepsy drug, and lead typical lives. The prognosis depends primarily on the type of seizure and the underlying brain pathology (Weinstein, 2002; Wong & Hockenberry-Eaton, 2001).

Muscular Dystrophies

The muscular dystrophies are the most common muscle diseases of childhood. They cause changes in the biochemistry and structure of the surface and internal membranes of the muscle cells and result in progressive degeneration and weakness of various muscle groups, disability, deformity, and sometimes death. For most of the neuromuscular disorders, which all have a genetic basis, the chromosomal location is known and the causal gene has been identified (Chance, Ashizawa, Hoffman, & Crawford, 1998).

Types of muscular dystrophy include limb-girdle, facioscapulohumeral, congenital, and Duchenne's (pseuodohypertrophic) muscular dystrophy (Wong & Hockenberry-Eaton, 2001). Figure 6-11 shows the differential distribution of paralysis with these dystrophies.

In *limb-girdle muscular dystrophy,* the initial muscles affected are the proximal muscles of the pelvis and shoulder girdles. The onset may occur anywhere from the first to the third decade of life, with progression usually slow but sometimes moderately rapid. The hereditary pattern is autosomal recessive, as with the congenital form (Dubowitz, 1999).

Facioscapulohumeral muscular dystrophy is autosomal dominant, and the onset usually occurs in early adolescence. Although the severity varies greatly among clients, involvement is primarily in the face, upper arms, and scapular region, as the name implies. Clinical manifestations include a slope to the shoulders, decreased ability to raise the arms above shoulder height, and decreased mobility in the facial muscles, resulting in a masklike appearance.

The most common and most severe form of muscular dystrophy is *Duchenne's muscular dystrophy.* It is inherited as an X-linked recessive disorder caused by a deficiency in the production of dystrophin. Because it is an X-linked disorder, the condition affects boys, and the incidence is 1 per 3,500 live male births. Dystrophin is a component of the plasma membrane of muscle fibers. Muscles cannot function and degenerate without dystrophin (Sarnat, 2004).

Children show typical development at birth, and symptoms usually begin to appear between the second and sixth years of life. Parents describe their child as having increasing difficulty climbing stairs and rising from a sitting or lying position. The child stumbles and falls excessively and tires easily. A distinctive characteristic of this form is the enlargement of calf muscles and sometimes of forearm and thigh muscles, giving the appearance of strong, healthy muscles. However, this

---

BOX 6-1 Emergency Treatment of Seizures

1 Time seizure episode.
2 Approach calmly.
3 Protect child during seizure:
- Do not attempt to restrain child or use force.
- If child is standing or sitting in wheelchair at beginning of attack, ease child down so that he or she will not fall; when possible, place cushion or blanket under child.
- Do not put anything in child's mouth.
- Loosen restrictive clothing.
- Prevent child from hitting hard on sharp objects that might cause injury during uncontrolled movements.
- Remove objects.
- Pad objects.
- Move furniture out of the way.
- Allow seizure to end without interference.
4 When seizure stops, check for breathing; if not present, use mouth-to-mouth resuscitation.
5 Check around mouth for evidence of burns or suspicious substances that might indicate poisoning.
6 Remain with child.
7 When child is able to move, seek help.

Adapted from Wong, D.L. (1997). *Whaley and Wong's essentials of pediatric nursing* (5th ed., p. 1023). St. Louis: Mosby.

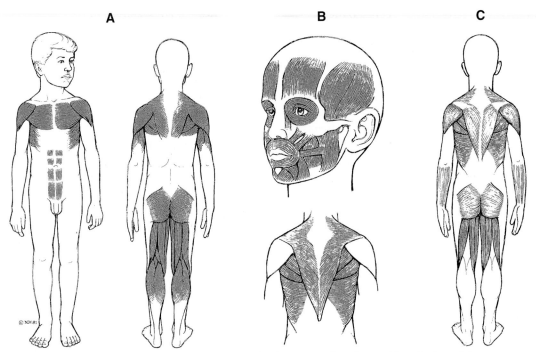

FIGURE 6-11 Initial muscle groups involved in muscular dystrophies. **A,** Pseudohypertrophic. **B,** Facioscapulohumeral. **C,** Limb-girdle. (From Wong, D.L. [1997]. *Whaley and Wong's essentials of pediatric nursing* [5th ed.]. St. Louis: Mosby.)

enlargement is caused by extensive fibrosis and proliferation of adipose tissue, which when combined with the other pathologic changes in the muscle tissue actually causes muscle weakness. This phenomenon is referred to as *pseudohypertrophy of muscles* (Sarnat, 2004).

Involvement begins in the proximal musculature of the pelvic girdle, proceeds to the shoulder girdle, and finally affects all muscle groups. As leg and pelvic muscles weaken, the child often uses his or her arms to "crawl" up the thighs into a standing position from a kneeling position. This maneuver is known as *Gower's sign* and is diagnostically significant (Figure 6-12). Independent ambulation is one of the first functions to be lost, and dependence on a wheelchair is common by 9 years of age. Gradually the simplest ADLs become difficult and then impossible. In the advanced stages of the disease, lordosis and kyphosis are common, as are contractures at various joints. Death, usually as a result of infection, respiratory problems, or cardiovascular complications, often occurs before the early twenties (Dubowitz, 1999).

Currently no treatment is available that arrests or reverses the dystrophic process, but antibiotic therapy and other advances in dealing with pulmonary complications have helped extend life expectancy. Steroids can help, but their use remains controversial because of their side effects. Myoblast transfer has been used on a trial basis. Although gene therapy is still in the preclinical trial phase, it is a promising option for treatment of Duchenne's and Becker's muscular dystrophies. Two types of treatment are being explored: the use of

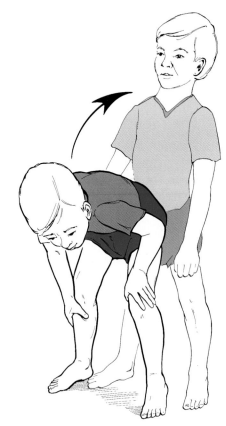

FIGURE 6-12 Child with Gower's sign.

adenovirus-mediated dystrophin gene transfer and upregulation of a natural dystrophin analog (Sarnat, 2004).

The goals of rehabilitation in patients with neuromuscular disease are to maximize and prolong independent function and locomotion, inhibit physical deformity, and provide access to full integration into society. A multidisciplinary team consisting of physicians, nurses, therapists, social and vocational counselors, and psychologists, among others, is ideal for managing the symptoms of these dystrophies. Stretching, ROM activities, timely surgical correction of spinal deformities and contractures, and bracing may improve or prolong ambulation and enhance functional use of the extremities. Moderate resistance (submaximal) weight lifting and aerobic exercise may improve strength and cardiovascular performance in slowly progressive neuromuscular diseases. For patients with advanced restrictive lung disease, positive pressure ventilation may improve breathing and comfort. Cardiac complications in some neuromuscular diseases can be severe and may require monitoring. Nutritional, psychologic, and vocational considerations should also be part of the management of neuromuscular disease. Major advances in biomedical and computer engineering continue to provide more functional equipment, enabling better strategies for improvement of quality of life (Hallum, 2001).

Congenital muscular dystrophies (CMDs) make up a heterogeneous group of muscle disorders with onset in utero or during the first year of life. Several forms of CMD show brain involvement in addition to the neuromuscular disorder (Voit, 1998). CMD is marked by hypotonia, generalized muscle weakness, and multiple contractures. Four categories have been identified: classic CMD I without severe impairment of intellectual functioning; CMD II, involving muscle and brain abnormalities; and the less severe types CMD III and IV, involving muscle, eye, and brain abnormalities (Sarnat, 2004). Associated problems include clubfoot, torticollis, diaphragmatic involvement, congenital heart and spinal defects. Often little or no progression of the disease is seen after childhood, and some functional improvement may be seen around this time (Dubowitz, 1999). The diagnosis is established by the presence of high serum levels of the muscle enzyme creatine kinase, by EMG analysis, and by examination of muscle tissue taken during biopsy (Sarnat). Clinical examination often reveals a "floppy" child with muscle weakness in the face, neck, trunk, and limbs; decreased muscle mass; and absent deep tendon reflexes (Dubowitz).

The use of orthopedic devices and adaptive equipment and activity can increase mobility, minimize contractures, delay spinal curvatures, and maximize independence in ADLs and thus in role functioning. Maintaining the child's independent mobility for as long as possible is a major goal. Children with CMDs appear to degenerate more rapidly once in a wheelchair. Because these children are generally aware of their situation, the therapist working with this child should also be prepared to work with the issues of death and dying. Genetic counseling for parents and female siblings and family support programs are also of value (Menkes, 2001).

All other disorders of muscles are usually called *myopathies.* Congenital myopathies are rare in infants; when they occur, they are usually caused by autosomal dominant patterns of inheritance but may also be caused by prolonged treatment with certain drugs, such as steroids. The symptoms are similar to those of the dystrophies, with proximal muscle weakness of the face, neck, and limbs. Congenital dislocation of the hip, scoliosis, seizures, and reduced cognitive skills may also be present. The diagnosis is made by muscle biopsy. Unlike the dystrophies, congenital myopathies progress slowly or not at all, which improves the prognosis (Menkes, 2001).

Neural Tube Defects and Spina Bifida

Neural tube defects (NTDs) are malformations that occur early in uterine development of the CNS. The three major forms of neural tube deficits are encephalocele, anencephaly, and spina bifida. *Encephalocele* is a result of brain protrusion in the occipital region of the brain. The overall incidence is approximately 2 per 1,000 births. These children typically have severe deficits, including MR, hydrocephalus, motor impairments, and seizures (Liptak, 2002). *Anencephaly* indicates a lack of neural development above the level of the brain stem; these children do not survive infancy. Females are three to seven times more likely to be affected than their male counterparts (Menkes, 2001).

Spina bifida is the term most commonly used to describe a congenital defect of the vertebral arches and spinal column. This defect may be mild, with the laminae of only one or two vertebrae affected and no malformation of the spinal cord, or it may involve an extensive spinal opening with an exposed pouch made up of cerebrospinal fluid (CSF) and the meninges *(meningocele)* or CSF, meninges, and nerve roots *(myelomeningocele).* Myelomeningocele is also called *spina bifida cystica,* as opposed to *spina bifida occulta,* in which no pouch is evident (Menkes, 2001; Morrissy & Weinstein, 2001) (Figure 6-13). This deficit appears to occur in the fourth week of prenatal development and can be identified by amniocentesis. The prevalence of neural tube deficits is falling primarily due to the ability to conduct prenatal screenings for NTD, the improvement in nutritional status, principally that of folic acid. Because the incidence of NTDs varies so widely it is assumed that both genetic and environmental factors play a part in vulnerability (Liptak, 2002). Recently the research suggests that a combination of heredity and a folic acid deficiency may

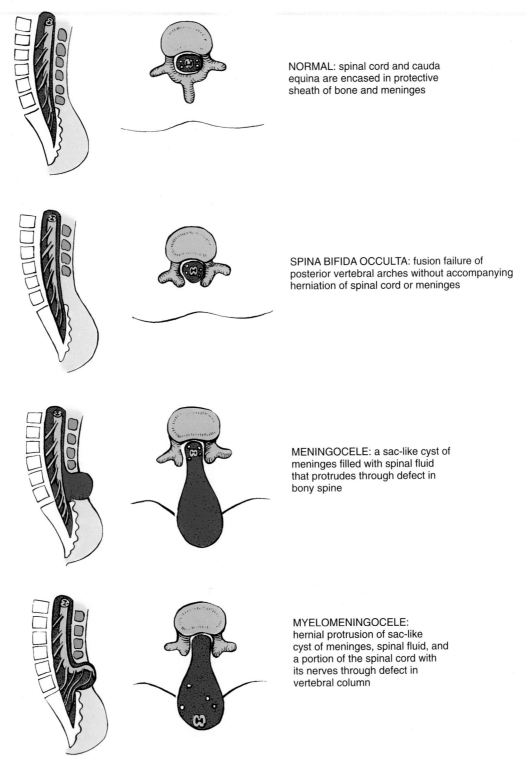

NORMAL: spinal cord and cauda equina are encased in protective sheath of bone and meninges

SPINA BIFIDA OCCULTA: fusion failure of posterior vertebral arches without accompanying herniation of spinal cord or meninges

MENINGOCELE: a sac-like cyst of meninges filled with spinal fluid that protrudes through defect in bony spine

MYELOMENINGOCELE: hernial protrusion of sac-like cyst of meninges, spinal fluid, and a portion of the spinal cord with its nerves through defect in vertebral column

FIGURE 6-13 Three forms of spina bifida. (From Wong, D.L. [1997]. *Whaley and Wong's essentials of pediatric nursing* [5th ed.]. St. Louis: Mosby.)

account for up to 50% of cases (Liptak, 2002). Studies have indicated that supplemental daily doses of folic acid can reduce the risk of NTDs by more than 50%. Even more convincing evidence for the role of folic acid is the ability of women to reduce their risk by 70% by taking the supplement when they are susceptible for recurrence

of an NTD. The incidence of spina bifida cystica is believed to be 0.2 to 4.2 per 1,000 live births. The CDC (2002) reported an annual rate of 900 babies born with spina bifida or meningocele in the United States.

The degree of impairment in NTDs depends on the level and degree of spinal cord involvement. This continuum of impairment can include no functional impairment, mild muscle imbalances and sensory losses, paraplegia, or even death in severe cases.

Many times in spina bifida occulta no external manifestations are visible, or the skin overlying the defect may be dimpled, pigmented, or covered with hair. Internally the spinal cord may be divided by a bony spur or congenital neoplasm, or there may be a slight bony malformation of one or more vertebrae (Liptak, 2002). Occasionally this area is slightly unstable, and some degree of neuromuscular impairment may occur, including mild gait deficits and bowel or bladder problems.

Spina bifida cystica is more serious and complex. A sac, or meningocele, visible above the bony defect characterizes spina bifida cystica. This sac is covered with skin and subcutaneous tissue and contains CSF, and although the meninges extend into the sac, the spinal cord remains confined to the spinal canal. In the neonatal period, great care must be taken not to rupture the sac and to prevent infection. Surgical skin closure is usually performed soon after birth to protect the cyst. In some cases part or all of the sac is removed (Menkes, 2001).

Spina bifida with myelomeningocele is the most severe form of spina bifida. In this form the sac may be covered with only a thin layer of skin, or the meninges and the spinal cord or nerve roots may protrude into the meningocele. Children with myelomeningocele usually display sensory and motor disturbances below the level of the lesion. Most lesions are in the thoracic or lumbar spine, resulting in lower extremity paralysis. Sensory dysfunction is variable. Some children also demonstrate hip, spinal, or foot deformities. Orthotic interventions include lightweight bracing, casting, orthopedic shoes, and assistive devices for ambulation. Bowel and bladder incontinence is often a problem. Family education in skin care, urology, and diet enhances the child's independence. Medication, bowel training, and intermittent catheterization may assist significantly in this area (Liptak, 2002).

Complications with these forms of spina bifida include meningitis and hydrocephalus. Infection is easily contracted because of environmental exposure of the meninges and spinal cord. Hydrocephalus is a common secondary complication that may be caused either by a developmental defect in the brain (e.g., aqueduct stenosis) or by slippage of the lower portion of the brain (and part of the cerebellum) through the foramen magnum, a condition known as *Arnold-Chiari syndrome* (Liptak, 2002; Menkes, 2001).

Hydrocephalus

Hydrocephalus is the result of a buildup of CSF in the ventricles of the brain. This occurs when an imbalance exists in the amount of CSF produced and the amount absorbed. Non-communicating ventricles that obstruct the outflow of CSF from the ventricles, an *Arnold-Chiari malformation,* or occasionally a tumor may produce this phenomenon.

In infants an early sign of the condition is enlarged head size. In an older child, whose head cannot grow, intracranial pressure increases. Definitive diagnosis may be made by sonography, computed tomography (CT), or magnetic resonance imaging (MRI) scans (Weinstein, 2002).

Clinical signs of hydrocephalus in infants include abnormal head growth with bulging fontanels, dilated scalp veins, and separated sutures; eyes that appear to deviate downward, producing a "sunset" appearance of the iris and visible sclera; and, after time, lethargy, irritability, and problems with reflexes, feeding, and tone. In older children, headache, irritability, development of strabismus or nystagmus, and cognitive changes may occur (Johnson, 2001).

The pressure produced by the hydrocephalus can result in visual and perceptual deficits, MR, and seizures and in extreme cases, death. Children with hydrocephalus may demonstrate sensory processing and perceptual problems. Often they exhibit fine motor delays in association with visual-perceptual impairment or dyspraxia. With problems in sensory, neuromotor, and perceptual performance areas, therapists often emphasize self-care, instrumental ADLs, and functional mobility skills (Schneider & Krosschell, 2001). If the hydrocephalus is caused by an obstruction, removal of the obstruction may alleviate the condition. The usual medical treatment for idiopathic hydrocephalus is placement of a ventriculoperitoneal (VP) shunt. This procedure (Figure 6-14) reduces the CSF pressure by means of a catheter that runs under the skin from one of the ventricles to the abdominal cavity, where the fluid can be safely absorbed. These shunts are usually effective but must be monitored regularly for signs of infection, clogging, kinking, or migration of the tube. Even with shunting, however, many of these children have cognitive, perceptual, visual, or other functional problems (Johnson, 2001).

Peripheral Nerve Injuries
Birth Injuries

Infants and children occasionally suffer traumatic injuries, perinatally and postnatally, that temporarily or permanently cause peripheral nerve impairment. For example, breech deliveries with after-coming arms can cause *brachial plexus lesions*. These infants may demonstrate weakness or wasting of the small muscles of the hands and sensory diminution in the area of the hand and arm served by this plexus (Wong & Hockenberry-Eaton, 2001). This condition, called *Erb-Duchenne palsy*, is typically unilateral and related to the upper brachial plexus only. It is usually a result of stretching of the

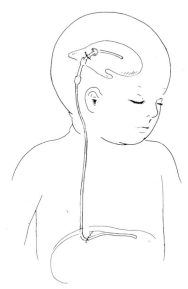

FIGURE 6-14 Ventriculoperitoneal shunt. Catheter is threaded subcutaneously from small incisions at the sites of ventricular and peritoneal insertions. (From Wong, D.L. [1997]. *Whaley and Wong's essentials of pediatric nursing* [5th ed., p. 1027]. St. Louis: Mosby.)

shoulder in extreme shoulder flexion (with the hand over the head). The condition is a common problem, and the incidence is 0.6 to 4.6 per 1,000 live births. Paralysis of the arm results and is often more pronounced in the shoulder musculature than in the hand. The child often holds his or her arm in a characteristic posture, with the shoulder adducted and internally rotated, elbow extended, forearm pronated, and wrist flexed. The prognosis depends on the extent of the damage to the nerves but can be good with early intervention. In *Klumpke's palsy,* or lower brachial plexus paralysis, the stretching injury generally is more severe. Klumpke's palsy results in paralysis of the hand and wrist muscles. A severe brachial palsy injury results in paralysis of the entire arm.

Partial immobilization and appropriate positioning to prevent contractures are required. Occupational therapy often involves fabrication of a sling that fits proximally around the humerus and passive and active assistive exercises. Later in infancy, resistive exercises may be recommended for development of optimal strength in the affected arm. If paralysis persists without improvement between 3 and 6 months of age, neuroplasty, neurolysis, end-to-end anastomosis, and nerve grafting are likely to be recommended (Stoll & Kliegman, 2004b; Trumble, 2000).

Traumatic Injury of Peripheral Nerves

In older children, injury to a peripheral nerve is usually caused by an accident, either through severing of the nerve or secondary to fractures, dislocations, excessive exercise, or occasionally medical treatments such as injections. Injuries of this type commonly occur to the radial, ulnar, and median nerves and the brachial plexus, lumbar plexus, peroneal nerves, or sciatic nerves (Trumble, 2000).

The diagnosis is made using a combination of techniques, such as family and medical histories, nerve conduction studies, observations of sensory and motor involvement, muscle biopsies, EMGs and, with serious accidents, surgical exploration.

Nerve injuries are categorized as class I, class II, or class III. A class III injury, the severest type, is a *neurotmesis,* which means the axon and endoneurium have been severed. A class II injury is referred to as an *axonotmesis,* meaning that the endoneurium is intact but the axon degenerates distal to the lesion. A class I injury is a *neurapraxia,* in which there is some degree of paralysis but no peripheral degeneration. Depending on the severity of the injury, impairments range from diminished strength, absence of deep tendon reflexes (DTRs), and impairment of sensation with spontaneous recovery to complete disruption of connective tissues, in which regeneration of the damaged nerves may not occur without surgical intervention.

Specific treatment depends on the extent, progression, location, and especially the cause of the nerve damage. In general, treatment includes rest, splinting, nerve and local anesthetic injections (medication injected into the injured nerve), and surgical intervention to relieve nerve compression or to repair the damaged nerve (Trumble, 2000).

TRAUMATIC BRAIN INJURIES

Traumatic brain injuries (TBIs) or *head injuries (HIs)* during childhood constitute a major medical and public health problem. Approximately 4,000 children die each year of head injuries in the United States. Approximately 1 in 500 children is seriously injured and must endure prolonged hospitalizations and lifelong complications to some degree (Adelson & Kochanek, 1998). Trauma is the leading cause of both morbidity and mortality in the pediatric population, and traumatic injury causes 50% of all childhood deaths (Michaud, Semel-Concepcion, Duhaime, & Lazar, 2002). Significant mortality rates have been reported for children with traumatic brain injury. Although children have better survival rates than adults with traumatic brain injury, the long-term sequelae and consequences are often more devastating in children because of their age and developmental potential (Mazzola & Adelson, 2002). The costs involved in the care of a child with severe traumatic brain injury, extended over the individual's lifetime, are significant.

Medical practitioners also have begun to recognize the importance of diagnosing minor head injuries, which may result in more subtle but persistent cognitive and functional impairments (American Academy of Pediatrics, 1999; CDC, 2002). According to the CDC, the most common causes of head injuries in young children, in order of frequency, are falls, motor vehicle accidents, assault or child abuse, and sports and recreation injuries (CDC). In older children, most head injuries are caused, in order of frequency, by motor vehicle accidents, sports-related injuries, and falls. As children reach adolescence, motor vehicle accidents remain the major cause of TBIs, followed by assault (primarily abuse and gunshot wounds), sports and recreation injuries, and falls.

Head traumas are classified by the nature of the force that causes the injury and the severity of the injury. Forces that cause head trauma are referred to as either *impact* or *inertial forces*. Impact forces result from the head striking a surface or a moving object striking the head; these forces most often cause skull fractures, focal brain lesions, and epidural hematomas. Inertial forces are typically the result of rapid acceleration and deceleration of the brain inside the skull, resulting in a shearing or tearing of brain tissue and nerve fibers. Most TBIs are the result of both types of forces. The severity of HIs is rated as a range, from relatively mild concussion to more serious injury (Michaud et al., 2002). Damage to nervous system tissue occurs both at the time of impact or penetration and through secondary damage caused by brain swelling, intracranial pressure, hematomas, emboli, and hypoxic brain conditions. Early medical intervention can prevent or at least minimize these secondary causes of nervous system damage (Adelson & Kochanek, 1998).

Loss of consciousness is a prime indicator of a significant head injury. TBI also is implicated if the child does not lose consciousness or loses it only momentarily at the time of injury but later develops symptoms of lethargy, confusion, severe headache, irritability, vomiting, or speech or motor impairment. If consciousness is lost longer than momentarily, immediate medical attention is indicated (Michaud et al., 2002).

Once the child's medical condition has been stabilized, the severity of brain injury is determined. An assessment tool often used for this purpose is the Glasgow Coma Scale (GCS) (Brain Trauma Foundation, 2000). The GCS rates several parameters, including eye opening (4 [spontaneous] to 1 [no response]), best motor response (6 [obeys] to 1 [no response]), and verbal response (5 [oriented] to 1 [no response]). The score range, therefore, is 3 to 15, and a score of 8 or lower is considered an indicator of severe TBI. Initial diagnostic procedures typically include MRI or CT scanning, EEG, angiography, and radiography to determine the extent and location of fractures (Michaud et al., 2002). Medical treatment for moderate and severe TBIs includes close monitoring and control of cerebral circulation and intracranial pressure through the use of sophisticated devices and control systems. If the intracranial pressure cannot be controlled by traditional means,

a large dose of barbiturate (e.g., phenobarbital) may be administered. If this fails to control the pressure, lowering the body temperature may help. Withdrawal from the barbiturate and body temperature treatments is difficult and may cause sleep disturbances, behavioral problems, apnea, and diminished intellectual functioning (Mazzola & Adelson, 2002).

Fortunately, most children who sustain a head injury have only a minor TBI (score of 13 to 15 on the GCS). Children with residual minor head injury deficits may require educational support, environmental modifications, and psychologic support. In most cases the prognosis for these children is very good (American Academy of Pediatrics, 1999).

Children who have sustained moderate or severe brain injuries typically follow a behavioral pattern of gradual and full return to consciousness. Depending on the severity of damage, the individual initially does not respond to any external stimuli or responds in a stereotypic manner. Only a small number of children remain in comas. At the first stage of recovery, children exhibit eye opening to external stimuli and generalized responses to noxious stimuli. The next stage of recovery can be the most difficult for family members because the individual is often agitated and combative; however, the child is rarely aware of his or her actions. As the agitation resolves, the child demonstrates increasingly appropriate responses to commands, ability to attend and concentrate, and recognition of family members. As the child progresses, intervention becomes more functional and goal oriented (Michaud et al., 2002).

An unfortunate perception of many health professionals is that children have better outcomes from severe TBI than adults; however, this belief is not substantiated by fact. The mortality rate for children with severe TBI (36% with a GCS score over 8) is similar to that for adults and, as do adults, these children make a guarded recovery (Adelson & Kochanek, 1998). Persistent deficits can vary widely; individuals who sustain moderate brain damage generally have fewer residual deficits. Performance skills deficits may include impairments in motor skills, process skills, and communication/interaction skills. Specific client factors likely to be involved are mental functions, sensory functions, and neuromusculoskeletal and movement-related functions. Typically, academic achievement is hindered, and the child requires modifications to the educational setting, including assistive technology and related services (American Academy of Pediatrics, 1999; Cassidy, Potoka, Adelson, & Ford, 2003; Haydel, 2003; Keenan et al., 2003; Teasdale & Engberg, 2003).

DEVELOPMENTAL DISABILITIES

This section addresses disorders found in childhood that are not specifically associated with one body system and that delay the child's developmental progress. In general, developmental disabilities are characterized by prenatal, perinatal, or early childhood onset. Some of the factors that negatively affect developmental outcomes are maternal in origin, and others are caused by infant complications. Chapter 20 discusses medical factors during and immediately after birth that place the infant at risk for long-term disability. Each of the developmental disabilities described in this section has the potential to affect several areas of the child's development and to impair the child's performance and roles.

Mental Retardation

Mental retardation is the most common developmental disability, affecting 0.8% to 3% of the population, depending on the definition used (Batshaw & Shapiro, 2002). Definitions of MR have three key factors: significantly impaired intellectual ability, usually measured on standardized psychoeducational tests; onset before 18 years of age; and impairment of the adaptive abilities necessary for independent living (i.e., communication, ADLs, instrumental activities of daily living, work, play/leisure, education, and social participation).

Formal testing and the history are used to make a diagnosis of MR. Testing usually includes intelligence quotient (IQ) testing and tests of adaptive behavior (basic reasoning, environmental knowledge, and developmentally appropriate daily living and self-maintenance skills). Although the use of IQ scores is controversial, significantly below-average scores remain a good predictor of future cognitive functioning. Fortunately, intelligence is composed of a wider range of skills than is demonstrated on IQ tests. In addition, as in typically developing children, the developmental outcomes of children with MR are significantly influenced by socioeconomic conditions, environmental events, having at least one parent who is highly committed to the child, and the individual's unique resilience (Horowitz & Haritos,

1998). A child is usually considered to have MR if he or she scores more than two standard deviations below the normative range for age. In the fourth edition of the *Diagnostic and Statistical Manual of Mental Disorders* (DSM-IV-TR), MR is classified into four levels: mild, moderate, severe, and profound (American Psychiatric Association [APA], 2000). Although this classification has changed over the years and is somewhat artificial (i.e., it does not always directly equate with function), it is commonly used to describe children with MR (Figure 6-15).

Intensive debate persists in the literature regarding the rate of development in individuals with MR and the ultimate potential of these individuals. These issues have significant implications for the identification and education of individuals with MR and their integration into society. The modes and strategies by which individuals with MR learn and the ways they differ in development are critical issues that must be resolved in order to facilitate education and the most appropriate therapeutic intervention (Burack, Hodapp, & Zigler, 1998). Children with mild MR have an IQ range of approximately 55 to 70. Characteristics include the ability to learn academic skills at the third to seventh grade level and the usual achievement of social and vocational skills adequate for living in the community with intermittent support. The employment rate for adults with mild MR is 80%, and 80% are married (Batshaw & Shapiro, 2002).

Children with moderate MR have an IQ range of approximately 40 to 55. These individuals require support to function in society. They are unlikely to progress past the second grade level in academics, but they can usually handle routine daily functions and do unskilled or semiskilled work in sheltered workshop conditions. A group home or supervised housing situation is usually the placement that families choose for these individuals as adults.

Children with severe MR have an IQ range of approximately 25 to 40. These individuals can usually learn to

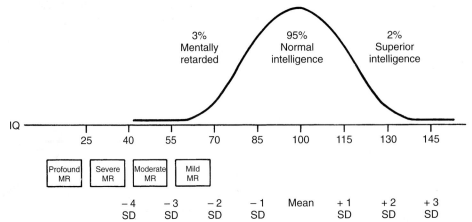

FIGURE 6-15 Criteria for determining the four degrees of severity in mental retardation (MR).

communicate, and they can be trained in basic health habits; however, they require extensive support and supervision to accomplish most tasks.

Children with profound MR have IQs below 25. These children need caregiver assistance for basic survival skills, and they usually have minimal capacity for sensorimotor or self-care functioning. Individuals with profound MR also often have interrelated neuromuscular, orthopedic, or behavioral deficits.

MR is a functional deficit that describes several disabilities. It can occur secondary to another condition or without apparent cause (Batshaw & Shapiro, 2002). These causes are usually categorized as (1) problems acquired in childhood (e.g., through toxins, trauma, or infection); (2) problems of fetal development and birth; (3) chromosomal problems; (4) CNS malformations; (5) congenital anomalies; and (6) neurocutaneous, metabolic, and endocrine disorders.

Approximately 80% of children with MR have additional problems. For example, it is estimated that approximately 50% have speech problems, 50% have ambulation problems, 20% have seizures, 25% have visual problems, and 40% have chronic conditions such as heart disease, diabetes, anemia, obesity, and dental problems (Burack et al., 1998).

Parents, physicians, and allied health professionals involved in well baby care and screening often express concerns about children with MR. Early signs of cognitive impairment include delays in meeting motor and speech milestones, unresponsiveness to handling and physical contact, reduced alertness or spontaneous play, feeding difficulties, and neurologic soft signs (e.g., balance, motor symmetry, perceptual motor skills, and fine motor skills). A formal diagnosis of MR generally is made when the child reaches school age because intellectual testing in preschool is limited by test sensitivity. Referrals for psychologic, educational, developmental, and speech and hearing evaluation may be made and then interpreted for the parents. Services must be determined, and parents, siblings, and other family members must be given support and advice (Batshaw & Shapiro, 2002; Hogan, Rogers, & Msall, 2000).

Today, health care professionals, educators, and the general public practice a philosophy of inclusion of individuals with MR. Beginning with early intervention, services and programs provide opportunities that enable these individuals to reach their maximal level of functioning in the least restrictive environment (Hogan et al., 2000).

Early programs for children with MR or delays usually focus on facilitating the attainment of developmental milestones; enriching the environment; developing self-help, language, and motor skills; and educating and supporting the parents. As the child grows, specific deficits may be addressed in special education programs. For the adolescent with MR, the development of vocational interests and skills, social skills and sex education, and community mobility skills are essential (Burack et al., 1998).

Autism and Pervasive Developmental Disorders

Pervasive developmental disorders (PDDs) constitute a broad class of conditions that reflect a range of deficits, of which autism is the most well-documented form. *Autism* is characterized by severe and complex impairments in reciprocal social interaction and communication skills and by the presence of stereotyped behavior, interests, and activities (APA, 2000). The onset typically occurs before 3 years of age, and the deficits persist throughout life. The most current prevalence rates indicate that PDDs are seen at an aggregate rate of 16.8 per 10,000 persons (Chakrabarti & Fombonne, 2001). Some surveys have suggested that the rate for all forms of PDD is about 3 per 1,000 people, but more recent surveys suggest that the estimate might be as high as 6 per 1,000 (Fombonne, 2003). These rates are almost twice as high as early epidemiologic reports of autism and may partly be the result of an increase in recognition and of the clarification of diagnostic criteria as opposed to a true increase in prevalence rates as suggested by popular news reports (Fombonne). The CDC (2002) estimates that approximately four times as many boys as girls have autism. Children with PDDs are found in families of all racial, ethnic, intellectual, and socioeconomic backgrounds. Besides autism, PDDs include atypical autism, Rett syndrome, other childhood disintegrative disorders, Asperger's syndrome, and pervasive developmental disorder–unspecified (APA, 2000).

The unusual combinations of sensory, communication, and behavioral characteristics seen with PDDs have significant negative effects on a child's ability to participate in home, school, and community activities. Particularly associated with autism are severe limitations in relating to others and the display of ritualistic, stereotypic behaviors. Since Kanner's original description of 11 children who had "extreme autistic aloneness," many theories on the cause of autism have been proposed (Kanner, 1943).

Neuroimaging studies have suggested that differences in cell density (i.e., brains are heavier) and reduced neuron size in areas critical to the trilogy of social-behavioral-communication disorders may be responsible for the impairments seen in PDDs (Rodier, 2000). Currently, autism is considered a biologic disorder of neurologic development. In typical development, connections in the brain are shaped by experience and learning; with PDDs, synaptic and dendritic growth occur without guidance in areas related to communication and interaction skills, therefore the correct migration and synaptic connections are not made (Chakrabarti & Fombonne, 2001).

Some theories hold that abnormal action of the genes that control myelination and the creation of synapses and dendritic connections may be responsible for incorrect selective molding and elimination of synaptic connections (Bespalova & Buxbaum, 2003; Burack et al., 1998; Kinnear, 2003). The areas primarily affected include the amygdala, cerebellum, right somatosensory cortex, and orbitofrontal cortex, as well as the cingulated gyri. Initial pathologic anomalies seem to occur at higher level cognitive processing pathways and involve the cerebral cortex as well (Towbin, Mauk, & Batshaw, 2002).

Neurochemical alterations also play a major role in autism. Studies consistently show elevated serotonin levels, and hypothalamic-pituitary-adrenal axis (HPA) dysfunctions and abnormalities in neuroendocrine functioning have been reported (Bauman, 1996; Rodier, 2000; Tsai, 1999). Although popular claims about the origins of autism abound, no evidence indicates that the disorder is correlated with diet or vaccinations (e.g., mumps, measles, and rubella vaccine) or that these affect the development or prevention of autistic disorders (Miller, 2003).

Autism often co-exists with neuropsychiatric disorders, including seizures, attention deficit hyperactivity disorder, affective disorders, anxiety disorders, obsessive-compulsive disorders and Tourette's syndrome (Mahoney et al., 1998).

The behavioral characteristics of autism are critical to the diagnosis of the disorder. These characteristics can be categorized into the following four subclusters of disturbances (APA, 2000):

1 Disturbances in social interactions
2 Disturbances in communication
3 Disturbances in behaviors
4 Disturbances of sensory and perceptual processing and associated impairments

Disturbances in social interactions affect the child's ability to establish meaningful relationships with people and inanimate objects. Although abnormalities in this area vary with age and in severity, they directly involve interactions that require initiative or reciprocal behavior from the child. Specific behaviors observed are poor or deviant eye contact, failure to develop peer relationships, delayed or inappropriate facial expression, apparent aversion to physical contact, lack of social reciprocity, delayed or absent anticipatory response to being picked up, and lack of spontaneous seeking of another to share enjoyment, an apparent preference for being alone.

Disturbances in communication may be thought of as a continuum from mild to severe. At the mild end of the continuum, normal language accompanied only by slight articulation or tonal deficits may be observed. At the severe end is a complete lack of speech (mute). Many other communication problems have been described at points along the continuum. For instance, much of the speech of children with autism is repetitive, or *echolalic,* in nature. Classic echolalia consists of parrot-like repetitions of phrases immediately after the child has been exposed to them; delayed or deferred echolalia consists of the repetition of phrases at a later time. Echolalic speech occurs out of social context and appears to have little or no communicative value. Other types of speech and language problems include syntax problems, atonal and arrhythmic speech, pronoun reversals, and lack of inflection and emotion during communication (Huebner, 1992).

Disturbances in behaviors are seen in the intolerance of deviation from routine, resistance to any type of change, and patterns of behaviors that are best categorized as stereotyped, perseverative, and lacking in representational or pretend play. In addition, bizarre attachments to unusual objects develop (e.g., intense interest in a vacuum cleaner or a sheet of paper versus stuffed animals or dolls). These patterns of behavior are obsessive rituals, from which any deviation is not tolerated (Towbin et al., 2002). Deviations from the routine, however slight, elicit intense temper tantrums.

Deviant motor patterns may involve the arms, hands, trunk, lower extremities, or entire body. Motor patterns in the upper extremities are common and include wiggling and flicking of the fingers, alternating flexion and extension of the fingers, and alternating pronation and supination of the forearm. Other motility patterns often seen include head rolling and banging, body rocking and swaying, lunging and darting movements, toe walking, dystonia of the extremities, involuntary synergies of the head and proximal segments of the limbs, and inability to perform two motor acts at the same time (Baird, Cass, & Slonims, 2003).

For almost 40 years, *disturbances of sensory and perceptual processing* have been reported in children with autism. These include abnormal responses to various visual, vestibular, and auditory stimuli. A. Jean Ayres describes two types of sensory processing problems in children with autistic behaviors. One type deals with the registration of or orientation to sensory input. It appears that in these children, the neurophysiologic processes that decide that sensory stimuli will be brought to the child's attention are working correctly at some times but not at others (Ayres & Tickle, 1980). Therefore the child reacts normally to sensory stimuli one minute, and the next minute (hour or day) he or she may overreact or under-react to the same stimuli.

The other sensory processing disturbance described by Ayres involves the control or modulation of a stimulus once it has entered the system. Again, the child with autistic behavior is believed to be capable of exerting control at some times but not at others, resulting in a child who processes tactile information normally at times and who, at other times, appears to be extremely hypersensitive (Ayres & Tickle, 1980).

Associated impairments in autism include MR, seizure disorders, and discontinuities in developmental rates. The fact that a large percentage of children with autism also suffer from cognitive deficiencies has been a controversial but relatively accepted issue. The cognitive deficiencies exhibited by children with autism are as disabling as those in children with MR, with the same long-term consequences. The incidence of seizure disorders in children with autism is high, and both tonic-clonic and complex partial seizures have been reported in this population (Towbin et al., 2002).

Although most children with autism have normal life expectancies, the functional prognosis is diverse. Some individuals with autism or other types of PDD live and work independently in the community; some are fairly independent, needing only minimal support for ADLs, whereas others continue to depend on support from family and friends. In general, the prognosis for children in the autism spectrum is closely related to communication skills and intelligence. Higher functioning children may become high-functioning adults with deficits in social interactions. The prognosis for independent functioning through behavioral and sensory interventions is encouraging (Cohen & Volkmar, 1997; Grandin, 1996).

Comprehensive intervention, including parental counseling, behavioral treatment, special education in highly structured environments, sensory integrative therapy, social skills training, speech-language therapy, medications, and family support, constitutes the best management for children with autism and other types of PDD (Towbin et al., 2002; Tsai, 1999). Various types of therapies have been advocated, including auditory integration training, dietary interventions, discrete trial training, medications, music therapy, and vision therapy. Despite wide use of these programs and the claims of benefits derived from them, most of these approaches lack rigorous scientific support. In general, studies to date indicate that individuals with autism respond best to a highly structured, specialized educational program that includes elements of communication therapy, social skills training, and sensory integration therapy (Cohen & Volkmar, 1997). The medications used for these children include sedatives, stimulants, major and minor tranquilizers, antihistamines, antidepressants, and psychotropic medications. It is believed that these medications work best when used in conjunction with an interdisciplinary special education program (Tsai, 1999). However, significant progress has been made in the efficacy and safety of pharmacotherapeutic agents, primarily the use of serotonin reuptake inhibitors.

Rett syndrome is an X-linked, dominant progressive neurologic disorder (i.e., it occurs exclusively in girls). It is caused by mutations in the gene MeCP2, which is responsible for coding the methyl-CpG-binding protein2, a protein critical to early brain development. This disorder is extremely rare, having a pooled estimated incidence across studies of 0.2 per 10,000 births. The presence of the abnormal gene on the X chromosome of the male embryo results in miscarriage (Baird, et al., 2003; Fombonne, 2003.) The condition is diagnosed by genetic analysis, and although its early symptoms are indistinguishable from those of autism, its progressive nature makes it unlike the other PDDs.

Development appears normal in children with Rett syndrome until about 6 months of age; thereafter the child demonstrates rapid degeneration in head growth, loss of hand skills, and poorly coordinated gait or trunk movements. Difficulties with social interaction are similar to those seen with autism, but are transient in nature. Initially there is a loss of social engagement but then social skills re-emerge later in the disorder. Microcephaly, spasticity, and seizures occur, and the child develops autistic-like behaviors such as hand mouthing, flapping, or wringing. Functional hand use disappears, and waking hyperventilation is characteristic. Children with Rett syndrome can survive for some time but are usually nonambulatory and nonverbal by late childhood. This is an incurable condition, but carbamazepine may be helpful for reducing symptoms and improving alertness (Towbin et al., 2002).

Asperger's syndrome can be distinguished from autism by the fact that these children do not exhibit clinically significant delays in language skills. The essential features of Asperger's syndrome are severe and sustained impairments in social interaction and the development of restricted, repetitive patterns of behavior, interests, and activities. The interference with functional daily living skills must be significant (APA, 2000). Children with Asperger's syndrome show typical cognitive development and age-appropriate self-help skills or adaptive behavior aside from social interaction impairments (Klin & Volkmar, 1997). Although language skills are age appropriate, individuals with Asperger's syndrome display idiosyncrasies in verbal communication, characterized by highly circumstantial utterances, long-winded and tangential accounts of events, failure to convey a clear thought, and one-sidedness. Often an obsessive interest in letters and numbers absorbs most of the person's attention and energy. In addition, these individuals display a lack of nonverbal communication and of empathy; they tend to intellectualize feelings and show a poor understanding of others' affect (Klin & Volkmar, 1997).

Epidemiologic studies suggest an overall incidence of 8.4 per 10,000 births, and the syndrome is five times more prevalent in boys. Treatment currently consists of supportive and symptomatic intervention. These services include special education programs, assistance with generalizing adaptive functioning to a wider variety of settings, problem-solving strategies, social skills training, speech and language skills training, and vocational training (Klin & Volkmar, 1997).

Attention Deficit Hyperactivity Disorder

Regarded as the most common childhood neurobehavioral disorder, *attention deficit hyperactivity disorder* (ADHD) is a heterogeneous behavioral disorder of uncertain cause that always is evident in childhood but that typically persists through adolescence and, for some, into adulthood (Elia, Ambrosini, & Rapoport, 1999). Because of past and recurring difficulties with strict definitions of ADHD, accurate prevalence data are difficult to determine (Barkley, 2003). Using DSM-IV-TR criteria as a standard, prevalence estimates for ADHD vary between 3% and 5% of the school-age population, or approximately 2 million children (APA, 2000). The disorder occurs approximately three times more often in boys than in girls.

The prevalence of ADHD subtypes may differ according to the source of referral, with hospital-based clinics, pediatric neurologists, and child psychiatrists treating predominantly a combined subtype and primary care practitioners treating a higher number of the inattentive subtype. Data synthesized from the National Ambulatory Medical Care Survey (NAMCS) (1990 to 1995) have documented a 2.8% rise in physician office visits among clients 5 to 18 years of age that resulted in a diagnosis of ADHD, supporting the perception that this diagnosis has dramatically increased in the past decade (Robison, Sclar, Skaer, & Galin, 1999). This increase is thought to be the result of better-defined diagnostic criteria and increased sensitivity of physicians to the diagnostic criteria (Greenhill, 1998).

Children with ADHD exhibit inattention, hyperactivity, and impulsivity that cause impairment in ADLs prior to 7 years of age. Inattention is demonstrated by failure to attend to details, difficulty sustaining attention during play, inability to listen actively to instructions or conversation, difficulty organizing tasks, and avoidance of tasks that require sustained attention. This child is easily distracted and is often forgetful in daily activities. Examples of hyperactivity are frequent fidgeting, inability to sit when remaining seated is expected (e.g., in a classroom), difficulty playing quietly, excessive talking, and being "constantly on the go." Impulsivity can be seen in the inability to wait one's turn, frequent and incessant interruptions, and blurting out of answers before a question is asked. Other related features include low frustration tolerance, sleep disorders, bossiness, excessive and frequent demands for attention, mood lability, demoralization, dysphoria, peer rejection, and poor self-esteem (Damico, Damico, & Armstrong, 1999). Children with ADHD are also at high risk for injuries associated with increased risk-taking behavior and impulsivity (DiScala, Lescohier, Barthel, & Li, 1998).

The symptoms vary in degree of impairment, frequency of occurrence, and pervasiveness across settings. They must occur "often" (to distinguish single symptoms from typical behavior observed in 48% to 52% of children) and across multiple settings (e.g., school, play, home, day care). The symptoms must persist for at least 6 months to a degree that is maladaptive and that subsequently interferes with all occupational activities, including self-care, academic performance, and peer relationships. In the past this disorder has been termed minimal brain dysfunction, hyperactive child syndrome, hyperkinetic reaction of childhood, and attention-deficit disorder with hyperactivity. However, the clinical description for these terms and criteria is now considered sufficiently similar to permit generalizations about cause and treatment (Barkley, 1998).

Over the past few decades, researchers have sought to develop and test theories about the etiology of ADHD. One theory that persists in popular literature is that ADHD is related to food allergies or food additives and the amount of sugar in a child's diet. The National Institutes of Health (NIH) concluded that there is no evidence that diet is responsible for the onset of ADHD (Wolraich, Milich, Stumbo, & Schultz, 1985) and in only 5% of children with ADHD is a restricted diet efficacious in reducing symptoms associated with this disorder. The current theories, widely supported but still under investigation, include genetic factors, neurologic factors, and neurochemical imbalances.

In neural imaging studies, a significant decrease in brain activity in the frontal parietal lobes, which inhibit impulsiveness and control attention, has been demonstrated in adults with ADHD; however, the primary cause of this decreased activity is still unknown (Barkley, 1998; Zametkin & Liotta, 1998). Studies of the heritability of this disorder are perhaps the best support that researchers have for linking ADHD with a neurobiologic etiology (Ballard et al., 1997; Faraone & Biederman, 1998; Garland, 1998; Zametkin & Liotta). It is clear that ADHD runs in families, and this may be one mechanism underlying ADHD symptoms. Siblings of children diagnosed with ADHD are five to seven times more likely to be diagnosed with ADHD as are children from unaffected families (Stein, Efron, Schiff, & Glanzman, 2002).

Three genes are hypothesized to be related to the onset of ADHD. Although these genes do not account for the majority of ADHD symptoms, the specific alleles of these genes may impart an increased susceptibility to ADHD (Stein et al., 2002). Neurochemical research into potential causes has failed to identify a single neurotransmitter that is responsible for the clinical deficits in ADHD (Greenhill, 1998). However, medications that influence neurotransmitter functioning are effective in treating some aspects of ADHD, leading researchers to believe that a neurochemical cause remains a viable theory. The selective availability of dopamine and norepinephrine are both candidates for a significant role in this disorder (Garland, 1998).

Two theories have been proposed for the cognitive impairments seen in ADHD. Barkley (1997) suggests that the symptoms seen in ADHD are a result of response inhibition, which prevents accurate self-regulation to environmental stimuli. He suggests that the response inhibition stems from underfunctioning of the orbital frontal cortex and its subsequent connections to the limbic system. Mercugliano (1999) holds that executive functioning deficits may underlie the observed behaviors in ADHD.

Two primary medical intervention strategies include stimulant pharmacotherapy (e.g., amphetamines, methylphenidate) and behavioral interventions. Pharmacotherapy allows 9 out of 10 children to focus and to be more successful at school, home, and play (Garland, 1998). There is no evidence that prolonged use of stimulant drugs is addictive, promotes addictive behavior in adolescence, makes children "high" or jittery, or sedates the child (Barkley, 1998). The realistic side effects of these drugs are weight loss, loss of appetite, interrupted sleep patterns and, in some children, slowed growth. Pharmacologic treatment seems to improve overactivity, attention span, impulsivity and self-control, compliance, physical and oral aggression, social interactions with peers, and academic productivity and accuracy (Greenhill, 1998; Zametkin & Ernst, 1999). Rarely, however, are medications alone sufficient to allow a child to function in most settings (Elia et al., 1999; Ingram, Hechtman, & Morgenstern, 1999). Deficits that seem to persist are those in reading skills, social skills, learning, academic achievement, and antisocial behavior (Ingram et al.; Zametkin & Ernst). Consequently, one or more behavioral interventions are typically needed. The most frequently recommended therapies include cognitive-behavioral therapy, behavior modification, educational interventions, social skills training, and psychotherapy (Damico et al., 1999; Elia et al.; Gillberg, 2003; Nemethy, 1997; Zametkin & Ernst). Although the definitive efficacy of any one strategy has not yet been determined, it is clear that a consistency in responses in all of the child's settings, the environmental adaptations, and counseling to alleviate low self-esteem contribute to improvement in learning and attainment of social skills (Gillberg). Occupational therapists can provide a multitude of successful strategies to the classroom for children with ADHD, including environmental adaptations, social skills training, self-management techniques, and interventions to enhance sensory modulation.

Learning Disabilities

The term *learning disabilities* describes a group of problems that affect a child's ability to master school tasks, process information, and communicate effectively. These disabilities are often not associated with a specific neurologic insult and may be accompanied by MR (Shapiro, Church, & Lewis, 2002). Learning disabilities are often associated with a variety of other neurologic problems (e.g., ADHD). Specific learning disabilities include auditory processing, language disabilities, and perceptual impairments.

Most children with a learning disability have average or above-average intelligence and adequate sensory acuity (are not blind or deaf) and have been provided with appropriate learning opportunities. Despite all these positive features, a significant discrepancy exists between the child's academic potential and his or her educational performance. The term *learning disability (LD)* includes conditions such as perceptual disabilities, dyslexia, and developmental aphasia. It does not include learning problems that stem from primary sensory deficits, MR, socioeconomic conditions, or psychosocial impairments. The National Joint Committee on Learning Disabilities defines *learning disability* as a generic term that refers to a heterogeneous group of disorders manifested by significant difficulties in the acquisition and use of listening, speaking, reading, writing, reasoning, or mathematic abilities (Hammill, 1990).

Although different studies and agencies report varying incidence figures, the figure most often given is approximately 4% to 5% of the school population, or about 2 million children. As with autism, more boys than girls are affected in this instance at a ratio of 4 : 1. In this case, however, some suggest that the gender difference is related to the tendency of girls not to exhibit oppositional defiant behavior and girls therefore are infrequently diagnosed (Shapiro et al., 2002).

A child with LD may display any number of the behaviors in the following nine categories:

1 *Disorders of motor function:* These include disorders both of motor skills and of motor activity level. Motor skills dysfunction may range from clumsiness, to poor performance in gross or fine motor skills, to problems planning new tasks (dyspraxia), to equilibrium deficits, to sensorimotor problems in a number of areas. Occasionally tics, grimaces, and choreoathetoid movements in the hands may be observed. The child may be described as always being in motion (hyperactive) or as being slow and lethargic (hypoactive).

2 *Educational disorders:* Educational disorders can occur in one or more academic subjects. Related educational skills that are often limited or delayed are copying from the blackboard, printing and cursive writing, organizing time and materials, understanding written and oral directions, symbolic confusion (reversing letters), cutting, coloring, drawing, and keeping place on the page.

3 *Disorders of attention and concentration:* Examples of these disorders include short attention span and other attention deficits, restlessness, impulsivity, and motor and verbal perseveration.

4 *Disorders of thinking and memory:* These types of disorders are characterized by difficulty with abstract reasoning and concept formation and by poor short- and long-term memory capabilities.

5 *Problems with speech and communication:* In these cases the child may show difficulty shifting topics of conversation; difficulty with "small talk"; difficulty with the sequencing of words, sentences, or sounds; slurred words; and articulation problems.

6 *Auditory difficulties:* Auditory difficulties associated with LD often stem from auditory perceptual and auditory memory problems and not from acuity (hearing) problems. Children with these types of problems are often the ones who cannot remember the oral directions just given to them (auditory memory), cannot sound words out or blend sounds into words (phonemic synthesis), cannot block out background noise (speech-in-noise), and cannot remember the sequencing of sounds, words, or numbers (auditory sequencing). These types of problems often affect school performance and should be explored by an audiologist who is familiar with the specific instruments and programs available to assess and treat auditory perceptual (central auditory processing) problems. The high incidence of allergies and ear infections in children with LD puts them at risk for auditory perceptual problems.

7 *Sensory integrative and perceptual disorders:* Children with LD often have various sensory integrative and perceptual disorders. Many of these children have difficulty with laterality and directionality concepts and tasks that require visual perception skills (Hammill, 1990).

8 *Psychosocial problems:* These disorders may be manifested as temper tantrums or antisocial behavior, and the child's social competencies may be delayed compared with his or her chronologic age and mental age. Many of these children are sensitive and decidedly at risk for poor self-esteem and for self-concept problems because they have the intelligence to know when they are being teased and to know the frustration of being good at some things and not at others.

9 *Specific learning difficulties that accompany the learning disability:* This is most frequently a specific reading disability (Shapiro et al., 2002).

Most children with LD retain some degree of disability as adults; however, most are contributing members of society. As with all disorders, the prognosis is affected by the severity of the disability. Therefore individuals with limited impairment should not be limited in their life and career skills, but those with severe LD may need vocational planning, counseling, and adaptations to ensure as high a level of social, emotional, and vocational functioning as possible.

The therapist's role in an intervention program for the child with LD may change as the child develops, depending on the nature and extent of the child's specific disability. With young children, sensory integration, play, and basic socialization and self-help skills may be addressed through early intervention and parent education. As the child progresses into school, sensory integration intervention may continue, but additional programs to promote social play, perceptual motor integration, and writing skills are indicated. By early adolescence the focus of evaluation and intervention shifts to independent living skills, psychosocial skills, and the development of compensatory and adaptive techniques, as well as vocational skills, interests, and habits.

Tourette's Syndrome

Tourette's syndrome (TS) is a pervasive disorder that affects neurologic and behavioral function. This condition is believed to be an autosomal dominant trait linked to a gene on chromosome 18, but the transmission pattern is still uncertain (Menkes, 2001). Dopamine dysfunction may be a factor. The prevalence of the condition varies geographically, but it is rare in African American children and occurs more frequently in boys than in girls. The onset of the syndrome may occur as early as 2 years of age, but it usually is seen during childhood or early adolescence and is by definition present before age 18 years. Approximately 5 per 10,000 children are affected by TS. Symptoms of the condition may appear in middle childhood, worsen for about 10 years, and then lessen somewhat. However, they usually continue throughout the individual's life, although there may be periods of remission (Johnston, 2004b; Menkes, 2001).

Most characteristic of TS are involuntary vocal and motor tics. Tics are sudden, nonrhythmic, rapid, and recurrent. At some time the child with TS has both vocal and motor tics. The child may also display obsessive and compulsive behavior with significant dysfunction in social, academic, or occupational skills. Hyperactivity, distractibility, and impulsivity are also quite common. Usually tics begin with simple motor movements of the head, including eye movements, grimacing, and shoulder shrugging. Vocal tics may begin with throat clearing, grunting, barking, sneezing, and coughing. As the disease progresses, complex behavioral tics, compulsive echolalia, and cursing may occur. In severe cases, self-mutilation may occur at times. Specific tics tend to appear, recur frequently for a period, and then fade, to be replaced by others (APA, 2000).

Tics may be suppressed voluntarily at some times, leading to problems in diagnosis and behavioral management; complex tics may be misinterpreted as emotional or behavioral disorders. Children who suppress tics may experience an "explosion" of tics in the later part of the day that may be accompanied by behavioral disturbances. Stress, anxiety, and anticipation of pleasant events can increase the frequency and intensity of tics and behaviors. Many of these children may also demonstrate ADHD, obsessive-compulsive disorders, or LD. These factors combine to impair social, school, and work functions.

Treatment includes clonidine and neuroleptic medication, such as haloperidol. However, these drugs have significant side effects that also may cause functional deficits. Children with obsessive-compulsive symptoms may also be treated with antidepressants. School- and play-based interventions may be necessary to address problems in writing, attention, and perceptual skills. Children may benefit from social skills and stress reduction programs, as well as understanding from and empathetic interactions with adults and peers. Additional time for testing may assist school performance (Johnston, 2004b).

Genetic and Chromosomal Abnormalities

Human beings normally have 23 pairs of chromosomes in each cell of the body, and each chromosome contains 250 to 2,000 genes. Smaller or larger numbers of chromosomes can cause significant developmental disabilities. These syndromes may present characteristic symptom patterns and can often be identified by chromosomal analysis of the child's body tissues. Genetic disorders range from addition or loss of an entire chromosome in each cell, to loss of part of a chromosome, to microdeletion of a number of contiguous genes within a chromosome. As a general rule, the larger the defect, the more severe the ensuing disorder (Batshaw, 2002). Analysis of the amniotic fluid may identify these children before they are born (Wong & Hockenberry-Eaton, 2001).

During cell division, chromosomes pass their identical genetic information to daughter cells. The two types of cell division are mitosis and meiosis. *Mitosis* creates two daughter cells from one parent cell. In *meiosis,* four daughter cells are created from one parent cell, with only 23 chromosomes passed on. Mitosis occurs in all cells, meiosis only in germ cells (i.e., it creates sperm and eggs). A number of events can occur during cell division that will adversely affect development.

One such event, *nondisjunction of autosomes* (i.e., unequal division of chromosomes during cell division) yields an excess or loss of chromosomal material. The most common condition is evidenced in the trisomy syndromes. The most common trisomy syndrome is *trisomy 21,* or *Down syndrome,* which is characterized by one additional chromosome 21. The egg that is fertilized has 23 chromosomes, and the resulting embryo has three copies of chromosome 21. This syndrome, found in approximately 1 in 660 newborns, causes specific mental and physical problems. Although a range of physical characteristics may be associated with Down syndrome, a few are common to most children, such as a short, stocky stature and a protruding abdomen. The head is often small and flattened at the back, and the eyes have an upward slant and abnormal epicanthal folds. Other common facial features include low-set ears, a flat nose, and often a mouth held slightly open with the tip of the tongue protruding. The extremities are shorter than normal, and the fingers and toes are usually broad and short. The palms of the hands typically have a single crease, known as the *simian crease* (Roizen, 2002).

Related health problems often include cardiovascular abnormalities, obesity, a higher incidence of respiratory infections and other infections caused by immune system inefficiency, thyroid deficiencies, gastrointestinal problems, and an apparent increase in the risk of leukemia (Roizen, 2002). Often visual acuity is poor and requires correction. One problem that is potentially dangerous to the child is atlantoaxial dislocation, which results in a tendency for dislocation between the first and second cervical vertebrae. A severe dislocation can result in spinal cord damage. If this dislocation is found through radiographic films, surgery may be performed, and the family may be given precautions about roughhouse play or participation in activities that put stress on this joint.

The life expectancy for children with Down syndrome has improved greatly over the past several years. Those without cardiac anomalies can be expected to live into late adulthood. However, it is common for these older individuals to develop a syndrome similar to Alzheimer's disease (Roizen, 2002).

Children with Down syndrome are usually recognized at birth by their facial characteristics. They frequently also have low muscle tone, hypermobile joints, and problems with sucking. A medical examination is performed to detect any related congenital cardiac and medical problems, which could extend the child's hospital stay. As the child grows, developmental delays in all areas of function are noted, although the degree can vary greatly from case to case. Motor planning skills, language, and cognitive skills develop slowly. Early intervention and special education, as well as support and education of the parents, help these children achieve their optimal function.

Other trisomies occur, but most of these are uncommon, and many of them result in abortion of the fetus or stillbirth. *Trisomy 18,* or *Edwards' syndrome,* occurs in approximately 1 in 3,000 births (Batshaw, 2002;

Menkes, 2001). These children have long, narrow skulls; low-set, malformed ears; a prominent occiput; small mouths and a weak cry; syndactyly and webbed neck; congenital heart and kidney malformations; severe MR; failure to thrive; and early death (Menkes, 2001). The survival rate beyond infancy is only about 10%.

Trisomy 13, or *Patau's syndrome,* occurs in 1 in 5,000 births (Menkes, 2001). Children with Patau's syndrome have multiple anomalies, including eye, ear, and nasal anomalies; cleft lip and palate; polydactyly and syndactyly; and microcephaly and neural tube defects. About 20% of these children survive, and most of these are severely retarded and have seizure disorders.

A decrease in the number of chromosomes (45 or less) also causes problems. Many fetuses with this genetic abnormality die early in gestation. One exception to this statement is children born with *Turner's syndrome,* which is found in approximately 1 in 5,000 girls and is caused by one missing sex chromosome. These babies may be born with webbing of the neck or congenital edema of the extremities and may have cardiac problems. Small stature, obesity, and underdeveloped ovaries, resulting in infertility and absence of secondary sexual characteristics, are symptoms that must be dealt with in the school-age child and adolescent with Turner's syndrome. Although visual perception problems are common, most of these children do not have MR, therefore their functional prognosis is good (Batshaw, 2002).

Other chromosomal abnormalities are caused by a missing portion of an individual chromosome (deletion) or by a portion of a chromosome breaking off and reattaching to another chromosome (translocation). The incidence of these events is lower than the chromosomal problems described, and because the amount of chromosomal material that is missing or duplicated varies, the resulting conditions are expressed differently. Problems common in these types of conditions are MR, abnormal brain development, and facial abnormalities.

Cri du chat syndrome is rare (1 in 50,000 live births) and is caused by deletion of part of chromosome 5. This condition is so named because this baby has a weak, mewing cry. These children have a small head and widely spaced, down-slanting eyes, cardiac abnormalities, failure to thrive, and microcephaly. They also have MR, hypotonia, and feeding and respiratory problems (Batshaw, 2002).

Nondisjunction of sex chromosomes, the most common type of which is *Klinefelter's syndrome,* is caused by an XXY sex chromosomal pattern. In this condition, the male is born with an extra X chromosome, derived primarily from the mother. This gives the child a total of 47 chromosomes instead of the usual 46. The syndrome occurs in approximately 1 in 500 live male births and results in a mild disorder that may not be recognized until adulthood. LDs and emotional and behavioral problems are characteristic of Klinefelter's syndrome.

Males with this syndrome are tall and slim, have small genitalia, and are infertile. An XYY chromosomal pattern occurs in 4 in 1,000 male births, and those with this pattern also are tall. These individuals may be expected to have mildly depressed IQ scores, tremors, reduced coordination, radioulnar synostosis, and an increased incidence of temper tantrums, impulsiveness, and inability to plan or to handle frustration and aggression (Wong & Hockenberry-Eaton, 2001).

The above syndromes represent the presence or absence of genes resulting from extra or deleted chromosomal material. Genetic disorders that stem from an abnormality in a single gene, of which there are an estimated 100,000 in the human genome (the set of all genes), can also occur. Genes are responsible for producing specific protein products and for regulating development and functions in the body.

Single-gene, or *mendelian trait,* genetic disorders are inherited abnormalities caused by abnormal genes that have had a negative effect on development (Batshaw, 2002). The four different patterns of single-gene inheritance are:

1 *Autosomal dominant inheritance,* in which an abnormal gene is present on one of the non-sex chromosomes. Usually this gene is directly passed from one of the parents to the child. On rare occasions the gene is not present in either the mother or the father, in which case it is known as a new, or "fresh," mutation. There is no carrier state; if the gene is present, the baby will have the abnormal characteristics. An example of an autosomal dominant illness is von Recklinghausen's disease (neurofibromatosis).

2 *Autosomal recessive inheritance,* in which an abnormal gene must be in a paired condition because it is less potent. This also exists on non-sex chromosomes. Commonly, both parents are carriers but have no symptoms of the illness. Examples of autosomal recessive illnesses are cystic fibrosis, phenylketonuria, Tay-Sachs disease, and diabetes. Many of the inherited diseases and illnesses have this pattern of inheritance, and in many instances the carrier states can be detected with various diagnostic procedures.

3 *X-linked inheritance,* in which the abnormal gene sits on the female sex chromosome, the X chromosome. Because this gene is recessive, in girls the normal gene on the second sex chromosome prevents expression of the disease. However, a boy who inherits the abnormal gene on his mother's X chromosome will be affected. Duchenne's muscular dystrophy and hemophilia (factor VIII deficiency) are examples of diseases inherited through this pattern.

4 *Polygenic,* or *multifactorial, inheritance,* which is a result of the interaction of heredity and the environment. Some congenital heart problems, cleft lip and palate, and meningomyelocele are examples of polygenic inheritance problems.

Fragile X syndrome accounts for one third of all X-linked causes of MR. This condition is most evident in boys, who have only one X chromosome. The prevalence is estimated at 0.4 to 0.8 per 1,000 boys and 0.2 to 0.6 per 1,000 girls. Genetic transmission of this disorder is complex, and outcomes can vary when the mother passes on the defective gene. The clinical manifestations become progressively more severe in subsequent generations of expression of fragile X syndrome. The underlying gene defect is the result of an abnormality of the X chromosome that causes a portion of the chromosome to become constricted; this defect has been named the *FMR1 gene*. The FMR1 gene affects body functions, primarily brain development. It is responsible for a protein that is important in brain development, and production of this protein is decreased. The progression in this disorder is due to the expanded section of DNA on the X chromosome, the sequence that is repeated is a series of three nucleotide bases, or a triplicate repeat of cytosine-guanine-guanine (CGG), at four fragile X locations. These mutations lead to a host of characteristics (Meyer & Batshaw, 2002).

In addition to MR, children with fragile X syndrome have craniofacial deformities, including elongated faces; prominent jaws and foreheads; large, protruding ears; a high-arched palate; hyperextensible joints; and flat feet. Other features, including prolapse of the mitral valve and enlarged testicles, become more pronounced with age. Some cognitive features seem to be preserved in males (e.g., simultaneous processing) even while they are identified as having MR with poor auditory memory and reception. Additionally, participation in daily living skills is preserved, whereas communication and social skills are impaired (Meyer & Batshaw, 2002; Wong & Hockenberry-Eaton, 2001). Speech tends to be echolalic, cluttered, and perseverative. Furthermore, these children may be identified as having PDDs because of the presence of stereotypic behavior, poor eye contact, unusual sensory stimuli responses, and lack of social skills (Wong & Hockenberry-Eaton).

Prader-Willi syndrome is associated with a defect in chromosome 15. This condition causes severe obesity, short stature, decreased muscle tone, a long face and slanted eyes, poor thermal regulation, and underdeveloped sex organs. Moderate MR and extreme food-seeking behaviors are classic signs. This condition occurs in 1 in 15,000 live births (Menkes, 2001).

Neurofibromatosis, or *von Recklinghausen's disease,* manifests in two forms, which have different genetic patterns. *Peripheral neurofibromatosis* (type 1) is the more common form; the other is *central neurofibromatosis* (type 2). The incidence is estimated at 1 in 3,000 to 5,000 live births, and the condition occurs more often in boys (Menkes, 2001). Neurofibromatosis causes multiple tumors, usually neurofibromas, on the central and peripheral nerves, café au lait spots on the skin, and vascular and visceral lesions. If these tumors occur in critical areas, they may cause death. Mild MR and LD are associated with the condition, as are speech disorders. Hypertension, optic gliomas (type 1), auditory tumors (type 2), skeletal anomalies, and short stature are also associated with the disease. Intervention for the condition may include surgical removal of dangerous or disfiguring lesions, reduction of symptoms, special education, and monitoring for cerebral tumors.

Williams syndrome has been traced to a microdeletion on chromosome 7 in the region of the gene that codes for elastin. Although the condition is rare (1 per 20,000 live births), its clinical features are dramatic. The syndrome yields a unique combination of cerebral maldevelopment and cardiovascular abnormalities. This inherited form of MR is characterized by mild mental retardation, yet striking preservation of musical aptitude, social skills, and writing, and an inability to draw even simple objects. The facial characteristics include a wide mouth, almond-shaped eyes, upturned nose, and small, pointed ears (Victor & Ropper, 2001). Sensitivity to auditory stimuli is paired with a delay in the acquisition of speech and deficits in visual, spatial, and motor skills. These individuals are virtually the converse of autism in their sociability and empathy.

Inborn Errors of Metabolism

Several genetic problems produce errors in the metabolism of environmental and internal substances. Left untreated, these conditions may cause serious disability and sometimes death. For some, early diagnosis allows treatment or prevention of these consequences, but for others, no known treatment has yet been found. For individuals with errors of metabolism, prenatal diagnosis and genetic counseling may be the only options.

Tay-Sachs disease is a degenerative nervous system disorder caused by the absence of an enzyme, called *hexosaminidase A,* that is usually found in the blood and major organs. This enzyme converts GM2 ganglioside, a product of nerve cell metabolism, into a nontoxic substance. Because this conversion does not take place in individuals with Tay-Sachs disease, the toxic substance builds up in the brain and other body organs, leading to brain damage.

Tay-Sachs disease is common in Jewish individuals whose ancestry can be traced to the Mediterranean region. Today, nearly 1 in 27 American Jews carries the Tay-Sachs gene (Menkes, 2001). Because Tay-Sachs disease is an autosomal recessive trait, both parents must be carriers of the abnormal gene for the disease to be passed to the child.

Carriers of Tay-Sachs disease can be detected by a simple blood test. In addition, through amniocentesis, the disease can be detected in the fetus by examination of the amniotic fluid for hexosaminidase A. This test, in addition to the relatively small and well-defined population in which the disease is primarily found, makes Tay-Sachs disease hypothetically a preventable condition.

Prevention is particularly important because Tay-Sachs disease is a devastating and fatal condition. Children with Tay-Sachs disease usually appear healthy at birth and develop normally for about 6 to 10 months. The child then becomes listless and regresses cognitively and motorically. A cherry red spot appears in both macular areas. Vision, hearing, and voluntary motor control loss occurs, and seizures appear, leading to death by the age of 3 years in most cases. There is no effective treatment for Tay-Sachs disease; medical and therapeutic efforts are essentially palliative and supportive (Menkes, 2001).

Research efforts are focusing on several treatment approaches that may someday offer help for children with Tay-Sachs disease. For example, the search continues for a substance that could substitute for hexosaminidase A or for a procedure to graft healthy cells into clients with Tay-Sachs disease so that the transplanted cells can produce hexosaminidase A. Research is also progressing in the transplantation of genes from normal into defective cells. Until an effective treatment is found, the best strategy is prevention through genetic counseling (Menkes, 2001).

Phenylketonuria (PKU) is an inborn error in the metabolism of phenylalanine, an amino acid commonly found in some proteins. This silent (i.e., produces acute toxicity) condition affects 1 in 15,000 children but is rare in individuals of Jewish origin and in African American children. These children predominantly have blond hair and blue eyes. If the condition is untreated severe cognitive and behavioral disabilities will develop and will, at times, mimic autism. The diagnosis can be made at birth with the Guthrie test. Treatment, which is effective, is dietary modification and involves withholding foods that have the precursors of phenylalanine to prevent toxic accumulation. It is believed that the restrictive diet must be maintained until age 10 years (Batshaw & Tuchman, 2002).

A similar condition, *galactosemia,* is the inability to convert galactose, a milk sugar, into glucose. Galactose builds up in the blood and causes hepatic and splenic dysfunction. If the condition goes untreated, the consequences include jaundice, vomiting and diarrhea, drowsiness and lethargy, cataracts, systemic infections, and death. Urine testing can detect the condition and is required for newborns in many states. Treatment involves a diet without galactose (no milk, milk products, or breast milk) and is usually effective in compliant children. In poorly controlled cases, some intellectual dulling, perceptual problems, tremors, choreoathetosis, and ataxia may be present (Wong & Hockenberry-Eaton, 2001).

Lesch-Nyhan syndrome is a progressive neuromuscular disease that is limited to boys and is characterized by an inability to metabolize purines. Children suffering from this condition appear normal for the first year but then experience significant MR, neuromotor degeneration, and spasticity, as well as a compulsive need to bite their lips and fingers and rub their faces. This behavior is involuntary and becomes self-mutilating if it goes unchecked. Vocal tics may also occur. Arthritis, anemia, and renal calculi are also common. Treatment usually includes protecting the child from self-mutilation, developmentally focused therapies, and medication to prevent secondary problems and to reduce mutilation. Naltrexone, an opioid antagonist, improves some of the clinical signs of this syndrome (Victor & Ropper, 2001).

DIABETES

Diabetes mellitus is a metabolic disorder of the pancreas in which the hormone insulin is secreted in insufficient amounts. Increased concentrations of glucose are found in the blood, and several systemic problems occur. The causes of diabetes are unknown, but the disease has a familial pattern and is now thought to be an autoimmune response to a viral infection in some cases (Wong & Hockenberry-Eaton, 2001).

There are two major types of diabetes. Type I results in the destruction of pancreatic beta cells, usually leading to absolute insulin deficiency. The onset usually occurs around age 10 but may occur earlier or later. This form of the disease tends to be more acute and requires the administration of insulin, carefully balanced with food intake and exercise, to provide adequate metabolic balance. Type II diabetes occurs more frequently in adults over 40 years of age. Type II is characterized by a resistance to insulin action, and it sometimes can be controlled by diet, exercise, or oral medications. Insulin may also be required in some stages of this form of diabetes. Maturity onset diabetes of the young is transmitted as an autosomal dominant disorder; it is characterized by the formation of structurally abnormal insulin that has decreased biologic activity. The onset typically occurs before 25 years of age, and the condition often can be controlled with dietary modifications and oral hypoglycemic agents (Wong & Hockenberry-Eaton, 2001).

Early symptoms of type I diabetes include polyuria, increased thirst, weight loss, and dehydration. Later symptoms may include acidosis, vomiting, hyperventilation, and coma (Alemzadeh & Wyatt, 2004). Overdose of insulin may cause insulin shock or hypoglycemia. Over many years, even with good care, microvascular lesions may occur in multiple organs and result in retinopathy that leads to blindness, nephropathy, and peripheral nerve damage. Sensory loss and increased infection, especially in the extremities, may occur. Individuals with diabetes are at increased risk for heart disease, and diabetic women are at increased risk for complications in pregnancy (Alemzadeh & Wyatt, 2004). Because this is a lifelong condition, the child and parents must be taught to administer insulin injections and to adjust and monitor blood glucose levels and life and dietary patterns. These children must also adjust to being drug dependent. This adjustment often is particularly difficult in adolescence.

The general goals of treatment are to ensure satisfactory growth and emotional development, help the child acquire some degree of normal life, resolve the symptoms, and prevent ketoacidosis and long-term sequelae, such as renal and cardiac damage and eye disease (Alemzadeh & Wyatt, 2004). Achievement of these goals is difficult, because a delicate balance must be maintained among so many factors, specifically exercise, nutritional intake, hormones, emotions, and many other internal and external influences on blood sugar levels.

TOXIC AGENTS

Prenatal Toxins

Several birth defects may be caused by adverse changes in the fetal environment. Substances and factors that negatively affect the developing fetus are called **toxic agents,** or *teratogens*. Drugs, radiation, and chemicals are the most common teratogens known to affect fetal development. Table 6-3 lists some common teratogens and their possible effects on the developing fetus. Several factors determine whether a teratogen will affect the fetus. The dosage, the gestational stage of the infant, and the specific sensitivity of the developing organs at the time of exposure to the teratogen are all factors that contribute to the outcome.

Alcohol-Related Birth Defects and Fetal Alcohol Syndrome

Alcohol-related birth defects (ARBDs), commonly referred to as *fetal alcohol syndrome (FAS)* or *fetal alcohol effects (FAE)*, are the most serious examples of a fetal syndrome caused by maternal exposure to a teratogen. FAS is a specific pattern of altered growth structure and function seen in infants of women who ingest high amounts of alcohol during pregnancy (Victor & Ropper, 2001). Infants with FAE, a milder form of FAS, may lack the distinct facial morphology and growth deficiencies but share many of the neurobehavioral deficits found in infants with FAS (Abel, 1998). The mechanism of injury includes a reduction in brain size, with the basal ganglia and cerebellum most impaired (Mattson, Riley, Gramling, Delis, & Jones, 1998).

TABLE 6-3 Effects of Common Teratogens on the Developing Fetus and Child

Substance	Effect on Fetus or Child
DRUGS	
Alcohol	Intrauterine growth retardation, mental deficiency, stillbirth. Infants may have complete fetal alcohol syndrome (including facial feature anomalies) or more mild fetal alcohol effects. They may experience withdrawal symptoms, mental retardation, hyperactivity, behavioral disorders, and learning disabilities.
Aspirin	In large amounts may be fatal or cause hemorrhagic manifestations
Cortisone	Possible factor in cleft palate
Caffeine	At extremely high levels, increased incidence of miscarriage and limb and skeletal malformations; mild intake shows no effect on the fetus
Dilantin	Fetal hydantoin syndrome (growth and mental deficiency, abnormalities of the face, anomalies of the hands)
Heroin, codeine, morphine	Hyperirritability, shrill cry, vomiting and withdrawal symptoms, decreased alertness and responsiveness to visual and auditory stimuli; can be fatal. Narcotic exposure has been associated with learning disabilities later in life.
Lysergic acid diethylamide (LSD)	Spontaneous abortion, chromosomal changes, suspected anomalies
Tetracycline	Staining of teeth, inhibition of bone growth
Thalidomide	Phocomelia, hearing loss, cardiac anomalies; can be fatal
Tobacco	Intrauterine growth retardation
Tranquilizers	All may cause withdrawal symptoms during neonatal period
Radiation therapy	Congenital anomalies, growth retardation, chromosomal damage, mental deficiency, stillbirth
CHEMICALS	
Methylmercury	Congenital abnormalities, growth retardation; can cause abortions
Pesticides (some types)	Congenital anomalies
Lead	Spontaneous abortion, intrauterine growth retardation, congenital anomalies, anemia; can be fatal

Modified from Klaus, M.H., & Farnaroff, A.A. (1979). *Care of the high-risk neonate.* Philadelphia: W.B. Saunders; Schuster, C.S., & Ashburn, S.S. (1986). *The process of human development: A holistic approach* (2nd ed.). Boston: Little, Brown.

Conservative estimates indicate that alcohol is the third leading cause of birth defects and the leading cause of MR. The incidence of FAS has been reported as 1 to 2 per 1,000 live births worldwide, and at least 1,200 children are born each year in the United States with this disorder. The estimate for children born with FAE is even higher, 3 to 5 per 1,000 live births worldwide (Sampson et al., 1997). The risk of FAS or FAE in children born to mild to moderate drinkers currently is the subject of controversy; some investigators show a high incidence of effects with even small amounts of alcohol, whereas others show few if any effects (Mattson & Riley, 1998). Investigators have demonstrated that the nature and extent of fetal injuries produced by alcohol depend on several factors, including (1) the amount of alcohol consumed per day, (2) the time during the pregnancy when the alcohol was taken, (3) other stressors experienced by the mother, (4) whether food was eaten near the time of alcohol consumption, (5) whether other substance abuse occurred during the pregnancy, and (6) the mother's general health (Coles, 1994; Jacobson, 1998).

Like other teratogens, alcohol causes a spectrum of defects that vary from severe physical and mental problems that are readily detectable at birth to more subtle learning problems that may not be detected until school age (Jacobson, 1998). The principal features of FAS include prenatal and postnatal growth deficiencies, a pattern of craniofacial malformations, and CNS dysfunction. Newborns typically are small for gestational age (SGA) and continue to show height, weight, and head circumference differences. The pattern of craniofacial malformations seen with FAS includes microcephaly, epicanthal folds, a long philtrum, short palpebral fissures, a flat midface, and a thin vermilion of the upper lip (Victor & Ropper, 2001) (Figure 6-16). Musculoskeletal problems include congenital dislocations, foot positional defects, cervical spine abnormalities, specific joint alterations, flexion contractures at the elbows, and tapering of the terminal phalanges. Many of these craniofacial and skeletal defects occur secondary to the effect of alcohol on brain development, and although craniofacial deficits may even recede with growth, microcephaly does not (Wunsch, Conlon, & Scheidt, 2002).

Although CNS dysfunction can vary, impairment of intellectual capacity is the disability most frequently noted with FAS. This impairment ranges from moderate MR to average intellectual function, with an average IQ of 70 being most recently cited (Mattson & Riley, 1998). Other notable CNS deficits include hyperactivity, attention deficits, vestibular problems, impulsivity, poor social skills, learning disabilities, memory deficits, and deficits in visuospatial-perceptual skills, as well as sensory problems affecting ocular, auditory, and possibly vestibular functioning (Church & Abel, 1998).

The prognosis for children with FAS or FAE varies with the extent and severity of the various malformations

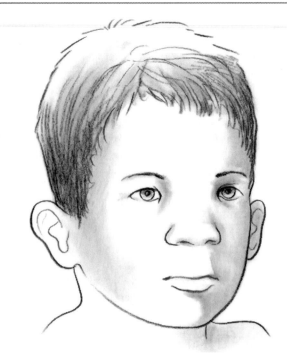

FIGURE 6-16 Typical facial features of a child with fetal alcohol syndrome (FAS).

and growth deficiencies. Two important factors are the severity of the maternal alcoholism and the quality and stability of the home environment (Abel, 1998). Studies of the long-term effects of FAS and FAE are just beginning to provide information about the influence of alcohol on the growth and development of the affected child. Size delays appear to continue for some time, with head circumference remaining smaller into middle childhood. The occupational performances of children with FAS or FAE show persistent delays in self-care, school activities, and play. Performance areas typically evaluated include mental function, interactions, sensory functions, and neuromusculoskeletal functions.

Families of children with FAS or FAE have multiple psychosocial issues, and the clinician must involve the entire family in the child's therapy program. Many health care professionals believe that with intensive family intervention (e.g., alcohol recovery programs for the mother and early intervention for the child) and with social, medical, and financial support, a better prognosis is possible. Hypothetically, FAS could be completely preventable if the public were educated to the deleterious effects of alcohol on unborn infants and behavior changed accordingly. The best that can be hoped for is a reduction in the number of newborns with FAS or FAE (Wunsch et al., 2002).

Cocaine and Opiates

The effects of cocaine, crack, and opiates on infants are of increasing concern to developmental specialists. Use of these drugs increased noticeably in the 1990s and continues to be a social concern, particularly the use of cocaine and "crack," a relatively cheap cocaine derivative. Also, maternal drug use is complicated by the tendency of these individuals to abuse other substances, such as alcohol and tobacco, and many mothers using these drugs are poorly nourished and receive less than adequate prenatal care. It is estimated that more than 100,000 infants each year are born to mothers who use drugs during pregnancy, although accurate counts are difficult because of the social and legal implications of reporting drug use (Wunsch et al., 2002; Zagon & Slotkin, 1992).

Cocaine is extremely addictive; it causes ecstatic "highs" and significant and prolonged "lows." Addiction to crack is said to be possible after one or two uses (Wunsch et al., 2002; Zagon & Slotkin, 1992). Cocaine increases the levels of norepinephrine, serotonin, and dopamine and has strong vasoconstrictive effects. It crosses the placenta and has similar effects in the fetus, and this vasoconstriction is believed to be damaging to the fetus. Use of opiates, heroin, or methadone by the mother results in an addicted infant who experiences drug withdrawal after birth.

The extent to which abuse of cocaine and other drugs causes developmental problems is still in question (Wagner, Katikaneni, Cox, & Ryan, 1998). Research in the area continues, but controlled studies are difficult to complete. Several general patterns are emerging. Babies born of addicted mothers are often SGA, with reduced head size and irritability and hypersensitivity to stimuli (Wagner et al.). Cocaine has been associated with congenital anomalies, limb deficiencies, cerebral hemorrhage, increased muscle tone, necrotizing enterocolitis, and rapid shifts of arousal state (Wong & Hockenberry-Eaton, 2001). Newborns who had been exposed to narcotics in utero go through active withdrawal, during which they are irritable, hypertonic, and poor feeders. Often they frantically suck on their hands. Motor coordination is reduced, and the activity level may be high. Respiratory distress has also been noted (Wagner et al.). These infants tend to require quiet, low-stimulus environments and may respond positively to swaddling. Parenting of these children can be difficult for several months.

The long-term effects are unclear. Some studies have found that by school age these children perform at age level expectations. However, others have reported performance problems, including hyperactivity and organizational problems, subtle learning and cognitive deficits, and play deficits. Furthermore, the mothers of these children often have few social supports and may be young or homeless or may remain addicted, and the children may be placed in foster care. Early intervention and school intervention programs may be necessary to identify, prevent, or minimize the long-term effects of the maternal substance abuse (Wunsch et al., 2002).

Heavy Metals

Heavy metal poisoning is a serious health concern. Because small children often put things in their mouths, they are at particular risk for poisoning by these substances (Victor & Ropper, 2001). Mercury can enter the body by means of ingestion or inhalation, resulting in *mercury poisoning,* which can cause tremors, memory loss, anorexia, weight loss, diarrhea, and acrodynia (painful extremities). Liquid mercury evaporates quickly and should be cleaned up immediately to prevent this problem.

Lead poisoning is usually caused by ingestion of environmental lead, such as the lead paint used in buildings before World War II. Lead paint has caused a significant problem in some inner city communities and in older houses that have been renovated (Mahaffey, 1992). Lead water pipes and some ceramic glazes have also been associated with lead poisoning.

A child may be acutely or chronically affected. Lead affects three body systems in particular: the renal, circulatory, and nervous systems. Renal damage occurs in the proximal tubules of the kidneys, resulting in abnormal excretion of important nutrients and impairment of vitamin D synthesis. Lead severely limits the body's ability to synthesize heme, leading to accumulation of alternate metabolites in the body and, ultimately, anemia (Wong & Hockenberry-Eaton, 2001). The most significant and irreversible effects of lead poisoning on the body occur in the nervous system. Fluid builds up in the brain, and intracranial pressure can reach life-threatening levels (Menkes, 2001). Cortical atrophy and lead encephalitis are usually associated with high blood levels of lead. This can lead to MR, paralysis, blindness, and convulsions. Low-level exposure has been associated with LDs, ADHD, hearing impairment, and milder intellectual deficits. Other lead poisoning symptoms include cramping, digestive difficulty, lethargy, headache, and fever (Menkes).

INFECTIOUS CONDITIONS

Maternal Infections

The fetus may be infected by a variety of organisms. Some of these infectious conditions are passed from the mother to the fetus during pregnancy (transplacental infections), and others are present in the vagina and are passed to the infant at birth (ascending infections). These infections invade the fetus at a time when it has a limited capacity to ward off disease and, in the case of transplacental infections, at a time when the infection may have a profound effect on the formation or growth and development of tissues and organs (Wong & Hockenberry-Eaton, 2001).

The most common maternal infections are the *STORCH infections* (i.e., syphilis, toxoplasmosis, rubella, cytomegalovirus, and herpes virus), which are also called *TORCH* or *TORCHS*. Each of these conditions is caused by a specific virus or bacterium and has a different set of characteristics. A summary of these five infections and their effects on the fetus can be found in Table 6-4. *Congenital syphilis* can be transmitted in the late stages of pregnancy or during delivery. It is the most virulent form of syphilis and requires isolation of the infected infant. The usual treatment for congenital syphilis is penicillin. Early-stage congenital syphilis is characterized by hepatitis, failure to thrive, neurologic involvement, fever, anemia, restlessness, irritability, and syphilitic rhinitis. Characteristic lesions may be present, and the hair and nails may be damaged. Osteochondritis at the joints and other bone abnormalities are relatively common. Because of residual damage from the infection, late-stage congenital syphilis is marked by bony and dental anomalies and visual and auditory deficits (Wong & Hockenberry-Eaton, 2001).

Toxoplasmosis can be contracted by the mother through ingestion of raw meat or contact with the feces of newly infected cats and can be transmitted to the fetus at any point during the pregnancy. Toxoplasmosis is also an increasingly common opportunistic infection in acquired immunodeficiency syndrome (AIDS) (McLeod & Remington, 2004). In the United States the incidence of toxoplasmosis is about 1.3 in 1,000 live births (McLeod & Remington). Stillbirth and death are common, but some newborns are asymptomatic. Children born with this condition are often severely mentally handicapped. Hydrocephalus, cerebral calcification, and chorioretinitis are classic symptoms. CP, seizures, cardiac and liver damage, and gastrointestinal problems are also found. Treatment with sulfonamides and pyrimethamine is usually initiated in infected mothers and children. Once acquired, the neurologic deficits related to the disease can be reduced but not eliminated by maternal treatment (McLeod & Remington).

Rubella, a common and fairly mild disease in children, can be devastating when contracted by a pregnant woman, particularly in the first trimester. With the advent of a preventive vaccine, congenital rubella syndrome has declined 99% in the past 25 years; however, the dangers to unvaccinated mothers are significant. Congenital defects, spontaneous abortion, and stillbirth may occur. Central processing and hearing loss, MR, microcephaly, and seizures are possible outcomes. Congenital heart defects, including patent ductus arteriosus, are characteristic, as are visual deficits, hepatomegaly, and splenomegaly (Maldonado, 2004). These children may be SGA and may suffer from numerous respiratory infections in infancy. Late-occurring symptoms include diabetes, encephalitis, hearing loss, and thyroid problems. Functionally, children with congenital rubella symptoms may be expected to have mixed developmental delays and hearing and vestibular deficits. The child's therapy program may need to be adjusted to accommodate cardiorespiratory effects (Maldonado, 2004).

Transmission of *cytomegalovirus* (i.e., cytomegalic inclusion disease) is similar to that for rubella, and the effects also are similar. This herpes-type viral infection may be transmitted before, during, or after birth. The infection may be active or latent in the newborn, therefore infection control precautions are appropriate for therapists working with these children. Clinical manifestations include low birth weight, sensorineural hearing loss, microcephaly, hepatomegaly, splenomegaly, and purpuric rash. Jaundice and hepatitis may also be present. Children with cytomegalovirus infection may be asymptomatic at birth. Symptomatic newborns have a poor prognosis with regard to neurologic deficits. These children often have learning disabilities and diminished cognitive skills (Wong & Hockenberry-Eaton, 2001).

The newborn most often contracts *congenital herpes* infection during or after delivery by a mother with herpes simplex infection, often genital herpes (Wong & Hockenberry-Eaton, 2001). Infected children frequently develop skin, mouth, or eye lesions within 6 to 10 days of contact, although some children do not develop overt symptoms. In the disseminated form, a sepsis-like picture presents itself, and the child may develop internal organ lesions and encephalitis with CNS involvement. Early signs are fever, lethargy, poor feeding, irritability, and vomiting. Infusion of antiviral agents may reduce the

TABLE 6-4 Intrauterine Infections (STORCH)

Infection	Cause	Type	Effects on Fetus
Syphilis	Parabacterial infection	A, T	Enlarged liver and spleen, jaundice, anemia, rash, rhinorrhea
Toxoplasmosis	Parasitic infection	T	Deafness, blindness, MR, seizures, pneumonia, enlarged liver and spleen
Rubella	Viral infection	T	Meningitis, hearing loss, cataracts, cardiac problems, MR, retinal defects
Cytomegalovirus	Viral infection	T	Hearing loss; in severe form, problems are similar to those seen with rubella
Herpes	Viral infection	A	Localized form: lethargy, rash, respiratory distress, jaundice, enlarged liver and spleen. Generalized form: virus attacks CNS, causing MR, seizures, and other problems.

STORCH, Syphilis, toxoplasmosis, rubella, cytomegalovirus, and herpes; *A*, ascending; *T*, transplacental; *MR*, mental retardation; *CNS*, central nervous system.

severity of this condition noticeably and has been known to prevent serious brain damage. Cesarean sections are sometimes used as a preventive measure for mothers with active lesions (Wong & Hockenberry-Eaton).

The sexually transmitted diseases *gonorrhea* and *chlamydia* are passed to the infant late in fetal development or during delivery. Both may result in eye infections, and gonococcal arthritis, septicemia, and meningitis may also occur. Fortunately, both infections respond well to antibiotic therapy if discovered early. Other maternal infections known to affect neonatal health are listeriosis, Lyme disease, hepatitis B, and AIDS, as well as infections caused by parvovirus, coxsackievirus, and varicella virus (chickenpox) (Wong & Hockenberry-Eaton, 2001).

Acquired Immunodeficiency Syndrome

Acquired immunodeficiency syndrome, which is caused by the human immunodeficiency virus (HIV), is a major health concern for all, including infants, children, and adolescents. Investigators estimate that as of 2000, about 1.4 million children worldwide under the age of 15 were infected with HIV. As many as 36 million people have the disease, and each year approximately 5 million new cases are detected. The transmission of HIV to children is primarily the result of perinatal contact with the mother (90% of the cases). In the United States, the mother to infant transmission rate is much lower, approximately 1% to 2%. Most perinatal transmission occurs in utero by transplacental passage of the virus, intrapartum through contact with infected maternal blood and cervical secretions, or postpartum through breast-feeding. HIV infection can be diagnosed between 1 and 6 months of age. Children with AIDS represent the most serious disease manifestations of HIV (Spiegel & Bonwit, 2002).

HIV infects and damages cells of the immune system, rendering the child vulnerable to life-threatening illnesses that do not affect children with normal immunity. HIV-positive newborns are often asymptomatic at birth. The interval from birth to the development of AIDS among perinatally affected infants varies widely. Evaluation of the most current data indicates that there is a subset of perinatally infected children who do not have significant disease for years after infection and a subset of children who develop the most serious manifestations of infection by 2 years of age (rapid progressors). The onset, which often occurs before 6 months of age, of serious clinical disease is a prognostic indicator of survival. Cases of rapid progression of the disease are currently under intensive study. Although investigators can identify the factors involved in rapid progression, they cannot yet offer reasons for this subset of pathogenesis (Langston et al., 2001).

Until the late 1990s the prognosis for children infected with HIV was grim. Although HIV infection is still ultimately fatal, the prognosis has clearly changed. An increasing proportion of children are surviving, and with the advent of the antiretroviral drug regimens, the mortality rate has dropped by 80%; this has converted HIV infection from a fatal disorder to a chronic illness in developed countries. The improvement in this prognosis is directly related to implementation of the highly active antiretroviral drugs (HARRT) to control replication in infants and to delay the progression of HIV infection to AIDS. Clinical management of HIV-infected children remains intensive, with recommendations for clinical evaluations and laboratory assessment to be completed every 3 months. Any viral or bacterial infection is considered a serious breach of immune system integrity and is carefully monitored. Recommendations for HIV-infected children are different; for example, inactivated vaccines are recommended for protection, and live vaccines are contraindicated.

The criteria for a diagnosis of HIV infection include positive results on two separate determinations or the presence of one or more AIDS-defining illnesses. Pediatric classifications for HIV infection are listed in two ways: one set of criteria for immune functioning and another set for clinical pathology.

Most HIV specialists believe that early and aggressive treatment for children with HIV should include antiretroviral drug therapy and administration of intravenous (IV) gamma globulin. These treatments decrease the viral load, preserve the immune system, extend the interval preceding the development of AIDS, and prolong survival. As indicated by the diagnostic features, infections are a common occurrence after HIV infection. Children tend to have a greater number of minor bacterial infections, including otitis media, urinary tract infections, and pneumonia. Fungal infections include oral candidiasis and candidal dermatitis. Children with recurrent infections may benefit from IV administration of gamma globulin. *Pneumocystis carinii pneumonia* (PCP) is the most common opportunistic infection seen in children. PCP prevention has become an important focus of care in both HIV and AIDS.

Although no cure currently exists for HIV infection or AIDS, antiretroviral drugs are successfully prolonging survival (Langston et al., 2001). The antiretroviral drugs commonly used in children fall into three categories: nucleoside transcriptase inhibitors, non-nucleoside reverse transcriptase inhibitors, and protease inhibitors. These drugs result in a significant slowing of progression of the disease and are associated with prolonged survival times. Therapy is started immediately after birth, and medical visits include monitoring of the HIV infection as well as routine care and immunizations. The goal of each class of drug is to prevent the virus from producing progeny. Other drugs are in development to prevent

HIV from infecting the CD4+ cells in the first place (Spiegel & Bonwit, 2002).

If the disease progresses to a severe level, suppression of the immune system, chronic respiratory illness, skin and other types of infection, and diarrhea often noticeably weaken infected children. These conditions often respond slowly to treatment (Wong & Hockenberry-Eaton, 2001). Developmental delays and degeneration may result in delayed or lost motor, speech, and independent living skills. Neurologic deficits, including ataxia, spasticity, rigidity, tremor, and seizures, may be expected as the disease progresses. Early intervention and rehabilitative and educational services are often indicated (Spiegel & Bonwit, 2002).

Interdisciplinary care is essential for the assessment and treatment of pediatric HIV infection. The team guides the family through well child visits, immunizations, nutritional support, antiretroviral therapy, adherence to medication regimens, monitoring of antiretroviral treatment, and coping with adverse drug reactions. Developmental assessment and educational programs may aid the child with multiple environmental influences, including socioeconomic factors, family environment, and failure to thrive. Other services that may need to be considered are social support, infection control at home and school, and possibly the need for placement outside the home (Spiegel & Bonwit, 2002; Wong & Hockenberry-Eaton, 2001).

Encephalitis and Meningitis

Encephalitis and meningitis, which are infections of the brain and its coverings, are frightening and sometimes dangerous. *Encephalitis*, or inflammation of the brain, may be caused by bacteria, spirochetes, or other organisms but usually is caused by a viral infection. The specific cause often is not identified clinically. The condition may be localized or may include the spinal cord or meninges. Infection of the brain may occur directly or secondary to another infection. Because mosquitoes spread several viral forms, a summer onset is common. Herpes simplex has also been associated disproportionately with encephalitis in young children (Wong & Hockenberry-Eaton, 2001).

The severity of these conditions varies with the cause. The onset may be sudden or gradual, and the condition often is difficult to distinguish from other infections. Symptoms include fever, headache, dizziness, stiff neck, nausea and vomiting, tremors, and ataxia. In severe cases, stupor, seizures, disorientation, coma, and death may occur. The diagnosis is based on environmental patterns of infection, clinical findings, EEG and MRI results, and laboratory examination of blood, brain tissue, or CSF. Treatment may include antibiotics if bacterial infection is suggested but is primarily supportive while the acute disease runs its course (Wong & Hockenberry-Eaton, 2001).

Unfortunately, encephalitis can result in mild to severe residual brain damage. The degree of damage depends on the child's age, the type of infection, and the care provided. Young children are at increased risk for neurologic complications. The health care staff must monitor the child's progress and neurologic status after the infection resolves. MR, LDs, behavior disorders, seizures, and neuromotor deficits are common. Neurorehabilitation techniques are applied to limit the disability, and compensatory interventions, including assistive technology, may help this child in school, play and, later, prevocational activities.

Meningitis is an infection of the meninges, the tissue covering the brain and spinal cord. Like encephalitis, meningitis may have a tubercular, fungal, protozoal, viral, or (most commonly) bacterial cause. Clinical manifestations of meningitis vary slightly in newborns, infants, older children, and adolescents, but the clinical picture is not unlike that for encephalitis. Headache, fever, and rigidity in the neck are classic signs. These may be accompanied by seizures, vomiting, spasticity, behavioral and arousal state changes and, in young children, bulging fontanels. In newborns, jaundice, cyanosis, hypothermia, and respiratory distress may also be present (Prober, 2004).

Diagnostic evaluation may include lumbar puncture, analysis of the CSF, and blood, throat, and nasal cultures. Treatment includes management of the underlying infection with antibiotics, hydration, maintenance of intracranial pressure, and treatment of symptoms and complications. Because many forms of the disease are highly contagious, the acutely ill client may be isolated. The child may be monitored for apnea and cardiac function. As with encephalitis, neuromotor, visual, auditory, seizure, and learning disorders may remain after the acute infection abates. Anticonvulsant and rehabilitative therapy is necessary to manage and remediate these sequelae (Prober, 2004).

NEOPLASTIC DISORDERS

Cancer is devastating for anyone, but it seems somehow even more insidious when it attacks children. The pain, fear, and life disruption it causes are chronic and affect the child, the child's family, and all those around the child. The major neoplastic disorders that children can acquire are discussed in this section.

Leukemia

Leukemia is a cancer of the blood-forming tissues. It is the most common form of cancer in children, occurring in 3 to 4 children per 100,000 in those less than 15 years of age. It occurs in boys more often than girls, almost always in white children, and most frequently in children with Down syndrome. The peak incidence occurs between 2 and 5 years of age. Two forms of leukemia recognized in children are acute lymphoid leukemia (ALL) and acute nonlymphoid leukemia (ANLL), also called acute myelogenous leukemia (AML) (Wong & Hockenberry-Eaton, 2001). The symptoms of these two forms of cancer are similar, but they react differently to treatment, with ALL having the more favorable response. The causes of leukemia are unknown, but immunologic and chromosomal factors have been associated with the condition.

Leukemia is characterized by the uncontrolled multiplication of immature white blood cells, which prevents the bone marrow from producing normal blood cells. Symptoms include loss of weight, night sweats, chronic fatigue, paleness, a high fever; repeated infections; purpura; and enlargement of the lymph nodes, spleen, and liver. Detection of lymphoblasts in a bone marrow specimen confirms the diagnosis. Blood counts are also taken.

The goal of medical management is to achieve a complete cure by inducing remission, eliminating cells in "sanctuaries" (e.g., the CNS), and maintaining the remission. Specifically, treatment is conducted in four phases. The first phase, *induction therapy*, is designed to rid the bone marrow and the rest of the body of the leukemic cells. In the second phase, c*entral nervous system (CNS) prophylaxis*, the intent is to consolidate the gains of remission by eliminating leukemic cells with different drugs. In the third phase, *intensification and consolidation*, chemotherapy is administered to treat small deposits of cells that remain after remission. The fourth phase, *maintenance* or *continuation therapy*, is aimed at killing cells in the sanctuary sites of the brain and spinal cord (Rudolph, Kamei, & Overby, 2002).

The prognosis for leukemia is much improved over recent years; a cure is obtained for most clients with ALL, and these children are expected to live relatively normal lives. Many go long periods with no recurrent signs. The prognosis for children with CNS involvement and ANLL is poorer but still hopeful, particularly with bone marrow transplantation. These children undergo long courses of treatment that can be painful and frightening, and recurrence of the disease and death remain possibilities that must be handled with support for the child's emotional capabilities (Rudolph et al., 2002).

Brain Tumors

Tumors of the brain and spinal cord are the most common tumors of solid tissues in children. Most of these tumors occur in the cerebellum and brain stem, with *medulloblastomas* and *astrocytomas* accounting for 30% of all childhood tumors. *Gliomas* and *ependymomas* (ventricular tumors) are also relatively common. The cause of brain tumors is unknown but is believed to be developmental or chromosomal in nature. Tumors may not become evident early in life because they usually are related to increases in intracranial pressure. In the young child the skull is soft enough to provide some accommodation for this phenomenon. The diagnosis is based on clinical signs and confirmed with CT scans, MRI imaging, EEG studies, and lumbar puncture.

Symptoms of brain tumors include recurrent and progressive headaches, vomiting (particularly in the morning), loss of coordination or strength, increased reflex activity, changes in behavior, seizures, and vital sign disturbances. Specific symptoms may relate to the location of the tumor. Treatment includes surgical removal of the tumor, radiation therapy, and chemotherapy. The prognosis varies with the type, size, and location of the tumor. The survival rate for astrocytomas (75%) is better than that for medulloblastomas (25% to 35%), which is better than that for glial cell tumors (20% to 30%). Survival with ependymomas varies from 15% to 60%, depending on the study (Wong & Hockenberry-Eaton, 2001). Recurrence of brain tumors is common, and surgery, chemotherapy, and radiation therapy may cause permanent brain damage. Children recovering from these tumors may require a broad spectrum of CNS-based rehabilitation to improve residual sensorimotor and cognitive function (Wong & Hockenberry-Eaton).

Hodgkin's Disease

Hodgkin's disease and other *lymphomas* are far less common than leukemia (15 per 1 million population) but are still significant. The condition is commonly a disease of later childhood and adolescence. This cancer of the lymphatic system is marked by painless adenopathy in the cervical region with or without fever. The child may also experience chills and night sweats, anorexia and weight loss, and general malaise. The diagnosis is made by histologic examination of the node. Blood studies may also show characteristic abnormalities. Four stages of the disease have been identified. In stage I, only one node is involved. Stage II demonstrates involvement on only one side of the diaphragm. In stages III and IV, progressively more organs are involved.

Treatment consists of radiation therapy, chemotherapy, or splenectomy. The prognosis is excellent for children in stages I, II, and III, with survival rates estimated at greater than 90%; however, clients with widespread disease have only a 65% to 75% survival rate (Wong & Hockenberry-Eaton, 2001).

Non-Hodgkin's lymphoma (NHL) occurs primarily in school-age children. These tumors are more common in boys and are a significant disorder for African American children. They may also occur as a second malignancy after Hodgkin's disease. The onset is acute and progression is rapid; most children have disseminated disease at diagnosis. Symptoms include abdominal pain, vomiting, anorexia, diarrhea, ascites, and distention of the abdomen. Fever, a palpable mass, and paraplegia may also be present. The diagnosis is made through a physical examination and analysis of laboratory results. Radiation therapy, chemotherapy, and surgery may be used to treat these conditions. The prognosis generally is excellent but varies with the degree of bone marrow and CNS involvement and with the number and size of tumors present. Survival past 24 months is considered a cure, and relapse is very rare past 2 years after treatment (Wong & Hockenberry-Eaton, 2001).

Bone Tumors

The two major tumors of the bone, osteosarcoma and Ewing's sarcoma, are relatively uncommon but result in physical disability. Most of these tumors occur in adolescence, more frequently in boys. For both cancers, survival depends on early diagnosis, before metastatic disease appears. The diagnosis is made by radiologic analysis, with each tumor having a characteristic pattern. Clinical signs include localized pain that may be relieved by a change in position, lumps, and a reduced activity level. Treatment is directed at control of the local tumor and systemic therapy to eradicate microscopic disease at distant sites. Preoperative chemotherapy is combined with surgery to reduce the bulk of the tumor, and postoperative chemotherapy optimizes the prognosis. If the tumor has not metastasized, the disease is cured in 65% to 75% of patients.

Osteosarcoma usually occurs at the end of the long bones, particularly the femur. Large spindle cells and malignant osteoid bone are formed next to the growth plate, and a painful mass develops. Frequently a secondary trauma at the site of the tumor brings the mass to light. Because osteosarcoma is resistant to radiation therapy, amputation is performed, if possible, followed by a course of chemotherapy. If metastases occur, they usually are found in the bones or lungs. In the absence of metastasis, the chance of survival is good but not certain. A child with osteosarcoma also requires prosthetic equipment and training after surgery (Salter, 1999).

Ewing's sarcoma occurs most often in the bones of the trunk but also in the long bones and skull. It does not form osteoid tissue, but rather produces small, round groups of cells. This condition spreads its metastases hematologically, particularly to the bones and lungs. Surgery is not performed routinely and often is done only late in treatment. Ewing's sarcoma responds well to radiation therapy, and chemotherapy is also routinely

prescribed. In the absence of metastases and for distal lesions, survival rates are good (60% to 70%). However, if metastases exist, the prognosis is poor (Rudolph et al., 2002).

BURNS

Major burn injury accounts for a large number of children who must undergo prolonged, painful, and restrictive hospitalizations. Countless other children suffer from minor burns. Thermal, electrical, chemical, and radioactive sources can cause burns, but thermal burns are by far the most common. Most burns can be attributed to accidents; however, 10% to 20% of hospital admissions for burns may be attributed to child abuse. Children under 3 years of age account for the majority of thermal burns, and of these, hot water and hot beverage scalds account for 50% to 60% of injuries (Murphy, Purdue, Hunt, & Hicks, 1997). About 30% of burns in older children are related to flame (e.g., match, gasoline, firecracker) or chemical burns. Short periods of high heat or long periods of low heat both can cause significant burns. Chemical burns can cause serious injury, but their effect often can be stopped with prompt emergency treatment. Electrical burns may damage not only the skin but also underlying bone, muscle, and nerve tissue along the conduction path. Further damage can be caused by smoke inhalation, respiratory failure, shock, and posttraumatic infection (Wong & Hockenberry-Eaton, 2001).

The criteria that determine the prognosis for survival of a child with a burn injury include the percentage of body area burned, the depth and location of the burn, the child's age, the causative agent, whether respiratory involvement is a factor, the length of the hospital stay, and whether other injuries are present (Murphy et al., 1997).

The percentage of area injured, in children, is assessed according to the total body surface area (TBSA) affected, either by the rule of nines in children older than 10 or by charts specifically designed to accurately estimate the body proportions involved in children of different ages (Murphy et al., 1997; Wong & Hockenberry-Eaton, 2001). The *rule of nines* ascribes 9% of the TBSA to the head and neck, 9% to each upper extremity, 18% to each lower extremity, 36% to the trunk (18% anterior and 18% posterior), and 1% to the perineum and genitals. In children under 10 years of age, the accuracy of TBSA estimations are improved through use of various charts to estimate the modified rule of nines (Figure 6-17). The mortality rate for children under 4 years of age with burns covering more than 30% of the TBSA is significantly higher than that for older children with a burn of the same size (46.9% versus 12.5%, respectively) (Morrow et al., 1996). Inhalation injuries are significantly correlated with death. In addition, major burns of

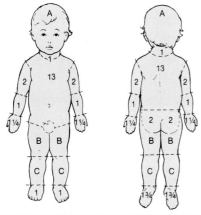

RELATIVE PERCENTAGES OF AREAS AFFECTED BY GROWTH

AREA	BIRTH	AGE 1 YR	AGE 5 YR
A = ½ of head	9½	8½	6½
B = ½ of one thigh	2¾	3¼	4
C = ½ of one leg	2½	2½	2¾

A

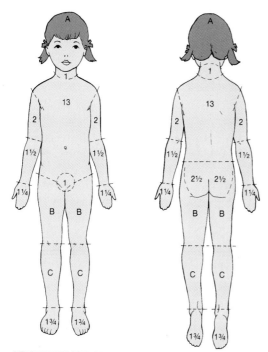

RELATIVE PERCENTAGES OF AREAS AFFECTED BY GROWTH

AREA	AGE 10 YR	AGE 15 YR	ADULT
A = ½ of head	5½	4½	3½
B = ½ of one thigh	4½	4½	4¾
C = ½ of one leg	3	3¼	3½

B

FIGURE 6-17 Estimation of distribution of burns in children. **A,** Children from birth to 5 years of age. **B,** Older children. (From Wong, D. [1999]. *Whaley and Wong's nursing care of infants and children* [6th ed.]. St. Louis: Mosby.)

less than 30% TBSA in children under 4 years of age may result in death despite excellent emergency and burn care.

The American Burn Association (2001) also classifies burns as minor, moderate, or severe. In minor burns, less than 10% of the TBSA is covered by a partial-thickness burn; these burns can be adequately treated on an outpatient basis. In a moderate burn, 10% to 20% of the TBSA is covered by a partial-thickness burn, and the child requires hospitalization. A major burn is considered to be any full-thickness burn or any burn injury in which more than 20% of the TBSA is covered by a partial-thickness burn (American Burn Association, 2001).

The depth of the burn is assessed according to the number of layers of tissue involved in the injury (Figure 6-18). *Superficial burns*, or first-degree burns, demonstrate minimal tissue damage, although they can be painful. In these burns the skin is red and dry, and healing typically occurs without scarring. *Partial-thickness burns*, or second-degree burns, involve the epidermis and dermis in varying degrees and can be further classified as deep or superficial burns. Superficial partial-thickness burns involve the epidermis and a portion of the dermis, but many of the dermal elements are left intact. Partial-thickness burns appear slightly raised, blistered, reddened, and moist, and they blanch to the touch. These are the most painful of burns and may result in some scarring, although superficial partial-thickness burns may heal spontaneously. In deep partial-thickness burns, both the epidermis and dermis are damaged, but the sweat glands and hair follicles of the dermis are left intact. In many cases a deep partial-thickness burn resembles a full-thickness burn. The appearance of these injuries is dry, soft, and waxy, with no edema or raised appearance. In *full-thickness burns*, or third- or fourth-degree burns, all layers of the skin are destroyed, as may be some of the underlying subcutaneous tissue (Figure 6-18). The appearance of full-thickness burns is hard, insensate, and leathery, with inflexible eschar. Some systems include a fourth-degree burn classification when the damage extends to underlying muscle, bone, and fascia. These burns may be charred, brown, or red; nerve endings and blood vessels may be damaged; and pain may not be present in the central area. Most third- and fourth-degree burns also have borders of second-degree burns that are painful (American Burn Association, 2001).

With a moderate or major burn, critical care focuses on maintenance of breathing if there is evidence of respiratory involvement, as well as immediate replacement of fluids, nutrition, and pain management. The intensive pathophysiologic response to a major burn creates a need to balance the amount of fluid replacement and nutrition carefully to compensate for the loss of blood, the presence of edema, and critical sodium or potassium changes. Sedation is needed to allow tolerance of treatment and for comfort. Pain management continues throughout treatment. Morphine combined with methadone, ketamine, propofol, and nitrous oxide have all demonstrated usefulness in pain management for victims of major burns (Wong & Hockenberry-Eaton, 2001).

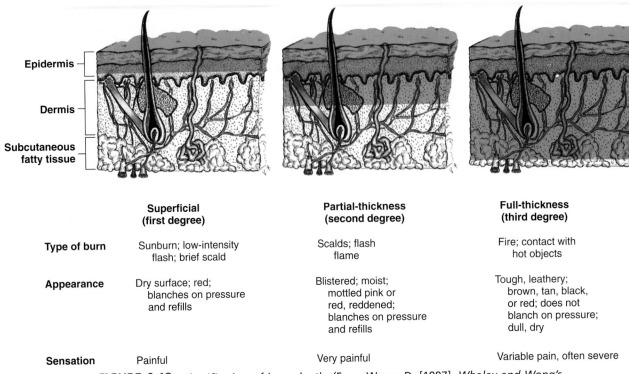

	Superficial (first degree)	Partial-thickness (second degree)	Full-thickness (third degree)
Type of burn	Sunburn; low-intensity flash; brief scald	Scalds; flash flame	Fire; contact with hot objects
Appearance	Dry surface; red; blanches on pressure and refills	Blistered; moist; mottled pink or red, reddened; blanches on pressure and refills	Tough, leathery; brown, tan, black, or red; does not blanch on pressure; dull, dry
Sensation	Painful	Very painful	Variable pain, often severe

FIGURE 6-18   Classification of burn depth. (From Wong, D. [1997]. *Whaley and Wong's essentials of pediatric nursing* [5th ed.]. St. Louis: Mosby.)

In addition to emergency care, prevention of secondary infection, wound débridement, and wound closure are critical. Application of antimicrobial agents to prevent secondary infection is an ongoing process until the wound is closed. A variety of topical antimicrobial agents are used to help prevent infection. Silver nitrate, silver sulfadiazine, mafenide acetate, nystatin, neomycin, povidone-iodine, and bacitracin are the most common (Wong & Hockenberry-Eaton, 2001). However, after a deep partial- or full-thickness burn, primary excision is often required before treatment with topical agents is effective. Physicians also are beginning to use growth hormone, which has been shown to enhance wound healing and decrease nutritional requirements (American Burn Association, 2001).

Débridement of necrotic tissue is essential to recovery. Hydrotherapy is used to remove debris, cleanse the wound, and allow increased range of motion (ROM) in all body parts. This is an extremely painful process that must be done twice a day, and typically the child must be sedated. Tissue is redressed with topical antimicrobial agents and gauze (Wong & Hockenberry-Eaton, 2001). Full-thickness, partial-thickness, or meshed skin grafts may be used to cover large burned areas. Wound healing procedures may need to be repeated if the grafts do not take. Skin grafting procedures using synthetic and animal skins have significantly improved the prognosis for skin healing. In severe burns, reconstructive surgeries often are needed to limit the long-term effects of burn injuries.

The team approach is essentially universal in burn care units in the United States. The American Burn Association has established guidelines for the personnel that make up a burn unit team (American Burn Association, 2001). The team consists of physicians with specialized training in burn care, nurses, occupational therapists, physical therapists, speech therapists, psychologists, and social workers. Occupational therapists are typically involved very early after the burn injury, often within 24 hours (Biggs, de Linde, Banaszewski, & Heinrich, 1998).

The major goals of burn rehabilitation are early skin coverage, correction of cosmetic damage, restoration of function, and integration back into the environment. During the acute period, positioning, hydrotherapy, splinting, active and passive ROM, and ADL modalities are used to prevent contractures and ensure optimal functional and physical outcomes. Many of these procedures are painful, and infection is a continued threat until all burned areas have been closed. During this period the child also experiences malaise and may be heavily sedated. Ongoing treatment goals include minimizing problems with scarring, optimizing active ROM, decreasing hypersensitivity, preventing contractures, ensuring good use of the hands, and optimizing skills for self-care and for home and school activities (Biggs et al., 1998). These goals include the use of various techniques, including fitting and maintenance of pressure garments, splinting, active and passive ROM, client and family education about scar formation, emotional support, massage to prevent hypertrophied scarring, and adaptation of ADLs.

Outcome measures used to determine successful burn rehabilitation include resumption of typical daily living skills (e.g., return to school), scar rating, and sensorimotor skills (e.g., ROM, gross and fine motor skills). Numerous rating scales have been developed to characterize or assess a scar. Reliable assessment of the scar surface (e.g., to evaluate healing) includes border height, thickness, and color of a scar (Yeong, 1997). Each of these four characteristics is rated from 1 to 4, with pictorial definitions used for each characterization; a composite score is then generated for the overall scar appearance

Scar appearance and location typically are believed to influence psychosocial adaptation. A scar on the face or neck has been correlated with lower self-esteem, less engagement in typical activities, and fewer interpersonal interactions; however, the accuracy of these beliefs is controversial (Wong & Hockenberry-Eaton, 2001). Ongoing scar massage techniques have been shown to be effective if initiated before the development of invasive hypertrophied scarring. Splinting continues to be used, primarily after limitations in ROM are noted, except for full-thickness or deep partial-thickness burns in which loss of ROM and the likelihood of scar contractures are greatest (Richard, Staley, Miller, & Warden, 1997). The process of scar remodeling, plastic surgery, and revision of skin grafts may require up to 2 years after a major injury.

Possibly more important measures are developmental and return to school outcomes. Developmental outcomes, especially language development and social skills, are delayed after burn injury in children, even if physical and functional skills are within normal limits (Gorga et al., 1999). Adjustment to school after a burn injury generally is successful regardless of the severity of the burn, provided the return to school reentry program is comprehensive (i.e., includes peer counseling, encouragement to return to school promptly, early contacts with the school, a comprehensive school plan, engagement of parents in reentry efforts, and social skills training) (Wong & Hockenberry-Eaton, 2001). Therapists can be involved in each step of the rehabilitation and return to school process, providing ongoing direct services, consultation, and monitoring.

SUMMARY

This chapter provided an overview of medical diagnoses in children who often receive occupational therapy services. Knowledge about the child's medical condition is important for developing appropriate intervention plans and for communicating with family and team members. Application of this information should consider that each

child's presentation of the diagnosis is unique and that the effect of the disease or disability on the child's function is highly influenced by environmental and developmental variables. The field of medicine continually expands, and the occupational therapist must stay abreast of new developments and current information. Best practice requires thorough research of each diagnosis incurred. To assist the student in researching the implication of the medical diagnoses discussed in this chapter, key references have been cited and should be consulted for additional information.

STUDY QUESTIONS

1 Describe the classification system for traumatic head injuries. How does such an injury affect the child's daily living function?

2 Describe osteogenesis imperfecta. What precautions should be taken in working with a child with this diagnosis?

3 Name two general goals of intervention for children with juvenile rheumatoid arthritis. What is the typical course of this disease?

4 Describe the pathology of two different neuromuscular conditions. Explain how impairment in functional performance results from the conditions.

5 List four functional performance consequences for children with cerebral palsy. Explain the difficulties that may be incurred in self-feeding in a child with (a) upper extremity spasticity and (b) upper extremity athetosis.

6 What are three impairments associated with myelomeningocele? Explain why a child with this diagnosis may have difficulty achieving independence in dressing.

7 Define *autism* and describe the primary problems that affect the autistic child's ability to engage in social play with peers.

8 The term *learning disabilities* is used to categorize a multitude of learning problems. Name two types of impairments classified as learning disabilities.

9 The common infections a mother can transmit to the fetus are called STORCH infections. What are these five infections? Briefly describe each.

10 List three types of cancer common to children. Explain the prognosis for each.

REFERENCES

Abel, E.L. (1998). *Fetal alcohol abuse syndrome*. New York: Plenum Press.

Adelson, P.D., & Kochanek, P.M. (1998). Head injury in children. *Journal of Child Neurology, 13* (1), 2-15.

Alemzadeh, R., & Wyatt, D.T. (2004). Diabetes mellitus in children. In R.E. Behrman, R.M. Kliegman, & H.B. Jenson (Eds.), *Nelson textbook of pediatrics* (pp. 1947-1972). Philadelphia: W.B. Saunders.

American Academy of Pediatrics (AAP). (1999). The management of minor closed head injury in children. *Pediatrics, 104,* 1407-1415.

American Burn Association. (2001). Guidelines for burn care. *Journal of Burn Care and Rehabilitation, 22* (5), 125-143.

American Psychiatric Association (APA) (2000). Diagnostic and Statistical Manual-Text Revision. Chicago, IL: Association.

Ayres, A.J., & Tickle, L.S. (1980). Hyperresponsivity to touch and vestibular stimuli as a predictor of positive response to sensory integration procedures by autistic children. *American Journal of Occupational Therapy, 34,* 375-381.

Baird, G., Cass, H., & Slonims, V. (2003). Diagnosis of autism. *British Medical Journal, 327* (7413), 488-493.

Ballard, S., Bolan, M., Burton, M., Snyder, S., & Martin, D. (1997). The neurological basis of attention deficit hyperactivity disorder. *Adolescence, 32,* 855-862.

Barkley, R.A. (1997). Inhibition, sustained attention, and executive functions: Constructing a unifying theory of ADHD. *Psychological Bulletin, 121,* 65-94.

Barkley, R.A. (1998). *Attention deficit hyperactivity disorder: A handbook for diagnosis and treatment* (2nd ed.). New York: Guilford.

Barkley, R.A. (2003). Issues in the diagnosis of attention-deficit/hyperactivity disorder in children. *Brain & Development, 25* (2), 77-83.

Batshaw, M.L. (2002). Chromosomes and heredity. In M.L. Batshaw (Ed.), *Children with disabilities* (pp. 3-26). Baltimore: Brookes.

Batshaw, M.L., & Shapiro, B. (2002). Mental retardation. In M.L. Batshaw (Ed.), *Children with disabilities* (pp. 287-305). Baltimore: Brookes.

Batshaw, M.L., & Tuchman, M. (2002). PKU and other inborn errors of metabolism. In M.L. Batshaw (Ed.), *Children with disabilities.* Baltimore: Brookes.

Bauman, M.L. (1996). Brief report: Neuroanatomic observations of the brain in pervasive developmental disorders. *Journal of Autism and Developmental Disorders, 26,* 199-203.

Bernstein, D. (2004). Congenital heart disease. In R.E. Behrman, R.M. Kliegman, & H.B. Jenson (Eds.), *Nelson textbook of pediatrics* (17th ed.). Philadelphia: W.B. Saunders.

Bespalova, I.N., & Buxbaum, J.D. (2003). Disease susceptibility genes for autism. *Annals of Medicine, 35* (4), 274-281.

Biggs, K.S., de Linde, L., Banaszewski, M., & Heinrich, J.J. (1998). Determining the current roles of physical and occupational therapists in burn care. *Journal of Burn Care and Rehabilitation, 19* (5), 442-449.

Boat, T.F. (2004). Cystic fibrosis. In R.E. Behrman, R.M. Kliegman, & H.B. Jenson (Eds.), *Nelson textbook of pediatrics* (pp. 1437-1450). Philadelphia: W.B. Saunders.

Brain Trauma Foundation. (2000). Glasgow Coma Scale. *Journal of Neurotrauma, 17* (6-7), 573-581.

Brook, M.M. (1998). The cardiovascular system. In R.E. Berhman & R.M. Kliegman (Eds.), *Nelson essentials of pediatrics* (3rd ed., pp. 497-544). Philadelphia: W.B. Saunders.

Burack, J.A., Hodapp, R.M., & Zigler, E. (1998). *Handbook of mental retardation.* New York: Cambridge University Press.

Butler, C., & Darrah, J. (2001). Effects of neurodevelopmental treatment for cerebral palsy: an AACPDM evidence report. *Developmental Medicine and Child Neurology, 43,* 778-790.

Cassidy, L.D., Potoka, D.A., Adelson, P.D., & Ford, H.R. (2003). Development of a novel method to predict disability after head trauma in children. *Journal of Pediatric Surgery, 38* (3), 482-485.

Centers for Disease Control and Prevention (CDC). (2002). *Metropolitan Atlanta congenital defects program.* Atlanta: Author.

Chakrabarti, S., & Fombonne, E. (2001). Pervasive developmental disorders in preschool children. *Journal of the American Medical Association, 285,* 3093-3099.

Chance, P.F., Ashizawa, T., Hoffman, E.P., & Crawford, T.O. (1998). Molecular basis of neuromuscular diseases. *Physical Medicine & Rehabilitation Clinics of North America, 9,* 49-81.

Church, M.W., & Abel, E.L. (1998). Fetal alcohol syndrome: Hearing, speech, language, and vestibular disorders. *Obstetrics and Gynecology Clinics of North America, 25,* 85-97.

Cohen, D.J., & Volkmar, F.R. (Eds.). (1997). *Handbook of autism and pervasive developmental disorders* (2nd ed.). New York: John Wiley & Sons.

Coles, C. (1994). Critical periods for prenatal alcohol exposure. *National Institutes of Health: Alcohol Health and Research World, 18* (1), 112-115.

Curry, C.R. (2002). An approach to clinical genetics. In R. Rudolph, R.K. Kamei, & K.J. Overby (Eds.), *Rudolph's fundamentals of pediatrics* (3rd ed.). New York: McGraw-Hill.

Damico, J., Damico, S., & Armstrong, M. (1999). Attention deficit hyperactivity disorder and communication disorders: Issues and clinical practices. *Child and Adolescent Psychiatric Clinics of North America, 8,* 37-60.

DiScala, C., Lescohier, I., & Barthel, M., & Li (1998). Injuries to children with attention deficit hyperactivity disorder. *Pediatrics, 102,* 1415-1421.

Dubowitz, V. (1999). Forty years of neuromuscular disease: a historical perspective. *Journal of Child Neurology, 14* (1), 26-28.

Elia, J., Ambrosini, P., & Rapoport, J. (1999). Treatment of attention deficit hyperactivity disorder. *New England Journal of Medicine, 34,* 780-788.

Emond, S., Camargo, C.J., & Nowak, R. (1998). 1997 National asthma education and prevention program guidelines: a practical summary for emergency physicians. *Annals of Emergency Medicine, 31,* 579-589.

Faraone, S., & Biederman, J. (1998). Neurobiology of attention deficit hyperactivity disorder. *Biological Psychiatry, 44,* 951-958.

Fombonne, E. (2003). Epidemiological surveys of autism and other pervasive developmental disorders: an update. *Journal of Autism and Developmental Disorders, 33* (4), 365-382.

Garland, E. (1998). Pharmacotherapy of adolescent attention deficit hyperactivity disorder: challenges, choices and caveats. *Journal of Psychopharmacology, 12,* 385-395.

Gillberg, C. (2003). Deficits in attention, motor control, and perception: A brief review. *Archives of Disease in Childhood, 88* (10), 904-910.

Gorga, D., Johnson, J., Bentley, A., Silverburg, R., Glassman, M., Madden, M., et al. (1999). The physical, functional, and developmental outcome of pediatric burn survivors from 1 to 12 months post-injury. *Journal of Burn Care and Rehabilitation, 20* (2), 171-178.

Grandin, T. (1996). *Thinking in pictures and other reports from my life with autism.* New York: Vintage Books.

Greenhill, L. (1998). Diagnosing attention deficit/hyperactivity disorder in children. *Journal of Clinical Psychiatry, 59* (Suppl 7), 31-41.

Haddad, G.G., & Fontan, J.J.P. (2004). Respiratory system. In R.E. Behrman, R.M. Kliegman, & H.B. Jenson (Eds.), *Nelson textbook of pediatrics* (pp. 1357-1385). Philadelphia: W.B. Saunders.

Hallum, A. (2001). Neuromuscular disease. In D. Umphred (Ed.), *Neurological rehabilitation.* St. Louis: Mosby.

Hammill, D.D. (1990). On defining learning disabilities: An emerging consensus. *Journal of Learning Disabilities, 23* (2), 31-41.

Haydel, M.J. (2003). Prediction of intracranial injury in children aged 5 years and older with loss of consciousness after minor head injury due to nontrivial mechanisms. *Annals of Emergency Medicine, 42* (4), 507-514.

Hemingway, C., Freeman, J.M., & Pillas, D.J., & Pyzik (2001). The ketogenic diet. *Pediatrics, 108,* 898-905.

Hogan, D.P., Rogers, M.L., & Msall, M.E. (2000). Functional limitations and key indicators of well-being in children with disability. *Archives of Pediatrics & Adolescent Medicine, 154* (10), 1042-1048.

Horowitz, P., & Haritos, C. (1998). The organism and understanding the environment. In J.A. Burack, R.M. Hodapp, & E. Zigler (Eds.), *Handbook of mental retardation and development* (pp. 20-40). New York: Cambridge University Press.

Huebner, R.A. (1992). Autistic disorder: a neuropsychological enigma. *American Journal of Occupational Therapy, 46,* 487-501.

Ingram, S., Hechtman, L., & Morgenstern, G. (1999). Outcome issues in ADHD: Adolescent and adult long-term outcome. *Mental Retardation and Developmental Disabilities, 5,* 243-250.

Jacobson, S.W. (1998). Specificity of neurobehavioral outcomes associated with prenatal alcohol exposure. *Alcoholism, Clinical & Experimental Research, 22* (2), 313-320.

Johnson, D.L. (2001). Hydrocephalus. In R.A. Hoekelman, H.M. Adam, N.M. Nelson, M. Weitzman, & M.H. Wilson (Eds.), *Primary pediatric care textbook* (pp. 1438-1457). St. Louis: Mosby.

Johnston, M.V. (2004a). Movement disorders. In R.E. Behrman, R.M. Kliegman, & H.B. Jenson (Eds.), *Nelson textbook of pediatrics* (17th ed., pp. 2019-2023). Philadelphia: W.B. Saunders.

Johnston, M.V. (2004b). Encephalopathies. In R.E. Behrman, R.M. Kliegman, & H.B. Jenson (Eds.), *Nelson textbook of pediatrics* (17th ed., pp. 2023-2029). Philadelphia: W.B. Saunders.

Kanner, L. (1943). Autistic disturbances of affective contact. *Nervous Child, 2,* 217-250.

Keenan, H.T., Runyan, D.K., Marshall, S.W., Nocera, M.A., Merten, D.F., & Sinal, S.H. (2003). A population-based study of inflicted traumatic brain injury in young children. *Journal of the America Medical Association, 290* (5), 621-626.

Kinnear, K.J. (2003). Purkinje cell vulnerability and autism: A possible etiological connection. *Brain & Development, 25* (6), 377-382.

Klin, A., & Volkmar, F.R. (1997). Asperger's syndrome. In D. Cohen & F. Volkmar (Eds.), *Handbook of autism and pervasive developmental disorders* (2nd ed., pp. 94-122). New York: John Wiley & Sons.

Langston, C., Cooper, E.R., & Goldfarb, J., et al. (2001). Human immunodeficiency virus–related mortality in infants and children. *Pediatrics, 107,* 328-338.

Leet, A.I., Dormans, J.P., & Tosi, L.L. (2002). Muscles, bones, and nerves. In M.L. Batshaw (Ed.), *Children with developmental disabilities.* Baltimore: Brookes.

Liptak, G.S. (2002). Neural tube defects. In M.L. Batshaw (Ed.), *Children with disabilities* (pp. 467-492). Baltimore: Brookes.

Loewen, P., Steinbok, P., Holsti, L., & MacKay, M. (1998). Upper extremity performance and self-care skill changes in children with spastic cerebral palsy. *Pediatric Neurosurgery, 29* (4), 191-198.

Mahaffey, K.R. (1992). Exposure to lead in childhood. *New England Journal of Medicine, 327,* 1308-1309.

Mahoney, W., Szatmari, P., MacLean, J., Bryson, S., Bartolucci, G., Walter, S., et al. (1998). Reliability and accuracy of differentiating pervasive developmental disorder subtypes. *Journal of the American Academy of Psychiatry, 37,* 278-285.

Maldonado, Y. (2004). Rubella. In R.E. Behrman, R. Kliegman, & H.B. Jenson (Eds.), *Nelson textbook of pediatrics* (pp. 1032-1034). Philadelphia: W.B. Saunders.

Mattson, S.N., & Riley, E.P. (1998). A review of neurobehavioral deficits in children with fetal alcohol syndrome or prenatal exposure to alcohol. *Alcoholism, Clinical & Experimental Research, 22* (2), 279-294.

Mattson, S.N., Riley, E.P., Gramling, L., Delis, D.C., & Jones, K.L. (1998). Neuropsychological comparison of alcohol-exposed children with or without physical features of fetal alcohol syndrome. *Neuropsychology, 12,* 146-153.

Mazzola, C.A., & Adelson, P.D. (2002). Critical care management of head trauma in children. *Critical Care Medicine, 30* (Suppl 11), S393-S401.

McLaughlin, J., Bjornson, K., Astley, S., Hays, R.M., Hoffinger, S.A., Armantrout, E.A., et al. (1998). Selective dorsal rhizotomy: Efficacy and safety in an investigator-masked, randomized clinical trial. *Developmental Medicine and Child Neurology, 40,* 220-232.

McLeod, R., & Remington, J.S. (2004). Toxoplasmosis. In R.E. Behrman, R.M. Kliegman, & H.B. Jenson (Eds.), *Nelson textbook of pediatrics* (pp. 1144-1154). Philadelphia: W.B. Saunders.

Menkes, J.H. (2001). *Textbook of childhood neurology.* Baltimore: Williams & Wilkins.

Mercugliano, M. (1999). What is ADHD? *Pediatric Clinics of North America, 46,* 831-843.

Meyer, G.A., & Batshaw, M.L. (2002). Fragile X syndrome. In M.L. Batshaw (Ed.), *Children with disabilities* (pp. 321-331). Baltimore: Brookes.

Michaud, L.J., Semel-Concepcion, J., Duhaime, A., & Lazar, M.F. (2002). Traumatic brain injury. In M.L. Batshaw (Ed.), *Children with disabilities* (pp. 525-545). Baltimore: Brookes.

Miller, M.L., & Cassidy, J.T. (2004). Juvenile rheumatoid arthritis. In R.E. Behrman, R.M. Kliegman, & H.B. Jenson (Eds.), *Nelson textbook of pediatrics* (17th ed., pp. 799-805). Philadelphia: W.B. Saunders.

Miller, T. (2003). Measles-mumps-rubella vaccine and the development of autism. *Seminars in Pediatric Infectious Diseases, 14* (3), 199-206.

Montgomery, R.R., & Scott, J.P. (2004). Hemorrhagic and thrombotic disease. In R.E. Behrman, R.M. Kliegman, & H.B. Jenson (Eds.), *Nelson textbook of pediatrics* (pp. 1651-1674). Philadelphia: W.B. Saunders.

Morrissy, R.T., & Weinstein, S.L. (2001). *Lovell and Winter's pediatric orthopaedics* (5th ed.). Philadelphia: Lippincott Williams & Wilkins.

Morrow, S.E., Smith, D.L., Cairns, B.A., Howell, P.D., Nakayama, D.K., & Peterson, H.D. (1996). Etiology and outcome of pediatric burns. *Journal of Pediatric Surgery, 31* (3), 329-333.

Murphy, J.T., Purdue, G.F., Hunt, J.L., & Hicks, B.A. (1997). Burn injury. In D.L. Levin & F.C. Morrissy (Eds.), *Essentials of pediatric intensive care* (pp. 1010-1021). New York: Churchill-Livingstone.

National Institutes of Health (NIH). (1997). *Expert panel report: Guidelines for the diagnosis and management of asthma* (No. 97-4051). Bethesda, MD: National Heart, Lung, and Blood Institute.

Nelson, C.A. (2001). Cerebral palsy. In D. Umphred (Ed.), *Neurological rehabilitation* (4th ed., pp. 259-286). St. Louis: Mosby.

Nemethy, M. (1997). Attention deficit/hyperactivity disorder: A guide to diagnosis and treatment. *Advance for Nurse Practitioners, 5,* 22-25, 29.

Park, M.K., & George, R. (2002). *Pediatric cardiology for practitioners* (4th ed.). St. Louis: Mosby.

Park, T.S., & Owen, J.H. (1992). Surgical management of spastic diplegia in cerebral palsy. *New England Journal of Medicine, 326,* 745-749.

Pellegrino, L. (2002). Cerebral palsy. In M.L. Batshaw (Ed.), *Children with disabilities* (pp. 443-466). Baltimore: Brookes.

Prober, C.G. (2004). Central nervous system infections. In R.E. Behrman, R.M. Kliegman, & H.B. Jenson (Eds.), *Nelson textbook of pediatrics* (pp. 2038-2047). Philadelphia: W.B. Saunders.

Rabinovitch, N., & Gelfand, E. (1998). New approaches to the treatment of childhood asthma. *Current Opinion in Pediatrics, 10,* 243-249.

Richard, R., Staley, M., Miller, S., & Warden, G. (1997). To splint or not to splint. *Journal of Burn Care and Rehabilitation, 18* (1), 64-71.

Robinson, L.K. (2004). Marfan syndrome. In R.E. Behrman, R.M. Kliegman, & H.B. Jenson (Eds.), *Nelson textbook of pediatrics* (17th ed., pp. 2338-2340). Philadelphia: W.B. Saunders.

Robison, L., Sclar, D., Skaer, T., & Galin, R. (1999). National trends in the prevalence of attention deficit/hyperactivity disorder and the prescribing of methylphenidate among school-age children: 1990-1995. *Clinical Pediatrics, 38,* 209-217.

Rodier, P.M. (2000). The early origins of autism. *Scientific American, 282* (2), 56-63.

Rogers, S.L., Coe, C.L., & Karaszewski, J.W. (1998). Immune consequences of stroke and cerebral palsy in adults. *Journal of Neuroimmunology, 91,* 113-120.

Roizen, N.J. (2002). Down syndrome. In M.L. Batshaw (Ed.), *Children with disabilities* (pp. 307-320). Baltimore: Brookes.

Rudolph, A.M., Kamei, R.K., & Overby, K.J. (2002). *Fundamentals of pediatrics* (3rd ed.). New York: McGraw-Hill.

Salter, R.B. (1999). *Textbook of disorders and injuries of the musculoskeletal system* (3rd ed.). Baltimore: Lippincott Williams & Wilkins.

Sampson, P., Streissguth, A., Bookstein, F., Little, R., Clarren, S., Dehaene, P., et al. (1997). Incidence of fetal alcohol syndrome and prevalence of alcohol-related neurodevelopmental disorder. *Teratology, 56,* 317-326.

Sarnat, H.B. (2004). Neuromuscular disorders. In R.E. Behrman, R.M. Kliegman, & H.B. Jenson (Eds.), *Nelson textbook of pediatrics.* Philadelphia: W.B. Saunders.

Schneider, J.W., & Krosschell, K.J. (2001). Congenital spinal cord injury. In D. Umphred (Ed.), *Neurological rehabilitation* (pp. 449-476). St. Louis: Mosby.

Shapiro, B., Church, R.P., & Lewis, M.E.B. (2002). Specific learning disabilities. In M.L. Batshaw (Ed.), *Children with disabilities* (pp. 417-442). Baltimore: Brookes.

Spiegel, H.M.L., & Bonwit, A.M. (2002). HIV infection in children. In M.L. Batshaw (Ed.), *Children with disabilities* (pp. 123-139). Baltimore: Brookes.

Stanley, F.J., Blair, E., & Alberman, E. (2000). *Cerebral palsies: Epidemiology and causal pathways* (Vol. 151). New York: Cambridge University Press.

Stein, M.A., Efron, L.A., Schiff, W.B., & Glanzman, M. (2002). Attention deficits and hyperactivity. In M.L. Batshaw (Ed.), *Children with disabilities* (pp. 389-416). Baltimore: Brookes.

Steinberg, M.H. (1996). Review: Sickle cell disease—present and future treatment. *Journal of Medical Science, 312* (4), 166-174.

Steinbok, P., Reiner, A., & Kestle, J.R. (1997). Therapeutic electrical stimulation following selective posterior rhizotomy in children with spastic diplegic cerebral palsy: A randomized clinical trial. *Developmental Medicine and Child Neurology, 39* (8), 515-520.

Stoll, B.J., & Kliegman, R.M. (2004a). Respiratory tract disorders. In R.E. Behrman, R.M. Kliegman, & H.B. Jenson (Eds.), *Nelson textbook of pediatrics* (17th ed.). Philadelphia: W.B. Saunders.

Stoll, B.J., & Kliegman, R.M. (2004b). Fetal and neonatal infant: Nervous system disorders. In R.E. Behrman, R.M. Kliegman, & H.B. Jenson (Eds.), *Nelson textbook of pediatrics* (17th ed., pp. 561-569). Philadelphia: W.B. Saunders.

Thompson, G.H. (2004). Bone and joint disorders. In R.E. Behrman, R.M. Kliegman, & H.B. Jenson (Eds.), *Nelson textbook of pediatrics* (17th ed., pp. 2251-2302). Philadelphia: W.B. Saunders.

Towbin, K.E., Mauk, J.E., & Batshaw, M.L. (2002). Pervasive developmental disorders. In M.L. Batshaw (Ed.), *Children with disabilities* (5th ed., pp. 365-387). Baltimore: Brookes.

Trombly, C.A., & Radomski, M.V. (Eds.). (2002). *Occupational therapy for physical dysfunction* (5th ed.). Baltimore: Williams & Wilkins.

Trumble, T.E. (2000). *Principles of hand surgery and therapy.* Philadelphia: W.B. Saunders.

Tsai, L.Y. (1999). Psychopharmacology in autism. *Psychosomatic Medicine, 61* (5), 651-665.

Victor, M., & Ropper, A.H. (2001). *Principles of neurology* (7th ed.). New York: McGraw-Hill.

Voit, T. (1998). Congenital muscular dystrophies: 1997 update. *Brain & Development, 20* (2), 65-74.

Wagner, C.L., Katikaneni, L.D., Cox, T.H., & Ryan, R.M. (1998). The impact of prenatal drug exposure on the neonate. *Obstetrics and Gynecology Clinics of North America, 25* (1), 169-194.

Weinstein, S. (2002). Epilepsy. In M.L. Batshaw (Ed.), *Children with disabilities* (5th ed., pp. 493-523). Baltimore: Brookes.

Wong, D.L. (Ed.). (2001). *Essentials of pediatric nursing* (5th ed.). St. Louis: Mosby.

Wunsch, M.J., Conlon, C.J., & Scheidt, P.C. (2002). Substance abuse. In M.L. Batshaw (Ed.), *Children with disabilities* (pp. 107-122). Baltimore: Brookes.

Yeong, E.K. (1997). Improved burn scar assessment with use of a new scar-rating scale. *Journal of Burn Care and Rehabilitation, 18* (4), 353-364.

Zagon, I.S., & Slotkin, T.A. (Eds.). (1992). *Maternal substance abuse and the developing nervous system.* San Diego: Academic Press.

Zametkin, A., & Ernst, M. (1999). Problems in the management of attention deficit hyperactivity disorder. *New England Journal of Medicine, 340,* 40-46.

Zametkin, A., & Liotta, W. (1998). The neurobiology of attention deficit/hyperactivity disorder. *Journal of Clinical Psychiatry, 59* (Suppl 7), 17-23.

SUGGESTED READINGS

Agency for Health Care Policy and Research, Sickle Cell Disease Guideline Panel. (1993). *Sickle cell disease: Screening, diagnosis, management, and counseling in newborns and infants* (No. 93-0562). Rockville, MD: Author.

American Psychiatric Association. (2000). *Diagnostic and statistical manual of mental disorders* (4th ed.). Washington, DC: Author.

Barnes, J., Abbot, N., Harkness, E., & Ernst, E. (1999). Articles on complementary medicine in the mainstream medical literature: an investigation of MEDLINE, 1966 through 1996. *Archives of Internal Medicine, 159,* 1721-1725.

Batshaw, M.L. (Ed.). (2002). *Children with disabilities* (5th ed.). Baltimore: Brookes.

Behrman, R.E., Kliegman, R.M., & Jenson, H.B. (Eds.). (2004). *Nelson textbook of pediatrics* (17th ed.). Philadelphia: W.B. Saunders.

Menkes, J.H., & Sarnat, H.B. (2000). *Textbook of child neurology* (7th ed.). Baltimore: Lippincott Williams & Wilkins

Morrissy, R.T., & Weinstein, S.L. (Eds.). (2001). *Lovell and Winter's pediatric orthopaedics* (5th ed.). Philadelphia: Lippincott-Raven.

Stedman, T. (2000). *Taber's cyclopedic medical dictionary* (27th ed.). Baltimore: Lippincott Williams & Wilkins.

Teasdale, T.W., & Engberg, A.W. (2003). Cognitive dysfunction in young men following head injury in childhood and adolescence: a population study. *Journal of Neurology, Neurosurgery, and Psychiatry, 74* (7), 933-936.

Wong, D.L., Hockenberry-Eaton, M., Wilson, D., Winkelstein, M.L., & Schwartz, P. (Eds.). (2001). *Wong's essentials of pediatric nursing* (6th ed.). St. Louis: Mosby.

Occupational Therapy Evaluation in Pediatrics

7 Purposes, Processes, and Methods of Evaluation

Katherine B. Stewart

KEY TERMS

Evaluation
Occupational profile
Analysis of occupa-
   tional performance
Screening
Comprehensive
   evaluation
Standardized tests
Norm-referenced
   measures

Skilled observations
Criterion-referenced
   measures
Reevaluation
Clinical research
Evaluation plan
Functionality
Ecologic assessments
Interview
Arena assessment

CHAPTER OBJECTIVES

1 Apply the Occupational Therapy Practice Framework to the evaluation process for children and
   their families.
2 Define the key terms used in pediatric occupational therapy evaluations.
3 List four primary reasons evaluations are
   conducted.
4 Discuss the variety of decisions pediatric occupational therapists make throughout the evaluation
   process.
5 Describe the specific steps pediatric occupational
   therapists follow in the process of evaluating
   children.
6 Describe the primary evaluation methods commonly used in pediatric occupational therapy.
7 Discuss the major factors therapists should consider when selecting evaluation methods and
   measures.
8 Apply the knowledge gained in this chapter to
   specific case studies of children who have or are
   at risk for disabilities.

Those who observe human behavior must be vigilant when examining the details of the behavior and when relating those details to each other in the context of that behavior. Occupational therapists involved in the evaluation of children face this challenge daily. To fully examine a child's occupational performance, the therapist evaluates the child's specific developmental skills and analyzes how his or her performance is influenced by the physical demands and social expectations of the home, school, and community environments. After identifying the areas of occupation most important to the child and the caregivers, the occupational therapist assesses the child's performance skills and performance patterns essential to his or her participation in the identified areas. To thoroughly evaluate the child's occupational performance, the occupational therapist must consider the context of the child, the demands of the activity, and the physical, cognitive, and psychosocial factors affecting the child.

The evaluation process is one of the most fundamental, yet complex, aspects of occupational therapy services. The American Occupational Therapy Association (AOTA) defines evaluation as "the process of obtaining and interpreting data necessary for understanding the individual, system, or situation (American Occupational Therapy Association" [AOTA], 1998). How the occupational therapist views this evaluation process, whether the therapist is open to new ways of understanding the child and family, which methods and measures the therapist selects to evaluate the child, and how the therapist interprets and documents the evaluation data all contribute to important decisions regarding the type and degree of occupational therapy intervention to be provided for the child and family.

This chapter describes the occupational therapy evaluation process for children. The first section provides a conceptual foundation for evaluating children based on the Occupational Therapy Practice Framework (AOTA, 2002). The second section outlines the purposes of evaluation and includes specific examples of evaluations commonly used in pediatric occupational therapy practice. The third section describes the evaluation process and illustrates it with a case example. The fourth section explains the general methods, measures, and principles used in selecting and administering pediatric occupational therapy evaluations.

TABLE 7-1 Methods and Measures for Kevin's Evaluation

Occupational Therapy Practice Framework	Methods and Measures
OCCUPATIONAL PROFILE	Initial teacher interview
	Initial phone interview with parent
	Direct observation of Kevin at school
	Interview with Kevin about his interests
ANALYSIS OF OCCUPATIONAL PERFORMANCE	
Activities of daily living	Battelle Developmental Inventory—Adaptive Domain
PLAY	Test of playfulness
Performance skills (motor and process)	Peabody Developmental Motor Scales (PDMS-2)
	Sensory Profile
Context(s)	Home Observation for Measurement of the Environment (Early Childhood HOME)
Activity demand	Skilled observation of Kevin performing a classroom activity
Client factor(s)	Developmental Test of Visual Perception (DTVP-2)

performance in the context of his home and school environments.

In summary, the occupational therapist carefully selects and administers various methods and measures to evaluate the child's participation in occupations, the child's performance of specific skills and activities, and the context or contexts in which the child performs everyday tasks.

Evaluation Purposes

Occupational therapists evaluate children and their environments to gather information helpful in making decisions about intervention services. This section discusses the decisions that therapists make during the various steps of careful screening and comprehensive evaluation of children who have or are at risk for disabilities.

The six primary purposes of occupational therapy evaluation are as follows:

1 To decide whether the child should be further evaluated using more comprehensive assessments
2 To decide whether the child is eligible for occupational therapy services
3 To assist in the diagnostic process
4 To develop an intervention plan
5 To evaluate the child's progress in therapy and determine whether further therapy is warranted
6 To research the efficacy of intervention services and clinical outcomes or to describe patterns of development and functional changes in children with specific diagnoses

Screening

The primary reason for screening children is to determine whether they warrant further, more comprehensive evaluation. Occupational therapists may participate in two levels of screening. The first level (type I) is a basic screening in which the child's general health (e.g., vision and hearing), growth (e.g., weight and height), and development (e.g., physical, social, language, and personal and adaptive skills) are checked. In some settings, such as public school programs, occupational therapists may participate in the screening of large numbers of children to determine which children should receive further testing. Public policies, including the Individuals with Disabilities Education Act (IDEA) (1997), Head Start, and Medicaid programs for children, mandate early screening to identify children at risk for disabilities. Some examples of type I screening of young children include the Ages & Stages Questionnaires (Bricker, Squires, & Mounts, 1995), the Bayley Infant Neurodevelopmental Screener (Aylward, 1999), the Denver Developmental Screening Test-II (Denver-II) (Frankenburg, & Dodds, 1992), and the (First STEp (Screening Test for Evaluating Preschoolers) (Miller, 1993).

More frequently, pediatric therapists are involved in the second level of child screening (type II). This type of screening usually occurs after a health care professional or teacher has identified the child as being at risk for developmental or functional deficits. One example of a type II measure is the Harris Infant Neuromotor Test (HINT), a new screening tool designed to identify neuromotor and behavioral concerns in at-risk infants between 3 and 12 months of age (Harris, Megens, Backman, & Hayes, 2003). At this point in the screening process, the therapist, sometimes with other interdisciplinary team members, determines whether the child is a candidate for more comprehensive testing in specific developmental or functional areas.

For example, type II screening of an older child might proceed as follows: A first grade teacher observes her

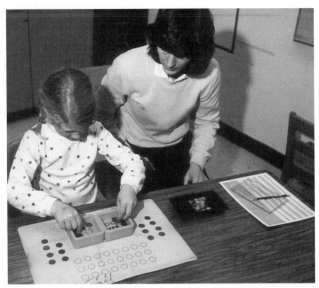

FIGURE 7-3 Child completing an item on the Bruininks-Oseretsky Test of Motor Proficiency.

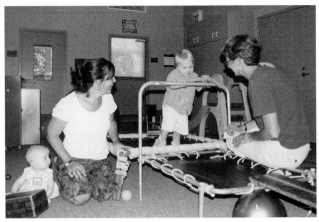

FIGURE 7-4 Therapist interviewing a parent about the child's preferred play activities.

student's unusual responses to everyday sensory experiences (e.g., finger painting) and his motor clumsiness on the playground at recess. The child is referred to the occupational therapist for screening to determine if he needs a more comprehensive evaluation. In this case, the therapist may choose the Short Sensory Profile (Dunn, 1999) and the Bruininks-Oseretsky Test of Motor Proficiency (Short Form) (Bruininks, 1978) (Figure 7-3) to screen the child and determine the need for further evaluation.

In addition to administering standardized screening tests, occupational therapists gather pertinent information from parents and teachers and through informal observations of a child's performance in his or her natural environments (e.g., classroom, playground, and home). Regardless of the setting and the level of screening (type I or type II), the therapist should consider the following points when screening children to determine whether further, more comprehensive evaluation is warranted.

1 Standardized screening tools are implemented whenever possible to ensure that the results of the screening are reliable and valid. Standardized tests require uniform procedures for administration and scoring. Chapter 8 provides more information on the use of standardized instruments.

2 In addition to standardized screening tools, the therapist gathers relevant information from the child and the child's teachers, parents, or other caregivers (Figure 7-4).

3 Information gathered during the screening process includes the child's performance across various developmental domains (e.g., motor, social, self-help) and in different environments to substantiate the need for further evaluation.

4 Screening tools should be carefully evaluated for their cultural validity, and the results should be interpreted cautiously when administered to children from diverse cultural backgrounds. A few instruments, such as the Miller Assessment for Preschoolers (Miller, 1988), have established norms for different ethnic populations.

Comprehensive Evaluation

In pediatric occupational therapy, a comprehensive evaluation of a child might be conducted for several reasons. Five reasons, or purposes (i.e., determination of eligibility for services, assistance in the diagnostic process, intervention planning, reevaluation, and clinical research) are discussed in this section. The therapist should keep in mind the purpose of the comprehensive evaluation because the purpose determines the different methods and measures that may be appropriate for the evaluation. Common assessment tools that occupational therapists use with children are listed in Appendix 7-A.

Eligibility Purposes

When children are evaluated for the purpose of determining their eligibility for services, standardized measures are used to ensure that the test results are reliable and valid. Many public school systems mandate the use of norm-referenced tests by school personnel, including occupational therapists, when qualifying students for special services. For example, in the Washington state public schools, children between 3 and 6 years of age must perform at least two standard deviations below the mean on a standardized norm-referenced test in one or more of the five developmental areas (including cognitive, social or emotional, physical, communication, and adaptive or self-help) to qualify in the developmentally delayed category (Washington Administrative Code, 1998).

Standardized, norm-referenced measures are helpful in determining how the individual child's performance compares with that of children in the normative sample. However, the therapist must use caution when interpreting the performance of a child with a disability on standardized tests. Often these instruments do not include children with disabilities in their standardization sample (Farran, 2000). For example, a child with Down syndrome may score more than two standard deviations below the mean for his or her chronologic age, but this standard score does not reveal how he or she performs relative to other children with Down syndrome.

The IDEA (1997) mandates that "Any assessment and evaluation procedures and materials that are used are selected and administered so as not to be racially or culturally discriminatory" (Section 303.323). Unfortunately, many measures that are standardized on the U.S. population have limited cultural validity for children who have recently immigrated to the United States and for children from ethnic groups not fully represented in the U.S. norms.

In summary, standardized tools have an important but limited function in the occupational therapy evaluation process. Some service systems may require their use for determining a child's eligibility. However, standard scores, when used alone, do not provide a complete picture of a child and may be misleading, particularly for children with established disabilities or those from diverse cultural or ethnic backgrounds.

Diagnostic Purposes

Often a child is referred to occupational therapy by another health care provider or educator to gain more information about why the child demonstrates performance deficits. This situation calls for a comprehensive evaluation by the occupational therapist. To assist in the diagnostic process, the therapist considers a combination of norm-referenced tools, caregiver interviews, and skilled observations. Skilled observations (Figures 7-5 and 7-6) are nonstandardized methods developed by therapists to gather objective data on the quality, frequency, and duration of the child's performance. The Evaluation Methods section in this chapter presents more specific information about the use of skilled observation. Box 7-1 provides a sample form for skilled observations of a child's neuromotor status. Scores from a norm-referenced measure provide the "anchor" for the child's developmental status relative to typically developing children. The therapist's skilled observations of a child's performance, however, provide rich information on the quality of performance and possible reasons for the child's delayed or deficient performance on the norm-referenced test. To illustrate how norm-referenced

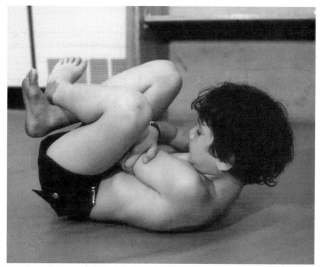

FIGURE 7-5 Skilled observation of a child in supine flexion.

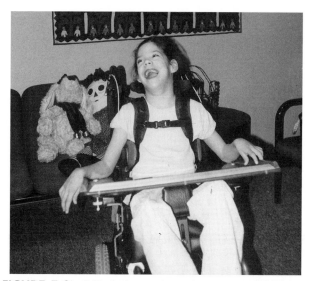

FIGURE 7-6 Skilled observation of a child's posture in a wheelchair.

measures are used in combination with nonstandardized, skilled observations, the following case example is provided.

Case Example. Jason is an 8-year-old boy with mild motor coordination deficits. The therapist administered a norm-referenced tool, the Sensory Integration and Praxis Tests (Ayres, 1989), to obtain standard scores on his sensory and motor performance (Figure 7-7). In addition, through skilled observations, the therapist obtained qualitative data regarding Jason's muscle tone, righting and equilibrium reactions, posture, and bilateral hand use. Combining this information enabled the examiners to understand Jason's sensory processing and sensory integration and helped them determine whether intervention was warranted.

BOX 7-1 Checklist for Skilled Observations of Neuromotor Status

As the child plays or moves, observe as many of the following functional gross and fine motor skills as possible. Note the child's posture, coordination, and transitional movement patterns. If a question or concern arises regarding the quality of movement or posture during functional gross and fine motor activities, examine the child's muscle tone, primitive reflexes, and automatic reactions by means of direct testing and physical handling.

FUNCTIONAL GROSS MOTOR SKILLS
- Sit (with or without support?)
- Pivot in prone (coordinated use of all four extremities?)
- Crawl (on stomach? in quadruped?)
- Stand (with or without support?)
- Cruise along furniture
- Walk (with or without support?)
- Ascend and descend stairs (with or without support? alternating feet?)
- Jump with both feet (in place? forward?)
- Run

TRANSITIONAL MOVEMENT PATTERNS
- Rolling (prone to supine, supine to prone) with rotation?
- Sit to prone with rotation?
- Prone to sit with rotation?
- Supine to sit with rotation?
- Pull to stand from half-kneel?
- Stand to sit with control?

FUNCTIONAL FINE MOTOR SKILLS
- Reach (bilateral? unilateral? arm preference?)
- Prehension patterns (whole hand grasp? partial hand grasp? digital grasp? pincer grasp?)
- Release of objects (support of hand on surface? well controlled?)
- Transfer of objects between hands
- Manipulation of objects within the hand
- Crossing midline of body
- Bilateral hand use
- Hand preference (hand dominance established?)
- Use of scissors (previous experience?)
- Use of writing utensil (crayon, marker, and pencil; note type and amount of pressure of grasp)
- Ability to button and use other fasteners on clothing
- Ability to use eating utensils

POSTURE (SYMMETRY AND ALIGNMENT)
- Supine
- Prone
- Sit
- Stand
- Prone extension
- Supine flexion

MUSCLE TONE
- At rest? During movement?
- Hypertonia? Hypotonia? Fluctuating tone?
- Abnormal tone in extremities? In trunk?
- Exaggerated stretch reflex (clonus)?
- Asymmetries?

RANGE OF MOTION
- Limitations in upper extremity joints?
- Limitations in lower extremity joints?
- Limitations from bone or soft tissue contractures?
- Asymmetries?

PRIMITIVE REFLEXES
- Asymmetric tonic neck reflex
- Symmetric tonic neck reflex
- Tonic labyrinthine reflex (prone? supine?)
- Walking reflex
- Neonatal positive support reflex in standing
- Grasp reflex
- Plantar reflex

AUTOMATIC REACTIONS
- Equilibrium reactions (head righting? trunk incurvation? extremity counterbalancing?)
- Protective arm extension reactions (forward? sideways? backward?)
- Asymmetries?

OCULOMOTOR SKILLS
- Ability to visually focus on object
- Ability to visually track a moving object
- Esotropia? exotropia? nystagmus?
- Peripheral vision

PHYSICAL AND STRENGTH ENDURANCE
- Physical strength to complete functional tasks
- Physical endurance to complete functional tasks

RESPONSE TO PHYSICAL HANDLING AND MOVEMENT ACTIVITIES
- Response to examiner's or caregiver's touch
- Response to activities that require movement through space (e.g., being carried or moved into different positions)

Intervention Planning Purposes

Another reason for an occupational therapist to conduct a comprehensive evaluation of a child is to determine the most appropriate intervention plan. When this is the primary reason for evaluation, the therapist considers evaluation methods that include in-depth observations of the child's performance and participation in his or her natural environments. Interviews with parents and other adults working with the child are another primary source of data regarding the child's performance and level of participation. For intervention planning, norm-referenced instruments may have limited value. Norm-referenced developmental assessments measure skills commonly seen in children who are typically developing; they do not necessarily measure what is critical for functional performance in children with disabilities. For example, several of the items on the Peabody Developmental Motor Scales-2 (Folio & Fewell, 2000) (PDMS-2) (Figure 7-8) require the stacking of 1-inch cubes (Folio & Fewell, 2000). Is this specific skill critical for the child's success on everyday tasks? A common mistake

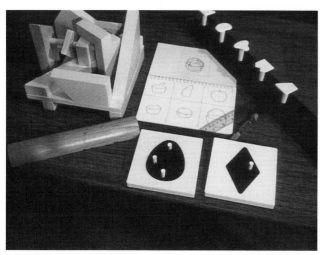

FIGURE 7-7 Materials for the Sensory Integration and Praxis Tests.

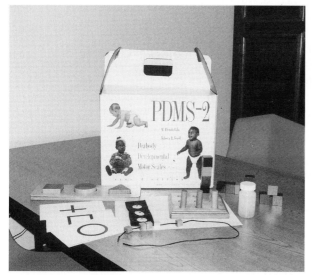

FIGURE 7-8 Fine motor materials from the Peabody Developmental Motor Scales (PDMS-2).

of therapists is to design intervention goals directly from norm-referenced test items. Unfortunately, this approach not only misses the mark with regard to writing functional outcomes, it may also invalidate the use of these test items during reevaluation because of the practice effect on the child.

Therapists should use criterion-referenced and curriculum-based assessments when the primary evaluation purpose is treatment planning. These measures provide information about specific skills important to the child's functional performance in activities of daily living, play, or school-related tasks. Some examples of criterion-referenced measures and curriculum-based assessments used by pediatric occupational therapists are the Hawaii Early Learning Profile (HELP) (Furuno, O'Reilly, Hosaka, Zeisloft, & Allman, 1984) the Assessment and Programming Systems for Infants and Young Children

(AEP) (Bricker, 1993), the Carolina Curriculum for Infants and Toddlers with Special Needs (Johnson-Martin, Jens, Attermeier, & Hacker, 1991), and the Transdisciplinary Play-Based Assessment (TPBA) (Linder, 1993). The Assessment of Motor and Process Skills (AMPS) (Fisher, 1999) and the School AMPS (Fisher & Bryze, 1997) are innovative observational assessments used by occupational therapists to measure the quality of a person's performance on goal-directed tasks. The School AMPS addresses functional performance issues in the classroom and provides information for effective programs and consultation in the school setting. An observational tool that measures an important dimension of children's play is the Test of Playfulness (Bundy, 1997). This criterion-based tool examines the key elements of playfulness: intrinsic motivation, suspension of reality, and internal locus of control. Occupational therapists working in rehabilitation settings may use the Functional Independence Measure for Children (WeeFIM) (Hamilton & Granger, 1991) to document clinical outcomes related to children's self-care, mobility, communication, and social problem solving.

Reevaluation Purposes

The fourth primary reason for a comprehensive evaluation is to reevaluate a child's performance so that progress can be measured and the need for continued therapy can be determined. The content and format of the reevaluation vary according to the specific purpose of the reevaluation. If a decision must be made on whether the child continues to qualify for special education services, the reevaluation probably will include a standardized, norm-referenced measure to ensure valid and reliable results. However, if the primary purpose of the reevaluation is to determine whether the child is making progress as a result of therapy, other measures, such as the specific functional goals and objectives written by the therapist during the initial phase of intervention, may be more appropriate and probably more sensitive to the developmental and functional changes in the child.

For example, an infant with Down syndrome may show a drop in scores on a standardized test over the course of the intervention year. However, these standard scores indicate only that the infant is developing at a slower rate compared with the test's normative sample. Measures of progress more sensitive to the developmental changes seen in this infant may be the long-term goals and short-term objectives written by the early intervention therapist. Short-term objectives are developed by therapists through careful task analysis, a process that lists specific target behaviors that lead sequentially to more advanced behaviors stated in the long-term goals.

It is important to emphasize that the process of reevaluation of children is ongoing and dynamic. Each time a therapist works with a child, the therapist evaluates his or her response to the therapeutic activities and assesses the child's performance on functional tasks. The therapist analyzes and interprets the data gathered during each therapy session to determine whether the intervention plan needs to be adjusted.

In summary, although a formal reevaluation of the child is conducted at specific times during the course of therapy services, the occupational therapist embeds evaluation probes within each therapy session.

Clinical Research

Instruments used in clinical research are carefully selected to measure the child's performance and behavior. A more complete discussion of standardized tests used for clinical research is presented in Chapter 8, but the following are a few of the major points:

1 Whether the research design includes a large group or a single subject, the instruments used must be reliable and valid measures of the dependent variable.
2 The measures used depend on the research design and can range from standardized, norm-referenced instruments, often used in large-group designs, to criterion-referenced instruments or therapy objectives operationally defined for single-subject research.
3 One of the most challenging steps in designing clinical research is finding an appropriate and accurate measure for documenting change in the subjects. Goal attainment scaling (GAS) is a technique used to evaluate the functional goal attainment of children receiving pediatric occupational therapy (King, McDougall, Palisano, Gritzan, & Tucker, 1999). GAS is an individualized, criterion-referenced measure of change that has been used to assess occupational therapy outcomes for children with learning disabilities (Young & Chesson, 1997) and children with traumatic brain injury (Mitchell & Cusik, 1998).

An important area of research in pediatric occupational therapy is the measurement of clinical outcomes to document the effectiveness of intervention programs. Law (1999) used a modified ICIDH-2 (WHO, 2001) framework (a predecessor to the ICF) to develop a computerized, self-directed software program designed to assist pediatric therapists in the selection of relevant and appropriate outcome measures for client, service, or program evaluation. With a database of 126 pediatric measures, this software program is an excellent resource for practitioners and researchers in occupational therapy who are conducting clinical outcome studies on children with disabilities.

EVALUATION PROCESS

The purpose of this section is to provide a logical sequence of steps that pediatric occupational therapists

can follow in the process of evaluating children. Kevin's case, discussed previously, is a good illustration of the evaluation process. Based on Kevin's occupational profile, the therapist identified several methods and measures to use to further evaluate Kevin's occupational performance. At this point the entry-level therapist may wonder where to begin. All the methods and measures listed in Table 7-1 do not need to be completed before occupational therapy can commence for Kevin. The process of evaluation in occupational therapy starts with the initial referral and continues for the duration of therapy services. The family and the rest of the team, including the occupational therapist, select specific evaluation areas that have priority for completion before developing an intervention plan and initiating therapy. Other areas of evaluation are completed as the child and family become better known to the therapist. The therapist, therefore, continually considers the new challenges the child must meet and other priorities that emerge for the family.

According to the Standards of Practice for Occupational Therapy, the occupational therapist (OT) and the occupational therapy assistant (OTA) have important but different functions in the evaluation of clients (AOTA, 1998). The OT is responsible for selecting evaluation methods and measures and interpreting and analyzing assessment data. The OTA, under the supervision of the OT, may contribute to the child's evaluation by administering some of the assessments and documenting some of the results.

To conduct thorough evaluations and provide accurate interpretation and documentation of evaluation results, therapists follow logical steps in the evaluation process. Figure 7-9 shows a flowchart for the evaluation sequence.

Referral

Children who have or are at risk for disabilities are referred to occupational therapists by health care providers, educators, and other professionals for evaluation of and intervention for occupational performance deficits. Often the child's diagnosis or deficits in specific developmental areas are listed on the referral form. To ensure that the referrals to occupational therapy are appropriate, it is critical that the occupational therapist be involved in the development of the referral format used in his or her work setting.

Development of the Child's Occupational Profile

Once a referral for therapy has been received, the therapist consults with parents, other caregivers, and professionals from other disciplines to determine which measures to use, the evaluation setting, and the sched-

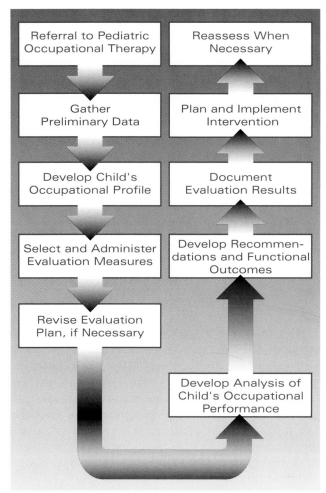

FIGURE 7-9 Flowchart for the evaluation process using the Occupational Therapy Practice Framework.

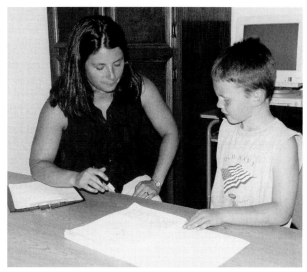

FIGURE 7-10 Administration of the Developmental Test of Visual Perception (2nd Ed.) (DTVP-2).

BOX 7-2 Checklist for Selection of Methods and Measures

1 Review reasons for referral.
2 Gather relevant medical, educational, and family histories (e.g., precautions for testing, need for interpreter, previous tests results).
3 Consider the caregiver's priorities regarding the child's functional skills.
4 Consider the developmental and chronologic age of the child.
5 Determine the theoretic frames of reference most appropriate for the evaluation of the child.
6 Consider the purpose of the evaluation, and select the most appropriate methods for the evaluation (see Table 7-2).
7 Consider the requirements of the agency for evaluation of children.
8 Identify available resources (e.g., child's caregiver, other professionals, instruments and test materials, time, and space).

ule for the occupational therapy evaluation activities. Most therapists find it helpful to formulate an evaluation plan based on the child's chronologic age, presenting problems, theoretic frame or frames of reference, parents' priorities regarding reasons for referral, availability of evaluation tools, type of service delivery model, and amount of time available for initial evaluation activities. The therapist lists the major concerns and the evaluation methods and measures that specifically assess those concerns. Box 7-2 provides a checklist of the important steps therapists take in the process of selecting appropriate methods and measures when evaluating children.

Kramer and Hinojosa described how philosophical foundations and theoretic frames of reference guide the occupational therapist in the selection, use, and interpretation of assessment measures (Kramer & Hinojosa, 1998). Kevin's case illustrates the application of theory to the evaluation process. As mentioned previously, the therapist hypothesized, based on Kevin's occupational profile, that his functional difficulties may be partly due to deficits in his foundational skills (e.g., sensory pro-

cessing and motor) and possibly due to some environmental factors. The therapist draws upon developmental theories and occupational therapy frames of reference (e.g., sensory integration, psychosocial, person-occupation-environment) to select methods and measures for Kevin's initial evaluation. The Battelle Developmental Inventory (BDI) (Newborg, Stock, Wnek, Guidubaldi, & Svinicki, 1988), the PDMS-2 (Folio & Fewell, 2000), and the Developmental Test of Visual Perception (2nd Ed.) (DTVP-II) (Hammill, Pearson, & Voress, 1998) (Figure 7-10) are measures based on developmental theories. The Sensory Profile (Dunn, 1999) is based on constructs consistent with theories of sensory processing. The Home Observation for Measurement of the Environment (HOME) (Caldwell & Bradley, 1984) is based on ecologic theories of psy-

TABLE 7-2   Selection of Appropriate Evaluation Methods

Purpose of Assessment	Evaluation Methods				
	Norm Referenced	Criterion Referenced	Skilled Observation	Interview	Checklists
Screening to determine need for further assessment	X		X	X	X
Comprehensive assessment to determine eligibility	X				
Comprehensive assessment to assist in diagnosis	X	X		X	
Comprehensive assessment to determine intervention plan		X	X	X	X
Reevaluation to monitor child's progress and determine need to continue therapy	X	X	X	X	X
Research to investigate clinical populations	X				

chosocial development. The Test of Playfulness (ToP) (Bundy, 1997) draws on theoretical constructs of human occupation.

As mentioned previously, the complete evaluation process occurs over time. Given the complexity of problems in children referred to pediatric occupational therapists, it may be difficult to formulate a comprehensive evaluation plan based on the limited referral information. It is expected, therefore, that the therapist will revise the initial evaluation plan after the child has been seen at least once by the therapist and more information has been gained regarding the caregiver's priorities and the child's developmental status. In the example of Kevin, the therapist learned from the parent phone interview that Kevin's mother is most concerned about his delayed toileting skills. The development of Kevin's occupational profile was based on interviews with his teacher and mother and on direct observations of Kevin at school (Box 7-3 presents Kevin's occupational profile).

Administration of Evaluation

Using the key information from the child's occupational profile, the therapist decides which methods and measures to administer to evaluate more fully the child's performance skills and the contexts that may be limiting his or her participation in everyday occupations. In Kevin's case, the therapist selected a series of methods and measures initially to evaluate his self-help skills, his motor development and neuromotor status, his behaviors related to sensory processing and modulation, and his home environment. Although the data from these methods and measures provide an initial picture of Kevin, the evaluation process is not over. For example, toward the end of the report in Box 7-3, the therapist recommends that further evaluation be administered to assess Kevin's playfulness and that skilled observation of Kevin printing his name at school be conducted to

analyze his performance on this important school-related task.

For most entry-level therapists in pediatrics, one of the most challenging aspects of the evaluation process is managing the child's behavior during administration of the evaluation measures, particularly when the measures are more formal, structured, and standardized. The evaluation of infants and young children in a structured situation is demanding for the children, the parents, and the therapist. Box 7-4 outlines several effective strategies therapists can use to manage young children's behavior during structured, standardized assessments. Chapter 8 offers a more in-depth discussion of competent administration of standardized tests and outlines some important ethical considerations for therapists in the use of standardized tests.

The administration of nonstandardized tools, skilled observations, environmental assessments, and interviews with the child's caregivers should receive the same careful attention and preparation by the occupational therapist as the standardized measures require. For some children a combination of standardized tests and nonstandardized measures is appropriate, but for many children with severe disabilities, norm-referenced tests are neither valid nor meaningful. In these cases, data gathered from nonstandardized measures provide the essential information for planning intervention. These evaluation methods, including naturalistic observation, other skilled observations, criterion-referenced measures, and interviews with the child's caregivers (e.g., teachers, parents, and daycare providers), are more fully described in the Evaluation Methods section.

Analysis of the Child's Occupational Performance

Once all the initial evaluation information on a child's performance has been gathered, the therapist analyzes

BOX 7-3 Initial Occupational Therapy Evaluation Report for Kevin

BACKGROUND INFORMATION

Kevin is a 5-year, 5-month-old African American boy, born on April 20, 1999, who has a history of developmental delay and attention deficit and hyperactivity disorder (ADHD). Approximately 6 months ago, Kevin's pediatrician, Dr. Mark Walker, placed him on medication to control his extreme hyperactivity. Kevin attends a developmental preschool program 5 half-days per week at Newport Elementary School. His classroom includes some nondisabled children and several children who exhibit mild to moderate developmental delays in speech and language, behavior, or motor skills. Kevin is the firstborn of three children in his family. He lives with both of his parents and his two younger brothers in a small home in a major urban area.

REFERRAL INFORMATION

Kevin was referred to occupational therapy on September 15, 2004, by his special education teacher, Mrs. Julie White, for a comprehensive evaluation to determine his need for occupational therapy intervention. Primary reasons for referral to occupational therapy include his fine and gross motor difficulties, possible visual-perceptual deficits, and poor social skills with peers.

OCCUPATIONAL PROFILE

A brief interview with Kevin's teacher revealed that he is having difficulty learning to print, making friends, and playing safely on playground equipment. The teacher reported that Kevin enjoys school and wants to do well on classroom tasks. In a telephone interview, Kevin's mother reported that he has problems dressing himself and also with toileting. She described her son as "difficult to manage" and reported that he often requires "punishment." Brief observation of and an interview with Kevin at school revealed that his primary interests include playing games on the classroom computer and running, jumping, and climbing at recess. He mentioned that he likes "wrestling" with his younger brothers at home and doesn't like "getting in trouble" at school or home.

Kevin's occupational profile suggests that he is having difficulty engaging in age-appropriate childhood occupations of play, self-help, and school-related tasks. These occupational performance difficulties may stem from underlying sensory processing and motor coordination deficits, as well as limitations in his home environment. The following assessments were conducted September 22-27, 2004, to analyze Kevin's occupational performance further in the context of his home and school environments.

ASSESSMENTS USED

Battelle Developmental Inventory (BDI)—Adaptive Domain (self-help)
Peabody Developmental Motor Scales (PDMS-2)
Skilled observations of Kevin's neuromotor status
Sensory profile
Developmental Test of Visual Perception (Revised) (DTVP-2)
Home Observation for Measurement of Environment (HOME) (Early Childhood version)

BEHAVIOR DURING STANDARDIZED ASSESSMENTS

Kevin was a friendly child who easily engaged in conversation with the examiner. He had significant difficulty attending to the structured test items, but when provided frequent social reinforcement and tangible rewards (e.g., stickers), he was able to complete most of the items presented on the standard measures. Kevin's hyperactivity and attention deficit limited his performance on some of the items, therefore his standard scores on the PDMS-2 and the DTVP-2 may underestimate his actual abilities.

ASSESSMENT RESULTS

Self-Help Skills

The Adaptive Domain of the Battelle Developmental Inventory (BDI) was administered to obtain a standard measure of Kevin's self-help skills. He had a developmental quotient of 65 and an age-equivalent score of 31 months. His overall performance fell into the 1st percentile rank (-2.33 SD), indicating significant delay.

During various dressing and eating activities, Kevin required extra structure from the examiner, including verbal and visual prompts. He independently took off and put on simple articles of clothing (e.g., hat, socks), but he needed physical assistance to put on his pants, shirt, and jacket. Kevin demonstrated his understanding of washing (with soap) and drying his hands, but he was easily distracted and required several verbal cues to stay on task. Kevin expressed his interest in learning how to toilet. His mother reported that he has several "accidents" during the day because "he is too busy to stop whatever he's doing and forgets to ask to go to the bathroom." At mealtime Kevin was able to drink from a regular cup without spilling and appropriately used his fork and spoon but not a table knife. He had difficulty remaining in his seat until his mealtime was over.

Motor Skills

The Peabody Developmental Motor Scales (PDMS-2) test was used to obtain a standard measure of Kevin's gross and fine motor abilities. He obtained a Motor Quotient of 71, placing him in the 3rd percentile compared with other children his age. He obtained a Gross Motor Quotient of 77 (6th percentile rank, -1.53 SD) and a Fine Motor Quotient of 67 (1st percentile rank, -2.33 SD). Kevin's subtest scores were:

PDMS-2 Subtests	Percentile Rank	Age-Equivalent Score (Months)	Standard Deviation (SD) Score
Stationary	16th	50	-1.00
Locomotion	25th	53	-0.67
Object manipulation (ball handling skills)	5th	33	-1.67
Grasping	5th	40	-1.67
Visual-motor integration	2nd	34	-2.00

Kevin preferred his right hand for most tasks that required the skilled use of a tool (e.g., crayons and scissors). He demonstrated hand tremors when attempting various fine motor tasks, but these tremors were not observed at rest. He moved impulsively and, even with verbal cues from the examiner, was unable to slow his movements. Kevin scored within age expectations on tasks requiring speed and agility but below average on tasks that required static balance (e.g., standing on one foot) and on gross motor tasks that required more precise coordination (e.g., throwing a ball at a target).

Neuromuscular Status

Skilled observations revealed muscle tone, range of motion, integration of primitive reflexes, and development of

Continued

BOX 7-3   Initial Occupational Therapy Evaluation Report for Kevin—cont'd

automatic reactions (righting and equilibrium responses and protective extension reactions) within the normal range. Posture and gait also appeared normal. His frequent falls and clumsiness on the playground appeared to be related more to his motor impulsivity and inattentiveness than to delayed equilibrium responses.

Sensory Responsivity

The Sensory Profile, a caregiver questionnaire, was used to obtain a standard measure of Kevin's sensory processing abilities and to evaluate possible contributions of sensory processing to his performance on everyday activities. Kevin's scores fell in the Definite Difference range ($\geq$2.0 SD) on factors of Sensory Seeking, Emotionally Reactive, Inattention/Distractibility, and Fine Motor/Perceptual. His sensory profile is consistent with that of other children diagnosed with attention deficit hyperactivity disorder.

Kevin's scores also fell in the Definite Difference range ($\geq$2.0 SD) on items measuring modulation related to body position and movement, and modulation of movement affecting activity level. His profile of scores suggests that his sensory reactivity and responsivity may be limiting his ability to regulate his behavior in accordance with some of the demands of his environment. This type of profile is common in children who are inconsistent in their responses to sensory input, reflecting their attempts simultaneously to respond to stimuli (e.g., they are distracted by extraneous input) and to protect themselves by reducing the sensory input (e.g., they avoid uncomfortable or frightening stimuli). When children have difficulty co-attending and are emotionally reactive, they often are hindered in the development of social relationships with peers.

Visual Perception

On the Developmental Test of Visual Perception (2nd Ed.) (DTVP-2), Kevin obtained a percentile rank of 21, indicating an overall performance in the low-normal range (−0.8 SD from the mean). His performance on each of the subtests varied significantly. His relative strengths were on the motor-reduced (visual perception) tasks, including the Spatial Relations and Figure-Ground subtests. His performance fell below average on the motor-enhanced (visual-motor integration) tasks, including the Eye-Hand Coordination and Copying subtests.

Home Observations

The Home Observation for Measurement of the Environment (Early Childhood Version) was used to assess the quantity and quality of social, emotional, and cognitive support available to Kevin at home. Although several strengths were observed related to parental affection toward Kevin and age-appropriate language stimulation, concerns were noted in the limited learning materials (e.g., few toys) and physical space (e.g., no space to play outdoors), as well as the limited variety of learning experiences available to him.

SUMMARY AND ANALYSIS OF OCCUPATIONAL PERFORMANCE

Kevin is a 5-year, 5-month-old boy with attention deficits and developmental delays who is currently enrolled in a developmental preschool program. This initial evaluation revealed that he is functioning more than 2 years below age expectations on self-help and fine motor tasks and at least 1 year below age level on the various gross motor skills. His neuromotor status, including muscle tone, equilibrium reactions, and posture, was within normal limits. His sensory profile revealed definite differences and was consistent with other children with ADHD. Some of his self-help delays and his difficulty modulating his behavioral responses during everyday routines may be partly due to his deficits in sensory processing (i.e., ability to register, process, and adapt to tactile, auditory, and movement stimuli). Kevin's overall performance on the DTVP-2 fell in the low-normal range. His scores were within normal limits on the visual-perceptual items but were below normal on items that required visual-motor integration. He is a friendly, charming boy who wants to do well, but his extreme hyperactivity and distractibility limit his physical and social performance in both his home and school environments.

RECOMMENDATIONS

Kevin would benefit from occupational therapy services in which intervention activities are carefully designed to enhance his social participation at school, to improve his motor performance on school-related tasks, and to facilitate his independence in dressing and toileting activities. Further assessment using the Test of Playfulness is recommended to obtain a more systematic measure of Kevin's playfulness. In addition, a skilled observation of Kevin learning to print will be conducted for an in-depth analysis of this important school-related task. The parents may benefit from suggestions for low-cost play materials and simple adaptations to Kevin's play environment at home. If there are any questions regarding this report, please contact this therapist at 123-4567.

---

the quantitative and qualitative data from standardized test results, skilled observations of the child's performance, caregiver interviews, and environmental assessments. When a standardized test is used, the therapist must carefully follow procedures outlined in the test manual regarding interpretation of the test results. When nonstandardized measures are used, the therapist must skillfully assess for patterns of strength and areas of concern across all measures. Often data obtained from nonstandardized measures can be instrumental in understanding the possible underlying reasons for a child's specific performance on standardized tests. To further illustrate this point, consider Kevin's case. His teacher noted his clumsiness on the playground at school, and his gross motor scores on the PDMS-2 were below average. However, after observing his performance across different settings (e.g., classroom, playground, and home), the therapist concluded that Kevin's attention deficit and high activity level, rather than a delay in his equilibrium responses, limited his motor performance (see Box 7-3).

Accurate and complete interpretation of all accumulated data is an important and demanding task in the evaluation process. The occupational therapist must be thorough in examining the details of a child's performance and viewing the child's behaviors in the context

BOX 7-4 Behavior Strategies for Testing Young Children

1 Be prepared. Know your testing procedures so well that you can focus on the child's behavior and performance, not on the test manual or your paperwork.

2 Be sensitive to the child's and the parents' physical and emotional needs. Whenever possible, adjust the pace of the examination to match the child's style and acknowledge any concerns the parents may express.

3 Be purposeful in carrying out the examination. Keep the situation friendly, interesting for the child, and informative for the parent.

4 Be sure that the testing room supports the child's optimal performance. The chair and table should be the appropriate size, and lighting should be sufficient. Remove all auditory and visual distractions. Use test materials attractive to children.

5 Build a rapport with the child before physically interacting with or handling him or her. Some children may do better starting with tabletop tasks in which the child sits across from the examiner and observes the situation before being handled physically for motor testing. Other children may do better if allowed to engage in a spontaneous play situation while the examiner focuses on the parent interview before directly testing the child. Be flexible and follow the child's lead whenever possible.

6 Use positive reinforcement that is meaningful to the child (e.g., praise, stickers, or a fun activity). Be sure to reinforce the child's effort rather than his or her success.

7 Begin and end with some easy items for the child. This helps the child feel more comfortable at the beginning and provides a positive ending to the test session for both the child and the parents.

8 Watch the complexity of your language. Be clear and concise in your instructions to the child. Consider using the parents' level of language complexity as a guide to what the child can understand.

9 Be organized. Keep the test materials arranged neatly in an area that is easily accessible to you but not to the child. It is sometimes helpful to have an attractive toy (not from the test kit) on the table or nearby for the child to play with while you are not directly testing him or her.

10 Try to develop reciprocal interactions with the child. When you first show a test object, allow the child to explore it briefly in his or her own way before you give the test instructions. This time provides an excellent opportunity for clinical observations. Then give the test instructions and allow the child to demonstrate his or her skill. If the child continues to be actively engaged with the object when you want to present a new item, it often is effective to present the new test object as you remove the old one.

of environmental demands and supports. Accurate and complete interpretation of evaluation data allows therapists to make sound clinical decisions, including whether the child would benefit from occupational therapy services and, if so, the appropriate frequency, duration, and type of therapeutic intervention. Once evaluation data have been analyzed, the therapist turns to the task of developing recommendations for the child.

Development of Recommendations Based on Evaluation Results

One of the first factors the therapist considers when developing recommendations based on evaluation results is the functionality of the recommendations. The term functionality refers to the relevance of the recommendation to the child's daily life (Notari & Bricker, 1990). When developing recommendations for a child, the therapist must always ask herself or himself the following two questions:

- Does this recommendation relate to the child's occupational performance?
- Is this recommendation relevant to the child's everyday function?

Writing therapy goals and objectives gives therapists the opportunity to think about and determine the most important skills a child needs to meet the demands of his or her environment or environments. Bundy (1991) suggests that functional outcomes for children should be viewed as an expression of possibilities—possibilities of what children may become with support from their families and therapists. The following examples illustrate how therapists can translate evaluation findings into functional, measurable treatment goals that are relevant to the everyday activities of children.

1 *Evaluation finding.* Because of poor fine motor release of objects, Jill was unable to stack 1-inch cubes on the PDMS-2.
   a *Inadequate treatment goal.* Jill will stack two 1-inch cubes, three out of four trials, by June 15, 2004.
   b *Functional goal.* After playing with small toys, Jill will independently pick up and place small toys in a container, three out of four trials, by June 15, 2004.

2 *Evaluation finding.* Because of increased muscle tone and poor reciprocal movements in the lower extremities, Ryan was unable to assume the half-kneel position on either leg when coming to stand, an item on the Gross Motor Function Measure (2nd Ed) (GMFM-II) (Russell et al., 1993).
   a *Inadequate treatment goal.* Ryan will maintain the half-kneel position for 30 seconds, three times over two consecutive therapy sessions, by June 15, 2005.
   b *Functional goal.* To participate in a self-help task at school, Ryan will step up with either leg on a 6-inch stool to use the classroom toilet without losing his balance, three out of four times, by June 15, 2005.

Another important component of the development of meaningful recommendations is focusing on the primary caregiver's priorities for the child and family. Hanft (1994) suggests that every recommendation from an occupational therapist to a parent of a child with special needs should be followed up with a question to the caregiver: "How will this suggestion work for you and your child?" For example, during a feeding evaluation in a child's home, a therapist observes a mother and her child who has athetoid cerebral palsy and failure to thrive. The therapist notes that the mother placed the child in an infant walker at mealtime. Because infant walkers have been declared unsafe by the American Academy of Pediatrics and because this particular child would benefit from a more stable seating device that provides trunk and head support for optimal oral-motor performance, the therapist might recommend that use of the infant walker be discontinued and that a special feeding seat be ordered. However, unless the therapist asks the mother what the implications of this recommendation are for the child and the family, the family members may not implement this important recommendation. In this case, additional history taking revealed that the child refused to be fed in any other position than in the walker, and the mother was more concerned about her child's adequate nutrition for growth than his feeding position. Based on the mother's input, the initial intervention goal should be for the child to demonstrate adequate oral-motor skills for physical growth. In this case, the therapist should add a recommendation to provide the parents with information about the safety of infant walkers and the importance of proper positioning when swallowing to prevent aspiration.

A third consideration of therapists when developing recommendations from evaluation findings is which service delivery model will meet the needs of the child and family. The range of service delivery models in which pediatric occupational therapists work has been defined as direct treatment, monitoring, and consultation (Dunn & Campbell, 1991). More recently, Dunn (2000) defined service delivery models as direct services, integrated or supervised therapy, and consultation. The therapist's recommendations should be consistent with the primary service delivery model. For example, if the therapist's primary role with the child is consultation, recommendations from the initial evaluation would center on how the parents and other adults working with the child can adapt the child's environment.

The therapist must be able to reconcile these three sometimes conflicting factors when developing meaningful recommendations for children. Years of experience can teach a therapist to negotiate through the maze of issues regarding the child, family, team, environments, and service delivery systems. Entry-level therapists, however, can use several basic strategies to help them become more competent in evaluating children:

1 Find a mentor who is experienced in working with children with various diagnoses and families from diverse backgrounds.
2 Be willing to search continually for new knowledge and resources that are relevant to working with children with special needs.
3 Be open to new ways of viewing children and families.
4 Learn to build effective communication and collaboration skills with team members, including the child's primary caregiver.

Documentation of Evaluation Results and Recommendations

The next step in the evaluation process is to provide written and oral reports on the evaluation findings and recommendations. The primary purpose of documenting the results of the pediatric occupational therapy evaluation is to describe to caregivers, physicians, teachers, and other individuals working with the child the child's current abilities and limitations on various functional tasks. McClain suggested that "Effective documentation is telling a true story with a particular style. It calls for the ordinary tasks of day-to-day experience to be succinctly stated in writing. The true story about any child who has a disability is not a simple tale" (p. 213).

When providing written documentation, the therapist must first consider for whom the reports are intended and then carefully construct reports that are understandable and useful to those individuals. The format and content of evaluation reports may vary significantly, depending on the referral concern, the complexity of the child's problem, and the regulations of the service delivery system in which the child is served (e.g., public school setting, hospital, or home health agency). In some situations, for eligibility purposes, written evaluation reports must also include specific standard scores documenting developmental delay. In all pediatric occupational therapy settings, documentation creates a chronologic record of the child's status, the occupational therapy services provided to the child, and the child's outcomes (AOTA, 2003).

As therapists write their reports, they should recognize that their words have great power. Therapists should carefully choose their words when documenting a child's evaluation results. Hanft (1989) cautions pediatric therapists that "words convey powerful personal images that can be positive and supportive or negative and destructive" (p. 5). Pediatric occupational therapists should use words that reflect positive attitudes toward children with disabilities. Unfortunately, therapy jargon is filled with technical terms that may not convey the intended message but may confuse or alienate parents. Therapists should always refer to the child first and to the disability as one characteristic of the child (e.g., a child with cerebral palsy; not a cerebral palsied child).

Box 7-3 provides a written example of how a therapist documented Kevin's evaluation findings and recommendations. An important point is that the therapist worded the report so that the information was helpful to Kevin's parents and teacher. The format and terminology of the evaluation report are consistent with the

Occupational Therapy Practice Framework (AOTA, 2002).

To summarize the major points discussed in the previous sections, occupational therapists should ask themselves the following questions about evaluations they have performed; that is, did the evaluation process:

1 Address the caregiver's concerns?
2 Use assessments that measured the child's engagement in occupations and activities and identified the factors that supported and hindered the child's occupational performance?
3 Use multiple methods of evaluation, including skilled observations, caregiver interviews, direct observations of the child in his or her natural environment, and standardized tools?
4 Fully recognize the influence of the child's cultural background on his or her evaluation performance and consider these cultural influences in the development of recommendations for the child?
5 Adhere properly to the administration procedures and ethical considerations when using standardized tests?
6 Recognize and acknowledge the child's strengths and interests in addition to areas of concern?
7 Result in a summary that contributed meaningful, user-friendly information about the child's functional abilities and disabilities?

This section described the evaluation process, including important sequential steps for conducting accurate, thorough evaluations of children and communicating evaluation findings to caregivers and other professionals working with the child. The next section provides additional, detailed information on the methods used in pediatric occupational therapy evaluations.

EVALUATION METHODS

Several evaluation methods are available to pediatric occupational therapists. The challenge for therapists is to determine which evaluation methods should be selected for a particular child or group of children. This section describes the primary evaluation methods commonly used in pediatric occupational therapy practice and discusses the major factors that therapists should consider when selecting a particular method or methods.

The starting point in the selection process is to identify clearly the purpose of the evaluation and to match appropriate evaluation methods with the identified purpose. For example, if the only purpose of the evaluation is to contribute to the determination of a child's eligibility for special education services in a public school setting, the primary evaluation method may be a norm-referenced, standardized test. However, if the primary purpose of the evaluation is to gain information useful for planning an intervention program for the child, the evaluation measures should include skilled observations of the child's functional performance and interviews with the child's caregivers. Often the initial evaluation of a

child serves more than one purpose, therefore therapists frequently use multiple measures and methods when conducting child evaluations.

Standardized Assessments

Norm-referenced measures are tests that have been developed by administering the test items to a sample of children (in a normative group) who are representative of the population to be tested. The child's score on a norm-referenced tool is compared with the scores of the normative group. To evaluate the usefulness of a norm-referenced measure, the pediatric occupational therapist should read the test manual carefully to learn how the norm-referenced scores were derived and the characteristics of the normative sample. The therapist using norm-referenced tests should also know how to interpret an individual child's scores accurately, including the standard score and the percentile rank. Chapter 8 provides a more in-depth discussion on the use of standardized tests, including norm-referenced and criterion-referenced measures.

Criterion-referenced measures are tests that consist of a series of skills in functional or developmental areas, usually grouped by age level. These tests compare the child's performance on each test item with a standard or criterion that must be met if the child is to receive credit for that item. Criterion-referenced tests are made up of items selected because of their importance to the child's school performance or everyday occupations. Because of their importance to the child's function, the items often become intervention targets when the child exhibits difficulty in successfully completing the items.

The primary advantage in using criterion-referenced tests is that the examiner obtains important information about the child's strengths and limitations on skills critical for function in everyday tasks. Some examples of criterion-referenced measures used in pediatric occupational therapy are HELP (Furuno et al., 1984), the revised Erhardt Developmental Prehension Assessment (Erhardt, 1994), and the Assessment and Programming System for Infants and Young Children (Bricker, 1993). Information gained from criterion-referenced tests is particularly helpful for assessment of the child's functional skills and for planning of appropriate intervention activities to enhance those skills (see Appendix 7-A).

Ecologic Assessments

Neisworth and Bagnato (1988) defined ecologic assessments as "the examination and recording of the physical, social, and psychological features of a child's developmental context." Consistent with the transactional approach (Sameroff & Fiese, 2000), ecologic assessments are also concerned with the interaction between the individual child and his or her environments (Figures 7-11 and 7-12).

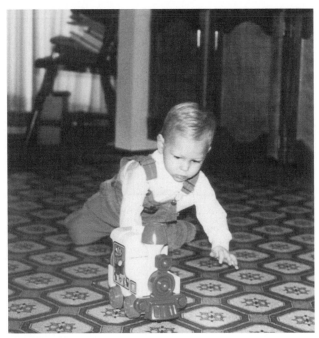

FIGURE 7-11 Observing a child playing in his natural environment.

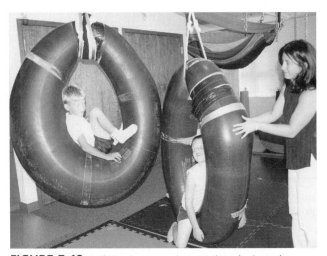

FIGURE 7-12 Observing peer interaction during play.

Pediatric occupational therapists are particularly interested in ecologic measures because these tools are a primary mechanism for obtaining data relevant to the child's performance context. An ecologic assessment of a child uses techniques that consider the cultural influences, socioeconomic status, and value system of the family or the physical demands and societal expectations of the child's environment. Some of these methods include naturalistic observations, interviews, and rating scales. Measures that contribute to ecologic evaluation and are often administered by occupational therapists include the Knox Preschool Play Scale (Knox, 1997), the revised HOME Inventory (Caldwell & Bradley, 1984),

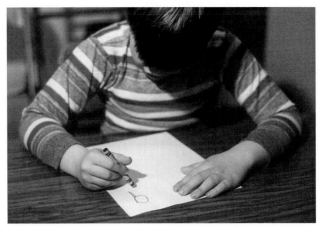

FIGURE 7-13 Skilled observation of a child performing a functional task at school.

and the TPBA (Linder, 1993). The SFA (Coster et al., 1998) is another example of an ecologic assessment.

Skilled Observation

An essential skill of the pediatric occupational therapist is the ability to observe keenly and accurately and record children's behavior in an objective manner. Although formal, standardized assessments are highly valued in pediatric practice, skilled observation of a child performing a functional task offers different but equally important information about the child's performance (Figure 7-13). According to Bailey and Wolery (1989), "Observation of children in familiar settings and routines allows more characteristic views of their abilities and may actually be more reflective of how children can be expected to perform even under the most optimal learning opportunities" (p. 256).

Dunn (2000) proposed that skilled observation is one of the essential tools available to occupational therapists. Dunn described the following key competencies required to conduct skilled observations: (1) Do not interfere with the natural course of events being observed; (2) Pay attention to the environmental features that support or limit a child's performance; and (3) Record the child's behavior in observable and neutral terms. When skilled observations are used in the evaluation process, therapists must select a systematic, objective recording procedure so that data collected are accurate and reliable. Clark and Miller (1996) proposed a problem-solving approach to functional assessments and data-based decision making for occupational therapists working with children in school settings. Using direct observations of the child's functional skills at school, the occupational therapist and other team members define the outcome behaviors and identify the relevant dimensions of those behaviors, design a useful data collection system to monitor the child's progress, and then use those data to make decisions about the child's intervention program.

A word of caution is due, however, about the use of skilled observations of the child in his or her natural environments. If the examiner is not experienced in observing children, he or she may not recognize key behaviors or patterns of behavior in the child and the meaning of those behaviors within the demands of the task and the environment. Therapists entering the field of pediatric occupational therapy should seek out master clinicians and mentors who are willing to help new therapists hone their skills at observing children and families.

Interviews

Another primary method used in pediatric occupational therapy evaluation is the interview with the child, the child's primary caregiver, the teacher, and other adults working with the child. Bailey and Wolery (1989) suggested that caregiver interviews regarding a child's development can serve several functions:

1 They allow the therapist to collect information about the child's skills from the parents' perspective.
2 They validate information collected through direct observations or testing by the professional.
3 They provide an opportunity for the parents to identify their values and priorities regarding the skills being evaluated by the therapist.

The Canadian Occupational Performance Measure (COPM) is a well-researched tool that uses a structured interview format to obtain information on children's performance and satisfaction in the areas of self-care, leisure, and productivity (Law et al., 1994). This tool was designed to help occupational therapists identify the priorities for intervention based on the primary caregivers' and the child's most important concerns (Chapter 15 presents more information on the COPM).

Interviews are best used with other evaluation methods that involve direct observation of the child. An important outcome of the interview is an accurate, meaningful exchange of information between the professional and the parent or other caregiver. When done well, interviews can provide an opportunity for building rapport between the therapist and the caregivers. They provide a unique opportunity for families to identify and discuss issues that are important to them. Interviews, therefore, are particularly useful when therapists are interested in the family's perceptions of a child's abilities, the influence of events (e.g., transitions in services) on the family, and the family's priorities for services. When interviews are conducted in a flexible, sensitive manner, parents and therapists are able to explore areas of concern as they arise.

Interviews may include closed- or open-ended questions or a combination of these. Specific questions, which are often closed-ended, allow the therapist to gather a predetermined set of information from a caregiver in a relatively short time. Unstructured interviews using open-ended questions allow caregivers to take the lead and set the priorities in the discussion. Open-ended questions invite the caregiver to elaborate on a topic and provide critical information about the child. Conducting an effective interview requires experience and sensitivity (Box 7-5). An important decision the therapist must make when conducting interviews with caregivers is whether the interview should be done in the presence of the child. Most parents are uncomfortable describing their child's deficits in front of the child, particularly if the child is over 3 years of age and aware of his or her difficulties. Therapists should carefully plan when, how, and where the interview or interviews should be conducted.

In summary, a skilled therapist conducts interviews with children (older than 3 years of age) and caregivers by carefully selecting questions and sensitively listening to the responses. Interviews offer a unique opportunity for an exchange of information among the child, the caregivers, and the therapist. During the interview, the therapist should reciprocate by providing caregivers with accurate, relevant information about the child's functional abilities, the intervention services, and community resources.

BOX 7-5 Basic Strategies for Conducting Effective Caregiver Interviews

1 Begin the session by clarifying the purpose of the interview with the caregiver in terms that are meaningful to him or her.
2 Be sensitive to the caregiver's physical and emotional needs throughout the evaluation.
3 Promote interaction by asking open-ended questions, and guide caregivers to where they may sit to participate fully in the conversation.
4 Through careful questioning, attempt to understand what is typical for the family regarding their values and cultural influences in raising their child.
5 Carefully plan when to take notes, preferably after the interview or when the caregiver is busy tending to the child.
6 Remain positive and realistic in your approach with caregivers and in the information you provide.
7 Be flexible throughout the interview, responding sensitively to the caregivers' questions and need for information. If you cannot answer a question, let them know and then figure out a plan with them to begin to find the needed information.
8 Use effective verbal and nonverbal communication skills. Often, nonverbal communication can override verbal information.
9 Avoid the use of therapy and medical jargon. If technical terms are used, be sure they are adequately explained.

Inventories and Scales

A variety of inventories and scales are used to gather data on a child's development, on caregiver-child interactions, or on the child's environments. Some published inventories, checklists, and scales are well developed instruments.

The Pediatric Evaluation of Disability Inventory (PEDI) is an evaluation of functional capabilities and performance in children 6 months to 7.5 years of age (Haley, Coster, Ludlow, Haltiwanger, & Andrellos, 1992). This assessment is one of the few inventories used by occupational therapists that is standardized with norms. The PEDI is administered through a structured interview with the parents or by professional judgment of clinicians and educators who are familiar with the child. It measures both capability and performance of functional activities in (1) self-care, (2) mobility, and (3) social function. The inventory consists of 197 functional skills items; the child is scored either 1 (has capability) or 0 (has not yet demonstrated capability, unable) on each item. Twenty additional items rate the amount of caregiver assistance required to complete key functional tasks. The PEDI was designed for use with young children who have a variety of disabling conditions, although the test's authors were primarily concerned with designing an instrument to be used with children who have physical disabilities. The authors completed a series of reliability and validity studies and developed criterion scores using Rasch analysis techniques. As a result, the PEDI stands as a well-developed, well-researched assessment tool for evaluating the functional performance and capabilities of children.

Rating scales may provide both quantitative and qualitative data. A rating system usually involves a number scale to rate the quality, degree, or frequency of a behavior. For example, the Caregiver/Parent-Child Interaction Feeding and Teaching Scales are designed to assess parent-child interactions in the context of feeding and teaching events (Sumner & Spietz, 1994). Figure 7-14 shows the type of data obtained using the feeding scale's rating system.

A parent, teacher, or other caregiver can complete some inventories and rating scales. For example, the Ages & Stages Questionnaires rely exclusively on parent report (Bricker, Squires, & Mounts, 1995). On this scale the items are clearly described, and many are illustrated so that parents can elicit specific behaviors from their children. After each item, parents check the appropriate box—"yes," "sometimes," or "not yet." The Developmental Profile II (DP-II) may be given by parent interview exclusively or by direct testing (Alpern, Boll, & Shearer, 1986). The Sensory Profile (Dunn, 1999) and the Infant/Toddler Sensory Profile (Dunn, 2002) are caregiver questionnaires that may be completed through a parent interview. A classroom teacher or parent can administer the Developmental Checklist for Pre-Dressing Skills (Dunn-Klein, 1983).

IV. COGNITIVE GROWTH FOSTERING	*YES*	*NO*
42. Caregiver provides child with objects, finger foods, toys, and/or utensils.		
43. Caregiver encourages and/or allows the child to explore the breast, bottle, food, cup, bowl, or the caregiver during feeding.		
44. Caregiver talks to the child using two words at least three times during the feeding.		
45. Caregiver verbally describes food or feeding situation to child during feeding.		
46. Caregiver talks to child about things other than food, eating, or things related to feeding.		
47. Caregiver uses statements that describe, ask questions, or explain consequences of behavior, more than commands, in talking to child.		
48. Caregiver verbally responds to child's sound within 5 seconds after child has vocalized.		
49. Caregiver verbally responds to child's movement within 5 seconds of child's movement of arms, legs, hands, head, trunk.		
50. Caregiver avoids using baby talk.		

FIGURE 7-14 Examples of items from the Caregiver/Parent-Child Interaction Feeding Scale.

Arena Assessments

The IDEA (1997) requires that evaluations of infants and children with disabilities be conducted, when appropriate, by a multidisciplinary team. However, the form and scope of the multidisciplinary evaluation vary widely, depending on the philosophy of the intervention program and the expertise of the professionals. For example, in some settings each professional provides an individual evaluation of the child or family, and the team members then meet to discuss evaluation findings and recommendations. Sometimes little or no communication occurs among team members before and during administration of the evaluation measures. In contrast, a team in another setting may use the transdisciplinary approach in which one primary team member conducts the evaluation of the child and family while other key team members contribute their expertise to the evaluation process through consultation.

The arena assessment uses a transdisciplinary approach that allows the child and primary caregiver to interact with one professional throughout the evaluation session while other professionals observe and, on occasion, directly test the child or interview the caregiver. An example of an arena assessment is the TPBA (Linder, 1993). This assessment places major emphasis on a team approach to the evaluation of young children. The purpose of the TPBA is to obtain developmental information on the child using multidimensional, functional observations of the child during a play session. Parents and professionals together plan, observe, and analyze the child's play session.

Arena assessment of feeding difficulties in children can also be an effective way to gather relevant information without overtesting the child or requiring the caregiver to participate in repeated interviews with different professionals. For example, an arena feeding assessment for a child with cerebral palsy and failure to thrive may include an occupational therapist, a nurse, and a nutritionist. One professional is designated the lead evaluator, depending on the primary referral concern. The occupational therapist may take the lead if the child has oral-motor deficits, such as chewing or swallowing difficulties, postural difficulties that create the need for external support of posture at mealtime, or fine motor difficulties that limit self-feeding skills. The nurse may take the lead in the evaluation process if the child exhibits behavioral difficulties, if the parent's caregiving skills appear limited, or if parent-child interactions are at risk. The nutritionist may take the lead if the child's diet needs careful analysis and if the family would benefit from specific information on types and amounts of food the child should eat. The benefit of an arena assessment of feeding is that the child and caregiver are subjected to the mealtime evaluation only once rather than several times. The arena assessment provides an opportunity for collaboration among parents and professionals to observe, discuss, and solve problems in critical areas together.

SUMMARY

Accurate, reliable evaluation of a child is one of the most challenging and rewarding services an occupational therapist can offer. This chapter described the purposes, processes, and methods of evaluation in pediatric occupational therapy. Having an understanding of the many purposes of evaluation and being able to carefully match appropriate methods and measures with those purposes are critical skills of the pediatric occupational therapist. Careful observation of the details of a child's performance on tasks and recognition of the importance of the context in which the child performs those tasks are also essential evaluation skills. Equally important in the evaluation process are the therapist's collaborative skills when working with the child's caregiver and other team members to gain an in-depth understanding of the child and his or her environments. An in-depth understanding of the child's occupational performance in natural contexts leads to the development of relevant, appropriate occupational therapy intervention plans and effective intervention strategies.

STUDY QUESTIONS

Case Study 1

Chelsea is an 8-month-old (corrected age) infant who was born at 32 weeks' gestation. Primary problems in the neonatal intensive care unit (NICU) included infant respiratory distress syndrome and neonatal abstinence syndrome secondary to maternal drug use. Cranial ultrasounds in the NICU indicated intraventricular hemorrhage. Chelsea is living with her mother, who is single, and her 2-year-old brother in a one-room studio apartment. Her mother is concerned because Chelsea is irritable throughout the day. She does not like her bath, nor does she enjoy being cuddled. Chelsea's pediatrician referred her for an occupational therapy evaluation because of her difficulty regulating her behavioral states, increased tone in her legs, and her delay in independent sitting.

1 Explain the primary purpose of the therapy evaluation for Chelsea.

2 Discuss the evaluation methods that would be appropriate for an initial evaluation of Chelsea and her family, and list two or three specific instruments.

3 What other professionals might be involved in Chelsea's case?

Case Study 2

Tin is a 2-year-old toddler with developmental delay of unknown cause. He is the firstborn of a newly immigrated family that had recently immigrated from Vietnam. The public health nurse administered the Denver Developmental Screening Test (2nd Ed) (Denver-II), which showed that Tin was functioning around the 18-month-old level in gross motor skills, near the 12-month-old level in fine motor and adaptive skills, and at the 10-month-old level in language skills. Tin and his family were referred to a community-based early intervention program. The occupational therapist working in the early intervention program serves on a team that includes a physical therapist, a speech pathologist, and an early childhood special educator. The team is preparing to meet with the family to develop the Individualized Family Service Plan.

1 What are some of the major points that the early intervention team should consider when assessing Tin and reporting evaluation information to the family?

2 Discuss the advantages and disadvantages of an arena assessment for Tin.

Case Study 3

Eva is a 6-year-old girl with mild cerebral palsy who has participated in early intervention and preschool programs since she was 2 years of age. Her cognitive abilities appear to be within the normal range. The early childhood staff reports that Eva has some difficulty following adult-directed activities and playing with her peers. Her parents are interested in enrolling her in a regular kindergarten class this year. She is currently being evaluated by the public school occupational therapist to determine if she is eligible for therapy in the school setting. Eva's previous therapist in the early intervention program administered the Peabody Developmental Motor Scales-II (PDMS-2) last year.

1 Given the primary purpose of the school occupational therapy evaluation, what methods and measures would be most appropriate for Eva's evaluation?

2 Discuss whether a norm-referenced or a criterion-referenced assessment should be used in this situation.

3 Discuss some important behavioral strategies that would be effective in evaluating Eva when using a standardized assessment.

4 In which natural environments should the therapist observe Eva to gain a better understanding of her occupational performance skills?

Case Study 4

Michael is a 9-year-old boy with sensory processing deficits and a learning disability. His mother reports that Michael has difficulty making friends in the neighbor-hood and following through with simple chores at home. Michael's teacher indicates that Michael continues to have difficulty in completing his written assignments and frequently disturbs his classmates while they are working. He has recently been referred to the school's occupational therapist, who was asked to determine if Michael would benefit from therapy.

1 What evaluation methods might be helpful in developing Michael's occupational profile?

2 Which measures would be most appropriate for a more in-depth analysis of Michael's occupational performance?

3 Write two functional, measurable therapy goals for Michael for this school year.

REFERENCES

Alpern, G., Boll, T., & Shearer, M. (1986). *Developmental Profile II*. Los Angeles: Western Psychological Services.

American Occupational Therapy Association (AOTA). (1998). Standards of practice for occupational therapy. *American Journal of Occupational Therapy, 52*, 866-869.

American Occupational Therapy Association (AOTA). (2002). Occupational therapy practice framework: Domain and process. *American Journal of Occupational Therapy, 56*, 609-639.

American Occupational Therapy Association (AOTA). (2003). *Guidelines for documentation of occupational therapy*. Available at www.aota.org/

Aylward, G.P. (1999). *Bayley infant Neurodevelopmental Screener*. San Antonio, Psychological Corporation.

Ayres, A.J. (1989). *Sensory Integration and Praxis Tests*. Los Angeles: Western Psychological Services.

Bailey, D.B., & Wolery, M. (1989). *Assessing infants and preschoolers with handicaps*. Columbus, OH: Merrill.

Bowden, S. (1995). Development of a research tool to enable children to describe their engagement in occupation. *Journal of Occupational Science Australia, 2* (3), 115-123.

Bricker, D. (Ed.). (1993). *Assessment, evaluation, and programming system*. Baltimore: Brookes.

Bricker, D., Squires, J., & Mounts, L. (1995). *Ages and stages questionnaires: a parent-completed, child-monitoring system* (2nd ed.). Baltimore: Brookes.

Bronfenbrenner, U. (1977). Toward an experimental ecology of human development. *American Psychologist, 32*, 513-531.

Bruininks, R. (1978). *Bruininks-Oseretsky test of motor proficiency*. Circle Pines, MN: American Guidance Service.

Bundy, A. (1991). Writing functional goals for evaluation. In C.B. Royeen (Ed.), *AOTA self-study series: School-based practice for related services* (pp. 7-30). Bethesda, MD: American Occupational Therapy Association.

Bundy, A. (1997). Play and playfulness: What to look for. In L.D. Parham & L.S. Fazio (Eds.), *Play in occupational therapy for children* (pp. 52-66). St. Louis: Mosby.

Caldwell, B.M., & Bradley, R.H. (1984). *Home observation for measurement of the environment* (rev. ed.). Little Rock, AR: University of Arkansas.

Clark, G.F., & Miller, L.E. (1996). Providing effective occupational therapy services: Data-based decision making in school-based practice. *American Journal of Occupational Therapy, 50* (9), 701-708.

Coster, W. (1998). Occupational-centered assessment of children. *American Journal of Occupational Therapy, 52* (5), 337-344.

Coster, W., Deeney, T., Haltiwanger, J., & Haley, S. (1998). *School Function Assessment*. San Antonio: Psychological Corporation.

Dunn, W. (1999). *Sensory Profile: User's manual*. San Antonio: Psychological Corporation.

Dunn, W. (Ed.). (2002). *Best practice occupational therapy in community service with children and families*. Thorofare, NJ: Slack.

Dunn, W. (2002). *Infant/toddler sensory profile: user's manual*. San Antonio: Psychological Corporation.

Dunn, W., Brown, C., & McGuigan, A. (1994). The ecology of human performance: A framework for considering the effect of context. *American Journal of Occupational Therapy, 48* (7), 595-607.

Dunn-Klein, M. (1983). *The developmental checklist for predressing Skills*. Tucson: Therapy Skill Builders.

Erhardt, R.P. (1994). *Erhardt Developmental Prehension Assessment* (revised). San Antonio: Psychological Corporation.

Farran, D.C. (2000). Another decade of intervention for children who are low income or disabled: what do we know now? In J.P. Shonkoff & S.J. Meisels (Eds.), *Handbook of early childhood intervention* (2nd ed., pp. 510-548). Cambridge, UK: Cambridge University Press.

Fisher, A.G. (1999). *Assessment of motor and process skills* (3rd ed.). Fort Collins, CO: Three Star Press.

Fisher, A.G., & Bryze, K. (1997). *School AMPS: School version of the assessment of motor and process skills*. Fort Collins, CO: Three Star Press.

Folio, M.R., & Fewell, R.R. (2000). *Peabody Developmental Motor Scales* (2nd ed.), Austin, TX: Pro-Ed.

Frankenburg, W., & Dodds, J. (1992). *Denver Developmental Screening Test-II*. Denver: Denver Developmental Materials.

Furuno, S., O'Reilly, K., Hosaka, C.M., Zeisloft, B., & Allman, T. (1984). *The Hawaii Early Learning Profile*. Palo Alto, CA: VORT.

Haley, S.M., Coster, W.J., Ludlow, L.H., Haltiwanger, M.A., & Andrellos, P.J. (1992). *Pediatric evaluation of disability inventory*. San Antonio: Psychological Corporation.

Hamilton, B.B., & Granger, C.U. (1991). *Functional Independence Measure for Children (WeeFIM)*. Buffalo, NY: Research Foundation of the State University of New York.

Hammill, D.D., Pearson, N.A., & Voress, J.K. (1998). *Developmental Test of Visual Perception* (2nd ed.). Austin, TX: Pro-Ed.

Hanft, B. (1989). How words create images. In B. Hanft (Ed.), *Family-centered care: an early intervention resource manual* (Unit 2, pp. 77-78). Bethesda, MD: American Occupational Therapy Association.

Hanft, B. (1994). The good parent: A label by any other name would not smell as sweet. *AOTA's Developmental Disabilities Special Interest Section Newsletter, 17* (2), 5.

Harris, S.R., Megens, A.M., Backman, C.L., & Hayes, V. (2003). Development and standardization of the Harris Infant Neuromotor Test. *Infants and Young Children, 16,* 143-151.

Individuals with Disabilities Education Act (IDEA) Amendments of 1997 (1997). (Public Law 105-17). USC 1400.

Johnson-Martin, N.M., Jens, K.G., Attermeier, S.M., & Hacker, B.J. (1991). *The Carolina Curriculum for Infants and Toddlers with Special Needs* (2nd ed.). Baltimore: Brookes.

King, G.A., McDougall, J., Palisano, R.J., Gritzan, J., & Tucker, M. (1999). Goal attainment scaling: its use in evaluating pediatric therapy programs. *Physical and Occupational Therapy in Pediatrics, 19* (2), 31-52.

Knox, S. (1997). Development and current use of the Knox Preschool Play Scale. In L.D. Parham & L.S. Fazio (Eds.). *Play in occupational therapy for children* (pp. 35-51). St. Louis: Mosby.

Kramer, P., & Hinojosa, J. (1998). Theoretical basis of evaluation. In J. Hinojosa & P. Kramer (Eds.), *Occupational therapy evaluation: obtaining and interpreting data* (pp. 17-28). Bethesda, MD: American Occupational Therapy Association, Inc.

Law, M. (2002). Participation in the occupations of everyday life. *American Journal of Occupational Therapy, 56* (6), 640-649.

Law, M.C. (1999). *All about outcomes: A program to help you organize your thinking about pediatric outcome measures*. Thorofare, NJ: Slack.

Law, M.C., Baptiste, S., McColl, M., Carswell, A., Polatajko, H., & Pollock, N. (1994). *Canadian Occupational Performance Measure* (2nd ed.). Ottawa, ON: Canadian Association of Occupational Therapy Publications.

Linder, T.W. (1993). *Transdisciplinary play-based assessment: a functional approach to working with young children*. Baltimore: Brookes.

McClain, L.H. (1991). Documentation. In W. Dunn (Ed.), *Pediatric occupational therapy: facilitating effective service provision* (pp. 213-244). Thorofare, NJ: Slack.

Miller, L.J. (1988). *Miller Assessment for Preschoolers*. San Antonio: Psychological Corporation.

Miller, L.J. (1993). *First STEp Screening Tool*. San Antonio: Psychological Corporation.

Missiuna, C. (1998). Development of "All About Me," a scale that measures children's perceived motor competence. *Occupational Therapy Journal of Research, 18* (2), 85-108.

Mitchell, T., & Cusik, A. (1998). Evaluation of a client-centred paediatric rehabilitation programme using goal attainment scaling. *Australian Journal of Occupational Therapy, 45* (1), 7-17.

Neisworth, J.T., & Bagnato, S.J. (1988). Assessment in early childhood special education: A typology of dependent measures. In S.L. Odom & M.B. Karnes (Eds.), *Early intervention for infants and children with handicaps: an empirical base* (pp. 23-49). Baltimore: Brookes.

Newborg, J., Stock, J.R., Wnek, L., Guidubaldi, J., & Svinicki, J. (1988). *Battelle Developmental Inventory, examiner's manual*. Chicago: Riverside.

Notari, A., & Bricker, D. (1990). The utility of a curriculum-based assessment instrument in the development of individualized education plans for infants and young children. *Journal of Early Intervention, 14,* 117-132.

Russell, D.J., Rosenbaum, P.L., Avery, L., & Lane, M. (2002). *Gross motor function measure*. User's manual. Cambridge: Cambridge University Press.

Sameroff, A.J., & Fiese, B.H. (2000). Transactional regulation: The developmental ecology of early intervention. In J.P. Shonkoff & S.J. Meisels (Eds.), *Handbook of early childhood intervention* (2nd ed., pp. 135-159). Cambridge, UK: Cambridge University Press.

Sturgess, J., Rodger, S., & Ozanne, A. (2002). A review of the use of self-report assessment with young children. *British Journal of Occupational Therapy, 65* (3), 108-116.

Sumner, G., & Spietz, A. (1994). *NCAST caregiver/parent-child interaction scales.* Seattle: NCAST Publications, University of Washington, School of Nursing.

Washington [State] Administrative Code (WAC). (1998). *Rules for the provision of special education: eligibility criteria for students with disabilities (WAC 392-172-114).* Olympia, WA: Office of Superintendent of Public Instruction.

World Health Organization (WHO). (2001). *ICF: International classification of functioning, disability and health.* Geneva: WHO.

Young, A., & Chesson, R. (1997). Goal attainment scaling as a method of measuring clinical outcomes for children with learning disabilities. *British Journal of Occupational Therapy, 60* (3), 111-114.

Young, N.L. (1997). *Activities Scale for Kids.* Toronto: Pediatric Outcomes Research Team, Hospital for Sick Children.

Young, N.L., Yoshida, K.K., Williams, J.I., Bombardier, C., & Wright, J.G. (1995). The role of children in reporting their physical disability. *Archives of Physical Medicine and Rehabilitation, 76* (10), 913-918.

SUGGESTED READINGS

American Occupational Therapy Association. (2001). *Pediatrics set: practice guideline series.* Bethesda, MD: AOTA.

Asher, I. (1996). *Occupational therapy evaluation tools: An annotated index* (2nd ed.). Bethesda, MD: American Occupational Therapy Association.

Dunn, W. (2000). *Best practice occupational therapy in community service with children and families.* Thorofare, NJ: Slack.

Mulligan, S. (2003). *Occupational therapy evaluation for children: A pocket guide.* Baltimore: Lippincott Williams & Wilkins.

Common Pediatric Assessments

The following list of pediatric assessments represents a small selection of a variety of measures used in occupational therapy. Occupational therapists working with infants, children, and adolescents should stay current with the research literature on pediatric measures and should carefully evaluate the reliability and validity of new instruments as they become available to practitioners.

Adolescent/Adult Sensory Profile

Brown, C., & Dunn, W. (2002)
This self-questionnaire for individuals 11 years of age or older measures possible contributions of sensory processing to the person's daily performance patterns. The classification system is based on normative information. www.sensoryprofile.com

Ages & Stages Questionnaires

Bricker, D., Squires, J., & Mounts, L. (1995)
These parent questionnaires were designed to screen children from birth to 5 years of age in communication, gross motor, fine motor, problem-solving, and personal-social development. www.brookespublishing. com/store/books/bricker-asq/index/htm

Alberta Infant Motor Scales (AIMS)

Piper, M.C., & Darrah, J. (1994). *Motor assessment of the developing infant.*
A norm-referenced measure designed to identify and monitor infants with gross motor delays from birth to 18 months of age. www.bmjbookshop.com

Assessment of Motor and Process Skills (AMPS)

Fisher, A.G. (1999)
This observational assessment is used to measure the quality of a person's performance on goal-directed tasks of domestic and personal activities of daily living.

Battelle Developmental Inventory (BDI)

Newborg, J., Stock, J.R., Wnek, L., Guidubaldi, J., & Svinicki, A. (1988)
A norm-referenced tool that measures the development of children from birth to 8 years of age. Domains assessed include personal-social, adaptive (self-help), motor, communication, and cognition. A short version is available for screening. www.riverpub.com

Bayley Scales of Infant Development (Second Edition)

Bayley, N. (1993)
This comprehensive, norm-referenced tool was designed to measure the cognitive and motor development of infants from 1 to 42 months of age. http://marketplace.psychcorp.com

Bruininks-Oseretsky Test of Motor Proficiency

Bruininks, R. (1978)
A norm-referenced measure of gross motor, upper limb, and fine motor proficiency in children 4.5 to 14.5 years of age. A short form is available for brief screening. www.agsnet.com

Canadian Occupational Performance Measure

Law, M.C., Baptiste, S., McColl, M., Carswell, A., Polatajko, H., & Pollock, N. (1994)
This interview tool helps identify the family's priorities for their child with special needs and assists in developing therapy goals with the child's primary caregivers. Distributed by the American Occupational Therapy Association. www.fhs.mcmaster.ca/canchild

Childhood Autism Rating Scale (CARS)

Schopler, E., Reichler, R.J., & Renner, B.R. (2002)
The CARS is an observational tool designed to identify children over 2 years of age who have mild, moderate,

or severe autism and to distinguish those children from children with developmental delay without autism. www.wpspublish.com

Denver Developmental Screening Test (Revised) (Denver-II)

Frankenburg, W., & Dodds, J. (1992)
The Denver-II is a standardized screening tool for children 1 month to 6 years of age who are at risk for developmental problems in the areas of personal-social, fine motor adaptive, language, and gross motor skills. www.denverii.com

Developmental Test of Visual Motor Integration (Fourth Edition) (VMI-4)

Beery, K.E., Buktenica, N.A., & Beery, N.A. (2004)
This standardized instrument was designed to identify visual-motor integration deficits in children ages 3 to 8 years (Short Form) and ages 3 to 18 (Long Form) that can lead to learning and behavior problems. www.pearsonassessments.com

Developmental Test of Visual Perception (Second Edition) (DTVP-2)

Hammill, D.D., Pearson, N.A., & Voress, J.K. (1993)
A norm-referenced tool that measures the visual perception and visual-motor integration skills in children 4 to 10 years of age. www.proedinc.com/store

Developmental Test of Visual Perception—Adolescent and Adult

Reynolds, C.R., Pearson, N.A., & Voress, J.K. (2002)
A battery of six subtests that measures different but interrelated visual-perceptual and visual-motor abilities in individuals 11 to 75 years of age. www.proedinc.com/store

Early Coping Inventory

Zeitlin, S., Williamson, G.G., & Szczepanski, M. (1988)
This observation instrument is used to assess coping-related behavior, including sensorimotor organization, reactive behaviors, and self-initiated behaviors, in children functioning at the 4-month to 36-month developmental level. www.ststesting.com/early.html#EAR

Erhardt Developmental Prehension Assessment (Revised)

Erhardt, R.P. (1994)
This observational tool was designed to measure components of arm and hand development in children who

have cerebral palsy or other neurodevelopmental disorders (all ages and cognitive levels). http://home.att.net/~rperhardtdp/home.html

Erhardt Developmental Vision Assessment

Erhardt, R.P. (1988)
This observational tool is used to assess the motor components of visual development (e.g., ocular pursuits) in individuals of all ages and cognitive levels with neurodevelopmental disorders (e.g., cerebral palsy). http://home.att.net/~rperhardt

Evaluation Tool of Children's Handwriting (ETCH)

Amundson, S.J. (1995)
A criterion-referenced tool designed to evaluate the manuscript and cursive handwriting skills of children in grades 1 through 6. www.alaska.net/~otkids/etch.htm

First STEP: Screening Test for Evaluating Preschoolers

Miller, L.J. (1993)
This standardized screening tool is used to identify children ages 2 years 9 months to 6 years 2 months who need in-depth diagnostic testing in the areas of cognition, communication, and motor development. http://marketplace.psychcorp.com

Functional Independence Measure for Children (WeeFIM)

Hamilton, B.B., & Granger, C.U. (1991)
This measure assesses the functional outcomes in children and adolescents with acquired or congenital disabilities. The WeeFIM was designed to document the need for assistance and the severity of disability in children functioning within the developmental level of 6 months to 7 years in the areas of self-care, mobility, and cognition. www.udsmr.org/Ped/Wee_Default.htm

Gross Motor Function Measure (Revised) (GMFM)

Russell, D., Rosenbaum, P., Avery, L., & Lane, M. (2002)
A clinical measure designed to evaluate change in gross motor function in children with cerebral palsy. The GMFM is appropriate for children whose motor skills are at or below those of a 5-year-old child without any motor disability. www.fhs.mcmaster.ca/canchild

Hawaii Early Learning Profile (HELP)

Furuno, S., O'Reilly, K.A., Hosaka, C.M., Zeisloft, B., & Allman, T.A.. (1984)

A curriculum-based assessment used with infants, toddlers, and young children and their families to identify developmental needs, determine intervention goals, and track children's progress. www.vort.com/profb3.htm

Home Observation for Measurement of the Environment (HOME)

Caldwell, B., & Bradley, R.H. (1984)

The initial version of this inventory, the Infant/Toddler HOME, was designed to measure the quality and quantity of stimulation and support available to a child from birth to 3 years of age in his or her home environment. More recent versions include the Early Childhood HOME (ages 3 to 6 years), the Middle Childhood HOME (ages 6 to 10 years), and the Early Adolescent HOME (ages 10 to 15 years).
www.ualr.edu/~coedept/ case/ent/home.html

Infant/Toddler Sensory Profile

Dunn, W. (2002)

This standardized tool is a judgment-based caregiver questionnaire designed to describe behavioral responses to various everyday sensory experiences in children from birth to 3 years of age. www.sensoryprofile.com

Knox Preschool Play Scale (Revised)

Knox, S. (1997)

This scale is a naturalistic observation tool used to assess play behaviors in children from birth to 6 years of age. The four parameters measured include space management, material management, pretense-symbolic, and participation. Available in Parham & Fazio (1997) *Play and Occupational Therapy for Children*. St. Louis: Mosby

Miller Assessment for Preschoolers (MAP)

Miller, L.J. (1988)

This norm-referenced tool was designed to identify children ages 2 years 9 months to 5 years 8 months who are at risk for mild to moderate developmental delays. The five domains measured include sensorimotor foundations, motor coordination, verbal and non-verbal skills, and performance on complex tasks.
http://marketplace.psychcorp.com

Motor-Free Visual Perception Test (MVPT-3)

Colarusso, R.R., & Hammill, D.D. (1995)

The MVPT-3 is a norm-referenced test used for individuals 4 to 70 years of age to assess visual-perceptual abilities that do not require motor involvement to make a response. www.academictherapy.com

NCAST Caregiver/Parent-Child Interaction Scales

Sumner, G., & Spietz, A. (1994)

These scales measure caregiver-child interactions during a feeding situation (with infants from birth to 12 months) and a teaching situation (with children from birth to 3 years). www.ncast.org/p-pci.asp

Peabody Developmental Motor Scales (2nd Edition) (PDMS-2)

Folio, M.R., & Fewell, R.R. (2000)

The PDMS-2 is a norm-referenced measure of gross and fine motor skills used for children from birth through 5 years of age. www.proedinc.com

Pediatric Evaluation of Disability Inventory (PEDI)

Haley S.M., Coster W.J., Ludlow, L.H., Haltiwanger, J.T., & Andrellos, P.J. (1992)

The PEDI is a standardized tool used to measure functional abilities (e.g., self-care, mobility, and social function) in children 6 months to 9 years of age. http://marketplace.psychcorp.com

Posture and Fine Motor Assessment of Infants

Case-Smith, J., & Bigsby, R. (2000)

This early intervention assessment tool is used to determine whether motor skills are delayed in infants 2 to 12 months of age. The criterion-referenced scores can be used to plan intervention and to document the infant's progress. http://marketplace.psychcorp.com

Quality of Upper Extremity Skills Test (QUEST)

DeMatteo, C., Law, M., Russell, D., Pollock, N., Rosenbaum, P., & Walter, S. (1992)

This outcome measure was designed to evaluate movement patterns and hand function in children with cerebral palsy from 8 months to 8 years of age. The four domains measured include dissociated movements, grasp patterns, protective extension reactions, and weight-bearing ability.

Available at the Neurodevelopmental Clinical Research Unit at McMaster University, Hamilton, Ontario, Canada.

School Function Assessment (SFA)

Coster, W., Deeney, T., Haltiwanger, J., & Haley, S. (1998)
The SFA is a judgment-based questionnaire designed to measure a student's performance of functional tasks that support his or her participation in the academic and social aspects of an elementary school program (kindergarten through grade 6). Three scales evaluate the student's level of participation, the type and amount of task supports needed, and his or her activity performance on specific school tasks.
http://marketplace.psychcorp.com

School Assessment of Motor and Process Skills (School AMPS)

Fisher, A.G., & Bryze, K. (1997)
The School AMPS is a naturalistic observation tool used to measure the student's schoolwork task performance in typical classroom settings during the student's typical school routines.

Sensory Integration and Praxis Tests (SIPT)

Ayres, A.J. (1989)
The SIPT are norm-referenced tests designed to measure the sensory integration processes that underlie learning and behavior in children 4 to 9 years of age. The 17 tests assess visual perception, somatosensory and vestibular processing, and various types of praxis. Extensive training is required to administer and interpret the SIPT. www.wpspublish.com

Sensory Profile

Dunn, W. (1999)
This caregiver questionnaire was designed to measure the frequency of behaviors related to sensory processing, modulation, and emotional responsivity to sensory input in children 3 to 12 years of age. www.sensoryprofile.com

Test of Playfulness (ToP)

Bundy, A. (1997)
This naturalistic observational tool measures three elements of playfulness in children of all ages: perception of control, source of motivation, and suspension of reality.

Available in Parham & Fazio (1997). *Play in occupational therapy for children.*

Test of Sensory Functions in Infants (TSFI)

DeGangi, G.A., & Greenspan, S.I. (1989)
The TSFI was designed to identify infants from 4 to 18 months of age who have sensory integrative dysfunction. Subdomains measured include reactivity to tactile deep pressure, visual-tactile integration, adaptive motor function, oculomotor control, and reactivity to vestibular stimulation. www.wpspublish.com

Test of Visual-Motor Skills (Revised) (TVMS-R)

Gardner, M.F. (1995)
The TVMS-R measures eye-hand coordination skills needed to copy geometric designs in children 3 to 13 years of age. www.academictherapy.com

Test of Visual-Motor Skills—Upper Level (TVMS-UL)

Gardner, M.F. (1992)
The TVMS-UL measures eye-hand skills needed to copy geometric designs in individuals 12 to 40 years of age. www.academictherapy.com

Test of Visual-Perceptual Skills (Non-Motor) (Revised) (TVPS-R)

Gardner, M.F. (1996)
The TVPS-R assesses visual-perceptual skills (e.g., discrimination, memory, spatial relations, form constancy, sequential memory, figure-ground and closure) in children 4 to 13 years of age. www.academictherapy.com

Test of Visual-Perceptual Skills (Non-Motor)—Upper Level (Revised) (TVPS-R:UL)

Gardner, M.F. (1997)
The TVPS-R:UL measures visual-perceptual skills in individuals 12 to 17 years of age. www.academictherapy.com

Toddler and Infant Motor Evaluation (TIME)

Miller, L.J., & Roid, G.H. (1994)
This standardized diagnostic assessment tool was designed to measure neuromotor changes in children who have atypical development. The tool is appropriate

for use with children who are functioning at or below 3.5 years. http://marketplace.psychcorp.com

Transdisciplinary Play-Based Assessment (TPBA)

Linder, T.W. (1993)
The TPBA is a naturalistic observation tool that uses an arena assessment approach in which early childhood professionals evaluate a child's development in cognitive, social-emotional, communication and language, and sensorimotor domains during play sessions. The TPBA can be used with children from infancy to 6 years of age in home- and center-based environments. www.pbrookes. com

Vineland Adaptive Behavior Scales (VABS)

Sparrow, S.S., Balla, D.A., & Cicchetti, D.V. (1984)
The VABS were designed to assess communication, daily living, socialization, and motor skills in individuals from birth to 18 years of age and in low-functioning adults. Different formats include an Interview Edition, a Survey Form, an Expanded Form, and a Classroom Edition. www.agsnet.com

Use of Standardized Tests in Pediatric Practice

Pamela K. Richardson

CHAPTER OBJECTIVES

1 List the characteristics of commonly used standardized pediatric tests.
2 Describe the differences between norm-referenced and criterion-referenced tests and give the purpose of each type of test.
3 Explain the descriptive statistics used in standardized pediatric tests.
4 Discuss the types of standard scores used in standardized pediatric tests.
5 Explain the concepts of reliability and validity
6 Discuss the importance of test validity.
7 Describe the procedures necessary to become a competent user of standardized tests.
8 Understand the ethical considerations involved in the use of standardized tests.
9 Demonstrate a knowledge of standardized test applications to information found in a case study.

What are standardized tests, and why are they important to occupational therapists? A test that has been standardized has uniform procedures for administration and scoring (Anastasi & Urbina, 1997). This means that examiners must use the same instructions, materials, and procedures each time they administer the test, and they must score the test using criteria specified in the test manual. A number of standardized tests are in common use. Most schoolchildren have taken standardized achievement tests that assess how well they have learned the required grade-level material. College students are familiar with the Scholastic Aptitude Test (SAT), the results of which can affect decisions on admission at many colleges and universities. Intelligence tests, interest tests, and aptitude tests are other examples of standardized tests frequently used with the general public.

Pediatric occupational therapists use standardized tests to help determine the eligibility of children for therapy services, to monitor their progress in therapy, and to make decisions on the type of intervention that would be most appropriate and effective for them. Standardized tests provide precise measurements of a child's performance in specific areas, and this performance is described as a standard score. The standard score can be used and understood by other occupational therapists and child development professionals familiar with standardized testing procedures.

Using anthropometric measurements and psychophysical testing to measure intelligence, Galton and Cattell developed the initial concept of standardized assessments of human performance late in the nineteenth century. The first widespread use of human performance testing was initiated in 1904, when the minister of public education in Paris formed a commission to create tests that would help to identify "mentally defective children," with the goal of providing them with an appropriate education. Binet and Simon developed the first intelligence test for this purpose. Terman and Merrill (1937) incorporated many of Binet's and Simon's ideas into the construction of the Stanford-Binet Intelligence Scale, which remains widely used today (Sternberg, 1990). Although intelligence was the first human attribute to be tested in a standardized manner, tests have been developed in the past 30 years that assess children's developmental status, cognition, gross and fine motor skills, language and communication skills, school readiness, school achievement, visual-motor skills, visual-perceptual skills, social skills, and other behavioral domains. Although the number and types of tests have changed radically since the time of Simon and Binet, the basic reason for using standardized tests remains the same: to identify children who may need special intervention or programs because their performance in a given area is outside the norm, or average, for their particular age.

The use of standardized tests requires a high level of responsibility on the part of the tester. The occupational therapist who uses a standardized test must be knowledgeable about scoring and interpreting the test, must know for whom the test is and is not appropriate, and must understand how to report and discuss a child's scores on the test. The tester must also be aware of the limitations of standardized tests in providing information about a child's performance deficits. This, in turn, requires a working knowledge of standardized testing concepts and procedures, familiarity with the factors that can affect performance on standardized tests, and awareness of the ethics and responsibilities of testers when using standardized tests.

The purpose of this chapter is to introduce pediatric standardized testing used by occupational therapists. The purposes and characteristics of standardized tests are discussed, technical information about standardized tests is presented, practical tips to help the student become a competent user of standardized assessments are given, and ethical considerations are explained. The chapter concludes with a summary of the advantages and disadvantages of standardized tests and a case study that incorporates the concepts presented in the chapter into a real life testing scenario. Throughout the chapter, several standardized assessments commonly used by pediatric occupational therapists are highlighted to illustrate the concepts of test administration, scoring, and interpretation.

PURPOSES

Standardized tests are used for several reasons. For example, a standardized test may be used as a screening tool to assess large numbers of children quickly and briefly and identify those who may have delays and are in need of more in-depth testing. Examples of screening tests frequently used by occupational therapists include the Miller Assessment for Preschoolers (MAP) (Miller,

1988), the revised Denver Developmental Screening Test (Denver-II) (Frankenburg & Dodds et al., 1990), and the FirstSTEp (Screening Test for Evaluating Preschoolers) (Miller, 1990).

Screening tests typically assess several developmental domains, and each domain is represented by a small number of items (Table 8-1). Screening tests generally take 20 to 30 minutes and can be administered by professionals or by paraprofessionals such as classroom aides, nurse's aides, or teaching assistants. Therapists who work in settings that primarily serve typically developing children (e.g., a public school system or Head Start program) may become involved in developmental screening activities. In addition, occupational therapists frequently use assessment tools to evaluate children with specific developmental problems. Therefore it is important for all therapists to be aware of the strengths and weaknesses of specific tests used in their settings. Although the screening tools mentioned are not discussed in greater depth, the concepts of developing, administering, scoring, and interpreting standardized tests (discussed later in this chapter) should also be considered when using screening tools.

Occupational therapists most frequently use standardized tests as in-depth assessments of various areas of occupation and performance skills. Standardized tests are used for three main purposes: (1) to assist in the determination of a medical or educational diagnosis, (2) to document a child's developmental and functional status, and (3) to aid the planning of an intervention program.

Assistance with Medical or Educational Diagnoses

A primary purpose of standardized tests is to assist in the determination of a diagnosis through use of normative scores that compare the child's performance with that of an age-matched sample of children. Standardized tests are frequently used to determine if a child has developmental delays or functional deficits significant enough to qualify the child for remedial services such as occupational therapy. Many funding agencies and insurance providers use the results of standardized testing as one

TABLE 8-1   Developmental Domains Assessed in Four Screening Tools

Screening Tool	Age Range	Domains Assessed
Denver Developmental Screening Test (Revised)	1 month to 6 years	Personal-social, fine motor adaptive, language, gross motor
Developmental Indicators for Assessment of Learning (Revised)	2.5 to 6 years	Motor, language, concepts
FirstSTEp: Screening Test for Evaluating Preschoolers	2 years, 9 months to 6 years, 2 months	Cognition, communication, physical, social and emotional, adaptive functioning
Miller Assessment for Preschoolers	2 years, 7 months to 5 years, 8 months	Foundations, coordination, verbal, nonverbal, complex tasks

criterion in the decision on whether a child will receive occupational therapy intervention. In school-based practice, standard scores are helpful for identifying specific student problems that may indicate that the involvement of an occupational therapist is appropriate. Funding approval for special services generally depends on documentation of a predetermined degree of delay in one or more developmental domains, and standardized test results are an important component of this documentation. The results of standardized testing performed by occupational therapists, when used in conjunction with testing done by other professionals, can help physicians or psychologists arrive at a medical or educational diagnosis.

Documentation of Developmental and Functional Status

Another purpose of standardized testing is to document a child's status. Many funding and service agencies require periodic reassessment to provide a record of a child's progress and to determine if the child continues to qualify for services. Standardized tests are often a preferred way of documenting progress because the results of the most current assessment can be compared with those of earlier ones. Periodic formal reassessment can also provide valuable information to the therapist working with the child. Careful scrutiny of a child's test results can help identify areas of greatest and least progress. This can assist the therapist in prioritizing intervention goals. Many parents are also interested in seeing the results of their child's periodic assessments. Standardized tests used in periodic assessments must be chosen carefully so that areas of occupation or performance skills addressed in the intervention plan are also the focus of the standardized testing.

A discussion about the child's progress in areas that may not be measured by standardized testing should accompany the discussion of test performance. Structured or unstructured observations of the child's play and self-care behavior, interviews with the caretaker about the child's home routine, the developmental and medical histories, and a review of pertinent medical or educational records are equally important components of the assessment process (see Chapter 7 for more information about the assessment process).

Planning of Intervention Programs

A third purpose of standardized testing is program planning. Standardized tests provide information about a child's level of function, and they help therapists determine the appropriate starting point for therapy intervention. Most commonly, criterion-referenced standardized tests are used as the basis for developing goals

and objectives for individual children and for measuring progress and change over time. Criterion-referenced tests are used extensively in educational settings and include such tools as the Hawaii Early Learning Profile (HELP) (Furuno et al., 1997); the Assessment, Evaluation, and Programming System for Infants and Children (Bricker, 1993); and the School Function Assessment (SFA) (Coster, Deeney, Haltiwanger, & Haley, 1998). Criterion-referenced tests are described in more detail in the following section.

CHARACTERISTICS

As stated earlier, standardized tests have uniform procedures for administration and scoring. These standard procedures permit the results of a child's tests to be compared either with his or her performance on a previous administration of the test or with the test norms developed by administration of the test to a large number of children.

Standardized tests characteristically include a test manual that describes the purpose of the test (i.e., what the test is intended to measure). The manual should also describe the intended population for the test. For pediatric assessments, this generally refers to the age range of children for whom the test was intended, but it may also refer to specific diagnoses or types of functional impairments. Test manuals also contain technical information about the test, such as a description of the test development and standardization process, characteristics of the normative sample, and studies done during the test development process to establish reliability and validity data. Finally, test manuals contain detailed information about the administration, scoring, and interpretation of the test scores.

Another characteristic of standardized tests is that they are composed of a fixed number of items. Items may not be added or subtracted without affecting the standard procedure for test administration. Most tests have specific rules about the number of items that should be administered to ensure a standardized test administration. These rules may differ significantly from test to test. For instance, the Bruininks-Oseretsky Test of Motor Proficiency (BOTMP) (Bruininks, 1978) specifies that the entire item set be administered regardless of the child's age. In contrast, the Bayley Scales of Infant Development (2nd Edition) (BSID-II) (Bayley, 1993) has a number of item sets corresponding to age bands (e.g., 22 to 24 months). Testers are instructed to begin testing at the age band corresponding to the child's chronologic age (or corrected age, if the child was born prematurely) and to move to a higher or lower age band, if necessary, depending on the child's performance. The decision to move to a different age band is made according to the number of items passed and failed at the initial age band,

and the decision rules are stated in the test manual. Box 8-1 explains how to compute ages corrected for prematurity.

A third characteristic of standardized tests is a fixed protocol for administration. The term *fixed protocol for administration* refers to the way each item is administered and the number of items administered. Generally, the protocol for administration specifies the verbal instruction or demonstration to be provided, the number of times the instructions can be repeated, and the number of attempts the child is allowed on the item. For some tests, instructions for each item are printed in the manual, and the tester is expected to read the instructions verbatim to the child without deviating from the text. However, other tests allow for more freedom of instruction, especially when the test involves a physical activity (Figure 8-1).

Standardized tests also have a fixed guideline for scoring. Scoring guidelines usually accompany the administration guidelines and specify what the child's performance must look like to receive a passing score on the item. Depending on the nature of the item, passing performance may be described using text, a picture, or a diagram. The administration and scoring guidelines for a test item from the BOTMP are shown in Figure 8-2. In this example, the instructions to be given to the child

---

BOX 8-1 Calculating the Chronologic and Corrected Age

Many standardized tests require that the examiner calculate the child's exact age on the date of testing. The method for calculating both the chronologic and the corrected age is presented below.

CALCULATING THE CHRONOLOGIC AGE
First, the date of testing and the child's birth date are recorded in the following order:

	Year	Month	Day
Date of testing	99	6	15
Birth date	95	3	10
Chronologic age	4	3	5

Beginning on the right (the Day category), the day, month, and year of the child's birth date are subtracted from the date of testing. In the above example, the child's chronologic age is 4 years, 3 months, 5 days at the time of testing.

The convention when calculating age is, if the number of days in the chronologic age is 15 or less, the month is *rounded down*. Therefore in the above example, the child's age would be stated as 4 years, 3 months, or 4-3. If the number of days in the chronologic age is between 16 and 30, the month is *rounded up*. If the above child's chronologic age had been 4 years, 3 months, 16 days, the chronologic age would be expressed as 4 years, 4 months, or 4-4.

Sometimes, "borrowing" is necessary to subtract the birth date from the date of testing correctly:

	Year	Month	Day
Date of testing	99	6	15
Birth date	95	10	22
Chronologic age	3	7	23

Begin with the Day category. Twenty-two cannot be subtracted from 15 without borrowing from the Month category. One month must be borrowed and placed in the Day category. One month equals 30 days; 30 is added to the 15 days in the Date of testing, giving a total of 45. Twenty-two is subtracted from 45, leaving 23 days. Moving to the Month category, 1 month has been borrowed by the Day category, leaving 5 months. Because 10 cannot be subtracted from 5, 1 year must be borrowed from the Year category. One year equals 12 months,

therefore 12 will be added to the 5 in the Month category for Date of testing, totaling 17. Ten is subtracted from 17, leaving 7 months. Moving to the Year category, 1 year has been borrowed by the Month category, leaving 98. Ninety-five can be subtracted from 98, leaving 3 years. Therefore this child's chronologic age is 3 years, 7 months, 23 days. Using the rounding convention discussed above, the month is rounded up, giving a chronologic age of 3 years, 8 months.

CALCULATING THE CORRECTED AGE
Corrected age is used for children who were born prematurely to "correct" for the number of weeks they were born prior to the due date. Generally, the age is corrected until the child turns 2 years old, although this convention can vary. Given 40 weeks' gestation as full term, the amount of correction is the difference between the actual gestational age at birth and the 40 weeks' full-term gestational age. Therefore a child born at 30 weeks' gestation is 10 weeks premature. Many practitioners consider 36 or 37 weeks or above to be full-term gestation, therefore children with a gestational age of 36 weeks or above do not receive a corrected age. Because there is some variation in how and when corrected age is used, it is wise for the therapist to learn the procedures of his or her facility and to adhere to them when calculating corrected age.

If the expected due date and birth date are both known, subtracting the birth date from the due date yields an exact measurement of prematurity.

	Year	Month	Day
Due date	98	9	20
Birth date	98	6	12
	—	3	8

This child is 3 months, 8 days premature. To calculate corrected age, subtract the prematurity value from the chronologic age:

	Year	Month	Day
Chronologic age	1	1	25
Prematurity	—	3	8
	—	10	17

The child's corrected age is 10 months, 17 days or, when rounded, 11 months.

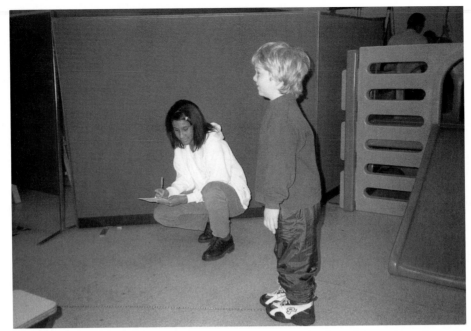

FIGURE 8-1 A therapist prepares to test a child on the broad jump item from the Bruininks-Oseretsky Test of Motor Proficiency.

are printed in bold type. Also included are the criteria for a passing score on the item, examples of incorrect responses, the number of trials and the time allowed for completion of the item. This example (Figure 8-2) describes how to present the item and what constitutes a passing score, as well as a diagram of what a passing performance looks like.

TYPES OF STANDARDIZED TESTS

The two main types of standardized tests are norm-referenced tests and criterion-referenced tests. Many pediatric occupational therapists use both types in their practices. Each type has a specific purpose, and it is important for testers to be aware of the purpose of the test they are using.

A norm-referenced test is developed by giving the test in question to a large number of children, usually several hundred or more. This group is called the normative sample, and *norms*, or average scores, are derived from this sample. When a norm-referenced test is administered, the performance of the child being tested is compared with the normative sample. The purpose of norm-referenced testing, then, is to determine how a child performs in relation to the average performance of the normative sample.

Test developers generally attempt to include children from a variety of geographic locations, ethnic and racial backgrounds, and socioeconomic levels so that the normative sample is representative of the population of the United States, based on the most recent U.S. Census data. Generally, the normative sample is composed of

children who have no developmental delays or conditions, although some tests include smaller subsamples of clinical populations as a means of determining whether the test discriminates between children whose development is proceeding normally and those who have known developmental delays.

Norm-referenced tests tend to be rather general in content and to cover a wide variety of skills. Some of the items may not have functional significance, but rather give an indication of the child's ability level in a particular domain. For example, the BOTMP includes a subtest, Bilateral Coordination. Items in this subtest involve tapping fingers and feet simultaneously, jumping and touching the feet, and performing running patterns with arms and legs. Although none of these activities are particularly functional in and of themselves, the standard score obtained from this subtest can tell the therapist whether a child has difficulty with bilateral coordination. If, in the therapist's clinical judgment, the bilateral coordination deficits affect the child's ability to appropriately engage in areas of occupation such as play, education, or activities of daily living, the therapist can select related functional activities to address the child's performance skill deficits.

Norm-referenced tests have standardized protocols for administration and scoring. The tester must adhere to these protocols so that each test administration is as similar as possible to that of the normative sample. This is necessary to compare any child's performance fairly with that of the normative sample.

Sometimes the examiner must deviate from the standard protocol because of special needs of the child

Touching Thumb to Fingertips — Eyes Closed

With eyes closed, the subject touches the thumb of the preferred hand to each of the fingertips on the preferred hand, moving from the little finger to the index finger and then from the index finger to the little finger, as shown below. The subject is given 90 seconds to complete the task once. The score is recorded as a pass or a fail.

Trials: 1

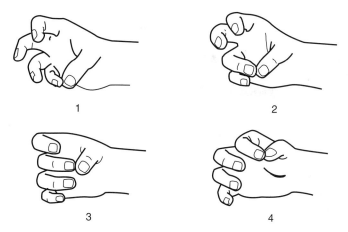

1   2

3   4

Administering and Recording

Have the subject sit beside you at a table. Have the subject extend the preferred arm. Then say, **You are to touch your thumb to each of the fingertips on this hand. Start with your little finger and touch each fingertip in order. Then start with your first finger and touch each fingertip again as you move your thumb back to your little finger** (demonstrate). **Do this with your eyes closed until I tell you to stop. Ready, begin.**

Begin timing. If necessary provide additional instruction. During the trial correct the subject and have the subject start over if he or she:
    a. Fails to maintain continuous movements
    b. Touches any finger except the index finger more than once in succession
    c. Touches two fingers at the same time
    d. Fails to touch fingers above the first finger joint
    e. Opens eyes

Allow no more than 90 seconds, including time needed for additional instruction, for the subject to complete the task once. After 90 seconds, tell the subject to stop.

On the Individual Record Form, record pass or fail.

FIGURE 8-2 Administration and scoring protocol for Bruininks-Oseretsky Test of Motor Proficiency, subtest 5, item 8. (From Bruininks, R.H. [1978]. *Bruininks-Oseretsky Test of Motor Proficiency*. Circle Pines, MN: American Guidance Service.)

being tested. For instance, a child with visual impairments may need manual guidance to cut with scissors, or a child with cerebral palsy may need assistance stabilizing the shoulder and upper arm to reach and grasp a crayon. If changes are made in the standardized procedures, the examiner must indicate this in the summary of assessment, and standard scores cannot be used to describe that child's performance in comparison with the normative sample.

Norm-referenced tests have specific psychometric properties. They have been analyzed by statisticians to obtain score distributions, mean or average scores, and standard scores. This is done to achieve the primary objective of norm-referenced tests: comparability of scores with the normative sample. A test under development initially has a much larger number of items than the final version of the test. Through pilot testing, items are chosen or rejected based partly on how well they statistically discriminate between children of different ages and/or abilities. Items are not primarily chosen for their relevance to functional skills. Consequently, some norm-referenced tests are not intended to link test performance with specific objectives or goals for intervention. Other norm-referenced tests, such as the Sensory Profile, are designed to specifically evaluate the effect of sensory processes on functional performance in daily life and, when combined with other evaluation and observation data, to allow therapists to develop intervention goals. A portion of the Sensory Profile questionnaire is presented in Figure 8-3.

A criterion-referenced test, by contrast, is designed to provide information on how children perform on specific tasks. The term *criterion referenced* refers to the fact that a child's performance is compared with a particular *criterion*, or level of performance of a particular skill. The goal of a criterion-referenced test is to determine which skills a child can and cannot accomplish, thereby providing a focus for intervention. In general the content of a criterion-referenced test is detailed and in some cases may relate to specific behavioral or functional objectives. The intent of a criterion-referenced test is to measure a child's performance on specific tasks rather than to compare the child's performance with that of his or her peers.

Many developmental checklists have been field tested and then published as criterion-referenced tests. The HELP is a good example of a developmental checklist designed to be used with children from birth to 3 years of age. It contains a large number of items in each of the domains of gross motor, fine motor, language, cognitive, social-emotional, and self-help skills. Each item correlates with specific intervention objectives. For instance,

if a child is not able to pass Fine Motor item 4.81, Snips with Scissors, a list of intervention ideas are presented in the HELP activity guide (Furuno et al., 1997). The activity guide is meant to accompany the test and is designed to help the therapist or educator by providing ideas for developmentally appropriate activities to address areas of weakness identified in the criterion-based assessment. The administration protocol for this item and the associated intervention activities are presented in Boxes 8-2 and 8-3.

Administration and scoring procedures may or may not be standardized on a criterion-referenced test. The HELP has standard procedures for administering and scoring each item. In contrast, the SFA is a judgment-based questionnaire completed by one or more school professionals familiar with the child's performance at school (Coster et al., 1998). Criteria for rating the child's performance on each item are provided. School professionals are encouraged to collaborate in determining ratings and to use these ratings as a basis for designing an intervention plan. Figure 8-4 shows a category of activity performance with the associated rating scale. Many other criterion-referenced tests take the form of checklists, in which the specific performance needed to receive credit on an item is not specified. Many therapist-designed tests for use in a particular facility or setting are nonstandardized, criterion-referenced tests.

Criterion-referenced tests are not subjected to the statistical analyses performed on norm-referenced tests. No mean score or normal distribution is calculated; a child

Sensory Processing				ALWAYS	FREQUENTLY	OCCASIONALLY	SELDOM	NEVER
Item			**A. Auditory Processing**					
👂	L	1	Responds negatively to unexpected or loud noises (for example, cries or hides at noise from vacuum cleaner, dog barking, hair dryer)					
👂	L	2	Holds hands over ears to protect ears from sound					
👂	L	3	Has trouble completing tasks when the radio is on					
👂	L	4	Is distracted or has trouble functioning if there is a lot of noise around					
👂	L	5	Can't work with background noise (for example, fan, refrigerator)					
👂	H	6	Appears to not hear what you say (for example, does not "tune-in" to what you say, appears to ignore you)					
👂	H	7	Doesn't respond when name is called but you know the child's hearing is OK					
👂	H	8	Enjoys strange noises/seeks to make noise for noise's sake					
			Section Raw Score Total					

Comments

FIGURE 8-3 A portion of the caregiver questionnaire for the Sensory Profile. (From Dunn, W. [1999]. *Sensory Profile user's manual*. San Antonio: Psychological Corporation.)

BOX 8-2 Administration and Scoring Protocol for Hawaii Early Learning Profile: Item 4.81—Snips with Scissors (23 to 25 Months)

Definition: The child cuts a paper edge randomly, one snip at a time, rather than using a continuous cutting motion.

Example observation opportunities: *Incidental*—May observe while the child is preparing for a tea party with stuffed animals or dolls. Demonstrate making fringe on paper place mats and invite the child to help. *Structured*—Using a half piece of sturdy paper and blunt scissors, make three snips in separate places along the edge of the paper while the child is watching. Exaggerate the opening and closing motions of your hand. Offer the child the scissors and invite him or her to make a cut. Let the child explore the scissors (if interested), helping him or her position the scissors in his or her hand as needed.

Credit: Snips paper in one place, holding the paper in one hand and scissors in the other (see also Credit Notes in this strand's preface).

From Parks, S. (1992). Inside HELP: Administration and reference manual for the Hawaii Early Learning Profile. Palo Alto, CA: Vort.

BOX 8-3 Administration and Scoring Protocol for Hawaii Early Learning Profile: Item 4.81— Activity Guide Suggestions

The child cuts with the scissors, taking one snip at a time rather than doing continuous cutting.
1 Let the child use small kitchen tongs to pick up objects and to practice opening and closing motions.
2 Let the child use child-sized scissors with rounded tips.
3 Demonstrate by placing your finger and thumb through the handles.
4 Position the scissors with the finger holes one above the other. Position the child's forearm in midsupination (i.e., thumb up). Let the child place his or her thumb through the top hole and the middle finger through the bottom hole. If the child's fingers are small, place the index and middle fingers in the bottom hole. The child will adjust his or her fingers as experience is gained.
5 Let the child open and close the scissors. Assist as necessary by placing your hand over the child's hand.
6 Let the child snip narrow strips of paper and use it for fringe in art work.
7 The different types of scissors available for children are a scissors with reinforced rubber coating on the handle grips; a scissors with double handle grips for your hand and the child's hand; a left-handed scissors; and a scissors for a prosthetic hook. Use the different types of child's scissors appropriately as required.

From Furuno, S., O'Reilly, K.A., Hosaka, C.M., Zeisloft, B., & Allman, T. (1985). *HELP activity guide*. Palo Alto, CA: Vort.

may pass all items or fail all items on a particular test without adversely affecting the validity of the test results. The purpose of the test is to learn exactly what a child can accomplish, not to compare the child's performance with that of the peer group. This goal is also reflected in the test development process for criterion-referenced tests. Items are generally chosen based on a process of task analysis or identification of important developmental milestones rather than for their statistical validity. Therefore the specific items on a criterion-referenced test have a direct relationship with functional skills and can be used as a starting point for generating appropriate goals and objectives for therapy intervention. To be useful for intervention planning, the summary scores from criterion-referenced tests should relate closely to the child's current pattern of performance (Fisher, 1993).

The characteristics of norm-referenced and criterion-referenced tests are compared in Table 8-2. As is shown in the table, some tests are both norm-referenced and criterion-referenced. This means that although the items have been analyzed for their ability to perform statistically, they also reflect functional or developmental skills that are appropriate for intervention. These tests permit the therapist to compare a child's performance with that of peers in the normative sample, and they also provide information about specific skills that may be appropriate for remediation.

The Peabody Developmental Motor Scales (2nd Edition) (PDMS-2) is an example of both a norm-referenced and a criterion-referenced test. Although the

PDMS-2 has been subjected to the statistical analyses used in norm-referenced tests, many individual items on the test also represent developmental milestones that can be addressed as part of the intervention plan. The SFA, although primarily a criterion-referenced test, provides a criterion score and standard error for each raw score based on a national standardization sample.

TECHNICAL ASPECTS

The following discussion of the technical aspects of standardized tests focuses on the statistics and test development procedures used for norm-referenced tests. Information on how standard scores are obtained and reported is included, as well as how the reliability and validity of a test are evaluated. It is the responsibility of the test author to provide initial data on test reliability and validity. However, these test characteristics are never definitively determined, and ongoing evaluation of validity and reliability are necessary. A knowledge of technical aspects of standardized tests is important to occupational therapists for the following reasons:
1 Therapists must be able to analyze and select standardized tests appropriately, according to the child's age and functional level and the purpose of testing.
2 Therapists must be able to interpret and report scores from standardized tests accurately.

Behavior Regulation

1. Displays appropriate restraint regarding self-stimulation (e.g., refrains from head banging, hand flapping).................	1	2	3	4
2. Accepts unexpected changes in routine...........	1	2	3	4
3. Refrains from provoking others..................	1	2	3	4
4. Uses nonaggressive words and actions..........	1	2	3	4
5. Maintains behavioral control in large groups of students (e.g., cafeteria, assemblies).............	1	2	3	4
6. Hears constructive criticism without losing temper..	1	2	3	4
7. Uses words rather than physical actions to respond when provoked or angry at others........	1	2	3	4
8. Seeks adult assistance, if necessary, when experiencing peer conflict, especially conflicts involving violence............................	1	2	3	4
9. Responds to/handles teasing in a constructive way...	1	2	3	4
10. Handles frustration when experiencing difficulties with school tasks/activities......................	1	2	3	4
11. Shows common sense in words and actions around bullies, gangs, or strangers....................	1	2	3	4
12. Resolves ordinary peer conflicts or problems adequately on his/her own without requesting teacher assistance...........................	1	2	3	4

Respondent's Initials	Behavior Regulation Raw Score	

Ratings Key for Activity Performance

1: Does not perform   **2:** Partial performance   **3:** Inconsistent performance   **4:** Consistent performance

FIGURE 8-4 One category of activity performance and corresponding rating scale for the School Function Assessment (SFA). (From Coster, W., Deeney, T., Haltiwanger, J., & Haley, S. [1998]. *School Function Assessment.* San Antonio: Psychological Corporation.)

TABLE 8-2 Comparison of Norm-Referenced and Criterion-Referenced Tests

Characteristic	Norm-Referenced Test	Criterion-Referenced Test
Purpose	Comparison of child's performance with normative sample	Comparison of child's performance with a defined list of skills
Content	General; usually covers a wide variety of skills	Detailed; may cover specific objectives or developmental milestones
Administration and scoring	Always standardized	May be standardized or nonstandardized
Psychometric properties	Normal distribution of scores; means, standard deviations, and standard scores computed	No score distribution needed; a child may pass or fail all items
Item selection	Items chosen for statistical performance; may not relate to functional skills or therapy objectives	Items chosen for functional and developmental importance; provides necessary information for developing therapy objectives
Examples	BSID-II; PDMS-2; BOTMP; PEDI	PDMS-2, PEDI, HELP, Gross-Motor Function Measure, SFA

BOTMP, Bruininks-Oseretsky Test of Motor Proficiency; *BSID-II,* Bayley Scales of Infant Development (Revised); *HELP,* Hawaii Early Learning Profile; *PDMS,* Peabody Developmental Motor Scales; *PEDI,* Pediatric Evaluation of Disability Inventory; *SFA,* School Function Assessment.

3 Therapists must be able to explain test results to caregivers and other professionals working with the child in a clear, understandable manner.

The following discussion of technical aspects of standardized tests focuses on the statistics and test development procedures used for norm-referenced tests. It includes information on (1) descriptive statistics, (2) standard scores, (3) correlation coefficients, (4) reliability, and (5) validity.

Descriptive Statistics

Descriptive statistics provide information about the characteristics of a particular group. Many human characteristics, such as height, weight, head size, and intelligence, are represented by a distribution called the *normal curve* (or *bell-shaped curve*) (Figure 8-5). The pattern of performance on most norm-referenced tests also follows this curve. The greatest number of people receive a score in the middle part of the distribution, with progressively smaller numbers receiving scores at either the high or the low end. Descriptive statistics also provide information about where members of a group are located on the normal curve. The two types of descriptive statistics are the measure of central tendency and the measure of variability.

The measure of central tendency indicates the middle point of the distribution for a particular group, or sample, of children. The most frequently used measure of central tendency is the *mean*, which is the sum of all the scores for a particular sample divided by the number of scores. It is computed mathematically using a simple formula

$$\bar{X} = \frac{\sum X}{n}$$

where Σ means to sum, X is each individual score, and n is the number of scores in the sample (the mean is also often called the average score).

Another measure of central tendency is the *median*, which is simply the middle score of a distribution. Half the scores lie below the median and half above it. The median is the preferred measure of central tendency when outlying or extreme scores are present in the distribution. The following distribution of scores is an example:

2 3 13 14 17 17 18

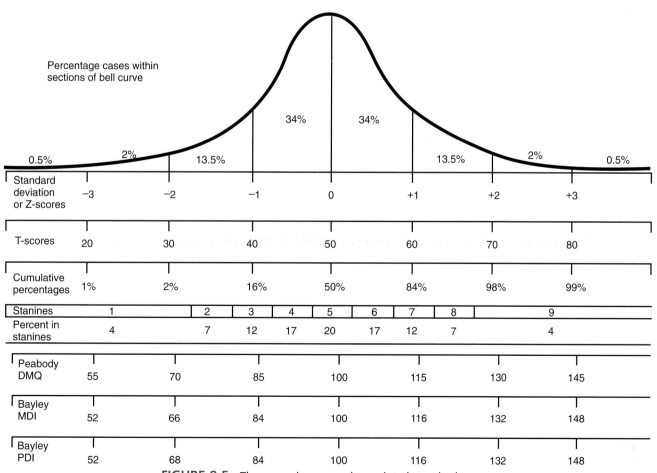

FIGURE 8-5 The normal curve and associated standard scores.

The mean score is 12 [i.e., (2 + 3 + 13 + 14 + 17 + 17 + 18) ÷ 7]. The median, or middle score, is 14. In this case the score of 14 is a more accurate representation of the middle point of these scores than is the score of 12 because the two low scores, or *outliers,* in the distribution pulled down the value of the mean.

The measure of variability determines how much the performance of the group as a whole deviates from the mean. Measures of variability are used to compute the standard scores used in standardized tests. As with measures of central tendency, measures of variability are derived from the normal curve. The two measures of variability discussed are the variance and the standard deviation.

The *variance* is the average of the squared deviations of the scores from the mean. In other words, it is a measure of how far the score of an average individual in a sample deviates from the group mean. The variance is computed using the following formula:

$$S^2 = \frac{\sum(X - \bar{X})^2}{n}$$

Where S^2 is the variance, $\sum(X - X)^2$ is the sum of each individual score minus the mean score, and n is the total number of scores in the group. The standard deviation is simply the square root of the variance. To illustrate, calculations are provided for the mean, the variance, and the standard deviation for the following set of scores from a hypothetical test:

$$17 \ 19 \ 21 \ 25 \ 28$$

To calculate the mean, the following equation is used:

$$\frac{(17 + 19 + 21 + 25 + 28)}{5} = 22$$

To calculate the variance, the mean must be subtracted from each score, and that value then must be squared:

$$17 - 22 = (-5)^2 = 25$$
$$19 - 22 = (-3)^2 = 9$$
$$21 - 22 = (-1)^2 = 1$$
$$25 - 22 = (3)^2 = 9$$
$$28 - 22 = (6)^2 = 36$$

The squared values are summed and then divided by the total number of scores:

$$25 + 9 + 1 + 9 + 36 = 80$$
$$80 \div 5 = 16$$

The variance of this score distribution is 16. The standard deviation is simply the square root of the variance, or 4.

The *standard deviation (SD)* is an important number because it is the basis for computing many standard scores. In a normal distribution (see Figure 8-5), 68% of the people in the distribution score within 1 SD of the mean (±1 SD); 95% score within 2 SD of the mean (±2 SD); and 99.7% score within 3 SD of the mean (±3 SD). In the score distribution with a mean of 22 and a standard deviation of 4, three of the five scores were within 1 SD of the mean (22 ± 4; a score range of 18 to 26), and all five scores were within 2 SD of the mean (22 ± 8; a score range of 14 to 30). The standard deviation, then, determines the placement of scores on the normal curve. By showing the degree of variability in the sample, the standard deviation reveals how far the scores can be expected to range from the mean value.

Standard Scores

Standardized tests are scored in several different ways. Scoring methods include Z-scores, T-scores, deviation intelligence quotient (IQ) scores, developmental index scores, percentile scores, and age-equivalent scores.

The *Z-score* is computed by subtracting the mean for the test from the individual's score and dividing it by the standard deviation, using the following equation:

$$Z = \frac{X - \bar{X}}{SD}$$

Using the score distribution above (i.e., 17 19 21 25 28), the person receiving the score of 17 would have a Z-score of $(17 - 22) \div 4 = -1.25$. The person receiving the score of 28 would have a Z-score of $(28 - 22) \div 4 = 1.5$. The negative value of the first score indicates that the Z-score value is below the mean for the test, and the positive value of the second score indicates that the Z-score value is above the mean. Generally, a Z-score value of −1.5 or less is considered indicative of delay or deficit in the area measured, although this can vary, depending on the particular test.

The *T-score* is derived from the Z-score. In a T-score distribution, the mean is 50 and the standard deviation is 10. The T-score is computed using the following equation:

$$T = 10(Z) + 50$$

For the two Z-scores computed above, the T-score values are as follows: for the first Z-score of −1.25, the T-score is $10(-1.25) + 50 = 37.50$. For the second Z-score of 1.5, the T-score is $10(1.5) + 50 = 65$. Note that all T-scores have positive values, but because the mean of a T-score distribution is 50, any number below 50 indicates a score below the mean. Because the standard deviation of the T distribution is 10, the first score of 37.50 is slightly more than 1 SD below the mean. The second score of 65 is 15 points, or 1.5 SD, above the mean.

Two other standard scores that are frequently seen in standardized tests are the *deviation IQ score* and the *developmental index score.* Deviation IQ scores have a mean of 100 and a standard deviation of either 15 or 16. These are the IQ scores obtained from such tests as the Stanford-Binet (Thorndike, Hagen, & Sattler, 1986) or the Wechsler Intelligence Scale for Children (WISC) (Wechsler, 1991). On these tests, individuals with IQ scores 2 SD below the mean (IQs of 70 and 68, respectively) are considered to be mentally retarded. Individuals with IQ scores 2 SD above the mean (IQs of 130 and 132, respectively) are considered gifted. Developmental index scores are used in developmental tests such as the PDMS-2 and the BSID-2. Like the deviation IQ scores, they have a mean of 100 and a standard deviation of 15 or 16. Children who receive a developmental index score of 2 SD below the mean (index score of 68 or 70) in one or more skill areas are considered to be in need of remedial services. In many cases children who receive developmental index scores lower than −1.5 SD (index score of 85) may also be recommended for remedial services.

Two other types of scores (i.e., percentile scores and age-equivalent scores) are frequently used in standardized tests. These are not standard scores in the strictest sense, because they are computed directly from raw scores rather than through the statistically derived measures of central tendency and variability. However, they give an indication of a child's performance relative to that of the normative sample.

The *percentile score* is the percentage of people in a standardization sample whose score is at or below a particular raw score. A percentile score of 60, for instance, indicates that 60% of the people in the standardization sample received a score that was at or below the raw score corresponding to the 60th percentile. Tests that use percentile scores generally include a table in the manual by which raw scores can be converted to percentile scores. These tables usually indicate at what percentile rank performance is considered deficient. Raw scores can be converted to percentile rank (PR) scores by a simple formula:

$$PR = \frac{\left(\begin{array}{c} \text{Number of people} \\ \text{below score} \end{array} + \begin{array}{c} \text{One half of} \\ \text{people at score} \end{array}\right) \times 100}{\text{Total number of scores}}$$

Using the previous sample data (i.e., 17 19 21 25 28), percentile ranks for the highest and lowest scores can be computed. The raw score of 17 is the lowest score in the distribution and is the only score of 17. Therefore the equation is as follows:

$$\frac{(0 + 0.5)}{5} \times 100 = \frac{0.5}{5} \times 100 = 10$$

The highest score in the distribution is 28, therefore four people have lower scores and one person received a score of 28. The equation is as follows:

$$\frac{(4 + 0.5)}{5} \times 100 = \frac{4.5}{5} \times 100 = 90$$

In this distribution, then, the lowest score is at the 10th percentile and the highest score is at the 90th percentile.

Although PR scores can be easily calculated and understood, they have a significant disadvantage: the percentile ranks are not equal in size across the score distribution. Distances between percentile ranks are much smaller in the middle of the distribution than at the ends; consequently, improving a score from the 50th to the 55th percentile requires much less effort than improving a score from the 5th to the 10th percentile (see Figure 8-5). As a result, an improvement in performance by a child functioning at the lower end of the score range may not be reflected in the PR score the child achieves. Other standard scores are more sensitive at measuring changes in the performance of children who fall at the extreme ends of the score distribution.

The *age-equivalent score* is the age at which the raw score is at the 50th percentile. The age-equivalent score generally is expressed in years and months; for example, 4-3 (i.e., 4 years, 3 months). It is a score that is easily understood by parents and caregivers who may not be familiar with testing concepts or terminology. However, age-equivalent scores have significant disadvantages. Although they may provide a general idea of a child's overall developmental level, it may be misleading to say, for example, that a 4-year-old is functioning at the 2.5-year level. The age-equivalent score may be more or less an average of several developmental domains, some of which may be at the 4.5-year level and some at the 1.5-year level. Therefore the child's performance may be highly variable and may not reflect that of a typical 2.5-year-old. In addition, because the age-equivalent score represents only the score that a child of a particular age who is performing at the 50th percentile would receive, a child who is performing within normal limits for his or her age but whose score is below the 50th percentile would receive an age-equivalent score below his or her chronologic age. This can cause parents or caregivers to conclude incorrectly that the child has delays. Age equivalents, then, are a type of standard score that can contribute to an understanding of a child's performance, but they are the least psychometrically sound, can be misleading, and should be used only with the greatest caution.

Correlation Coefficients

Test manuals often report correlation coefficients when describing the test's reliability and validity. A correlation coefficient tells the degree or strength of the relationship between two scores or variables. Although the standard scores are used to compute individual scores, correlation coefficients are used to determine the relationship between scores from one measurement and those from another. Correlation coefficients range from −1.00 to +1.00. A correlation coefficient of 0.00

indicates that no relationship exists between the two variables measured. Any relationship that occurs is strictly by chance. The closer the correlation coefficient is either to −1.00 or to +1.00, the stronger is the relationship between the two variables. A negative correlation means that a high score on one variable is accompanied by a low score on the other variable. A positive correlation means that a high score on one variable is accompanied by a high score on the other variable and that a low score on one variable is accompanied by a low score on the other variable.

Examples of two variables that generally have a fairly high positive correlation are height and weight. Taller individuals are also generally heavier than shorter individuals. However, this is not always true. Some tall individuals are light, and some short individuals are heavy. Consequently, the correlation between height and weight for a given population is a positive value, but it is not a perfect 1.00. Examples of two variables that are unrelated are eye color and height. The correlation coefficient for these two variables for any population is close to zero, because a person's eye color cannot be predicted by the individual's height.

An example of two variables that have a negative correlation might be hours spent studying and hours spent watching television. A student who spends many hours studying probably watches fewer hours of television, and a student who watches many hours of television probably spends fewer hours studying. Hence, a negative relationship exists between these two variables. As one variable increases, the other decreases. Several different correlation coefficients may be calculated, depending on the type of data used. Some correlation coefficients commonly used in test manuals include the Pearson Product-Moment Correlation Coefficient or Pearson r, the Spearman Rank-Order Correlation Coefficient, and the Intraclass Correlation Coefficient (ICC).

Why are correlation coefficients important? As the following sections on reliability and validity illustrate, correlation coefficients are important tools for evaluating the properties of a test. Knowledge of test characteristics helps testers know how best to use a test and makes them aware of the strengths and limitations of individual tests.

Reliability

The reliability of a test describes the consistency or stability of scores obtained by one individual when tested on two different occasions with different sets of items or under other variable examining conditions (Anastasi & Urbina, 1997). For instance, if a child is given a test and receives a score of 50 and 2 days later is given the same test and receives a score of 75, the reliability of the test is questionable. The difference between the two scores is called the *error variance* of the test, which is a result of random fluctuations in performance between the two

testing sessions. Some amount of random error variance is expected in any test situation because of variations in such things as the child's mood, fatigue, or motivation. Error variance can also be caused by environmental characteristics such as light, temperature, or noise. However, it is important that error variance caused by variations in examiners or by the characteristics of the test itself be minimal. Confidence in the scores obtained requires that the test have adequate reliability over a number of administrations and low error variance.

Most standardized tests evaluate two or three forms of reliability. The three forms of reliability most commonly used in pediatric standardized tests are (1) test-retest reliability, (2) interrater reliability, and (3) standard error of measurement (SEM).

Test-Retest Reliability

Test-retest reliability is a measurement of the stability of a test over time. It is obtained by giving the test to the same individual on two different occasions. In the evaluation of test-retest reliability for a pediatric test, the time span between test administrations must be short to minimize the possibility of developmental changes occurring between the two test sessions. However, the time span between tests should not be so short that the child may recall items administered during the first test session, thereby improving his or her performance on the second test session (this is called the *learning,* or *practice, effect*).

Generally, the time span between testing sessions is no more than 1 week for infants and very young children and no more than 2 weeks for older children. During the process of test development, test-retest reliability is evaluated on a subgroup of the normative sample. The size and composition of the subgroup should be specified in the manual. The correlation coefficient between the scores of the two test sessions is calculated. This coefficient is the measure of the test-retest reliability. A test that has a high test-retest reliability coefficient is more likely to yield relatively stable scores over time. That is, it is affected less by random error variance than is a test with a low test-retest reliability coefficient. When administering a test with a low test-retest reliability coefficient, the examiner has less confidence that the score obtained is a true reflection of the child's abilities. If the child were tested at a different time of day or in a different setting entirely, different results might be obtained.

A sample of 175 infants was evaluated twice within 2 weeks (about 4 days apart) to assess the test-retest reliability of the BSID-II (Bayley, 1993). Correlation coefficients were high but not perfect (0.83 for the Mental Scale and 0.77 for the Motor Scale). The performance of a young child often varies within short periods because it is highly influenced by variables such as mood, hunger, sleepiness, and irritability. The test-retest reliability coefficients for 50 children tested twice within 1 week with the PDMS-2 ranged from 0.73 for the Fine Motor Quotient and 0.84 for the Gross Motor Quotient for 2- to 11-month-old children to 0.94 for the Fine Motor Quotient and 0.93 for the Gross Motor Quotient for 12- to 17-month-old children (Folio & Fewell, 2000).

To evaluate the test-retest reliability of the Developmental Test of Visual Perception, Second Edition (DTVP-II), 88 students were tested twice within 2 weeks (Hammill, Pearson, & Voress, 1993). The correlation coefficients for the test's subsections ranged from 0.80 to 0.93. The reliability for the total test scores was 0.95.

These three examples of good to excellent test-retest reliability are typical examples of pediatric sensorimotor tests. The rapid and variable development of young children and the practice effect are two factors that negatively influence the tests' stability over time. The test-retest reliability of a test is critical to the use of the results as a measure of progress or of intervention efficacy.

Interrater Reliability

Interrater reliability refers to the ability of two independent raters to obtain the same scores when scoring the same child simultaneously. Interrater reliability is generally measured on a subset of the normative sample during the test development process. This is often accomplished by having one rater administer and score the test while another rater observes and scores at the same time. The correlation coefficient calculated from the two raters' scores is the interrater reliability coefficient of the test. It is particularly important to measure interrater reliability on tests for which the scoring may require some judgment on the part of the examiner.

Although the scoring criteria for many test items are specific on most tests, to a certain extent, scoring depends on individual judgment, and scoring differences can arise between different examiners. A test that has a low interrater reliability coefficient is especially susceptible to differences in scoring by different raters. This may mean that the administration and scoring criteria are not stated explicitly enough, requiring examiners to make judgment calls on a number of items. Alternatively, it can mean that the items on the test call for responses that are too broad or vague to permit precise scoring.

No universal agreement has been reached regarding the minimum acceptable coefficient for test-retest and interrater reliability. The context of the reliability measurement, the type of test, and the distribution of scores are some of the variables that can be taken into account when determining an acceptable reliability coefficient. One standard suggested by Anastasi and Urbina (1997) and used by a number of examiners is 0.80.

Not all tests have test-retest or interrater reliability coefficients that reach the 0.80 level. Lower coefficients indicate greater variability in scores. When examiners use a test that has a reliability coefficient below 0.80, scores must be interpreted with great caution. For example, if one subtest of a test of motor development has test-retest reliability of 0.60, the examiner who uses it to measure change over time must acknowledge that a portion of the apparent change between the first and second test administration is a result of the error variance of the test.

Interrater reliability was assessed for the BSID-II using 51 children 2 to 30 months of age. Items were administered and scored by one examiner and simultaneously scored by an observer. The interrater reliability coefficients were 0.96 for the Mental Scale and 0.75 for the Motor Scale. The correlation coefficient for the Motor Scale seemed to be lower because these items involved manipulation of the infant to score, placing the observer at a disadvantage (Bayley, 1993).

Interrater reliability for the PDMS-2 was evaluated using a slightly different method. Sixty completed test protocols were randomly selected from the normative sample and were independently scored by two examiners. The resulting correlation coefficients were 0.97 for the Gross Motor Composite and 0.98 for the Fine Motor Composite (Folio & Fewell, 2000). It should be noted that this method of determining reliability is not based on two independent observations of the child's performance but on review of completed scoring protocols. Hence, potential error related to the way examiners interpreted and applied the scoring criteria to determine scores on individual items was not addressed. This could result in spuriously high interrater reliability coefficients. In a test such as the DTVP-II, in which scores are based on a written record of the child's response, interrater reliability is excellent. When two individuals scored 88 completed DTVP-II protocols, the interscorer reliability was 0.98 (Hammill et al., 1993).

When individual subtests of a comprehensive test have a low reliability coefficient, it is generally not recommended that the standard scores from the subtests be reported. Often the reliability coefficient of the entire test is much higher than that of the individual subtests. One reason for this is that reliability increases with the number of items on a test. Because subtests have fewer items than the entire test, they are more sensitive to fluctuations in the performance or scoring of individual items. When this occurs, it is best to describe subtest performance qualitatively, without reporting standard scores.

Standard scores can be reported for the total, or comprehensive, test score. Examiners should consult the reliability information in the test manual before deciding how to report test scores for individual subtests and for the test as a whole. The interrater reliability coefficients reported in the manual are estimates based on the context and conditions under which they were studied by the test developers. This reliability coefficient is an estimate; interrater reliability may vary when children are tested in different contexts or when examiners have differing levels of training and experience.

Examiners can exert some control over the interrater reliability of tests they use frequently. It is good practice for examiners to check interrater reliability with more experienced colleagues when learning a new standardized test before beginning to administer the test to children in the clinical setting. Also, periodic checking of interrater reliability with colleagues who are administering the same standardized tests is a good practice. Some simple methods for assessing interrater reliability are discussed in more detail later in the chapter.

Standard Error of Measurement

The *standard error of measurement (SEM)* is a statistic used to calculate the expected range of error for the test score of an individual. It is based on the range of scores an individual might obtain if the same test were administered a number of times simultaneously, with no practice or fatigue effects. Obviously, this is impossible; the SEM, therefore, is a theoretic construct. However, it is an indicator of the possible error variance in individual scores.

The SEM creates a normal curve for the individual's test scores, with the obtained score in the middle of the distribution. The child has a higher probability of receiving scores in the middle of the distribution than at the extreme ends. The SEM is based on the standard deviation of the test and the test's reliability (usually the test-retest reliability). The SEM can be calculated using the following formula:

$$SEM = SD\sqrt{(1-r)}$$

where *SEM* is the standard error of measurement, *SD* is the standard deviation, and *r* is the reliability coefficient for the test. Once the SEM has been calculated for a test, that value is added to and subtracted from the child's obtained score. This gives the range of expected scores for that child, a range known as the *confidence interval.* The SEM corresponds to the standard deviation for the normal curve: 68% of the scores in a normal distribution fall within 1 SD on either side of the mean, 95% of the scores fall within 2 SD on either side of the mean, and 99.7% of the scores fall within 3 SD on either side of the mean. Similarly, a child receives a score within 1 SEM on either side of his or her obtained score 68% of the time; a score within 2 SEM of the obtained score 95% of the time; and a score within 3 SEM of the obtained score 99.7% of the time.

Generally, test manuals report the 95% confidence interval. As can be seen by the equation above, when the SD of the test is high or the reliability is low, the SEM increases. A larger SEM means that the range of possible scores for an individual child is much greater (i.e., a larger confidence interval) and consequently that there is a greater degree of possible error variance for the child's score. This means that the examiner is less confident that any score obtained for a child on that test represents the child's true score.

An example may help to illustrate this point. Two tests are given, both consisting of 50 items and both testing the same skill area. One test has an SD of 1.0 and a test-retest reliability coefficient of 0.90. The SEM for that test is calculated as follows:

$$SEM = \sqrt{(1-0.90)}$$
$$SEM = 0.32$$

The second test has an SD of 5.0 and a test-retest reliability coefficient of 0.75. The SEM for that test would be calculated as follows:

$$SEM = 5\sqrt{(1-0.75)}$$
$$SEM = 2.5$$

Using the SEM, a 95% confidence interval can be calculated for each test. A 95% confidence interval is 2 SEM, therefore test 1 has a confidence interval of ±0.64 points from the obtained score, or a total of 1.28 points. Test 2 has a confidence interval of ±5 points, or a total of 10 points. If both tests were available for a particular client, an examiner could use test 1 with much more confidence that the obtained score is truly representative of that individual's abilities and is not caused by random error variance of the test.

Occupational therapists that use standardized tests should be aware of how much measurement error a test contains so that the potential range of performance can be estimated for each individual. Currently, the trend is to report standardized test results as confidence intervals rather than as individual scores (Dietz, 1989; Gregory, 2000). The score tables for the BSID-II include confidence intervals for each index score. According to Bayley, "the reporting of confidence intervals also serves as a reminder that the observed score contains some amount of measurement error" (Bayley, 1993, p. 192).

Consideration of the SEM is especially important when the differences between two scores are evaluated (e.g., when the progress a child has made with therapy over time is evaluated) (Anastasi & Urbina, 1997). If the confidence intervals of the two test scores overlap, it may be incorrect to conclude that any change has occurred. For instance, a child is tested in September and receives a raw score of 60. The child is tested again in June with the same test and receives a raw score of 75. Comparison of the two raw scores would seem to indicate that the child has made substantial progress. However, the scores should be considered in light of an SEM of 5.0. Using a 95% confidence interval (the 95% confidence interval is 2 SEM on either side of the obtained score), the confidence interval for the first score is 50 to 70, and the confidence interval of the second score is 65 to 85.

Based on the two test scores, it cannot be conclusively stated that the child has made progress because the confidence intervals overlap. It is conceivable that a substantial amount of the difference between the first and second scores is a result of error variance rather than actual change in the child's abilities. (See Cunningham-Amundson and Crowe [1993] for a more in-depth discussion of the use of the SEM in pediatric assessment, particularly the effect of the SEM in the interpretation of test scores and the qualification of children for remedial services.)

Validity

Validity is the extent to which a test measures what it says it measures (Anastasi & Urbina, 1997). For example, it is important for testers to know that a test of fine motor development actually measures fine motor skills and not gross motor or perceptual skills. The validity of a test must be established with reference to the particular use for which the test is being considered (Anastasi & Urbina, 1997). For instance, a test of fine motor development is probably highly valid as a measure of fine motor skills. It is less valid as a measure of visual-motor skills and has low validity as a measure of gross motor skills.

The information on validity reported in test manuals has been obtained during the test development process. In addition, after a test becomes available commercially, clinicians and researchers continue to evaluate validity and to publish the results of their validation studies. This information about test validity can help examiners make decisions about appropriate uses of standardized tests. The four categories of validity are construct-related validity, content-related validity, criterion-related validity, and Rasch analysis.

Construct-Related Validity

Construct-related validity is the extent to which a test measures a particular theoretic construct. Some constructs frequently measured by pediatric occupational therapists include fine motor skills, visual-perceptual skills, self-care skills, gross motor skills, and functional performance at home or school. There are many ways to determine construct validity, a few of which are discussed in this chapter.

One method of establishing construct validity involves investigating how well a test discriminates among different groups of individuals. For instance, a developmental test (e.g., BSID-II, PDMS-2, and BOTMP) is expected to differentiate between the performance of older and younger children. Older children should receive higher scores than younger children, providing clear evidence of developmental progression with advancing age. Because these tests are also intended to discriminate typically developing children from children with developmental delays, children in specific diagnostic categories should receive lower scores than children with no documented deficits.

For example, during the development process for the Sensory Profile (Dunn, 1999), the sensory processing patterns of children in the following clinical groups was evaluated: attention deficit hyperactivity disorder, autism/pervasive developmental disorder, fragile X disorder, sensory modulation disorder, and other disabilities. The scores for children in each of these groups differed from that of the standardization sample, with the score ranges for all factors generally lower than those for the standardization sample. This indicates that the Sensory Profile is able to differentiate children with typical sensory processing from those who have sensory processing differences. In addition, score patterns for various clinical groups were identified, allowing therapists to compare client scores with those of the corresponding clinical group. Subsequent research using the Sensory Profile has identified differences in sensory processing scores for children with Asperger's syndrome (Dunn, Myles, & Orr, 2002).

Factor analysis can be used as another method of establishing construct-related validity. *Factor analysis* is a statistical procedure for determining relationships between test items. In a test of motor skills that includes gross motor items and fine motor items, factor analysis is expected to identify two factors on which items showed the strongest correlation, one composed mostly of gross motor items and one composed mostly of fine motor items. Factor analysis of the Sensory Integration and Praxis Tests (SIPT) (Ayres, 1989) resulted in identification of four primary factors. The constructs that emerged from the analysis demonstrated that the test primarily measures praxis (motor planning). The constructs measured were visual-perceptual skills (related to praxis); somatosensory-praxis skills; bilateral integration and sequencing of movements; and praxis on verbal command (Ayres & Marr, 1991). Factor analysis helped establish the functions that are measured by the SIPT and that can be used to interpret the results of testing individual children.

The third method of establishing construct-related validity requires repeated administration of a test before and after a period of intervention. For example, a group of children is given a test of visual-perceptual skills and subsequently receives intervention focused on improving those skills. They are then retested with the same test and the difference in scores is analyzed. A rise in test scores supports the assertion that the test measured visual-perceptual skills and provides evidence of construct-related validity.

Content-Related Validity

Content-related validity is the extent to which the items on a test accurately sample a particular behavior domain. For instance, to test self-care skills, it is impractical to ask a child to perform every conceivable self-care activity. A sample of self-care activities must be chosen for inclusion on the test, and conclusions can be drawn about the child's abilities on the basis of the selected items. Examiners must have confidence that self-care skills are adequately represented so that accurate conclusions regarding the child's self-care skills can be made. Test manuals should show evidence that the authors have systematically analyzed the domain being tested. Content validity is established by review of the test content by experts in the field who reach some agreement that the content is, in fact, representative of the behavioral domain to be measured.

Criterion-Related Validity

Criterion-related validity is the ability of a test to predict how an individual performs on other measurements or activities. To establish criterion-related validity, the test score is checked against a criterion, an independent measure of what the test is designed to predict. The two forms of criterion-related validity are concurrent validity and predictive validity.

Concurrent validity describes how well test scores reflect current performance. The degree of relationship between the test and the criterion is described with a correlation coefficient. Most validity correlation coefficients range from 0.40 to 0.80; a coefficient of 0.70 or above indicates that performance on one test can predict performance on a second test.

Concurrent validity is examined in the test development process to determine the relationship between a new test and existing tests that test a similar construct. For instance, during the development of the Sensory Profile, children were scored with both the Sensory Profile and the School Function Assessment (SFA). The SFA was chosen because some aspects of children's performance at school depend on sensory processing and modulation (Dunn, 1999). High correlations between SFA performance items and the Fine Motor/Perceptual factor on the Sensory Profile were expected, because both tests address hand use. In addition, the SFA socialization and behavior interaction sections were expected to correlate highly with the modulation sections and factors on the Sensory Profile, because problems with regulating sensory input could result in problems with generating appropriate responses. The scores on the two tests were compared for a random sample of 16 children enrolled in special education programs. Portions of the correlational data are presented in Table 8-3. The correlations are negative because of the different scoring systems on the two tests; lower scores are desirable on the SFA but undesirable on the Sensory Profile.

As Table 8-3 shows, there are areas of moderate to high correlation and areas of low correlation between the two tests. Factor 9, which consists of items describing product-oriented behaviors, correlated strongly with three sections of the SFA. Factors 3, 6, and 8 on the Sensory Profile contain items that indicate low responsiveness, whereas Factor 5 contains items indicating over-responsiveness. These four factors correlated moderately with the Behavioral Regulation and Positive Interaction sections of the SFA, suggesting relationships between sensory processing and modulation, and children's social/behavioral repertoires (Dunn, 1999). This pattern of correlation coefficients supports the research hypotheses about relationships between the constructs measured

---

TABLE 8-3 Correlations between the Sensory Profile and the School Function Assessment

	School Function Assessment			
	Behavioral Regulation		Positive Interaction	
Sensory Profile				
FACTOR	**ADAPTATIONS**	**ASSISTANCE**	**ADAPTATIONS**	**ASSISTANCE**
1 Sensory Seeking	−0.434	−0.436	−0.095	−0.328
2 Emotionally Reactive	−0.372	−0.360	−0.245	−0.282
3 Low Endurance/Tone	−0.584*	−0.721*	−0.584*	−0.716*
4 Oral Sensory Sensitivity	−0.199	−0.320	.007	−0.300
5 Inattention/Distractibility	−0.582*	−0.584*	−0.495	−0.373
6 Poor Registration	−0.615*	−0.340	−0.348	−0.388
7 Sensory Sensitivity	−0.452	−0.478	−0.546*	−0.388
8 Sedentary	−0.551*	−0.554*	−0.545*	−0.368
9 Fine Motor/Perceptual	−0.502	−0.720†	−0.703†	−0.681†

Modified from Dunn, W. (1999). *Sensory Profile user's manual* (p. 54). San Antonio: Psychological Corporation.
*Correlation is significant at the 0.05 level (2-tailed).
†Correlation is significant at the 0.01 level (2-tailed).

by the two tests and also supports the validity of the Sensory Profile as a measure of sensory processing and modulation.

In contrast to concurrent validity, *predictive validity* identifies the relationship between a test given in the present and some measure of performance in the future. Establishing predictive validity is a much lengthier process than establishing other forms of validity because often several years must elapse between the first and second testing sessions. The predictive validity of a test often is not well documented until it has been in use for several years.

An area of interest to many pediatric occupational therapists has been the ability of developmental tests to predict which young children, identified as high risk because of premature birth, medical complications, or developmental concerns, will require special therapeutic or educational interventions as they become older. Prediction of outcomes necessitates testing of children early in life and subsequent testing of their developmental, physical, academic, or cognitive status several months or years later.

The Miller Assessment for Preschoolers (MAP) (Miller, 1988) is used frequently for preschool screening purposes, and several longitudinal studies have been conducted to establish the predictive validity of this instrument. A followup study of the MAP standardization sample 4 years after screening found moderate relationships between MAP total scores and WISC scores (correlation coefficients of 0.45 to 0.50) and Woodcock-Johnson Psycho-Educational Battery scores (Woodcock & Johnson, 1977) (correlations of 0.35 to 0.38), suggesting that the MAP adequately predicted intelligence and academic performance 4 years later (Miller, Lemerand, & Cohn, 1987). A more recent predictive study followed 15 preschoolers classified as being at risk based on MAP scores and 15 preschoolers classified as not being at risk. When tested 5 to 7 years after the initial screening with the MAP, the at-risk group demonstrated significantly poorer performance on visual-motor, cognitive, reading, and handwriting tests, as well as reduced overall school functional status (Parush, Winokur, Goldstand, & Miller, 2002). These studies lend support to the validity of the MAP in predicting later academic performance.

One final point about criterion-related validity: the meaningfulness of the comparison between a test and its criterion measure depends on both the quality of the test and the quality of the criterion. In the above example of predictive validity, the comparison of the MAP with the various intelligence and performance tests rests on the assumption that these tests are adequate measures of the constructs they claim to measure. If any of the tests were found to measure these criteria inaccurately, the validity of the MAP would also be in question. Because no single measure of criterion-related validity provides conclusive evidence of the test's validity, multiple investigations should be undertaken. Important standardized assessments undergo extensive evaluation of validity after publication. The resulting information helps the test user decide when and with whom the test results are most valid.

In summary, validity is an important but sometimes elusive concept that rests on a number of judgments by authors of the tests, users of the tests, and experts in the field of occupational therapy. It is important to remember that validity is not an absolute and that a test that is valid in one setting or with one group of children may not be valid for other uses. Test users must not assume that because a test has been developed and published for commercial distribution, it is universally useful and appropriate. An examiner must apply his or her clinical knowledge and experience, knowledge of normal and abnormal development, and understanding of an individual child's situation when deciding whether a test is a valid measure of the child's abilities.

Rasch Model of Measurement

The Rasch models of measurement (Andrich, 1988) have been used to develop item scaling for several tests developed recently in the field of occupational therapy. The SFA, the Pediatric Evaluation of Disability Inventory (PEDI) (Haley, Coster, Ludlow, Haltiwanger, & Andrellos, 1992), and the Assessment of Motor and Process Skills (AMPS) (Fisher, 2003a and 2003b) have used Rasch methodology in the test development process. Rasch methodology has also been used to develop a school version of the AMPS (School AMPS) (Atchison, Fisher, & Bryze, 1998; Fisher, Bryze, & Atchison, 2000).

A test instrument developed using Rasch methodology must meet several assumptions (Coster et al., 1998). The construct being measured (e.g., activities of daily living) can be represented as a continuous function with measurement covering the full range of possible performance from dependent to independent. The instrument (or individual scale of the instrument) measures one characteristic (or construct) of performance, and each item represents a sample of the characteristics measured. The scale provides estimates of item difficulty that are independent of the sample of persons tested, and an individual's ability estimate is independent of the specific items tested.

The Rasch model generates a hierarchical ranking of items on the test from easiest to most difficult, creating a linear scale of items from ordinal observations. With the items ranked along the continuum within each skill area, an individual's performance can be compared to an item's difficulty rather than against a normative sample. The ranking of items creates an expected pattern of mastery of items; the model predicts that more difficult items on the continuum are mastered only after easier items have been. Therefore therapists who administer an assessment tool developed using Rasch methodology generally can assume that the most appropriate goals for intervention will be the items and/or skills immediately above the items successfully passed by the client.

Occupational therapy tests developed using Rasch methodology emerge from a different philosophical base than traditional standardized tests. The two main methods of data collection are naturalistic observation and parent/teacher/caregiver report. The tasks observed are the ones the child engages in daily (e.g., schoolwork, self-care, social participation, mobility) rather than items administered in a controlled testing situation. Intervention recommendations can be generated directly from the child's observed and/or reported performance and participation. This approach to assessment is known as a *top-down approach* (Coster, 1998) because it focuses on children's participation in occupations; the *bottom-up approach* of traditional standardized tests, on the other hand, focuses on specific performance skills such as motor coordination, strength, or visual perception.

Tests developed using the Rasch model are not considered norm-referenced tests because individual performance is not compared against that of a normative sample. However, the Rasch model provides an objective measure of performance that can be linked directly to desired occupational performance outcomes. The Rasch model has been applied to a variety of rating scales and traditional measurement instruments to assess disablement and functional status (Grimby et al., 1996; Roth et al., 1998). It is a model that can be used alone or in conjunction with traditional test development and measurement theory to produce measurement tools that provide a clearer connection between the assessment process and intervention planning.

BECOMING A COMPETENT TEST USER

The amount of technical information presented here might make the prospect of learning to administer a standardized test seem daunting. However, potential examiners can take a number of specific steps to ensure that they administer and score a test reliably. These steps also help examiners interpret test results accurately so that they provide a valid representation of each child's abilities. This section discusses the process of learning to administer and interpret any standardized test, be it a screening tool or a comprehensive assessment.

Choosing the Appropriate Test

The therapist's first step is to decide which test, or tests, to learn. A number of standardized tests used by pediatric occupational therapists address a wide age span and a number of different performance skills and areas of occupation. The examiner must decide which tests most likely will meet the assessment needs of his or her particular work setting and of the children served in that setting. For instance, an occupational therapist working in an early intervention setting might use the BSID-II or the Alberta Infant Motor Scale (AIMS) (Piper & Darrah, 1994). A therapist working in preschools might use the MAP or the PDMS-2. A therapist working in a school-based setting might use the SFA, the School AMPS, or BOTMP. Instruments such as the PEDI or the AMPS can be used in a variety of settings. Selected pediatric standardized assessments are summarized in Table 8-4.

A number of other standardized tests are available that assess more specialized areas of function, such as the SIPT, the Developmental Test of Visual-Motor Integration (Beery, 1997), the Sensory Profile, or the DTVP-II. Examiners should consult with other therapists working in their practice settings to determine which tests are most commonly used. In addition, they should examine the characteristics of the children referred to them for assessment to determine which tests are most appropriate.

Learning the Test

Once a decision has been made about which test to learn, the therapist should read the test manual carefully. In addition to administration and scoring techniques, the technical attributes of the test should be studied. Particular attention should be paid to the size and composition of the normative sample, the reliability coefficients, the validation data, and the intended population for the test. The examiner should determine the standardized administration procedures and whether they can be altered for children with special needs. He or she should also understand how the scores should be reported and interpreted if the standardized procedure is changed.

It may also be appropriate to consult other sources for information about a test. *The Fifteenth Mental Measurements Yearbook* (Plake, Impara, & Spies, 2003) and *Tests in Print VI* (Murphy, Plake, Impara, & Spies, 2002) publish descriptions and critical reviews of commercially available standardized tests written by testing experts. These resources can also be accessed online through most university library systems. In addition, published studies of the validity or reliability of tests relevant to pediatric occupational therapists appear throughout the occupational therapy literature.

The next step in learning a test is to observe it being administered by an experienced examiner. If possible, the therapist should also discuss administration, scoring, and interpretation of the test results. One observation may suffice; however, it may be helpful to watch several

TABLE 8-4   Summary of Selected General Pediatric Standardized Tests

Test	Age Range	Domains Tested	Standard Scores Used	Time to Administer
Bayley Scales of Infant Development (2nd Ed.) (BSID-II)	1 to 42 months	*Mental scale:* Cognitive, language, and personal-social *Psychomotor scale:* Gross motor skills, fine motor skills, quality of movement, sensory integration, perceptual-motor integration *Behavior rating scale:* Social interactions, orientation toward environment and objects, interests, activity level, need for stimulation	Developmental index scores Percentile-rank scores Developmental age-equivalent scores	25 to 60 minutes, depending on child's age
Peabody Developmental Motor Scales (2nd Ed.) (PDMS-2)	1 to 84 months	*Gross motor scale:* Reflexes, balance, locomotor, nonlocomotor, receipt and propulsion *Fine motor scale:* Grasping, hand use, eye-hand coordination, manual dexterity	Percentile rank scores Z-scores T-scores Age-equivalent scores Developmental motor quotient scores Sealed scores	45 to 60 minutes for total test; 20 to 30 minutes for each scale
Bruininks-Oseretsky Test of Motor Proficiency (BOTMP)	4.5 to 14.5 years	*Gross motor subtest:* Running speed and agility, balance, bilateral coordination, strength, upper limb coordination *Fine motor subtest:* Response speed, visual-motor control, upper limb speed, dexterity	Subtest and total test Standard score Percentile rank score Stanine score Age-equivalent scores	45 to 60 minutes for long form; 15 to 20 minutes for short form
Pediatric Evaluation of Disability Inventory (PEDI)	6 months to 7 years	Social function, self-care, mobility; each domain is scored in functional skills, caregiver assistance, and modifications.	Normative standard score Scaled score	45 to 60 minutes when scoring by parent report
School Function Assessment (SFA)	Kindergarten to grade 6	Participation, Task Supports (divided into five assistance and five adaptations scales), and Activity Performance, which is divided into physical tasks (12 scales) and cognitive and/or behavioral tasks (nine scales).	Criterion scores for each scale; cutoff scores identified for kindergarten to grade 3 and for grade 4 to grade 6 for each scale	Varies; can be completed by one or more respondents; total time is 1½ to 2 hours, or 5 to 10 minutes per scale
Assessment of Motor and Process Skills (AMPS)	3 years and up	Quality of motor and process skills in the performance of instrumental and basic activities of daily living (ADLs)	ADL ability measure; logit scores for motor and process scales	30 to 40 minutes
School Assessment of Motor and Process Skills (School AMPS)	3 to 11 years (can be administered as a criterion-referenced test for children over 11 years)	Quality of occupational performance of school motor and process skills in five classroom tasks Pen/pencil writing, drawing and coloring, cutting and pasting, computer writing, manipulative	Logit scores for motor and process scales	30 to 40 minutes

administrations of the test to children of different ages and abilities. Observation is an excellent way to learn how other examiners deal with the practical aspects of testing (e.g., arranging test materials, sequencing test items, handling unexpected occurrences, and managing behavior). A discussion with the examiner about the interpretation of a child's performance can also be extremely helpful for acquiring an understanding of how observed behaviors are translated into conclusions and recommendations.

Once these preparatory activities have been completed, the learner should practice administering the test. Neighborhood children, friends, or relatives can be recruited to be "pilot subjects." It is a good idea to test several children whose ages are similar to those for whom the test is intended. Testing children, rather than adults, provides the realism of the mechanical, behavioral, and management issues that arise with a clinical population (Figure 8-6).

Checking Interrater Reliability

When possible, an experienced examiner should observe the testing and simultaneously score the items as a check of interrater reliability. A simple way to assess interrater agreement is to use *point-by-point agreement* (Kazdin, 1982). With this technique, one examiner administers and scores the test while the other observes and scores. The two examiners then compare their scores on each item (Figure 8-7). The number of items on which the examiners assigned the same score is then added up.

Interrater agreement then is computed using this formula:

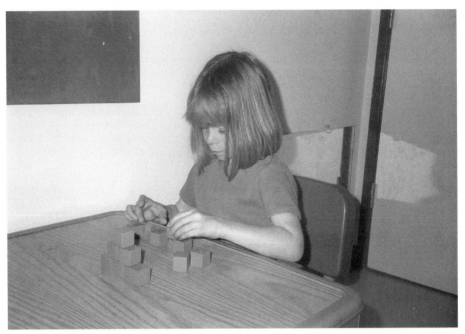

FIGURE 8-6   A child performs a fine motor item from the PDMS-2.

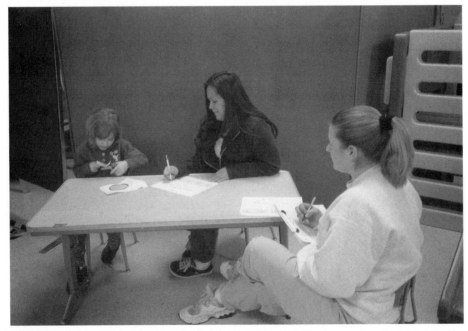

FIGURE 8-7   Two therapists check their interrater reliability by scoring the same testing session.

$$\text{Point-by-point agreement} = \frac{A}{A+D} \times 100$$

where *A* equals the number of items on which there was agreement and *D* equals the number of items on which there was disagreement.

The following example illustrates point-by-point agreement.

Two examiners score a test of 10 items. The child receives either a pass (+) or fail (−) for each item. The scores for each examiner are shown in Table 8-5. According to the data, the raters agreed on 7 of the 10 items. They disagreed on items 2, 7, and 9.

Their point-by-point agreement would be calculated as follows:

$$\frac{7}{7+3} = 0.70 \times 100 = 70\% \text{ Point-by-point agreement}$$

TABLE 8-5 Raters' Scores for Point-by-Point Agreement

Item	Rater 1	Rater 2
1	+	+
2	+	−
3	+	+
4	−	−
5	−	−
6	+	+
7	−	+
8	−	−
9	−	+
10	+	+

This means that the examiners agreed on the scores for 70% of the items. To benefit from this exercise, the two examiners should discuss the items on which they disagreed and their reasons for giving the scores they did. A new examiner may not understand the scoring criteria and may be making scoring errors as a result. The experienced examiner can help clarify scoring criteria. This procedure helps bring the new examiner's administration and scoring techniques in line with the standardized procedures.

The point-by-point agreement technique can also be used for periodic reliability checks by experienced examiners, and it is particularly important if the examiners may be testing the same children at different times. No universally agreed-on standard exists for a minimum acceptable level for point-by-point agreement. However, 80% is probably a good guideline. Examiners would be well advised to aim for agreement in the range of 90% if possible. Organization of the testing environment and materials can improve reliability by creating a standard structured environment.

Selecting and Preparing the Optimal Testing Environment

The testing environment should meet the specifications stated in the test manual. Generally, the manual specifies a well-lighted room free of visual or auditory distractions. If a separate room is not available, a screen or room divider can be used to partition off a corner of the room. An example of an appropriate test setup is shown in Figure 8-8.

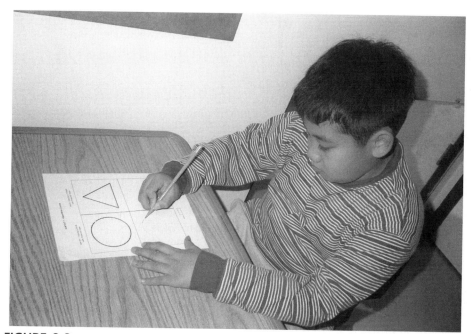

FIGURE 8-8 A child completes a portion of the visual-motor subtest of the Bruininks-Oseretsky Test of Motor Proficiency.

Testing should be scheduled at a time when the child is able to perform optimally. For young children, caregivers should be consulted about the best time of day for testing so that the test session does not interfere with naps or feedings. Older children's school or other activities should be considered in the scheduling of assessments. For instance, a child who has just come from recess or a vigorous physical education session may have decreased endurance for gross motor activities.

The test environment should be ready before the child arrives. Furniture should be appropriately sized so that children sitting at a table can rest their feet flat on the floor and can comfortably reach items on the table. If a child uses a wheelchair or other adaptive seating, he or she should be allowed to sit in the equipment during testing. Infants or young children generally are best seated on the caregiver's lap unless particular items on the test specify otherwise. The examiner should place the test kit where he or she can easily access the items but not where the child can see the kit or get into it. Often a low chair placed next to the examiner's chair is a good place to put a test kit.

Each examiner should consider what adaptations are necessary to administer the test efficiently. In many cases a test manual is too large and unwieldy to have at hand during testing, and the score sheet does not provide enough information about administration and scoring criteria. Examiners have developed many ways to meet this need. A common method is a cue card, on which the examiner records specific criteria for administration and scoring, including the instructions to be read to the child. This can be accomplished by making a series of note cards, putting color codes on a score sheet, or developing a score sheet with administration information.

Administering Test Items

Most important, the examiner must be so familiar with the test that his or her attention can be focused on the child's behavior and not on the mechanics of administering the test. This is a critical part of preparation, because much valuable information can be lost if the examiner is unable to observe carefully the quality of the child's responses because he or she instead must devote energy to finding test materials or looking through the test manual. In addition, young children's attention spans can be short, and the examiner must be able to take full advantage of the limited time the child is able to attend to the activities.

Familiarity with the test also allows the examiner to change the pace of activities if necessary. The child can be given a brief break to play, have a snack, or use the bathroom while the examiner interviews the caregiver or jots down notes. Most standardized tests have some flexibility about the order or arrangement of item sets, and an examiner who knows the test can use this to his or her advantage. Sometimes, because of the child's fatigue or behavior or because of time constraints, a test cannot be administered completely in one session. Most tests provide guidelines for administering the test in two sessions, and examiners should be familiar with these guidelines before starting to test.

Evaluating the Clinical Usefulness of the Test

The final area of preparation is to evaluate the clinical usefulness of the test. The learner should discuss the test with colleagues: What are its strengths and weaknesses? What important information does it give? What information needs to be collected through other techniques? For which children does it seem to work especially well and for which is it an especially poor choice? Can it be adapted for children with special needs? Does it measure what it says it measures? Do other tests do a better job of measuring the same behavioral domain? Is it helpful for program planning or program evaluation? An ongoing dialog is an important way to ensure that the process of standardized testing meets the needs of the children, families, therapists, and service agencies that use the tests. The steps to becoming a competent user of standardized tests are summarized in Box 8-4.

ETHICAL CONSIDERATIONS IN TESTING

All pediatric occupational therapists who use standardized tests in their practice must be aware of their responsibilities to the children they evaluate and their families. Anastasi and Urbina (1997) have discussed several ethical issues relevant to standardized testing, including (1) examiner competency, (2) client privacy, (3) communication of test results, and (4) cultural bias.

Examiner Competency

Examiner competency was discussed in detail in the previous section. However, it is important to reemphasize

---

BOX 8-4   Steps to Becoming a Competent Test User

1. Study the test manual.
2. Observe experienced examiners; discuss your observations.
3. Practice using the test.
4. Check interrater agreement with an experienced examiner.
5. Prepare administration and scoring cue sheets.
6. Prepare the testing environment.
7. Consult with experienced examiners about test interpretation.
8. Periodically recheck interrater agreement.

here that examiners must achieve a minimal level of competency with a test before using it in practice. Along with knowing how to administer and score a test, a competent examiner should know for whom the test is intended and for what purpose. This also means knowing when it is *not* appropriate to use a particular standardized instrument. The examiner should be able to evaluate the technical merits of the test and should know how these characteristics may affect the administration and interpretation of the test. The examiner also should be aware of the many things that can affect a child's performance on a test, such as hunger, fatigue, illness, or distractions, as well as sources of test or examiner error.

The competent examiner draws conclusions about a child's performance on a standardized test only after considering all available information about the child. Such information can include the results of nonstandardized tests, informal observations, caregiver interviews, and reviews of documentation from other professionals. It is extremely important to put a child's observed performance on standardized testing in the context of all sources of information about the child; this ensures a more accurate and meaningful interpretation of standard scores.

Client Privacy

The Privacy Rule of the Health Insurance Portability and Accountability Act (HIPAA) mandates that all recipients of health care services be notified of their privacy rights; that they have access to their medical information, including provision of copies at their request; and that they be notified of any disclosure of medical information for purposes other than treatment or billing. For minor children, the parent or legal guardian must provide consent prior to initiation of any evaluation or intervention procedures. Agencies have different forms and processes for obtaining consent, and examiners must be aware of the procedures for their particular institution. Informed consent generally is obtained in writing and consists of an explanation of the reasons for testing, the types of tests to be used, the intended use of the tests and their consequences (i.e., program placement or qualification for remedial services), and the testing information that will be released and to whom it will be released. Parents/guardians should be given a copy of the summary report and should be informed about who will receive the additional copies. If test scores or other information will be used for research purposes, additional consent procedures must be followed.

Verbal exchanges about the child should be limited. Although it is often necessary to discuss a case with a colleague for the purposes of information sharing and consultation, it is not acceptable to have a casual conversation about a particular child in the elevator, lunchroom, or hallway. If others overhear the conversation, a violation of confidentiality could result.

Communication of Test Results

Reports should be written in language that is understandable to a nonprofessional, with a minimum of jargon. Each report should be objective in tone, and the conclusions and recommendations should be clearly stated. When the results of tests are discussed, the characteristics of the person receiving the information should be taken into account.

Speaking with other professionals and speaking with family members require different communication techniques. When sharing assessment results with family members, the examiner should be aware of the general level of education and, in the case of bilingual families, the level of proficiency with English. Even if family members have a reasonable capability in the English language, it may be a good idea to have an interpreter available. Often the family members most skilled in English act as interpreters. However, this may not be the optimal arrangement for sessions in which test results are discussed because of the technical nature of some of the information. The ideal interpreter is one who is familiar with the agency and the kinds of testing and services it offers and who has developed techniques for helping examiners offer information in an understandable and culturally meaningful way.

When presenting information to family members, examiners must also consider the anticipated emotional response. A parent who hears that his young child has developmental delays may be emotionally devastated. Therefore the information should be communicated sensitively. Every child has strengths and attributes that can be highlighted in the discussion of his or her overall performance. The examiner should also avoid any appearance of placing blame on the parent for the child's difficulties, because many parents are quick to blame themselves for their child's problems. The tone of any discussion should be objective, yet positive, with the emphasis placed on sharing information and making joint decisions about a plan of action.

Cultural Bias

A number of authors have discussed the cultural bias inherent in standardized tests (Anastasi & Urbina, 1997; Leavitt, 1999; Lynch & Hanson, 1992; Polgar, 2003). Tests developed primarily on a white, middle-class population may not be valid when used with children from diverse cultural backgrounds. It is important for examiners to be aware of the factors that may influence how children from diverse cultures perform on standardized tests.

Children who have not had any experience with testing may not understand the unspoken rules about test taking. They may not understand the importance of doing a task within a time limit or of following the examiner's instructions. They may not be motivated to perform well on tasks because the task itself has no intrinsic meaning to them. The materials or activities may be seen as irrelevant, or the child, having had no experience with the kinds of materials used in the tests, may not know how to interact with them. Establishing a rapport may be difficult either because of language barriers or because of a cultural mismatch between the child's social interaction patterns and those of the examiner. If the examiner is aware of these potential problems, steps can be taken to minimize possible difficulties.

The caregiver or an interpreter can be present to help put the child more at ease. The caregiver can be questioned about the child's familiarity with the various test materials; this information can help the examiner determine whether the child's failure to perform individual items is the result of unfamiliarity with the materials or of inability to complete the task. The caregiver can also be shown how to administer some items, particularly those involving physical contact or proximity to the child. This may make the situation less threatening for the child. However, if these adjustments are made, standard procedure has been violated, and it may be inappropriate to compute a standard score. Even so, the test can provide a wealth of descriptive information about the child's abilities.

Standardized tests should be used cautiously with children from diverse cultures. Occupational therapists who find themselves frequently evaluating children from cultural or ethnic groups that are underrepresented in the normative samples of most standardized tests may want to consider developing "local norms" on frequently used instruments that reflect the typical patterns of performance among children of that culture. This information can help provide a more realistic appraisal of children's strengths and needs. Several studies have attempted to establish cultural norms for pediatric standardized tests, both in the United States and internationally (Chow, Henderson, & Barnett, 2001; Crowe, McClain, & Provost, 1999; Katz, Kizony, & Parush, 2002; Kerfeld, Guthrie, & Stewart, 1997). In addition, observation of the child in a variety of contexts and communication with the family, caregivers, and others familiar with the child are essential to the assessment process.

Clearly, when using standardized tests, occupational therapists must have a number of skills beyond the ability simply to administer test items. Professional communication skills are essential when administering tests and reporting information. Awareness of family and cultural values helps put the child's performance in a contextual framework. An understanding of the professional and ethical responsibilities involved in dealing with sensitive and confidential information is also extremely important. A competent examiner brings all these skills into play when administering, scoring, interpreting, and reporting the results of standardized tests.

ADVANTAGES AND DISADVANTAGES OF STANDARDIZED TESTING

Standardized tests have allowed occupational therapists and other professionals to develop a more scientific approach to assessment, and the use of tests that give statistically valid numeric scores has helped give the assessment process more credibility. However, standardized tests are not without their drawbacks. The following section discusses the advantages and disadvantages of using standardized tests, along with suggestions on how to make test results more accurate and meaningful.

Advantages

Standardized tests have several characteristics that make them a unique part of the assessment inventory of pediatric occupational therapists. For example, they are tests that in general are well known and commercially available. This means that a child's scores on a particular test can be interpreted and understood by therapists in other practice settings or geographic locations.

Standard scores generated by standardized tests allow testers from a variety of professional disciplines to "speak the same language" when it comes to discussing test scores. For example, a child may be tested by an occupational therapist for fine motor skills, by a physical therapist for gross motor skills, and by a speech pathologist for language skills. All three tests express scores as T-scores. An average T-score is 50. The child receives a fine motor T-score of 30, a gross motor T-score of 25, and a language T-score of 60. It is apparent that although this child is below average in both gross and fine motor skills, language skills are an area of strength; in fact, they are above average. These scores can be compared and discussed by the assessment team, and they can be used to identify areas requiring intervention and areas in which the child has particular strengths.

Standardized tests can be used to monitor developmental progress. Because they are norm referenced according to age, the progress of a child with developmental delays can be measured against expected developmental progress compared with the normative sample. In this way, occupational therapists can determine if children receiving therapy are accelerating their rate of development because of intervention. Similarly, children who are monitored after discharge from therapy can be assessed periodically to determine whether they are maintaining the expected rate of developmental progress or are beginning to fall behind their peers without the assistance of intervention.

Disadvantages

The 1997 amendments to the Individuals with Disabilities Education Act (IDEA) place a greater emphasis on functional assessments than did the original legislation. Standard scores obtained from norm-referenced tests cannot be substituted for the results of functional performance assessments and may not assist in the development of functional goals (Clark & Coster, 1998).

Because most standardized tests assess performance skills (e.g., balance, bilateral coordination, and visual-motor skills) rather than occupational performance areas (e.g., play, activities of daily living, social participation, and educational or prevocational activities), the intervention goals generated as a result of standardized assessment frequently address these performance components instead of the child's functional performance in the environmental context. As a result, occupational therapy intervention that relies solely on the results of these standardized tests may not adequately address a child's occupational performance in a meaningful way.

The importance of assessing standardized testing results within the child's performance context is discussed in Chapter 7. A standardized test cannot stand alone as a measure of a child's abilities. Clinical judgment, informal or unstructured observation, caregiver interviews, and data gathering from other informants are all essential parts of the assessment process. These less-structured evaluation procedures are needed to provide meaning and interpretation for the numeric scores obtained by standardized testing.

Several other considerations must be taken into account when standardized tests are used. For example, a test session provides only a brief "snapshot" of a child's behavior and abilities. The performance a therapist sees in a 1-hour assessment in a clinic setting may be different from that seen daily at home or at school. Illness, fatigue, or anxiety, or lack of familiarity with the test materials, the room, or the tester can adversely affect a child's performance. The tester must be sensitive to the possible impact of these factors on the child's performance.

A competent tester can do a great deal to alleviate a child's anxiety about testing and to ensure that the experience is not an unpleasant one. However, any test situation is artificial and usually does not provide an accurate indication of how the child performs on a daily basis. Therefore it is important for the therapist to speak to the child's parent, caregiver, or teacher at the time of testing to determine whether the observed behavior is truly representative of the child's typical performance, and the representativeness of the behavior must be taken into account when the child's test scores are interpreted and reported.

Another concern about standardized tests is the rigidity of the testing procedures themselves. Standardized tests specify both particular ways of administering test items and, in many cases, exactly what instructions the tester must give. Children with problems as diverse as hearing impairment, attention deficit, muscle weakness, or lack of coordination may not have an opportunity to perform optimally given these administration requirements. Many therapists believe that the standard score obtained by a standardized test administration is strongly affected by the child's particular deficits and does not accurately reflect the child's true abilities. Although this issue is not addressed by all standardized tests, some provide guidelines for administering the test under nonstandard conditions. For example, the PDMS provides case illustrations of how the test can be adapted for children with vision impairment and cerebral palsy. The BSID-II and the Sensory Profile provide normative data for several clinical groups. Piper and Darrah (1994), in developing the AIMS, used infants who were preterm or born with congenital anomalies, as well as those who were full term and those who did not have an unusual diagnosis.

It is important to reiterate that although it is permissible to alter the administration procedures of most tests to accommodate children's individual needs, the child's performance cannot be expressed as a standard score. Rather, the purpose of the testing is to provide a structured format for describing the child's performance. The test manual should always be consulted for guidelines on alterations in test procedures.

Three standardized tests have been developed specifically for use with children who have physical disabilities: the PEDI, the Gross Motor Function Measure (GMFM) (Russell, Rosenbaum, Avery, & Lane (2002), and the SFA. A unique characteristic of the PEDI is that it measures the amount of caregiver assistance and environmental modifications required for children to perform specific functional tasks. This provides a way to assess the level of independence and the quality of performance of children whose disabilities may prevent them from ever executing a particular task normally. The GMFM is a criterion-referenced test that measures the components of a gross motor activity that a child with cerebral palsy can accomplish. It is meant to provide information necessary for designing intervention programs and measuring small increments of change. The SFA is a criterion-referenced test to be used with children who have a variety of disabling conditions. The SFA evaluates the child's performance of occupational roles in the context of daily life, specifically the performance of functional tasks that support participation in the academic and social aspects of an elementary school program. These instruments are part of a new wave of tests designed by and for occupational and physical therapists, and they show promise for addressing the specific assessment and program-planning needs of pediatric therapists.

Case Study

Caitlin is a 5.5-year-old kindergarten student referred for occupational therapy assessment by her teacher, Mrs. Clark. Mrs. Clark notes that Caitlin appears to be having a great deal of difficulty learning to write; she holds her pencil awkwardly and exerts either too much or not enough pressure on the paper. She complains of fatigue during writing and coloring activities. On the playground and in physical education (PE) classes, she has difficulty keeping up with the rest of the class. She falls frequently, appears uncoordinated, and has difficulty learning new motor skills. On several occasions she has complained of minor ailments; Mrs. Clark believes that she does this to avoid participating in PE. Mrs. Clark would like to know whether any underlying problems may be causing Caitlin's school difficulties and whether any special help is needed.

Debra received the occupational therapy referral. She spoke to Caitlin's parents before initiating her assessment and obtained additional information. She discovered that Caitlin received physical therapy briefly as an infant because of low muscle tone and slow achievement of developmental milestones. Although Caitlin appeared to make good progress in therapy, she continued to lag behind her peers. Her parents were particularly worried about her ability to cope with the increase in writing assignments in first grade and about whether other children would accept her if she continued to struggle in school. They did not have much free time but were willing to consider some home activities to help Caitlin develop additional skills. They declined Debra's offer for them to be present at the testing session, citing concerns about Caitlin's behavior when they were present. However, they asked to meet with Debra after Caitlin's evaluation.

Debra considered Caitlin's age (5.5 years) and the areas of concern cited by Mrs. Clark and Caitlin's parents (gross and fine motor skills and social adjustment) in choosing which standardized test to use. She decided to administer the PDMS-2, along with clinical observations of Caitlin's posture, muscle tone, strength, balance, motor planning, hand use and hand preference, attention, problem-solving skills, and visual skills. She also asked Caitlin's teacher to complete the SFA to provide information on Caitlin's performance of functional school-related behaviors.

Test Results

Caitlin came enthusiastically to the testing session, which was scheduled at midmorning to avoid possible effects of fatigue or hunger. She attended well, although she needed encouragement for the more challenging items. By the end of the session she complained of fatigue, but Debra believed she was able to get a representative sample of Caitlin's motor skills and that the scores obtained were reliable.

On the PDMS-2 Caitlin received a gross motor quotient of 81, placing her at the 10th percentile for her age. Her fine motor quotient was 76, placing her at the 5th percentile. In the gross motor area, ball skills were an area of relative strength for Caitlin, but she had difficulty with balance activities and activities involving hopping, skipping, and jumping. In the fine motor area, Caitlin used a static tripod grasp on the pencil, frequently shifting into a fisted grasp if the writing task was challenging. Based on the small number of visual-motor items on this test, visual-perceptual skills appeared to be an area of strength, whereas tasks involving speed and dexterity were particularly difficult.

Debra found that Caitlin had low muscle tone overall, particularly in the shoulder girdle and hands, and strength was somewhat decreased overall. Caitlin's endurance was poor; for many tasks she performed well initially, but her performance deteriorated as she continued. Motor planning difficulties were evident in the way she handled test materials and moved about the environment. She had difficulty devising alternate ways to accomplish tasks that were challenging for her and required Debra's manual guidance to complete some tasks. She became frustrated to the point of tears on two occasions, and she needed encouragement to continue when this occurred.

Debra obtained a functional profile on the SFA based on Mrs. Clark's responses to the items on the test. On the scales of recreational movement, using materials, clothing management, written work, and task behavior and/or completion, Caitlin received scores below the cutoff for her grade level. Other scales were within grade-level expectations, with strengths in the scales of memory and understanding, following social conventions, and personal care awareness.

Observations and Recommendations

According to her scores on the PDMS-2, Caitlin had mild delays in her gross motor skills and mild to moderate delays in her fine motor skills. Although Debra believed that the PDMS-2 gave a good indication of what Caitlin could do under optimal circumstances (i.e., a nondistracting environment, individual attention and encouragement, and structuring of tasks to maximize success and minimize frustration), she also thought it did not represent the level of performance that would be seen over the course of a typical day.

She observed Caitlin in her classroom and discovered that Caitlin avoided fine motor and gross motor activities whenever possible and completed writing and drawing activities rapidly, resulting in poor quality of the end product. She was near tears after experiencing frustration with her attempts at an art activity. SFA results indicated that her performance of tasks involving fine and gross motor coordination and task organization was below grade-level expectations.

Debra and Mrs. Clark met with the school psychologist, the school principal, and Caitlin's parents to determine a plan of action. The SFA was used to facilitate collaborative problem solving by helping to identify which specific areas of school function could be targeted in the classroom and which skills should be identified as functional outcomes.

The team determined that Debra would provide recommendations to Mrs. Clark about classroom modifications and activities that would increase Caitlin's success and build her motor skills. The team members also collaborated to design strategies and routines that could be used at school and at home to improve Caitlin's on-task behavior and ability to manage daily tasks at school.

Debra provided a pencil gripper and a chair that fit Caitlin better and allowed better positioning for writing. She provided Mrs. Clark with ideas for appropriate activities and ways of teaching Caitlin new motor skills. Debra provided Caitlin's parents with suggestions for family-oriented activities that would improve general strength and endurance (e.g., bicycle riding and swimming) and provided specific ideas for ways they could build Caitlin's fine motor skills at home. She also agreed to be available to Mrs. Clark for periodic informal consultation. It was agreed that a reassessment would be scheduled at the end of the school year so that the team could make a decision about further intervention and program planning for the next school year.

SUMMARY

Standardized testing, specifically the PDMS-2 and SFA, provided a helpful framework for Debra's assessment of Caitlin and gave specific information about areas of strength and difficulty. Debra made use of her clinical observations and information gathering from a variety of sources to recommend interventions she felt would be beneficial, efficient, and relatively easy to implement. The standardized scores helped her identify Caitlin's problems in fine and gross motor skills, and the test items provided activities that revealed the challenges Caitlin faced when performing motor tasks. However, if Debra had simply relied on the standardized test scores, she would not have acquired the breadth of knowledge that led to her decision-making process for developing intervention options.

This example illustrates the important roles of both standardized testing and other methods of data collection in arriving at meaningful and realistic conclusions about children's intervention needs and modes of service delivery.

STUDY QUESTIONS

1 For what testing purposes is a criterion-referenced test preferred? A norm-referenced test?

2 Brandon, who is 2 years old, is being evaluated with a standardized test. He refuses to attempt several items, throws test materials, and repeatedly tries to leave the test area. Brandon's mother states that this behavior is not typical and that she knows he is able to do many of the tasks presented to him. What statement can be made about the reliability of the test results? What strategies might be used to maximize the quantity and quality of information obtained during the test session?

3 Carmen, who is 9 years old, is scheduled for her periodic formal school reassessment. Previous testing, with the PDMS-2, was done when Carmen was 6. Now that Carmen is beyond the age range of the PDMS-2, what tests can be used, and how can the scores from these tests be compared with her previous test scores?

4 Jared, who is 7 years old, is given a standardized test and receives a raw score of 83. Therapy services are provided to Jared for 6 months. On reevaluation he receives a score of 98 on the same standardized test. The SEM of the test is 4.0. Using the 95% confidence interval, what is the potential range of scores for Jared for each testing session? What can be concluded about the effect of the therapy he has been given?

5 A therapist has just purchased a newly published test of visual-motor skills and is interested in how a child's performance on this test will relate to his or her handwriting skills. What information would the therapist look for in the test manual to find the answer to this question?

6 A therapist is learning to administer a standardized test. He or she checks the interrater agreement on the test with another therapist who frequently uses the instrument. Their point-by-point agreement on the test is 65%. What strategies can they use to improve interrater agreement, and what level of agreement should they aim to achieve?

7 A child is referred to a therapist for assessment. When the child and her mother arrive, the therapist discovers that their English skills are

extremely limited. Knowing that the test he or she plans to use requires that the child be given verbal instructions, how should the therapist proceed? How should the therapist discuss the results?

8 A therapist is reviewing a new test. The test manual reports a concurrent validity of 0.85 with another well-known and well-regarded test that is used frequently by the therapist's department and other agencies in the area. What additional information should the therapist look for when deciding which of these two tests to administer?

9 A 3-year-old boy with possible developmental delays is referred to a therapist. No other information is available on the referral note, but the therapist knows that the child was recently screened in his preschool program. What information can the therapist obtain that would help him or her to decide what areas to test and at what approximate developmental level to begin testing?

10 Given the following referral information, state which standardized tests and nonstandardized evaluation techniques should be used to assess this child:

Natalie was 3 years, 3 months old at the time of her referral. She was born at 35 weeks' gestation to a mother who used cocaine and marijuana throughout her pregnancy. Natalie had mild respiratory distress in the first few days of life. She has had chronic middle ear infections and currently has ear tubes. She had early difficulties with sucking and is a picky eater.

Natalie's mother entered a drug treatment program during a subsequent pregnancy and has been drug free and sober for 1.5 years. Natalie lives with her mother and two siblings in a small apartment. Her mother states that Natalie is "different" from her other children and that she has difficulty controlling Natalie's behavior. Natalie seems to be bright, but she is active and easily frustrated with fine motor activities. She has frequent temper tantrums, refuses to nap, and wakes several times during the night.

A public health nurse has been involved with the family since Natalie's birth, and she and Natalie's mother agree that some additional intervention may be necessary. Natalie is scheduled to enter a Head Start preschool program, and the nurse and Natalie's mother would like recommendations for both home and school strategies.

REFERENCES

Anastasi, A., & Urbina, S. (1997). *Psychological testing* (7th ed.). New York: Prentice Hall.

Andrich, D. (1988). *Rasch models for measurement.* Beverly Hills, CA: Sage Publications.

Atchison, B.T., Fisher, A.B., & Bryze, K. (1998). Rater reliability and internal scale and person response validity of the School Assessment of Motor and Process Skills. *American Journal of Occupational Therapy, 52,* 843-850.

Ayres, A.J. (1989). *Sensory Integration and Praxis Test manual.* Los Angeles: Western Psychological Corporation.

Ayres, A.J., & Marr, D. (1991). Sensory Integration and Praxis Tests. In A. Fisher, E. Murray, & A. Bundy (Eds.), *Sensory integration: Theory and practice* (pp. 201-233). Philadelphia: F.A. Davis.

Bayley, N. (1993). *Bayley Scales of Infant Development* (2nd ed.). San Antonio: Psychological Corporation.

Beery, K.E. (1997). *Developmental Test of Visual-Motor Integration: Administration, scoring, and teaching manual* (4th revision). Los Angeles: Western Psychological Services.

Bricker, D. (Ed.). (1993). *AEPS measurement for birth to three years.* Baltimore: Brookes.

Bruininks, R.H. (1978). *Bruininks-Oseretsky Test of Motor Proficiency.* Circle Pines, MN: American Guidance Service.

Chow, S.M.K., Henderson, S.E., & Barnett, A.L. (2001). The Movement Assessment Battery for Children: A comparison of 4-year-old to 6-year-old children from Hong Kong and the United States. *American Journal of Occupational Therapy, 55,* 55-61.

Clark, G.F., & Coster, W.J. (1998). Evaluation, problem solving and program evaluation. In J. Case-Smith (Ed.), *Occupational therapy: Making a difference in school system practice.* Bethesda, MD: American Occupational Therapy Association.

Coster, W. (1998). Occupation-centered assessment of children. *American Journal of Occupational Therapy, 52,* 337-344.

Coster, W., Deeney, T., Haltiwanger, J., & Haley, S. (1998). *School function assessment.* San Antonio: Psychological Corporation.

Crowe, T.K., McClain, C., & Provost, B. (1999). Motor development of Native American children on the Peabody Developmental Motor Scales. *American Journal of Occupational Therapy, 53,* 514-518.

Cunningham-Amundson, S.J., & Crowe, T.K. (1993). Clinical applications of the standard error of measurement for occupational and physical therapists. *Physical and Occupational Therapy in Pediatrics, 12* (4), 57-71.

Deitz, J.C. (1989). Reliability. *Physical and Occupational Therapy in Pediatrics, 9* (1), 125-147.

Dunn, W. (1999). *Sensory Profile user's manual.* San Antonio: Psychological Corporation.

Dunn, W., Myles, B.S., & Orr, S. (2002). Sensory processing issues associated with Asperger syndrome: A preliminary investigation. *American Journal of Occupational Therapy, 56,* 97-102.

Fisher, A.G. (2003a). *Assessment of Motor and Process Skills. Vol. 1: Development, standardization, and administration manual* (5th ed.). Fort Collins, CO: Three Star Press.

Fisher, A.G. (2003b). *Assessment of Motor and Process Skills. Vol. 2: User manual* (5th ed.). Fort Collins, CO: Three Star Press.

Fisher, A.G., Bryze, K., & Atchison, B.T. (2000). Naturalistic assessment of functional performance in school settings: Reliability and validity of the School AMPS scales. *Journal of Outcome Measurement 4*, 504-522.

Fisher, W.P. (1993). Measurement-related problems in functional assessment. *American Journal of Occupational Therapy, 47*, 331-338.

Folio, M.R., & Fewell, R.R. (2000). *Peabody Developmental Motor Scales* (2nd ed.). Austin: Pro-Ed.

Frankenburg, W.K., & Dodds, J.B. (1990). *Denver II Developmental Screening Test.* Denver: Denver Developmental Materials.

Furuno, S., O'Reilly, K.A., Hosaka, C.M., Inatsuka, T.T., Allman, T.L., & Zeisloft, B. (1997). *The Hawaii Early Learning Profile.* Palo Alto, CA: Vort.

Gregory, R.J. (2000). *Psychological testing: History, principles and applications* (3rd ed.). Needham Heights, MA: Allyn & Bacon.

Grimby, G., Andren, E., Holmgren, E., Wright, B., Linacre, J.M., & Sundh, V. (1996). Structure of a combination of functional independence measure and instrumental activity measure items in community-living persons: A study of individuals with cerebral palsy and spina bifida. *Archives of Physical Medicine and Rehabilitation, 77*, 1109-1114.

Haley, S.M., Coster, W.J., Ludlow, L.H., Haltiwanger, J.T., & Andrellos, P.J. (1992). *Pediatric Evaluation of Disability Inventory: Development, standardization and administration manual.* San Antonio: Psychological Corporation.

Hammill, D.D., Pearson, N.A., & Voress, J.K. (1993). *Developmental Test of Visual Perception* (2nd ed.). Austin: Pro-Ed.

Katz, N., Kizony, R., & Parush, S. (2002). Visuomotor organization and thinking operations of school-age Ethiopian, Bedouin, and mainstream Israeli children. *Occupational Therapy Journal of Research, 22*, 34-43.

Kazdin, A.E. (1982). *Single-case research designs.* New York: Oxford University Press.

Kerfeld, C.I., Guthrie, M.R., & Stewart, K.B. (1997). Evaluation of the Denver-II as applied to Alaska Native children. *Pediatric Physical Therapy, 9*, 23-31.

Leavitt, R.L. (1999). Cross-cultural rehabilitation: An international perspective. London: W.B. Saunders.

Lynch, E.W., & Hanson, M.J. (Eds.) (1992). *Developing cross-cultural competence: A guide for working with young children and their families.* Baltimore: Brookes.

Miller, L.J. (1988). *Miller Assessment for Preschoolers: MAP manual* (rev. ed.). San Antonio: Psychological Corporation.

Miller, L.J. (1990). *First STEp screening tool.* San Antonio: Psychological Corporation.

Miller, L.J., Lemerand, P.A., & Cohn, S.H. (1987). A summary of three predictive studies with the MAP. *Occupational Therapy Journal of Research, 7*, 378-381.

Murphy, L.L., Plake, B.S., Impara, J.C., & Spies, R.A. (Eds.). (2002). *Tests in print VI.* Lincoln, NE: Buros Institute of Mental Measurements.

Parush, S., Winokur, M., Goldstand, S., & Miller, L.J. (2002). Prediction of school performance using the Miller Assessment of Preschoolers (MAP): A validity study. *American Journal of Occupational Therapy, 56*, 547-555.

Piper, M.C., & Darrah, J. (1994). *Motor assessment of the developing infant.* London: W.B. Saunders.

Plake, B.S., Impara, J.C., & Spies, R.A. (Eds.). (2003). *The fifteenth mental measurements yearbook.* Lincoln, NE: University of Nebraska Press.

Polgar, J.M. (2003). Critiquing assessments. In B. Crepeau, E.S. Cohn, & B.A. Boyt Schell (Eds.), *Willard and Spackman's occupational therapy* (10th ed., pp. 299-313). Philadelphia: Lippincott Williams & Wilkins.

Roth, E.J., Heinemann, A.W., Lovell, L.L., Harvey, R.L., McGuire, J.R., & Diaz, S. (1998). Impairment and disability: Their relation during stroke rehabilitation. *Archives of Physical Medicine and Rehabilitation, 79*, 329-335.

Russell, D., Rosenbaum, P., Avery, L.M., & Lane, M. (2002). *Gross Motor Function Measure* (GMFM-66 and GMFM-88) User's manual. Cambridge: Cambridge University Press.

Sternberg, R.J. (1990). *Metaphors of mind: Conceptions of the nature of intelligence.* Cambridge, UK: Cambridge University Press.

Terman, L.M., & Merrill, M.A. (1937). *Measuring intelligence.* Boston: Houghton Mifflin.

Thorndike, R.L., Hagen, E.P., & Sattler, J.M. (1986). *Technical manual, Stanford-Binet Intelligence Scale* (4th ed.). Chicago: Riverside.

Wechsler, D. (1991). *Wechsler Intelligence Scale for Children.* San Antonio: Harcourt.

Woodcock, R.W., & Johnson, M.B. (1977). *Woodcock-Johnson Psycho-Educational Battery.* Hingham, PA: Teaching Resources.

Occupational Therapy Intervention: Performance Areas

Development of Postural Control

Deborah S. Nichols

KEY TERMS

Neuromotor control
Development of postural control
Righting reactions
Protective reactions
Equilibrium

Balance
Antigravity movements
Reactive postural control
Anticipatory postural control

CHAPTER OBJECTIVES

1 Describe the development of postural control systems and the influence of that development on gross- and fine-motor development.

2 Discuss atypical development of postural control and its influence on the development of gross- and fine-motor skills.

3 Identify appropriate assessment tools available for the evaluation of postural control.

4 Identify appropriate treatment techniques for facilitating reactive and anticipatory postural control.

5 Apply the knowledge gained in this chapter to specific case studies of children with postural control deficits.

Early child development is characterized by the emergence of a series of motor milestones (rolling, crawling, creeping, and walking), which parents track and brag about to their friends and therapists use to identify developmental delays. However, underlying these observable milestones is the emergence of postural control, which is the ability to maintain body alignment while upright in space. Thus, postural development and motor development are inextricably linked.

Postural control requires the development of both muscle strength, which allows for antigravity movements, and proximal-axial muscle control, which results in dynamic patterns of co-contraction and mature postural reactions. In the past, therapists conceptualized postural and motor development as a hierarchy in which high-level brain structures (i.e., the cortex) control and mediate the functions of lower-level brain structures (i.e., the brainstem). Under the hierarchical model of neuromotor control, postural and motor development was thought to be determined by maturation of the nervous system, resulting in the emergence of increasingly advanced reflex patterns and eventually voluntary movement as higher levels of the nervous system developed (Woollacott, Shumway-Cook, & Williams, 1989). In addition, postural control was considered to mirror motor development and proceed in a cephalocaudal and proximodistal manner (Bly, 1983; Connor, Williamson, & Siepp, 1978).

More recently, research has suggested (1) an interplay between higher and lower system control; (2) control of complex movements, not just reflexes, at low levels of the nervous system; and (3) an overlap in the emergence of proximal versus distal control as well as head and trunk control. All of these contradict the hierarchical model. Furthermore, the hierarchical model of motor development does not adequately explain the high level of variability in child development (e.g., why some babies roll at 4 months and others at 6 months, or why some babies roll leading with their head and others leading with their legs).

The system theories of motor control, and more specifically dynamic systems theory, have also been used to explain motor development and have influenced the way that therapists view development. System theories recognize that postural and motor development result from more than maturation of a hierarchically organized nervous system. These theories acknowledge the importance of muscle strength, body mass, sensory processing, behavior, cognition, and environmental constraints on motor and postural development. According to dynamic systems theory, motor behavior, including postural control, emerges from an interaction between the systems of the body, the environment in which the movement takes place, and the task that the infant/child is trying to perform. This begins to answer the question of why babies develop at such variable rates (e.g., why a baby born weighing 10 pounds may acquire motor milestones at a later age than a baby born weighing 7 pounds or why an active baby might acquire motor milestones faster than a less active baby). Systems theories begin to provide explanations of these phenomena based on the interaction of internal body systems, the task, and the environment (Bernstein, 1967; Thelen, 1995).

As developmental theorists attempted to apply dynamic systems theory to the emergence of motor behavior, a key concern was the relationship of what had previously been thought of as a hard-wired nervous system (a system with genetically preprogrammed connections) to the variability of a dynamic system. Neuronal selection theory was developed to explain the emergence of motor behavior within this newly conceived plastic or dynamic nervous system. According to neuronal selection theory, the connections of the nervous system emerge in synchrony with motor behavior such that connections between various aspects of the nervous system (motor, sensory, behavioral, cognitive) are strengthened as a certain motor behavior is practiced. During motor development, new connections are strengthened and old connections weaken as new behaviors emerge (walking) and old behaviors diminish (crawling) (Edelman, 1987; Sporns, Tononi, & Edelman, 2000; Thelen, 1995).

This chapter uses these developmental theories to explain the development of and assessment and intervention for postural and motor function in children. It includes descriptions of the development of antigravity movement, postural reactions and control, sensory processing associated with reactive postural control and anticipatory postural control, and the interaction of postural control development and motor milestone acquisition. Evaluations of all of these components of posture are described, and intervention strategies for improving postural control, and indirectly motor development, are provided.

DEVELOPMENT OF ANTIGRAVITY MOVEMENT

An important aspect of postural control is the development of antigravity movement. Margaret Rood proposed a four-stage sequence in the development of movement: (1) mobility, (2) stability, (3) mobility superimposed on stability, and (4) skill (Stockmeyer, 1967) (Figure 9-1). The stage of mobility is characterized by the development of antigravity movement. This stage is followed by the development of muscle co-contraction at the proximal joints, producing stability sufficient for the maintenance of weight-bearing postures. Once stability is achieved, the child superimposes movement on this stability, characterized by Rood as proximal movement on a fixed distal limb component. An example of this behavior is the infant who assumes a quadruped position and then begins to rock back and forth (proximal movement on a fixed distal limb component, the hands and knees).

The last stage is characterized by skill or the ability to combine stability and mobility in non–weight-bearing postures (e.g., reach, grasp, and manipulation) (Stockmeyer, 1967). Rood's model suggests that the development of postural control and movement is integrated.

An important component of the development of mobility and stability is the development of antigravity movement. Pountney, Mulcahy, and Green (1990) identified six levels in the development of antigravity movement, which were associated with more mature movement patterns, in both the prone and supine positions (Figures 9-2 and 9-3). Using this sequence, the child develops an increased ability to move against gravity with all body parts, demonstrated by a shift from lateral movements to midline movements as antigravity muscle strength is achieved. The newborn infant is asymmetric, with the head turned to the side and arm and leg movements occurring in the lateral plane. Over the course of the first few months, there is movement of the center of gravity from the upper body toward the pelvis, which is associated with increased freedom of movement of the head and extremities, allowing head control and extremity weight bearing to develop. This progression also includes a dissociation of the body segments so that the infant can roll segmentally, lift one leg, and reach across midline with one hand. Accordingly, the progression from one level to the next involves changes in head control, trunk control, and extremity movement and, therefore, does not follow a strict cephalocaudal progression. In addition, the change from one level to the next coincides with the integration of the preceding level in both prone and supine positions.

The emergence of head control also contributes to the child's ability to explore the environment visually. Early tracking by infants younger than 5 months is characterized almost exclusively by eye movement and is thus limited to the excursion of the eyes. As head control emerges, the 5-month-old infant begins to use head movement, sometimes without accompanying eye movement to track objects. Over the next several months, infants begin to couple head and eye movements as they track visually (Bertenthal & Von Hofsten, 1998; Von Hofsten & Rosander, 1996).

Pountney et al. (1990) also describe similar changes in neck and trunk extension, including increased scapular stabilization, in the acquisition of independent sitting. The posture of a 1-2 month infant when placed in a sitting position is one of total trunk flexion. This stage is followed by one in which the child exhibits increasing trunk extensor strength but has difficulty grading the activation of the back extensor muscles. When placed in a sitting position, the 3-5 month old child frequently activates the back extensors without sufficient co-activation of the trunk flexors and, as a result, falls backward. At this time the child uses upper-extremity weight

PROGRESSION OF MOTOR DEVELOPMENT

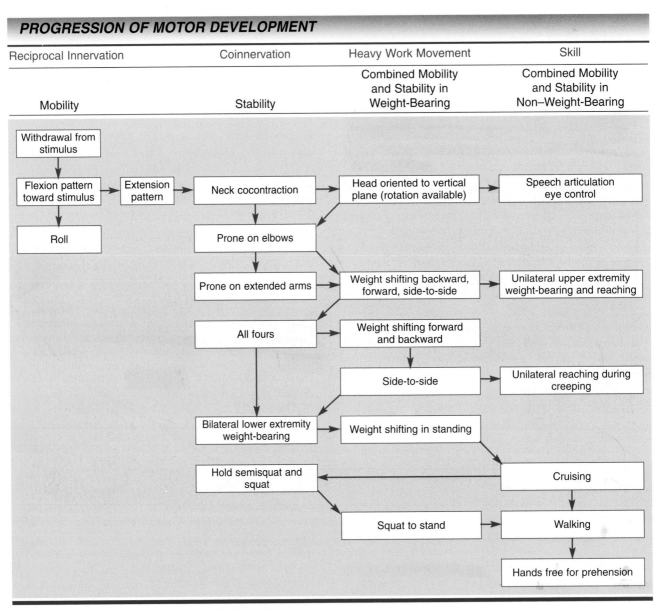

FIGURE 9-1 Rood's developmental progression.

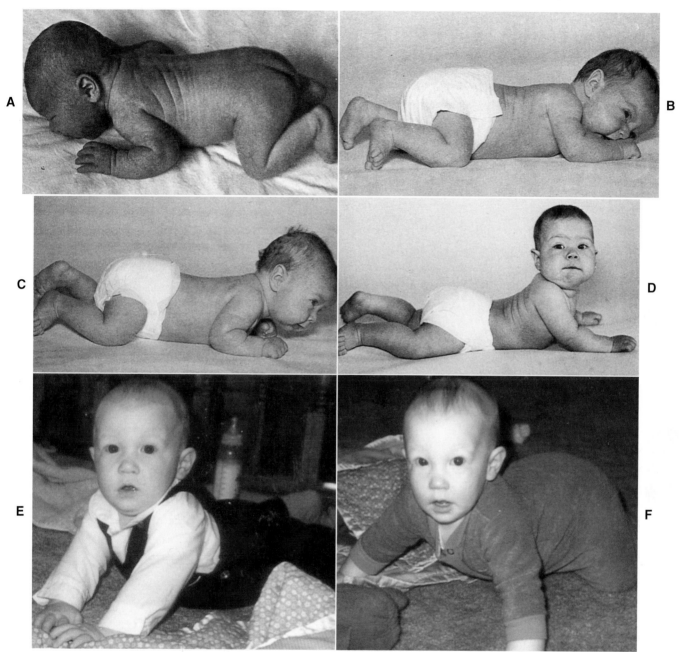

FIGURE 9-2   Prone development of antigravity movement. **A,** Level 1: "Top heavy." Weight bearing is through chest, shoulders, and face. Pelvis is posteriorly tilted, hips and knees are flexed, and shoulder girdle is retracted. Posture is asymmetric, and head is to one side. **B,** Level 2: Child settles when placed. Weight bearing is through chest and upper abdomen. Shoulder girdle is retracted, shoulders are flexed and adducted, head is to one side, and child is beginning to lift head from floor but not sustaining. Posture is asymmetric, and bottom is moving laterally as head turns side to side. **C,** Level 3: Child maintains prone position with neutral pelvis, and shoulder girdle is beginning to protract. Symmetric weight bearing is through abdomen, lower chest, knees, and thighs. Child maintains head lift from floor. Child has no lateral weight shift and therefore often topples into supine position when lifting head and chest. **D,** Level 4: Pelvis is anteriorly tilted but not "anchoring." Shoulder girdle is protracted, and child bears weight through abdomen and thighs, varying between forearm and hand propping with shoulders elevated. Head and upper trunk movement is dissociated from lower trunk, allowing lateral trunk flexion with lateral weight shift (a beginning of pivoting). Unilateral leg is kicking, and hand and foot play is midline. **E,** Level 5: Pelvis is anteriorly tilted, shoulder girdle is protracted with hand propping, extended elbows, and lumbar spine extension. Weight bearing is through iliac crest, thighs, and lower abdomen. Deft pivoting with lateral trunk flexion and moving backward on floor. Child rolls purposefully from prone to supine position. **F,** Level 6: Free movement of pelvis and shoulder girdle. Child begins to bear weight on all fours, rocking on all fours.

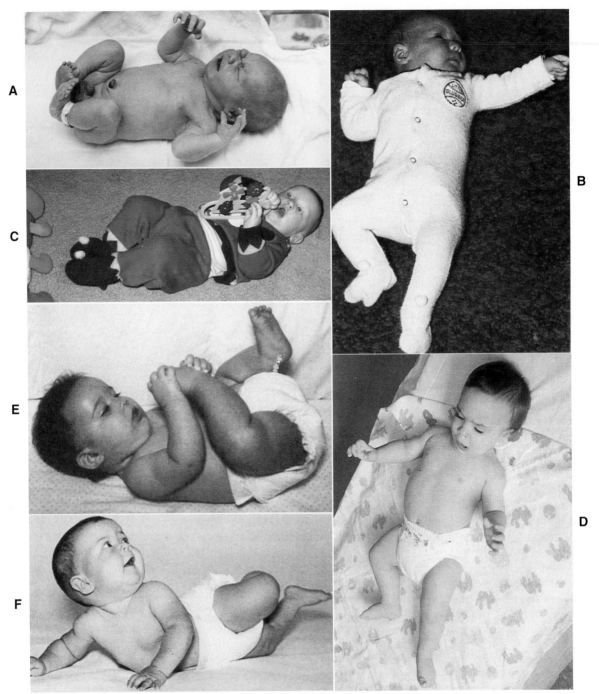

FIGURE 9-3 Supine development of antigravity movement. **A,** Level 1: Child is unable to maintain supine position when placed, except momentarily, and then position is asymmetric. Child rolls into and maintains side-lying position (body follows head, turning in a total body movement). Weight bearing is through lateral aspect of head, trunk, and thigh. **B,** Level 2: Child settles when placed on back ("top heavy"). Weight bearing is through upper trunk and head. Posture is asymmetric (head is to one side), and child has difficulty turning it side-to-side. Bottom moves laterally as the head is turned, resulting in a "corkscrew" appearance. **C,** Level 3: Child maintains supine position with neutral pelvic tilt, hip abduction, and shoulder girdle in neutral position. Posture is symmetric but "top heavy." Chin is tucked (not retracted) and head is in midline and able to move freely from side to side without lateral movement of bottom. Child is able to track objects visually and make eye contact. Child begins unilateral grasp to side of body and takes fist and objects to mouth. Child may roll into prone position. **D,** Level 4: Symmetry of posture and movement is first seen at level 4. Shoulders are flexing and adducting, allowing midline play above chest with hands and feet together. Posture is symmetric, and weight bearing is through upper trunk and pelvis. "Free" pelvic movement is beginning, allowing child to touch knees with flexed hips (but not toes). Child begins to be able to shift weight laterally and raise leg unilaterally, indicating independence of limbs from trunk. Adept finger movements toward end of this stage. **E,** Level 5: Free movement of shoulder girdle and pelvis on trunk. Pelvis has full range of movement, allowing child to play with toes with legs extended and to roll into side-lying position. Child is functional in side-lying position and can return to supine position. Child plays between these postures. Efficient limb movement (hand play and prehensile feet) crossing midline. **F,** Level 6: Pelvic and shoulder girdle move freely. Child is able to roll into prone position by achieving side-lying position (level 5) and then anteriorly tilting pelvis on trunk and extending hips.

bearing (propping) to maintain a sitting position. Finally, the child develops sufficient strength of the trunk muscles to allow upright sitting. These changes in the development of antigravity trunk extension with reciprocal trunk flexion and the emergence of sitting stability are depicted in Figure 9-4.

As stated previously, the development of postural control is tightly linked to the acquisition of motor milestones. The center of gravity is initially located toward the head and then moves toward the pelvis. This shift frees the upper body from providing static stability to demonstrating dynamic mobility as the child moves in and out of upper-extremity weight-bearing positions. As the center of gravity moves to the pelvis, the child demonstrates increased independence in extremity movement and dissociation of body parts, including rotation through the trunk and pelvis. When the child first attempts new postures against gravity, he or she tends to stiffen the trunk to achieve the stability needed. For example, when the child begins to sit and stand, he

or she shows minimal rotation. With practice and experience the child uses rotation in each new posture. This rotation increases movement opportunities for the child and enables him or her to make transitions from one posture to another (e.g., sitting to quadruped) (Connor et al., 1978). The approximate ages of motor milestone acquisition are depicted in Table 9-1. Although an age range is provided for each skill, individual development is highly variable, and thus many factors should be taken into account when using age ranges to evaluate motor development.

The development of antigravity muscle strength has also been found to coincide with the development of higher-level balance and motor skills. In addition, there is an interaction between the posture of the child, the weight of the limb and body, and the emergence of antigravity movement. Newborns demonstrate infantile stepping, involving antigravity hip flexion, which "disappears" typically during the second month and reemerges during the fifth or sixth month before the

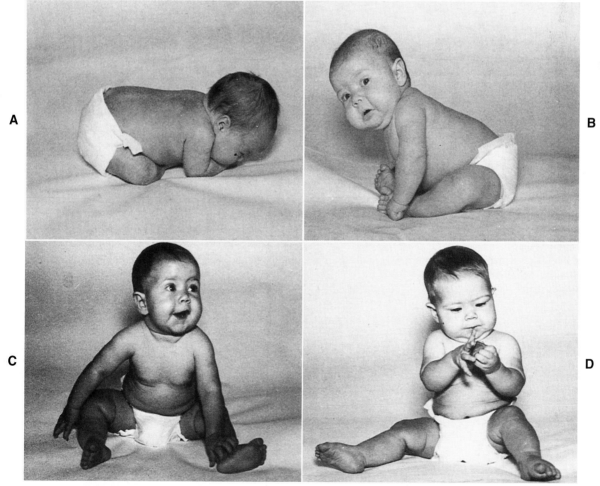

FIGURE 9-4   Development of antigravity movement in sitting. **A,** Total flexion posture of infant. **B,** Bursts of back extensor activity results in falling backward. **C,** Increased upper extremity strength allows stability in sitting with upper-extremity weight bearing. **D,** Mature sitting posture associated with antigravity trunk and neck extensor strength.

TABLE 9-1 Ages of Motor Milestone Acquisition

Motor Milestone	Age in Months
HEAD CONTROL	
Prone	
Lifts head to 45°	2
Lifts head to 90°	4
Supine	
Maintains in midline	2
Lifts	6
ROLLING	
Prone to supine	
Without rotation	4-6
With rotation	6-9
Supine to prone	
Without rotation	5-7
With rotation	6-9
SITTING	
Unsustained with arm support	4-5
Sustained with arm support	5-6
Unsustained without arm support	6-7
Sustained without arm support	7-9
MOBILITY	
Crawling	7-9
Creeping	9-11
Cruising	9-13
Walking	12-14

emergence of cruising and walking. Hierarchic theorists explained this change in behavior as secondary to maturation of higher brain centers with the subsequent inhibition of lower brain centers. Thelen and Fisher (1982) related the loss of stepping behavior to an increase in the weight of the legs (primarily because of an increase in subcutaneous fat, not muscle), which prevents the demonstration of stepping during these early months. As further evidence of this relationship, they found that infants supported in a standing position in water continued to display stepping. In addition, they explored the relationship between supine kicking and infantile stepping and identified that the pattern of movement was the same (Thelen & Fisher, 1983). Thus, the inability of 2- to 5-month-old infants to step seems to be because of the increased weight of the legs and not to a reorganization or maturation of the nervous system. This is further substantiated by more recent research on treadmill stepping in infants who no longer exhibit infantile stepping nor independent stepping on a stable surface; when placed on a treadmill with support under the armpits, these infants will demonstrate reciprocal stepping movements with similar kinematics to adult walking (Thelen & Ulrich, 1991).

The interaction between postural development and the development of motor skill might best be exemplified by examination of reaching behavior. Midline head control in supine emerges in infants between 9 and 15 weeks of age and precedes active reaching in supported sitting by 4 to 5 weeks. During this 4- to 5-week prereaching stage, the infant begins to reorganize proximal muscle activation with increased activity in the trapezius and deltoid muscles and decreased reliance on biceps and triceps activity, which allows stabilization of the head in preparation for the reach and occurs 1 to 2 weeks prior to active reaching (Thelen & Spencer, 1998). As the infant acquires independent sitting, reach when sitting is initially characterized by highly variable trunk and lower extremity activity, which is often insufficient to stabilize the infant, resulting in a loss of balance and falling during the reach. The 8-month-old baby when sitting is able to coordinate postural activity to reach in forward and lateral directions and remain stable. By 15 months, the toddler is able to anticipate how his or her center to gravity will be displaced by the reach and initiate postural activity prior to the reach that is consistent to the magnitude and velocity of the displacement (Van der Fitts, Otten, Klip, Van Eykern, & Hadders-Algra, 1999).

Additional support for the interaction of antigravity muscle strength and motor development was found in a study of children between 4 and $5\frac{1}{2}$ years of age (Sellers, 1988). The children's abilities to maintain the antigravity postures of prone extension and supine flexion, which require substantial antigravity muscle strength, were highly correlated with static balance (e.g., single limb stance) and dynamic balance capabilities (e.g., balance beam activities). Therefore the development of antigravity movement is strongly associated with the development of higher levels of postural control, balance, and movement. Furthermore, the weight of the children was related to the acquisition of antigravity movement. These associations have relevance when asking why the motor development of a baby born weighing 10 pounds might be slower than that of a baby born weighing 7 pounds.

EMERGENCE OF POSTURAL REACTIONS

The development of postural reactions (i.e., righting, protective, and equilibrium) has been reported to occur in a predictable sequence with reactions first appearing in the prone position, followed by supine, sitting, quadruped, and standing. Success in the development of these reactions in earlier positions may be a prerequisite for their development in later positions (Connor et al., 1978).

A series of righting reactions develops in the first year of life and serves to maintain head alignment with the body and upper-body alignment with the lower body. When rotation is imposed on the body, these reactions realign the segments of the body. These reactions also maintain body alignment during forward flexion of the trunk and prone suspension (Barnes & Crutchfield, 1990).

The neck on body righting reaction is observed in two forms. In the immature infant, turning of the head to the side results in a log roll to the side-lying position; in the mature form, turning of the head produces a segmental roll. The body on body righting reaction is similar; rotation of the infant's hips stimulates a log roll of the upper body in the immature form and a segmental roll of the upper body in the mature form to realign the body segments. The body on head righting reaction serves to influence head position in response to a part of the body touching a support surface. In the prone position, the tactile input from the stomach touching the support surface stimulates head lifting; alternately, touching the back to the support surface when lying supine also elicits neck flexion and head lifting.

Two other righting reactions give the infant experiences of full body extension and full body flexion. The Landau reaction results in maintenance of body alignment during prone suspension, produced by neck, trunk, and leg extension. When the child is pulled to a sitting position, the development of antigravity neck flexion is associated with the child's ability to maintain head and trunk alignment against the pull of gravity, which is sometimes referred to as the *flexion righting reaction* and is demonstrated in Figure 9-5. Table 9-2 provides approximate ages when righting reactions emerge.

Orientation of the body in space involves the maintenance of an upright posture under both static and dynamic conditions. This ability is often called balance. The earliest form of body orientation is observed in two vertical righting reflexes: the optical righting reflex and the labyrinthine righting reflex. These two reflexes realign the head vertically when the body is displaced and

TABLE 9-2	Age of Postural Reactions Acquisition
Balance Reactions	**Age (months)**
RIGHTING REACTIONS	
Neck on body	
Immature	Birth
Mature	4-5
Body on body	
Immature	Birth
Mature	4-5
Body on head	
Prone (partial)	1-2
Mature	4-5
Supine	5-6
Landau	
Immature	3
Mature	6-10
Flexion	
Partial (head in line)	3-4
Mature (head forward)	6-7
Vertical	
Partial (head in line)	2
Mature (head to vertical)	6
PROTECTIVE REACTIONS	
Forward	6-7
Lateral	6-11
Backward	9-12
EQUILIBRIUM REACTIONS	
Prone	5-6
Supine	7-8
Sitting	7-10
Quadruped	9-12
Standing	12-21

are mediated, respectively, by the visual and vestibular systems. The maintenance of balance also involves the child's ability to respond adequately to external disturbances (e.g., a push or trip) or self-generated movements (e.g., reaching).

Responses to external disturbances are reactive or compensatory and are classified as equilibrium or protective reactions. These reactions emerge in lower-level positions (supine and prone) when the infant is 4 to 6 months of age. They continue to develop in more upright positions throughout the first 5 years. Equilibrium reactions, often called *tilting reactions* because of the way they are tested, return the child's body to a vertical position after displacement. When the child is supine on a tiltboard, a lateral tilt to the right elicits trunk incurvation to the left, righting of the head, and abduction of the left arm and leg. These same movements are associated with equilibrium reactions in prone, sitting, quadruped, and standing to lateral tilt positions. Figure 9-6 demonstrates equilibrium reactions to lateral displacements in sitting, quadruped, and standing positions. In addition, when the child is in upright postures (e.g.,

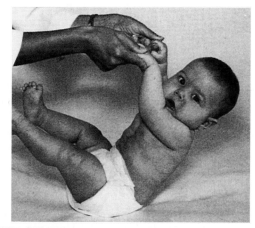

FIGURE 9-5 Flexion response. The development of antigravity neck strength is first associated with the ability to maintain the head aligned with the body when pulled to a sitting position.

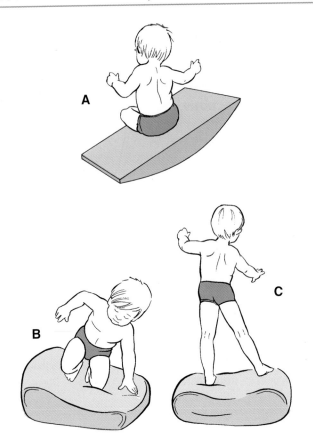

FIGURE 9-6 Equilibrium reactions in sitting (**A**), quadruped (**B**), and standing (**C**).

theories, which posit simultaneous and overlapping development of higher- and lower-level brain areas and corresponding motor functions.

Kinematic analysis of postural activity during the acquisition of sitting balance has delineated the progression of muscle activity necessary to maintain sitting in the presence of forward and backward displacement. In infants who are not sitting independently, a perturbation elicits a postural response in the trunk muscles; however, this response often incorporates only partial recruitment of appropriate muscles, is highly variable, and is not modulated to match the magnitude of the displacement. However, the response initiated is not simply a stretch response to a change in hip position as it occurs even when there is no change in the length of the hip or trunk muscles (i.e., when the infant is seated in a chair on a platform that moves forward and backward or in a chair that is tipped backward or forward) (Hadders-Algra, Brogren, & Forssberg, 1996a, 1998; Hirschfeld & Forssberg, 1994). By 9-10 months, the degree of variability has diminished and the complete pattern to forward displacement, which induces a loss of balance backward, is consistent (neck flexion, abdominal, and rectus femoris contraction) and associated with inhibition of the opposing muscles. The response to backward displacement (neck, trunk, and hip extension) remains more variable, which may be due to the increased stability in the forward direction (Hadders-Algra et al., 1996a).

sitting or kneeling), tilting in anterior or posterior directions results in a corrective movement in the opposite direction to the tilt (i.e., posterior to an anterior displacement), returning the body to an upright position. Protective reactions differ from equilibrium reactions in that they protect the infant from a fall rather than correct a displacement. Therefore these reactions are characterized by extension of the extremities to "catch" the child as he or she falls, and they occur in the direction of the fall.

Haley (1986) assessed the emergence of a series of righting, protective, and equilibrium reactions in infants between 2 and 10 months of age. Righting reactions emerged first in all positions, at least in their immature forms, before the development of any protective or equilibrium reactions in these postures. However, the development of protective and equilibrium reactions was overlapping within a given posture and between postures. For example, protective reactions in the sitting position developed at the same time as the equilibrium reactions. In addition, equilibrium reactions began to develop in higher-level positions (e.g., quadruped) and continued to be refined in lower-level positions (e.g., supine) simultaneously (Haley). These findings are inconsistent with a hierarchic explanation of motor development but are easily explained through systems

NATURE VERSUS NURTURE IN THE EMERGENCE OF POSTURAL CONTROL AND MOTOR MILESTONES

Historically, the emergence of postural reactions was attributed to the maturation of the nervous system as predicated on the hierarchic model of motor control. Although the debate on the effects of nature and nurture raged in the areas of cognitive and language development, little attention has been paid to the role of experience on motor development. However, there is substantial evidence for the role of experience in development of postural control and acquisition of motor milestones.

First, the amount of experience that a child has in a given posture has been found to influence the development of mature postural reactions as evidenced by patterns of muscle activation. Woollacott, Debu, and Mowatt (1988) found that infants younger than 5 months of age demonstrated inadequate or absent neck and trunk muscle activation patterns to linear translations in supported sitting. However, infants 6 to 8 months of age who had experience in independent sitting demonstrated appropriate activation patterns of the neck and trunk muscles to the same translations. Subsequent findings by Hadders-Algra et al., (1996a, 1996b, 1998) have identified the emergence of these postural responses by 5-6 months, prior to the acquisition of independent sitting. However, training of postural behavior through reaching activities at the edge of balance loss was found to accelerate the development of postural control as demonstrated by earlier modulation of muscle activity to the displacement, increased co-contraction of postural muscles, and a distal to proximal activation pattern consistent with older infants (Hadders-Algra et al., 1996b). Similar differences in the standing position were identified between infants who had not yet developed independent stance and those who had. In addition, young children tend to demonstrate larger amplitude of muscle activation and greater variability in the activation patterns (Shumway-Cook & Woollacott, 1985a; Williams, Fisher, & Tritschler, 1983). Thus, the maturation of the nervous system can set the foundation for the emergence of these reactions, but postural reactions appear to be related to both experience in a given position and to neuronal maturation.

The development of motor skills also appears dependent on experience in given postures. Research has found that infants who sleep in the prone position roll from prone to supine earlier than infants who sleep in either the side-lying or supine position. Additionally, some infants whose primary sleeping position was supine rolled from supine to prone before rolling from prone to supine (Jantz, Blosser, & Fruechting, 1997). Thus, the sleeping position of an infant, or more likely the time that the child spends in either the prone or supine position, influences the emergence of rolling.

Evidence of the influence of experience on motor development suggests that training, practice, and experience can affect motor skill acquisition. Practicing reaching, with emphasis on reaching to the side and semi-backward, facilitates the development of postural muscle activity in sitting in infants between 5 and 9 months of age (Hadders-Algra et al., 1996b, 1997). Similarly, infants who practiced stepping on a treadmill between 3 and 7 months of age were found to demonstrate an increase in stepping behavior (Thelen & Ulrich, 1991; Vereijken & Thelen, 1997). Findings such as these support the interactive nature of neuromotor maturation and environmental experience.

SENSORY SYSTEMS ASSOCIATED WITH POSTURAL CONTROL

Three sensory systems contribute to the child's awareness of orientation in space: the visual system, the vestibular system, and the somatosensory system. The visual system provides a representation of the vertical plane that is dependent on the objects in the visual field. The child's somatosensory system provides input from proprioceptors, mechanoreceptors, and cutaneous receptors, which supply information about limb position and support surface characteristics. The vestibular system provides a constant gravitational reference for postural orientation with which the child compares visual and somatosensory input. When the three sensory systems provide disparate information, a feeling of disequilibrium results. Discrepancies between the visual and somatosensory cues are decided in favor of the vestibular system (Horak & Nashner, 1986; Nashner, 1990).

As the infant matures, the relative influence of the sensory systems on postural control changes. Newborns demonstrate the ability to orient to a visual stimulus and are capable of tracking a moving object by turning the head if it is supported (Bullinger, 1981). Initially, infants appear to rely more on visual than somatosensory information in developing postural control. Eventually, and with experience in each new posture, this reliance on vision is transferred to reliance on somatosensory cues (Woollacott, 1988; Woollacott, Shumway-Cook, & Williams, 1989). Studies document that the vestibular system is able to detect accurately postural disturbances at an early age (Jouen, 1984). Infants as young as 4 months of age make appropriate postural responses when they are tilted with their vision occluded. This early maturation of the vestibular system seems to be critical to the development of postural control. However, despite the integrity of the vestibular system early in life, when visual inputs are available, infants and young children tend to rely on them. This dominance of visual input is seen in each transitional state as the child acquires motor milestones. Thus, the child first uses visual information to make postural adjustments in sitting. He or she later relies on vestibular and somatosensory input. Similar changes occur in the quadruped and standing positions (Woollacott, 1988). The time course of this transition in standing is long; it is not until 6 or 7 years of age that children appear to switch from a reliance on visual inputs to a reliance on somatosensory inputs similar to that of adults (Shumway-Cook & Woollacott, 1985b).

EMERGENCE OF ANTICIPATORY POSTURAL CONTROL

In addition to the automatic reactions described in the preceding paragraphs, postural control also involves the programming of postural muscle activation in association with volitional movement. This activation occurs in a feed-forward manner. *Feed-forward* refers to the anticipatory strategies that are observed in the postural adjustments that the individual makes before voluntary movements. These postural adjustments can be observed before the onset of arm, hand, or whole-body movements. This type of anticipatory control is dependent on the child's experience with the task and the environment in which the task takes place. It is also dependent on adequate postural muscle strength. The effect of anticipatory muscle activation is the creation of a stable base on which movement can take place (Bouisset & Zattara, 1981; Forssberg & Nashner, 1982).

Infants as young as 10 months of age demonstrate anticipatory responses to an arm reach in the sitting position, yet these responses are inconsistent until the infant is independent while sitting and has had considerable experience with reaching in this position (von Hofsten, 1986); by 15 months, most infants demonstrate consistent anticipatory responses (Van der Fitts, Otten, Klip, & Hadders-Algra, 1999). Van der Heide Otten, van Eykern, & Hadders-Algra (2003) found that the adult form of anticipatory control during reaching was not consistently observed until 11 years of age. Investigations of reaching in standing have also identified the emergence of anticipatory postural activation by 12 to 15 months of age (Forssberg & Nashner, 1982). By 4 years of age, children demonstrate a pattern similar to that found in adults when reaching while standing (Hayes & Riach, 1989). Again, there is an interaction between development and experience. Children must play within a given posture, disturbing their own balance as they reach for toys, lean in all planes, and right themselves for feed-forward control to develop. In therapy sessions, anticipatory control may be facilitated through practice activities.

DEVELOPMENTAL CHANGES IN POSTURAL SWAY AND MUSCLE ACTIVATION

Postural sway is the natural movement of the center of gravity within the base of support in any upright position. When standing, a child or an adult is not perfectly still but demonstrates a normal oscillatory movement from side to side and forward and back. With recent advances in technology, this postural sway has been evaluated and quantified by using several different techniques. Several studies have examined postural sway in children and have identified a developmental progression. Young children demonstrate significantly more postural sway than older children, with more variability between children and with less influence from closing the eyes (Forssberg & Nashner, 1982; Foudriat, DiFabio, & Anderson, 1993; Riach & Hayes, 1987). In studies that used the Pediatric Clinical Test of Sensory Integration for Balance (P-CTSIB) (Crowe, Deitz, Richardson, & Atwater, 1990; Deitz, Richardson, Atwater, Crowe, & Odiorne, 1991; Richardson, Atwater, Crowe, & Deitz, 1992), mature levels of postural sway in static standing emerge somewhere around 13 years of age. Children between 5 and 7 years of age demonstrate greater sway than younger children, which may be attributable to the transition that occurs at this age between dominance of

the visual system and dominance of the somatosensory system for the control of balance in standing (Deitz, et al.; Riach & Hayes, 1987; Shumway-Cook & Woollacott, 1985b).

The muscle activity elicited also varies with age in children. In young children, significantly greater amplitudes of muscle activity are used to maintain a posture than in older children (Berger, Quintern, & Dietz, 1985; Haas, Diener, Bacher, & Dichgans, 1986). Thus, young children tend to use more muscles than do older children to maintain balance, and they require a greater degree of muscle contraction than do older children. With experience in a given posture, there is a natural refinement in the muscle activity needed to maintain the posture (Shumway-Cook & Woollacott, 1985b; Williams, Fisher, Tritschler, 1983; Woollacott & Sveistrup, 1992).

OTHER INFLUENCES ON MOTOR AND POSTURAL CONTROL DEVELOPMENT

Systems theorists and motor learning theorists have sparked interest in the influence of other systems, outside of the neuromotor system, on the development of postural control and motor milestones. As mentioned previously, maturation of the musculoskeletal system influences the development of posture and movement because antigravity muscle strength and muscle co-contraction are necessary for the emergence of upright postures and higher-level motor skills. There also is an interaction between the weight of a body segment and the ability to move against gravity (Thelen & Fisher, 1982, 1983).

ASSESSMENT OF POSTURAL CONTROL

The assessment of postural control takes different forms, depending on the age of the child and the nature of the postural control dysfunction. In young children, postural assessment is linked to motor milestones and the development of antigravity movement and appropriate postural reactions. In children who have acquired ambulation, postural assessment has typically focused on higher-level balance capabilities, such as single-limb stance and balance beam activities, and the acquisition of play skills (ball throwing, kicking, and jumping). Although an indirect measure of postural control, these milestones are dependent on the development of adequate feed-forward postural control. More recently, evaluations of standing balance have begun to examine the functioning of sensory systems associated with balance function, the development of appropriate muscle synergies in response to perturbations, and the development of stability under various testing conditions.

Assessment of Righting, Equilibrium, and Protective Reactions

Righting Reactions

The *righting reactions* (neck on body, body on body, body on head, Landau, flexion, and vertical) are assessed through handling of the infant. The relative ages of emergence of these reflexes in their mature form are depicted in Table 9-2.

1 To elicit the *neck on body reaction*, the child's head is manually turned to the side and the rolling response is observed. As stated previously, the immature response is a log roll to realign the body, and the mature response is a segmental roll.

2 The *body on body reaction* is evaluated in a similar fashion; the child's hips are rotated to the side and the upper body is observed. The immature response is a log roll, and the mature response is a segmental roll.

3 The *body on head reaction* is observed as the child is placed prone on a support surface. In the partial response, the child lifts his or her head vertically 45°; in the full response, the child raises the head vertically in midline (90°) and is able to maintain this upright position.

4 The *Landau reaction* is observed in prone suspension; the examiner supports the child under the abdomen and looks for extension of both the neck and lower extremities. An immature response may be noted for the Landau; young infants may keep the head in line with the body before being able to demonstrate the mature response of head, trunk, and lower-extremity extension.

5 The *flexion response* is assessed by pulling the child to sitting from the supine position and is considered present if the child can maintain the head in alignment with the body without any initial head lag.

6 The *vertical reactions (labyrinthine and optical)* are typically evaluated by supporting the infant under the arms and suspending him or her vertically. Then the infant is laterally tilted about 45°; the reaction is considered present if the infant rights his or her head vertically. The *labyrinthine reaction* is tested either with a blindfold covering the eyes or in a dark room. Testing with the eyes open is considered to evaluate *optical righting* because vision dominates vestibular input in young infants (see the previous section on sensory development). A partial response to vertical righting is often observed, characterized by the maintenance of the head in line with the body, which is considered an immature response (Barnes & Crutchfield, 1990).

Therapists and researchers have begun to question the relative importance of evaluating righting reactions and what the presence or absence of righting reactions indicates. Although the emergence of mature responses is associated with a normally developing nervous system, delay in developing these reactions provides little insight into the cause. Delayed or deficient reactions can be secondary to neuromotor dysfunction, musculoskeletal abnormalities, or sensory system dysfunction.

Equilibrium Reactions

Testing *equilibrium* and protective reactions has typically taken the form of placing the child on a tiltboard or other unstable surface (e.g., ball or bolster). The child's responses to displacement are observed in lateral, anterior, posterior, and diagonal directions. All appropriate developmental positions are used (prone, supine, sitting, quadruped, kneeling, and standing).

An alternate form of testing involves observation of the child's response to manual displacement from a stationary support surface (i.e., the child is pushed in a given direction). A typical equilibrium reaction is characterized by movements of the trunk and extremities that oppose the imposed displacement and bring the center of gravity back within the base of support. For example, when the child is sitting, a posterior displacement results in contraction of the abdominal, neck flexor, hip flexor, and hamstring muscles to produce a forward movement of the body. Conversely, an anterior push or tilt is associated with neck, trunk, and hip extension; and hamstrings may activate to maintain the seated position. Similarly, lateral displacements are associated with trunk incurvation toward the elevated side if tilted or toward the pushed side if pushed. The child should rotate the upper body toward the elevated (pushed) side and often will extend the extremities on the elevated or pushed side (see Figure 9-6). These responses to lateral tilting are consistent with those seen in all positions. Tilting in a diagonal direction is associated with increased trunk and neck rotation to oppose the movement. These rotary movements combine with trunk flexion when the child is tilted backward and trunk extension when he or she is tilted forward.

Adequate flexibility, muscle strength, and experience with postural disturbance in a given position are necessary for mature equilibrium responses. Thus, neuromotor maturation alone does not account for the emergence of these responses.

Protective Reactions

Protective reactions, sometimes called *parachute reactions*, are also elicited by displacement on a tilting surface or manual displacement on a stable surface. These reactions differ from equilibrium reactions in that they are designed to protect the infant from a fall rather than to correct the displacement. Therefore these reactions are characterized by extension of the extremities to "catch" the child as he or she falls and occur in the direction of the fall. Forward protective reactions can be tested by suspending the child and then moving him or her forward toward a support surface. A positive response includes arm extension and abduction sufficient to stop the forward movement. Testing while the child is sitting also involves displacement in any direction sufficient to elicit arm extension to stop the movement. The amount of displacement needed to elicit a protective reaction must be greater in degree than that used to elicit an equilibrium reaction (Figure 9-7).

Neuromotor Assessment

Neuromotor assessments have been designed to evaluate the emergence and progression of postural reactions. Most neuromotor assessments include some, but not all, of the postural reactions in their assessment of motor milestones. Examples include the Infant Neurological International Battery (INFANIB) (Ellison, 1994), Alberta Infant Motor Scale (AIMS) (Piper & Darrah, 1994), Test of Infant Motor Performance (TIMP) (Campbell, Kolobe, Osten, Lenke, & Girolami, 1995), and the Postural and Fine Motor Assessment (Case-Smith & Bigsby, 2000). The TIMP is a comprehensive test of motor and postural control in infants under 4 months of age (32 weeks gestational age to 16 weeks). It is designed to measure postural control important to

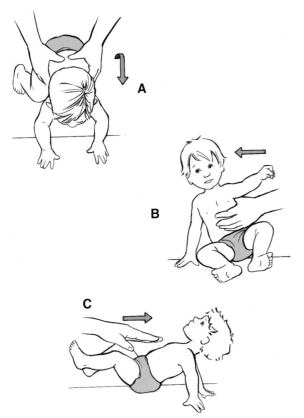

FIGURE 9-7 Protective reactions forward (**A**), lateral (**B**), and backward (**C**).

functional activities such as how the infant is able to change positions and stabilize his head when handled. The scale consists of 59 items divided into two sections: elicited and observed. The elicited section items assess the infants' motor response to handling according to standardized procedures (i.e., response to specific vestibular, proprioceptive input). Behaviors are rated on a 4, 5, or 6-point hierarchical scale. The observed scale items rate spontaneous behaviors as present or not. The TIMP has been well developed and extensively studied. Studies of construct validity have shown it to be of ecological relevance (Murney & Campbell, 1998), sensitive to age-related changes (Campbell et al.), and able to identify infants at risk for developmental dis-ability (Campbell & Hedeker, 2001). Other studies have demonstrated that the TIMP has concurrent and predictive validity with the AIMS (Campbell, Kolobe, Wright, & Linacre, 2002) and has ability to predict future motor function using the Bruininks Oseretsky (Flegel & Kolobe, 2002).

The Alberta Infant Motor Scale (AIMS) is an observational assessment scale constructed to measure gross motor maturation in infants from birth through independent walking. It is a criterion referenced scale of 58 items that rate the infant's posture and motor function in four positions: prone, supine, sitting, and standing. Each item describes three aspects of motor performance: weight bearing, posture, and antigravity movements. The infant's least and most mature observed posture and motor skill are identified. The items between the infant's highest and lowest performance are determined to be the infant's window of emerging skills and may be an appropriate focus for intervention (Piper & Darrah, 1994). Each skill observed receives one point; all of the items present are summed as the infant's total score. The AIMS was originally developed using a sample of 506 infants, birth through 18 months. The scale demonstrates high intrarater and interrater reliability (ICC = .97-.99) and high concurrent validity with the Bayley Scales of Infant Development (r = .78 and .90) at 6 and 12 months (Jeng, Yau, Chen, & Hsiao, 2000).

Assessment of Antigravity Movement

The emergence of antigravity movement is assessed in most developmental tests through the appearance of motor milestones such as prone and supine head control and reaching. The six levels of prone and supine postural development described by Pountney and colleagues (1990) can be used to plot an infant's progression. In addition, the AIMS (Piper & Darrah, 1994), the TIMP (Campbell et al., 1995), and the Posture and Fine Motor Assessment (Case-Smith & Bigsby, 2000) have sections that address antigravity movement and the emergence of antigravity postures.

Assessment of Sensory Organization

The initial evaluation of the child should include testing of sensory systems to determine function. The testing of optical and labyrinthine righting in infants begins to explore the integrity of these systems for use in the control of balance. As described previously, these reactions are typically tested with the infant vertically suspended because this position is believed to assess vestibular system function while eliminating somatosensory input. However, in optical righting, with the eyes open, the vestibular system operates in conjunction with the eyes and may provide the essential input for balance control. Therefore the testing procedure for optical righting does not effectively evaluate the infant's ability to use visual information to orient his or her body in space.

Few clinical assessments that validly measure sensory organization are available. The Sensory Integration and Praxis Tests (SIPT) (Ayres, 1989) were designed for evaluation of sensory integrative function, including sensory organization, balance, and praxis. The SIPT is described in Chapter 11.

Primarily developed for research purposes, posturography provides a method for analyzing the separate and combined influences of the sensory systems on standing balance (Nashner, 1990). Although this sophisticated test is not often available to clinicians, the method of analysis is helpful in understanding how the interactions of the sensory systems contribute to postural stability and upright stance. Posturography typically involves testing under six conditions, also involving sensory deprivation and conflict, using a computerized force platform system on which the child stands. The platform can be stable or sway referenced (moves as child sways such that the ankle joint remains in the same position). A curtainlike structure surrounds the child's entire visual field and can also be sway referenced. The six testing conditions are (1) eyes open, stable platform; (2) eyes closed, stable platform; (3) sway-referenced visual surround, stable platform; (4) eyes open, sway-referenced platform; (5) eyes closed, sway-referenced platform; and (6) sway-referenced visual surround and platform (Nashner). This type of evaluation requires expensive equipment, but it is often used to assess vestibular dysfunction in adults and has been used with children (Forssberg & Nashner, 1982; Horak, Shumway-Cook, Crow, & Black, 1988; Nashner, Shumway-Cook, & Marnin, 1983; Shumway-Cook, Horak, & Black, 1987).

Interpretation of posturography involves the examination of sway and the duration of time that the child can maintain each position. Children who have difficulty with a given condition demonstrate increased sway or lose their balance. Difficulty with condition 2 reflects an overreliance on the visual system. Although children and adults demonstrate a slight increase in sway in this condition, children as young as 4 years of age have had no difficulty in maintaining stance for 30 seconds. Condition 3 examines the child's ability to remain standing in the presence of inaccurate visual cues but with accurate somatosensory and vestibular cues. Conditions 4 through 6 require stance in the presence of inaccurate somatosensory cues and varying visual input (present, absent, or conflicting). Individuals with sensory organization problems have difficulty with all conditions in which conflicting sensory cues are present (conditions 3 through 6). However, the last two conditions require the individual to rely on vestibular information only; therefore difficulties with only conditions 5 and 6 are typical of individuals with vestibular disorders. In testing with young children, a developmental progression occurs with an increase in stability between 3 and 6 years of age; 6-year-old children responded similarly to adults across conditions (Foudriat, DiFabio, & Anderson, 1993). However, even 3- and 4-year-old children were able to disregard misleading sensory inputs to maintain stance but with increased sway (Foudriat et al., 1993; Richardson et al., 1992).

Assessment of Higher-Level Balance Skills

More advanced balance skills are typically evaluated through parts of gross motor tests. Typical test items include single-limb stance (standing on one foot), balance beam activities involving stance and ambulation, and other walking balance activities (walking heel-to-toe or walking in a straight line). For the most part, assessment of these skills involves timed tests of static stance capabilities (how long the child can stand on one foot) or frequency counts (how many consecutive heel-to-toe steps the child can take). The Bruininks-Oseretsky Test of Motor Proficiency can be used to examine these areas in children $4\frac{1}{2}$ to $14\frac{1}{2}$ years of age (Bruininks, 1978). The Gross Motor Scale of the Peabody Development Motor Scales (PDMS) (Folio & Fewell, 2000) includes several items for children between 4 and 6 years of age that rate balance reactions in higher-level positions (e.g., on the balance beam, in single-limb stance, or hopping).

The Gross Motor Function Measure (GMFM) (Russell, Rosenbaum, Avery, & Lane, 2002) is a criterion referenced measure that assesses a child's balance and motor function in progressively higher level positions. The GMFM was developed to evaluate change in gross motor function in children with cerebral palsy. The original scale consists of 88 items that rate (1) lying and rolling, (2) sitting, (3) crawling and kneeling, (4) standing, and (5) walking, running, and jumping. The GMFM items are scored one a 4-point scale through observation of a child's performance. Reliability (Gowland et al., 1995) and validity (Bjornson, Graubert, Buford, & McLaughlin, 1998; Russell et al., 1994) have been established. Researchers have used the GMFM with children with cerebral palsy to measure the effectiveness of intrathecal baclofen (Almeida, Campbell, Girolami, Penn, & Corcos, 1997), horseback riding (Sterba, Rogers, France, & Vokes, 2002), and strength training (MacPhail & Kramer, 1995).

A shorter version of the scale (GMFM-66) has been developed to improve its efficiency and scalability (i.e., creating an interval scale). The test-retest reliability and construct validity of the GMFM-66 have been studied and are comparable to the reliability and validity of the GMFM-88. The test is most sensitive to changes in children under 5 years old (Russell et al., 2000).

Assessment of Anticipatory Postural Control

Assessment of anticipatory postural control is accomplished through the observational skills of the therapist. Children who have delays in anticipatory postural control will typically exhibit general delays in motor control. Children with limited anticipatory control have difficulty reaching, catching, or throwing in any posture. These activities involve sequential displacements of the child's center of gravity and require that postural tone remain activated (preset) for the child to be successful. An overreliance on protective reactions is another indication that anticipatory control is ineffective or limited. For example, a child who loses his or her balance when he or she attempts a reach may be demonstrating poor feed-forward control.

ATYPICAL POSTURAL DEVELOPMENT

Postural development is associated with maturational and experiential changes in the sensorimotor, musculoskeletal, and cognitive systems. Therefore abnormal functioning of any of these systems can result in atypical postural development.

Persistence of Primitive Reflexes

Primitive reflexes are present at or soon after birth and disappear during the first year of life. The traditional hierarchic model proposed that these reflexes were controlled at lower levels of the central nervous system (CNS), and that reflex integration was associated with maturation of patterns mediated by higher centers (i.e., the higher centers inhibited the expression of these reflexes by the lower centers) (Bobath & Bobath, 1954; Taylor, 1931; VanSant, 1993). The reemergence of these reflex patterns after brain injury in children and adults lends support to this concept.

The movement patterns of many children with cerebral palsy and children who have incurred traumatic brain injury are influenced by primitive reflex activity, including the asymmetric tonic neck, symmetric tonic neck, and tonic labyrinthine reflexes. The persistence of these reflexes or their reemergence after brain injury has been associated with delayed postural reflex development (i.e., righting, protective, and equilibrium reactions) (Bobath & Bobath, 1954; Shumway-Cook, 1989). However, in a study of 156 typically developing children, Bartlett (1997) found that the emergence of motor milestones did not relate to the presence or absence of primitive reflexes. Thus, in the typically developing infant the emergence of motor milestones can be independent of the integration of primitive reflexes. However, damage to the developing nervous system may result in persistence of primitive reflexes and disrupted neuromotor control, both of which may influence the acquisition of postural reactions and motor milestones.

Abnormal Muscle Tone, Motor Control, and Force Generation

Damage to the CNS is associated with many changes in motor control, including changes in muscle tone, motor planning, and patterns of movement. The adequate development of postural reactions has also been linked to the presence of normal muscle tone (Bobath, 1966). Conversely, the presence of abnormal muscle tone in the form of hypertonia, hypotonia, athetosis, or rigidity (i.e., in cerebral palsy) has been associated with deficits in postural control mechanisms. Children with cerebral palsy demonstrate limitations in postural reactions, antigravity movement, proximal muscle cocontraction, and stability in upright postures (Bly, 1983; Bobath, 1966; Perin, 1989). Fedrizzi et al. (2000) followed children with cerebral palsy from the ages of 12 months through 41 months to examine the emergence of postural control. They report that children with diplegia typically are able to assume a symmetrical prone prop position on extended arms with the head inline with the spine, but triplegic children are not; however, the timetable for the acquisition of these skills is variable and delayed. Postural control for the children at 12 months remained asymmetric; however, they were able to rotate the head but not the trunk and demonstrated consistent leg hyperextension. By 41 months, most of the children with diplegia were not only able to maintain a prone prop position with extended arms but were also able to manipulate an object by rotating the trunk and weight bearing on one arm. In addition, leg hyperextension had diminished and was primarily noted distally. Furthermore, the acquisition of these more mature postural skills was correlated with visual acuity and general cognitive functioning. Finally, the ability to demonstrate a mature sequence of prone postural control was predictive of later independent sitting.

According to Bly (1983), the inability to develop antigravity movement and stability combined with the need to move results in fixing, or locking, of various body segments, which provides some stability but also blocks more mature movement patterns, such as head control, extremity mobility, and dynamic weight bearing. Repeatedly using limited patterns of movement suggests that children with poor stability limit the degrees of freedom within the system by stabilizing, or locking, certain body segments. Furthermore, the continued use of this type of movement pattern can increase the stability of the pattern and limit the acquisition of other patterns of movement (Kamm, Thelen, & Jensen, 1990).

Children, who lack antigravity muscle strength and therefore stability, learn to provide stability through the fixing (blocking) of certain joints (e.g., the neck in hyperextension to maintain the head upright in sitting). This fixing, in turn, limits the variety of movements that the child can produce. The child who achieves upright head control by hyperextending the neck and elevating the shoulders while sitting limits his or her ability to develop protection and equilibrium reactions, reaching skill in sitting, and independent neck and trunk movements. Over time the abnormal movement pattern becomes more stable, limiting the development of more mature patterns of movement and making the pattern difficult to change.

In addition to the delay or inability to develop antigravity movement and stability, many children with abnormal tone associated with cerebral palsy demonstrate hyperreflexia, which is characterized by exaggerated monosynaptic reflexes (e.g., deep tendon reflexes such as the patellar tendon reflex). These reflexes are hyperexcitable and are associated with activation of both the agonist and antagonist muscles. In response to tapping of the patellar tendon, both the quadriceps muscle and hamstrings would be activated. As a result, the child is unable to make a selective, graded movement.

In many children with cerebral palsy, muscle groups adjacent to those stimulated are activated as well; this response is termed *overflow*. Overflow is often seen in young, typically developing children and decreases after the first year of life. Normal overflow is not as widespread and does not involve as many muscles as the atypical overflow observed in children with cerebral palsy (Leonard, Hirschfeld, & Forssberg, 1988). Because stretching of a spastic muscle activates this same monosynaptic reflex, this overflow pattern can be expected to occur in such activities as extending the arm quickly to protect from a fall. In the child with cerebral palsy the reflex activates the biceps, shoulder, and wrist muscles and results in failure to stop the fall effectively. In children with spasticity, the development of effective protective reactions is typically delayed and often absent (Bobath & Bobath, 1954).

Although abnormal tone and changes in reflex activity are often the most observable alterations in motor function associated with brain injury, adults and children with CNS injuries also demonstrate alterations in motor planning and force generation. Motor planning requires the ability to use sensory feedback from a movement to determine its effectiveness and the efficiency of the muscles activated and the movement produced. In addition, motor planning requires that the child be able to interpret the demands of the task accurately, using sensory and cognitive systems. Deficits in sensory systems and the interpretation of sensory feedback also accompany CNS damage (see section on alterations in sensory function). Furthermore, successful movements require sufficient antigravity control, appropriate motor unit recruitment, and grading of muscle contraction in both agonist and antagonist muscles. Children with CNS damage display difficulties in motor unit recruitment and grading of muscle contractions (see the later section on the organization of the motor response). Thus, the presence of abnormal muscle tone coupled with motor planning and force generation difficulties may delay or prevent the development of antigravity control necessary for mature movement patterns.

Delays in the development of postural control have been described in conjunction with ligamentous laxity and decreased muscle strength in children with Down syndrome (Fetters, 1991). Musculoskeletal abnormalities are also associated with cerebral palsy and other developmental disabilities (e.g., arthrogryposis and muscular dystrophy). Contractures secondary to spasticity or soft tissue abnormalities can restrict movement and thereby disrupt the efficacy of postural reactions; thus, changes in musculoskeletal alignment and joint biomechanics can reduce the child's ability to exhibit adequate protective reactions. Adequate muscle strength is also necessary to produce joint stability and adequate equilibrium reactions; therefore, conditions that result in diminished muscle strength (e.g., muscular dystrophy and cerebral palsy) may be associated with deficits in postural control.

The development of equilibrium reactions is affected by the presence of musculoskeletal abnormalities, and the need for these reactions is altered. In any position there are limits to how far the child can lean before a fall occurs. These limits are referred to as *the limits of stability* (Nashner, 1990). Because these limits of stability are decreased in children or adults with musculoskeletal limitations, it takes a smaller movement to elicit a loss of balance. A movement such as lifting the arm to reach for a toy may be sufficient to displace the child's center of gravity outside of the limits of stability and thereby elicit a fall. If the musculoskeletal change is asymmetric (e.g., in the child with hemiplegia), the decrease in the limits of stability occurs only on the side of the musculoskeletal abnormality (Nashner, 1990). Thus, in a child with unilateral weakness, the limits of stability on the involved side are decreased. To compensate, the child moves his or her center of gravity toward the sound side to minimize the chance of falling, resulting in asymmetric postures.

Altered Sensory Function or Integration

Postural control, according to Horak and Shumway-Cook (1990), "relies on (1) intact peripheral sensory pathways, and (2) the ability of the CNS to extract appropriate sensory information relevant to gravity, the surface, and visual environments" (p. 110). Postural control requires intact perception of visual, vestibular, and somatosensory stimulation and the ability to determine the best source of information under the existing environmental conditions, particularly when conflicting sensory inputs are presented (e.g., unstable support surface resulting in inaccurate somatosensory inputs). When children with impairments in visual, somatosensory, or vestibular processing are required to resolve conflicting sensory input, they demonstrate deficits in postural control. Children with visual impairments typically demonstrate deficits in both static and dynamic balance skills when compared with sighted children (Johnson-Kramer, Sherwood, Frech, & Canabal, 1992; Ribaldi, Rider, & Toole, 1987). Similarly, about 60% of children with hearing impairments also demonstrate abnormal vestibular function and deficits in balance activities that rely on vestibular integrity. However, children with loss of one sensory system are able to compensate in most conditions by use of the two remaining systems (Horak et al., 1988).

Shumway-Cook (1989) reported that children with impaired hearing and hypothesized vestibular dysfunction demonstrated normal postural reactions under conditions in which the sensory inputs were consistent but had difficulty in situations in which the sensory inputs were conflicting (e.g., on a moving platform with visual input that remained unchanged despite postural sway). This inability to interpret conflicting inputs and organize an appropriate response appears to be secondary to abnormalities within the central processes at the level of the cerebellum, brainstem, or cortex (Shumway-Cook). Children with a variety of other diagnoses, including cerebral palsy and learning disabilities, have been reported to have deficits in the selection of appropriate sensory inputs for postural control (Horak et al., 1988; Nashner, Shumway-Cook, & Marin, 1983; Shumway-Cook et al., 1987). Children with ataxic or diplegic cerebral palsy have demonstrated similar deficits in sensory organization under conditions of conflicting sensory cues (Nashner et al., 1983). Because the accurate interpretation of sensory cues from the environment is necessary for effective motor planning to occur, deficits in sensory processing and integration are expected to affect the acquisition of mature postural control and mature patterns of movement necessary for motor milestone acquisition.

Organization of the Motor Response

The child's motor response to tilt on an unstable surface or displacement of his or her center of gravity results in activation of the appropriate muscle groups to compensate for the loss of balance. An effective response to this displacement requires muscle activation that is accurately timed and of sufficient amplitude to reestablish the child's center of gravity. Abnormalities in the motor response result in inaccurate patterns of muscle activation and errors in the timing or amplitude, limiting the child's ability to maintain an upright posture.

A delay in the onset of muscle activity has been reported in children with Down syndrome (Shumway-Cook & Woollacott, 1985a) and children with cerebral palsy (both hemiplegic and ataxic) (Nashner et al., 1983; Shumway-Cook, 1989). This delay can result in use of an ineffective movement strategy when the child's center of gravity is displaced. In addition to a delay in the onset of muscle activity, children with cerebral palsy demonstrate patterns of muscle activation that are ineffective for maintaining postural control. The child may activate distal rather than proximal muscles, resulting in a stiffening of extremities instead of dynamic axial cocontraction. Additionally, overflow contractions that do not effectively contribute to the equilibrium response are observed (Leonard, Hirschfeld, & Forssberg, 1988; Nashner et al.).

For example, in the development of sitting balance, children with hypertonia demonstrate an immature response to posterior displacement, characterized by activation of the neck flexors first, followed by the abdominals and hip flexors; this is the same pattern displayed by young infants prior to the acquisition of independent sitting (Brogren et al., 1996; 1998). Typically developing children, after they have acquired sitting, activate these muscles in the reverse order (hip flexors, abdominals, and neck flexors). In addition, children with hypertonia tend to have difficulty modulating their response to the level of the displacement and often simultaneously activate the antagonistic muscles, making the response less effective (Brogren et al., 1998). In subsequent research, children with diplegia were found to have better control when sitting with their legs crossed than with their legs extended; the crossed-leg position was also preferred by most of the children with cerebral palsy, suggesting that the children assume a more stable position to accommodate their deficits in stability and protective responses (Brogren, Forssberg, & Hadders-Algra, 2001).

Similarly, in the development of standing balance, children with cerebral palsy tend to have greater amplitude of sway, difficulty modulating their postural response to the displacement generated by their own sway, increased co-activation of leg muscles rather than a distal to proximal activation pattern, and a reliance on hip movement to maintain stability during quiet stance (Burtner & Woollacott, 1999; Ferdjaliah, Harris, Smith, & Wertsch, 2002; Rose et al., 2002). Children with cerebral palsy demonstrate a crouched posture that increases during instability, and they have a tendency to go up on their toes when displaced (Burtner & Woollacott). These limitations in stability are further complicated by the use of ankle-foot orthoses (AFOs) to correct ankle and foot abnormalities. In a study of children with and without cerebral palsy, all children demonstrated limited gastrocnemius activation, a disorganization of muscle recruitment, increased mobility at the knee, and decreased use of the ankle strategy when wearing rigid AFOs. This compounded the findings of increased co-activation, crouched posturing, and increased activation of a "toes-on" posture that the children with cerebral palsy demonstrated without the AFOs. The wearing of dynamic AFOs minimized the impact of the bracing on the balance response for both groups of children; thus, standing stability may be facilitated by the use of dynamic rather than rigid AFOs (Burtner & Woollacott).

High-level motor skills require appropriate anticipatory control in addition to the selection of appropriate movement strategies. Thus, when a child wants to throw a ball, he or she needs to activate appropriate muscles on the back of the body to counteract the forward momentum created by the throw, or he or she will fall forward as the ball is released. Again, children with CNS damage may demonstrate ineffective anticipatory control, thus limiting the effectiveness of their movements. Similar to the preceding discussion of postural reactions, children with CNS damage may activate too many muscles, select the wrong muscles for activation, or have difficulty with matching the strength of the postural muscle activation needed for the ongoing movement. They may also demonstrate poor motor unit recruitment when trying to move postural muscles, resulting in timing of the anticipatory response that is not tied to the ongoing movement. These deficits in the planning or implementation of anticipatory control may limit the child's ability to acquire advanced motor skills. In the case of a child throwing a ball, too little postural activity or inaccurately timed trunk extension results in him or her falling forward as the ball is released; too much postural activity may result in limited shoulder excursion during the throw and thus an unsuccessful throw. Evaluation of advanced motor skills should also take into account the presence and effectiveness of anticipatory postural control.

INTERVENTION

This chapter describes intervention as it relates to basic posture and movement. Subsequent chapters address the integration of postural control as a foundation for skilled activity performance. Specific occupational therapy approaches to intervention with children who have neuromotor or musculoskeletal problems are presented elsewhere in this text.

Intervention, based on a systems view of motor development, should take into account the many influences contributing to the movement, including the task requirements, the neuromotor system, the environment in which the intervention takes place, and the motivation of the child. Motor learning theories acknowledge that motor skills do not simply develop as a course of maturation and that motor function involves more than subcortical sensory experiences. A motor pattern is the result of learning and practice with a permanent change in skill. Therapists who use motor learning theories stress the important role of motivation and volition in learning new skills (VanSant, 1994).

An individual learns a new motor skill from the intrinsic and extrinsic feedback received in association with the movement (Adams, 1971). *Intrinsic feedback* refers to the sensory information generated from the action or the perceptual experience. *External feedback* refers to the response of the environment produced because of the action (knowledge of results). The therapist's response to the child's accomplishment or achievement reinforces the learner's "knowledge of results." The child's knowledge of the effects and results of his or her own movements is critical to learning and generalizing motor skills.

Although feedback appears important to learning new movements, not all movement is based on somatosensory feedback. Some is generated and carried out without feedback (e.g., rapid movements such as throwing a ball). Schmidt (1988) hypothesized that recall and recognition schema are the basis for learning new motor skills. The schema are a set of rules learned about movement that are applied and generalized to new situations. The learner recognizes the relationships between the environment conditions, task requirements, and previously learned movements. In this theoretic context, movement is the solution to a motor problem; skill allows the generalization of this solution to multiple problems similar to the original. The outcome of performance and the sensory feedback help the learner establish new motor skills based on an understanding of the relationships between environmental conditions, task requirements, and previously learned movements. Thus, although sensory feedback may not be required as the movement is carried out, it is used in the production of the "next" movement.

Motor learning theories emphasize the importance of practice and sensory feedback combined with knowledge of results. Implications of these theories on practice have been postulated and are currently topics of research. One implication is that random practice reinforces learning more than blocked practice. Blocked practice involves extended periods of repetitious movements with consistent reinforcement provided throughout the practice session. In random practice, an activity is practiced under constantly changing conditions (e.g., therapist changes direction and distance in practice of reach), and practice of one task (e.g., reaching) is interspersed with practice of other tasks (e.g., in-hand manipulation, placing of the object). Performance is reinforced on an intermittent or random schedule.

Feedback during practice is also important to learning. High levels of feedback appear to be detrimental rather than helpful when learning a new motor task. Giving intermittent feedback and reducing feedback as the skill is achieved are ideal ways to reinforce learning (feedback frequency should be higher early in skill acquisition and taper as the child learns the task). Another tenet of motor learning theory is that errors during practice are important for learning, allowing the learner to compare the internal and external feedback from the unsuccessful movement with those of the successful movement.

When applying a motor learning practice model, handling of the child is viewed from several aspects:

1 Handling becomes a type of feedback by providing sensory cues for the movement. Early in the acquisition of a motor skill, higher levels of feedback are thought to facilitate movement, and therapist input, such as tapping a muscle to focus attention on its recruitment, may facilitate the development of the movement. However, feedback during every attempt, including handling, is thought to be detrimental because it may encourage the child to rely on that input rather than his or her own sensory feedback for planning and performing the movement.

2 Handling the child changes the demands of the task (i.e., decreasing the need for anticipatory control or changing the amount of force needed to produce the movement) and may result in ineffective motor learning. If the child learns to move only with assistance of the therapist's hands, he or she may not be able to produce the same movement in the absence of handling.

3 Handling typically decreases the number of errors produced by the child in attempting to move. If errors are important to learning, then preventing errors through too much handling may impair motor learning.

Handling should be used judiciously. A small number of assisted repetitions may allow the child to "feel" the movement and facilitate motor learning. Thus, although handling should be done with caution, it may still play a roll in facilitating movement acquisition.

Another aspect of motor learning is the role of part versus whole practice. In tasks that have identifiable components (e.g., picking up a block and placing it in a container), the individual parts can be practiced; however, the practice of parts of a skill should be followed by practice of the entire skill for motor learning to occur. In many skills the parts are interrelated and therefore inseparable. Thus, practicing components of the task appears to be ineffective. For example, when reaching for a glass, the amount of finger opening, the force of the grip, and the force of the arm movement are predicated on the expected weight of the glass and how full it is. Thus, practicing opening the hand in the absence of gripping the glass may not facilitate the task of grasping the glass and bringing it to the mouth. Therefore the learning of the skill parts may best occur within the context of whole skill practice. These principles regarding learning and the system theories that relate postural development to the function of neurophysiologic and biomechanical variables in the child are the basis for the intervention activities described in the following section.

Motor learning theory has become the cornerstone for treatment of children with postural control limitations as well as other disorders in the past few decades; the principles of motor learning are, therefore, incorporated into the treatment program. Recently, the neurodevelopmental treatment (NDT) approach has also incorporated the principles of motor control and motor learning theories into its therapeutic principles. As described, the primary differences between strict motor learning interventionists and NDT practitioners appears to be the emphasis placed on "precise therapeutic handling" techniques as espoused by NDT practitioners (Howle, 2002).

Treatment of Musculoskeletal Abnormalities

To prepare the child to work on postural control, limitations in joint range of motion and problems in postural alignment need to be addressed (Effgen, 1993). Contractures or joint limitations secondary to spasticity or soft tissue changes often result in poor postural alignment (e.g., anterior or posterior pelvic tilt that blocks trunk rotation). Decreased range of motion limits mobility and decreases the base of support. As a result, adequate equilibrium and protective reactions do not develop, and the child is limited in everyday play, self-care, and school activities.

A variety of inhibition techniques can be used to reduce muscle tone and improve range of motion. Most techniques focus on improving the child's range of motion and flexibility of the spine with the expected result of improved postural alignment and increased postural flexibility. Therapeutic techniques to increase muscle elongation are also used to help the child achieve extension of the extremities. Adequate arm and leg extension are needed for the development of protective extension responses. In particular, full knee and hip extension are required as a base for effective equilibrium responses in stance.

Facilitation of Antigravity Movement

As previously described, normal postural control requires antigravity control in prone, supine, and upright postures. With the development of antigravity trunk flexion and extension, the child achieves upright positions that allow for the development of skilled movements. When a child has not developed sufficient strength in the neck and trunk musculature to move against gravity, he or she is limited in activities such as prone extension and coming to sitting. These movements can be modified to diminish the pull of gravity so that the child can successfully practice the positions and movements to increase neck and trunk strength. Use of a therapeutic ball or a wedge provides some assistance against gravity and reduces the range in which the child must move against gravity. A pull-to-sit activity can then be done from an incline or a ball (Figure 9-8). With the child's head and trunk positioned on an inclined surface, less neck and trunk flexion is required to accomplish pull-to-sit activity. The degree of incline is gradually decreased as the child gains neck flexor strength.

An alternative method for eliciting neck flexion is to help the child move from sitting toward the supine position. The therapist gradually lowers the child backward from the sitting position until the child starts to lose head control. The therapist then assists the child in returning to a sitting position. This activity requires neck flexor control in both directions (lowering from and returning to the sitting position). If the child does not have sufficient strength to perform either of these activities, neck and trunk flexion can be initiated in the side-lying position where gravity is eliminated and then progressed to the coming-to-sitting activities. Moving the child in lateral weight shifts, while sitting, also increases neck strength in a gravity-reduced plane. The therapist's support at the shoulders, trunk, and pelvis is necessary to allow isolation of the neck and trunk flexors. As the child's strength increases, the therapist introduces diagonal weight shifts that produce rotation. Diagonal or angular movements activate the transverse neck and trunk muscles (e.g., the oblique abdominal muscles) that are required in mature equilibrium responses.

Similarly, neck and trunk extension can be elicited by working with the child in a variety of activities in the prone position over a ball, bolster, or wedge. When the child is positioned in a prone position on an inclined surface, the pull of gravity is reduced, allowing for more effective use of neck and trunk extension. Toys or the parent's voice is used to motivate the child to raise his or her head while the therapist moves him or her in small ranges of anterior and posterior weight shift to stimulate a righting response. As the child's control of head and trunk extension improves, the degree of incline is gradually decreased. Engaging the child in reaching activities with one or both hands can facilitate antigravity trunk extension in the prone position (Figure 9-9). The

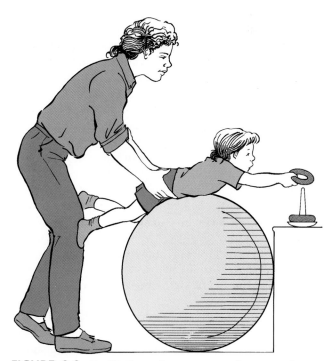

FIGURE 9-9 Facilitation of prone extension over therapeutic ball. Key point of control is at pelvis.

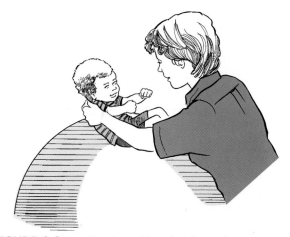

FIGURE 9-8 Facilitation of head righting from therapeutic ball. Other inclined surface could be used. Therapist supports child's shoulders, scapula, and trunk to encourage isolated activation of neck muscles.

therapist's handling should again provide stability so that specific extensor muscle activity is elicited and overflow contractions are inhibited (Bobath & Bobath, 1964; Perin, 1989; Sternat, 1993).

In addition to the traditional activities described previously, biofeedback devices are increasingly used with children who have muscular and neuromuscular disorders. Biofeedback can provide the needed feedback to the child about successful and unsuccessful muscle activation or positioning. In addition, it can provide the motivation for the child to attempt the activity. One example of biofeedback is a mercury switch strapped to the child's head and activated with upright head movement. Using this switch, the child can turn on the radio, tape recorder, or other battery-powered toy using simple head movements. Kramer, Ashton, and Brander (1992) found the mercury head switch to be effective in improving head control in prone and sitting positions over an 8-week period. Thus, for some children, biofeedback can be used during therapy sessions or in a home-based program as a tool to increase the child's motivation and improve antigravity movement.

Facilitation of Postural Reactions

The therapist can facilitate postural reactions using activities that displace the center of gravity and require corrective or protective responses. The speed, range, and direction of displacement determine whether righting or equilibrium responses are elicited. As mentioned previously, rapid movements in greater ranges elicit protective extension responses. These activities can also be performed on therapeutic balls, bolsters, equilibrium boards, or any other unstable surfaces (Figure 9-10).

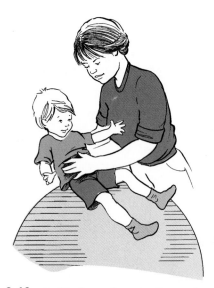

FIGURE 9-10 Facilitation of protective and equilibrium reaction to displacement on therapeutic ball.

Reaching activities with the child positioned on an unstable surface can facilitate the development of these reactions because the child will displace his or her center of gravity during the reach, requiring a compensatory response. Initially, the therapist provides pelvic stability (e.g., with his or her hands) as a base from which the child can begin to produce the desired response. As postural reactions improve, this support is reduced and finally eliminated. Then the child practices skills unsupported on a stable surface, using first a wide base of support (most of his or her legs and buttocks are in contact with the supporting surface) and later a smaller base of support (only the buttocks are in contact with the surface). Placing the child in a sitting position on an unstable surface will refine postural reactions. During advanced practice of these activities, the therapist moves the surface using a variety of speeds, ranges (degrees of tilt), and rhythms. Safety and protection of the child's fall become increasingly important as greater challenges to balance are imposed on the child. In addition to activities on an unstable surface, reaching activities that require the child to shift weight facilitate the development of equilibrium and righting reactions (Bobath & Bobath, 1964; Effgen, 1993; Perin, 1989). During all of these activities, a high level of task variability can facilitate the learning process.

Mature postural control and the motor patterns associated with these abilities develop through experience with the conditions in which they are required. Therefore the therapist provides the child with a variety of experiences that demand the use of postural reactions (VanSant, 1991). The therapist's role is to present a task that is sufficient for these motor patterns to be expressed, motivate the child such that the activity is fun and meaningful, and provide feedback to the child about the appropriateness of the motor response. As skills develop, the child is encouraged to evaluate his or her own responses (Effgen, 1993). As described in the section on facilitating antigravity movement, biofeedback can be used as a method for reinforcing postural responses by providing additional feedback to the child. Research has demonstrated its successful use to increase head righting and control in the prone and supine positions (Kramer, Ashton, & Brander, 1992) and to improve weight shift and ankle motion during walking (Conrad & Bleck, 1980; Seeger & Caudrey, 1983).

Standing balance control can also be addressed through use of movable force platform systems. In a simple study of balance training in standing, Shumway-Cook, et al. (2003) found that training on a movable force platform, consisting of repetitive forward and backward translations, for 5 days produced a decrease in the induced sway and a quicker response time that persisted up to 30 days following the completion of training. Although this is only one study, it does suggest that postural stability can be trained through the experience of repetitive perturbations.

Facilitation of Sensory Organization

As discussed previously, many children with developmental disorders demonstrate deficits in the organization of sensory inputs for use in balance. When sensory organization seems to be the basis for difficulty in postural control, it also becomes the focus of intervention. The therapist creates experiences with altered surfaces or visual contexts that match the identified needs of the child (Shumway-Cook, Horak, & Black, 1987). For example, children who demonstrate immature equilibrium responses when relying only on the somatosensory system benefit from activities that challenge this system, such as ball, bolster, or tilt board activities in a darkened room or with vision occluded (e.g., with the use of a blindfold). These activities should be designed so that the child does not feel threatened by the disruption of his or her vision and by the progress from easier positions to more complex positions (e.g., sitting to standing). Conversely, children with difficulty balancing when relying on visual information in the presence of conflicting somatosensory cues should benefit from practice of activities on unstable surfaces that challenge the somatosensory system. Movement on a surface padded with foam or covered with sand challenges balance with ambiguous information to the proprioceptive system. Combining the conflicting visual and somatosensory cues should require reliance on the vestibular system and would be appropriate to facilitate vestibular function in children with deficits in this area.

Facilitation of Anticipatory Postural Control

Facilitation of anticipatory postural control requires that the child experience the need for this control. Reaching, catching, and throwing activities can be used to identify deficits in anticipatory control and to facilitate its use. Again, the therapist needs to set up a task that requires anticipatory control. Practice with weight shifting may be necessary before practice of the displacing activity. Initially, this may be enhanced by handling, but as soon as possible the handling must be diminished and then curtailed. When the child experiences success or failure in independent performance of the task, the knowledge of results reinforces learning of the task (Schmidt, 1988). Experiences in reaching with and without handling allow the child to evaluate and learn from the sensory input during anticipatory weight shift (e.g., to recognize errors in anticipatory postural control). Varying the direction, speed, and magnitude of the displacing activity is also important so that the child is required to reassess the

intended movement and impose the appropriate anticipatory response (Van Sant, 1994). Reaching for a variety of objects of different size and weight at a variety of positions with a different goal (throwing, placing, bringing to the mouth) should provide sufficient variability to facilitate motor learning.

SUMMARY

This chapter described the development of postural control as influenced by the neuromotor, somatosensory, vestibular, and musculoskeletal systems. The importance of experience, sensory feedback, and practice to the development of effective postural control was explained using motor learning theories. Through in-depth understanding of the influence of multiple systems and experience to a child's development of dynamic upright postures, the therapist can successfully design interventions for children with postural instability.

Case Study 1

Marcy was diagnosed with spastic diplegic cerebral palsy. She was born at 32 weeks' gestation, weighing 2 pounds 11 ounces. Her hospital stay was complicated by respiratory distress syndrome and a grade II intraventricular hemorrhage.

Assessment

At $2\frac{1}{2}$ years of age, Marcy presented with spasticity in all four extremities, greater in the legs than in the arms. She demonstrated hypotonicity in the trunk. Her head control was good in all positions, but she continued to demonstrate an immature neck flexion response when pulled to sit. While sitting, she demonstrated a posterior pelvic tilt with weight bearing primarily on her sacrum and her trunk flexed forward. She could free one hand for play but required one hand for support to maintain sitting. She lacked antigravity back extension sufficient for sitting without arm support. Forward protective reactions were present, and lateral protective reactions were developing (i.e., they remained inconsistent). Protective and equilibrium reactions backward were absent. Marcy was motivated to move about her environment using a type of commando crawl movement of the arms with her legs tightly scissored (i.e., adducted). She was unable to assume or maintain the quadruped position.

Interpretation

Marcy demonstrated gross motor skills at the 6- to 7-month age level. She also demonstrated delayed development of antigravity head and trunk control and delayed development of protective and equilibrium reactions. Her movement patterns were influenced by spasticity with overflow into synergistic and antagonistic muscles.

Intervention

Intervention focused on developing antigravity neck and trunk strength, facilitating protective and equilibrium reactions, and developing independent sitting without arm support. Antigravity neck flexion was facilitated by lowering from a sitting to a supine position and practicing small lateral weight shifts in sitting. Antigravity neck and trunk extension were promoted through activities that involve moving from a side-lying to a prone position on a large therapy ball. The movement of the ball was used to facilitate postural extension. Reaching activities while sitting on a ball or bolster were used to facilitate trunk strength and the development of trunk righting and equilibrium and protective reactions.

Case Study 2

John, who has Down syndrome, was enrolled in a preschool program at 5 years of age. His teacher reported that he frequently fell and had difficulty keeping up with the other ambulatory children in the class. He avoided situations that required walking on unstable surfaces such as gravel or stepping over obstacles. Prior testing found vision and vestibular function to be within normal limits.

Assessment

John presented with a mild degree of hypotonia, ligamentous laxity, and joint hypermobility at all peripheral joints. He walked with a stiff-legged, flat-foot gait characterized by minimal hip and knee flexion, knee recurvatum during stance, and an absent heel-strike. He did not achieve either a prone extension or supine flexion posture. On the Gross Motor Scale of the PDMS, John scored at the 30-month age level. Testing using posturography revealed that John had difficulty with balance when conflicting sensory input was given and seemed to rely too heavily on vision to maintain his balance.

Interpretation

John exhibited generalized hypotonia and immature movement patterns while standing associated with decreased antigravity muscle strength. John demonstrated a gross motor delay with function limited in activities of jumping and single-limb stance such as hopping, skipping, and alternating feet on walking up or down steps (the activities that John failed on the PDMS). The results of the posturography suggested that John had difficulty with the organization of sensory cues for use in balance, resulting in difficulty under conditions of conflicting sensory cues from either the visual or somatosensory system.

Intervention

Intervention focused on developing antigravity muscle strength and facilitating the organization of sensory cues. Activities to increase antigravity extension included (1) reaching while prone on a ball or bolster, (2) pushing from a wall and holding onto rubber tubing while being pulled around the room prone on a scooter board, and (3) reaching and throwing while lying prone in a hammock swing. Activities to increase supine flexion included (1) moving from the supine position to sitting on an inclined surface and (2) reaching while sitting on the therapy ball.

Activities that challenged the sensory organization system were helpful in facilitating the ability to deal with conflicting sensory cues, including walking on foam, sand, grass, or thick carpet in various visual conditions such as eyes closed, dim lighting, and conflicting conditions (e.g., the conflict dome). In addition, standing activities that challenged the postural system facilitated more mature balance reactions. These activities included walking up and down stairs with an alternating step pattern, stepping over obstacles of various heights and widths, and kicking a ball. The use of a movable force platform system to induce forward and backward displacements would also challenge the postural system to facilitate more mature balance reactions.

STUDY QUESTIONS

1 What are the roles of the visual, vestibular, and somatosensory systems in balance control? How do these roles change in the developing child?
2 What is the difference between compensatory postural reactions and anticipatory postural control? How can each of these be evaluated?
3 How is postural control affected by abnormalities of the musculoskeletal system, alterations in muscle tone, and abnormal motor pattern selection? How can intervention address these limitations?

REFERENCES

Adams, J.A. (1971). A closed loop theory of motor learning. *Journal of Motor Behavior, 3,* 110-150.

Almeida, G.L., Campbell, S.K., Girolami, G.L., Penn, R.D., & Corcos, D.M. (1997). Multidimensional assessment of motor function in a child with cerebral palsy following intrathecal administration of baclofen. *Physical Therapy, 77,* 751-764.

Ayres, A. (1989). *Sensory Integration and Praxis Tests.* Los Angeles: Western Psychological Services.

Barnes, M., & Crutchfield, C. (1990). *Reflex and vestibular aspects of motor control, motor development and motor learning.* Atlanta: Stokesville.

Bartlett, D. (1997). Primitive reflexes and early motor development. *Developmental and Behavioral Pediatrics, 18* (1), 151-156.

Berger, W., Quintern, J., & Dietz, V. (1985). Stance and gait perturbation in children: Developmental aspects of compensatory mechanisms. *Electroencephalographic Clinical Neurophysiology, 61,* 385-395.

Bernstein (1967). The coordination and regulation of movements, London: Pergamon.

Bertenthal, B., & Von Hofsten, C. Eye, head and trunk control: The foundation for manual development. (1998). *Neuroscience and Biobehavioral Reviews, 22* (4), 515-520.

Bjornson, K.F., Graubert, C., Buford, V., & McLaughlin, J.F. (1998). Validity of the Gross Motor Function Measure. *Pediatric Physical Therapy, 10,* 43-47.

Bly, L. (1983). *The components of normal movement during the first year of life and abnormal development.* Oak Park, IL: Neurodevelopmental Treatment Association.

Bobath, B., & Bobath, K. (1954). A study of abnormal postural reflex activity in patients with lesions of the central nervous system. *Physiotherapy, 40,* 1-30.

Bobath, K. (1966). The motor deficit in patients with cerebral palsy. *Clinics in Developmental Medicine, 23,* 1-54.

Bobath, K., & Bobath, B. (1964). The facilitation of normal postural reactions and movements in the treatment of cerebral palsy. *Physiotherapy, 21,* 3-19.

Bouisset, S., & Zattara, M. (1981). A sequence of postural movements precedes voluntary movement. *Neuroscience Letters, 22,* 263-270.

Brogren, E., Forssberg, H., & Hadders-Algra, M. (2001). Influence of two different sitting positions on postural adjustments in children with spastic diplegia. *Developmental Medicine and Child Neurology, 43,* 534-546.

Brogren, E., Hadders-Algra, M., & Forssberg, H. (1996). Postural control in children with spastic diplegia: Muscle activity during perturbations in sitting. *Neuroscience and Biobehavioral Reviews, 38,* 379-388.

Brogren, E., Hadders-Algra, M., & Forssberg, H. (1998). Postural control in sitting children with cerebral palsy. *Neuroscience and Biobehavioral Review, 22* (4), 591-596.

Bruininks, R. (1978). *Bruininks-Oseretsky Test of Motor Proficiency.* Examiners Manual, Circle Pines, MN: American Guidance System.

Bullinger, A. (1981). Cognitive elaboration of sensorimotor behavior. In G. Buttorworth (Ed.), *Infancy and epistemology: An evaluation of Piaget's theory.* London: Harvester Press.

Burtner, P., & Woollacott, M. (1999). Stance balance control with orthoses in a group of children with spastic cerebral palsy. *Developmental Medicine and Child Neurology, 41,* 748-757.

Campbell, S.K., & Hedeker, D. (2001). Validity of the Test of Infant Motor Performance for discriminating among infants with varying risk for poor motor outcome. *Journal of Pediatrics, 139,* 546-551.

Campbell, S.K., Kolobe, T.H.A., Osten, E.T., Lenke, M., & Girolami, G.L. (1995). Construct validity of the Test of Infant Motor Performance. *Physical Therapy, 75,* 585-596.

Campbell, S.K., Kolobe, T.H.A., Wright, B.D., & Linacre, J.M. (2002). Validity of the Test of Infant Motor Performance for prediction of 6-, 9-, and 12-month scores on the Alberta Infant Motor Scale. *Developmental Medicine and Child Neurology, 44,* 263-272.

Case-Smith, J., & Bigsby, R. (2000). *Posture and Fine Motor Assessment of Infants: Parts I and II.* San Antonio, TX: Psychological Corporation.

Connor, F., Williamson, G., & Siepp, J. (1978). *Program guide for infants and toddlers with neuromotor and other developmental disabilities.* New York: Teachers College Press.

Conrad, L., & Bleck, E. (1980). Augmented auditory feedback in the treatment of equinus in children. *Developmental Medicine and Child Neurology, 22,* 713-718.

Crowe, T., Deitz, J., Richardson, P., & Atwater, S. (1990). Interrater reliability of the pediatric clinical test of sensory interaction for balance. *Physical and Occupational Therapy in Pediatrics, 10* (4), 1-27.

Deitz, J., Richardson, P., Atwater, S., Crowe, T., & Odiorne, M. (1991). Performance of normal children on the Pediatric Clinical Test of Sensory Interaction for Balance. *Occupational Therapy Journal of Research, 11* (6), 336-356.

Edelman, G.M. (1987). *Neural Darwinism,* New York: Basic Books.

Effgen, S. (1993). Developing postural control. In B. Connolly & P. Montgomery (Eds.), *Therapeutic exercise in developmental disabilities.* Hixson, TN: Chattanooga Group.

Ellison, P. (1994). *The INFANIB: A reliable method for the neuromotor assessment of infants.* Tucson, AZ: Therapy Skill Builders.

Fedrizzi, E., Pagliano, E., Marzarole, M., Fazzi, E., Maraucci, I., Furhanetto, A., & Fachin, P. (2000). Developmental sequence of postural control in prone position in children with spastic diplegia. *Brain and Development, 22,* 436-444.

Ferdjullah, M., Harris, G., Smith, P., & Wertsch, J. (2002). Analysis of postural control synergies during quiet standing in healthy children and children with cerebral palsy. *Clinical Biomechanics, 17,* 203-210.

Fetters, L. (1991). Cerebral palsy: Contemporary treatment concepts. In M. Lister (Ed.), *Contemporary management of motor control problems proceedings of the II step conference.* Alexandria, VA: Foundation for Physical Therapy.

Flegel, J., & Kolobe, T.H.A. (2000). Predictive validity of the Test of Infant Motor Performance as measured by the Bruininks-Oseretsky Test of Motor Proficiency at school age. *Physical Therapy, 82,* 762-771.

Folio, M., & Fewell, R. (2000). *Peabody Developmental Motor Scales* (2nd ed.). Austin, TX: Pro Ed.

Forssberg, H., & Nashner, L. (1982). Ontogenetic development of postural control in man: Adaptation to altered support and visual conditions during stance. *Journal of Neuroscience, 2* (5), 545-552.

Foudriat, B., DiFabio, R., & Anderson, J. (1993). Sensory organization of balance responses in children 3-6 years of age: A normative study with diagnostic implications. *International Journal of Pediatric Otorhinolaryngology, 27,* 255-271.

Gowland, C., Boyce, W.F., Wright, V., Russell, D.J., Goldsmith, C.H., & Rosenbaum, P.L. (1995). Reliability of the Gross Motor Performance Measure. *Physical Therapy, 75*, 597-602.

Haas, G., Diener, H., Bacher, M., & Dichgans, J. (1986). Development of postural control in children: Short-, medium-, and long-latency EMG responses of leg muscles after perturbation of stance. *Experimental Brain Research, 64*, 127-132.

Hadders-Algra, M., Brogren, E., & Forssberg, H. (1996a). Ontogeny of postural adjustments during sitting in infancy variation, selection, and modulation. *Journal of Physiology, 493* (1), 273-288.

Hadders-Algra, M., Brogren, E., & Forssberg, H. (1996b). Training affects the development of postural adjustments in sitting infants. *Journal of Physiology, 493* (1), 289-298.

Hadders-Algra, M., Brogren, E., & Forssberg, H. (1997). Nature and nurture in the development of postural control in human infants. *Acta Pediatric Supplement, 422*, 48-53.

Hadders-Algra, M., Brogren, E., & Forssberg, H. (1998). Development of postural control-differences between ventral and dorsal muscles. *Neuroscience and Biobehavioral Reviews, 22* (4), 501-506.

Haley, S. (1986). Sequential analyses of postural reactions in nonhandicapped infants. *Physical Therapy, 66* (4), 531-536.

Hayes, K., & Riach, C. (1989). Preparatory postural adjustment and postural sway in young children. In M. Woollacott & A. Shumway-Cook (Eds.), *Development of posture and gait across the life span*. Columbia: University of South Carolina Press.

Hirshfeld, H., & Forssberg, H. (1994). Epigenetic development of postural responses for sitting during infancy. *Experimental Brain Research, 97*, 528-540.

Horak, F., & Nashner, L. (1986). Central programming of posture control: Adaptation to altered support-surface configurations. *Journal of Neurophysiology, 55*, 1368-1381.

Horak, F., & Shumway-Cook, A. (1990). Clinical implications of posture control research. In P. Duncan (Ed.), *Balance proceedings of the APTA forum*. Alexandria, VA: American Physical Therapy Association.

Horak, F., Shumway-Cook, A., Crowe, T., & Black, F. (1988). Vestibular function and motor proficiency in children with hearing impairments and in learning disabled children with motor impairments. *Developmental Medicine and Child Neurology, 30*, 64-79.

Howle, J. (2002). *Neuro-developmental treatment approach: Theoretical foundations and principles of clinical practice.* Laguna Beach, CA: The North American Neuro-Developmental Treatment Association.

Jantz, J., Blosser, C., & Fruechting, L. (1997). A motor milestone change noted with a change in sleep position. *Archives of Pediatric and Adolescent Medicine, 151*, 565-568.

Jeng, S.F., Yau, K-I, T., Chen, L-C., & Hsiao, S-F. (2000). Alberta Infant Motor Scale: Reliability and validity when used on preterm infants in Taiwan. *Physical Therapy, 80*, 168-178.

Johnson-Kramer, C., Sherwood, D., Frech, R., & Canabal, M. (1992). Performance and learning of a dynamic balance task by visually impaired children. *Clinical Kinesiology, 1*, 3-6.

Jouen, F. (1984). Visual-vestibular interactions in infancy. *Infant Behavior and Development, 7*, 135-145.

Kamm, K., Thelen, E., & Jensen, J. (1990). A dynamical systems approach to motor development. *Physical Therapy, 70* (12), 763-775.

Kramer, J., Ashton, B., & Brander, R. (1992). Training of head control in the sitting and semi-prone position. *Child Care, Health, and Development, 18*, 365-376.

Leonard, C., Hirschfeld, A., & Forssberg, H. (1988). Gait acquisition and reflex abnormalities in normal children and children with cerebral palsy. In B. Amblard, A. Berthoz, & F. Clarae (Eds.), *Posture and gait development, adaptation, and modulation.* New York: Elsevier Science.

MacPhail, A., & Kramer, J.F. (1995). Effect of isokinetic strength training on functional ability and walking efficiency in adolescents with cerebral palsy. *Developmental Medicine and Child Neurology, 37*, 763-775.

Murney, M.E., & Campbell, S.K. (1998). The ecological relevance of the Test of Infant Motor Performance: Elicited Scale items. *Physical Therapy, 78*, 479-489.

Nashner, L. (1990). Sensory, neuromuscular, and biomechanical contributions to human balance. In P. Duncan (Ed.), *Balance proceedings of the APTA forum*. Alexandria, VA: American Physical Therapy Association.

Nashner, L., Shumway-Cook, A., & Marin, O. (1983). Stance posture control in selected groups of children with cerebral palsy: Deficits in sensory organization and muscular coordination. *Experimental Brain Research, 49*, 393-409.

Perin, B. (1989). Physical therapy for the child with cerebral palsy. In J. Techlin (Ed.), *Pediatric physical therapy*. Philadelphia: J.B. Lippincott.

Piper, M., & Darrah, J. (1994). *Motor assessment of the developing infant*. Philadelphia: W.B. Saunders.

Pountney, T., Mulcahy, C., & Green, E. (1990). Early development of postural control. *Physiotherapy, 76* (12), 799-802.

Riach, C., & Hayes, K. (1987). Maturation of postural sway in young children. *Developmental Medicine and Child Neurology, 29*, 650-658.

Ribaldi, H., Rider, R., & Toole, T. (1987). A comparison of static and dynamic balance in congenitally blind, sighted, and sighted blindfolded adolescents. *Adapted Physical Activity Quarterly, 4*, 220-225.

Richardson, P., Atwater, S., Crowe, T., & Deitz, J. (1992). Performance of preschoolers on the pediatric clinical test of sensory interaction for balance. *American Journal of Occupational Therapy, 46* (9), 793-800.

Rose, J., Wolff, D., Jones, V., Bloch, D., Gelhert, J., & Gamble, J. (2002). Postural balance in children with cerebral palsy. *Developmental Medicine and Child Neurology, 44*, 58-63.

Russell, D.J., Rosenbaum, P.L., Avery, L.M., & Lane, M. (2002). *Gross Motor Function Measure (GMFM-66 and GMFM-88) user's manual*. Cambridge: Cambridge University Press.

Russell, D.J., Avery, L.M., Rosenbaum, P.L., Raina, P.S., Walter, S.D., & Palisano, R.J. (2000). Improved scaling of the gross motor function measure for children with cerebral palsy: evidence of reliability and validity, *Physical Therapy, 80*, 873-885.

Russell, D.J., Rosenbaum, P.L., Lane, M., Gowland, C., Boyce, W.F., & Plews, N. (1994). Training uses in the Gross Motor Function Measure: Methodological and practical issues, *Physical Therapy, 74*, 630-636.

Schmidt, R. (1988). *Motor control and learning* (2nd ed.). Champaign, IL: Human Kinetics.

Seeger, B., & Caudrey, D. (1983). Biofeedback therapy to achieve symmetrical gait in children with hemiplegic cerebral palsy: Long term efficacy. *Archives of Physical Medicine and Rehabilitation, 64,* 160-162.

Sellers, J. (1988). Relationship between antigravity control and postural control in young children. *Physical Therapy, 68* (4), 486-430.

Shumway-Cook, A. (1989). Equilibrium deficits in children. In M. Woollacott & A. Shumway-Cook (Eds.), *Development of posture and gait across the life span.* Columbia: University of South Carolina Press.

Shumway-Cook, A., Horak, F., & Black, F. (1987). A critical examination of vestibular function in motor impaired learning disabled children. *International Journal of Otorhinolaryngology, 14,* 21-30.

Shumway-Cook, A., & Woollacott, M. (1985a). Dynamics of postural control in the child with Down syndrome. *Physical Therapy, 9,* 1315-1322.

Shumway-Cook, A., & Woollacott, M. (1985b). The growth of stability: Postural control from a developmental perspective. *Journal of Motor Behavior, 17* (2), 131-147.

Shumway-Cook, A., Hutchinson, S., Kartin, D., Price, R., & Woollacott, M. (2003). Effect of balance training on recovery of stability in children with cerebral palsy. *Developmental Medicine & Child Neurology, 45,* 591-602.

Sporns, O., Tononi, G., & Edelman, G.M. (2000). Connectivity and complexity: The relationship between neuroanatomy and brain dynamics. *Neural Networks, 13,* 909-922.

Sterba, J.A., Rogers, B.T., France, A.P, & Vokes, D.A. (2002). Horseback riding in children with cerebral palsy: Effect on gross motor function. *Developmental Medicine and Child Neurology, 44,* 301-308.

Sternat, J. (1993). Developing head and trunk control. In B. Connolly & P. Montgomery (Eds.), *Therapeutic exercise in developmental disabilities.* Hixson, TN: Chattanooga Group.

Stockmeyer, S. (1967). An interpretation of the approach of Rood to the treatment of neuromuscular dysfunction. *American Journal of Physical Medicine, 46,* 900-956.

Taylor, J. (1931). *Selected writings of John Hughlings Jackson* (Vol. II). London: Holder & Stoughton.

Thelen, E. (1995). Motor development: A new synthesis. *American Psychologist, 50* (2), 79-95.

Thelen, E., & Fisher, D. (1982). Newborn stepping: An explanation for a "disappearing reflex." *Developmental Psychology, 18,* 760-775.

Thelen, E., & Fisher, D. (1983). The organization of spontaneous leg movements in newborn infants, *Journal of Motor Behavior, 15,* 353-377.

Thelen, E., & Spencer, J.P. (1998). Postural control during reaching in young infants: A dynamic systems approach. *Neuroscience and Biobehavioral Reviews, 22* (4), 507-514.

Thelen, E., & Ulrich, B.D. (1991). Hidden skills: A dynamic systems analysis of treadmill stepping during the first year. *Monographs of the Society for Research in Child Development, 56* (1, Serial No. 223).

Van der Fitts, I., Otten, E., Klip, A., Van Eykern, L., & Hadders-Algra, M. (1999). The development of postural adjustments during reaching in 6- to 18-month old infants. *Experimental Brain Research, 126,* 517-528.

Van der Heide, J., Otten, B., van Eykern, L., & Hadders-Algra, M. (2003). Development of postural adjustments during reaching in sitting children. *Experimental Brain Research, 151,* 32-45.

VanSant, A. (1991). Neurodevelopmental treatment and pediatric physical therapy: A commentary. *Physical Therapy, 3* (3), 137-140.

VanSant, A. (1993). Concepts of neural organization and movement. In B. Connolly & P. Montgomery (Eds.), *Therapeutic exercise in developmental disabilities.* Hixson, TN: Chattanooga Group.

VanSant, A. (1994). Motor control and motor learning. In D. Cech & S. Martin (Eds.), *Functional movement development across the life span.* Philadelphia: W.B. Saunders.

Vereijken, B., & Thelen, E. (1997). Training infant treadmill stepping: The role of individual pattern stability. *Developmental Psychobiology, 30,* 89-102.

Von Hofsten, C. (1986). The emergence of manual skills. In M. Wade & A. Whiting (Eds.), *Motor development in children: Aspects of coordination and control.* Boston: Martinus Nijhoff.

Von Hofsten, C., & Rosander, K. (1996). The development of gaze control and predictive tracking in young infants. *Vision Research, 36,* 81-96.

Williams, H., Fisher, J., & Tritschler, K. (1983). Descriptive analysis of static postural control in 4, 6, and 8 year old normal and motorically awkward children. *American Journal of Physical Medicine, 62* (1), 12-26.

Woollacott, M. (1988). Posture and gait from newborn to elderly. In B. Amblard, A. Berthoz, & F. Clarae (Eds.), *Posture and gait development, adaptation, and modulation.* New York: Elsevier Science.

Woollacott, M., Debu, B., & Mowatt, M. (1988). Neuromuscular control of posture in the infant and child: Is vision dominant? *Journal of Motor Behavior, 19* (2), 167-186.

Woollacott, M., Shumway-Cook, A., & Williams, H. (1989). The development of posture and balance control in children. In M. Woollacott & A. Shumway-Cook (Eds.), *Development of posture and gait across the lifespan.* Columbia: University of South Carolina Press.

Woollacott, M., & Sveistrup, H. (1992). Changes in the sequencing and timing of muscle response coordination associated with developmental transitions in balance abilities. *Human Movement Science, 11,* 23-36.

10 Development of Hand Skills

Charlotte E. Exner

Visual-motor integration
Fine motor coordination
Fine motor skills
Dexterity
Hand skills
Reach
Grasp
Carry
Voluntary release
In-hand manipulation
Bilateral hand use

CHAPTER OBJECTIVES

1 Describe the typical development of hand skills in children.
2 Identify factors that contribute to typical or atypical development of hand skills.
3 Explain the implications of hand skill problems for children's occupational performance, particularly in the areas of play, activities of daily living, and school performance.
4 Describe typical problems with children's development of hand skills.
5 Describe frames of reference and theories that the therapist can use in structuring intervention plans for children with hand skill problems.
6 Identify evaluation tools and methods useful in assessing hand skills in children.
7 Describe intervention strategies for assisting children in improving or compensating for problems with hand skills.

Hand skills are critical to interaction with the environment. The hands allow action through human contact and contact with objects. Hands are the "tools" most often used to accomplish work and play and to perform activities of daily living. The child who has a disability affecting hand skills has less opportunity to take in sensory information from the environment and to experience the effect of his or her actions on the world.

COMPONENTS OF HAND SKILLS

Effective use of the hands to engage in a variety of occupations depends on a complex interaction of hand skills, postural mechanisms, cognition, and visual perception. The term visual-motor integration refers to the interaction of visual skills, visual-perceptual skills, and motor skills. The term hand skills is used interchangeably with the terms fine motor coordination, fine motor skills, and dexterity. Because this chapter refers only to skills of the hands that are needed to attain and manipulate objects, the more specific term *hand skills* is used.

Although most therapists assume that the development of hand skills depends on adequate postural functions and sufficient visual-perceptual and cognitive development, these areas are not discussed in detail in this chapter. Hand skills are patterns that normally rely on both tactile-proprioceptive and visual information for accuracy. However, the child can accomplish these skills without visual feedback if somatosensory functions provide adequate information. The patterns include reach, grasp, carry, and voluntary release, as well as the more complex skills of in-hand manipulation and bilateral hand use. Briefly, these patterns can be defined as follows:

- Reach: Extension and movement of the arm for grasping or placing objects
- Grasp: Attainment of an object with the hand
- Carry: Transportation of a hand-held object from one place to another; also referred to as "moves" and "lifts" in the Occupational Therapy Practice Framework (AOTA, 2002, p. 621)
- Voluntary release: Intentional letting go of a hand-held object at a specific time and place
- In-hand manipulation: Adjustment of an object in the hand after grasp
- Bilateral hand use: Use of two hands together to accomplish an activity

In this discussion, the term *hand-arm* refers to the interactive movement and stabilization of different parts of the hand and arm to accomplish a fine motor task.

Visual skills constitute the use of extraocular muscles to direct eye movements. These skills include the ability to visually fix on a stationary object and the smooth, accurate tracking of a moving target. *Visual-perceptual skills* involve the recognition, discrimination, and processing of sensory information through the eyes and related central nervous system (CNS) structures. Visual-perceptual skills include the identification of shapes, colors, and other qualities; the orientation of objects or shapes in space; and the relationship of objects or shapes to one another and to the environment (see Chapter 12).

CONTRIBUTIONS OF CONTEXT FACTORS TO HAND SKILLS

For occupational therapists, a knowledge of context factors is critical for understanding, evaluating, and providing intervention for hand skill problems. Social and cultural factors, in particular, are likely to play important roles in the acquisition and use of various hand skills. Social factors that can affect the development of hand skills include socioeconomic status, and gender and role expectations. Like culture, social factors are less likely to affect the development of more basic hand skills but may have a greater influence on skills needed for complex manipulation of objects and tool use. For example, children who live in conditions of poverty may not have the exposure to writing utensils, scissors, and other materials common to children from middle-class environments.

Verdonck and Henneberg (1997) studied differences in performance on the Box and Block Test of Manual Dexterity in two groups of South African children between 6 and 17 years of age. The groups reportedly differed only in socioeconomic status and rural versus urban living environments. Children from the middle-class urban area performed significantly better than those from the poor rural area. Yim, Cho, and Lee (2003) found that school-age Korean children had somewhat less strength in palmar and lateral pinch than Western children.

The objects that are important to the child's cultural group influence the development of object manipulation. Because tools that are important in one culture may not be available in another, children may not have the opportunity to develop some tool-specific skills. For example, eating utensils vary from chopsticks to forks and spoons. Scissors use may be important for school performance in some cultures but not in others.

In addition, the age at which children are expected to achieve skill in object manipulation can vary. Safety concerns influence parents in some cultural groups to delay introduction of a knife to their child, whereas parents in other cultural groups encourage independence in knife use. Some cultures introduce children to the use of writing materials before 1 year of age. Other cultures do not provide children with these materials until they can be expected to adhere to requirements such as using them only on paper (rather than on the wall or on clothing).

Culture also influences the perception of children's need for manipulative materials. Linked to this is the cultural group's view of the importance of play. Play materials that provide opportunities for the development of manipulative skills (e.g., building sets, beads, puzzles, and table games) are highly valued in some cultural groups, whereas in other groups, play with gross motor objects (e.g., balls and riding toys) or play with animals is more valued. Some cultural groups do not view children's play as important, therefore few play materials of any type are available.

Although the types of activities encouraged can promote the development of specific skills, acquisition of the basic hand skills of reach, grasp, release, and manipulation does not rely on the availability of any particular materials; rather, it relies on reasonable exposure to a variety of materials with the opportunity to handle them.

CONTRIBUTIONS OF CLIENT FACTORS TO HAND SKILLS

A variety of client factors play a critical role in the development of hand skills. Although therapists usually give motor issues the most attention, many dimensions of development significantly influence effective hand use, including the child's visual skills, somatosensory functions, sensory integration (SI), visual perception, cognition and, as discussed above, social factors and culture. As children mature, they begin to coordinate visual skills with hand skills effectively, and later they combine hand-eye coordination with visual-perceptual skills (Ayres, 1958).

SENSORY FUNCTIONS

Visual Skills

Visual skills play a major role in the development of hand function (Bertenthal & von Hofsten, 1998; Jeannerod, 1994; von Hofsten, 1991). Vision is particularly important for learning new motor skills. At about 4 months of age, infants begin to move their hands under visual control as they reach for an object and make differentiated finger movements. The visuomotor development required for accurate reach matures by approximately 6 months of age. The infant's visual-motor coordination continues to refine, and by 9 months of age, the infant guides his or her hand movements using visual-somatosensory integration (i.e., these sensory inputs are combined and compared as the infant anticipates and plans movement). Vision is also important as the infant learns new fine motor skills or when an activity requires highly precise and accurate movements (e.g., stringing small beads or putting together a puzzle).

Somatosensory Functions

The relationship between somatosensory functions of the hands and hand skills is strong. Good hand skills are associated with good somatosensory functioning. However, good somatosensory functioning does not necessarily yield good hand skills.

The role of somatosensory information and feedback is critical to development in many areas of children's hand skills, particularly those involving isolated movements of the fingers and thumb. Typical infants develop the ability to match *haptic perception* (knowledge of objects gathered by means of active touch) of some three-dimensional objects with visual perception within the first 6 months of life (Stillwell & Cermak, 1995). Bushnell and Boudreau (1999) reported that children as young as 2.5 years of age can identify common objects by touch alone and that children 5 years of age demonstrate good haptic recognition of unfamiliar objects. Many aspects of haptic perception, such as identification of three-dimensional common objects and perception of spatial orientation, are well developed by 6 years of age. The adolescent has fully developed the refinement of haptic perception and the ability to discriminate all aspects of object characteristics through touch (Stillwell & Cermak, 1995).

The fingertips gather precise information about many types of object qualities. Children with impaired control of finger movement have limited access to somatosensory information. Initiating and sustaining grasp force requires tactile and proprioceptive input and integration (Gordon & Duff, 1999; Johansson & Westling, 1988). The ability to sustain objects in the hand (i.e., to prevent objects from dropping) is primarily related to intact somatosensory functioning (Gordon & Forssberg, 1997). Gordon and Duff also noted that tactile information is critical for anticipating the amount of force needed to grasp and lift an object. Apparently a minimum amount of tactile awareness, as measured by two-point discrimination, is needed for functional development of these fine motor skills.

Somatosensory functioning is difficult to study in children, particularly in young children and those with disabilities. In testing, the performance of these children varies from one session to another, which further complicates the assessment process. Given that the link between somatosensory functioning and hand skills is a strong one, further investigation of the relationship between tactile functioning and various hand skills will support the development of new intervention approaches for these children.

Sensory Integration

The types of SI problems most likely to influence hand use are sensory registration problems, tactile hypersensitivity, poor tactile discrimination, and dyspraxia. Children with poor sensory registration engage in few activities involving hand skills. The child with tactile defensiveness is likely to avoid contact with certain materials, thus limiting exposure to various objects. Motor-planning deficits and clumsiness are associated with poor tactile and proprioceptive functioning. Praxis problems based on poor tactile and proprioceptive processing are referred to as *somatodyspraxia* (Ayres, 1989).

Visual Perception and Cognition

Perceptual development and cognitive development are difficult to isolate from each other, particularly as they relate to object-handling skills in children; for this reason, these areas are addressed together. The development of hand skills allows for more complex interaction with objects, and perceptual and cognitive development allows the child to know the possibilities available for object use and interactions.

The child's perception of object characteristics, movement speed required, and power needed affects his or her ability to effectively control objects (Elliott & Connolly, 1984). The child acquires knowledge about objects through object manipulation.

During the first 6 months, the infant uses visual and tactile stimuli to guide fine motor development and begins to develop an awareness of object placement in space. In the second half of the first year, the infant adjusts the actions of the hand in response to object characteristics, such as size, shape, and surface qualities (Corbetta & Mounoud, 1990). Ruff, McCarton, Kurtzber, and Vaughan (1984) emphasized the importance of object manipulation in infants between 6 and 12 months of age for learning object characteristics, because this learning was believed to be important for concept and language development. Infants demonstrate their perceptual and cognitive skills when reaching for objects. By 9 to 10 months of age, infants adapt their arm positions to horizontal versus vertical object presentations and shape their hands appropriately for convex and concave objects.

During the second year, infants learn to relate objects to one another with more accuracy and purpose. Before 18 months of age, infants modify their movement approach in anticipation of the weight of the object (Bushnell & Boudreau, 1999; Corbetta & Mounoud, 1990).

Exner and Henderson (1995) discussed the interaction of cognition and hand skill development. Like perceptual development, cognitive development influences and is supported by the development of hand skills.

For example, changes in attentional control and the development of problem-solving strategies are seen in the gradual improvement in infants' ability to handle two objects simultaneously. Without this development in cognition, bilateral skills would not be possible. The infant must be able to attend to two objects simultaneously to be able to bang objects together, stabilize an object with one hand while manipulating with the other, and manipulate two or more objects simultaneously (e.g., in buttoning or tying). Because attention and planning demands are greater for two-handed activities than for one-handed activities, bilateral skill development lags behind unilateral skill development (Bushnell & Boudreau, 1999; Corbetta & Mounoud, 1990).

NEUROMUSCULOSKELETAL AND MOVEMENT-RELATED FUNCTIONS

Functions of Joints and Bones

The integrity of the hand is an important consideration in hand function. Children with congenital hand anomalies may be missing one or more digits, a condition that significantly affects the variety of possible prehension patterns. Refined finger movements and in-hand manipulation skills may also be limited or absent. Severe congenital anomalies can affect bilateral hand use. Involvement of the thumb has a more significant effect on the development of hand function than impairment of any other digit.

Joint range of motion (ROM) has a significant effect on the positioning of the arm for hand use and on reaching and carrying skills. Effective hand function also depends on adequate mobilization of distal muscle groups that control palmar arches. Limitations in range can occur as a result of abnormal joint structure, muscle weakness, or joint inflammation. Any of the problems that reduce range of motion are likely to affect a child's ability to grasp larger objects or to flatten the hand to stabilize materials.

Muscle Functions

Muscle functions include muscle power (strength), muscle tone, and muscle endurance. Sufficient strength is necessary to initiate all types of grasp patterns and to maintain these patterns during lifting and carrying. Children's grasp strength gradually increases through the preschool years (Lee-Valkow, Aaron, Eladoumikdachi, Thornby, & Netscher, 2003; Link, Lukens, & Bush, 1995), the elementary school years (Yim, Cho, & Lee, 2003), and adolescence (Mathiowetz, Weimer, & Federman, 1986; Smits-Engelsman, Westenberg, & Duysens, 2003). This increase allows them to engage in activities with objects of increasing weight. Children with poor strength may be unable to initiate the finger exten-

sion or the thumb opposition pattern necessary before grasp. They also may not have the flexor control to hold a grasp pattern. Many children with diminished strength are unable to use patterns that rely on the intrinsic muscles for control and therefore are unable to use thumb opposition or metacarpophalangeal (MCP) joint flexion with interphalangeal (IP) joint extension. Children with fair strength may be able to initiate a grasp pattern but may be unable to lift an object against gravity while maintaining the grasp. Endurance during an activity can be a problem for children with mildly diminished strength, particularly in situations in which they must use a sustained grasp pattern or hold an object against resistance (e.g., during eating with utensils, coloring, handwriting, and scissors activities).

Tone in muscle groups affects the stability of parts of the arms and hands during activities and the types of movements possible. Damage to the CNS causes tonal abnormalities, which can affect joint ROM and, in general, decrease speed of movement. Increased tone results in loss of ROM, whereas decreased tone results in exaggerated joint ROM and decreased stability. Children with fluctuating tone typically have full ROM, but they can maintain joint stability only at the extreme end of a joint position (full flexion or full extension). In addition, movements are less controlled and often are random or unrelated to the task.

GENERAL DEVELOPMENTAL CONSIDERATIONS

Developmental principles are further described in Chapter 4. Two principles with particular application to hand skill development are the development of movement patterns from mass to specific and of motor control from proximal to distal. Two additional principles are discussed in this section; specifically, that mature movement patterns are characterized by integrated stability and mobility and that involuntary movement patterns precede associated movements that developed into isolated, voluntary movement and coordinated action.

The mass-to-specific principle of development means that less-differentiated movement patterns precede discrete, highly specialized skills. For example, the infant uses all fingers in early grasping and later uses only the specific number of fingers needed for object contact.

The proximal-to-distal principle means that development initially occurs proximally (in the head and trunk) and gradually progresses toward the distal parts of the body (hands and feet). In using this principle to guide treatment, some therapists suggest that intervention for hand skills should be deferred until postural control matures.

Clinicians have interpreted this relationship to mean that improvement in postural control results in improvement in hand skills and/or that intervention should be sequential, proceeding from proximal to distal control. However, several clinical research studies (Case-Smith, Fisher, & Bauer, 1989; Wilson & Trombly, 1984) and some authors (Pehoski, 1992, 1995) have questioned this principle. The clinical studies have yielded weak correlations between postural or proximal control and hand function (approximately $r = 0.20$ to 0.35). Case-Smith and colleagues stated that "the correlations between the proximal and distal motor functions would be markedly higher if proximal motor control was necessary for the development of distal motor skill" (p. 661). The relationship between proximal and distal control is a functional or biomechanical one in which postural control is necessary for placement of the hand in space and support of the hand during its execution of skills. Case-Smith and co-workers emphasized that "therapists should not assume that proximal control is a necessary precursor to fine motor skill; they should, however, assume that treating proximal weakness may affect distal function" (p. 661). However, the degree of proximal control does not necessarily determine the child's degree of distal control.

Pehoski (1992, 1995) used work by Lawrence and Kuypers (1968) to explain why distal control is not directly linked to proximal control. Two motor systems are used in upper extremity control. One system is responsible for postural control and proximal control, including integrated body-limb and body-head movements. This system comprises primarily the ventromedial brain stem pathways that synapse primarily with interneurons to trunk and proximal muscles (Pehoski, 1992, 1995). In contrast, the corticospinal track system originates in the primary motor cortex, and its fibers directly synapse with the motoneurons for hand muscles. The latter system allows for isolated finger movements, which are needed for a precise pincer grasp and fine manipulation (Pehoski, 1992, 1995). Thus development of upper extremity skills and hand skills occurs because of proximal *and* distal control mechanisms, rather than as a result of one proximal *to* distal mechanism.

Refined movements also depend on the ability to combine patterns of stability and mobility effectively (Bobath, 1978). The child must develop the ability to stabilize the trunk effectively and maintain it in an upright position without relying on the frequent use of one or both arms to maintain balance. In addition, the child sequentially develops patterns of stability and mobility in the scapulohumeral, elbow, and wrist joints; this permits arm use independent of, but effectively used with, trunk movement. Eventually the ability to use stability and mobility in the hand emerges.

For normal functioning, joints must be able to stabilize at any point in the normal range of movement and to move within small, medium, or large segments of range. At times during arm-hand activities, the proximal joints are more stable. Grasp is an example of this because the arm is stable while the fingers are moving. However, in carrying, the distal joints are stable while the arm is moving. In mature handwriting, the elbow, forearm, and wrist joints are relatively stable and the shoulder and finger joints are mobile.

An important sequence in the development of motor control is the use of straight movement patterns before the emergence of controlled rotation patterns. For example, the infant first develops controlled stability and mobility in basic flexion and extension of the shoulder, elbow, and wrist. This is followed by control of internal and external rotation of the shoulder and pronation and supination of the forearm.

In typical development the infant gradually learns to use both sides of the body well together and to use each side of the body independently of the other. Initially the infant uses his or her arms in asymmetric patterns that are not coordinated. Movements of one arm often elicit reflexive, nonpurposeful reactions in the other arm. Gradually the infant develops the ability to move the two arms together in the same pattern. As skilled use of symmetric hand and arm patterns is refined, the infant begins to use the two arms independently of one another for different parts of an activity. For example, one hand stabilizes an object while the other hand manipulates it. Overflow and associated movements gradually decrease to allow separate but coordinated action of the two hands.

DEVELOPMENT OF HAND SKILLS

As in all areas of occupational therapy, the therapist must supplement academic study of hand skill development and treatment with observations of typical infants and children and of children with differences in development. Imitating each of the normal and abnormal movements and patterns described in the following text also helps clarify the descriptions provided.

Reach

Rosblad (1995) stated that "in a reaching movement, the goal is to transport the hand to the target, with precision in both time and space" (p. 81). Thus the development of reaching is described in terms of the changes that take place in the control and speed of the hand's movement toward the object and the preparation of the hand for grasp.

The arm movements of the newborn are asymmetric. However, even in the first several days of life, the infant shows increasing visual regard of objects close to him or her and activation of the arms in response to objects (von Hofsten, 1982). Over the next few months the arms become active and the infant swipes or bats at objects with the arm abducted at the shoulder. Reach with an extended arm is likely to occur between approximately 12 and 22 weeks of age (Thelen et al., 1993). Objects are rarely grasped and then only by accident. If grasped, they are released at random, generally in association with arm movements.

Gradually a midline orientation of the hands develops. Initially the hands are held close to the body. Soon, with an increased desire for visual regard of the hands and greater proximal arm stability, the child holds the hands further away to view them. This pattern precedes the onset of symmetric bilateral reaching, which usually occurs first in the supine and then in the sitting position. At this stage, the child initiates reach with humeral abduction, partial shoulder internal rotation, forearm pronation, and full finger extension.

As the infant shows increasing dissociation of the two body sides during movement, unilateral reaching begins. Abduction and internal rotation of the shoulder are less prominent in reach. The hand opens in preparation for grasping the object and is usually more open than necessary for the size of the object.

As scapular control and trunk stability mature, the infant begins to use shoulder flexion, slight external rotation, full elbow extension, forearm supination, and slight wrist extension during reaching. Active supination of the forearm is not seen until some external rotation is used to stabilize the humerus. In addition, well-controlled elbow extension evolves as the rotation elements are developing. Mature reach is usually seen with sustained trunk extension and a slight rotation of the trunk toward the object of interest. Over the next few years, the child refines this unilateral reaching pattern, increasing the accuracy of arm placement and the grading of finger extension as appropriate to the size of the object (Figure 10-1), as well as the timing of the various movement elements. The quality of reach with grasp continues to mature until approximately 12 years of age, at which time the child prepares the hand with the optimal hand opening for the object size at the initiation of reach (Kuhtz-Buschbeck, Stolze, Johnk, Boczek-Funcke, & Illert, 1998). Before this age the child needs to use visual monitoring for accuracy in hand opening during reach.

Grasp Patterns
Classification

Napier (1956) proposed two basic terms to describe hand movements: prehensile and nonprehensile. *Nonprehensile movements* involve pushing or lifting an object with the fingers or the entire hand. In contrast, *prehensile movements* involve grasp of an object and may be subdivided according to the purpose of the grasp: precision or power. *Precision grasps* involve opposition of the thumb to fingertips. *Power grasps* involve the use of the

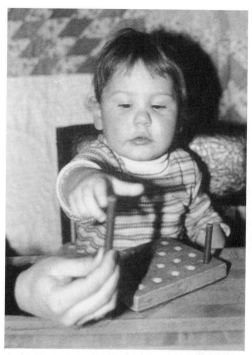

FIGURE 10-1 This typically developing child demonstrates reach with trunk rotation, full elbow extension, slight forearm rotation, and wrist stability, yet some degree of excess finger extension before grasp. (Photograph courtesy Ed Exner, Greensburg, Penn.)

entire hand. In a power grasp, the thumb is held flexed or abducted to other fingers, depending on control requirements.

In most cases the activity and the object's characteristics determine the grasp pattern used. Small objects are generally held in a precision grasp, primarily because of the large amount of sensory feedback available through the fingertips and the control used to move them. Medium objects can be held with either pattern, and large objects are held with a power grasp. Napier (1956) noted a frequent interplay between precision and power handling of different objects based on needs within an activity.

Weiss and Flatt (1971) described a slightly different method of classification. Grasps with no thumb opposition include hook grasp, power grasp, and lateral pinch. Patterns that use thumb opposition include tip and palmar pinches. The palmar pinch category is divided into standard, spherical, cylindrical, and disk grasps.

The *hook grasp* is used when strength of grasp must be maintained to carry objects. For this grasp, the transverse metacarpal arch is essentially flat, the fingers are adducted with flexion at the IP joints, and flexion or extension occurs at the MCP joints (Weiss & Flatt, 1971) (Figure 10-2). The thumb can be flexed over the fingers if additional power is needed. Observation of this pattern provides an indication of the child's ability to sustain wrist extension during finger flexion.

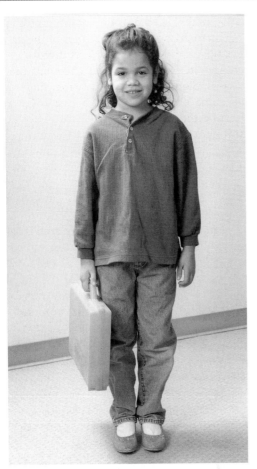

FIGURE 10-2 Hook grasp used to carry a child's art case. (Photograph courtesy Kanji Takeno, Towson University.)

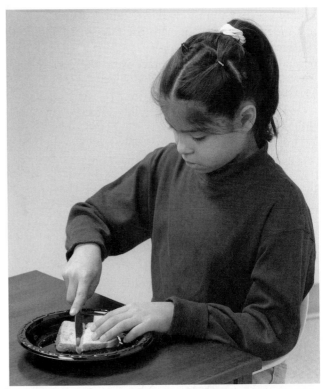

FIGURE 10-3 Power grasp with the right hand, used in cutting bread. (Photograph courtesy Kanji Takeno, Towson University.)

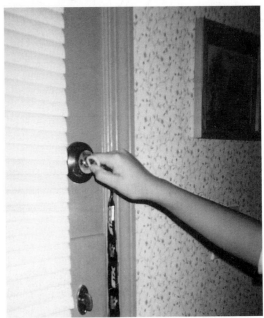

FIGURE 10-4 Lateral pinch with the right hand, used to open a lock on a door.

In contrast, the *power grasp* often is used to control tools or other objects. Oblique object placement in the hand, flexion of the ulnar fingers, less flexion with the radial fingers, and thumb extension and adduction facilitate precision handling with this grasp (e.g., for brushing the hair). Thus the child stabilizes the object with the ulnar side of the hand and controls the object for position and use with the radial side of the hand (Weiss & Flatt, 1971) (Figure 10-3). Observation of this pattern allows for notation of the degree of radial-ulnar dissociation in the hand that the child can use and his or her control of thumb adduction with extension.

Lateral pinch is used to exert power on or with a small object. Partial thumb adduction, MCP flexion, and slight IP flexion are characteristics of this pattern. Although the index finger is slightly flexed, it is more extended than the other fingers. The pad of the thumb is placed against the radial side of the index finger at or near the distal interphalangeal (DIP) joint (Figure 10-4). This pattern involves controlling the index finger while adducting and flexing the thumb.

There are two types of standard pinches. Opposition of the thumb to the index finger pad only describes the *pad-to-pad, two-point pinch* (Smith & Benge, 1985) or

pincer grasp (Gesell & Amatruda, 1947) (Figure 10-5). Opposition of the thumb simultaneously to the index and middle finger pads, which provides increased stability of prehension, describes the *three-point pinch* (Smith & Benge, 1985) or *three-jaw chuck grasp* (Erhardt, 1982)

(Figure 10-6). In both cases, the thumb forms an oval or a modified oval shape with the fingers. In addition, the forearm is slightly supinated, which frees the thumb and radial fingers from contact with the surface and allows for an optimal view of the object. Observation of this pattern allows for notation of the child's ability to control objects with the radial finger pads while controlling thumb opposition.

Opposition of the thumb tip and the tip of the index finger, forming a circle, describes a *tip pinch* (Figure 10-7). All joints of the index finger and thumb are partly flexed. This pinch pattern is used to obtain small objects.

Observation of this grasp provides information about the child's ability to dissociate the two sides of the hand and to use the tips of the index finger and thumb.

Differences in hand posture characterize the other palmar grasps. Significant wrist extension, finger abduction, and some degree of flexion at the MCP and IP joints describe the *spherical grasp* (Figure 10-8). Stability of the longitudinal arch is necessary to use this pattern to grasp large objects. The hypothenar eminence lifts to assist the cupping of the hand for control of the object (Weiss & Flatt, 1971). Observation of this grasp pattern suggests the child's ability to balance control of the intrinsic and extrinsic hand muscles.

In the *cylindrical grasp*, the transverse arch is flattened to allow the fingers to hold against the object. The fingers are only slightly abducted, and IP and MCP joint flexion is graded according to the size of the object. When additional force is required, more of the palmar surface of the hand contacts the object (Weiss & Flatt, 1971) (Figure 10-9). Observation of this pattern allows for observation of palmar arch control during handling of a relatively large object.

A *disk grasp* has finger abduction that is graded according to the size of the object held, hyperextension of the MCP joints, and flexion of the IP joints (see Figure 10-9) (Weiss & Flatt, 1971). The wrist is more flexed when objects are larger, and only the pads of the fingers contact the object. The amount of thumb extension also increases with object size. The transverse metacarpal arch is flattened in this prehension pattern. This pattern involves dissociation of flexion and extension movements and use of a combination of wrist flexion with MCP extension and IP flexion.

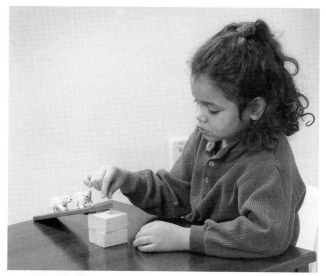

FIGURE 10-5 Pincer grasp, used to place "food" for the climbing polar bears. (Photograph courtesy Kanji Takeno, Towson University.)

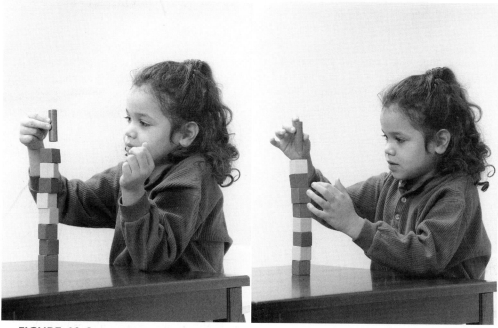

FIGURE 10-6 This child uses variations of a three-jaw chuck grasp with her right hand, depending on task demands. (Photograph courtesy Kanji Takeno, Towson University.)

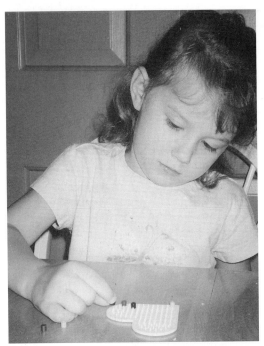

FIGURE 10-7 Tip pinch with the right hand, used to complete a bead craft project. Normal radial grasps, such as the tip pinch, are accompanied by slight forearm supination.

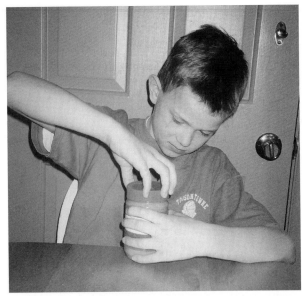

FIGURE 10-9 This child uses a cylindrical grasp with his left hand and a disk grasp with his right hand to open a jar. Note the grading of finger abduction with the left hand to provide adequate stability to the jar.

Sequential Development of Grasp Patterns

Several developmental trends affect the particular type of grasp pattern an infant is able to use at any time. The sequences shown in Box 10-1 interact and overlap. The infant's growing interest in objects, desire to attain them, and desire to explore them and relate them to other objects influence these motor sequences. Haptic development and visual-perceptual development contribute to the infant's ability to shape the hand appropriately for the object and to approach the object with optimal orientation of the arm and hand.

Another aspect of motor development that contributes to the infant's use of increasingly mature and more varied patterns is the ability to use internal stability throughout the upper extremity, forearm supination, and thumb opposition. Thumb activity and control are necessary to allow for patterns other than palmar grasp. Hirschel, Pehoski, and Coryell (1990) discussed the influence of increasing arm stability on the infant's use of a mature pincer grasp. The ability to stabilize the wrist in a slightly extended position is important for grasp patterns that use distal (fingertip) control. Slight forearm

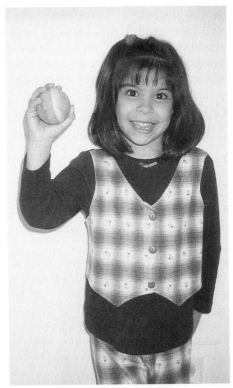

FIGURE 10-8 Spherical grasp, used in preparation to throw a ball.

BOX 10-1 Sequential Development of Grasp

1 Ulnar grasp, palmar grasp, radial grasp
2 Palmar contact, finger surface contact, finger pad contact (Hohlstein, 1982)
3 Use of long finger flexors, use of intrinsic muscles with extrinsic muscles (long flexors and extensors)

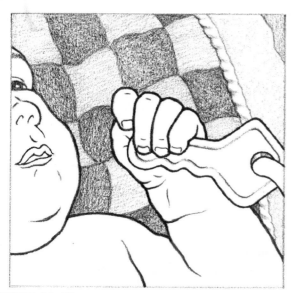

FIGURE 10-10 Ulnar-palmar grasp. The index finger and thumb are not used in this pattern.

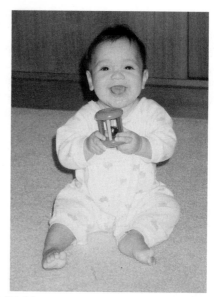

FIGURE 10-11 This baby uses a radial-digital grasp with both hands to hold a toy for shaking and mouthing.

supination is important because it positions the hand so that the thumb and radial fingers are free for active object exploration, and it allows the infant to view his or her fingers and thumb during grasp.

A typical sequence can be seen during the infant's first 6 months. Initially the infant appears to have no voluntary hand use. The hands alternately open and close in response to various sensory stimuli. Gradually the traction response and grasp reflex decrease, and a voluntary palmar grasp begins to emerge (Figure 10-10). By approximately 6 months the infant progresses to being able to use a radial palmar grasp. Case-Smith, Bigsby, and Clutter (1998) found a marked increase in grasp skill between 4 and 5 months of age. They noted less change between 5 and 6 months of age.

The second 6 months is a key period for the development of hand skills. The ability to grasp a variety of objects increases significantly between 6 and 9 months of age. During this time, grasp patterns with active thumb use emerge. Crude raking of a tiny object is present by about 7 months of age, and by 9 months of age the infant is able to attain a tiny object on the finger surface and with the thumb. By 8 to 9 months of age, the infant holds a larger object between the thumb and the radial fingers (Figure 10-11) and readily varies the grasping pattern according to the shape of the object. Case-Smith et al. (1998) noted a particularly dramatic increase in skill between 8 and 9 months of age. However, at this time intrinsic muscle control is not effective because the infant does not use grasp with MCP flexion and IP extension. Between 9 and 12 months of age, refinement occurs in the ability to use thumb and finger pad control for tiny and small objects. More precise preparation of the fingers before initiation of grasp, more inhibition of the ulnar fingers, and slight

wrist extension and forearm supination are characteristics of this refinement.

After 1 year of age, further refinement occurs in grasp patterns that were seen earlier, and more sophisticated patterns emerge. Between 12 and 15 months of age, the infant's ability to hold crackers, cookies, and other flat objects identifies an increasing control of the intrinsic muscles. Although studies are limited in terms of grasp development for patterns other than the pincer grasp, between 18 months and 3 years of age, most children with typical development acquire the ability to use a disk grasp, a cylindrical grasp, and a spherical grasp with control. Control of a power grasp continues to develop through the preschool years. The pattern for a lateral pinch may be present by 3 years of age, but children generally do not use this pattern with power until later in the preschool years. Overall grasp patterns for a variety of objects are well developed by 5 years of age, but those involving tools may continue to mature into the early school years.

In addition to quality of grasp, strength of grasp continues to increase throughout childhood. Lee-Valkow, Aaron, Eladoumikdachi, Thornby, and Netscher (2003) reported on the development of grip and pinch strength in typical preschool-age children. They noted significant increases in strength for palmar grip, key (lateral) pinch, and tripod (three-point) pinch for children between 3 and 4 years of age and 4 and 5 years of age. The increase in strength was greater between 4 and 5 years than between 3 and 4 years in both preferred and nonpreferred hands. Yim, Cho, and Lee (2003) found increases in grip, lateral pinch, palmar pinch, and tip pinch across the age range in 7- to 12-year-old Korean children; they also reported significant differences in grip strength between boys and girls in each age group for both right and left hands. They noted that right-handed girls were stronger than left-handed girls in grip strength and lateral pinch with both hands. In a study of isometric strength of the index finger, Smits-Engelsman, Wilson, Westenberg, and Duysens (2003) found that isometric force increased gradually during the 5- to 10-year-old age span, reflecting corticospinal system maturation. Compared to 10- to 12-year-olds, adults exhibited greater use of alternative strategies for selecting and monitoring force needed in an activity.

In-Hand Manipulation Skills
Classification

In-hand manipulation includes five basic types of patterns: finger-to-palm translation, palm-to-finger translation, shift, simple rotation, and complex rotation (Exner, 1992). All skills require the ability to control the arches of the palm (Figure 10-12). Long, Conrad, Hall, and Furler (1970) described translation as a linear movement of the object from the palm to the fingers or from the fingers to the palm; the object stays in constant contact with the thumb and fingers during this pattern. The fingers and thumb maintain grasp but move into and out

of MCP and IP flexion and extension. In contrast, Exner's description of the pattern of finger-to-palm translation notes that the object is grasped with the pads of the fingers and thumb and then is moved into the palm (Exner, 1992). The finger pad grasp is released so that the object rests in the palm of the open hand or is held in a palmar grasp at the conclusion of the pattern. The object moves in a linear direction in the hand, and the fingers move from an extended position to a more flexed position during the translation. An example of this skill is picking up a coin with the fingers and thumb and moving it into the palm of the hand.

Palm-to-finger translation is the reverse of finger-to-palm translation (Exner, 1992). However, palm-to-finger translation requires isolated control of the thumb and use of a pattern beginning with finger flexion and moving toward finger extension (see Figure 10-12). This pattern is more difficult for the child to execute than finger-to-palm translation. An example of this skill is moving a coin from the palm of the hand to the finger pads before placing the coin in a vending machine.

Shift involves linear movement of the object on the finger surface to allow for repositioning of the object on the pads of the fingers (Exner, 1992). In this pattern the fingers move just slightly at the MCP and IP joints, and

A   B   C

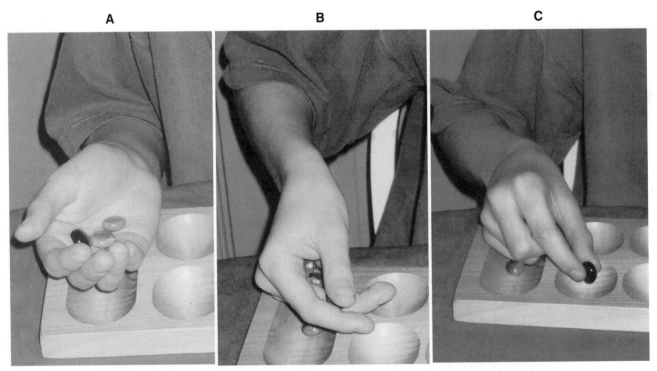

FIGURE 10-12 A, The child shows the ability to keep the palm in a cupped position to hold several stones for a game. The forearm is in almost full supination. **B,** Palm-to-finger translation with stabilization is initiated for one of the stones while the other stones are retained in the palm. The translation movement produced by the fingers is accompanied by forearm rotation into midposition. **C,** Palm-to-finger translation with stabilization is completed for one stone. The other stones are retained in the hand by flexion of the ulnar fingers. The forearm moves toward pronation to assist with placement of the stone on the game board.

the thumb typically remains opposed or adducted with MCP and IP extension throughout the shift. The object usually is held solely on the radial side of the hand. Examples of this skill include separating two pieces of paper that are weakly stuck together, moving a coin from a position against the volar aspect of the DIP joints to a position closer to the fingertips (e.g., so that the coin can be easily inserted into the slot of a vending machine), and adjusting a pen or pencil after grasp so that the fingers are positioned close to the writing end of the tool. This skill is used frequently in dressing tasks such as buttoning, fastening snaps, lacing shoes, and putting a belt through belt loops.

The two patterns of rotation are simple rotation and complex rotation. Simple rotation involves the turning or rolling of an object held at the finger pads approximately 90 degrees or less (Exner, 1992). The fingers act as a unit (little or no differentiation of action is shown among them), and the thumb is in an opposed position. Examples of simple rotation include unscrewing a small bottle cap, reorienting a puzzle piece in the hand by turning it slightly before placing it in the puzzle, and picking up a small peg and rotating it from a horizontal to a vertical position for insertion into a pegboard.

Complex rotation involves the rotation of an object 180 to 360 degrees once or repetitively (Exner, 1992). During complex rotation the fingers and thumb alternate in producing the movement, and the fingers typically move independently of one another. An object may be moved end over end, such as in turning a coin or a peg over or in turning a pencil over to use the eraser.

In-hand manipulation skills can occur with only one object in the hand or with two or more objects in the hand. (Skills involving only one object in the hand are described in a previous section.) For example, a child typically unscrews a bottle lid with no other objects in his or her hand. However, these skills may be used when the child is holding other objects in the hand. For example, a child may have two or more pieces of cereal in his or her hand but brings only one piece out to the finger pads before placing it in the mouth (see Figure 10-12). The term *with stabilization* refers to the use of an in-hand manipulation skill while other objects are stabilized in the hand. This activity therefore is described as involving palm-to-finger translation with stabilization, whereas unscrewing the bottle lid is simple rotation. In-hand manipulation skills done with stabilization are more difficult than the same skill done without the simultaneous stabilization of other objects in the hand.

Developmental Considerations

Motor skill prerequisites for in-hand manipulation include the following:

- Movement into and stability in various degrees of supination

- Wrist stability
- Opposed grasp with thumb opposition and object contact with the finger surface (not in the palm)
- Isolated thumb and radial finger movement
- Control of the transverse metacarpal arch
- Dissociation of the radial and ulnar sides of the hand
- Successive increases and decreases in fingertip forces (Eliasson & Gordon, 2000)

Children who are unable to use in-hand manipulation skills are likely to substitute other patterns. Substitution patterns are part of the typical strategies used in acquiring in-hand manipulation skills; however, their use does not necessarily represent abnormal fine motor control. Typical patterns a child uses when he or she shows very limited in-hand manipulation are (1) changing of hands (putting the object in the other hand for use) and (2) transferring from hand to hand (moving the object from one hand to the other and back to the hand that held it first). The child uses these patterns after the initial grasp when he or she realizes that the object in the hand needs to be repositioned for use but that the object cannot readily be adjusted in that hand. The child therefore moves the object to the other hand (and perhaps back to the first hand) to adjust the position. For example, a child picks up a crayon or marker with the right hand but is unable to shift it to place the fingers near the writing end, therefore he or she grasps the object with the left hand and then transfers it back to the right hand with the fingers appropriately positioned. Some children preplan for this by picking up the crayon with the non-preferred hand and changing it to the preferred hand.

Therapists observe several skills in children who are beginning to use in-hand manipulation skills or are preparing for the use of these skills. The substitutions or precursors involve supporting the object while the hand is changing position on it. The type of support the child uses depends on the type of in-hand manipulation skill being used. Infants typically engage in bilateral manipulation of objects by moving an object between the two hands. As the child moves the object between the hands, he or she turns and repositions it within the hands. Children use this strategy, called a *hand assist*, to substitute for palm-to-finger translation or rotation. In this case the object does not leave the hand that grasped it initially, but the other hand helps with repositioning of the object. The child uses movement of the fingers to assist with repositioning of the object, as opposed to only grasp and release of the object. Sometimes children use other surfaces or other parts of the body to provide support for the manipulation. Children commonly use assist strategies for shift and complex rotation.

Ongoing research is directed toward determining a sequence for the development of in-hand manipulation skills (Exner, 1990a; Pehoski, Henderson, & Tickle-Degnen, 1997a, 1997b). Based on these research studies, the following developmental traits have emerged. By approximately 12 to 15 months of age, infants use finger-to-palm translation to pick up and "hide" small pieces of food in their hands. By 2 to 2.5 years of age, children use palm-to-finger translation and simple rotation with some objects. Complex rotation skills are observed in children at 2.5 to 3 years of age, although this age group often has difficulty with them. By 4 years of age, children consistently use complex rotation without using an external support (Pehoski, Henderson, & Tickle-Degnen, 1997a). Children between 3.5 and 5.5 years of age develop skills in rotating a marker (regardless of its initial orientation) and shifting it into optimal position for coloring and writing (Exner, 1990a; Humphry, Jewell, & Rosenberger, 1995). Shift typically is evident but inconsistent in children 3 and 3.5 years old (Exner, 1990a).

After 3 years of age the child uses in-hand manipulation skills with greater proficiency and consistency. Dropping of objects during in-hand manipulation tasks decreases through the preschool years (Pehoski et al., 1997b). Lee-Valkov et al. (2003) reported data on preschool-age children's object manipulation speed, as gathered with the Functional Dexterity test (a pegboard with short pegs approximately 1 inch in diameter). The test was administered to both hands, and scoring was based on the amount of time needed to rotate and place 16 pegs; 5-second scoring penalties were added to the time score for use of substitution patterns or for dropping. Children obtained slightly higher scores with their preferred hands, and the amount of time needed to complete the test decreased by approximately 7 to 8 seconds each year.

By 6 years of age, children develop the ability to use a variety of in-hand manipulation skills with stabilization (Exner, 1990a; Pehoski et al., 1997b). Between 6 and 7 years of age, children more consistently use combinations of in-hand manipulation skills that must be used in an activity (e.g., palm-to-finger translation with stabilization followed by complex rotation with stabilization).

Ongoing research by Exner and others suggests that children continue to refine in-hand manipulation skills up to approximately 9 to 10 years of age and continue to develop speed of skill use through 12 years of age. Yim, Cho, and Lee (2003) used the Nine-Hole Pegboard test to evaluate dexterity skills (complex rotation skills) in Korean children without disabilities between the ages of 7 and 12 years. In comparing their data for 12-year-olds with data for adults obtained by Kellor, Rost, Silberberg, Iversen, and Cummings (1971), they found that the girls' mean time scores were approximately the same as those for the youngest adults, but that the 12-year-old boys' mean time scores were slightly slower. The difference may reflect a cultural difference or possibly the continuing development of object manipulation speed during adolescence.

The ability to use a skill with one type of object is not always associated with an ability to use the skill with another size or shape of object. For example, the child may be able to use simple rotation to turn a small peg but may not be able to use simple rotation to orient a crayon for coloring. In general, small objects (e.g., smaller diameter crayons) are easier for children to manipulate than slightly larger objects (e.g., larger diameter crayons) or tiny objects. Tiny objects require precise fingertip control, whereas medium-sized and larger objects require control with more fingers.

In addition to object characteristics and the need for in-hand manipulation skill with or without stabilization, other factors can contribute to a child's use of these skills with particular materials; such factors include the cognitive-perceptual demands of the activity, the child's interest in the manipulative materials or the activity, and the child's motor-planning skills. Problems in any of these areas, or in processing tactile-proprioceptive information or visual acuity, can affect development of in-hand manipulation skills. Data collected by Lee-Valkov et al. (2003) suggest that dexterity in typical preschool children is not significantly correlated with grip or pinch strength. However, it should be noted that typical children were likely to have grip and pinch strength generally within normal limits. Markedly diminished strength could have a negative effect on in-hand manipulation skills.

Carry

Carrying ("moving" and "lifting") involves a smooth combination of body movements accompanied by stabilization of an object in the hand. When carrying involves objects used in most occupational activities, small ranges of movements are used and adjusted in accordance with the demands of the activity. Co-contraction in the more distal joints of the wrist and hand often is present. The child must be able to hold the forearm stable while in any degree of rotation, and he or she must be able to modify the forearm and wrist positions during the carry so that the object remains in an optimal position. Similarly, the child must be able to use shoulder rotation movements simultaneously with shoulder flexion and abduction so that appropriate object orientation is maintained.

Voluntary Release

Voluntary release, like grasp, depends on control of arm and finger movements. To place an object for release, the arm must move into position accurately and then stabilize as the fingers and thumb extend. Gordon, Lewis,

Eliasson, and Duff (2003) refer to the two components of voluntary release as *replacement* and *release*.

Initially the infant does not voluntarily release an object; objects either drop involuntarily from the hand or must be forcibly removed from the hand. As the infant's nondiscriminative responses to tactile and proprioceptive stimuli decrease and visual control and cognitive development increase, volitional control of release emerges. With increases in the mouthing of objects and bringing of both hands to midline and playing with them there, the infant begins to transfer objects from one hand to another. Initially the child stabilizes the object in the mouth during transfers or pulls it out of one hand with the other. Soon the infant begins to freely transfer the object from one hand to another. The receiving hand stabilizes the object, and the releasing hand is fully opened.

By 9 months of age, the infant begins to release objects without stabilizing then with the other hand. The arm is fairly extended during release (Connor, Williamson, & Siepp, 1978). The infant exhibits increasing humeral control as he or she moves the arm to drop objects in different locations. The next step is the development of elbow stability in various positions, and the infant begins to release with the elbow in some degree of flexion. The therapist may stabilize the arm or hand on the surface during release. At about 1 year of age, the child can release objects with shoulder, elbow, and wrist stability; however, the MCP joints remain unstable during this pattern, therefore the infant continues to show excess finger extension (Figure 10-13). Gradually the child develops the ability to release objects into smaller containers (Figure 10-14) and to stack blocks

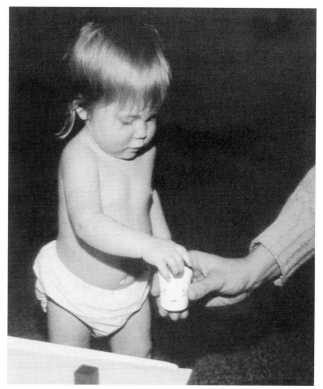

FIGURE 10-14   The child's shoulder, elbow, and wrist are stable, and less finger extension occurs with release. The child visually monitors release of the object into a small container. (Courtesy Kennedy Kreiger Institute, Baltimore, MD.)

(Figure 10-15). The release pattern is refined over the next few years until the child can release small objects with graded extension of the fingers, indicating control over the intrinsic hand muscles. These skills also illustrate the integration of perceptual, cognitive, and sensory skills with motor skills. For example, Eliasson and Gordon (2000) reported that typical children between 7 and 13 years of age demonstrate the ability to effectively modulate the timing of the decreases in force with which they grasp a lighter object and a heavier object to allow for appropriate timing in voluntary release.

Bilateral Hand Use ("Coordinates")

As discussed previously, the normal infant progresses from asymmetry to symmetry to differentiated asymmetric movements, which are used in bilateral hand activities. Asymmetry is a characteristic of movement patterns until almost 3 months of age. Symmetric patterns predominate between 3 and 10 months of age, when bilateral reach, grasp, and mouthing of the hands and objects are primary activities. Control of these movements originates proximally at the shoulders, allowing the hands to engage at midline. By 9 to 10 months of age, the infant can hold one object in each hand and

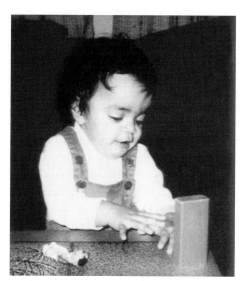

FIGURE 10-13   Full finger extension and some wrist movement occur with voluntary release. Note the visual regard of the object being released.

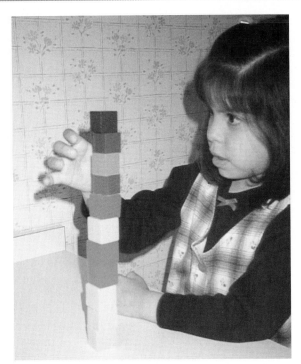

FIGURE 10-15 Stability of the shoulder, elbow, forearm, wrist, and fingers combines with perceptual development to promote accurate placement of objects. This 5-year-old is able to use forearm supination to midposition with controlled finger extension. In this challenging task, only slight overextension of the fingers occurs.

bang them together (see Figure 10-11). This ability to hold an object in each hand at the same time is critical for further bilateral skill development. By 10 months of age, bimanual action is well differentiated, with one hand grasping the object and the other manipulating parts of it (Fagard & Jacquet, 1989). More complex bilateral skills depend on this ability.

Bimanual activity emerges first as reciprocal or alternating hand movements, then as simultaneous hand movements. By 17 to 18 months of age, infants frequently use role-differentiated strategies (i.e., one hand stabilizes or holds the materials and the other manipulates or activates them) (Ramsey & Weber, 1986). For these skills to emerge, the infant must be able to dissociate the two sides of the body and begin to use the two hands simultaneously for different functions. Effective stabilization of materials also depends on adequate shoulder, elbow, and wrist stability.

Between 18 and 24 months of age, the child begins to develop skills that are precursors to simultaneous manipulation. Bilateral skill refinement depends heavily on continuing development of reach, grasp, release, and in-hand manipulation skills. Skills in visual-perceptual, cognitive, and motor areas become more integrated, leading to the child's effective use of motor planning for task performance. The child demonstrates simultaneous manipulation at 2 to 3 years of age (Connor et al., 1978).

The mature stage of bilateral hand use, which is the ability to use opposing hand and arm movements for highly differentiated activities (e.g., cutting with scissors) begins to emerge at about 2.5 years of age. The child applies and refines the patterns from each stage of bilateral hand use in a variety of activities throughout childhood.

Ball-Throwing Skills

Ball-throwing skills reflect the child's ability to use voluntary release skills. In throwing a small ball, the child must sequence and time movements throughout the entire upper extremity. The child must bring the arm into a starting position, then prepare for projection of the ball into space by moving the trunk with the scapulohumeral joint, stabilizing the shoulder while beginning to extend the elbow, stabilizing the elbow while moving the wrist from extension to a neutral position, and simultaneously forcefully extending the fingers and thumb.

Children progress through a series of skill levels before they can smoothly sequence these movements and project the ball to the desired location. By 2 years of age, the child should be able to throw a ball forward and maintain balance so that his or her body does not also move forward (Sheridan, 1975). At this age the child uses extensor movements to fling the ball but is unable to sustain shoulder flexion during the toss (Folio & Fewell, 2000). The child can dissociate trunk and arm movement but cannot dissociate humeral and forearm movements. By 2.5 to 3 years of age, the child can aim the ball toward a target and project the ball approximately 3 feet forward. This ability to control the direction of the ball to some degree implies that the child can control the humerus so that the elbow is in front of the shoulder when the ball is released. Thus the shoulder has sufficient stability to support controlled elbow and finger movement. By 3.5 years of age, the child is able to throw the ball 5 to 7 feet toward a target with little deviation from a straight line (Folio & Fewell). To accomplish this accuracy, the child positions his or her elbow in front of the shoulder before the ball is released.

Further refinement of ball-throwing skills continues over the next few years. Distance and accuracy improve as the child gains scapulohumeral control, the ability to sustain the humerus above the shoulder, and the ability to control the timing of elbow, wrist, and finger extension. Thus at approximately 5 years of age, the child is able to use an overhand throw to hit a target 5 feet away fairly consistently. Children between 6 and 7 years of age are able to hit a target 12 feet away by using an overhand throw (Folio & Fewell, 2000). Underhand throws to contact a target are also possible in children 5 years of age or older. This skill requires the ability to move the humerus into flexion while sustaining full external rotation.

Tool Use

Connolly and Dalgleish (1989) defined a *tool* as "a device for working on something . . . tools serve as extensions of the limbs and enhance the efficiency with which skills are performed" (p. 895). They defined *tool use* as "a purposeful, goal-directed form of complex object manipulation that involves the manipulation of the tool to change the position, condition or action of another object" (Connolly & Dalgleish, p. 895). Tool-use skills are more complex than other hand skills, because the child must use a tool, rather than the hand, to act on objects.

The development of skill in using tools is critical to a variety of self-care, play and leisure, and school and work tasks. Skills in tool use for eating and play typically begin to emerge during the second year, after the child has mastered the basic skills of reach, grasp, and release. The skills emerge concurrently with in-hand manipulation skills, which are necessary for the progression of tool use skills beyond grasp and release proficiency. In-hand manipulation skills allow the tool to be adjusted in the hand after it has been grasped.

A key factor in the acquisition of tool-use skills is the high degree of interaction of these skills and cognitive development. Connolly and Dalgleish (1989) emphasized that an individual needs to know both what he or she wants to do (the intentional aspect of the task) and how he or she can accomplish it (the operational aspect of the task). Both of these elements require development of the child's cognitive skills and operational aspects of the child's motor skills.

As with any new skill, when the child is developing tool use, the therapist sees inconsistencies in the child (even in the same session). The therapist is likely to record multiple strategies for children who are beginning to use a particular skill. Thus "inconsistency" in the strategy used to perform a skill should be considered an important stage in the skill acquisition process. As skill acquisition progresses, practice allows the skill to progress from being performed with a high level of attention to being performed at a more automatic level. With such practice, performance becomes faster, more accurate, and smoother. Practice typically is necessary for a skill to become functional for execution in daily life tasks.

Researchers have studied the acquisition of children's skills in the use of three tools: drawing and writing, scissoring, and eating. Of these, most of the research has focused on drawing and writing tool use (see Chapter 17 for a description of this type of tool use).

Schneck and Battaglia (1992) described the development of scissors skills in young children. This skill emerges when the child first learns to place his or her fingers in the holes and to open and close the scissors. Early cutting is actually snipping, a process of closing the scissors on the paper with no movement of the paper and with no ability to repetitively open and close the scissors while flexing the shoulder and extending the elbow to move across the paper. Three-year-old children may use a pronated forearm position or a forearm-in-midposition placement (Schneck & Battaglia, 1992), or they may alternate between the two forearm positions. By 4 years of age, children typically hold both forearms in midposition for the cutting activity.

The Peabody Developmental Motor Scales has established the following typical sequence for scissors skills (Folio & Fewell, 2000):

- By 2 years of age, children can snip with scissors.
- By 2.5 years of age, most children can cut across a 6-inch piece of paper.
- By 3 to 3.5 years of age, they can cut on a line that is 6 inches long.
- By 3.5 to 4 years of age, they can cut a circle.
- By 4.5 to 5 years of age, they can cut a square.

More complex cutting skills develop between 6 and 7 years of age. Other factors the therapist should consider when assessing a child's skill in cutting include the width of the line to cut on, the size of the paper, the size of the design to be cut, and the complexity of the design.

The child's grasp on the scissors changes over time. The thumb position in one hole remains consistent, but the finger positions change according to the child's level of maturation and the type of scissors used (Schneck & Battaglia, 1992). In a mature grasp, which may not be achieved until after 6 years of age, the child has the middle finger in the lower hole of the handle, the ulnar two fingers flexed (inside or outside the lower hole, depending on its size), and the index finger positioned to stabilize the lower part of the scissors (Myers, 1992; Schneck & Battaglia).

The general ages at which a child learns to use various utensils in eating are as follows: a spoon by 18 months of age, a fork by 2.5 years of age, and a knife by 6 years of age (Henderson, 1995). However, documentation regarding how these skills are acquired and how various components of movement interact to produce skill is limited. To address this issue, Connolly and Dalgleish (1989) conducted a longitudinal study on development of spoon use skills in infants between 11 and 23 months of age. They analyzed videotapes of the infants' grasp patterns on the spoon; the placement of the spoon in the hand; movements used in filling the spoon, bringing it to the mouth, clearing the spoon, and taking it out of the mouth; and visual monitoring of the pattern, timing, and use of the nonpreferred hand in the eating process. They found that the mean number of grasp patterns decreased between 11 and 17 months of age and that most infants 17 months of age or older showed a clear hand preference for eating.

The infants used 10 different grasp patterns, but none of them used an adult pattern. The most commonly used pattern was a transverse palmar grasp with all four fingers flexed around the handle of the spoon. The next two most commonly used patterns were ones in which the fingers were flexed but the handle was on the finger surface rather than in the palm. In 17- to 23-month-old infants, this pattern was accompanied by some degree of index finger extension, which is a precursor to manipulation of the spoon's orientation in the hand and is similar to a power grasp. The infants became increasingly efficient in spoon use during this period and improved their visual monitoring of the process.

Another component in the development of tool use in children is the role of the assisting hand. In handwriting and coloring, the assisting hand plays an important role in stabilizing the paper. However, in using scissors and eating, the assisting hand is likely to be much more active. In cutting, this hand must hold the paper and orient it through rotation by moving in the same or the opposite direction as the hand with the scissors. In eating, the child's assisting hand may be involved in a variety of activities, depending on the child's age and the utensils used. Connolly and Dalgleish (1989) found that infants between 18 and 23 months of age showed significantly more involvement of the assisting hand in stabilizing a dish during spoon feeding than did infants between 12 and 17 months of age. Learning to use a knife entails learning to stabilize food with one hand or with another tool while the child uses the preferred hand with the knife for spreading or cutting.

RELATIONSHIP OF HAND SKILLS TO CHILDREN'S OCCUPATIONS

Hand skills are vital to the child's interaction with the environment. Engagement in most occupations requires object handling, almost all of which is accomplished with the hands. Usually greater impairment of hand use results in the need for increased adaptations if the child is to develop daily life skills. Children with a wide variety of types of disabilities are likely to have difficulty with hand function. These disabilities include cerebral palsy (Fedrizzi, Pagliano, Andreucci, & Oleari, 2003; Hanna et al., 2003), developmental coordination disorder (Mandich, Polatajko, & Rodger, 2003), attention deficit hyperactivity disorder (Pitcher, Piek, & Hay 2003), and mental retardation and epilepsy (Beckung, Steffenburg, & Uvebrant, 1997). As Mandich et al. noted, "Incompetence in everyday activities [has] serious negative effects for the children" (p. 583).

Play

Although infants engage with people and objects through their visual and auditory senses, these are distant senses and do not readily bring the infant key information, which can be gained only through touch. Ruff (1980) described object handling with visual exploration as essential for an infant to learn object properties. The interaction of touching and looking helps enhance the infant's ability to integrate sensory information and to learn that objects remain the same regardless of visual orientation. Typically this object handling in infants is called *play* because it is purposeful and done with pleasure.

With increasing age, until at least the early school years, a great deal of play depends on competence in fine motor skills. These skills are reflected in the child's interest in activities such as cutting with scissors, dressing and undressing dolls, putting puzzles together, constructing with various types of building materials and model sets, participating in sand play, completing craft projects, and engaging in imaginary play with objects. Playing video games and using computers also require fine motor control. Some children may pursue play and leisure activities through organized groups such as the Girl Scouts or Boy Scouts and 4-H clubs, which tend to have projects requiring manual skills as a key component of their programs.

Activities of Daily Living

Activities of daily living also depend on the child's ability to use all types of hand skills. According to Henderson, the specific skills needed for skill development in this area are "(1) abilities in grip, (2) the use of two hands in a complementary fashion, (3) the ability to use the hands in varied positions with and without vision, (4) the execution of increasingly complex action sequences, and (5) the development of automaticity" (Henderson, 1995, p. 181). Case-Smith (1996) found that speed of object rotation using in-hand manipulation skills, grasp strength, motor accuracy, and tool handling were each significantly positively correlated with self-care skills in preschool-age children receiving occupational therapy services.

Dressing skills involve complex grasp patterns and in-hand manipulation skills in the use of fasteners, but the ability to use all types of bilateral skills and a variety of grasp patterns is useful for putting on and removing shirts, shoes, socks, and pants. The ability to put on jewelry relies on the ability to use delicate grasp patterns and in-hand manipulation.

Bathing, showering, and other personal hygiene skills depend on the child's increasing fine motor skills in handling slippery objects (e.g., soap). In addition, these skills are likely to be needed when an individual is in a standing position, such as when putting toothpaste on a toothbrush (Figure 10-16), brushing the teeth, shaving, or applying makeup. A high level of skill in tool use is needed for complex hygiene activities such as shaving, applying makeup, using tweezers, cutting nails, and styling hair (using barrettes, rubber bands, a curling iron, a brush, and a hair dryer).

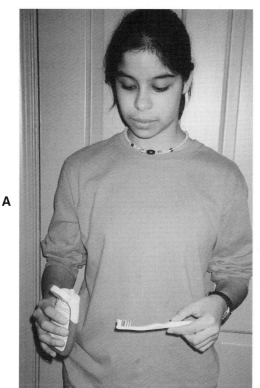
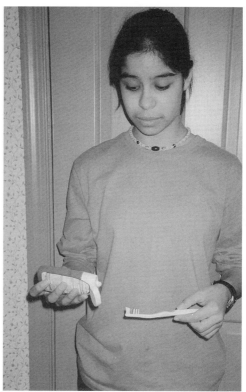

FIGURE 10-16 **A,** Different grasp patterns are used in preparation for putting tooth-paste on a toothbrush. The child uses just-right force to stabilize the toothbrush with a modified power grasp (with supination to midposition) while using a cylindrical grasp on the toothpaste container. **B,** The child has used forearm supination and the in-hand manip-ulation skill of simple rotation to position the toothpaste container for application of the toothpaste to the toothbrush.

Eating skills rely on refinement of the ability to use forearm control with a variety of grasp patterns and tools. The ability to use both hands together effectively is necessary for spreading and cutting with a knife, opening all types of containers, pouring liquids, and preparing food. In-hand manipulation skills are used to adjust eating utensils (Figure 10-17) and finger foods in the hand, to handle a napkin, and to manipulate the opening of packaged food and utensils.

School (Formal Educational Participation)

Independent functioning in the school environment requires effective fine motor skills. The preschool classroom presents children with a variety of manipulative activities, including the use of crayons, scissors, small building materials, and puzzles, as well as simple cooking and art projects. During kindergarten and the early elementary school years, children should be able to use fine motor skills most of the school day. McHale and Cermak (1992) found that 45% to 55% of the school day for first and second grade children is spent in fine motor activi-ties. Fourth grade children spend approximately 30% of their school day participating in fine motor tasks. The primary fine motor activities in all of these grades are paper-pencil tasks. Any writing activity includes preparing one's paper, using an eraser, and getting writing tools in and out of a box. Other typical fine motor activities in children's classrooms include cutting with scissors, folding paper, using paste and tape, carrying out simple science projects, assuming responsibility for managing one's own snack and lunch items, and organizing and maintaining one's desk. Children also need computer skills in most elementary classrooms.

Older children and adolescents need fine motor skills for science projects, vocational courses (e.g., woodworking, metal shop, and home economics), art classes, music classes (other than vocal music), managing a high volume of written work and notebooks, keyboarding, and maintaining a locker. Greater speed (e.g., in writing and keyboarding) and greater strength (e.g., for physical education and vocational courses) are required. Adolescents should be able to demonstrate consistent hand skills that they can execute quickly in a variety of situations.

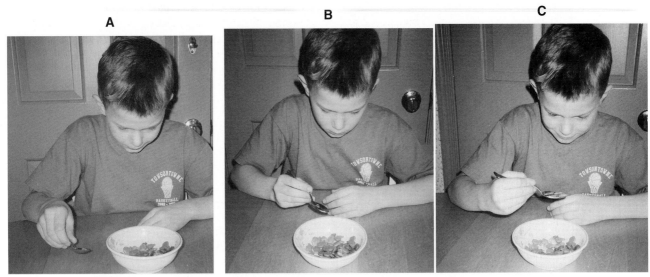

FIGURE 10-17 **A,** The child grasps the spoon from the table surface with a radial-digital grasp. The forearm is slightly supinated. **B,** He uses the in-hand manipulation skill of complex rotation to move the handle of the spoon from the palmar surface of his hand toward the web space between the index finger and thumb. Isolation and differentiation of the index finger and thumb are needed to produce this rotation. Forearm movement toward midposition assists. **C,** The child completes spoon positioning in his hand by moving the spoon so that the end of the handle is stabilized in the web space. Additional flexion of the metacarpophalangeal (MCP) joints of the fingers while extension of the interphalangeal (IP) joints is sustained assists with optimal positioning for eating.

GENERAL MOTOR PROBLEMS THAT AFFECT HAND SKILLS

Regardless of the nature of the disability a child may have, he or she is likely to have impaired hand skills. Impairment of basic hand function (reach, grasp, carry, and release) in early childhood precludes emergence of more advanced hand skill and bilateral hand use. This section presents problems that may be observed as major or minor in any child with hand skill difficulties.

One of the more common problems is *inadequate isolation of movements.* Children who demonstrate significant problems in this area tend to use total patterns of flexion or extension throughout the upper extremities, and they are unable to combine wrist extension with finger flexion or elbow flexion with finger extension. Similarly, the child may be unable to perform differentiated motions with each arm and hand. Inadequate isolation of movements is handicapping even in early infancy because it affects the most basic reach and grasp skills. More subtle problems may be seen in children who have difficulty isolating wrist and finger movements.

Another common problem is *poorly graded movement,* which may refer to movements not effectively graded in terms of range or strength. Eliasson and Gordon (2000) use the term *poor force scaling* to refer to difficulties in appropriately adjusting the force needed for grasp or release. In children with disabilities, usually the extent of a movement is too great for the task, which impairs accu-

racy of performance. This problem occurs when joint stability in the hand or proximal to the hand is not effective. For example, the child may be unable to hold the elbow in approximately 90 degrees of flexion and the wrist in neutral position during a grasp activity. Thus when initiating the grasp, the child may overflex the fingers in an attempt to obtain the object before the arm posture is lost. Children with poorly graded movements lack the ability to use the middle ranges of movement effectively; instead, during attempts at hand use they hold one or more joints in a locked position of full flexion or full extension (Figure 10-18). Typical patterns that children use to increase their stability include internal rotation of the shoulder, elbow extension, and hyperextension and/or abduction of the MCP joints (Figure 10-19). Problems with grading of movement are typically associated with tactile sensory problems, abnormal tone, and/or muscle weakness. The child with sensory problems has difficulty perceiving and evaluating feedback and therefore cannot accurately plan the extent of movements or force needed for a task. Gordon and Duff (1999) found that "spasticity may limit the ability to finely grade the fingertip force to the object's properties" (p. 590).

Insufficient force may interfere with grasp control. Problems with force have been noted in children with developmental coordination disorder (Wilson, Maruff, Ives, & Currie, 2001) and in children with cerebral palsy (Gordon & Duff, 1999). Difficulties with regulation of

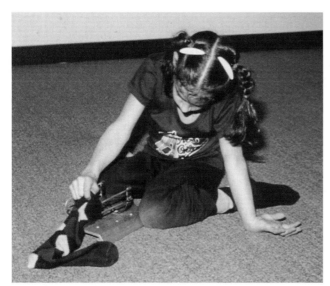

FIGURE 10-18 This child, who has involuntary movement, demonstrates the attempt to find stability by locking her elbows in extension and by elevating her right shoulder during hand use. She also has difficulty isolating upper extremity movements and using the two hands together at midline. (Courtesy Kennedy Kreiger Institute, Baltimore, MD.)

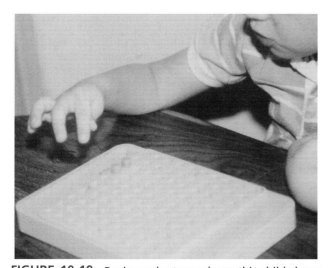

FIGURE 10-19 During voluntary release this child shows overextension and increased abduction of the fingers, with hyperextension at the MCP joints of the ulnar fingers. He also shows adduction of the thumb rather than slight abduction.

force may be due to poor tactile discrimination and/or spasticity (Gordon & Duff). Muscle weakness has also been suggested as a problem for individuals with cerebral palsy (Damiano & Abel, 1998); weakness could contribute significantly to insufficient force.

Poor timing of movements can also be a problem. Improper timing of muscle contractions leads to the use of movements that are too fast or too slow for the intended purpose. Movements that are too fast also tend

to be poorly graded. Eliasson and Gordon (2000) describe difficulties in children with spastic hemiplegic cerebral palsy relative to the timing of "transitions between phases [and] sequential generation of forces" as needed for grasp and release of objects (p. 228). During voluntary release, children with increased tone are likely to place an object very quickly, then have slowed movement of the fingers away from the object (Eliasson & Gordon).

Wilson et al. (2001) similarly reported difficulties with timing of movements in children with developmental coordination disorder. Tone problems or muscle weakness are often the underlying factors in movement that is too slow. Poor coordination of agonist and antagonistic muscles and poor tactile discrimination are likely to be key factors in impaired timing of actions (Eliasson & Gordon, 2000). Speed and accuracy demands, particularly when these skills are required to place an object on an unstable surface, lead to increased difficulty with motor timing and regulation of force (Gordon et al., 2003). Instability at joints can contribute to disordered sequences of hand and arm movements. For example, wrist extension may not be combined with the reach for an object but instead may occur after the grasp.

A fourth problem that affects hand function is a *disorder in bilateral integration of movements*. This affects both the normal symmetric and asymmetric movements needed to develop and use hand functions. Some children are unable to bring both hands to midline effectively or to maintain the use of both hands at midline long enough to accomplish a task. Other children can hold objects symmetrically at midline but are unable to dissociate arm movements; they therefore have difficulty with activities that require reciprocal or simultaneous bilateral hand use.

Many children have difficulty with hand use because of *limitations in trunk movement and control*. CNS dysfunction or generalized muscle weakness can impair development or effective use of equilibrium reactions. Therefore the child may use one or both arms for support in maintaining sitting or standing positions. This significantly limits bilateral hand use and may limit the development of fine motor skills in the hand that the child most often uses for support.

Children with trunk instability or abnormal posture have difficulty with smooth, accurate placement of the hand and arm being used for a fine motor task. When the trunk is postured in flexion, functional ROM in the arm is limited (Figure 10-20). Conversely, arching of the trunk is accompanied by hyperextension of the humerus. The latter pattern typically causes one of three patterns of shoulder and elbow positioning: external rotation with elbow flexion, neutral rotation with elbow flexion, or internal rotation with elbow extension. Posturing in any of these arm patterns affects the development of hand skills. Similarly, lateral trunk flexion causes the child to

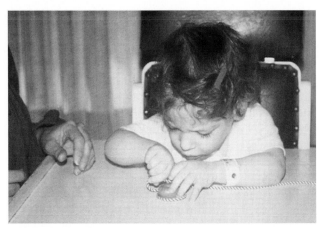

FIGURE 10-20 Poor trunk stability affects the upper extremity range of motion that this child can use. Note the right forearm pronation and wrist flexion. The child is unable to use a three-jaw chuck, or pincer, grasp effectively on the materials. However, she demonstrates awareness of the need to use both hands in this manipulative activity and good visual monitoring of the materials. (Courtesy Kennedy Kreiger Institute, Baltimore, MD.)

lean to one side and thus affects the child's ability to use the arm on the flexed side.

The problems discussed in this section can contribute to the child's use of *compensatory patterns of movement.* In an effort to increase function, the child seeks another pattern to substitute for movements impaired by the primary problem. For example, the child with weakness or instability may learn to use lateral trunk flexion to increase the height of the opposite arm during reach, or a child with increased tone may compensate for limited finger extension by using a wrist tenodesis (flexion) action. Although these patterns are functional for certain tasks, continued use of compensatory movements may hinder the development of higher level skills.

OTHER FACTORS THAT AFFECT HAND SKILLS IN CHILDREN WITH DISABILITIES

Somatosensory Problems

Somatosensory problems can produce significant problems with hand function, even when motor control is good (Pehoski, 1995), and poor hand skills can contribute to the child obtaining a limited amount of somatosensory information. Children with poor tactile discrimination receive less feedback about how their fingers move together and independently of one another. In addition, poor tactile discrimination has been found to be associated with difficulty anticipating the force needed in grasp, modulating the force needed for grasp, and transitioning from grasp to lift (Gordon & Duff, 1999).

Children with cerebral palsy are likely to have tactile discrimination problems as well as motor control problems. Several studies of tactile dysfunction in children with cerebral palsy were conducted in the 1950s and 1960s. These studies verified the presence of a variety of tactile discrimination problems in the hands of a high percentage of children with this disorder (Kenney, 1963; Monfraix, Tardieu, & Tardieu, 1961; Twitchell, 1965). Recent studies of children with spastic hemiplegia have resulted in similar findings. Cooper, Majnemer, Rosenblatt, and Birnbaum (1995) found that eight of the nine children with spastic hemiplegia whom they tested had bilateral sensory deficits. Yekutiel, Jariwala, and Stretch (1994) found that 51% of the 55 children with cerebral palsy whom they tested had sensory deficits on two-point discrimination and/or stereognosis. In a study of 25 children with spastic hemiplegia, Krumlinde-Sundholm and Eliasson (2002) found that 18 had impairment of the hemiplegic hand in two-point discrimination at 3 mm and more than half had difficulty with two-point discrimination at 7 mm. For approximately one third of these children, tactile problems were noted in all five tests of tactile discrimination in the hemiplegic hand. A marked difference in stereognosis was seen between testing with common objects (11 showed impairment) and testing with flat shapes (of 10 objects, 24 children showed the ability to identify five or fewer). Some researchers have found that children with hemiplegia have deficits in the less (non) involved upper extremity as well as the hemiplegic hand (Cooper et al., 1995).

Although some researchers note that the degree of tactile problems is not always associated with the degree of motor impairment (Cooper et al., 1995), Krumlinde-Sundholm and Eliasson (2002) found a strong relationship between impairment in sensation and dexterity in the more impaired hand of children with spastic hemiplegia (correlations between dexterity and two-point discrimination and stereognosis were 0.60 to 0.71). They noted that bilateral hand skills were less associated with the level of tactile discrimination. Differences in these study findings may be associated with differences in tactile testing methodologies and sample sizes. Children with cerebral palsy tend to need more trials than nondisabled children to match tactile and proprioceptive information with force for grasp and lift of objects (Eliasson, 1995).

Children with milder problems also are at risk for somatosensory problems that affect hand skills. Case-Smith (1991) studied the relationship between both tactile defensiveness and tactile discrimination and in-hand manipulation skills in 50 children between 4 and 6 years of age. In this sample, which included 80% nondysfunctional children, those having problems with either tactile defensiveness or decreased tactile discrimination showed no significant problems with performing the in-hand manipulation tasks presented. However, those who had both tactile discrimination problems and tactile defensiveness had difficulty performing the in-hand manipulation tasks that were timed. Their performances were significantly less efficient than those of the children in the other groups.

Tactile problems have been identified in other populations as well. Children with developmental coordination disorder appear to have tactile problems, because they have difficulty with feed-forward strategies (Smits-Engelsman, Wilson, Westenberg, & Duysens, 2003) and with planning for intentional actions that depend on the anticipation of force and timing (Wilson, Maruff, Ives, & Currie, 2001). These strategies and plans of action rely on knowledge of object properties that probably is gained through tactile information. In addition, Beckung, Steffenburg, and Uvebrant (1997) identified sensorimotor impairments in a majority of the children they studied who had mental retardation and epilepsy.

Learned Nonuse Phenomenon in Children with Hemiplegia

Sterr, Freivogel, and Schmalohr (2002) conducted a study to assess available use in the more involved arm-hand of a sample of 21 children, adolescents, and young adults with hemiplegia. Their research was based on several other studies with adults with learned nonuse as a result of strokes. They found that "the learned nonuse model predicts that even if the residual movement capacities of the hemiparetic arm should allow the person to carry out activities of daily living . . . that arm is not, in fact, used in the real-life situation" (Sterr et al., 2002, p. 1727). The difference between these individuals' available movement skills and the use of them in spontaneous situations was significant. The authors concluded that the limited use of the hemiplegic arm was not primarily due to the motor disability, but rather that limited integration of that arm-hand into functional activities seemed to be due to learned nonuse.

Differences in Developmental Trends between Children with and without Disabilities

Although information about normal development of hand skills can be useful to therapists in understanding difficulties with functioning and/or in guiding intervention planning, therapists also need to recognize that normal developmental sequences may not apply to children with some types of disabilities. For example, in a longitudinal study by Hanna et al. (2003), hand function in children with cerebral palsy generally improved in early childhood and then began to decline. They found somewhat different patterns of development with

children who had mild, moderate, and severe impairments and for children with hemiplegic cerebral palsy and with quadriplegic cerebral palsy. Hand skills increased more slowly in children with greater degrees of motor impairment. In general, the children with quadriplegic cerebral palsy showed more decrease in quality of functioning over time than did the children with hemiplegia. Overall the highest quality of functioning was found at the average age of 46 months, and the highest scores on the PDMS Fine Motor Scale were achieved at approximately 5 years of age.

ANALYSIS OF HAND SKILL PROBLEMS

A sample analysis of an occupational performance problem in the area of constructive play that is at least partly caused by hand skill difficulties is presented in Box 10-2. In this example the therapist has identified two

---

BOX 10-2   Problem: Inability to Engage Effectively in Constructive Play (Performance Problems, Body Function Factors, and Causes)

1 Lacks in-hand manipulative skills
   a Unstable wrist in neutral position or extension, uses wrist flexion; possible causes:
      (1) Decreased tone in wrist extensors
      (2) Increased tone in wrist flexors
   b Unstable metacarpophalangeal (MCP) joints; possible causes:
      (1) Poor co-contraction in finger joints
      (2) Increased pull of extensor digitorum
   c Inability to identify finger being touched because of decreased tactile discrimination
   d Lack of midrange movements of finger joints; possible causes:
      (1) Decreased proprioception
      (2) Poor co-contraction of MCP and interphalangeal (IP) flexors and extensors
      (3) Tightness in intrinsics and long finger flexors
2 Breaks materials, often by dropping and crushing them
   a Inability to sustain finger pad grasp; possible causes:
      (1) Poor tactile or proprioceptive awareness
      (2) Poor co-contraction of muscle groups
   b Excessive finger flexion in grasp; possible causes:
      (1) Poor proprioceptive awareness of size and weight of object
      (2) Increased finger flexor tone
      (3) Associated reactions
      (4) Inactivity in intrinsics
   c Ineffective bilateral handling; possible causes:
      (1) Unstable grasp because of poor wrist extension caused by increased flexor tone
      (2) Overflow in one upper extremity
      (3) Learned nonuse

main performance problems: lack of ability to manipulate materials after grasp and breakage of materials being handled ("manipulates" and "calibrates" [AOTA, 2002, p. 621]). The therapist then attempts to determine how sensory functions, neuromusculoskeletal and movement-related functions, and mental functions contribute to this performance limitation. Muscle and movement functions associated with this problem may include difficulties with wrist and MCP joint stability, limited midrange movement control, lack of isolated finger movement, and excessive use of flexion. Based on evaluation findings and the therapist's frames of reference, specific impairments are identified.

Theories and Frames of Reference Used in Assessment and Intervention for Hand Skill Problems

This section defines the theories or frames of reference most commonly used in the assessment of and intervention for children who have problems with hand skills. Selected theories that describe specific intervention strategies are discussed.

Biomechanical Frame of Reference

The biomechanical frame of reference is used primarily in assessing and treating children with limitations in ROM, strength, or endurance that affect their hand skills. It is used to explain difficulties in arm use for reach caused by problems in postural alignment or impaired ability to use the arms against gravity (Colangelo, 1999). Biomechanics helps the therapist understand the principles involved in tenodesis grasping patterns and the relationship of intrinsic and extrinsic muscle control for grasp and in-hand manipulation patterns. Activities are designed based on these principles of hand function. Splinting for hand problems most often relies on the biomechanical frame of reference.

Developmental Frame of Reference

The developmental frame of reference focuses on describing the sequences of skills as they are observed in typically developing children. For example, this frame of reference is used to describe children's grasp progression from an ulnar grasp pattern to a pincer grasp pattern. This frame of reference is also used in developmental curricula that present tasks in a sequential order and are grouped under age levels. In planning intervention for hand skill problems, occupational therapists often rely on an understanding of the developmental sequences of skills that children typically follow; these sequences may be used as a basis for sequencing goals and treatment. At other times the therapist makes a decision not to use the typical sequence of skill acquisition. This frame of reference also helps the therapist understand how hand skills relate to other developmental skills.

Neurodevelopmental Treatment Frame of Reference

The neurodevelopmental treatment frame of reference focuses on understanding the child's difficulties with postural tone, postural control, and stability and mobility and presents interventions to address these areas of difficulty (Schoen & Anderson, 1999). Although the therapist uses this frame of reference most often to address the development of equilibrium and controlled movement against gravity, it also includes methods to improve arm and hand motor control (Boehme, 1988; Danella & Vogtle, 1992). Certain splinting techniques use neurodevelopmental treatment principles.

Sensory Integration Frame of Reference

The sensory integration frame of reference addresses the importance of sensory functioning and the integration of sensory processing to allow for adaptive responses. Occupational therapists can use this frame of reference to describe hand skill problems caused by problems with integrating tactile or proprioceptive information. Children with sensory integration problems that affect hand function may demonstrate problems with motor-planning and sequencing actions despite relatively good motor control. They may have difficulty differentiating among the specific sensory qualities of objects. The therapist can use this frame of reference in assessing and treating children who demonstrate somatodyspraxia, a problem characterized by difficulties with praxis and with the processing of tactile and proprioceptive information.

Motor Learning Theory

Therapists are increasingly using motor learning theory in occupational therapy practice. When using this theory, the therapist focuses on the child's acquisition of specific motor skills and how the learning of these motor skills occurs. The therapist assists the child in acquiring these skills through structure and feedback and provides him or her with structured practice to refine the skills. The type of practice the therapist uses and the feedback he or she gives the child while practicing are important. The therapist can use motor learning theories to assist the child with developing a particular grasp pattern or in-hand manipulation skill or with developing speed in a motor skill, such as buttoning.

Behavioral Theory

Behavioral theory focuses on reinforcement of children's performances through specific feedback. In contrast to the motor learning theory, this acquisitional theory usually emphasizes tasks or functional activities that involve more than motor components. Therapists often structure activities by using *backward chaining,* in which the child performs the last step of the desired skill first, and then other elements of the skills are added in a backward order so that the first step of the process is learned last. For example, in teaching shoe tying, the therapist first directs the child to pull the loops of the bow tight. The therapist eventually adds each step of the process to the sequence until the last step involves beginning to form the bow. In addition, therapists typically provide positive verbal feedback for the child to indicate success with performance of the task or a component of it. Therapists often let the child choose an activity that he or she will complete after doing a nonpreferred activity.

Cognitive Orientation to Daily Occupational Performance

Cognitive orientation to daily occupational performance (CO-OP) emphasizes problem-solving strategies and guided discovery of child- and task-specific strategies (Miller, Polatajko, Missiuna, Mandich, & Macnab, 2001). This type of intervention focuses on the child identifying the specific occupational task to be learned and then discovering strategies for performing the task. The child is expected to reflect on the strategies used. Mandich, Polatajko, Missiuna, and Miller (2001) have explored the use of this approach with children with developmental coordination disorder.

EVALUATION OF HAND SKILLS IN CHILDREN

The occupational therapist evaluates a child's hand skills when the evidence is sufficient to suggest that problems with performance of occupational skills are at least partly attributable to the child's problems with hand skills. A hand skill evaluation should not be performed simply to obtain information about the child's fine motor skills. The therapist first must have evidence suggesting that the child has a problem with at least one area of occupational performance. Parents, teachers, and the child often are the best sources of information about difficulties with participation in the family and the community, and this information can be obtained through the development of an occupational profile.

Screening for Hand Skill Problems

When a problem with occupational performance has been identified, the therapist needs to continue gathering information on the child's performance of specific daily life activities. As part of this process, the therapist determines whether it is reasonable to carry out a full evalua-

tion of fine motor and hand skill performance. This information must include data about the child's age and general information about motor skills, cognitive and perceptual skills, sensory processing, social situation and skills, and emotional functioning, as well as contexts that affect the child. The therapist can obtain screening information from parents, teachers, the child, and other professionals or from reports of other professionals.

Screening of hand skills can include observation of the skills noted in Table 10-1. This list of observations of fine motor skills includes reach, grasp, release, in-hand manipulation, and bilateral skills. It is not a standardized test, nor is it meant to replace administration of standardized tests to a child. However, because few standardized tests include assessment of specific hand skills, the therapist can use this list to record his or her observations about the child's quality of hand skills. Sections of this chapter covering the normal development of various hand skills can be used as a basis for determining whether the child has difficulty with a particular skill.

The information gathered through screening can help determine whether further observation of the child's hand skills is necessary or whether the therapist should administer a standardized test. In addition, parents or teachers and the child may find these tasks useful for delineating areas that are difficult for the child and those at which the child may be more successful. Discussion of observations during or after the screening often serves as a basis for collaborative intervention planning to address the areas of difficulty.

The activities listed in Table 10-1 are appropriate for use in screening a child's hand skills. Because some skills are inappropriate for younger children, an "X" designates the age group for which any activity may be used. When a skill emerges within a particular age group, ages are listed rather than an "X." For block stacking, the number represents the number of blocks a child in that age group should be able to stack. The therapist can vary the materials used for some of the items so that he or she can assess many of these skills during a mealtime, dressing, hygiene, or play activity. For all categories except Bilateral Skills and Tool Use, the therapist should ask the child to perform the activities both with the right hand and with the left hand. Evaluation of both hands is important, because subtle difficulties may not be readily apparent. For example, Gordon et al. (2003) found mild problems in the timing of voluntary release components in the noninvolved hand of children with hemiplegia.

Evaluation Content

A child with occupational performance problems who shows difficulties on screening for hand skills should be further evaluated so that the characteristics of the problem and the situations in which the child's

TABLE 10-1 Screening Activities for Hand Skills

Activities	Age Groups			
	6-12 mo	1-2 yr	3-5 yr	6+ yr
REACH				
Move both arms in full range of motion	X	X	X	X
Reach to midline, extended elbow	X	X	X	X
Reach across midline		X	X	X
GRASP				
Use full palmar grasp	X	X	X	X
Use radial-digital grasp	9 mo	X	X	X
Use standard pincer grasp	10 mo	X	X	X
Use spherical grasp		X	X	X
Use intrinsic-plus grasp		X	X	X
Use power grasp on tool			X	X
RELEASE				
Release object freely	X	X	X	X
Release 1-inch object into container		X	X	X
Stack 1-inch blocks*		2-6 blocks	9-10 blocks	10 blocks
Release tiny object into small hole		X	X	X
Throw small ball at least 3 feet			X	X
IN-HAND MANIPULATION				
Manipulate object between two hands	X	X	X	X
Use finger-to-palm translation, small object[†]		X	X	X
Use palm-to-finger translation				
One object[†]		2 yr	X	X
Two to three objects[†]		2 yr	X	X
With coin			X	X
Unscrew bottle top		2 yr	X	X
Use shift to separate magazine pages or cards			X	X
Roll piece of clay into a ball[‡]			X	X
Pick up marker or crayon using rotation			4 yr	X
Shift on marker or pencil			5 yr	X
Rotate pencil to use eraser and back				X
BILATERAL SKILLS				
Hold or carry large ball with two hands	X	X	X	X
Stabilize paper during coloring or writing			X	X
Hold paper during scissors use			X	X
Manipulate paper during scissors use				X
TOOL USE				
Use scissors to cut				
Line			3 yr	X
Simple shapes			4 yr	X
Complex shapes				X
Scribble with marker	X			
Copy appropriate forms		X		X
Handwriting appropriate for grade				X

*Block stacking allows for assessment of arm stability in space, spatial orientation of the objects, and controlled finger extension. Voluntary release of objects other than blocks may be used. Screening should include placement of objects when arm is not supported and placement that requires precision.

[†]An object that is not flat should be used, such as small pieces of cereal (appropriate for children under 3 years or those who still mouth objects), small beads, or small pegs.

[‡]A piece of clay approximately $\frac{1}{4}$-inch thick and 1 inch in diameter is placed in the palm of the child's hand. The child is asked to form the clay into a ball without using the other hand or the table surface. Palm to finger translation, finger to palm translation, simple rotation, and sometimes complex rotation may be observed.

performance is optimal can be carefully delineated. For example, the therapist may need to determine (1) whether the child is able to use any type of functional grasp, (2) if wrist extension is possible in any grasp patterns, (3) the situations under which voluntary release are most feasible for the child, (4) the types of objects that are easiest for the child to handle when using the in-hand manipulation skill of simple rotation, and (5) whether the child is able to stabilize materials better when the materials are closer to or farther from his or her body.

When determining the child's performance in the area of hand skills and potential reasons for any problems, the occupational therapist often uses a variety of standardized and nonstandardized assessments. All children should receive an assessment of hand skills in activities such as dressing, eating, hygiene skills, school activities, and play activities. The therapist can perform other standard testing if it will yield information that (1) documents the child's current status, allowing the therapist to determine later whether the child has shown progress in hand skills, maintained the same skills, or lost skills; (2) aids in the determination of the causes of the child's hand skill problems; (3) aids in the determination of the child's potential for improvement in hand skills; and (4) supports the planning of intervention strategies.

Analysis of the identified hand skills problem involves administration of specific assessments or scales that define the basis of the problem and the extent of the impairment. The following outline presents examples of tools and methods used to assess the underlying impairments associated with hand skill difficulties and delays.

1 Measurement of active and passive ROM (especially important for children who have weakness or increased muscle tone)
2 Evaluation of strength
   - Muscle testing (general and/or specific)
   - Grip and pinch strength testing
3 Evaluation of tactile and proprioceptive functioning using standard assessment of tactile discrimination or two-point discrimination and finger identification with vision occluded
4 Assessment of postural alignment and postural stability, including stability and mobility of the hand
5 Administration of a standardized general developmental test that includes a fine motor section for young children (see Appendix 7-A)
   - Hawaii Early Learning Profile (HELP)
   - Bayley Scales of Infant Development (2nd Ed.) (BSID-II)
6 Administration of a developmental motor test
   - PDMS Fine Motor Scale
   - Bruininks-Oseretsky Test of Motor Proficiency (BOTMP)
7 Administration of a standardized test of fine motor skills for older children and adolescents

- Purdue Pegboard Test (Mathiowetz, Rogers, Dowe-Keval, Donohoe, & Rennells, 1986)
- Bruininks-Oseretsky Test of Motor Proficiency
8 Administration of a visual-motor integration test
   - Test of Visual-Motor Skills (TVMS)
   - Developmental Test of Visual-Motor Integration (VMI)
9 Assessment of hand skills in prevocational or work tasks (important for adolescents)

GUIDELINES FOR INTERVENTION

Setting Goals

Several factors affect the types of goals developed in the area of hand skills and in other areas of the child's functioning: the child's occupational performance problems, the contexts in which the skills are needed, the types of problems in the hand skill area, the therapist's frame of reference, and the setting in which services are to be provided. For some children, developmental sequences of skills influence the selection of goals, but for the child with a motor disability, other factors affect the goals established and the strategies selected for intervention. These factors include the types of occupational performance skills the child needs, the complexity and severity of the child's problems, and the human and nonhuman resources available to support the intervention program.

A child's goals generally are developed through a process of team and family collaboration. In that context, the therapist must be realistic in the number and types of goals that he or she can recommend relative to other goals for the child. In addition, the therapist must consider hand skill goals that are feasible for the child to accomplish. Such goals may be limited for children with severe disabilities. In all cases the therapist must link hand skill goals to the child's ability to engage in occupational activities more effectively. For some children the most appropriate focus of intervention is the development of skills in using adaptive equipment and strategies for accomplishing skills needed in activities of daily living. For children who show readiness to develop better quality or more complex hand skills, intervention can focus on acquisition of these skills. Factors to consider in planning intervention for hand skills problems are discussed in the following sections.

Sequencing of Intervention Sessions

When the therapist provides direct services to improve hand and arm function, he or she usually carries out in the following sequence:
1 Preparation
   - Positioning of the child
   - Attention to postural tone issues

- Improvement of postural control (pelvic, shoulder, head)
2 Development of hand skills
    - Promotion of isolated arm and hand movements, such as external rotation, supination, and wrist extension
    - Enhancement of reach, grasp, carry, and release skills
    - Enhancement of in-hand manipulation skills
    - Facilitation of bilateral hand use skills
    - Generalization of skills (integration of hand skills into functional activities)

Not all children need all the steps in this sequence. In addition, intervention for all areas is rarely done in one session.

Preparation for Hand Skill Development

Many children require preparation of the total body in each treatment session before the therapist can address intervention for specific hand skill problems. In addition to intervention to improve motor function, the therapist should pay specific attention to the child's sensory functioning. The therapist can provide tactile and proprioceptive input to the arms and hands to enhance sensory awareness and discrimination. Lotion, toys, the child's own clothing or, preferably, active movements of the child's hands, with or without assistance, can provide stimuli. Children have greater tactile sensitivity when performing an activity that involves active touching rather than being touched (Haron & Henderson, 1985). The therapist should also encourage visual awareness of the hands with tactile and proprioceptive input.

Interventions to increase strength may improve skilled hand use in children with certain disabilities. Focus on strength needs to be addressed carefully in children with tone problems, because a primary focus on strength would diminish focus on coordination, which seems to be the primary problem in these children. Damiano and Abel (2003) reported on the use of strength training to support functioning in children with cerebral palsy. They researched strengthening for walking and found that the children they assessed had marked muscle weakness. With a controlled program of strengthening, the children's strength improved, as did the quality of some components of walking. However, caution is required in applying these results to hand skills, because strengthening programs to enhance arm and hand function of children with cerebral palsy have not yet been researched.

In another study that focused on strengthening, Weaver, Gardner, Triolo, and Betz (1990) used neuromuscular electrical stimulation (NMES) with toddlers who had arthrogryposis that significantly affected their arm and finger strength and movement. The NMES resulted in several positive changes in functions of the fingers, including greater ROM at the various finger joints. Associated changes in the developmental level of the children's grasp patterns occurred as well, resulting in the use of a more radial and distal grasp rather than an ulnar-palmar pattern. The authors suggest that NMES may be a positive addition to other interventions for this population.

Positioning of the Child

In selecting the positioning of the therapist and the child for fine motor intervention, the therapist must consider the optimal position for eliciting the particular skills desired in that child and the position in which the child will use the skills. When these positions are different, the therapist must consider whether to use only one position at this time and introduce the other position later or to use both positions concurrently. For example, the child may be able to bring both hands to midline and to reach with the greatest elbow extension in the side-lying position. However, for functional use the child may need to be able to contact a switch on a surface while in an adapted sitting position. In an intervention session the therapist initially may work with the child in the side-lying position, then move to a supported sitting position to help the child generalize the skills to a functional position. Eventually the therapist may work with the child primarily in a supported sitting position. The therapist almost always needs to specifically address carryover of skills across positions with the child, often through activities developed collaboratively with the parents or the teacher.

The therapist can use certain body positions to elicit specific hand skills. The supine position is effective for working with children on arm movements and visual regard of the hands during movement. The prone position on the forearms is appropriate for addressing shoulder stability and co-contraction in 90-degree elbow flexion, dissociation of the two sides of the body during weight bearing on one arm while manipulating with the other, gross bilateral manipulation of objects, and visual regard of the hands. Side-lying can be an effective position for encouraging unilateral arm movement to bat at an object and for hand-to-hand play. Visual regard of the hands and objects is difficult to address in the side-lying position.

Sitting at a table is often the position in which children are most likely to use fine motor skills. For optimal hand use, children need a stable chair with adequate foot support. Even young children without motor disabilities benefit from sitting in furniture that fits appropriately. Smith-Zuzovsky and Exner (2004) found that typical young children had significantly better in-hand manipulation skills when seated in chairs and at a table fitted to them (Figure 10-21) than when seated in chairs and at a table that were slightly too large. They suggest that

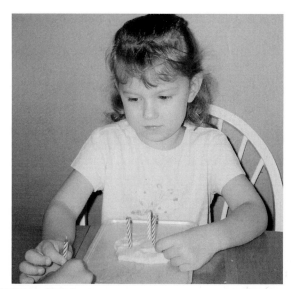

FIGURE 10-21 This child is seated at a table that is an appropriate height for tabletop activities. She can effectively place her arms on the surface without elevating her shoulders. Arm support on the surface, elbow flexion, and handing her the candles in a vertical position rather than having her grasp them from a table surface encourages the child's use of forearm supination and fingertip control during grasp and placement of the candles on the clay birthday cake. (Courtesy Kanji Takeno, Towson University.)

appropriately fitted furniture may enhance hand function by means of its effect on proximal stability and/or by allowing the child to focus more on the manipulative tasks and less on postural readjustments. A study by Wingrat and Exner (2003) supported the theory that classroom chair size affects posture and attention. They found that typical young children's sitting posture and on-task classroom behaviors were enhanced when they were in chairs appropriate to their size compared with their performance when seated in standard but slightly too large classroom chairs.

For children with disabilities, seated positioning for hand function activities requires specific attention. The therapist should not expect a child who cannot yet sit independently to work on sitting stability while working on hand skills. Such children need adaptations for sitting (e.g., lateral supports and chest straps) when working on hand skills. A tray or table surface should be a work surface rather than a support surface. The table or tray should be only slightly above elbow height, because a lower table promotes use of body flexion and a higher surface promotes use of abduction and internal rotation of the arms. The therapist also may provide activities with the child sitting on the floor or in a chair without a table, particularly when working on reaching skills or gross bilateral skills.

For children with mild to moderate motor involvement, standing may be an appropriate position for treatment of some hand skills. Many daily living skills that rely on hand skills are most commonly done while standing, such as brushing the teeth, zipping and buttoning clothing, shaving, applying makeup, and cooking. For children who have substantial difficulties with standing, the therapist should use this position only after the child has mastered the skills in a sitting position.

Improvement of Postural Tone and Control

The child with increased tone throughout the body may need overall inhibition of tone before participating in hand skill activities. Slow rotary movements using small ranges of motion between internal and external shoulder rotation and between forearm pronation and supination can help inhibit tone (Finnie, 1975). Upper extremity weight bearing is particularly useful as a treatment technique for improving postural control and improving stability in the scapulohumeral area. The therapist can also use upper extremity weight bearing to encourage the child to maintain elbow co-contraction and some degree of wrist extension while engaging in slight weight shifting (Boehme, 1988; Danella & Vogtle, 1992). The therapist provides proprioceptive input during weight bearing. For most children the primary focus is on helping the child increase overall stability rather than concentrating on achieving full elbow, wrist, or finger extension. The therapist can carry out weight-bearing activities with the child in the prone position on the forearms, the prone position on extended arms, the side-sitting position, or the long-sitting position, depending on the child's skill level (Boehme, 1988).

For the child who has tightness in wrist flexion, a position of upper extremity weight bearing on hands with the arms extended often is difficult if not impossible to achieve. The most appropriate positions for these children to use for weight bearing include prone on the forearms and side-lying. The therapist can help the child position the wrists in neutral position, and some therapists use splints during weight bearing to assist with wrist and hand positioning (Kinghorn & Roberts, 1996).

Finger flexion is permitted during weight bearing as long as the thumb is not in an abnormal position. If the child's thumb is tightly adducted and flexed, the therapist should use handling techniques before weight bearing. The therapist can use his or her own hand to provide firm pressure over the first metacarpal joint and relax the child's hand through slow, small, rotary and flexion-extension movements. Mildly and moderately involved children often can work toward maintaining full finger extension during weight bearing.

Using a multiple-baseline single-subject design, Barnes (1986, 1989a, 1989b) found that children with cerebral palsy demonstrated increased use of wrist extension and finger extension after upper extremity weight bearing. The weight bearing increased wrist extension during these activities but did not affect grasp and voluntary release quality and skill. Kinghorn and Roberts (1996), who conducted a single-subject study of weight bearing with splinting for a child with cerebral palsy, did not find significant changes in objective measures of tone, positioning, or function. However, family members reported improved functioning.

Development of Hand Skills

When addressing hand skill development in children, the therapist must select activities that are interesting and appropriately challenging to the child. To support skill development, the therapist must be able to repeat these activities. Therefore toys and games with many pieces and eating activities can be particularly useful and enjoyable. Engaging in play while addressing hand skills can have important benefits, including motivating the child to engage in activities repeatedly and building his or her play repertoire (Couch, Dietz, & Kenny, 1998; Tobias & Goldkopf, 1995). Recent research suggests that the use of cognitive strategies to encourage awareness of elements of task performance may be helpful for enhancing the performance of children with developmental coordination disorders (Candler & Meeuwsen, 2002; Miller et al., 2001).

Promotion of Isolated Arm and Hand Movements

The therapist may choose to address specific movements in the upper extremity apart from specific hand skills. For example, the therapist may assist the child in using elbow flexion-extension, supination-pronation, or wrist flexion-extension movements before integrating these movements into reaching, grasping, or releasing patterns. Helping children generalize the movement patterns they have practiced and learned into a functional activity is an important aspect of motor learning theory. Such an approach is most successful with children who can follow verbal instructions and participate actively in working on specific hand skills. The therapist can use games or songs to practice the use of these movements. The therapist needs to emphasize specific movements and, in the same treatment session, use them in a functional context.

Supination control is one of the areas of greatest difficulty for children with disabilities, particularly those with tone problems. Abnormal posturing at the trunk, shoulder, elbow, or wrist often compensates for difficulties in initiating or sustaining forearm supination. Supination is easiest to use when the elbow is fully flexed and most difficult to use with full elbow extension. The therapist therefore can use activities that position the elbow in greater than 90 degrees of flexion to facilitate supination. Examples of such activities include finger feeding, holding a kaleidoscope, and putting lotion on the face.

If the child can initiate supination but has poor control of this pattern, he or she can benefit from activities with the elbow held in 90 degrees of supination with the forearm stabilized on a surface and an object presented vertically (see Figure 10-21). Gradually the therapist moves materials to encourage the child to use more elbow extension while maintaining the supinated position. Children with more severe involvement may be able to achieve only about 30 degrees of supination, the minimum amount needed to handle materials on a table effectively. The therapist should encourage children with less motor impairment to obtain and use at least 90 degrees of supination to accomplish functional activities such as drinking, eating with utensils, or turning a doorknob. Supination is critical for successful, smooth use of in-hand manipulation skills. In these activities it also is helpful to facilitate supination in the nonpreferred arm so that that hand can stabilize materials more effectively.

Enhancement of Reach Skills

Problems

Children with neuromotor disabilities exhibit typical problems in reach that limit range and control. Examples of problems in reach include the following:

- Use of abduction and internal rotation to initiate reach
- Use of shoulder elevation and lateral trunk flexion to increase the height of the arm for reaching
- Inability to coordinate the degree of hand opening or the hand position with the timing of the reach
- Difficulty maintaining an upright body posture when reaching forward or across the midline

Goals. The following list presents examples of goals the therapist can use for children with a variety of levels of disability. The goals are in approximate order of difficulty, although difficulty using any one pattern can vary with the individual child. All the goals in this example are associated with increasing the child's independence in morning hygiene skills. Some children may attain more limited independence in morning hygiene activities. Sample applications of the specific objects that could be the focus of the goals are indicated in parentheses below. The goals are that the child will:

1 Maintain visual regard of the (soap, faucet handle, comb) while making hand contact

2 Bring the hand into contact with hygiene items (soap, toothpaste, towel) presented in various planes

3 Attain hygiene items needed (soap, toothpaste, toothbrush, comb) located near the body but in various planes while sustaining sufficient finger extension to allow for grasp

4 Pick up objects (a towel, the toilet lid) presented at midline by reaching with both hands together (forearm may be pronated)

5 Attain large objects (e.g., a towel) in a variety of locations using both hands and incorporating appropriate forearm positioning

6 Attain hygiene items (toothbrush, toothpaste, shampoo bottle, safety razor) using appropriate hand positioning for grasp combined with a mature reaching pattern

7 Pick up and place items (toothbrush, washcloth, makeup items) in various locations on a bathroom sink or counter, crossing the midline with an erect trunk posture and humeral external rotation, elbow extension, and forearm supination to midposition

8 Attain items from all levels in a cabinet or closet (including reaching above the head) with control

Intervention Strategies. When the child initiates little movement or is unable to open the hand during arm movement, the primary focus of intervention is on controlled initiation of arm movements. This includes using various types of arm movements and being able to place and hold the arm to allow for contact with objects. This type of reaching goal is a priority for children with extremely limited movement control or strength and those with a degenerative disease process that results in skill regression. These movements are important for contact with others, and the child can use them to activate switches for toys and electronic equipment.

To facilitate arm movements and contact with objects, the therapist must identify the best position to promote postural stability and visual regard. The most commonly used position is sitting, with attention given to head and trunk control, visual regard, and visual tracking. However, the therapist also can use the supine and side-lying positions effectively.

Children with severe motor involvement need toys and materials that are easy to activate and that have no "failure" elements. Such toys include play foam, beans, rice, musical toys activated by light touch, and soap bubbles. The therapist usually can obtain the best results through proximal handling at the shoulders and upper arms while assisting the child with movements of either or both arms. The initial emphasis is on general arm movement, then on hand and arm placement, and finally on finger extension during arm movement as a precursor for reach with grasp.

When children are able to contact objects with some control, the therapist should introduce structured activities to assist the child in using elements of a more mature reaching pattern. Gradually these elements are combined to promote a smooth, direct reach. The therapist needs to determine the placement of objects in relation to the child's body so that the child can use the best reaching pattern possible. From that position the therapist can begin to vary object placement and orientation. For example, because presentation of objects at shoulder height often results in the child reaching with internal rotation and elbow flexion, initial presentation of objects

at a level below the child's shoulder may facilitate the use of shoulder flexion and neutral rotation. Gradually the child can raise objects higher as she or he develops more control. The therapist can use activities that require lateral reaching with shoulder abduction and slight external rotation before encouraging reaching with shoulder flexion.

The therapist should also encourage the child to reach behind his or her body, combining humeral hyperextension with controlled internal rotation and various elbow positions. Many children have difficulty with this posterior reaching pattern, which is required in dressing and other daily living skills. Some children can use neutral to slight external shoulder rotation in combination with humeral flexion if the therapist provides them with a minimal amount of handling at the humerus or elbow and appropriate object orientation (Figure 10-22). However, if such handling techniques are required for a child to use a mature reaching pattern, the therapist should present objects somewhat to the side or in front of the shoulder initially and then gradually toward the midline. To encourage reaching that incorporates neutral to slight external rotation of the shoulder and forearm supination, the therapist should orient the objects vertically. Horizontal orientation of an object encourages the use of forearm pronation.

Children with muscle weakness are better able to reach objects when they can use a table or tray surface at or slightly above elbow height. The therapist can use mobile arm suspension systems to support and assist

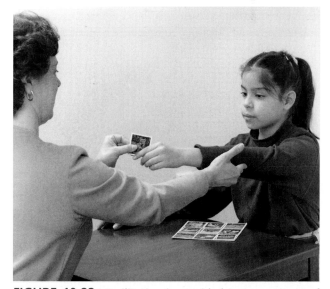

FIGURE 10-22 Facilitation is provided to prompt use of slight humeral external rotation and forearm supination. The object is held vertically to assist this reaching pattern. A lotto card game is used to engage the child and allow for repetition of the pattern. (Courtesy Kanji Takeno, Towson University.)

the child who has muscle strength rated as fair-minus or less.

The therapist should provide objects that have high color contrast or bright, solid colors to children with visual impairment. In cases of severe visual impairment, objects can combine both auditory stimuli and varied textures. If the child has not developed the ability to search for objects, the therapist should provide materials in a confined space or tied to strings so that the child can easily retrieve them when they are dropped.

Enhancement of Grasp Skills

Problems

The following are problems in the development of effective grasp (Figure 10-23 illustrates some of the following problems):

- Fisting or finger flexion that prevents hand opening
- Wrist flexion (often with ulnar deviation) in combination with finger extension
- Excessive forearm pronation, which interferes with the use of radial finger grasp patterns
- Thumb adduction in grasps that should use opposition, often with MCP or IP flexion

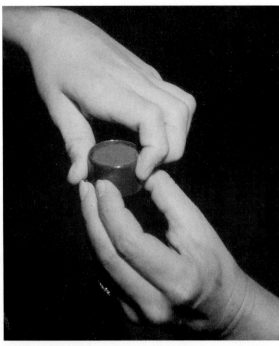

FIGURE 10-23 When this child combines reach with grasp, he demonstrates significant difficulties with effective hand positioning. Note the slight wrist flexion, the thumb adduction with IP joint extension, and the finger MCP joint hyperextension with IP flexion that he uses in an attempt to achieve stability with this grasp. The arm positioning in abduction and internal rotation contribute to use of this grasp pattern.

- Inability to use thumb abduction and adduction with MCP and IP extension
- Inability to initiate or sustain thumb opposition
- Inability to use grasp patterns that involve control of the intrinsic finger muscles
- Inability to vary grasp in accordance with object characteristics and activity demands

Goals.   The following examples of goals can be used for children with a variety of levels of disability. The goals are in approximate order of difficulty, although difficulty using any one pattern can vary with the individual child Some children may develop grasp only up to one of the lower levels identified here, whereas others may be able to attain the higher level skills. To illustrate how the goals associated with grasp may be integrated with occupations of the child or adolescent, sample occupations are identified for each grasp. The goals are that the child will:

1 (Put on clothing, pick up a towel, play a game with large game pieces) using a sustained grasp with the arm in a variety of positions
2 (Hold hard finger foods, pick up clothing, play with a car set) using a finger surface grasp on a variety of objects
3 (Eat finger foods, use math manipulatives, play a game with small pieces, do a puzzle) using a finger pad grasp with thumb opposition on small objects
4 (Prepare a meal, perform dressing tasks, perform hygiene tasks) using an opposed thumb and fingertip grasp pattern in accordance with object shapes and characteristics
5 (Use a key to open a door, build with construction toys) using an effective lateral pinch grasp pattern
6 (Handle computer materials such as paper and disks and file papers in folders; eat a cracker or sandwich) using finger pads to hold thin, flat objects
7 (Brush the teeth, use a knife, comb the hair, and use a safety razor) using a power grasp

Intervention Strategies.   For children with delays and functional difficulties in grasp, the therapist needs to match preparation techniques, such as positioning, handling, or strengthening, to the child's problem. Some children fist their hands or refuse to grasp objects because of tactile hypersensitivity, which also can influence the ability to maintain grasp. If this problem is present, grading tactile input from well tolerated to more difficult to tolerate is helpful. Initially, the child best tolerates firm objects with smooth surfaces and contours.

Tactile discrimination problems can contribute to grasp problems. Poor discrimination can affect dynamic use of grasp patterns and regulation of pressure in grasp. Problems with regulating pressure are seen as the child either holding objects with excessive force or dropping objects. Most children benefit from graded sensory input and attention to sensory discrimination as part of the intervention for grasp skills. Having the child actively explore the sizes, shapes, and textures of objects can precede emphasis on grasp in a treatment session.

In planning intervention that addresses grasp problems, the therapist, when selecting objects, should keep in mind the child's interests, sensory needs, and motor skills. Properties to consider include the size, shape, color, weight, and texture of objects.

Children with Severe Disabilities. Children with severe disabilities need to develop an effective palmar grasp and, if possible, grasp patterns using the finger surface. If possible the therapist should stress the abilities to initiate grasp and sustain grasp with the arm in a variety of positions. If the child is unable to open the hand readily for grasp, the therapist may explore whether changing the child's body position would be helpful. The side-lying position may reduce stress on overall body posture and may make it possible for the child to open the hand more easily. In supported sitting, the child may find opening the hand easier if the therapist places an object below the seat of the chair and lateral to the child's body. Boehme (1988) described other handling techniques that may assist the child with hand opening. The therapist should follow these techniques with movement of the open hand across objects and surfaces as a way of increasing the child's sustained hand opening and object interaction.

For the child who can independently open the hand but who shows wrist flexion with grasp, the therapist can emphasize wrist extension with grasp by positioning objects above the table surface or at chest height. Once the child can sustain wrist extension, the therapist can assist or encourage him or her to move the arm while maintaining grasp of an object. Sample activities using this skill include using a small stick to hit a suspended balloon or to break soap bubbles blown by the therapist, touching pictures on a wall or mirror with a stick, or holding onto clothing items while they are pulled up or down.

The child with a severe disability can wear a splint or other orthotic device during treatment and at other times of the day. Splinting techniques that may be useful in supporting hand function during treatment are described later in this chapter. Many of these children need adaptations to materials to support their performance of activities at home, school, and play. Use of standard materials may not be possible. Built-up handles that accommodate a palmar grasp pattern and larger objects, such as game pieces and blocks, may be used instead of smaller ones. Adapted page turners for books, switches for toys, and computer adaptations may be necessary to give the child some independence in play and school activities.

Children with Moderate Disabilities. Children with moderate disabilities are able to grasp but have difficulty with functional use of a variety of grasp patterns. They have problems in forearm control, wrist extension,

thumb opposition, and control of the MCP and IP joints (see Figure 10-23). Grasp may be initiated with wrist flexion. Grasp goals for these children usually are designed to address the use of opposed grasp patterns and grasp patterns in which the hand effectively accommodates to objects.

The selection of objects for use in developing opposed grasp patterns is critical. The child must be able to use objects in the context of an activity that is interesting and meaningful to the child and that has elements the child can repeat. Games and imaginary play materials can provide opportunities for repetitive presentation of objects to the child. The child can use opposed grasps with medium-sized, small, and tiny objects. Children often can demonstrate better thumb and finger control with small or medium-sized objects that have well-defined edges. Tiny objects require too much precision, such that the child often resorts to a more primitive grasping pattern. In fact, skill in using a pincer grasp usually is less critical for the child's functional performance of daily life tasks than skill in using and varying a three-finger opposed grasp pattern. Once the child begins to acquire an opposed grasp pattern, the therapist can vary the objects by size, shape, texture, and weight.

The research findings of Case-Smith et al. (1998) support the clinical observation that object characteristics are important in eliciting specific grasp patterns, particularly when these patterns are emerging. To develop an opposed grasp pattern, the therapist can begin working on grasp alone rather than reach and grasp. The child's arm should be well stabilized when objects are presented. Having the wrist in a neutral or slightly extended position is critical; if appropriate, the therapist can stabilize the volar surface of the child's forearm on the table surface and give support over the dorsum of the forearm. The therapist should present objects in line with the shoulder and not at midline, because midline positioning has a tendency to encourage the use of pronation. With objects presented in line with the shoulder, neutral rotation of the humerus is encouraged (versus internal rotation), and slight forearm supination is likely to occur. The therapist holds the object with his or her fingers and presents the object directly to the child's fingers (Figure 10-24). After grasp, the child carries the object to a nearby container or surface. Practice of this strategy for grasp, carry, and release using a variety of objects is needed for the child to integrate this skill.

Once the child is able to use this pattern well, the therapist can move to the next skill level. At this level the therapist places the object in his or her cupped hand (just under the child's hand and in line with the child's shoulder), so that the object is stable, and asks the child to grasp the object (Figure 10-25). When the therapist uses this strategy, the child needs to use more internal

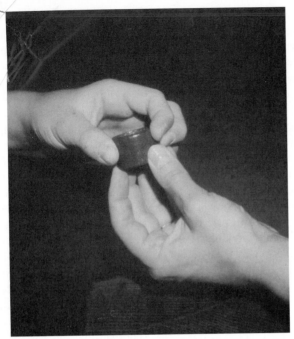

FIGURE 10-24 The child shows the ability to use a controlled radial-digital grasp pattern with the wrist in a neutral position, thumb opposition, and appropriate finger flexion when he is not asked to combine reach with grasp. Note that the therapist's grasp of the object helps ensure that the child will grasp the object with his fingertips. Her grasp also assures that the object remains stable while the child initiates the grasp pattern.

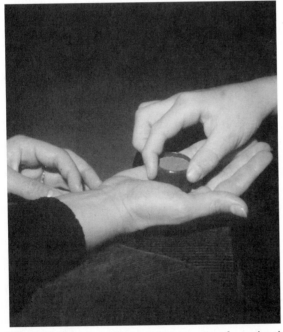

FIGURE 10-25 The child practices grasping from the therapist's hand. His arm is stabilized on his leg during this grasp. The therapist's hand provides some degree of stability to prevent the object from moving during initiation of grasp.

stability of the arm and some degree of prepositioning of the fingers before grasp.

As the child develops skill in grasping from the therapist's hand, the therapist can begin to place an object on the table surface. As at the prior two levels, the object is in line with the child's shoulder, not at midline. The therapist may need to stabilize the object or place it on a nonskid surface for the child who does not have sufficient arm stability to grasp without unintentionally moving the object.

After the child is able to grasp from the table surface with the object in line with the shoulder, the therapist can begin to move the object further away on the table surface, above the table surface, and closer to midline. In this way the therapist is structuring activities to combine reach with grasp. This requires the child to stabilize the arm in space while controlling finger movements. The therapist may use a variety of these object placements in a therapy session to elicit the child's best skills. Different object placements may be needed with various sizes and shapes of objects.

Using principles of motor learning theory, the therapist systematically varies object placement and the size and weight of objects during intervention activities. Varying the input enables the child to develop more adaptable, flexible skills that can be generalized to a variety of situations. Duff and Gordon (2003) noted that 7- to 14-year-old children with hemiplegic cerebral palsy were able to demonstrate anticipatory control (i.e., the ability to adjust the force needed to lift an object) with novel objects, given the ability to practice these grasp-lift patterns. Their findings suggest that these children can develop an awareness of the object properties and the adjustment in force needed by practicing grasping and lifting objects of similar size but different weights. In addition, this ability may be achieved through practice of several grasp-lift repetitions with objects that have the same weight followed by repetitions with objects that have a different weight, or the weights of the objects can be varied randomly in a practice session (Duff & Gordon). The therapist can assess the type of repetition that seems to have the most positive effect for a particular child. Further study will be needed to determine children's retention of these skills over time.

Children with Mild Disabilities. Children with mild disabilities typically have difficulty with small ranges of movements in supination and wrist extension. Sustained control with the intrinsic muscles of the hand may be difficult for these children to achieve. Fingertip control in grasp often is poor, as is the ability to control the palmar arches and to achieve radial-ulnar dissociation of movements within the hand. Some children substitute use of the middle finger for the index finger in attempting a pincer grasp (Figure 10-26); typical children may use this pattern occasionally, but children with tone problems (high or low) tend to use it frequently because

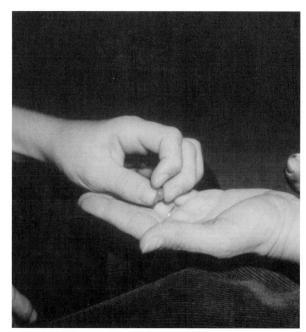

FIGURE 10-26 The child uses a substitution for a standard pincer grasp or tip pinch. Note that with slight adduction of the thumb, the pad of the thumb is more aligned with the middle finger than the index finger. The index finger is slightly too flexed to participate in the grasp.

of instability with the index finger and/or difficulty controlling the thumb in true opposition. Thus the thumb aligns more directly with the middle finger. This pattern can be functional for activities with tiny objects, but if the index cannot be used effectively with the middle finger, stable three-jaw chuck grasp patterns are not available for the child.

Goals for grasp skills for these children usually focus on the use of a variety of grasp patterns, with accommodation of the grasp pattern to the object characteristics. These patterns include use of an effective pincer grasp and lateral pinch grasp pattern; use of a grasp with MCP flexion and IP extension to hold thin, flat objects; and/or use of a power grasp on a variety of tools in daily living tasks. The standard and lateral pinch patterns and the grasp for thin, flat objects require wrist stability and use of the intrinsic muscles.

The therapist can use a variety of treatment strategies with children who are working on these skills, including verbal cueing and structuring of activities to elicit intrinsic muscle activity. Sample activities include holding all fingers in adduction and extension while rolling out clay, using finger abduction to stretch rubber bands placed around two or more fingers, playing finger games that require isolation and small ranges of finger movements, holding or hiding objects in a cupped hand, and squeezing clay or other objects between the pad of the thumb and the pads of one or more fingers.

Development of a power grasp relies on the development of radial-ulnar dissociation and the ability to extend

the index finger and thumb during ulnar finger flexion. Emphasis on radial-ulnar dissociation in the hand and on grasp with MCP flexion and IP extension is helpful as a precursor to the power grasp pattern. To address radial-ulnar dissociation, the therapist structures activities in which the child holds two objects in one hand and releases one at a time; holds an object in the ulnar side of the hand with the ring and little fingers while grasping and releasing with the radial fingers and thumb; and engages in activities that develop finger-to-palm translation with stabilization skills. In addressing the power grasp in functional activities, the therapist carefully selects the type of tool the child handles. Tools that have a narrow surface for index finger contact are particularly difficult for children to control. The therapist can use verbal cues, stickers, or dots on the handles of the tools to encourage appropriate finger placement. The child may need built-up handles to facilitate performance initially.

Enhancement of Carrying Skills

The child must maintain grasp of an object during the carry phase. The therapist, therefore, must attend to the child's ability to vary all joint positions in the arm while sustaining grasp and must emphasize wrist extension with sustained finger flexion. The therapist should be especially attentive to the child's use of compensatory trunk movements and to difficulty dissociating arm and trunk movements. If these are present, the child may need intervention to improve sustained trunk control in the midline and trunk rotation with arm movements. The use of adapted equipment to support the trunk in a symmetric, erect posture is helpful for many children. The therapist also may need to stabilize the shoulder to prevent scapular elevation.

The therapist can use facilitation of arm movements in a manner similar to that described for reaching to encourage carrying patterns of shoulder rotation, graded elbow movements, and forearm supination. Most children with increased tone or stability problems have more difficulty carrying small or thin objects. Use of objects that are larger in diameter, such as those adapted with built-up handles, can promote wrist extension and management of objects during carrying.

Enhancement of Voluntary Release Skills
Problems

Therapists usually combine treatment for voluntary release problems with intervention for grasp. Children who have difficulty releasing objects may exhibit the following:

- Fisting and tight finger flexion
- Difficulty with sustained arm position during object placement and release

- Difficulty combining wrist extension with finger extension
- Inability to use slight forearm supination to allow for release in small areas or near other objects and with visual monitoring of the placement
- Overextension of the fingers in release, limiting control of specific object placement

In their study of 7- to 13-year-old children with hemiplegic cerebral palsy, Eliasson and Gordon (2000) reported specific difficulties with both the placement phase and the release phase of object voluntary release. The children's replacement "is abrupt," they said, "and their force coordination is impaired, resulting in a prolonged and uncoordinated release of the grasp" (p. 232).

Goals. The following are examples of goals the therapist can use for children with a variety of levels of disability. These goals specifically define the size of an area in which the child can release the object (e.g., into a container with a 4-inch opening) or the height of a surface on which the child can release the object (e.g., a stack of six cubes). The following goals incorporate these commonly used measures of voluntary release skill. The goals are in approximate order of difficulty, although difficulty using any one pattern can vary with the individual child. The therapist should integrate these goals with the child's functional goals. The goals are that the child will:

1 Release objects into a container placed on the floor (e.g., pick up toys to put away [hard objects may be easier to use than soft objects])
2 Release objects into a container placed on a table surface with the container at arm's length from the child's body to encourage wrist extension with finger extension (e.g., put objects into and take them out of a container)
3 Release objects into a container at the midline while using wrist extension (e.g., put pens and pencils into a basket after a group activity)
4 Release tiny objects into a container with a small opening (e.g., put nails or screws into a container after a project or put beads into a container for a beaded art project)
5 Place objects within 1 inch of other objects without making other objects move or fall (e.g., place game board pieces during a game, set the table with utensils)
6 Release unstable, lightweight objects while keeping them in an upright position (e.g., place objects on a desk at school and paper cups on the lunch table)
7 Release objects without visual monitoring (e.g., put a toothbrush into container, pencils into a container, paper on a desk)

Intervention Strategies. Intervention focuses on one or more of the following areas, depending on the child's problems: hand opening for object release, arm placement and stability for release, and accuracy of object placement. Releasing patterns correlate with grasping patterns. A child who uses a palmar grasp will use full finger extension to release the object. A child who uses a pincer grasp can use voluntary release with good control of the intrinsic muscles as balanced with the extrinsic muscles.

When the child shows excessive finger flexion (fisting), initial treatment for voluntary hand opening focuses on the child's ability to move the arm while maintaining some finger extension. Splinting may be helpful in supporting the child's wrist or facilitating increased wrist and finger extension. In children with fisting, asking the child to place the object into a container increases the child's fisting. Some children have success releasing to the side of their body because movement away from the midline decreases the pronation-flexion posturing, thus increasing the hand fisting.

If the child can accomplish this level of voluntary release, he or she can attempt release of large and medium-sized objects into a container with a large opening that is placed on the floor. For some children, transfer of objects from hand to hand is a reasonable strategy for encouraging release with object stabilization.

Children who can voluntarily open their hands but who use tenodesis patterns may benefit from intervention to increase voluntary finger extension while maintaining the wrist in a neutral position. For some children, structured activities and handling are effective; other children benefit from wearing a dorsal wrist splint. A therapist can have the child wear a splint during part of the therapy session and encourage finger extension through a variety of activities, including voluntary release. The therapist can use similar activities after splint removal.

Children who use wrist flexion with voluntary release may benefit from structured activities in which a container for objects is placed slightly lateral to the child's midline and at a sufficient distance from the child's body that the child needs to extend the elbow (Figure 10-27). This level of control is similar to that of an infant who releases objects with the arm held in a total extension pattern. Over time, the therapist can move the target containers closer to the child's body, requiring gradually increasing elbow flexion with wrist extension for release of objects. Sometimes the therapist can facilitate this pattern if he or she sets the containers at an angle. Once the child can release medium-sized objects into a container at the midline while maintaining wrist extension to at least a neutral position, the therapist can reduce the size of the container opening.

Children with overextension of the fingers during voluntary release may benefit from activities described previously that address the development of intrinsic muscle control. They also may need intervention to

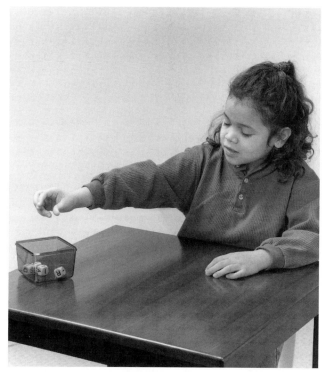

FIGURE 10-27 Positioning materials to elicit elbow extension during release encourages the child's use of wrist extension. (Courtesy Kanji Takeno, Towson University.)

improve somatosensory awareness of their hands. Activities for these children often incorporate the use of lightweight materials and objects that vary in size and stability. Verbal cueing of the child to attend to object and hand placement and graded activities to facilitate increasing accuracy and visual monitoring of materials are often helpful. Also, Gordon et al. (2003) observed that tasks that required increased accuracy (including object placement on a relatively unstable surface) could be used to encourage children with hemiplegia to slow their movements. Instruction was helpful to the children in encouraging faster movements (Gordon et al.). Based on findings from their studies, these researchers suggested that different speeds be used during voluntary release activities and that "practicing release tasks with the noninvolved hand first or practicing with bimanual tasks may enhance performance and should be studied" (Gordon et al., p. 247). In addition, the work of Eliasson and Gordon (2000) suggests that repetition of object release in which the object's weight remains constant over a number of trials allows children with hemiplegic cerebral palsy to learn to adjust the release of grasp. These findings provide support for the use of activities for voluntary release in which repetition and timing can be adjusted. Games of various types are often very effective for this purpose and are selected for the child's cognitive level as well as the motor level.

Enhancement of In-Hand Manipulation Skills

Problems

Children who have difficulty with in-hand manipulation skills drop objects, use surfaces for support during manipulation, or are slow in the execution of skills (Exner, 1990a). Case-Smith (1993) found empirical support for these problems in her study of children with and without fine motor delays. These problems are associated with tactile problems (Case-Smith, 1991). Praxis and motor control problems, particularly of the intrinsic muscles, also may be a major cause of limited in-hand manipulation skill development. Attentional and cognitive problems contribute to these problems in some children. Problems that limit in-hand manipulation include the following:

- Limited finger isolation and control
- Inability to effectively cup the hand to hold objects in the palm
- Inability to hold more than one object in the hand at the same time
- Insufficient stability for controlling object movement at the finger pads, resulting in objects being dropped frequently

Goals. The following are examples of goals the therapist can use for children with a variety of levels of in-hand manipulation skill. The goals are in approximate order of difficulty, although difficulty using any one pattern can vary with the individual child. The activities are examples of activities the child may need that depend upon in-hand manipulation skills. The goals are that the child will:

1 (Move coins, finger foods) into the palm of the hand by demonstrating finger-to-palm translation
2 (Move several coins, pieces of finger foods) into the palm of one hand by using finger-to-palm translation with stabilization skills
3 (Adjust coins for placement into a bank, paper for placement into the printer, playing cards for a game) using shift skills
4 (Adjust eating utensils, a toothbrush while cleaning the teeth) using simple rotation skills
5 (Eat small finger foods, setup/clean up a game board) using palm-to-finger translation (and palm-to-finger translation with stabilization)
6 (Play with a building set, put caps onto markers) using simple rotation with stabilization skills
7 (Erase with a pencil, handle containers or lids used in hygiene skills) using complex rotation skills

Intervention Strategies. The therapist's assessment of the causes of the child's problems and the therapist's determination of the child's potential for acquiring specific in-hand manipulation skills influence intervention goals and strategies. Many children with moderate and severe disabilities who lack the necessary prerequisite skills cannot develop in-hand manipulation skills. Children with mild disabilities usually can develop at least lower level in-hand manipulation skills.

Specific activity suggestions are given in Box 10-3. The following sections provide suggestions for strategies therapists can use with children with different levels of skills. Exner (1995) provides additional information on treatment of in-hand manipulation skills.

Children with No In-Hand Manipulation Skills. The therapist may encourage the child with no in-hand manipulation skills or only finger-to-palm translation to manipulate objects between the two hands and use support surfaces to assist in object manipulation. Use of these strategies can help the child begin to move the fingers actively over object surfaces. The therapist can use objects such as cubes that have pictures on all sides,

---

BOX 10-3 In-Hand Manipulation Treatment Activities

PREPARATION ACTIVITIES

1 Activities involving general tactile awareness
   - Using crazy foam
   - Using shaving cream
   - Applying hand lotion
   - Finger painting
2 Activities involving proprioceptive input
   - Weight bearing (e.g., wheelbarrow, activities on a small ball)
   - Pushing heavy objects (e.g., boxes, chairs, benches)
   - Pulling (e.g., tug-of-war)
   - Pressing different parts of the hand into clay
   - Pushing fingers into clay or therapy putty
   - Pushing shapes out of perforated cardboard
   - Tearing open packages or boxes
   - Playing clapping games
3 Activities involving regulation of pressure
   - Tearing edges off computer paper
   - Rolling clay into a ball
   - Squeezing water out of a sponge or washcloth
   - Pushing snaps together
4 Activities involving tactile discrimination
   - Playing finger games and singing songs
   - Playing finger identification games
   - Discriminating among objects with the objects stabilized
   - Discriminating among shapes with the shapes stabilized
   - Writing on the body and identifying the shape, letter, or object drawn
   - Discriminating among textures

SPECIFIC IN-HAND MANIPULATION ACTIVITIES

1 Translation (fingers to palm)
   - Getting a coin out of a change purse
   - Hiding a penny in the hand (magic trick)
   - Crumpling paper
   - Picking up a small piece of food and bringing it into the palm
2 Translation (fingers to palm with stabilization)
   - Getting two or more coins out of a change purse, one at a time
   - Taking two or more chips off a magnetic wand, one at a time
   - Picking up pegs or paper clips one at a time and holding two or more in the hand at one time
   - Picking up several utensils one at a time and holding two or more in the hand at one time
3 Translation (palm to fingers)
   - Moving a penny from the palm to the fingers
   - Moving a chip to the fingers to put on a magnetic wand
   - Moving an object to put it into a container
   - Moving a food item to put it in the mouth

4 Translation (palm to fingers with stabilization)
   - Holding several chips to put on a wand, one at a time
   - Handling money to put it into a bank or soda machine
   - Putting one utensil down when holding several
   - Holding several game pieces (chips, pegs, or markers)
5 Shift
   - Turning pages in a book
   - Picking up sheets of paper, tissue paper, or dollar bills
   - Separating playing cards
   - Stringing beads (shifting string and bead as string goes through the bead)
   - Shifting a crayon, pencil, or pen for coloring or writing
   - Shifting paper in the nonpreferred hand while cutting
   - Playing with Tinker Toys (long, thin pieces)
   - Moving a cookie while eating
   - Adjusting a spoon, fork, or knife for appropriate use
   - Rubbing paint, dirt, or tape off the pad of a finger
6 Shift with stabilization
   - Holding a pen and pushing the cap off with the same hand
   - Holding chips while flipping one out of the fingers
   - Holding fabric in the hand while attempting to button or snap
   - Holding a key ring with the keys in hand, shifting one for placement in a lock
7 Simple or complex rotation (depending on object orientation)
   - Removing or putting on a small jar lid
   - Putting on or removing bolts from nuts
   - Rotating a crayon or pencil with the tip oriented ulnarly (simple rotation)
   - Rotating a crayon or pencil with the tip oriented radially (complex rotation)
   - Removing a crayon from the box and preparing it for coloring
   - Rotating a pen or marker to put the top on it
   - Rotating toy people to put them in chairs, a bus, or a boat
   - Rotating a puzzle piece for placement in the puzzle
   - Feeling objects or shapes to identify them
   - Handling construction toy pieces
   - Turning cubes that have pictures on all six sides
   - Constructing twisted shapes with pipe cleaners
   - Rotating a toothbrush or eating utensils during use
8 Simple or complex rotation with stabilization
   - Handling parts of a small shape container while rotating the shape to put it into the container
   - Holding a key ring with keys, rotating the correct one for placement in the lock

kaleidoscopes, and textured toys. When the child can effectively move the fingers over objects, the therapist can introduce finger-to-palm translation activities in the context of "hiding the object" games using various objects. Finger isolation games can be useful, and the therapist should incorporate the thumb into these activities. The child should be assisted in developing and functionally using a variety of grasp patterns, including those that combine flexion at the MCP joints with extension at the IP joints. The therapist can use tactile discrimination and proprioception activities to enhance awareness of fingers and areas of the palm of the hand.

Children with Beginning In-Hand Manipulation Skills. Children who can use finger-to-palm translation and beginning simple rotation, or shift, or palm-to-finger translation skills can work on refining these skills, expanding their repertoire of skills used without stabilization, and beginning their ability to stabilize objects in the ulnar side of the hand while manipulating with the radial fingers.

Object selection for in-hand manipulation skills with these children is important. Objects that do not roll and that are small (not tiny) are often the easiest for the child to handle. Examples include dice-sized cubes, nickels, game pieces, and other small toys. With larger objects, the child must involve all fingers in the manipulation and must use more hand expansion, therefore these objects are more difficult for the child to handle. With tiny objects, the child must have excellent tactile discrimination and fingertip control, which also makes these objects more difficult to handle than small objects.

The therapist structures the presentation of objects to assist the child in using a particular in-hand manipulation skill and often cues the child in the use of the skill. In a study of preschool children without disabilities who had emerging in-hand manipulation skills, Exner (1990b) found that use of verbal cues or demonstration of skills had a positive effect on the children's scores (as a group). However, children with lower scores showed more improvement with cues than children with higher scores. These findings suggest that verbal cueing may be an important component of intervention for in-hand manipulation skills. The CO-OP approach encourages the therapist to provide verbal cues and the child to select his or her own goals and strategies and to talk his or her way through an activity as methods of increasing coordination and motor planning.

In addressing palm-to-finger translation, the therapist first places the object on the middle phalanx of the child's index finger. When the child is able to move the object from this position out to the pads of the fingers, the therapist places the object on the volar surface of the proximal phalanx of the index finger. Later the therapist places the object in the palm of the child's hand to promote thumb isolation and control to move the object.

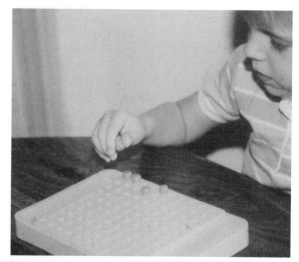

FIGURE 10-28 The peg has been placed in the child's hand upside down to encourage rotation prior to placement in the game board.

The therapist can structure simple rotation skills by placing the object in the child's hand (in a radial grasp pattern) and asking the child to turn it upright (Figure 10-28). Pegs and peglike objects (e.g., candles and objects that look like little people) can be helpful in developing these skills.

Finger-to-palm translation with stabilization is the one skill with stabilization that is likely to be feasible for these children. This child often can facilitate this skill during finger-feeding activities and in play with coins. The therapist first encourages the child to hold one object in the hand while picking up and hiding another. After the child can manage two objects, the therapist can progress to using three or more objects.

Children with Basic In-Hand Manipulation Skills. For children with basic in-hand manipulation skills, the therapist emphasizes the development of complex rotation skills (Figure 10-29) and the use of stabilization with the other skills. The therapist introduces small and medium-sized objects and emphasizes use of the skills in a variety of functional activities, including dressing, hygiene, and school tasks. The child practices combinations of skills, such as finger-to-palm translation, palm-to-finger translation, and simple rotation. The therapist also can stress speed of skill use by timing skills and reporting the speed to the child. Children who are working at this level of skill typically respond well to verbal cueing for strategies to use in performing skills and to feedback about the effectiveness and speed of their skills.

Facilitation of Bilateral Hand Use Skills

Problems

Difficulties with bilateral hand use result from a combination of problems, of which motor factors are only one

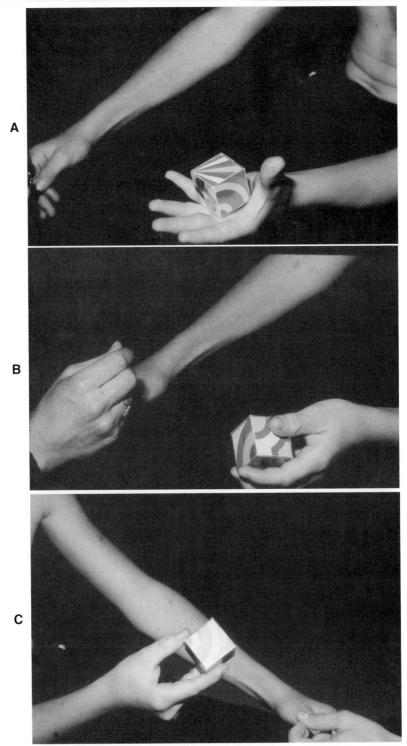

FIGURE 10-29 **A,** The child is forming a picture with a set of puzzle blocks. He is encouraged to find the side of the block that fits the design being constructed. The therapist has placed the correct side of the block against the palm of his hand so that he must use complex rotation to find it. **B,** Prior to using the in-hand manipulation skill of complex rotation, the child must use palm-to-finger translation to move the block toward the distal finger surface. In that process the block begins to be turned. **C,** Having identified the correct side, the child shifts the object out to the pads of the fingers prior to placement with the other blocks.

component. Some children with significant cognitive delays cannot attend to two objects simultaneously, therefore reciprocal hand use or stabilization with one hand combined with object handling by the other hand is not possible. Deficits in integration of the two body sides may be present, and impaired sensation may contribute to a lack of attention to one body side. Lack of bilateral motor experience, as in children with hemiplegia or brachial plexus injuries, can cause children to approach all tasks in a one-handed manner. Other problems include the following:

- The child cannot effectively sustain both hands at the midline.
- The child has difficulty using supination during bilateral activities.
- The child has overflow movements and associated reactions in one upper extremity when using the other.

Goals. The following are examples of goals the therapist can use for children with a variety of levels of disability. These goals fit the categories of gross symmetric bilateral skills, stabilizing or manipulating with one hand while manipulating with the other hand, and bilateral simultaneous manipulation. The following goals show increasing levels of difficulty that are consistent with a developmental approach. This progression in skills may not be appropriate for children with significant weakness or motor problems on one body side. The goals are that the child will:

1 Push large objects using both hands together
2 Lift and carry large objects using both hands
3 Lift and carry medium-sized objects using both hands
4 (Color, write, hold a puzzle board) demonstrating the ability to stabilize materials on a table surface with one open hand while the other hand manipulates materials
5 (Hold the handle of a small pan while pretending to cook, hold the edge of a puzzle box while putting pieces away, hold the handle of a small pail while filling with water) demonstrating the ability to stabilize materials using a palmar grasp while the other hand manipulates materials
6 (Hold a cup while pouring liquid into it, hold a slice of bread while spreading butter on it, hold a marker box while putting the markers away) demonstrating the ability to stabilize materials using a variety of grasp patterns while the other hand manipulates materials (Figure 10-30)
7 (Button, tie shoes, fix hair, do a mechanical project) demonstrating the ability to manipulate objects with both hands simultaneously (Figure 10-31).

Treatment goals vary depending on the severity of the child's disability and the level of skills the child is expected to acquire. The therapist must consider the child's need and potential for gross symmetric hand use,

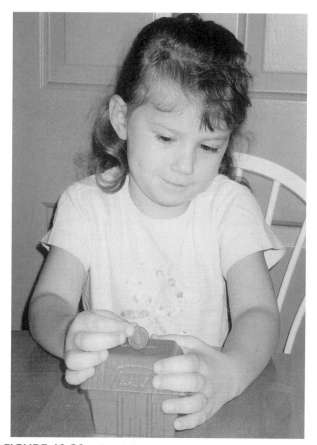

FIGURE 10-30 This child shows the bilateral skill of stabilizing with a refined grasp with her left hand while placing a penny in the bank with her right hand. Note the appropriate use of force in holding both objects.

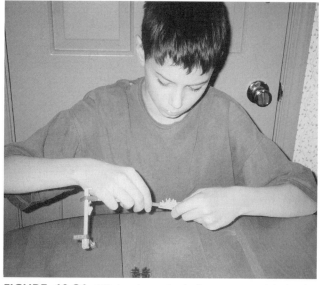

FIGURE 10-31 Bilateral manipulation occurs with both hands in this construction activity. The child uses modifications of the power grasp with different forearm positions on the right and left while connecting two parts of the toy.

stabilizing with one hand while manipulating with the other, and bilateral simultaneous manipulation.

Intervention Strategies

Children with Severe Disabilities

Treatment of the child with significantly increased tone or marked asymmetry focuses on promoting the child's ability to stabilize materials with the more involved hand while manipulating with the more proficient hand. Activities that require stabilization with grasp are often easier for these children than are symmetric bilateral skills or stabilization without grasp. However, the child can accomplish stabilization without grasp as long as he or she can use the hand in a fisted position with the wrist in neutral to slight extension. Symmetric bilateral hand use may receive some attention, particularly if these activities serve to increase awareness of one arm and to increase movement and/or control of that arm. Simultaneous bilateral manipulation skills usually are inappropriate for these children unless the therapist can use adaptations.

Special handling techniques can promote the child's ability to stabilize objects while manipulating them or to use gross bilateral skills. The therapist can sit behind the child and stabilize both shoulders to help the child bring and keep both hands at the midline. The therapist should also encourage trunk rotation so that the child can cross the midline effectively.

Toys and materials selected for bilateral activities must require both hands to be used, particularly in the early phases of treatment. Initially the child may be more successful with gross bilateral skills if he or she can sustain grasp and keep the forearms pronated, such as in holding a stick horizontally to hit a balloon. For the child who is working on stabilizing with one hand while manipulating with the other, presenting objects on a slippery surface may require the child to use one hand as a stabilizer. Objects that have handles are useful when the therapist is working on stabilization with grasp. Activities that are simple for the manipulating hand can allow the child to focus on the role of the stabilizing hand.

Usually the therapist places materials for bilateral skill development at the midline. However, the therapist and the child should explore other positions if midline positioning is not optimal.

If a child cannot successfully stabilize materials and does not show potential for this skill in the near future, the therapist should consider adaptations. Nonskid surfaces and other devices can assist in stabilization of materials for table activities.

Children with Moderate Disabilities.
Intervention for children with low tone or some degree of involuntary movement can approximate the normal sequence of bilateral hand skill development. Therapy initially focuses on improving symmetry and stability and proceeds through developing the child's skills in stabilizing with and without grasp. Children at this skill level may

benefit from working on a slightly unstable surface to prompt spontaneous stabilization of materials during manipulation. The child may need adaptations for certain highly demanding activities (e.g., handwriting) in which one hand must be an effective stabilizer. Generally, simultaneous bilateral manipulation is not feasible for these children.

Children with Mild Disabilities.
Children with mild disabilities may require further refinement of gross symmetric bilateral skills and stabilizing with one hand while manipulating with the other. These children can also develop or improve their simultaneous bilateral manipulation skills. To enhance development of simultaneous bilateral manipulation skills, the therapist carefully selects, grades, and structures a variety of activities that elicit these skills. The therapist may also use functional activities of daily living to facilitate development of these skills.

Children with Muscle Weakness.
Children with muscle weakness can often manage simultaneous manipulation activities well because little hand strength and movement of the arms against gravity are required. These children often need assistance or adaptations to develop the ability to stabilize materials with one hand because this demands more strength in the stabilizing arm. The child may be able to accomplish gross symmetric bilateral skills only on table surfaces that provide arm support.

Group Intervention for Children with Hand Skill Problems.
Often occupational therapy intervention for children with hand skill problems is provided on an individual basis. However, small group intervention can have many benefits and may be considered at the least as a supplement to individual intervention. Bumin and Kayihan (2001) reported on a study comparing individual and group treatment of children with spastic diplegia; the average age was 7 years. Intervention consisted of one group of children receiving individual treatment identified as being sensory-motor-perceptual in nature (which included sensory, gross and fine motor, and visual-perceptual activities). Children in another group were placed into small groups of four children per group and were provided with the same treatment activities. The control group children received a home program. The children receiving direct intervention had treatment across a 3-month period for $1\frac{1}{2}$ hours per session 3 days a week. Outcomes were assessed using the Southern California Sensory Integration Test (SCSIT) and the Physical Ability Test, which includes activities of daily living. The differences between pre- and post-test results were statistically significant for all of the SCSIT subtests, except Manual Form Perception, for both the group of children treated individually and the group that received small group treatment. The children who received the home program showed significant differences between pre- and post-test scores for only four of the 11 SCSIT

subtests. All three groups of children showed significant change from pre- to post-test on the Physical Ability Test, but the effect size was much smaller in the control group than in the other two groups. The authors concluded that both individual and group treatment were effective for this sample of children.

Small group intervention can allow for focus on a number of skills in addition to sensory and motor factors. The social context of the small group allows children to observe and learn from one another and to practice leadership skills, depending on the opportunities created by the therapist. In addition, small groups support turn-taking and communication skills. Many children are more willing to engage in repetition of actions (which is very beneficial for some hand skills) in a gamelike atmosphere in a small group than in an individual session with a therapist. In addition, some games benefit from having more players than just the child and the therapist.

In structuring for small group therapy sessions that focus on enhancing the development of hand skills, the therapist should consider the cognitive and interactional skills of the children as well as their hand skill problems. However, sessions that use play/leisure- or work-based activities are particularly amenable to modification for inclusion of other children. In contrast, intervention that focuses on improved use of hand skills in activities of daily living often is more appropriately carried out in individual sessions.

Generalization of Skills into Functional Activities

Most children do not readily generalize skills from isolated activities to everyday life activities without assistance. The therapist therefore should present activities to the child who has hand or arm function problems in a meaningful context and should seek ways in which the child can practice specific fine motor skills in everyday activities. For example, the child can carry out reaching program activities during dressing and hygiene training or while playing with a toy that has many different parts. The therapist can incorporate grasp activities into independent eating and vocational readiness tasks. The child can facilitate in-hand manipulation by using materials from his or her pencil or crayon box or by building with construction toys. The therapist can structure voluntary release into a game that uses moveable pieces. The child can develop bilateral hand use through meal preparation activities, play, and schoolwork. Many other combinations are possible to help the child develop mature function of hand or arm skills, with increasing competence in daily life activities. Work by Mandich, Polatajko, and Rodger (2003) supports the clear importance of addressing occupational performance and social participation, in that parents of children with mild motor problems (developmental coordination disorder) report a

substantial negative impact on their children's activities of daily living. These authors emphasize that children need to have the opportunity to choose the activity-oriented goals for their intervention. Such goals are important in supporting the children's involvement in social settings.

RESEARCH ON INTERVENTION FOR HAND SKILL PROBLEMS

Studies on the efficacy of fine motor and hand skill intervention in children increasingly are providing information that is useful in the determination of intervention strategies and the planning of occupational therapy programs. However, currently almost all studies have looked at the short-term benefits of intervention. Longer term and longitudinal studies are just beginning to emerge.

Case-Smith has conducted a number of studies designed to assess the effectiveness of school-based occupational therapy on improvement in children's hand skills. In a study designed to assess the outcomes of occupational therapy programs for 26 preschool-age children who were treated during one school year, Case-Smith (1996) found that the children showed significant change in several aspects of fine motor skills, including in-hand manipulation skills, motor accuracy, and tool use. In addition, the children showed significant improvement in their self-care skills. In a follow-up study with a larger group of preschool-age children with problems and a group of children without problems, Case-Smith, Heaphy et al. (1998) compared children who received services with those without problems. The children who received services made significant progress in the areas of in-hand manipulation skills and motor accuracy. The researchers also found that more consultation was significantly associated with the children's improvement in some fine motor skills.

A subsequent study by Case-Smith (2002) included 38 children of elementary school age (7 to 10 years old) who had handwriting difficulties. Data were collected regarding the children's in-hand manipulation skills as well as their handwriting skills. As a group, the 29 children who had received occupational therapy services across the school year (i.e., a 7-month period) showed more improvement in in-hand manipulation speed than the group of nine children who did not receive occupational therapy. The occupational therapists who provided the services to these children reported that they included object manipulation activities in their weekly 30-minute treatment sessions with the children. This study, as well as Case-Smith's 1998 study, is particularly valuable in supporting intervention for in-hand manipulation problems in children in that even in studies in which the intervention was not highly controlled (in which different therapists provided treatment activities that varied based on the child's needs), in-hand manipulation skills have been shown to improve. Such studies suggest that children with mild involvement can make significant changes in these skills with occupational therapy intervention. Further studies are needed to determine more specifically the impact of such improvement on occupational performance in the children.

A study by Schoemaker, Niemeijer, Reynders, and Smits-Engelsman (2003), similarly supports intervention for children with mild disabilities. Children with developmental coordination disorder were placed in a treatment group (n = 10) and a control group (n = 5). The experimental group received 18 treatment sessions of "a task-oriented treatment program based upon recent insights from motor control and motor learning research," and the control group did not receive treatment (p. 155). The children who received treatment improved significantly in handwriting quality and performance on the Movement Assessment Battery for Children (ABC).

Miller et al. (2001) and Candler and Meeuwsen (2002) discussed the potential effectiveness of use of a problem-solving strategy and self-discovery with children who have developmental coordination disorder. In this approach, the therapist guides the child's exploration of alternative strategies. As Candler and Meeuwsen noted, "Children with developmental coordination disorder can implicitly recognize and respond to environmental cues important to task performance" (p. 434). These children do not necessarily benefit from highly specific cueing of their performance.

Other studies have been conducted on treatment effectiveness in children with more substantial motor disabilities. Boyd, Morris, and Graham (2001) conducted a comprehensive literature review of interventions for children with upper extremity problems. Fedrizzi, Pagliano, Andreucci, and Oleari (2003) conducted a longitudinal study with 31 children with spastic hemiplegia in which they assessed the children for grip skill and use of the more involved hand in bilateral activities. From the time of the initial referral to age 4, the children received individual therapy two or three times a week, then from 4 to 7 years, the children received small group treatment (three or four children per group). Therapy focused on improvement of hand skills through the use of motor learning principles in play and activities of daily living. These authors' findings support intervention focused on use of the hemiplegic hand in functional activities for these children. In fact, the greatest improvements in grasp were found to occur during the years of small group treatment (ages 4 to 7). However, this change may have been due to developmental readiness for improvement in grasp at that time; further study would be needed to determine whether the change was associated with the specific treatment. The authors noted that use of the more involved hand was more impaired in spontaneous bilateral activities than when used alone in grasp-

ing skills. The children in their study with the most severe motor disabilities (a small number of children) tended to deteriorate in grasp skill as they approached adolescence. These authors recommended monitoring of children with more severe involvement in this age group for potential additional treatment.

CONSTRAINT-INDUCED MOVEMENT THERAPY FOR CHILDREN WITH CEREBRAL PALSY

Children with hemiplegic cerebral palsy tend to show more limitation in bilateral hand use than in grasp skill (Fedrizzi et al., 2003). Sterr, Freivogel, and Schmalohr (2002) verified the differences in available movement/ skill versus spontaneous use in children and young adults with hemiplegia. They found that although these individuals were able to use their involved hand, they tended not to do so and that they believed they had more limited ability to use their hands than they actually had. Therapists therefore have often sought a variety of strategies to increase spontaneous use of this hand.

Taub's research (e.g., Taub, Aswatte, & Pidiki, 1999) has provided the basis for clinical application of constraint-induced movement therapy, which is now used with adults with hemiplegia and is being explored with children in a number of clinical settings. A key characteristic of this therapy is the use of some method of restraint of the less involved arm and hand to promote use of the more involved arm and hand. Implementation of this intervention with children varies in the method used to restrict movement in the less involved arm and hand, in the amount of intervention provided during the restriction of movement, and the number of days or weeks of restriction. Some researchers report using a splint on the less involved hand (Crocker, MacKay-Lyons, & McDonnell, 1997; Glover, Mateer, Yoell, & Speed, 2002); others report using casting of the less involved arm and hand (DeLuca, Echols, Ramey, & Taub, 2003; Willis, Morello, Davie, Rice, & Bennett, 2002). In the studies (which may reflect clinical practice models), some children were provided with no additional specific intervention (Crocker et al., 1997; Willis et al., 2002); others received additional therapy sessions during the days of restricted movement of the less involved hand (Glover et al.); and still others received 6 hours of intervention per day during the casting (DeLuca et al.). The most common time frame reported in the research studies was 3 to 4 weeks (Crocker et al.; DeLuca et al.; Willis et al.). The one factor that appeared to be relatively constant in implementation of this intervention is restriction of the less involved hand for at least 6 waking hours a day.

Crocker and others (1997) used a single case study approach to study the effectiveness of this approach with a 2-year-old child. Outcomes immediately after splinting and 2 weeks later included more arm-hand use with better quality, as demonstrated in play, finger feeding, and PDMS Fine Motor Test results. Six months later, additional improvement was noted.

Glover et al. (2002) assessed constraint-induced movement in a 19-month-old child. Changes noted were significant in frequency of arm-hand use, accuracy of movements, and strength. Spontaneous use in bilateral activities and quality of reaching and voluntary release were evident, but grasp was not substantially improved. Although spasticity was diminished immediately upon discontinuation of the constraint-induced movement program, it did return gradually. At $2\frac{1}{2}$ months after intervention, spontaneous use remained improved.

Another case study to assess constraint-induced movement therapy was conducted by DeLuca et al. (2003) with a 15-month-old girl. However, in this study, the researchers provided another session of this therapy 5 months after the end of the first session. Positive changes in the child's arm-hand use and major changes in the spontaneity of her use of the more involved hand resulted. She showed significant improvement in occupational performance activities appropriate for her age.

A group comparison study of constraint-induced movement therapy with children between the ages of 1 and 8 years was conducted by Willis et al. (2002). All children received the casting, but half of the children received casting during each of two month-long intervention periods. Based on testing with the PDMS, the children who were casted improved approximately 10 points more than those who were not casted during each of the study time periods. The results were sustained in the first group casted when these children were tested 6 months after conclusion of their casting period. All parents of the children casted also documented improvement.

Constraint-induced movement therapy, therefore, seems to be a potential adjunct to other interventions for children with asymmetric motor involvement due to CNS dysfunction. All children studied showed improvement in one or more aspects of neuromusculoskeletal and movement-related functions, performance skills, and occupational performance. However, some authors noted the parents' concern, at least initially with the constraint regarding the loss of independence in activities they previously could accomplish since the children were unable to use their preferred hand (DeLuca et al., 2003) and because of the children's level of frustration (Glover et al., 2002). However, the parents also noted substantial improvements in their children's functioning as a result of participation in this type of intervention. Therefore psychosocial support for the parents and the child seems imperative with constraint-induced movement therapy.

Further research is needed to assess the following elements of constraint-induced movement therapy:

- The best type of constraint to be used
- Benefits for different age groups of children
- How characteristics of the child's disability may affect the length of this particular program
- Appropriate levels of intervention to facilitate use of the more involved upper extremity while the child is wearing the constraint

SPLINTING

Splinting is often a component of occupational therapy intervention for children with hand function problems. Children who have one or more of the following problems may benefit most:

- Sustained abnormal posturing
- Increased tone or markedly decreased tone
- Limitations in movement of the hand
- Limitations in functional skills secondary to problems with hand functions

Children with severe motor disability associated with CNS dysfunction may benefit from splinting to reduce tone or improve mobility and functional skills. The child with minimal involvement secondary to CNS damage may have more difficulty with thumb use than with wrist or finger control. This child may need a thumb splint to diminish flexor muscle tone or to provide thumb MCP stability so that function is enhanced.

The following sections provide an overview of splinting for children with disabilities. Gabriel and Duvall-Riley (2000) provide additional information on the selection of splints and more specific details about construction of a wide variety of splints for children.

Precautions and Indications for Splint Use

Precautions for splint use are always in order, particularly for nonverbal children who may have poor sensation. These factors make them vulnerable to skin irritation and pressure problems. Children may be unable to report sensory problems during or after splint application, therefore the therapist must carefully instruct the child's parents regarding the wearing schedule, possible problems, and postural changes to note.

Static splints generally are worn for shorter periods than splints that allow hand movement. Initially children may tolerate wearing a splint for only 5 to 10 minutes. Usually the therapist can gradually increase these periods. If the child has increased tone, maximum wearing time for a static splint is usually 6 to 8 hours per day. However, if splints allow some hand movement and the therapist uses them to aid accomplishment of functional activities, the child may tolerate them for additional hours. Children generally wear night splints all night, but they should spend at least a part of each 24-hour period without the splints.

Not all children with increased tone need night resting splints. In many cases their hands are more relaxed during sleep, and their parents can arrange their arms and hands in neutral position. Children who have neutral positioning at night generally are at less risk for the development of contractures. However, the child who shows abnormal hand posturing during the day but not at night may require daytime splint application to increase function.

Boehme (1988) noted that some children have learned to use abnormal patterns of wrist flexion and ulnar deviation or thumb adduction to accomplish their daily activities. If a splint inhibits this pattern, the child may compensate by using another abnormal position of the hand or arm. Therefore before the therapist applies a splint, he or she must determine whether functional skill patterns that the child is using will be lost. Often the therapist needs to increase the frequency of intervention sessions when children are wearing splints so that they can develop better patterns of hand use.

Types of Splints Used with Children

Splints are categorized as those that allow hand movement and those that do not. *Static splints* include resting pan splints, other volar and dorsal full hand and wrist splints, spasticity reduction splints, and thumb positioning splints. *Dynamic splints* assist the child with a particular wrist, finger, or thumb movement. A *neurophysiologically based* splint may provide stimulation to the hand or arm or assist with stabilization of one or more joints during hand or arm activities.

Doubilet and Polkow (1977) and Snook (1979) reported case studies suggesting that *spasticity reduction splints* help decrease tone in adults. McPherson (1981) examined the effectiveness of Snook's spasticity reduction splint in five adolescents with severe disabilities. Splint-wearing time was gradually increased from 15 minutes the first day to 2 hours daily by the fourth week. The outcome measure was passive muscle tone at the wrist, which was documented on a daily basis through use of a scale that measured pounds of force when the individual assumed wrist flexion. During the 4 weeks of splint application, the subjects' wrist tone decreased significantly. When they did not wear the splints for a week, their tone increased again.

When the therapist applies spasticity reduction splints, he or she should take care to control the thumb MCP joint. Distal force on the thumb can result in stretching or even rupture of the ulnar collateral ligament of the thumb's MCP joint (Phelps & Weeks, 1976) and subluxation of the MCP joint. Because children with spasticity usually demonstrate marked thumb adduction, distal control of the thumb moves the MCP and IP joints into hyperextension; therefore control at the car-

pometacarpal (CMC) joint is needed to abduct and extend the first metacarpal CMC joint.

Resting pan splints may provide more support to and control of the thumb than some of the spasticity reduction devices. However, the therapist should plan and monitor splints carefully for reactions at the wrist and fingers. Children with increased tone may not tolerate the classic position for a resting hand splint, in which the wrist is in 20 to 30 degrees of extension and the fingers are in slight flexion. The child with moderately increased tone may have more tolerance for a resting splint that holds the wrist in neutral position and the fingers in slight flexion. However, if flexor spasticity is severe, splinting that begins with the wrist in marked flexion and emphasizes slightly increased finger extension (out of full fisting) may be most effective. Initially the therapist should stabilize the wrist position in just slightly more extension than the child normally achieves. The therapist then adjusts or reconstructs splints to position the wrist, thumb, and fingers. In general, the therapist increases extension at only the wrist *or* fingers at one time to prevent the occurrence of flexion or extension deformities in the fingers.

The therapist may use other *volar splints*, such as the wrist support splint, with children who respond to control of wrist flexion but who do not need or cannot tolerate positioning of the fingers or thumb simultaneously. Wrist support splints allow the child to use the hand to perform functional activities, and the therapist may adjust them periodically to promote a progression of controlled finger extension during activities. The volar wrist splint should control ulnar deviation.

Controversy regarding the use of dorsal versus volar static splints is long-standing and has yet to be resolved. From a functional perspective, dorsal splints are most effective with children with muscle weakness or mild to moderately increased tone. The therapist uses the dorsal splint shown in Figure 10-32 on children with high tone and on those with low tone to hold the wrist in a neutral position. The splint provides support to the palmar arch. Although the child cannot use extreme wrist flexion, the therapist may use a small degree of wrist flexion in functional activities. Because no splint material contacts the volar surface of the hand and forearm, this splint interferes less with controlled arm use on a surface than a volar splint would. Children have responded favorably to this splint. However, dorsal static splints have limited use in controlling abnormal finger position in children with CNS deficits.

The therapist uses thumb splints when a child has difficulty with thumb control but can adequately coordinate movements in other parts of the wrist and hand or when thumb control is the greatest problem. Exner and Bonder (1983) reported a study of short opponens thumb splint use with 12 children who had cerebral palsy

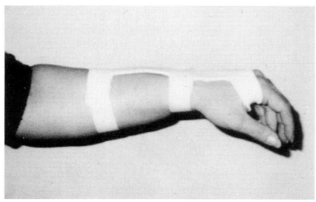

FIGURE 10-32 Dorsal splint to support the wrist in extension for stability or to control a mild to moderate pull into flexion. The hand section can be molded to support the palmar arch.

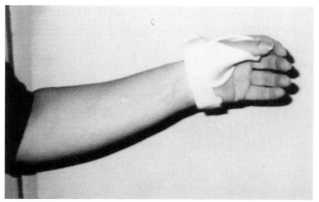

FIGURE 10-33 Short opponens thumb splint made of a thermoplastic material. A similar design can be made with Neoplush.

with spastic hemiplegia. These splints controlled the thumb over the first metacarpal joint and extended onto the distal phalanx (Figure 10-33). The researchers used the splints 8 hours daily for 6 weeks. After this program, two children showed improvement in bilateral hand use and three children showed improved grasp. Some children found that wearing the splints on the nonpreferred hand interfered with stabilization of materials that could not be grasped. In clinical use, the splint is beneficial in improving children's functional use of their hands.

The therapist can use a soft splint to enhance thumb control in children with mildly increased tone. Neoprene or Neoplush is a commonly used material for soft splints. Use of the opponens splint pattern described previously is suitable when higher tone is present (Figure 10-34). The McKie splint (McKie, 2003) is a soft thumb splint designed specifically for use with children. In a small study of four young children with cerebral palsy, this splint was found to have a positive effect on grasp and supination. The author notes that the children also showed improvement in use of the hand in play activities.

Gabriel and Duvall-Riley (2000) reported on the use of a weight-bearing splint for children who need additional wrist and/or finger-thumb support to allow for more effective weight bearing. This splint is usually designed to extend from the forearm to the fingertips. It positions the child's wrist in approximately 90 degrees of wrist extension and the fingers in appropriate extension. The child wears this splint only during weight-bearing activities.

Other orthotic devices are available for children with increased tone or contractures. The positioning of children who have suffered head injuries to prevent loss of range is particularly important during extensive comatose, semicomatose, and recovery periods. The therapist

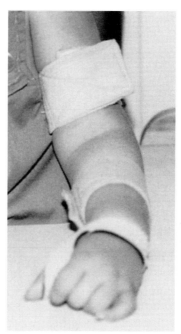

FIGURE 10-34 A Neoplush thumb splint is worn with orthokinetic cuffs on the forearm and upper arm. Both orthokinetic cuffs are designed to promote extension and inhibit flexion. The active area of the cuff on the forearm is over the wrist and finger extensors. The active area on the cuff on the upper arm is over the triceps.

uses inflatable air (pneumatic) splints (Hill, 1988) to decrease tone, maintain and increase joint range, and stimulate somatosensory function.

Some therapists use casting with children who exhibit spasticity and contractures secondary to cerebral palsy or head injury (Hill, 1994; Yasukawa, 1992; Yasukawa & Hill, 1988). Casting may be used with children in an effort to enhance ROM and/or movement quality (Teplicky, Law, & Russell, 2002). Tona and Schneck (1993) conducted a single subject study using upper extremity casting. Their findings were positive regarding the effectiveness of the approach for that child. Law et al. (1997) conducted a well-designed group experimental study to determine the effects of standard occupational therapy treatment on young children's use of hand skills compared to an intervention program with upper extremity casting and intensive neurodevelopmental treatment. The study was conducted over a 10-month period. The children in the study appeared to benefit as much from standard occupational therapy treatment as from the more intensive treatment coupled with casting. Russell and Law (2003) noted that casting of the arm and hand may be useful for decreasing tone, increasing ROM, or enhancing movement but that these changes may not result in improved occupational performance. Changes in these areas, as well as the changes in biomechanical areas, need to be assessed in research studies.

Teplicky, Law, and Russell (2002) emphasized the need for additional research on the question of hand splinting in children who have suffered a traumatic head injury as well as those with cerebral palsy. In particular, they noted that although a number of studies have been reported in the literature, replication studies have not been conducted. Studies with groups of children and studies that replicate other research are needed to support clinical decision making regarding splinting and casting in children (Teplicky et al., 2002).

SUMMARY

This chapter presented a description of the components of hand and arm function that are instrumental in the performance of play, self-maintenance, schoolwork, and vocational readiness activities. Factors that influence the development of hand function and types of problems in hand and arm use were discussed. The normal sequences of development for basic skills of reach, grasp, release, and carry, as well as advanced functions of in-hand manipulation and bilateral hand use, were presented. Intervention strategies for development of various hand skills were described, as were appropriate uses of splinting with children. The therapist should always frame assessment of and intervention for hand and arm function problems in the context of the child's daily environments and his or her play, school, and activities of daily living.

STUDY QUESTIONS

1 What are the major considerations for intervention with an adolescent who has spastic hemiplegia; who demonstrates elbow flexion, forearm pronation, and fisting in the nonpreferred hand; and who is having difficulty completing manual dexterity tasks in his or her vocational readiness program?

2 A 5-year-old girl with marked involuntary movements of her arms and poor postural stability would like to feed herself. What aspects of arm and hand function would the therapist assess to determine if she can do this with or without adaptive equipment? What intervention strategies would the therapist use to promote the most effective grasp of the spoon and cup and achievement of the plate-to-mouth pattern? What types of splinting might the therapist consider?

3 A 6-year-old boy has a diagnosis of autism. He does not sustain eye contact with objects and shows limited hand contact with objects. How would the therapist begin to determine treatment priorities for him? What strategies would the therapist use to assess his hand skills and factors contributing to the limited use? Are in-hand manipulation skills a priority to address in treatment? Why or why not?

4 An 8-year-old boy has illegible handwriting. How may problems with bilateral hand use and in-hand manipulation skills interact with short attention span and somatosensory problems to contribute to his handwriting difficulties?

5 What aspects of reach, grasp, release, and bilateral hand use should the therapist address with a 15-month-old infant who has Down syndrome, associated limited hand function, and cognitive skills at the 8- to 10-month level?

6 A 10-year-old girl sustained a head injury 2 months ago. Before the accident she was left-hand dominant. She is now alert but has some memory deficits and motor planning problems. She has a left elbow contracture and shows moderately increased tone in wrist flexion, thumb adduction, and finger flexion. What types of splinting should the therapist consider? How can the therapist determine whether the splinting devices are effective treatment?

REFERENCES

American Occupational Therapy Association (AOTA). (2002). Occupational therapy practice framework: Domain and process. *American Journal of Occupational Therapy, 56,* 609-639.

Ayres, A.J. (1958). Ontogenetic principles in the development of arm and hand function. *American Journal of Occupational Therapy, 8,* 95-99.

Ayres, A.J. (1989). *Sensory Integration and Praxis Tests manual.* Los Angeles: Western Psychological Services.

Barnes, K.J. (1986). Improving prehension skills of children with cerebral palsy: A clinical study. *Occupational Therapy Journal of Research, 6* (4), 227-239.

Barnes, K.J. (1989a). Direct replication: Relationship of upper extremity weight bearing to hand skills of boys with cerebral palsy. *Occupational Therapy Journal of Research, 9,* 235-242.

Barnes, K.J. (1989b). Relationship of upper extremity weight bearing to hand skills of boys with cerebral palsy. *Occupational Therapy Journal of Research, 9,* 143-154.

Beckung, E., Steffenburg, U., & Uvebrant, P. (1997). Motor and sensory dysfunctions in children with mental retardation and epilepsy. *Seizure, 6,* 43-50.

Bertenthal, B., & von Hofsten, C. (1998). Eye, head and trunk control: The foundation for manual development. *Neuroscience and Biobehavioral Reviews, 22* (4), 515-520.

Bobath, B. (1978). *Adult hemiplegia: Evaluation and treatment* (2nd ed.). London: Heinemann.

Boehme, R.H. (1988). *Improving upper body control: An approach to assessment and treatment of tonal dysfunction.* Tucson: Therapy Skill Builders.

Boyd, R.N., Morris, M.E., & Graham, H.K. (2001). Management of upper limb dysfunction in children with cerebral palsy: A systematic review. *European Journal of Neurology, 8* (Suppl. 5), 150-166.

Bumin, G., & Kayihan, H. (2001). Effectiveness of two different sensory integration programmes for children with spastic diplegic cerebral palsy. *Disability and Rehabilitation, 23* (9), 394-399.

Bushnell, E.W., & Boudreau, J.P. (1999). Exploring and exploiting objects with the hands during infancy. In K.J. Connolly (Ed.), *The psychobiology of the hand* (pp. 144-161). London: Cambridge University Press.

Candler, C., & Meeuwsen, H. (2002). Implicit learning in children with and without developmental coordination disorder. *American Journal of Occupational Therapy, 56,* 429-435.

Case-Smith, J. (1991). The effects of tactile defensiveness and tactile discrimination on in-hand manipulation. *American Journal of Occupational Therapy, 45,* 811-818.

Case-Smith, J. (1993). Comparison of in-hand manipulation skills in children with and without fine motor delays. *Occupational Therapy Journal of Research, 13,* 87-100.

Case-Smith, J. (1996). Fine motor outcomes in preschool children who receive occupational therapy services. *American Journal of Occupational Therapy, 50,* 52-61.

Case-Smith, J. (2002). Effectiveness of school-based occupational therapy intervention on handwriting. *American Journal of Occupational Therapy, 56,* 17-25.

Case-Smith, J., Bigsby, R., & Clutter, J. (1998). Perceptual-motor coupling in the development of grasp. *American Journal of Occupational Therapy, 52,* 102-110.

Case-Smith, J., Fisher, A.G., & Bauer, D. (1989). An analysis of the relationship between proximal and distal motor control. *American Journal of Occupational Therapy, 43,* 657-662.

Case-Smith, J., Heaphy, T., Marr, D., Galvin, B., Koch, V., & Ellis, M.G., et al. (1998). Fine motor and functional outcomes in preschool children. *American Journal of Occupational Therapy, 52,* 788-796.

Chakarian, D.L., & Larson, M. (1991). The effects of upper extremity weight bearing on hand function in children with cerebral palsy. *NDTA Newsletter,* 4-5.

Colangelo, C.A. (1999). Biomechanical frame of reference. In P. Kramer & J. Hinojosa (Eds.), *Frames of reference for pediatric occupational therapy* (pp. 233-305). Philadelphia: Lippincott Williams & Wilkins.

Connolly, K., & Dalgleish, M. (1989). The emergence of a tool-using skill in infancy. *Developmental Psychology, 25,* 894-912.

Connor, F.P., Williamson, G.G., & Siepp, J.M. (1978). Movement. In *Program guide for infants and toddlers.* New York: College Press.

Cooper, J., Majnemer, A., Rosenblatt, B., & Birnbaum, R. (1995). The determination of sensory deficits in children with hemiplegic cerebral palsy. *Journal of Child Neurology, 10,* 300-309.

Corbetta, D., & Mounoud, P. (1990). Early development of grasping and manipulation. In C. Bard, M. Fleury, & L. Hay (Eds.), *Development of eye-hand coordination across the life span* (pp. 188-213). Columbia: University of South Carolina.

Couch, K.J., Dietz, J.C., & Kenny, E.M. (1998). The role of play in pediatric occupational therapy. *American Journal of Occupational Therapy, 52,* 111-117.

Crocker, M.D., MacKay-Lyons, M., & McDonnell, E. (1997). Forced use of the upper extremity in cerebral palsy: A single case design. *American Journal of Occupational Therapy, 5,* 824-833.

Damiano, D., & Abel, M.F. (1998). Functional outcomes of strength training in spastic cerebral palsy. *Archives of Physical Medicine and Rehabilitation 79,* 119-125.

Danella, E., & Vogtle, L. (1992). Neurodevelopmental treatment for the young child with cerebral palsy. In J. Case-Smith & C. Pehoski (Eds.), *Development of hand skills in the child* (pp. 91-110). Rockville, MD: American Occupational Therapy Association.

DeLuca, S.C., Echols, K., Ramey, S.L., & Taub, E. (2003). Pediatric constraint-induced movement therapy for a young child with cerebral palsy: Two episodes of care. *Journal of the American Physical Therapy Association, 83,* 1003-1013.

Doubilet, L., & Polkow, L.S. (1977). Theory and design of a finger abduction splint for the spastic hand. *American Journal of Occupational Therapy, 31* (5), 320-322.

Duff, S.V., & Gordon, A.M. (2003). Learning of grasp control in children with hemiplegic cerebral palsy. *Developmental Medicine and Child Neurology, 5* (11), 746-757.

Eliasson, A.C. (1995). Sensorimotor integration of normal and impaired development of precision movement of the hand. In A. Henderson & C. Pehoski (Eds.), *Hand function in the child* (pp. 40-54). St. Louis: Mosby.

Eliasson, A.C., & Gordon, A.M. (2000). Impaired force coordination during object release in children with hemiplegic cerebral palsy. *Developmental Medicine and Child Neurology, 42,* 228-234.

Elliott, J.M., & Connolly, K.J. (1984). A classification of manipulative hand movements. *Developmental Medicine and Child Neurology, 26,* 283-296.

Erhardt, R.P. (1982). *Erhardt Developmental Prehension Assessment.* Tucson: Therapy Skill Builders.

Exner, C.E. (1990a). In-hand manipulation skills in normal young children: A pilot study. *Occupational Therapy Practice, 1* (4), 63-72.

Exner, C.E. (1990b). The zone of proximal development in in-hand manipulation skills of nondysfunctional 3- and 4-year-old children. *American Journal of Occupational Therapy, 44,* 884-891.

Exner, C.E. (1992). In-hand manipulation skills. In J. Case-Smith & C. Pehoski (Eds.), *Development of hand skills in the child* (pp. 35-45). Rockville, MD: American Occupational Therapy Association.

Exner, C.E. (1995). Remediation of hand skill problems in children. In A. Henderson & C. Pehoski (Eds.), *Hand function in the child.* St. Louis: Mosby.

Exner, C.E., & Bonder, B.R. (1983). Comparative effects of three hand splints on the bilateral hand use, grasp, and arm-hand posture in hemiplegic children: A pilot study. *Occupational Therapy Journal of Research, 3,* 75-92.

Exner, C.E., & Henderson, A. (1995). Cognition and motor skill. In A. Henderson & C. Pehoski (Eds.), *Hand function in the child* (pp. 93-110). St. Louis: Mosby.

Fagard, J., & Jacquet, A.Y. (1989). Onset of bimanual coordination and symmetry versus asymmetry of movement. *Infant Behavior and Development, 12,* 229-236.

Fedrizzi, E., Pagliano, E., Andreucci, E., & Oleari, G. (2003). Hand function in children with hemiplegic cerebral palsy: Prospective follow-up and functional outcome in adolescence. *Developmental Medicine and Child Neurology, 45,* 85-91.

Finnie, N.R. (1975). *Handling the young cerebral palsied child at home* (2nd ed.). New York: E.P. Dutton.

Folio, R.M., & Fewell, R. (2000). *Peabody Developmental Motor Scales–Revised.* Chicago: Riverside.

Gabriel, L., & Duvall-Riley, B. (2000). Pediatric splinting. In B. Coppard (Ed.), *Introduction to splinting: A critical reasoning & problem solving approach* (pp. 396-443). San Diego: Technical Books.

Gesell, A., & Amatruda, C.S. (1947). *Developmental diagnosis.* New York: Harper & Row.

Glover, J.E., Mateer, C.A., Yoell, C., & Speed, S. (2002). The effectiveness of constraint-induced movement therapy in two young children with hemiplegia. *Pediatric Rehabilitation, 5,* 125-131.

Gordon, A.M., & Forssberg, H. (1997). Development of neural mechanisms underlying grasping in children. In K.J. Connolly & H. Forssberg (Eds.), *Neurophysiology and neuropsychology of motor development.* London: MacKeith Press.

Gordon, A.M., Lewis, S.R., Eliasson, A.C., & Duff, S.V. (2003). Object release under varying task constraints in children with hemiplegic cerebral palsy. *Developmental Medicine and Child Neurology, 45,* 240-248.

Gordon, A.W., & Duff, S.V. (1999). Relation between clinical measures and fine manipulative control in children with hemiplegic cerebral palsy. *Developmental Medicine and Child Neurology, 41,* 586-591.

Hanna, S.E., Law, M.C., Rosenbaum, P.L., King, G.A., Walter, S.D., & Pollock, N., et al. (2003). Development of hand function among children with cerebral palsy: Growth curve analysis for ages 16 to 70 months. *Developmental Medicine and Child Neurology, 45,* 448-455.

Haron, M., & Henderson, A. (1985). Active and passive touch in developmentally dyspraxic and normal boys. *Occupational Therapy Journal of Research, 5,* 101-112.

Henderson, A. (1995). Self-care and hand skill. In A. Henderson & C. Pehoski (Eds.), *Hand function in the child* (pp. 164-183). St. Louis: Mosby.

Hill, J. (1994). The effects of casting on upper extremity motor disorders after brain injury. *American Journal of Occupational Therapy, 48,* 219-224.

Hill, S.G. (1988). Current trends in upper extremity splinting. In R. Boehme (Ed.), *Improving upper body control* (pp. 131-164). Tucson: Therapy Skill Builders.

Hirschel, A., Pehoski, C., & Coryell, J. (1990). Environmental support and the development of grasp in infants. *American Journal of Occupational Therapy, 44,* 721-727.

Hohlstein, R.R. (1982). The development of prehension in normal infants. *American Journal of Occupational Therapy, 36*(3), 170-176.

Humphry, R., Jewell, K., & Rosenberger, R.C. (1995). Development of in-hand manipulation and relationship with activities. *American Journal of Occupational Therapy, 49,* 763-774.

Jeannerod, M. (1994). The hand and the object: The role of posterior parietal cortex in forming motor representations. *Canadian Journal of Physiology and Pharmacology, 72,* 535-541.

Johansson, R.S., & Westling, G. (1988). Coordinated isometric muscle commands adequately and erroneously programmed for the weight during lifting tasks with precision grip. *Experimental Brain Research, 71,* 59-71.

Kellor, Rost, Silberberg, Iversen, & Cummings (1971). Hand strength and dexterity. *American Journal of Occupational Therapy, 25,* 77-83.

Kenney, W.E. (1963). Certain sensory defects in cerebral palsy. *Clinical Orthopedics, 27,* 193-195.

Kinghorn, J., & Roberts, G. (1996). The effect of an inhibitive weight-bearing splint on tone and function: A single case study. *American Journal of Occupational Therapy, 50,* 807-815.

Krumlinde-Sundholm, L., & Eliasson, A.C. (2002). Comparing tests of tactile sensibility: Aspects relevant to testing children with spastic hemiplegia. *Developmental Medicine and Child Neurology, 44,* 604-612.

Kuhtz-Buschbeck, J.P., Stolze, H., Johnk, K., Boczek-Funcke, A., & Illert, M. (1998). Development of prehension movements in children: A kinematic study. *Experimental Brain Research, 122,* 424-432.

Law, M., Russell, D., Pollock, N., Rosenbaum, P., Walter, S., & King, G. (1997). A comparison of intensive neurodevelopmental therapy plus casting and a regular occupational therapy program for children with cerebral palsy. *Developmental Medicine and Child Neurology, 39,* 664-670.

Lawrence, D.G., & Kuypers, H.G. (1986). The functional organization of the motor system in monkey. I and II. *Brain, 91,* 1-36.

Lee-Valkov, P.M., Aaron, D.H., Eladoumikdachi, F., Thornby, J., & Netscher, D.T. (2003). Measuring normal hand dexterity values in normal 3-, 4-, and 5-year-old children and their relationship with grip and pinch strength. *Journal of Hand Therapy, 16,* 22-28.

Link, L., Lukens, S., & Bush, M.A. (1995). Spherical grip strength in children 3 to 6 years of age. *American Journal of Occupational Therapy, 49,* 318-326.

Long, C., Conrad, P.W., Hall, E.A., & Furler, S.L. (1970). Intrinsic-extrinsic muscle control of the hand in power grip and precision handling. *Journal of Bone and Joint Surgery, 52A,* 853-913.

Mandich, A.D., Polatajko, H.J., & Rodger, S. (2003). Rites of passage: Understanding participation of children with developmental coordination disorder. *Human Movement Science, 22,* 583-595.

Mandich, A.D., Polatajko, H.J., Missiuna, C., & Miller, L.T. (2001). Cognitive strategies and motor performance in children with developmental coordination disorder. *Physical and Occupational Therapy in Pediatrics, 20,* 125-143.

Mathiowetz, V., Rogers, S.L., Dowe-Keval, M., Donohoe, L., & Rennells, C. (1986). The Purdue Pegboard: Norms for 14- to 19-year-olds. *American Journal of Occupational Therapy, 40,* 174-179.

Mathiowetz, V., Weimer, D.M., & Federman, S.M. (1986). Grip and pinch strength: Norms for 6- to 19-year-olds. *American Journal of Occupational Therapy, 40,* 705-711.

McHale, K., & Cermak, S.A. (1992). Fine motor activities in elementary school: Preliminary findings and provisional implications for children with fine motor problems. *American Journal of Occupational Therapy, 46,* 898-903.

McKie Splints. (2003). *Grasp study: spastic cerebral palsy.* Retrieved December 31, 2003, from http://www.mckiesplints.com/research1.htm

McPherson, J.J. (1981). Objective evaluation of a splint designed to reduce hypertonicity. *American Journal of Occupational Therapy, 35,* 189-194.

Miller, L.T., Polatajko, H.J., Missiuna, C., Mandich, A.D., & Macnab, J.J. (2001). A pilot trial of a cognitive treatment for children with developmental coordination disorder. *Human Movement Science, 20,* 183-210.

Monfraix, C., Tardieu, G., & Tardieu, C. (1961). Disturbances of manual perception in children with cerebral palsy. *Developmental Medicine and Child Neurology, 22,* 454-464.

Myers, C.A. (1992). Therapeutic fine motor activities for preschoolers. In J. Case-Smith & C. Pehoski (Eds.), *Development of hand skills in the child* (pp. 47-59). Rockville, MD: American Occupational Therapy Association.

Napier, J.R. (1956). The prehensile movements of the human hand. *Journal of Bone Joint Surgery, 38B,* 902-913.

Pehoski, C. (1992). Central nervous system control of precision movements of the hand. In J. Case-Smith & C. Pehoski (Eds.), *Development of hand skills in the child* (pp. 1-11). Rockville, MD: American Occupational Therapy Association.

Pehoski, C. (1995). Cortical control of skilled movements of the hand. In A. Henderson & C. Pehoski (Eds.), *Hand function in the child* (pp. 3-15). St Louis: Mosby.

Pehoski, C., Henderson, A., & Tickle-Degnen, L. (1997a). In-hand manipulation in young children: Rotation of an object in the fingers. *American Journal of Occupational Therapy, 51,* 544-552.

Pehoski, C., Henderson, A., & Tickle-Degnen, L. (1997b). In-hand manipulation in young children: Translation movements. *American Journal of Occupational Therapy, 51,* 719-728.

Phelps, R.E., & Weeks, P.M. (1976). Management of thumb-in-palm web space contracture. *American Journal of Occupational Therapy, 30,* 543-556.

Pitcher, T.M., Piek, J.P., & Hay, D.A. (2003). Fine and gross motor ability in males with ADHD. *Developmental Medicine and Child Neurology, 45,* 525-535.

Ramsey, D.S., & Weber, S. (1986). Infant's hand preference in a task involving complementary roles for the two hands. *Child Development, 57,* 300-307.

Rosblad, B. (1995). Reaching and eye-hand coordination. In A. Henderson & C. Pehoski (Eds.), *Hand function in the child* (pp. 81-92). St. Louis: Mosby.

Ruff, H.A. (1980). The development of the perception and recognition of objects. *Child Development, 51,* 981-992.

Ruff, H.A., McCarton, C., Kurtzber, D., & Vaughan, H.G. Jr. (1984). Preterm infants' manipulative exploration of objects. *Child Development, 55,* 1166-1173.

Russell, D., & Law, M. (2003). *Casting-splinting-orthoses.* Retrieved December 30, 2003 from http://www-fhs.mcmaster.ca/canchild/publications/keepcurrent/KC95-2.html

Schneck, C., & Battaglia, C. (1992). Developing scissors skills in young children. In J. Case-Smith & C. Pehoski (Eds.), *Development of hand skills in the child* (pp. 79-89). Rockville, MD: American Occupational Therapy Association.

Schoemaker, M.M., Niemeijer, A.S., Reynders, K., & Smits-Engelsman, B.C. (2003). Effectiveness of neuromotor task training for children with developmental coordination disorder: A pilot study. *Neural Plasticity, 10,* 155-163.

Schoen, S., & Anderson, J. (1999). Neurodevelopmental treatment frame of reference. In P. Kramer & J. Hinojosa (Eds.), *Frames of reference for pediatric occupational therapy* (pp. 49-86). Baltimore: Williams & Wilkins.

Sheridan, M.D. (1975). *From birth to five years: Children's developmental progress.* Atlantic Highlands, NJ: Humanities Press.

Smith, R.O., & Benge, M.W. (1985). Pinch and grasp strength: Standardization of terminology and protocol. *American Journal of Occupational Therapy, 39,* 531-535.

Smith-Zuzovsky, N., & Exner, C.E. (2004). The effect of seated positioning quality on typical 6- and 7-year-old children's object manipulation skills. *American Journal of Occupational Therapy, 58,* 380-388.

Smits-Engelsman, B.C., Westenberg, Y., & Duysens, J. (2003). Development of isometric force and force control in children. *Cognitive Brain Research, 17,* 68-74.

Smits-Engelsman, B.C., Wilson, P.H., Westenberg, Y., & Duysens, J. (2003). Fine motor deficiencies in children with developmental coordination disorder and learning disabilities: An underlying open-loop control deficit. *Human Movement Science, 22,* 495-513.

Snook, J.H. (1979). Spasticity reduction splint. *American Journal of Occupational Therapy, 33,* 648-651.

Sterr, A., Freivogel, S., & Schmalohr, D. (2002). Neurobehavioral aspects of recovery: Assessment of the learned nonuse phenomenon in hemiparetic adolescents. *Archives of Physical Medicine and Rehabilitation, 83,* 1726-1731.

Stillwell, J.M., & Cermak, S.A. (1995). Perceptual functions of the hand. In A. Henderson & C. Pehoski (Eds.), *Hand function in the child* (pp. 55-80). St. Louis: Mosby.

Tachdjian, M.O., & Minear, W.I. (1958). Sensory disturbances in the hands of children with hemiplegia. *Journal of the American Medical Association, 155,* 628-632.

Taub, E., Aswatte, G., & Pidiki, R. (1999). Constraint-induced movement therapy: A new family of techniques with broad application to physical rehabilitation—a clinical review. *Journal of Rehabilitation Research and Development, 36,* 237-251.

Teplicky, R., Law, M., & Russell, D. (2002). The effectiveness of casts, orthoses, and splints for children with neurological disorders. *Infant and Young Children, 15,* (1), 42-50.

Thelen, E., Corbetta, D., Kamm, K., Spencer, J.P., Schneider, K., & Zernicke, R.F. (1993). The transition to reaching: Mapping intention and intrinsic dynamics. *Child Development, 64,* 1058-1098.

Tobias, M.V., & Goldkopf, I.M. (1995). Toys and games: Their role in hand development. In A. Henderson & C. Pehoski (Eds.), *Hand function in the child* (pp. 223-254). St. Louis: Mosby.

Tona, J.L., & Schneck, C.M. (1993). The efficacy of upper extremity inhibitive casting: A single-subject pilot study. *American Journal of Occupational Therapy, 47,* 901-910.

Twitchell, T.E. (1965). The automatic grasping responses of infants. *Neuropsychologics, 3,* 247-259.

Verdonck, M.C., & Henneberg, M. (1997). Manual dexterity of South African children growing in contrasting socioeconomic conditions. *American Journal of Occupational Therapy, 51,* 303-306.

von Hofsten, C. (1982). Eye-hand coordination in the newborn. *Developmental Psychology, 18,* (3), 450-461.

von Hofsten, C. (1991). Structuring of early reaching movements: A longitudinal study. *Journal of Motor Behavior, 23,* (4), 280-292.

Weaver, S., Gardner, E.R., Triolo, R.J., & Betz, R.R. (1990). Improvement of hand function in children with arthrogryposis following neuromuscular electrical stimulation (NMES): A preliminary report. *Journal of the Association of Children's Prosthetic-Orthotic Clinics, 25,* (2), 32.

Weiss, M.W., & Flatt, A.E. (1971). Functional evaluation of the congenitally anomalous hand. II. *American Journal of Occupational Therapy, 25,* 139-143.

Willis, J.K., Morello, A., Davie, A., Rice, J.C., & Bennett, J.T. (2002). Forced-use treatment of childhood hemiparesis. *Pediatrics, 110,* 94-96.

Wilson, B., & Trombly, C.A. (1984). Proximal and distal function in children with and without sensory integrative dysfunction: An EMG study. *Canadian Journal of Occupational Therapy, 51,* 11-17.

Wilson, P.H., Maruff, P., Ives, S., & Currie, J. (2001). Abnormalities of motor and praxis imagery in children with DCD. *Human Movement Science, 20,* 135-159.

Wingrat, J., & Exner, C.E. (2003). The impact of school furniture on fourth grade children's on-task and sitting behavior in the classroom: A pilot study. (under review)

Yasukawa, A. (1992). Upper extremity casting: Adjunct treatment for the child with cerebral palsy. In J. Case-Smith & C. Pehoski (Eds.), *Development of hand skills in the child* (pp. 111-123). Rockville, MD: American Occupational Therapy Association.

Yasukawa, A., & Hill, J. (1988). Casting to improve upper extremity function. In R. Boehme (Ed.), *Improving upper body control* (pp. 165-188). Tucson: Therapy Skill Builders.

Yekutiel, M., Jariwala, M., & Stretch, P. (1994). Sensory deficit in the hands of children with cerebral palsy: A new look at assessment and prevalence. *Developmental Medicine and Child Neurology, 36,* 619-624.

Yim, S.Y., Cho, J.R., & Lee, I.Y. (2003). Normative data developmental characteristics of hand function for elementary school children in Suwon area of Korea: Grip, pinch, and dexterity study. *Journal of Korean Medical Science, 18,* 552-558.

WEB SITES

Children's Hemiplegia and Stroke Association. (2002). *Handsplints.* Retrieved December 30, 2003, from http://www.hemikids.org/handsplints.htm

Children's Hemiplegia and Stroke Association. (2002). *Occupational Therapy.* Retrieved December 30, 2003, from http://www.hemikids.org/occupational.htm

Comfy Splints. (2000). *Pediatric Comfy Splints.* Retrieved December 31, 2003, from http://www.comfysplints.com/pediatric.htm

McKie Splints. (no date). *About us.* Retrieved December 31, 2003, from http://www.mckiesplints.com/about.htm

The Joe Cool Company. (no date). *Manufacturers of soft pediatric thumb abduction splints and gloves.* Retrieved December 31, 2003, from http://www.joecoolco.com

SUGGESTED READINGS

Ager, C.L., Olivett, B.L., & Johnson, C.L. (1984). Grasp and pinch strength in children 5 to 12 years old. *American Journal of Occupational Therapy, 38,* 107-113.

Blackwell, P.L. (2000). The influence of touch on child development: Implications for intervention, *Infants and Young Children, 13,* 25-39.

Blashy, M.R.M., & Fuchs, R.L. (1959). Orthokinetics: A new receptor facilitation method. *American Journal of Occupational Therapy, 13,* 226-234.

Bruni, M. (1998). *Fine motor skills in children with Down syndrome: A guide for parents and professionals.* Bethesda, MD: Woodbine House.

Cermak, S.A., & Larkin, D. (2002). *Developmental coordination disorder.* Albany, NY: Delmar.

Duff, S.V. (1995). Prehension. In D. Cech & S. Martin (Eds.), *Functional movement development across the life span* (pp. 313-353). Philadelphia: W.B. Saunders.

Eliasson, A.C., Gordon, A.M., & Forssberg, H. (1991). Basic co-ordination of manipulative forces of children with cerebral palsy. *Developmental Medicine and Child Neurology, 33,* 661-670.

Henderson, A., & Pehoski, C. (1995). *Hand function in the child.* St. Louis: Mosby.

Hogan, L., & Uditsky, T. (1998). *Pediatric splinting: Selection, fabrication, and clinical application of upper extremity splints.* San Antonio: Therapy Skill Builders.

Jensen, G.D., & Alderman, M.E. (1963). The prehensile grasp of spastic diplegia. *Pediatrics, 31,* 470-477.

Kopp, C.B. (1974). Fine motor abilities of infants. *Developmental Medicine and Child Neurology, 16,* 629-636.

Latch, C.M., Freeling, M.C., & Powell, N.J. (1993). A comparison of the grip strength of children with myelomeningocele to that of children without disability. *American Journal of Occupational Therapy, 47,* 498-503.

Magill, R.A. (1998). 1997 McCloy Research Lecture: Knowledge is more than we can talk about: Implicit learning in motor skill acquisition. *Research Quarterly for Exercise and Sport, 69,* (2), 104-110.

Mandich, A.D., Polatajko, H.J., Macnab, C., & Miller, L.T. (2001). Treatment of children with developmental coordination disorder: What is the evidence? *Physical and Occupational Therapy in Pediatrics, 20,* (2/3), 51-68.

Mandich, A.D., Polatajko, H.J., Missiuna, C., & Miller, L.T. (2001). Cognitive strategies and motor performance in children with developmental coordination disorder. *Physical and Occupational Therapy in Pediatrics, 20,* (2/3), 125-143.

Missiuna, C., Mandich, A.D., Polatajko, H.J., & Malloy-Miller, T. (2001). Cognition orientation to daily occupational performance (CO-OP). I. Theoretical foundations. *Physical and Occupational Therapy in Pediatrics, 20,* (2/3), 69-81.

Ruff, H.A. (1982). Role of manipulation in infants' responses to invariant properties of objects. *Developmental Psychology, 18,* 682-691.

Sugden, D.A., & Keogh, J.F. (1990). *Problems in movement skill development.* Columbia: University of South Carolina.

CHAPTER 11 Sensory Integration

L. Diane Parham ■ Zoe Mailloux

KEY TERMS

Sensory nourishment
Adaptive responses
Neural plasticity
Sensory processing
Sensory modulation
Underresponsiveness
Sensory registration
Sensation seeking
Overresponsiveness
Sensory discrimination

Vestibular-
  proprioceptive
  problems
Praxis
Dyspraxia
Classical sensory inte-
  gration treatment
Compensatory skill
  development

CHAPTER OBJECTIVES

1 Explain the neurobiologic concepts that are basic to an individual's sensory integrative function.

2 Explain the link between sensory input from the environment and the child's adaptive response.

3 Describe the development of sensory integration from prenatal life through childhood.

4 Explain the clinical picture and hypothesized basis for problems in underresponsiveness, overresponsiveness, and sensory discrimination.

5 Describe vestibular-proprioceptive problems and the types of behaviors that children with these problems often demonstrate.

6 Define developmental dyspraxia, and identify examples of behaviors that might be observed in a young child with dyspraxia.

7 Relate the sensory integration frame of reference to childhood occupation and the Occupational Therapy Practice Framework

8 Discuss the clinical evaluation of sensory integration within a top-down assessment process.

9 Identify and describe tests, interviews, and instruments used to evaluate sensory integration.

10 Define and explain classical sensory integrative treatment, and discuss limitations and benefits of using such an intervention approach.

11 Explain some considerations for determining that individual therapy should focus on compensatory skill development.

12 Describe group therapy programs and consultative models, and explain the benefits and limitations of using these models in combination with, or instead of, classical treatment.

13 Identify the expected outcomes of an occupational therapy program using a sensory integrative approach.

14 Discuss the published research on the effectiveness of sensory integration.

The term sensory integration holds special meaning for occupational therapists. In some contexts it is used to refer to a particular way of viewing the neural organization of sensory information for functional behavior. In other situations this term refers to a clinical frame of reference for the assessment and treatment of people who have functional disorders in sensory processing. Both of these meanings originated in the work of A. Jean Ayres, an occupational therapist and educational psychologist whose brilliant clinical insights and original research revolutionized occupational therapy practice with children.

Ayres's ideas ushered in a new way of looking at children and understanding many of the developmental, learning, and emotional problems that arise during childhood. Her innovative practice and groundbreaking research met a tremendous amount of resistance within the profession when introduced in the late 1960s and 1970s. Today, the treatment methods that she pioneered continue to be questioned and investigated, but there is little doubt that her perspective has had a profound influence on occupational therapy practice. The presence of sensory integration concepts in nearly all of the chapters of this book attests to the extent to which these ideas have affected the thinking of pediatric occupational therapists. Furthermore, the research base of the sensory integration frame of reference is extensive. More research has been conducted in the area of sensory integration than in any other area of occupational therapy.

This chapter provides an in-depth orientation to this fascinating aspect of occupational therapy practice. The reader will gain a general sense of how sensory integration as a brain function is related to everyday occupations. Following is a description of how sensory integration is manifested in typically developing children and in relation to the daily-life problems of children who experience difficulty with sensory integration. The history of research on sensory integrative dysfunction is reviewed to give the reader a perspective on how this field came into being, what the major constructs are, and how they have changed—and continue to change—over time. Sensory integration, as a clinical frame of reference, is described by identifying types of sensory integrative dysfunction, reviewing approaches to clinical assessment, and outlining the characteristics of both direct and indirect modes of intervention. The issue of effectiveness research is addressed. Case examples of children who have been helped by occupational therapists using sensory integrative principles are presented.

SENSORY INTEGRATION IN CHILD DEVELOPMENT

One of the most distinctive contributions that Ayres made to understanding child development was her focus on sensory processing, particularly with respect to the proximal senses (vestibular, tactile, and proprioceptive). From the sensory integration viewpoint, these senses are emphasized because they are primitive and primary; they dominate the child's interactions with the world early in life. The distal senses of vision and hearing are critical and become increasingly more dominant as the child matures. Ayres believed, however, that the body-centered senses are a foundation on which complex occupations are scaffolded. Furthermore, when Ayres began her work, the vestibular, tactile, and proprioceptive senses were virtually ignored by scholars and clinicians who were interested in child development. She devoted her career to studying the roles that these forgotten senses play in development and in the genesis of developmental problems of children.

Ayres's (1972b) basic assumption was that brain function is a critical factor in human behavior. She reasoned, therefore, that knowledge of brain function and dysfunction would give her insight into child development and would help her understand the developmental problems of children. However, Ayres also had a pragmatic orientation that sprang from her professional background as an occupational therapist. She was concerned particularly with how brain functions affected the child's ability to participate successfully in daily occupations. Consequently, her work represents a fusion of neurobiologic insights with the practical, everyday concerns of human beings, particularly children and their families.

As Ayres developed her ideas about sensory integration, she used terms such as *sensory integration, adaptive response,* and *praxis* in ways that reflected her orientation. A glossary of terms that are commonly used within the framework of sensory integration theory is presented in Appendix 11-A. It may be helpful to the reader to refer to these definitions frequently while reading this chapter.

Ayres coined some of the terms in Appendix 11-A, whereas other terms were drawn from the literature of other fields. When Ayres borrowed a term from another field, however, she imparted a particular meaning to it. For example, Ayres did not use the term *sensory integration* to refer solely to intricate synaptic connections within the brain, as neuroscientists typically do. Rather, she applied it to neural processes as they relate to functional behavior. Hence, her definition of sensory integration is the "organization of sensation for use" (Ayres, 1979, p. 5). It is the inclusion of the final clause "for use" that is Ayres's hallmark, because it ties sensory processing to the person's occupation.

Ayres introduced a new vocabulary of sensory integration theory and synthesized important concepts from the neurobiologic literature to organize her views of child development and dysfunction. Many of these ideas were first published in her classic book, *Sensory Integration and Learning Disorders* (Ayres, 1972b). Later she wrote a book for parents, *Sensory Integration and the Child* (Ayres, 1979, 2004), outlining the behavioral changes that can be observed in a child as sensory integration develops. Major points made in these books regarding neurobiologic concepts in relationship to development and the ontogeny of sensory integration are presented in the following sections.

NEUROBIOLOGICALLY BASED CONCEPTS

Sensory Nourishment

Sensory input is necessary for optimal brain function. The brain is designed to constantly take in sensory information, and it malfunctions if deprived of it. Sensory deprivation experiments conducted in the 1950s and 1960s make it clear that without an adequate inflow of sensation, the brain generates its own input in the form of hallucinations and subsequently distorts incoming sensory stimuli (Solomon et al., 1961). If adequate sensory stimulation is not available at critical periods in development, brain abnormalities and resulting behavioral disorders occur (Hubel & Wiesel, 1963; Jacobs & Schneider, 2001; Kolb & Whishaw, 1985). It is now well established that serious impairments in cognitive, social, and emotional functioning often result when infants and young children are institutionalized in environments that are impoverished with respect to availability of a wide range of sensory experiences, the presence of a nurturing caregiver, and opportunities for sensory-motor exploration (Cermak, 2001; Provence & Lipton, 1962).

Ayres (1979) considered sensory input to be *sensory nourishment* for the brain, just as food is nourishment for the body. Wilbarger (1984), a colleague of Ayres, built on this concept with her notion of the *sensory diet* designed specially for the child with sensory integrative dysfunction. The therapeutic sensory diet provides the optimal combination of sensations at the appropriate intensities for an individual child. For most typically developing children, the sensory diet does not require conscious monitoring by caregivers. The environment continuously "feeds" the child a variety of nourishing sensations in the flow of everyday life.

As critical as input is to the developing brain, the mere provision of sensory stimulation is limited in value. Too much stimulation can generate stress that is detrimental to brain development and may reduce the person's subsequent ability to cope with stress (Gunnar & Barr, 1998). To have an optimal effect, the child must actively organize and *use* sensory input to act on the environment.

Adaptive Response

A child does not passively absorb whatever sensations come along. Rather the child actively selects those sensations that are most useful at the time and organizes them in a fashion that facilitates accomplishing goals. This is the process of *sensory integration*. When this process is going well, the child organizes a successful, goal-directed action on the environment, which is called an adaptive response. When a child makes an adaptive response, he or she successfully meets some challenge presented in the environment. The adaptive response is possible because the brain has been able to efficiently organize incoming sensory information, which then provides a basis for action (Figure 11-1).

Adaptive responses are powerful forces that drive development forward. When a child makes an adaptive response that is more complex than any previously accomplished response, the brain attains a more organized state and its capacity for sensory integration is enhanced. Thus, sensory integration leads to adaptive responses, which in turn result in sensory integration that is more efficient.

Ayres (1979) provides the example of learning to ride a bicycle to illustrate this process. The child must integrate sensations, particularly from the vestibular and proprioceptive systems, to learn how to balance on the bicycle. The senses must accurately and quickly detect when the child begins to fall. Eventually, perhaps after many trials of falling, the child integrates sensory information efficiently enough to make the appropriate weight shifts over the bicycle to maintain balance. This is an adaptive response, and once made, the child is able to balance more effectively on the next attempt to ride the bike. The child's nervous system has changed and now is more adept at bicycle riding.

In making adaptive responses the child is an active doer, not a passive recipient. Adaptive responses come from within the child. No one can force a child to respond adaptively, although a situation may be set up

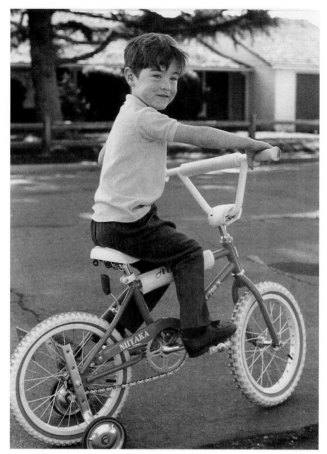

FIGURE 11-1 Adaptive responses help the child acquire skills such as riding a bicycle. Although training wheels reduce the challenge for this boy, his nervous system must integrate vestibular, proprioceptive, and visual information adequately to successfully steer the bicycle while it is moving. (Courtesy of Shay McAtee.)

that is likely to elicit adaptive responses from the child. For typically developing children and for most children with disabilities, there is an innate drive to develop sensory integration through adaptive responses. Ayres (1979) called this *inner drive* and speculated that it is generated primarily by the limbic system of the brain, a structure known to be critical in both motivation and memory. Ayres designed therapeutic activities and environments to engage the child's inner drive (elicit adaptive responses) and, in so doing, advance sensory integrative development and the child's occupational competence.

Neural Plasticity

It is thought that when a child makes an adaptive response, change occurs at a neuronal synaptic level. This change is a function of the brain's neural plasticity. Plasticity is the ability of a structure and concomitant function to be changed gradually by its own ongoing activity (Ayres, 1972b). It is well established in the neuroscientific literature that when organisms are permitted to explore interesting environments, significant increases in dendritic branching, synaptic connections, synaptic efficiency, and size of brain tissue result (Jacobs & Schneider, 2001). These changes are most dramatic in a young animal and probably represent a major mechanism of brain development, although it is clear that such manifestations of plasticity are characteristic of optimal brain functioning throughout the lifespan (Bach-Y-Rita, 1981).

Studies of the effects of enriched environments on animals indicate that the essential ingredient for positive brain changes is that the organism actively interacts with a meaningful and challenging environment (Bennett, Diamond, Krech, & Rosenzweig, 1964; Jacobs & Schneider, 2001). Passive exposure to sensory stimulation does not produce these same positive changes (Dru, Walker, & Walker, 1975). It can be hypothesized from these findings that adaptive responses activate the brain's neuroplastic capabilities. Furthermore, the brain's plasticity makes it possible for an adaptive response to increase the efficiency of sensory integration at a neuronal level.

Schaaf (1994) used the activity of learning to ride a bicycle to illustrate how neuroplasticity may be manifested in child behavior. She pointed out that a child first practices the basic skill of maintaining balance on the bicycle. Once this is mastered, the child uses it repeatedly in riding up and down the sidewalk for hours. After this is mastered, the child looks for greater challenges, such as riding up and down hills or jumping curbs. Schaaf interpreted these behaviors using concepts of developmental plasticity. First the child solidifies the necessary neural pathways for bike riding and then later enhances or modifies these pathways by creating challenging environments. Schaaf further drew a parallel between this process and the opportunities that are afforded a child during sensory integrative treatment.

Central Nervous System Organization

Ayres (1972b) looked to the organization of the central nervous system (CNS) for clues as to how children organize and use sensory information and how sensory integration develops over time. At the time that she was developing her theory, *hierarchic* models of the CNS dominated thinking in the neurosciences.

Hierarchic models view the nervous system in terms of vertically arranged levels, with the spinal cord at the bottom, the cerebral hemispheres at the top, and the brainstem sandwiched in between. These levels are interdependent yet reflect a trend of ascending control and specialization. Thus, the cerebral cortex at the top of the hierarchy is highly specialized and analyzes precise details of sensory information. Ordinarily the cortex assumes a directive role over lower levels of the hierarchy. For example, the cortex may command lower centers to "ignore" certain stimuli deemed unimportant. This process is called *descending inhibition* and is critical in enabling higher brain functions to work efficiently (Ayres, 1972b). The lower levels of the CNS, however, have functions that are more diffuse, primitive, less specialized, and yet potentially more pervasive in influence compared with those of the higher levels. One of the important responsibilities of the lower levels is to filter and refine sensory information before relaying organized sensory messages upward to the cerebral cortex. Thus, cortical centers are dependent on lower centers for the receipt of essential, well-organized sensory information to analyze in preparation for the planning of action. According to hierarchic views, the higher levels of the CNS superimpose functions that are more sophisticated on the lower levels, but these do not replace the important lower-level functions (Ayres).

Ayres (1972b) believed that critical aspects of sensory integration are seated in the lower levels of the CNS, particularly the brainstem and thalamus. Most of the CNS processing of vestibular information occurs in the brainstem, and much somatosensory processing takes place there and in the thalamus. One of the basic tenets of Ayres's theory is that, because of the dependence of higher CNS structures on lower structures, increased efficiency at the levels of the brainstem and thalamus enhance higher-order functioning (Ayres). This view is in sharp contrast to mainstream neuropsychology and education, which tend to emphasize the direct study and remediation of high-level, cortically directed skills such as reading and writing.

In adopting a hierarchic view of the CNS, Ayres (1972b) also assumed that the CNS develops hierarchically from bottom to top, with spinal and brainstem structures maturing before higher-level centers. At the time that Ayres was developing her theory, this was somewhat speculative although generally accepted by neuroscientists. In research conducted in more recent years, the use of positron electron tomography (PET) scans on infants has provided direct support for the notion that brain development proceeds in a bottom-to-top direction (Chugani & Phelps, 1986).

The hierarchic approach to CNS functioning and development led Ayres to emphasize the more primitive vestibular and somatosensory systems in her work with young children. These systems mature early and are seated in the lower CNS centers (particularly the brainstem, cerebellum, and thalamus). Using the logic of hierarchy, Ayres reasoned that the refinement of primitive functions, such as postural control, balance, and tactile perception, provides a sensorimotor foundation for higher-order functions, such as academic ability, behavioral self-regulation, and complex motor skills (e.g., those required in sports). Thus, she viewed the developmental process as one in which primitive body-centered functions serve as building blocks upon which complex cognitive and social skills can be scaffolded. This view undergirds a basic premise of the therapy approach that she developed: by enhancing lower-level functions related to the proximal senses, one might have a positive influence on higher-level functions.

On some points Ayres (1972b) departed from a strictly hierarchic view of the CNS. For example, she noted that each level of the CNS can function as a self-contained sensory integration system. Therefore the brainstem has the capacity to independently direct some sensorimotor patterns without being directed by the higher-level cortex. Furthermore, the sensory integrative process involves the brain working as a whole, not simply as a series of hierarchically controlled messages, as rigid hierarchic models might suggest. These ideas are more consistent with the view of some contemporary biologists that the brain is a *heterarchic* system. A heterarchy is a system in which different parts may assume the controlling role in different situations; control does not always flow in a top-down direction (Salthe, 1985). Ayres was ahead of her time in suggesting that the brain does not operate exclusively as a hierarchy but has holistic characteristics. These heterarchic notions strengthened her view that functions considered primitive were worthy of serious consideration in therapy.

SENSORY INTEGRATIVE DEVELOPMENT AND CHILDHOOD OCCUPATIONS

Ayres (1979) believed that the first 7 years of life is a period of rapid development in sensory integration. She drew this conclusion not only from her many years of observing children, but also from research in which she gathered normative data on tests of sensory integration (Ayres, 1972b). By the time most children reach 7 or 8 years of age, their scores on standardized tests of sensory integrative capabilities reflect almost as much maturity as an adult's.

Development, from a sensory integrative standpoint, occurs as the CNS organizes sensory information and adaptive responses with increasing degrees of complexity. Sensory integration, of course, enables adaptive responses to occur, which in turn promote the *development of sensory integration* and the emergence of occupational engagement and social participation (Parham, 2002; Spitzer & Roley, 2001). As this process unfolds in infancy, the developing child begins to attach meaning to the stream of sensations experienced. The child becomes increasingly adept at shifting attention to what he or she perceives as meaningful, tuning out that which is irrelevant to current needs and interests. As a result the child can organize play behavior for increasing lengths of time and gains control in the regulation of emotions.

Inner drive leads the child to search for opportunities in the environment that are "just right challenges." These are challenges that are not so complex that they overwhelm or induce failure, nor so simple that they are routine or disinteresting. The just right challenge is one that requires effort but is accomplishable for the child. Because there is an element of challenge, a successful adaptive response engenders feelings of mastery and a sense of oneself as a competent being.

It is fascinating to watch this process unfold. Most children require no adult guidance or teaching to acquire basic developmental skills such as manipulating objects, sitting, walking, and climbing. Little if any step-by-step instruction is needed to learn daily occupations such as playing on playground equipment, dressing and feeding oneself, drawing and painting, and constructing with blocks. These achievements seem to just happen. They are the product of an active nervous system busily organizing sensory information and searching for challenges that bring forth behaviors that are more complex, all shaped within the context of a world saturated with sociocultural expectations and meanings (Parham, 2002).

In the following sections, developmental hallmarks of sensory integration are identified and connected to the occupational achievements of childhood. The proximal senses dominate early infancy and continue to exert their influence in critical ways as the visual and auditory systems gain ascendancy. Although there is some variability across children in the sequence in which developmental achievements unfold during the first year of life, this variability becomes increasingly apparent after this first year. By kindergarten age, skills vary tremendously among children because of differences in environmental opportunities, familial and cultural influences, personal experiences, and genetic endowment. It is important to keep in mind that, throughout development, sensory integrative processes contribute to the child's construction of his or her identity, but many other influences are powerful as well—the family and cultures that shape the child's occupational routines, the interpretations given to the child's behaviors by others, the child's talents and abilities, and even chance events that carry special meaning to the child (Parham, 2002).

Prenatal Period

The first known responses to sensory stimuli occur early in life, at approximately $5\frac{1}{2}$ weeks after conception (Humphrey, 1969). These first responses are to tactile stimuli. Specifically, they involve reflexive avoidance reactions to a perioral stimulus (e.g., the embryo bends its head and upper trunk away from a light touch stimulus around the mouth). This is a primitive protective reaction. It is not until about 9 weeks' gestational age that an approach response (moving of the head toward the chest) occurs (Humphrey, 1969), probably as a function of proprioception.

The first known responses to vestibular input in the form of the Moro reflex also appear at about 9 weeks' postconception. The fetus continues to develop a repertoire of reflexes such as rooting, sucking, Babkin, grasp, flexor withdrawal, Galant, neck righting, Moro, and positive supporting in utero that are fairly well established by the time of birth. Thus, when the time comes to leave the uterus, the newborn is well equipped with the capacity to form a strong bond with a caregiver and to actively participate in the critical occupation of nursing. These innate capacities require rudimentary aspects of sensory integration that are built into the nervous system. However, even in this earliest period of development, environmental influences, such as maternal stress, may have a significant impact on the quality of sensory integrative development. For example, Schneider and her colleagues (1992, 1998) found that infant rhesus monkeys born to mothers who had experienced stress in early pregnancy had signs of diminished responses to vestibular input, such as impaired righting responses, weak muscle tone, and attenuated postrotary nystagmus.

Neonatal Period

Touch, smell, and movement sensations are particularly important to the newborn infant, who uses these to maintain contact with a caregiver through nursing, nuzzling, and cuddling. Tactile sensations, especially, are critical in establishing a primary attachment relationship with a caregiver and fostering feelings of security in the infant. This is just the beginning of the important role that the tactile system plays in a person's emotional life because it is directly involved in making physical contact with others (Figure 11-2). Proprioception is also critical in the mother-infant relationship, enabling the infant to mold to the adult caregiver's body in a cuddly manner. The phasic movements of the infant's limbs generate additional proprioceptive inputs. Together, all of these tactile and proprioceptive inputs set the stage for the eventual development of body scheme (the brain's map of the body and how its parts interrelate).

The vestibular system is fully functional at birth, although refinement of its sensory integrative functions, particularly its integration with visual and proprioceptive systems, continues through childhood. Of all the sensory systems, the vestibular system is the first to mature (Maurer & Maurer, 1988). Most caregivers who use rocking and carrying to soothe and calm the infant instinctively appreciate the influence of vestibular stimuli on the infant's arousal level. Ayres (1979) pointed out that sensations such as these, which make a child contented and organized, tend to be integrating for the child's nervous system.

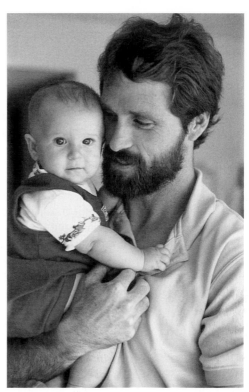

FIGURE 11-2 Tactile sensations play a critical role in generating feelings of security and comfort in the infant and are influential in emotional development and social relationships throughout the life span. (Courtesy of Shay McAtee.)

Experiences that activate the vestibular sense have other integrating effects on the infant as well. Being lifted into an upright position against the caregiver's shoulder is known to increase alertness and visual pursuit (Gregg, Hafner, & Korner, 1976). While being held in such a position, the young infant's vestibular system detects the pull of gravity and begins to stimulate the neck muscles to raise the head off the caregiver's shoulder. This adaptive response reaches full maturation within 6 months. In the first month of life, head righting may be minimal and intermittent with much wobbling, but it will gradually stabilize and become firmly established as the baby assumes different positions (first when the baby lies in a prone position and later in the supine position).

The visual and auditory systems of the newborn are immature. The newborn orients to some visual and auditory inputs and is particularly interested in human faces and voices, although meaning is not yet attached to these sensations. Visually the infant is attracted to high-contrast stimuli, such as black and white designs, and the range of visual acuity for most stimuli is limited to approximately 10 inches. The infant's visual acuity and responsiveness to visual patterns expand dramatically over the first few months of life (Maurer & Maurer, 1988). During this time the infant begins to use eye contact to relate to the caregiver, further strengthening the bond between them.

Stimulation in each of the sensory systems potentially affects the infant's state of arousal. The infant's capacity to behaviorally adapt to changing sensations is another important aspect of sensory integrative development—the development of self-regulation. It is relatively easy to overstimulate young infants, for example, with changes in water temperature, changes in body position, or an increases in auditory or visual stimuli (Schaaf & Anzalone, 2001). However, as sensory integration develops, the older child is better able to self-regulate his or her responses to changing stimuli by initiating behaviors that will be calming and soothing (such as thumb sucking or cuddling with a favorite blanket) or exciting and energizing (such as jumping or singing) (Reeves, 2001). This process of self-regulation begins in the neonatal period and develops throughout early childhood.

First 6 Months

By 4 to 6 months of age, a shift occurs in the infant's behavioral organization. The sensory systems have matured to the extent that the baby has much greater awareness and interest in the world, and developing vestibular-proprioceptive-visual connections provide the beginnings of postural control. During the first half of the first year, the infant begins to show a strong inner drive to rise up against gravity (Figure 11-3), and this drive is evident in much of the baby's spontaneous play. Body positions during the first 6 months characteristically involve the prone position, with gradually increasing extension from the neck down through the trunk and arms gradually bearing more weight to help push the chest off the floor. By 6 months of age, many infants spend a great deal of time in the prone position with full

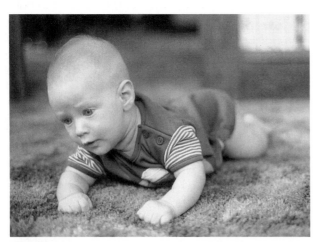

FIGURE 11-3 Strong inner drive to master gravity is evident in this infant's efforts to lift his head and shoulders off the floor. This is an early form of the prone extension posture. (Courtesy of Shay McAtee.)

active trunk extension, and most are able to sit independently, at least if propped with their own hands. These body positions usually are the infant's preferred positions for play and are reflective of the maturing lateral vestibulospinal tract. Head control is well established by 6 months of age and provides a stable base for control of eye muscles. This, of course, reflects the growing integration of vestibular, proprioceptive, and visual systems, which becomes increasingly important in providing a stable visual field as the baby becomes mobile.

Somatosensory achievements at this time are particularly evident in the infant's hands. The infant uses tactile and proprioceptive sensations to grasp objects, albeit with primitive grasps. Touch and visual information are integrated as the baby begins to reach for and wave or bang objects. The infant has a strong inner drive to play with the hands by bringing them to midline while watching and touching them. Connections between the tactile and visual systems pave the way for later hand-eye coordination skills. In addition, midline hand play is a significant milestone in the integration of sensations from the two sides of the body.

By now, neonatal reflexes no longer dominate behavior; the baby is beginning to exercise voluntary control over movements during play. The earliest episodes of motor planning occur as the infant works to produce novel actions. This becomes evident as the infant handles objects and begins to initiate transitions from one body position to another, as in rolling from prone position to supine. Although reflexes play a role in such actions (such as grasp and neck righting reflexes), the infant's actions have a goal-directed, volitional quality and are not stereotypically reflex bound. The emergence of intentionality is a marker of the beginning of occupational engagement.

Second 6 Months

Another major transition occurs during the latter half of the first year. Infants become mobile in their environments, and by the first birthday they can willfully move from one place to another, many walking while others creep or crawl. These locomotor skills are the product of the many adaptive responses that have gone before, resulting in increasingly more sophisticated integration of somatosensory, vestibular, and visual inputs.

As the infant explores the environment, greater opportunities are generated for integrating a variety of complex sensations, particularly those responsible for developing body scheme and spatial perception. The child learns about environmental space and about the body's relationship to external space through sensorimotor experiences.

During the second 6 months after birth, tactile perception becomes further refined and plays a critical role in the child's developing hand skills. The infant relies on precise tactile feedback in developing a fine pincer grasp, which is used to pick up small objects. Proprioceptive information is also an important influence in developing manipulative skills, and now the baby experiments with objects using a variety of actions. These somatosensory-based adaptive responses contribute to development of motor planning ability. Further development of midline skills is also apparent as the baby easily transfers objects from one hand to the other and may occasionally cross the midline while holding an object.

Through the first year, auditory processing plays a significant role in the infant's awareness of environment, especially the social environment. Auditory information is integrated with tactile and proprioceptive sensations in and around the mouth as the infant vocalizes. The fruits of this process begin to blossom in the latter half of this first year, when the infant begins to experiment with creating the sounds of the language used by caregivers. Vocalizations such as consonant-vowel repetitions ("baba" and "mamama") are common. Parents often attach meaning to these infant vocalizations and strongly encourage them, thus leading the infant also to attach meaning to these sounds. By their first birthday, many infants have a small vocabulary of words or word-like sounds that they use meaningfully to communicate desires to caregivers.

Another major landmark toward the end of the first year is beginning independence in self-feeding. This complex achievement requires refined somatosensory processing of information from the lips, the jaw, and inside the mouth to guide oral movements in the chewing and swallowing of food. Taste and smell sensations are also integral to this process, but self-feeding involves more than the mouth. All of the acquired sensory integrative milestones involving hand-eye coordination are important to self-feeding. The infant at this period of life uses the fingers directly to feed him or herself and to explore the textures of foods. At this stage, use of a utensil such as a spoon is not very functional and is messy because motor planning skills have not progressed to the point that the child can manipulate the utensil successfully. However, many infants begin to demonstrate a drive to use the spoon in self-feeding by the end of the first year. For many contemporary American infants, use of a spoon is the first real experience in using a tool (Figure 11-4).

The occupation of dining, then, begins to emerge in infancy as sensory integrative abilities mature, allowing the child to engage in self-feeding. As an occupation, dining in its fullest sense goes far beyond the physical, sensorimotor act of feeding. Dining usually takes place within a social context, whether at a family dinner at home or in a formal restaurant, so social standards for acceptable behavior and etiquette become increasingly important as the child develops. Furthermore, partaking

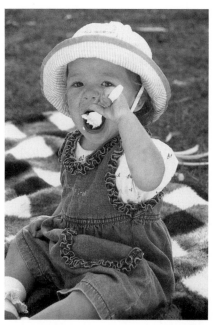

FIGURE 11-4 Because somatosensory processing and visual-motor coordination strongly influence self-feeding skills, sensory integration is an important contributor to the development of dining, a fundamental occupation. (Courtesy of Shay McAtee.)

in a meal and sharing certain types of food gradually come to take on powerful symbolic meanings. The sensory integrative underpinnings of the dining experience influence how the child experiences mealtimes and how others view the child as a dining partner, thus playing a role in shaping the social and symbolic aspects of this vitally important occupation.

Second Year

As the child moves into the second year, the basic vestibular-proprioceptive-visual connections that were laid down earlier continue to refine, resulting in growing finesse in balance and fluidity of dynamic postural control. Discrimination and localization of tactile sensations also become much more precise, allowing for further refinement of fine motor skills.

Increasingly complex somatosensory processing contributes to the continuing development of body scheme. Ayres (1972b) hypothesized that as body scheme becomes more sophisticated, so does motor planning ability. This is because the child draws on knowledge of how the body works to program novel actions (Figure 11-5). Throughout the second year, the typically developing toddler experiments with many variations in body movements. Imitation of the actions of others contributes further to the child's movement repertoire. In experiencing new actions, the child generates new sensory experiences, thus building an elaborate base of information from which to plan future actions.

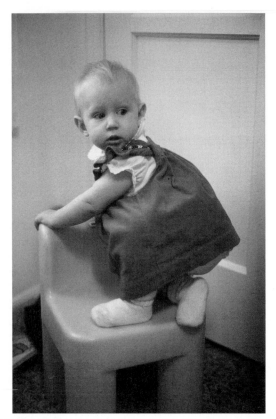

FIGURE 11-5 As motor planning develops during the second year of life, the infant experiments with a variety of body movements and learns how to transition easily from one position to another. These experiences are thought to reflect the development of body scheme. (Courtesy of Shay McAtee.)

While motor planning ability becomes increasingly more complex in the second year, another aspect of praxis, ideation, begins to emerge. Ideation is the ability to conceptualize what to do in a given situation. Ideation is made possible by the cognitive ability to use symbols, first expressed gesturally and then vocally during the second year of life (Bretherton et al., 1981). Symbolic functioning enables the child to engage in pretend actions and to imagine doing actions, even actions that the child has never before done. By the end of the second year, the toddler can join several pretend actions in a play sequence (McCune-Nicolich, 1981). Furthermore, the 2-year-old child demonstrates that he or she has a plan before performing an action sequence, either through a verbal announcement or through a search for a needed object (McCune-Nicolich, 1981). Thus, a surge in practic development occurs in the second year as the child generates many new ideas for actions and begins to plan actions in a systematic sequence.

The burgeoning of praxis abilities plays an important role in the development of self-concept. Infant psychiatrist Daniel Stern (1985) suggests that the sense of an integrated core self begins in infancy as an outcome of the volition and the proprioceptive feedback involved in motor planning. The consequences of the child's voluntary, planned actions add to the developing sense of self as an active agent in the world. As praxis takes giant leaps during the second year, so does this sense of self as an agent of power. The child feels in command of his or her own life when sensory integration allows the child to move freely and effectively through the world (Ayres, 1979).

Third through Seventh Years

The child's competencies in the sensorimotor realm mature in the third through seventh years of life, which Ayres (1979) considered a crucial period for sensory integration because of the brain's receptiveness to sensations and its capacity for organizing them at this time. This is the period when sensorimotor functions become consolidated as a foundation for higher intellectual abilities. Although further sensory integrative development can and usually does occur beyond the eighth birthday, the changes that take place are likely to be far more limited than those that occurred earlier.

In the third through seventh years, children have strong inner drives to produce adaptive responses that not only meet complicated sensorimotor demands but also sometimes require interfacing with peers. The challenges posed by children's games and play activities attest to this complexity. In the visual-motor realm, sophistication develops through involvement in crafts, drawing and painting, constructional play with blocks and other building toys, and video games (Figure 11-6). Children are driven to explore playground equipment by swinging, sliding, climbing, jumping, riding, pushing, pulling, and pumping. Toward the end of this period they enthusiastically grapple with the motor planning challenges posed by games such as jump rope, jacks, marbles, and hopscotch. It is also during this period that children become expert with cultural tools such as scissors, pencils, zippers, buttons, forks and knives, pails, shovels, brooms, and rakes (Figure 11-7). Many children begin to participate in occupations that present sensorimotor challenges for years to come, such as soccer, softball, karate, gymnastics, playing a musical instrument, and ballet. Furthermore, children develop the ability to organize their behavior into more complex sequences over longer time frames. This makes it possible for them to become more autonomous in orchestrating daily routines, such as getting ready for school in the morning, completing homework and other school projects, and performing household chores.

As children participate in these occupations, they must frequently anticipate how to move in relation to changing environmental events by accurately timing and sequencing their actions (Fisher, Murray, & Bundy,

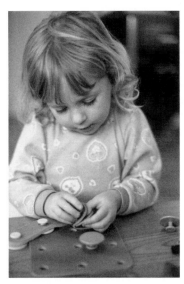

FIGURE 11-6 Adaptive responses involved in this activity require precise tactile feedback and sophisticated praxis. During activities such as this one, the preschooler becomes adept at handling tools and objects that are encountered in daily occupations throughout life. (Courtesy of Shay McAtee.)

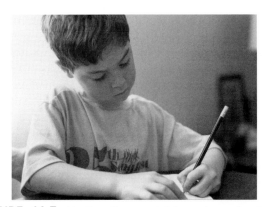

FIGURE 11-7 By the time a child reaches school age, sensory integrative capacities are almost mature. The child now can devote full attention to the demands of academic tasks because basic sensorimotor functions, such as maintaining an upright posture and guiding hand movements while holding a tool, have become automatic. (Courtesy of Shay McAtee.)

1991). This is particularly challenging in sports when peers, with their often unpredictable moves, are involved. Their bodies are challenged to maintain balance through dynamic changes in body position. In fine motor tasks, children must efficiently coordinate visual with somatosensory information to guide eye and hand movements with accuracy and precision while maintaining a stable postural base.

Children meet these challenges with varying degrees of success. Some are more talented than others with respect to sensory integrative abilities, but most children eventually achieve a degree of competency that allows

them to fully participate in the daily occupations that they are expected to do and wish to do at home, in school, and in the community. Furthermore, most children experience feelings of satisfaction and self-efficacy as they master those occupations that are heavily dependent on sensory integration.

WHEN PROBLEMS IN SENSORY INTEGRATION OCCUR

Unfortunately, not every child experiences competency in sensory integration. When some aspect of sensory integration does not function efficiently, the child may experience stress in the course of everyday occupations because processes that should be automatic or accurate are not. It may be stressful, for example, to simply maintain balance when sitting in a chair, to get dressed in the morning before school, to attempt to play jump rope, or to eat lunch in a socially acceptable manner. The child is aware of these difficulties and becomes frustrated by frequent failure when confronted with ordinary tasks that come easily for other children. Many children with sensory integrative problems develop a tendency to avoid or reject simple sensory or motor challenges, responding with refusals or tantrums when pushed to perform. If this becomes a long-term pattern of behavior, the child may miss important experiences, such as playing games with peers, which are critical in building feelings of competency, mastering a wide repertoire of useful skills, and developing flexible social strategies. Thus, the capacity to participate fully in the occupations that the child wants to do and needs to do is compromised.

Often behavioral, social, academic, or motor coordination concerns are cited when a child with a sensory integrative dysfunction is referred to occupational therapy. The occupational therapist needs to evaluate whether a sensory processing problem may underlie these concerns. The therapist then must decide on a course of action to help the child move toward the goal of greater success and satisfaction in doing meaningful occupations. These challenges to the therapist—to identify a problem that may be hidden and to figure out how to best help the child—were the challenges to which Ayres devoted most of her career.

As mentioned previously, Ayres turned to the neurobiologic literature to give her insight into understanding children's learning and behavior problems. Ayres also took on the responsibility of conducting research to develop her theory of sensory integration. In doing so, she produced a diagnostic system for clinical evaluation of children through the use of standardized tests. She also conducted research that was designed to evaluate the effectiveness of her treatment methods. After each study, Ayres always returned to her theory to revise and refine it in light of research findings. While she was doing this, she maintained a private practice; thus, she had many years of firsthand, clinically based experience on which to ground her theoretic work.

The following sections examine the research that Ayres conducted to identify different types of sensory integrative dysfunction in children. The general categories of sensory integrative dysfunction that concern clinicians today, based on research findings and clinical experience, are discussed. The field of sensory integration continues to be a dynamic field that changes as future research generates new findings and as future experiences of clinicians generate new ways of interpreting those findings.

RESEARCH BASE FOR SENSORY INTEGRATIVE DYSFUNCTION

Throughout her professional career, Ayres was guided by her keen observation skills and her search to reach a deeper understanding of the clinical problems that she encountered in practice. To begin answering the questions that arose as she worked with children, Ayres initiated the process of developing standardized tests of sensory integration during the 1960s. She originally developed these tests solely as research tools to aid in theory development. At the time, she was working with children with learning disabilities, many of whom she suspected had covert difficulties processing sensory information, and she sought to uncover the nature of whatever sensory integrative difficulties might exist. It was after her initial efforts at research using her tests that other therapists asked to have access to the tests, instigating their publication by Western Psychological Services.

The first group of tests Ayres created was published as the Southern California Sensory Integration Tests (SCSIT) (Ayres, 1972c). These were later revised and renamed the Sensory Integration and Praxis Tests (SIPT) (Ayres, 1989). Normative data were collected on a regional scale for the SCSIT and on a national scale for the SIPT. The tests were designed to measure aspects of visual, tactile, kinesthetic, and vestibular sensory processing as well as motor planning abilities.

Using first the SCSIT and later the SIPT with samples of children, Ayres used a statistical procedure called *factor analysis* to develop a typology of sensory integrative function and dysfunction. Tables 11-1 and 11-2 summarize results of her factor analytic studies, along with results of several studies conducted by other researchers. In factor analysis, sets of test scores are grouped according to their associations with one another. The resulting groups of associated test scores are called *factors*. Ayres interpreted the factors that emerged from her studies as representative of neural substrates underlying learning and behavior in children. For example, in her 1965 study, Ayres found that the tactile tests correlated highly with the motor planning tests,

forming a factor. She hypothesized that there is an ability called *motor planning* that is dependent on somatosensory processing and influences one's interactions with the physical world. *Apraxia* is the term she used to identify a disorder in this ability. In her later work, she subsumed the notion of motor planning under the construct of praxis and replaced the term *apraxia* with dyspraxia when referring to children.

In her last set of analyses with the SIPT, just before her death in 1988, Ayres used both factor analysis and another statistical technique called *cluster analysis,* which groups together children with similar SIPT profiles (see Table 11-1). This approach was used to further carve out diagnostic groupings of children that might be useful clinically. Today, consideration of both factor analysis and cluster groupings is a critical component in the interpretation of a child's SIPT scores.

Through the years as Ayres conducted her studies with different groups of children, she continually revisited her theory, bringing along new hypotheses based on new research results. Of particular interest were the patterns that recurred despite being generated from different samples of children. Among the most consistent findings was that children who had been identified as having learning or developmental problems often displayed difficulties in more than one sensory system. Ayres (1972b) interpreted this finding in light of the neurobiologic literature on intersensory integration, which indicates that the sensory systems tend to function synergistically with each other rather than in isolation. Thus, the idea of intersensory integration as critical to human function became one of the major tenets of sensory integration theory.

Another finding, which emerged in early studies and in later SIPT studies, was that some patterns of scores were seen only in groups of children who had been identified as having disorders. In other words, some factors were not evident in typically developing children at any age. This led to the proposal that the sensory integrative disorders associated with these particular patterns were representative of neural dysfunction rather than developmental lag.

Yet another recurrent pattern was a relationship between tactile perception and praxis scores. This association appeared repeatedly in her studies and led Ayres to theorize that the tactile system contributes importantly to the development of efficient practic functions. The robustness of this finding across many studies influenced Ayres to emphasize the relationship between the tactile system and praxis, a relationship that has become a cornerstone of sensory integration theory.

Throughout her research, several patterns emerged that Ayres suspected were related to a discrete involvement of cortical rather than brainstem or intersensory dysfunction. Ayres came to view these types of problems

Text continued on p. 374

TABLE 11-1 Purpose, Methods, Results, and Contributions of Studies of Sensory Integrative Patterns

Year	Author	Purpose	Instruments	Hypothesis	Analysis	Subjects	Results	Contribution to Theory
1965	Ayres, A.J.	Identify relationships among sensory perception, motor performance, laterality in normal and children with perceptual problems. Establish construct and discriminant validity	Early versions of the SCSIT, additional perceptual-motor and laterality tests, also freedom from hyperactivity and tactile defensiveness.	Test results would identify factors for children with and without dysfunction. Normal and dysfunctional children will demonstrate different factors.	Thirty-three tests. Two behavioral parameters. Analysis of difference between group means. Q- and R-technique factor analysis.	n = 100 dysfunctional n = 50 normal Dysfunctional children had learning or behavioral disorders.	Tests discriminated between normal and dysfunctional groups. Five patterns detected: apraxia, dysfunction form and space perception, deficit bilateral integration, visual figure-ground perception, tactile defensiveness	Established discriminant validity of early versions. Most children demonstrated more than one factor, therefore factors related. Sensory integration-clusters were not by sensory systems Praxis and tactile functions linked Tactile defensiveness, hyperactivity, distractibility linked Cognitive aspects deemphasized Eye-hand agreement not discriminative. Empirical support for syndromes.
1966a	Ayres, A.J.	Explore perceptual-motor relationships in a normal sample and compare with prior studies. Establish construct validity.	Frostig tests, early versions of the SCSIT. Also freedom from hyperactivity and tactile defensiveness.	That factors would emerge.	Seventeen tests. R-technique factor analysis (simplified matrix).	n = 92 Formed normal distribution, 10% abnormal, three with mild cerebral palsy.	Praxis accounted for most variance. Motor planning, kinesthesia, tactile functions, motor accuracy, bilateral coordination. Visual perception factor: Ayres Space Test, Frostig.	More support for praxis syndrome. Visual component without motor element. Perceptual-motor functions correlate as a whole in normative sample. Kinesthesia closer to tactile than visual perception as in prior study.
1966b	Ayres, A.J.	Provide an understanding of whether syndromes represent dysfunction or developmental lag. Establish construct validity.	Nearly the same as 1966a.	That variation in perceptual-motor abilities would be small in a group of typical children.	Sixteen tests Two behavioral parameters. R-technique factor analysis.	n = 64 Adopted, all normal on Gesell.	Visual motor ability accounted for most variation. Praxis and tactile perception were least variable. Hyperactivity, distractibility, tactile defensiveness factor. Factors weak because of lack of variance in performance of normal children.	Suggested that low scores in praxis and tactile perception represent developmental deviation, not delay. Little systematic variation when tests given to normal children. Tactile defensiveness-hyperactivity may have a maturational component.

TABLE 11-1 Purpose, Methods, Results, and Contributions of Studies of Sensory Integrative Patterns—cont'd

Year	Author	Purpose	Instruments	Hypothesis	Analysis	Subjects	Results	Contribution to Theory
1969	Ayres, A.J.	To provide an in-depth analysis of dysfunctional patterns in children with learning handicaps. Establish construct validity.	Sixty-four tests and observations: SCSIT, psycholinguistic, intelligence, auditory, postural-ocular reactions, academic achievement.	Brain functions involve several levels and will cluster accordingly.	Q-technique factor analysis.	n = 36 Educationally handicapped children.	Five factors identified: Auditory language, sequencing; postural and bilateral integration; right hemisphere dysfunction; apraxia; tactile defensiveness.	Hints to left hemisphere dysfunction.
1971	Ayres, A.J.	To identify predictors of severity of sensory integrative syndromes.	Forty-eight tests and observations: SCSIT, psycholinguistic, intelligence, eye-hand usage, postural responses.	That predictive equations would emerge.	Ten-step regression equations for each syndrome calculated.	n = 140 Educationally handicapped children.	Presence of more than one type of disorder was the norm. Prone extension best predictor of postural-bilateral integration. Imitation of postures best predictor of praxis.	Somatosensory and praxis linked again. Elucidated best predictors of syndromes. As many children may have apraxia as have postural and bilateral coordination problems.
1972	Ayres, A.J.	To further analyze and refine factors. Establish construct validity	Same as above.	That similar factors as presented previously would emerge.	R-technique factor analysis.	n = 148 Educationally handicapped children.	Six factors identified: Form and space perception; auditory language; postural ocular; motor planning; reading, spelling, and IQ; hyperactivity, tactile perception.	Further confirmed left hemisphere dysfunction. Reconfirmed syndromes found in other samples of learning-disabled children.
1977	Ayres, A.J.	To further analyze interrelationships (add SCPNT) so that differential diagnosis can be further refined.	SCSIT SCPNT, postural-ocular and lateralization measures, dichotic listening, ITPA, intelligence, academic achievement. Flowers-Costello (auditory).	That clusters would continue to be refined.	Series of R-technique factor analyses (not all measures entered each time).	n = 128 Learning-disabled children	Five major domains identified: Somatosensory-motor planning; auditory-language, postural-ocular, eye-hand coordination; postrotary nystagmus.	Further elucidated nature of interhemispheric integration. Role of vestibular system clarified.
1987	Ayres, A.J.	To continue to attempt to differentiate types of sensory integration dysfunction.	SCSIT, SCPNT, selected ITPA test, sentence repetition. Clinical observation of	Is praxis a unitary function? Would computer-generated clusters match those that had	Screen plot factor analyses, correlation coefficients. Comparison of test profiles of children with diagnoses.	n = 182 Learning or behavior disorders.	Praxis tests were related with one another. Visual tests correlated with tactile tests	Suggestion of a general somatopractic function. Further verified close association of tactile score and praxis.

Year	Author	Purpose	Tests	Hypothesis	Method	Sample	Results	Conclusions
			New praxis tests as well as many of the tests that had been used in past studies. prone extension, supine flexion, ocular pursuits. Preliminary versions of newly designed praxis tests: Sequencing Praxis, Praxis on Verbal Command, Oral Praxis, block building test	been identified clinically and through factor analysis?	Use of computer generated clusters.		Somatovisual-practic factor identified. Tactile scores and praxis related; short duration postrotary nystagmus; statistical association with praxis.	Computer-generated clusters were not meaningful.
1989	Ayres, A.J.	Factor analyses: to clarify the nature of the constructs measured by the Sensory Integration and Praxis Tests (SIPT).	SIPT (17 tests)	That factors related to those of the SCSIT would emerge.	Principal components analysis.	Three analyses: n = 1750. Normative sample. n = 125. Learning or sensory integrative disorders. n = 293 Combined sample of learning or sensory integrative disorders and matched children from normative sample.	Visuopraxis and somatopraxis factors emerged in all three analyses. Bilateral integration and sequencing factor and praxis on verbal command factor seen only in dysfunctional sample. Other factors related to vestibular and somatosensory processing identified.	Expanded understanding of vestibular-bilateral disorders to include sequencing element. Somatopraxis factor reinforced previous findings linking tactile perception and praxis. Visuopraxis factor provided support for previous visual-motor linkages.
1989	Ayres, A.J.	Cluster analyses: to assist in identifying children in need of different types of remediation or services.	SIPT (17 tests)	That meaningful diagnostic groupings would emerge.	Agglomerative cluster analysis, Ward's method.	n = 293. Same sample as above, combined dysfunctional and normative.	Six cluster groups identified: Low average bilateral integration and sequencing, generalized sensory integrative dysfunction, visuo- and somatodyspraxia, low average sensory integration and praxis, dyspraxia on verbal command, high average sensory integration and praxis.	Children with and without dysfunction can be differentiated on the basis of SIPT profiles. Identified specific SIPT profile that may be characteristic of left hemisphere dysfunction.
2000	Mulligan, S.	To explore subgroupings of children referred for SIPT testing and to	SIPT	That cluster groups similar to those identified by Ayres (1989) would emerge.	Agglomerative cluster Analysis, Ward's method.	n = 1961 children assessed with the SIPT between 1989 and 1993.	Five cluster groups identified: generalized sensory integration dysfunction and	Demonstrated many similarities with Ayres's cluster analysis, with some differences.

TABLE 11-1 Purpose, Methods, Results, and Contributions of Studies of Sensory Integrative Patterns—cont'd

Year	Author	Purpose	Instruments	Hypothesis	Analysis	Subjects	Results	Contribution to Theory
		provide information about the validity of the six cluster groups identified in the SIPT manual.					dyspraxia-severe, dyspraxia, generalized sensory integration dysfunction and dyspraxia-moderate, low average bilateral integration and sequencing, average sensory integration and praxis.	Supports evidence of bilateral integration and sequencing deficit, dyspraxia on verbal command, and more general dyspraxia. More helpful in identifying degree of dysfunction rather than type, as this sample did not include a normative sample as did Ayres's analysis.
1998	Parham, L.D.	To examine whether sensory integrative measures are predictive of school achievement, when intelligence and other factors are taken into account, concurrently and over a 4-year period.	SIPT, converted into 3 factor scores: Praxis, visual perception, and somatosensory. Intelligence, reading, and math achievement. Socioeconomic status.	That sensory integrative performance at ages 6-8 years is related to achievement concurrently and predictively 4 years later. That sensory integrative performance at ages 10-12 is not related to achievement.	Multiple regression analyses.	n = 91, of whom 43 were identified as learning disabled. Children were 6-8 years old initially, 10-12 years old at follow-up	When controlling for IQ sensory integration: at ages 6-8 significantly correlated with math, but not reading; at ages 6-8 significantly predicted math and reading 4 years later; at ages 10-12 significantly predicted math and reading at same age. Strong relationships between praxis and math achievement identified.	Supported the hypothesis that sensory integration, especially praxis, is related to achievement when taking IQ into account. Sensory integration continues to contribute to achievement at middle school age.

CFA, Confirmatory factor analysis; *SIPT*, Sensory Integration and Praxis Tests; *SEM*, structural equation modeling.
Ayres, A.J. (1965). Patterns of perceptual-motor dysfunction in children: a factor analytic study. *Perceptual and Motor Skills, 20*, 335-368.
Ayres, A.J. (1966a). Interrelationships among perceptual-motor functions in children. *American Journal of Occupational Therapy, 20* (2), 68-71.
Ayres, A.J. (1966b). Interrelationships among perceptual-motor abilities in a group of normal children. *American Journal of Occupational Therapy, 20* (6), 288-292.
Ayres, A.J. (1969). Deficits in sensory integration in educationally handicapped children. *Journal of Learning Disabilities, 2* (3), 44-52.
Ayres, A.J. (1971). Characteristics of types of sensory integrative dysfunction. *American Journal of Occupational Therapy, 25* (7), 329-334.
Ayres, A.J. (1972). Types of sensory integrative dysfunction among disabled learners. *American Journal of Occupational Therapy, 26* (1), 13-18.
Ayres, A.J. (1977). Cluster analyses of measures of sensory integration. *American Journal of Occupational Therapy, 31* (6), 362-366.
Ayres, A.J., Mailloux, Z., & Wendler, C.L.W. (1987). Development apraxia: is it a unitary function? *Occupational Therapy Journal of Research, 7* (2), 93-110.
Ayres, A.J. (1989). *Sensory Integration and Praxis Tests manual.* Los Angeles: Western Psychological Services.
Mulligan, S. (2000). Cluster analysis of scores of children on the Sensory Integration and Praxis tests. *Occupational Therapy Journal of Research, 20*, 256-270.
Parham, L.D. (1998). The relationship of sensory integrative development to achievement in elementary students: Four-year longitudinal patterns. *Occupational Therapy Journal of Research, 18*, 105-127.

TABLE 11-2 Factors and Clusters Identified in Research

Date of Study	Author	Dyspraxia	Deficit in Visual Perception and Visual-Motor Functions	Deficit in Vestibular, Postural, and Bilateral Integration	Deficit in Auditory and Language Functions	Somatosensory	Miscellaneous
1965: 100 dysfunctional, 50 normal	Ayres, A.J.	Tactile tests Motor planning (imitation of posture, motor accuracy, Grommet) Eye pursuits	Frostig tests Kinesthesia Manual form Perception Ayres's Space Test	Right-left discrimination Avoidance crossing midline Rhythmic activities	Not tested	Poor tactile perception Hyperactive-distractible behavior Tactile defensiveness	Figure-ground a separate factor Eye-hand agreement not related to perceptual-motor dysfunction
1966a: Normal distribution of Gesell developmental quotients	Ayres, A.J.	Accounted for most variance Motor planning Tactile and kinesthesia Motor accuracy Figure-ground Frostig tests	Figure-ground Frostig spatial relations Ayres' Space Test		Not tested	Low association of tactile defensiveness with praxis factor	Identified two main factors in normal sample: General perceptual-motor (somatosensory and motor) Visual perception
1966b: Only normal children	Ayres, A.J.		Frostig tests Ayres's Space Test Motor Accuracy Figure-ground	Integration two sides of body and tactile perception	Not tested	Tactile defensiveness and hyperactivity—may be a maturational factor involved	Visual-motor ability accounted for most variation in normal children Poor motor planning—tactile perception not seen in normal children
1969: Educationally handicapped children	Ayres, A.J.	Tactile Motor planning	Most SCSIT; visual tests not included in analysis Possible right hemisphere dysfunction: eye movement deficits, better right- than left-sided function	Bilateral integration Postural reactions Reading and language problems	Possible left hemisphere dysfunction: Auditory-language Reading achievement Auditory and visual-motor sequencing	Tactile defensiveness and hyperactivity—loaded together but not a separate factor	
1972: Educationally handicapped children	Ayres, A.J.	Motor planning Hyperactivity Tactile defensiveness (more emphasis On motor than tactile)	Position in space ITPA visual closure Space Visualization Design copying Tactile tests	Poor ocular control Excessive residual primitive postural responses Relatively good left-hand coordination	Auditory language Intelligence	Hyperactivity-distractibility Tactile perception	Reading-spelling load together Motor accuracy highly associated with all parameters

TABLE 11-2 Factors and Clusters Identified in Research—cont'd

Date of Study	Author	Dyspraxia	Deficit in Visual Perception and Visual-Motor Functions	Deficit in Vestibular, Postural, and Bilateral Integration	Deficit in Auditory and Language Functions	Somatosensory	Miscellaneous
1977: Learning disabled children	Ayres, A.J.	*Analysis 5:* Imitation of postures Composite tactile Kinesthesia	*Analysis 3:* Four SCSIT visual tests Manual form Perception	Bilateral integration symptom did not load *Analysis 5:* Prone extension Composite postural Flexion posture Composite tactile Kinesthesia Bilateral integration symptom did not load	*Analysis 5:* Composite language (ITPA) Dichotic listening Flowers-Costello (auditory)	Not measured	Visual tests have strong cognitive component (loaded with IQ on Analysis 2) SVCU associated with lateralization indices Motor accuracy loaded separately on all
1989: Children with learning disorders and sensory integrative deficits and children from normative sample of SIPT	Ayres, A.J.	Somatopraxis (Oral Praxis, Postural Praxis, Graphesthesia) Visuo- and somatodyspraxia cluster	Visuopraxis (Constructional Praxis, Design Copying, Space Visualization, Figure-Ground)	Bilateral integration and sequencing (Sequencing Praxis, Bilateral Motor Coordination, Standing and Walking Balance) Low average bilateral integration and sequencing cluster	Praxis on Verbal Command Dyspraxia on verbal command cluster (high Postrotatory Nystagmus with low Praxis on Verbal Command)	Not measured	High functioning group identified within normative sample Generalized dysfunction group identified within group with learning disorders and sensory integrative dysfunction

1998: 10,475 children primarily with mild learning, behavior, or motor problems.	Mulligan, S.	Dyspraxia (Oral Praxis, Postural Praxis, and Praxis on Verbal Command); Also suggests generalized practic function underlying all other factors.	Visual Perceptual Deficit (Design Copying, Constructional Praxis, Space Visualization, Manual Form Perception, Figure Ground Perception)	Bilateral Integration and Sequencing Deficit (Sequencing Praxis and Bilateral Motor Coordination)	Not tested	Tactile tests and kinesthesia
2000	Mulligan, S.	Three patterns of dyspraxia identified, differentiated most by severity	Low scores in all visual perception and visual practic tests grouped with severe dyspraxia pattern	Bilateral integration and sequencing confirmed as a pattern (SWB, GRA, DC, PPr, KIN, SPr, Opr). Like Ayres's BIS pattern, this cluster had the lowest mean average on PRN of the 5 clusters identified	Similarity to dyspraxia on verbal command pattern noted on one of the dyspraxia clusters	Low tactile and KIN scores present on three dyspraxia clusters in comparison to BIS and average SI patterns	Unlike Ayres's (1989) cluster analysis, high SI functions did not emerge. This is because Ayres included a group of children without dysfunction in her study, whereas this study analyzed a sample that predominately was clinically referred

ITPA, Illinois Test of Psycholinguistic Abilities; SCSIT, Southern California Sensory Integration Test; SVCU, Space Visualization Contralateral Use.

Ayres, A.J. (1965). Patterns of perceptual-motor dysfunction in children: A factor analytic study. Perceptual and Motor Skills, 20, 335-368.
Ayres, A.J. (1966a). Interrelationships among perceptual-motor functions in children. American Journal of Occupational Therapy, 20 (2), 68-71.
Ayres, A.J. (1966b). Interrelations among perceptual-motor abilities in a group of normal children. American Journal of Occupational Therapy, 20 (6), 288-292.
Ayres, A.J. (1969). Deficits in sensory integration in educationally handicapped children. Journal of Learning Disabilities, 2 (3), 44-52.
Ayres, A.J. (1972). Types of sensory integrative dysfunction among disabled learners. American Journal of Occupational Therapy, 26 (1), 13-18.
Ayres, A.J. (1977). Cluster analyses of measures of sensory integration. American Journal of Occupational Therapy, 31 (6), 362-366.
Ayres, A.J. (1989). Sensory Integration and Praxis Tests manual. Los Angeles: Western Psychological Services.
Mulligan, S. (1998). Patterns of sensory integration dysfunction: A confirmatory factor analysis. American Journal of Occupational Therapy, 52, 819-828.
Mulligan, S. (2000). Cluster analysis of scores of children on the Sensory Integration and Praxis tests. Occupational Therapy Journal of Research, 20, 256-270.

as different than those classified as sensory integrative disorders and less likely to be responsive to the treatment techniques that she was developing. An example is the association of low Praxis on Verbal Command scores with high postrotary nystagmus scores. Praxis on Verbal Command is the only test on the SIPT with a strong language comprehension component. Postrotary nystagmus is a test that may reflect cortical dysfunction if scores are extremely high. In this example, it is hypothesized that an underlying cortical dysfunction, possibly involving the left hemisphere (where language centers are located), is responsible for the pattern of scores. Ayres did not view this particular pattern as a sensory integrative dysfunction, although it could be detected by her tests.

As Bundy and Murray (2002) pointed out, the limitations of Ayres's factor analytic studies include small sample sizes in relation to the number of tests studied, and the repetition of exploratory techniques with different groups of tests in her studies, instead of using confirmatory factor analysis to replicate results using the same group of tests. It is important to note, however, that similar factors did recur across her studies despite these limitations (see Tables 11-1 and 11-2). Furthermore, many of the factors were replicated recently by Mulligan (1998) in a confirmatory factor analytic study of more than 10,000 children. The robustness of some of these factors across many studies strengthens the hypothesis that they reflect underlying patterns of function.

Ayres conducted her factor and cluster analyses to shed light on the types of sensory integrative dysfunctions that children experience, yet she did not view the resulting typologies as specific diagnostic labels to pin on individual children. Rather, the typologies were seen as general patterns exhibited time after time by groups of children who were struggling in school or with some other aspect of behavior or development. They provide the therapist with relevant information to consider when conducting clinical assessments. They do not provide prefabricated slots in which to fit children. Ultimately, the important job of interpreting an individual child's pattern of scores in relation to his or her unique life situation lies in the purview of the therapist's judgment.

SENSORY INTEGRATIVE DISORDERS

The results of research, combined with the experiences of clinicians and the work of scholars in the field, have generated many different ways of conceptualizing sensory integrative disorders over the past 30 years. The complexity of this domain can be initially confusing to the novice therapist, but it is also one of the most intriguing aspects of the field. The term *sensory integrative*

disorder does not refer to one particular type of problem but to a heterogeneous group of disorders that are thought to reflect subtle, primarily subcortical, neural dysfunction involving multisensory systems. These disorders affect human behavior in ways that are often difficult to interpret unless seen through the eyes of someone with special training in sensory integration.

Most discussions of sensory integrative problems assume normal sensory receptor function. In other words, sensory integrative disorders involve central, rather than peripheral, sensory functions. This assumption has been supported in several well-designed studies. For instance, Parush, Sohmer, Steinberg, and Kaitz (1997) found that the somatosensory-evoked potentials of children with attention-deficit hyperactivity disorder (ADHD) differ from those of typically developing children with respect to indicators of central tactile processing but not in peripheral receptor responses. Many of the children with ADHD in this study were also identified as having tactile defensiveness, a sensory integrative problem. In another study, researchers found that children with learning disabilities, compared with nondisabled children, had impaired postural responses involving central integration of vestibular, proprioceptive, and visual inputs, whereas measures of peripheral receptor functions were normal (Shumway-Cook, Horak, & Black, 1987). Thus, when sensory integrative disorders involving the vestibular system are discussed, these problems are generally thought to be based within CNS structures and pathways (i.e., the vestibular nuclei and its connections) rather than the vestibular receptors (i.e., the semicircular canals, utricle, or saccule). This has been a point of confusion in some studies in which measures of peripheral vestibular receptor functioning were used inappropriately to evaluate Ayres's concept of central vestibular dysfunction (e.g., Polatajko, 1985). Wiss (1989) has provided an excellent discussion of this issue in relation to vestibular processing. The same point could apply to other sensory systems as well. In this chapter, the discussions of sensory integrative problems assume that peripheral function is normal.

As noted previously, different conceptualizations of sensory integrative disorders have been generated over the years. Although perfect consensus on how to categorize sensory integrative dysfunctions does not exist, clearly there are recurring themes across all authors. Distinct but overlapping taxonomies of sensory integrative dysfunction include, for example, those of Clark, Mailloux, and Parham (1989); Fisher, Murray, and Bundy (1991); and Kimball (1999). More recently, Bundy, Lane, and Murray (2002) presented a taxonomic model that depicts sensory integrative dysfunction as manifested in two major ways: poor sensory modulation and poor praxis. For the purposes of this chapter, we discuss sensory integrative problems as falling into four general categories:

1 Sensory modulation problems
2 Sensory discrimination and perception problems
3 Vestibular-proprioceptive problems
4 Praxis problems

The first of these four categories corresponds to Bundy, Lane, and Murray's category of sensory modulation. The latter three categories can be thought of as subsumed under their category of praxis. We find it helpful to discuss these four areas as distinct patterns because, although they very often coexist, we occasionally find that a child is experiencing problems that are specific to just one of these patterns. Because each pattern sometimes appears as a discrete problem area that calls for particular considerations when planning intervention, we find it useful pragmatically to consider each of these as a special category with characteristic features. We discuss each of these categories in turn next.

Sensory Modulation Problems

Sensory modulation refers to CNS regulation of its own activity (Ayres, 1979). With respect to sensory systems, this term is used to refer to the tendency to generate responses that are appropriately graded in relation to incoming sensory stimuli, rather than underreacting or overreacting to them. Cermak (1988) and Royeen (1989) hypothesized that there is a continuum of sensory responsivity, with hyporesponsivity at one end and hyperresponsivity at the other. An optimal level of arousal and orientation lies in the center of the continuum (Figure 11-8). This is where most activity falls for most individuals, although everyone experiences fluctuations across this continuum of sensory responsivity in the course of a day. In the continuum model, dysfunction is indicated when the fluctuations within an individual are extreme or when an individual tends to function primarily at one extreme of the continuum or the other. The individual who tends to function at the extremely underresponsive end of the continuum may be said to have diminished sensory registration. This person fails to notice sensory stimuli that elicit the attention of most people. At a less severe degree of underresponsiveness, the individual notices sensory stimuli, but is slow to respond or seems to crave intense sensory input. At the opposite extreme of the continuum is the overresponsive individual with sensory defensiveness. This person is overwhelmed and overstressed by ordinary sensory stimuli.

Originally, Ayres (1979) thought of sensory registration problems as different in nature from sensory modulation problems such as tactile defensiveness. Soon after she introduced the concept of sensory registration, however, other experts in the field of sensory integration suggested that sensory registration and tactile defensiveness might be related through common underlying limbic system functions (Dunn & Fisher, 1983; Royeen & Lane, 1991). This idea contributed to the continuum model shown here. Experts soon found that this simple continuum model did not adequately address the complexity of child behaviors, however. For example, Royeen and Lane (1991) hypothesized that the relationship between underresponsiveness and overresponsiveness may be circular instead of linear, because a child who is extremely defensive may be overloaded to the point of shutting down and becoming underresponsive. Previously, we have criticized the continuum model as overly simplistic because sensory modulation very likely is influenced by the individual's history of personal experiences and interpretation of the situation, as well as interactions among multiple neural systems (Parham & Mailloux, 2002).

Recently, Dunn (1997, 2001) presented a conceptual model that takes into account the potential roles of various neural processes in generating patterns of underresponsiveness and overresponsiveness (see Figure 11-9). In her model, four main patterns represent individual differences in sensory responding: low registration, sensation seeking, sensitivity to stimuli, and sensation avoiding. These patterns are hypothesized to emerge from individual differences in the neural processes of habituation, sensitization, threshold, and maintenance of homeostasis. The person who falls in the low-registration

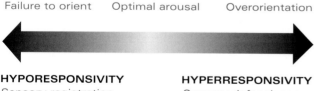

Failure to orient   Optimal arousal   Overorientation

HYPORESPONSIVITY   **HYPERRESPONSIVITY**
Sensory registration   Sensory defensiveness
problem

FIGURE 11-8 Continuum of sensory responsivity and orientation. (Modified from Royeen, C.B., & Lane, S.J. [1991]. Tactile processing and sensory defensiveness. In A.G. Fisher, E.A. Murray, & A.C. Bundy [Eds.], *Sensory integration: Theory and practice.* Philadelphia: F.A. Davis.)

	Responding/Self-Regulation Strategies	
Thresholds/Reactivity	Passive	Active
High	Low Registration	Sensory Seeking
Low	Sensory Sensitivity	Sensory Avoiding

FIGURE 11-9 Dunn's Model of Sensory Processing. (Adapted from Dunn, W. [1997]. The impact of sensory processing abilities on the daily lives of young children and families: A conceptual model. *Infants and Young Children, 9* [4] 23-25.)

quadrant of the model is underresponsive due to a high threshold for reactivity and therefore needs to have a high level of intensity in environmental stimuli in order to notice and attend. The person who falls in the sensation-seeking quadrant is also considered underresponsive with regard to high threshold but expresses this behaviorally by actively seeking out intense sensory input. The sensory sensitivity and sensation avoiding quadrants represent overresponsive patterns. Individuals who fall in the sensory sensitivity quadrant have heightened awareness of, and are distracted by, sensory stimuli due to a low threshold, but they tend to passively cope with these sensations. In contrast, those who are sensation avoiding not only have heightened awareness of sensory stimuli but actively attempt to avoid the ordinary sensations that they experience as noxious. One of the most important contributions of this model is that it can be used to consider what kinds of work and play or leisure environments present an optimal match for an individual's sensory modulation characteristics (Dunn, 2001).

In another new model that addresses the complexity of sensory modulation, Miller, Reisman, McIntosh, and Simon (2001) differentiate between physiologic and behavioral elements of what they call sensory modulation disorders (SMDs). Their ecological model includes both external and internal dimensions affecting sensory modulation (Figure 11-10). External dimensions identified are culture, environment, relationships, and tasks,

whereas internal dimensions are sensory processing, emotion, and attention. The external dimensions highlight the importance of context, while the internal dimensions focus on enduring differences among individuals. In this model, external and internal dimensions are interlinked through multidirectional, rather than linear, relationships and must be viewed together to design interventions for children with SMDs.

These models of sensory modulation help us to organize the complex information that is relevant to understanding children with difficulties in overresponding or underresponding to sensory information in everyday situations. We continue to have many unanswered questions about modulation. For example, some research indicates that many children frequently demonstrate behavioral characteristics of both underresponding and overresponding, often within the same sensory system (Lai, Parham, & Johnson-Ecker, 1999). This may be particularly the case for children with autism (Lee, 1999). Also, we have clinical evidence that some children are overresponsive in one sensory system, but underresponsive in another. Our existing models do not yet do an adequate job of explaining these phenomena. Nevertheless, these models are important because they provide a foundation upon which research programs can be built to explicate the complex issues that are involved. Today, research on patterns of sensory modulation and their manifestations in everyday activities is an area of focused

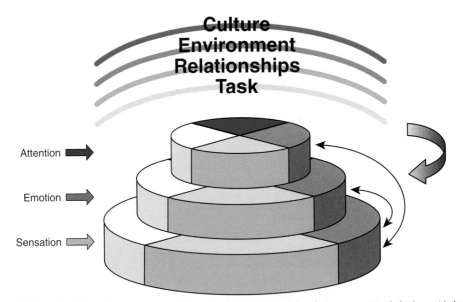

FIGURE 11-10 Miller et al.'s (2001) Ecological Model of Sensory Modulation. Light shading = underresponsivity

Medium shading = normal responsivity (a match between the external and internal dimensions)

Dark shading = overresponsivity

Black = lability, severe overresponsivity alternating with severe underresponsivity. (From Miller, L.J., Reisman, J.E., McIntosh, D.N., & Simon, J. [2001]. An ecological model of sensory modulation: Performance of children with Fragile X syndrome, autistic disorder, attention-deficit/hyperactivity disorder, and sensory modulation dysfunction. In S.S. Roley, E.I. Blanche, & R.C. Schaaf [Eds.], *Understanding the nature of sensory integration with diverse populations* [pp. 57-88]. San Antonio, TX: Therapy Skill Builders.)

investigation in occupational therapy (Baranek, Foster, & Berkson, 1997; Dunn, Myles, & Orr, 2002; Miller, Reisman, McIntosh, & Simon, 2001).

Although we have much to learn about sensory modulation, a general consensus exists among sensory integration experts regarding the behaviors that characterize different kinds of sensory modulation difficulties. We turn now to the classic descriptions of each of these problems.

Sensory Registration Problems

As noted previously in this chapter, sensory integration is the "organization of sensory input for use" (Ayres, 1979, p. 184). However, before sensory information can be used functionally, it must be registered within the CNS. When the CNS is working well, it knows when to "pay attention" to a stimulus and when to "ignore it." Most of the time this process occurs automatically and efficiently. For example, a student may not be aware of the noise of traffic outside the window of a classroom while listening to a lecture, instead focusing his or her attention on the sound of the lecturer's words. In this situation, the student registers the auditory stimuli generated by the lecturer but not the stimuli generated by the traffic. The process of sensory registration is critical in enabling efficient function so that people pay attention to those stimuli that enable them to accomplish desired goals. Simultaneously, if the process is working well, energy is not wasted attending to irrelevant sensory information.

Traditionally, occupational therapists, beginning with Ayres (1979), have used the term *sensory registration problem* to refer to the difficulties of the person who frequently fails to attend to or register relevant environmental stimuli. This kind of problem is often seen in individuals with autism, but it may also be seen in other individuals with developmental problems. When a sensory registration problem is present, the child often seems oblivious to touch, pain, movement, taste, smells, sights, or sounds. Usually more than one sensory system is involved, but for some children one system may be particularly affected. Sometimes the same child who does not register relevant stimuli may be overfocused on irrelevant stimuli; this is commonly seen in children with autism. It is also common for children with severe developmental problems, such as autism, to lack sensory registration in some situations but react with extreme sensory defensiveness in other situations.

Safety concerns are frequently an important issue among children with sensory registration problems. For example, the child who does not register pain sensations has not learned that certain actions naturally lead to negative consequences, such as pain, and therefore may not withdraw adequately from dangerous situations. Instead of avoiding situations likely to result in pain, the child may repeatedly engage in activities that may be injurious, such as jumping from a dangerous height onto a hard surface or touching a hot object. Other children with sensory registration problems may not register noxious tastes and smells that warn of hazards. Similarly, sights and sounds such as sirens, flashing lights, firm voice commands, and hand signals or signs that are meant to warn of perils go unheeded if not registered. This can be a life-endangering problem in some circumstances (e.g., when a child steps in front of a moving car).

A sensory registration problem interferes with the child's ability to attach meaning to an activity or situation. Consequently, in severe cases, the child lacks the inner drive that compels most children to master ordinary childhood occupations (e.g., the child who is generally unmotivated to engage in play activities or to practice skills). Therefore the long-term effects on the child's development can be profound.

It is thought that the lack of inner drive in children with autism and severe underresponsivity renders them among the most challenging children to treat using a sensory integrative approach. These children can benefit from individual occupational therapy, but gains may be slow to develop (Ayres & Tickle, 1980). Both clinical experience and research indicate that sensory registration can be enhanced in these children through vestibular stimulation, particularly linear stimulation, and proprioceptive input, particularly when it involves joint compression and traction (Ayres, 1979; Slavik, Kitsuwa-Lowe, Danner, Green, & Ayres, 1984).

Sensation-Seeking Behavior

Some children register sensations yet are underresponsive to the incoming stimuli. These children seem to seek intense stimulation in the sensory modalities that are affected. The child who is hyporesponsive to vestibular stimuli may seek large quantities of intense stimulation when introduced to suspended equipment in a clinic setting. This child registers the vestibular sensations and usually shows signs of pleasure from the sensations, but the input does not affect the nervous system to the extent that it does for most other children. The underresponsive child may not become dizzy or show any autonomic responses in response to intense stimulation that would be overwhelming for most peers. This is called *hyporesponsivity* because it refers to the underlying mode of sensory processing rather than to observable motor behavior. Although the child may appear to be active motorically, the child is not reacting to intense vestibular stimuli to the degree that most children do. In everyday settings, these children often appear to be restless, motorically driven, and thrill seeking.

Some children seem to seek greater-than-average amounts of proprioceptive input. Typically these children often seek active resistance to muscles, deep touch pressure stimulation, or joint compression and traction (e.g., by stomping instead of walking; intentionally falling or bumping into objects, including other people, or pushing against large objects). They may tend to use strong ballistic movements such as throwing objects forcefully. Some of these children may not seem to register the positions of body parts unless intense proprioceptive stimulation is present.

Some children who seek large amounts of proprioceptive input demonstrate signs of tactile defensiveness or gravitational insecurity. Because proprioception is thought to have an inhibitory effect on tactile and vestibular sensations, these children may be seeking increased proprioceptive input in order to help themselves modulate the overwhelming touch and movement sensations that they often experience.

The behaviors generated by sensation-seeking children may be disruptive or inappropriate in social situations. Safety issues frequently are of paramount concern, and often these children are labeled as having social or behavioral problems. A challenge for the occupational therapist working with these children may be to identify strategies by which they can receive the high levels of stimulation that they seek without being socially disruptive, inappropriate, or dangerous to themselves or others.

Overresponsiveness

At the opposite end of the sensory modulation continuum are problems associated with overresponsiveness, sometimes called hyperresponsivity or sensory defensiveness. The child who is overresponsive is overwhelmed by ordinary sensory input and reacts defensively to it, often with strong negative emotion and activation of the sympathetic nervous system. This condition may occur as a general response to all types of sensory input, or it may be specific to one or a few sensory systems.

The term *sensory defensiveness* was first introduced by Knickerbocker (1980) and later used by Wilbarger and Wilbarger (1991) to describe sensory modulation disorders involving multisensory systems. Sensory modulation problems include overreactions to touch, movement, sounds, odors, and tastes, any of which may create discomfort, avoidance, distractibility, and anxiety. Most of the research-based and clinical knowledge regarding overresponsiveness is related to the tactile and vestibular systems.

Tactile Defensiveness. Tactile defensiveness involves a tendency to overreact to ordinary touch sensations (Ayres, 1964; 1972b; 1979). It is one of the most commonly observed sensory integrative disorders involving sensory modulation. Individuals with tactile defensiveness experience irritation and discomfort from sensations that most people do not find bothersome. Light touch sensations are especially likely to be disturbing. Common irritants include certain textures of clothing, grass or sand against bare skin, glue or paint on the skin, the light brush of another person passing by,

the sensations generated when having one's hair or teeth brushed, and certain textures of food. Common responses to such irritants include anxiety, distractibility, restlessness, anger, throwing a tantrum, aggression, fear, and emotional distress.

Common self-care activities such as dressing, bathing, grooming, and eating are often affected by tactile defensiveness. Classroom activities such as finger painting, sand and water play, and crafts may be avoided. Social situations involving close proximity to others, such as playing near other children or standing in line, tend to be uncomfortable and may be disturbing enough to lead to emotional outbursts. Thus, ordinary daily routines can become traumatic for children with tactile defensiveness and for their parents. Teachers and friends are likely to misinterpret the child with tactile defensiveness as being rejecting, aggressive, or simply negative.

It is difficult for individuals with tactile defensiveness to cope with the fact that others do not share their discomforts and may actually enjoy situations that they find so upsetting. For a child with this disorder, who may not be able to verbalize or even recognize the problem, the accompanying feelings of anxiety and frustration can be overwhelming and the influence on functional behavior is likely to be significant.

An occupational therapist working with a child who is tactually defensive must become aware of the specific kinds of tactile input that are aversive and the kinds that are tolerated well by that particular child. Usually light touch stimuli are aversive, especially when they occur in the most sensitive body areas such as the face, abdomen, and palmar surfaces of the upper and lower extremities. Generally, tactile stimuli that are actively self-applied by the child are tolerated much better than stimuli that are passively received, as when being touched by another person. Tactile stimuli may be especially threatening if the child cannot see the source of the touch. Most individuals with tactile defensiveness feel comfortable with deep touch stimuli and may experience relief from irritating stimuli when deep pressure is applied over the involved skin areas.

Knowledge of these characteristics of tactile defensiveness helps the occupational therapist identify strategies that help the child and others who interact with the child to cope with this condition. For example, the occupational therapist may recommend to the teacher that if the child needs to be touched, it should be done with firm pressure in the child's view, rather than with a light touch from behind the child.

Gravitational Insecurity. Gravitational insecurity is a form of overresponsiveness to vestibular sensations, particularly sensations from the otolith organs, which detect linear movement through space and the pull of gravity (Ayres, 1979). Children with this problem have an insecure relationship to gravity characterized by excessive fear during ordinary movement activities. The gravitationally insecure child is overwhelmed by changes in head position and movement, especially when moving backward or upward through space. Fear of heights, even those involving only slight distances from the ground, is a common problem associated with this condition.

Children who display gravitational insecurity often show signs of inordinate fear, anxiety, or avoidance in relation to stairs, escalators or elevators, moving or high pieces of playground equipment, and uneven or unpredictable surfaces. Some children are so insecure that only a small change from one surface to another, as when stepping off the curb or from the sidewalk to the grass, is enough to send them into a state of high anxiety or panic.

Common reactions of children with gravitational insecurity include extreme fearfulness during low-intensity movement or when anticipating movement and avoidance of tilting the head in different planes (especially backward). They tend to move slowly and carefully, and they may refuse to participate in many gross motor activities. When they do engage in movement activities such as swinging, many of these children refuse to lift their feet off the ground. When threatened by simple motor activities, they may try to gain as much contact with the ground as possible or they may tightly clutch a nearby adult for security. These children often have signs of poor proprioception in addition to the vestibular overresponsiveness.

Playground and park activities are often difficult for children with gravitational insecurity, as are other common childhood activities such as bicycle riding, ice skating, roller skating, skateboarding, skiing, and hiking. Ability to play with peers and to explore the environment is therefore significantly affected. Functioning in the community may also be affected when the child needs to use escalators, stairs, and elevators.

A distinction can be made between gravitational insecurity and a similar condition called *postural insecurity*. Postural insecurity was the term Ayres originally used to refer to all children with fears related to movement. Over the years, however, it became clear that some children moved slowly and displayed fears of movement not because of a hyperresponsivity to vestibular input but because they lacked adequate motor control to perform many activities without falling. The fears of these children, then, seemed to be based on a realistic appraisal of their motor limitations. The term *posturally insecure* is used to refer to these children.

Often it is difficult to discern whether a child's anxiety is based on sensory overresponsivity or limited motor control because these two conditions can, and often do, coexist in the same child. Sometimes, however, the distinction is clear. Children with mild spastic diplegia, for example, commonly have postural but not gravitational insecurity. These children typically (and appropriately) react with anxiety when faced with a minimal climbing task; however, they may show pleasure at receiving vestibular stimulation, including having the head radically tilted in different planes as long as they are securely held and do not have to rely on their own motor skills to maintain a safe position.

Overresponsiveness in Other Sensory Modalities. Hyperresponsivities in other sensory systems can also have a significant influence on a person's life. For example, overreactions to sounds, odors, and tastes are often problematic for children with heightened sensitivities. These types of problems, like overresponsiveness to touch and movement, may create discomfort, avoidance, distractibility, and anxiety. Most people interpret the raucous sounds found at birthday parties, parades, playgrounds, and carnivals as happy sounds, but these can be overwhelming to a child with auditory defensiveness. A visually busy and unfamiliar environment may evoke an unusual degree of anxiety in a child with visual defensiveness. Similarly, the variety of tastes and odors encountered in some environments may be disturbing to a child with overresponsivity in these systems.

Sensory Discrimination and Perception Problems

Sensory discrimination and perception allow for refined organization and interpretation of sensory stimuli. Some types of sensory integrative disorders involve inefficient or inaccurate organization of sensory information (e.g., difficulty differentiating one stimulus from another or difficulty perceiving the spatial or temporal relationships among stimuli). A classic example involving the visual system is the older child with a learning disability who persists in confusing a *b* with a *d*. A child with an auditory discrimination problem may be unable to distinguish between the sounds of the words *doll* and *tall*. A child with a tactile perception problem may not be able to distinguish between a square block and a hexagonal block using touch only, without visual cues.

Some children with perceptual problems have no difficulty with sensory modulation. However, modulation problems often coexist with perceptual problems. It makes sense that these two types of problems are associated. A child who often does not register stimuli probably has deficit perceptual skills because of a lack of experience interacting with sensory information. Conversely, the child who has sensory defensiveness may exert a lot of energy trying to avoid certain sensory experiences. Defensive reactions may make it difficult to attend to the detailed features of a stimulus and thereby may impede perception.

Discrimination or perception problems can occur in any sensory system. They are best detected by standardized tests, except in the case of proprioception, which is difficult to measure in a standardized manner.

Professionals in many fields, such as neuropsychology, special education, and speech pathology, are trained to evaluate perceptual problems, and their focus usually is on the visual and auditory systems. In contrast, occupational therapists are unique in their emphasis on somatosensory perception.

Tactile Discrimination and Perception Problems

Poor tactile perception is one of the most common sensory integrative disorders. Children with this disorder have difficulty interpreting tactile stimuli in a precise and efficient manner. For example, they may have difficulty localizing precisely where an object has brushed against them or using stereognosis to manipulate an object that is out of sight. Fine motor skills are likely to suffer when a tactile perception problem is present, especially if tactile defensiveness is also present (Case-Smith, 1991).

As discussed previously in this chapter, the tactile system is a critical modality for learning during infancy and early childhood. Tactile exploration using the hands and mouth is particularly important. If tactile perception is vague or inaccurate, the child is at a disadvantage in learning about the different properties of objects and substances. It may be difficult for a child with such problems to develop the manipulative skills needed to efficiently perform tasks such as connecting pieces of constructional toys, fastening buttons or snaps, braiding hair, or playing marbles. Inadequate tactile perception also interferes with the feedback that is normally used to precisely guide motor tasks such as writing with a pencil, manipulating a spoon, or holding a piece of paper with one hand while cutting with the other.

Tactile perception is associated with visual perception (Ayres, Mailloux, & Wendler, 1987); thus, it is fairly common to see children with problems in both of these sensory systems. Not surprisingly, these children tend to have concomitant problems with hand-eye coordination. One of the most striking findings in the factor analytic studies of sensory integration tests is the link between tactile perception and motor planning, which recurred in different studies (Ayres, 1965, 1966a, 1966b, 1971, 1972a, 1977; Ayres, Mailloux, & Wendler, 1987; Mulligan, 1998). These findings led Ayres to hypothesize that tactile perception is an important contributor to the ability to plan actions. She speculated that the tactile system is responsible for the development of body scheme, which then becomes an important foundation for praxis.

Ordinarily, tactile perception operates at such an automatic level that, when it is impaired, compensation strategies take a great deal of energy. An example of this is the child who cannot make the subtle manipulations needed to fasten a button without looking at it. Because this child needs to use compensatory visual guidance, the task of buttoning, which is usually performed rapidly and automatically, becomes a tedious, tiring, and frustrating task. The necessity of using such compensatory strategies throughout the day tends to interrupt the child's ability to focus on the more complex conceptual and social elements of tasks and situations.

Proprioception Problems

Another type of perceptual problem involves proprioception, which arises from the muscles and joints to inform the brain about the position of body parts. This is a difficult area to research because direct measures of proprioception are not available. However, the experience of many master clinicians indicates that many children have serious difficulties interpreting proprioceptive information.

Children who do not receive reliable information about body position often appear clumsy, distracted, and awkward. As with poor tactile perception, these children must often rely on visual cues or other cognitive strategies (e.g., use of verbalizations) to perform simple aspects of tasks, such as staying in a chair or using a fork correctly. Other common attributes of children with poor proprioception include using too much or too little force in activities such as writing, clapping, marching, or typing. Breaking toys, bumping into others, and misjudging personal space are other ramifications of poor proprioception, which have strong social implications.

Many children with proprioception problems seek firm pressure to their skin or joint compression and traction. These sensation-seeking behaviors may be an attempt to gain additional feedback about body position, or they may reflect a concomitant hyporesponsiveness to tactile and proprioceptive sensations. In any case, if these behaviors are done in socially inappropriate ways or at inopportune times, such as leaning on another child during circle time or hanging from a doorway at school, the child's behavior may be misinterpreted as being willfully disruptive.

Visual Perceptual Problems

Visual perception is an important factor in the competent performance of many constructional play activities and fine motor tasks. Tests are available to measure figure-ground perception, spatial orientation, depth perception, and visual closure, to name just a few of the many aspects of visual perception that have been of concern to professionals in many disciplines.

Problems with visual perception are commonly seen in children with sensory integrative disorders, particularly when poor tactile perception or dyspraxia is present (Ayres, 1989; Ayres, Mailloux, & Wendler, 1987). Whereas some children have only a specific visual perception problem without any other sign of a sensory integrative dysfunction, many others have difficulties in visual perceptual abilities as a component of broader sensory integration difficulties. Henderson, Pehoski, and Murray (2002) point out the many relationships between visual spatial abilities and functions such as grasp, balance, locomotion, construction, and cognition. As these authors note, low scores on test of visual perception can occur for a variety of reasons and in some cases will represent a problem that therapists would not view as reflective of a sensory integrative disorder. A classic sensory integrative treatment approach, as described later in this chapter, is inappropriate for these children, although an occupational therapist might choose to work with the child using another treatment approach, such as visual perception training, use of compensatory strategies, or skill training in specific occupations.

Other Perceptual Problems

Many other dimensions of perception and sensory discrimination exist. For example, perception of movement through space involves the integration of vestibular, proprioceptive, and visual integration and may be affected in children with vestibular-proprioceptive problems. Auditory perception is an important function that may be involved in some children with sensory integrative disorders. Central auditory processing disorders recently have received increasing attention in the literature, and some authors have suggested that more attention should be given to the role of the auditory system in the sensory integration literature (Burleigh, McIntosh, & Thompson, 2002). However, since so much of the function of the auditory system is related to the functions of hearing, speech, and language, this area of study in sensory integration may be most appropriately pursued in collaboration with speech-language pathologists and audiologists. Although auditory perception problems are not usually considered to be a type of sensory integrative dysfunction when seen in isolation, difficulties with auditory perception and language development often coexist with signs of sensory integrative dysfunction. The relationship between these processes warrants further research.

Vestibular-Proprioceptive Problems

In her research, Ayres identified a pattern of problems thought to reflect inefficient central vestibular processing. The clinical signs related to this type of problem involve the motor functions that are outcomes of vestibular processing, such as poor equilibrium reactions and low muscle tone, particularly of the extensor muscles, which are strongly influenced by the vestibular system. These disorders are assessed using informal and formal clinical observations and standardized test scores.

Different names have been applied to vestibular processing problems at different points in time because of the changing patterns of research findings. In her early factor analytic studies, Ayres identified a linkage between postural-ocular mechanisms and integration of the two sides of the body. Clinically, she called the related dysfunction a disorder in "postural and bilateral integration," and she noted that it often occurred in children with learning disabilities, especially those with reading disorders (Ayres, 1972b). Additional problems commonly seen in this disorder include low muscle tone, immature righting and equilibrium reactions, poor right-left discrimination, and lack of clearly defined hand dominance.

Later in the 1970s, Ayres included the Southern California Postrotary Nystagmus Test (SCPNT) (Ayres, 1975) in her research as a more specific measure of vestibular processing. This test continues to be used and is part of the SIPT. Based on analysis of SCPNT scores, Ayres (1978) identified a vestibular processing component to the postural and bilateral integration (PBI) disorder. At this point she replaced the old PBI concept with the term *vestibular-bilateral integration (VBI)* disorder. One of the main characteristics of this problem was depressed postrotary nystagmus scores, suggesting inefficient central processing of vestibular input. Also characteristic were other signs of vestibular-related dysfunction, such as low muscle tone, postural-ocular deficits, and diminished balance and equilibrium reactions. In addition, poor bilateral coordination was implicated in VBI.

Factor and cluster analyses using the SIPT led to further evolution of the concept of vestibular processing disorders. The SIPT studies identified a *bilateral integration and sequencing (BIS)* factor characterized by poor bilateral coordination and difficulty sequencing actions, which Ayres (1989) proposed was influenced primarily by vestibular functioning. Building on Ayres's ideas, Fisher (1991) suggested that poor vestibular-proprioceptive processing is the basis for a type of sensory integrative dysfunction characterized by poor bilateral and sequencing. She used the term *vestibular-proprioceptive* to emphasize the fact that these two sensory systems work so closely together that their functions are intertwined.

In addition, Fisher (1991) introduced an interesting new concept in relation to the BIS pattern: the notion of *projected action sequences*. A projected action sequence involves anticipating how to move as one's spatial relationship to the environment changes, as when running to kick a ball or catching a moving ball. Fisher suggested that difficulty with projected action sequences is related to poor vestibular-proprioceptive processing, and, furthermore, that such deficits are a form of motor planning disorder. Thus, Fisher proposed a formal link between vestibular processing and praxis through the production of bilateral and sequenced movements.

Following Fisher's work, other experts recently addressed the *BIS* pattern as a mild form of praxis disorder that generally is associated with vestibular-proprioceptive difficulties and characterized by problems with bilateral coordination as well as anticipatory actions (Bundy & Murray, 2002; Koomar & Bundy, 2002; Reeves & Cermak, 2002). These authors also acknowledge that there may be a subset of children with BIS problems who do not have sensory integrative difficulties, in much the same way that children with isolated visual or auditory perception problems are not thought to have a sensory integration disorder.

Despite the variety of ways that have been used to describe vestibular-proprioceptive problems, certain classic clinical signs are common to all. In general, many children with these problems do not have a severe level of dysfunction, so the problem is easy to overlook. These children often exhibit poor equilibrium reactions, lower-than-average muscle tone, particularly in extensor muscles, poor postural stability, a tendency toward slouching, and difficulty in keeping the head upright. Inefficiency of the vestibular-ocular pathways may adversely affect function when directing head and eye movements while moving, as when watching a rolling soccer ball while running to kick it. Impaired balance and equilibrium reactions are likely to affect competence in performing activities such as bicycle riding, roller-skating, skiing, and playing games like hopscotch. Poor bilateral integration interferes with these activities as well. In addition, poor bilateral integration makes activities such as cutting with scissors, buttoning a shirt, or doing jumping jacks especially challenging. Bilateral integration difficulties are sometimes manifested in delays in body midline skill development, such as hand preference, spontaneous crossing of the body midline, and right-left discrimination. Neural connections between the vestibular centers in the brainstem and the reticular activating system also put children with vestibular processing disorders at risk for problems with attention, organization of behavior, communication, and modulation of arousal.

Praxis Problems

Praxis is the ability to conceptualize, plan, and execute a nonhabitual motor act (Ayres, 1979). Problems with praxis are often referred to as dyspraxia. When the term *dyspraxia* is used in regard to children, it usually refers to a condition characterized by difficulty with praxis that cannot be explained by a medical diagnosis or developmental disability and that occurs despite ordinary environmental opportunities for motor experiences. When Ayres originally wrote about dyspraxia, she used the term *developmental apraxia* (Ayres, 1972b). However, because the term *apraxia* is often associated with brain damage in adults, she later replaced this term with *developmental dyspraxia* (Ayres, 1979, 1985). The prefix *developmental* implies that the condition emerges in early childhood development and is not the result of traumatic injury.

As noted previously, Ayres was struck with the relationship between tactile perception and praxis that emerged in study after study. She hypothesized that good tactile perception contributes to development of an accurate and precise body scheme, which serves as a reservoir of knowledge to be drawn on when planning new actions. Her interest in praxis appeared to grow over time, as is evident in the number of praxis tests included in the SIPT as opposed to the older SCSIT. When Ayres (1989) discussed praxis in relation to her SIPT studies, she introduced the idea that praxis problems may be manifested in different forms, not all of which are sensory integrative in nature. She coined the term *somatopraxis* to refer to the aspect of praxis that is sensory integrative in origin and grounded in somatosensory processing. At the same time she introduced the term *somatodyspraxia* to refer to a sensory integrative deficit that involves poor praxis and impaired tactile and proprioceptive processing. By definition, somatodyspraxia involves a disorder in tactile discrimination and perception. Cermak (1991) noted that not all children with developmental dyspraxia demonstrate poor tactile perception. The term *somatodyspraxia* applies only to those who do.

The child with somatodyspraxia typically appears clumsy and awkward. Novel motor activities are performed with great difficulty and often result in failure. Transitioning from one body position to another and sequencing and timing the actions involved in a motor task may pose a great challenge. These children typically have difficulty relating their bodies to physical objects in environmental space. They often have difficulty accurately imitating actions of others. Directionality of movement may be disturbed, resulting in toys being broken unintentionally when the child forcefully pushes an object that should be pulled. Many of these children have difficulties with oral praxis, which may affect eating skills or speech articulation.

Some children with dyspraxia have problems with *ideation* (i.e., they have difficulty generating ideas of what to do in a novel situation). When asked to simply play, without being given specific directions, these children may not initiate any activity or they may initiate activity that is habitual and limited or seems to lack a goal. Typical responses, for example, are to wander aimlessly; to perform simple repetitive actions such as patting or pushing objects around; to randomly pile up objects with no apparent plan; or for the more sophisticated child, to wait to observe others doing an activity and then imitate them rather than initiating an activity independently. May-Benson (2001) expanded on the role of ideation in praxis, highlighting the role of language and the social environment and reviewing the neuroanatomical foundations for this important function.

For children with dyspraxia, skills that most children attain rather easily can be excessively challenging (e.g., donning a sweater, feeding oneself with utensils, writing the alphabet, jumping rope, and completing a puzzle). These skills can be mastered only with high motivation on the part of the child, coupled with a great deal of practice, far more than most children require. Participation in sports is often embarrassing and frustrating, and organization of schoolwork may be a problem of particular concern. Children who have somatodyspraxia and are aware of their deficits often avoid difficult motor challenges and may attempt to gain control over such situations by assuming a directing or controlling role over others.

Praxis is best evaluated using the SIPT, which is sensitive to difficulties in this area. However, parent interview and informal observations provide critical pieces in the assessment process. In fact, these are essential in evaluating ideation because currently available standardized tests are extremely limited in their measurement of this aspect of praxis.

Secondary Problems Related to Sensory Integrative Dysfunction

As we have already shown, sensory integration difficulties often impose some limitation on the quality of the child's participation in occupations that he or she wants to do, or needs to do as a member of a family, classroom, or community. How others respond to the child's struggles may have a powerful effect on the child's developing competence. In addition, the child's willingness to grapple with challenging experiences will influence his or her occupational life over the years (Parham, 2002). Unfortunately, a number of secondary problems often arise in conjunction with sensory integration problems. These secondary problems may actually have a more powerful impact on the child's life outcomes than the original sensory integration difficulty. In some cases, what started out as a minor sensory integration difficulty can become magnified into a major barrier to life satisfaction. Following is an explanation of several of these indirect, but significant, influences on the child and family.

First, sensory integrative dysfunction is an "invisible" disability (i.e., not directly and easily detected by the casual observer) that is easily misinterpreted. Sensory integrative disorders can fluctuate in severity from one time to another within the same child. Moreover, the severity of dysfunction and the ways that dysfunction is expressed vary tremendously from one individual to another. This makes it difficult to predict which situations cause problems for a particular child, how much discomfort results, and when distress is likely to occur. Parents and teachers of children with these disorders often find the unpredictability of the child's behavior to be frustrating and difficult to understand. As a result, sensory integrative problems are frequently misinterpreted as purely behavioral or psychological issues. Consequently, the child may be punished or responded to inappropriately, which may lead to chronic feelings of hopelessness as the child comes to think of her or himself as bad or incapable.

A second indirect effect of sensory integrative dysfunction on the child's life is its negative influence on skill development secondary to limited participation in childhood occupations. The child who avoids finger painting because of tactile defensiveness or who rarely attempts climbing on the jungle gym because of dyspraxia misses more than these singular experiences. The child also misses experiences that hone underlying functions such as tactile discrimination, hand strength and dexterity, shoulder stability, balance and equilibrium, hand-eye coordination, bilateral coordination, ideation, and motor planning. If the child misses a substantial amount of such experiences over time, the gap between the child's sensorimotor skills and the skills of peers may grow.

In addition to interference with the development of sensorimotor functions, interactions important to the development of communication and social skills may not occur. Thus, some children with sensory integrative disorders may lack the ability to play successfully with peers partially because they have not been able to participate fully in the play occupations in which sensory, motor, cognitive, and social skills emerge and develop. The fear, anxiety, or discomfort that accompanies many everyday situations is also likely to work against the expression of the child's inner drive toward growth-inducing experiences. Therefore lack of experience and diminished drive to participate compound the direct effects of a sensory integrative disorder. Consequently, the development of competence in many domains of development may be seriously compromised.

A third indirect effect of sensory integrative dysfunction is the undermining of self-esteem and self-confidence over time. Children with sensory integrative dysfunction are often aware of their struggles with commonplace tasks, so it is natural for them to react with frustration. Frustration is likely to mount as the child observes peers mastering these same tasks effortlessly. Chronic frustration can negatively affect and detract from the child's feelings of self-efficacy. Instead, the child may develop feelings of helplessness. This leads to further limitations in the child's experiences because the child becomes less likely to attempt challenging activities.

ASSESSMENT OF SENSORY INTEGRATIVE FUNCTIONS

Assessment of sensory integration, like all other areas addressed in occupational therapy, requires a multifaceted approach because of the need to understand presenting problems, not only in relation to the individual who is being assessed, but also with respect to the family and environments in which that individual lives. Assessment by the occupational therapist begins with a general exploration of the occupations of the child and family, focusing on their concerns and hopes in relation to the child's participation in routine activities. A variety of tools are needed to help the therapist identify whether a sensory integrative disorder is a factor in the child's life and, if so, what the nature of the problem is and whether any intervention should be recommended. Assessment tools employed by occupational therapists using a sensory integration perspective include interviews and questionnaires, informal and formal observations, standardized tests, and consideration of services and resources available to and appropriate for the family. Roley (2002) provided an excellent discussion of how this process of assessment is consistent with the guidelines laid out in the Occupational Therapy Practice Framework adopted by the American Occupational Therapy Association (2002).

Interviews and Questionnaires

The potential need for an occupational therapy assessment of sensory integration usually arises with a referral from someone who knows the child and something about the problems that the child is experiencing. Therefore the time of referral is often ideal for initiating the assessment process. The referral source, family members, and others who work with the child may all be valuable sources of information through interview or questionnaire (Figure 11-11). This initial phase of evaluation identifies the presenting problems, or main concerns, about the child and begins the process of determining whether a sensory integrative dysfunction is a significant influence on the child's ability to function.

During the initial interview, as the parent, teacher, psychologist, physician, or other referral source describes the child's difficulties, the therapist may gather important information by probing to uncover hidden signs of sensory integrative dysfunction that may be present. For example, the teacher may report that the child is always fighting while standing in line and cannot seem to stay seated during reading circle time. Further questioning by the therapist may disclose signs of possible tactile defensiveness that might explain the child's behavior but were not considered important by the teacher who is unfamiliar with this condition. A parent may be able to provide critical information about the child's development, which may be helpful in identifying early signs of

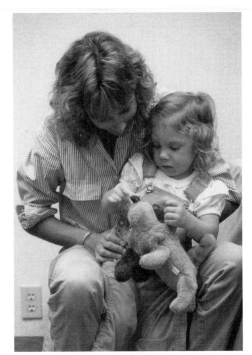

FIGURE 11-11 Because parents know their child better than anyone else, they are invaluable sources of information to the therapist, especially in beginning phases of the assessment process. (Courtesy of Shay McAtee.)

sensory integrative dysfunction. For instance, parents may have noticed that it always takes their child longer than others to learn new tasks, such as cutting with scissors or riding a tricycle; this is a possible sign of dyspraxia. Another important role of the interview is to uncover alternative explanations of the child's difficulties that may rule out sensory integrative dysfunction, such as when a recent emotional crisis (e.g., a divorce or death) coincides with the onset of problems. Miller and Summers (2001) provided examples of the kinds of questions one might ask in a parent interview.

Questionnaires, checklists, and histories given by caregivers and other adults who know the child well are other means for gathering information that aid in identifying presenting problems, estimating how long they have been a concern, and clarifying the priorities of the family. One such instrument is a sensory history or similar questionnaire. Originally developed by Ayres as an unpublished questionnaire, this type of instrument asks parents questions regarding specific child behaviors indicative of sensory integrative dysfunction, and parents respond by rating the child using a Likert-style scale. In the past decade, the reliability and validity of these types of questionnaires have been evaluated with encouraging results. Currently, three such questionnaires are the most extensively researched: the Sensory Profile (Dunn, 1999), the Evaluation of Sensory Processing (ESP) (Parham & Ecker, 2002), and the Sensory Rating Scale (Provost, 1991). The Sensory Profile is available in versions for infants and toddlers (Dunn, 2002) and children in early and middle childhood (Dunn, 1999), as well as for adolescents and adults (Brown & Dunn, 2002).

Behavior checklists and other questionnaires that address classroom performance are often a convenient way to elicit information from teachers (Carrasco & Lee, 1993). An additional way to gather information in the initial phases of assessment is through clinical records, including reading previous reports from other professionals and reviewing medical histories.

It may be useful to talk with the child directly when possible. Royeen and Fortune (1990, 2002) developed a child questionnaire for the assessment of tactile defensiveness, called the Touch Inventory for Elementary School-Aged Children (TIE). Children with enough verbal skills to discuss their own abilities, perceptions, and difficulties can sometimes provide invaluable insight into their condition through such a questionnaire-based interview. The Alert Program (Williams & Shellenberger, 1994), a group intervention program for older children and adults, includes a self-assessment of sensory preferences that can be adapted for assessment of younger children to help them identify and communicate their characteristic sensory responses.

The information garnered through the initial interview process is used to decide whether further assessment is warranted and, if so, which evaluation procedures are most appropriate. This information is also critical in interpreting the final pool of information gathered through assessment and in prioritizing goals for the child in light of the main concerns of the family.

Informal and Formal Observations of the Child

Direct observation of the child is essential to the evaluation of sensory integration. Informal observations, clinical observations, and standardized testing are commonly used.

Informal Observations

Informal observation of the child in natural settings, such as a classroom, playground, or home, is informative and should be done whenever feasible. Informal observation will influence the conclusion as to whether a sensory integrative disorder is present and will, perhaps more importantly, indicate how the child's difficulties are interfering with daily occupations. For example, an experienced therapist can often detect signs of poor body awareness by observing the child at school. Such signs may include exerting too much pressure on a pencil, standing too close to classmates in line, misstepping when climbing on a jungle gym, and sitting in an ineffective position in a chair while doing class assignments. Teachers may not necessarily report these behaviors to

the therapist if they perceive them as typical signs of inattentiveness or clumsiness.

Informal observation of the child in the clinical setting can also be useful in that it shows how the child responds to situations that are novel or unpredictable. A child with dyspraxia may have a great deal of difficulty figuring out how to mount an unfamiliar climbing structure in the clinic, even though performance is adequate on similar tasks at home or at school where the child has practiced them. The novelty of the clinical therapy room elicits responses from children that may be diagnostically relevant. For children with good ideation and sensory processing abilities, the endless opportunities afforded by sensory integration equipment in the clinic can be exhilarating. For the child with a disorder like dyspraxia, the same environment may be confusing, puzzling, or frustrating. A child with gravitational insecurity may be terrified by the prospect of equipment that moves, whereas a child with autism may be distressed by the clinic environment because of its unpredictability and discrepancy from familiar settings. Parham (1987) has provided some guidelines for organizing informal observations in the clinic, with special attention to issues related to praxis. Although her suggestions are focused on the assessment of preschoolers, they can also be applied to older children and may be particularly helpful in evaluating older children who are unable to cooperate with standardized testing.

Clinical Observations

Formal observations that are highly structured and similar to test items are often used in an occupational therapy assessment of sensory integration. Usually referred to as *clinical observations*, these typically involve a set of specific tasks, reflexes, and signs of nervous system integrity that are associated with sensory integrative functioning. Ayres (1965, 1966a, 1966b, 1969, 1971, 1972d, 1977) included measures of such formal observations in her factor analytic studies, along with standardized tests. She also developed a set of clinical observations that she used in clinical practice. These unpublished, nonstandardized evaluation tools were intended to supplement standardized test scores and subsequently were revised and expanded upon by many other therapists over the years (Blanche, 2002; Bundy, 2002; Dunn, 1981; Wilson, Pollock, Kaplan, & Law, 2000). Examples of some of the most commonly used clinical observations are described in Box 11-1.

One of the difficulties in using clinical observations as an assessment tool is that administration and scoring criteria have not been standardized. This means that they are administered using different procedures from one clinician to another. Furthermore, most of them lack any normative data to aid in interpretation of any scores that might be obtained. Some, but not all, clinical observations have research behind them to inform interpretation

BOX 11-1 Examples of Commonly Used Clinical Observations

- *Crossing body midline:* A movement that has a tendency to occur when using the hand to reach for or manipulate an object in contralateral space. This tendency typically emerges during toddlerhood and early childhood and is related to the development of hand preference. Delays in midline crossing may be related to inadequate hand preference and bilateral integration.
- *Equilibrium reactions:* Automatic postural and limb adjustments that occur when the body's center of gravity shifts its base of support. These adjustments serve to restore the body's center of gravity over its base of support so that balance is maintained or restored. Difficulties with equilibrium reactions are associated with vestibular processing problems.
- *Muscle tone:* The readiness of a muscle to contract. Force with which a muscle resists being lengthened.
- *Prone extension:* Ability to assume and hold an "airplane" position (neck, upper body, and hips extended to lift head, arms, and legs off the floor) while lying prone. Difficulty maintaining this position for 30 seconds is related to inefficient vestibular processing in children 6 years of age and older.
- *Supine flexion:* Ability to assume and hold a curled position (neck, upper body, hips, and knees flexed so that knees are drawn close to the head) while lying supine. Difficulty maintaining this position for 30 seconds is related to poor praxis in children 6 years of age and older.

(e.g., Dunn, 1981; Gregory-Flock & Yerxa, 1984; Magalhaes, Koomar, & Cermak, 1989; Wilson et al., 2000). Occupational therapists must rely on the information from these studies, as well as their personal expertise and judgment, to interpret the results of clinical observations. Without the requisite data in hand, occupational therapists are cautioned to avoid overinterpretation of clinical observations in light of the lack of standardized procedures and inadequate information regarding expected performance across age, gender, and other demographically related groups.

It is perhaps most problematic that most clinical observations address motor functions that may be strongly affected by conditions other than sensory integrative dysfunction. Therefore, the therapist must master advanced knowledge of sensory integration theory before meaningful interpretations of these observations can be made.

Standardized Testing

Occupational therapists frequently use standardized tests to evaluate sensory integration. Although most relevant tests are not labeled as tests of sensory integration per se, they do include items or subtests from which inferences regarding sensory integration may be drawn. For example, the Miller Assessment for Preschoolers (Miller, 1988) includes tests of stereognosis, tactile perception, and some vestibular functions. Many tests, such as

the Bruininks-Oseretsky Test of Motor Proficiency (Bruininks, 1978), measure aspects of fine and gross motor skills (such as bilateral coordination) that are related to sensory integrative functions. Other tests, such as the Developmental Test of Visual Motor Integration (Beery, 1997), provide specific information related to visual-perceptual and perceptual-motor skills.

Some tests geared toward the broader evaluation of occupation, such as the School Function Assessment (SFA) (Coster, Deeney, Haltwanger, & Haley, 1998) are useful for identifying the extent to which sensory integrative disorders may be affecting the child's participation in occupations within specific settings. When the child being assessed is suspected of having a sensory integrative disorder, tests such as the SFA are most effectively used along with specific measures of sensory integration. When combined, these tests identify the functional problems to target in intervention and the reasons for the child's difficulties.

Although several tests are available that contribute incidental information regarding sensory integrative functions, the SIPT are the only set of standardized tests designed specifically for in-depth evaluation of sensory integration. The SIPT evolved from a series of tests that Ayres developed in the 1960s (Ayres, 1963, 1964, 1966a, 1966b, 1969) and later published as the SCSIT (Ayres, 1972c) and the SCPNT (Ayres, 1975). The standardization process used in the development of the SIPT was rigorous, involving normative data on approximately 2000 children in North America and extensive reliability and validity studies (Ayres, 1989). Its 17 tests measure tactile, vestibular, and proprioceptive sensory processing; form and space perception and visuomotor coordination; bilateral integration and sequencing abilities; and praxis (Ayres & Marr, 1991). A list of the 17 tests and the functions measured by each is presented in Table 11-3.

The SIPT require about 2 hours to administer and another 30 to 45 minutes to score. Raw scores may be translated into standard scores by the therapist using a computer diskette available from the publisher. Alternatively, raw scores may be sent to the publisher, Western Psychological Services, for an analysis using the normative data. After normative scores are obtained, the therapist critically examines them to determine if patterns of sensory integrative dysfunction are evident. Not only are patterns of test scores scrutinized, but also the observations that the therapist has made of child behavior during testing are considered in interpreting test scores. Finally, test scores and test behaviors are integrated with all other sources of information from the assessment in reaching a conclusion regarding the status of sensory integrative functioning.

Because it is a standardized test, the SIPT must be administered with strict adherence to standardized procedures (Figure 11-12). Specialized training is required

TABLE 11-3 Functions Measured by the Sensory Integration and Praxis Tests

Function	Description
Space visualization	Motor-free visual space perception; mental manipulation of objects
Figure-ground perception	Motor-free visual perception of figures on a rival background
Manual form perception	Identification of block held in hand with visual counterpart or with block held in other hand
Kinesthesia	Somatic perception of hand and arm position and movement
Finger identification	Tactile perception of individual fingers
Graphesthesia	Tactile perception and practic replication of designs
Localization of tactile stimuli	Tactile perception of specific stimulus applied to arm or hand
Praxis on verbal command	Ability to motor-plan body postures on the basis of verbal directions without visual cures
Design copying	Visuopractic ability to copy simple and complex two-dimensional designs, and the manner or approach one uses to copy designs
Constructional praxis	Ability to relate objects to each other in three-dimensional space
Postural praxis	Ability to plan and execute body movements and positions
Oral praxis	Ability to plan and execute lip, tongue, and jaw movements
Sequencing praxis	Ability to repeat a series of hand and finger movements
Bilateral motor coordination	Ability to move both hands and both feet in a smooth and integrated pattern
Standing and walking balance	Static and dynamic balance on one or both feet with eyes opened and closed
Motor accuracy	Hand-eye coordination and control of movement
Postrotary nystagmus	Central nervous system processing of vestibular input assessed through observation of the duration and integrity of a vestibuloocular reflex

Reprinted from Mailloux, Z. (1990). An overview of the Sensory Integration and Praxis Tests. *American Journal of Occupational Therapy, 44,* 589-594.

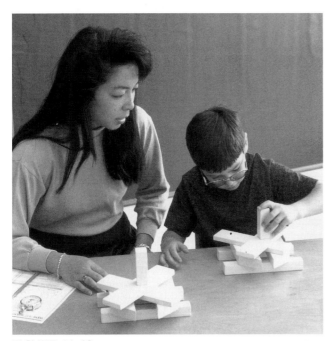

FIGURE 11-12 The Constructional Praxis Test is one of 17 tests of the Sensory Integration and Praxis Tests (SIPT). The SIPT must be administered individually with strict adherence to standardized procedures. (Courtesy of Shay McAtee.)

to administer and interpret the SIPT. It is a complex set of tests and, unlike most published tests, cannot be self-taught by simply reading the manual. In addition to formal training for the SIPT, it is strongly recommended that therapists practice administration of the tests with children who do not have any known problems and with children who have recognized difficulties. With this experience and training, the therapist can administer the tests in a manner that produces reliable scores while allowing for observation of behaviors that provide additional information about the child's sensory integration and praxis abilities.

Consideration of Available Services and Resources

In addition to the information that is gathered about the child, an occupational therapy assessment of sensory integration should take into consideration the services and resources that are available to the child. Information regarding the type of services that the child is currently receiving, how he or she is responding to these services, and what services, programs, and resources are available to the child need careful consideration in light of the purpose and findings of the evaluation before recommendations can be formulated. For example, an occupational therapist may be asked to provide a reevaluation of a child who has been receiving occupational therapy for several years. If the child continues to demonstrate significant sensory integrative dysfunction and has shown a diminishing response to treatment using a classical sensory integration approach, the recommendations would be different than if the child no longer showed evidence of a significant sensory integrative dysfunction.

Similarly, a child who lives in an area where no occupational therapists are qualified to provide classical sensory integration intervention needs a different program recommendation than a child who has easy access to this type of service. Understanding family aspirations and values, as well as resources in terms of funding, transportation, time, and available caregivers, are also critical in identifying what kinds of services are most helpful to the child and family. These issues are just as important to the assessment process as the within-child factors that are addressed in a sensory integration evaluation.

Interpretation of Assessment Findings

Once all of the information from interviews, questionnaires, informal and formal observations, standardized tests, and consideration of available services and resources has been collected, the occupational therapist must integrate and interpret these data to reach meaningful conclusions and appropriate recommendations for the individual child. Conclusions and recommendations should be framed with an overriding concern for the occupations of the child and family and the contexts that influence occupational engagement (Roley, 2002). Burke (2001) advocate the strategy of creating a narrative, or story, to form an integrated understanding of the child and family in order to focus assessment and intervention planning on issues that are most meaningful and important to them. In creating such a narrative, the therapist not only generates a picture of the child and family in the present, but also imagines how changes might unfold over the next few years. Parham (2002) has called this a "future-oriented, top-down" approach to assessment.

One of the important steps in this process is to evaluate whether a sensory integrative dysfunction is a contributor to the occupational challenges of the child. To do this, data are classified into categories that either support or refute the presence of particular types of sensory integrative dysfunction. After a detailed analysis of the constellation of assessment findings, a hypothesis is generated as to whether a sensory integrative dysfunction appears to be present. If a sensory integrative dysfunction is thought to be present, the type of disorder is tentatively identified.

It is critical to relate the assessment findings to the presenting problems and initial concerns of the family or referral source. For example, an assessment may uncover signs of tactile defensiveness in a child described by the parents as destructive and impulsive. The evaluating therapist explains how tactile defensiveness may be related to the child's behavior problems. Because sensory integrative problems are not commonly recognized, the therapist usually includes an explanation of how the assessment findings are linked to the daily life experiences and occupations of the child and family.

If an assessment leads to a recommendation for intervention, it generally includes an estimate of the duration of time that the child should receive therapy, some indication of prognosis, and a statement regarding expected areas of change. The anticipated gains can be further clarified through the establishment of specific goals and objectives. The format in which goals are specified is often a function of the setting in which therapy is delivered. For example, a school district may tend to include certain types of goals as part of an individualized education plan, whereas a hospital setting may lean toward more medically related outcomes. Whatever the case, goals should be established in a manner that is culturally relevant for the family and considers the needs and wishes of the individual child.

SENSORY INTEGRATIVE DYSFUNCTION INTERVENTION

Planning an occupational therapy program for a child with a sensory integrative disorder requires the same careful analysis that is used when applying any theoretic framework in clinical practice. The constellation of child and family characteristics is analyzed in relation to the occupations of the individuals involved. Intervention is designed to focus on engagement in occupation in order to support the participation of the child in the everyday contexts of his or her life (AOTA, 2002). In a sensory integration approach to intervention, the unique ways in which sensory integrative problems affect engagement and participation in the occupations of the particular child and his or her family provide the cornerstone upon which decisions regarding treatment are made (Roley, 2002). Intervention is continually planned and evaluated in relation to the occupations that the child wants and needs to do in the contexts of home, school, and community.

The assessment process aids the therapist in deciding whether any intervention is recommended and, if so, in what format: individual therapy, group sessions, collaborative problem solving with parents and teachers, or consultation. Regardless of the form in which intervention is delivered, theory-based concepts regarding the nature of sensory integration are applied whenever a sensory integrative approach is selected. Six guiding principles from Ayres's work (1972b, 1979, 1981) are summarized in Box 11-2. The key ideas behind these principles were introduced previously in this chapter in the sections on sensory integrative development and sensory integrative disorders.

Making decisions regarding the manner in which occupational therapy should be provided for children with sensory integrative disorders requires a great deal of expertise that is developed through advanced training and years of practice. The field of sensory integration is a complex, specialized area of occupational therapy practice that demands that the therapist synthesize informa-

BOX 11-2   Guiding Principles from Sensory Integration Theory

1 Sensory input can be used systematically to elicit an adaptive response.
2 Registration of meaningful sensory input is necessary before an adaptive response can be made.
3 An adaptive response contributes to the development of sensory integration.
4 Better organization of adaptive responses enhances the child's general behavioral organization.
5 More mature and complex patterns of behavior are composed of consolidations of more primitive behaviors.
6 The more inner-directed a child's activities are, the greater the potential of the activities for improving neural organization.

tion from many sources. Because it is a dynamically changing field of practice, it is important that the therapist stays abreast of new developments in sensory integration theory, practice, and research. These sources of information, in combination with the unique situation of the child and family being helped, all influence the decision of whether to intervene and, if so, how. In the following section, three of the primary methods of service delivery are described: individual therapy, group sessions, and consultation. Most of the time in clinical practice, these forms of intervention are used in combination rather than as the sole service delivery method. They may also be used with interventions based on other frames of reference, such as neurodevelopmental treatment or training of in-hand manipulation, as long as the underlying assumptions of the interventions are mutually compatible.

Individual Therapy

Individual occupational therapy for a sensory integrative disorder is the most intensive form of intervention. Individual therapy is usually recommended as the most effective way to initially help a child gain improved capabilities when sensory integrative problems are interfering with the child's occupations at home, in play, at school, or in the community. Individual occupational therapy for sensory integrative disorders can generally be classified into two categories: classical sensory integration treatment and compensatory skill development.

Classical Sensory Integrative Treatment

In this section, the term classical sensory integration treatment refers to the kind of individual occupational therapy that Ayres developed specifically to remediate sensory integrative dysfunction in children. Although she originally designed this therapy for children with learning disabilities (Ayres, 1972b), she and many other expert clinicians have used this kind of intervention, along with compensatory approaches and consultation, to help children with other kinds of problems as well, including autism (Mailloux, 2001; Mailloux & Roley, 2002).

In designing this specialized form of occupational therapy, Ayres was influenced by the neurobiologic literature, which shows that nervous systems have plasticity or changeability. Plasticity is particularly characteristic of the developing young child. This led Ayres to hypothesize that the neural systems that impair function may be remediable, especially in the young child. Accordingly, she set out to design therapy that capitalized on the plasticity of the nervous system to remediate sensory integrative dysfunction. This is *not* to say that sensory integrative treatment cures conditions such as learning disability, autism, or developmental delays. Rather, the intent is to improve the efficiency with which the nervous system interprets and uses sensory information for functional use. Therefore in a classical sensory integration approach, therapy is aimed at promoting underlying capabilities to the greatest degree possible.

Classical sensory integrative treatment has several defining characteristics. It is virtually always applied on an *individual* basis because the therapist must adjust therapeutic activities moment by moment in relation to the individual child's interest in the activity or response to a specific challenge or sensory experience (Clark et al., 1989; Kimball, 1999; Koomar & Bundy, 2002). This requires the therapist to continually focus attention on the child while being mindful of opportunities in the environment for eliciting adaptive responses. The therapist's decisions regarding how and when to intervene involve a delicate interplay between the therapist's judgment regarding the potential therapeutic value of an activity and the child's motivation to do the activity. The therapist does not use a "cookbook" approach in providing this therapy (e.g., by entering the therapy situation with a predetermined schedule of activities that the child is required to follow). Rather, the therapist enters into a relationship with the child that fosters the child's inner drive to actively explore the environment and to master challenges posed by the environment.

Treatment involves a *balance between structure and freedom* (Ayres, 1972b, 1979), and its effectiveness is contingent on the proficiency of the therapist in making judgments regarding when to step in to provide structure and when to step back and allow the child to choose activities. The therapist's job is to create an environment that evokes increasingly complex adaptive responses from the child. To accomplish this, the therapist respects the child's needs and interests while taking opportunities to help the child successfully meet a challenge. An example is a child who needs to develop more efficient righting and equilibrium reactions and chooses to sit and swing on a platform swing. The therapist may allow the child to swing awhile to become accustomed to the vestibular sensations. Once the child seems comfortable, the therapist steps in to jiggle the swing to stimulate the desired responses. However, if the child responds to this challenge with signs of anxiety or fear, the therapist needs to intervene quickly to help the child feel safer. For example, the therapist might set an inner tube on the swing to provide a base to stabilize the lower part of the child's body and increase feelings of security while the child's upper body is free to make the required righting reactions. Therapeutic activities thus emerge from the interaction between therapist and child. Such individualized treatment can be fully realized only when there is a one-to-one ratio between therapist and child (Figure 11-13).

The emphasis on the *inner drive* of the child is another key characteristic of classical sensory integration therapy (Ayres, 1972b, 1979; Clark et al., 1989; Koomar & Bundy, 2002). Self-direction on the part of the child is encouraged because therapeutic gains are maximized if the child is fully invested as an active participant. However, this is not to say that the child is permitted to engage in free play with no adult guidance. The optimal therapy situation is one in which a balance is struck

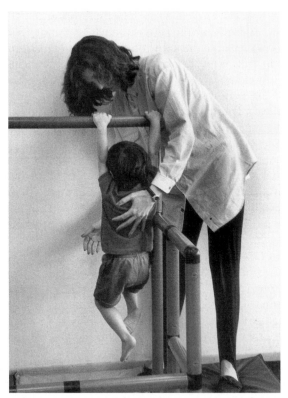

FIGURE 11-13 Classical sensory integration treatment requires the therapist to attend closely to the child on a moment-by-moment basis to ensure that therapeutic activities are individually tailored to changing needs and interests of the child. (Courtesy of Shay McAtee.)

between the structure provided by the therapist and some degree of freedom of choice on the part of the child (Ayres, 1972b, 1981). Drawing on the child's interests and imagination is often a key to encouraging a child to exert more effort on a difficult task or to stay with a challenging activity for a longer time. However, because children with sensory integrative problems do not always demonstrate inner drive toward growth-inducing activities, it is often necessary to modify activities and to find ways to entice a child toward interaction. A high degree of directiveness often is needed when working with children with autism or other children whose inner drive is limited. Occasionally a therapist may use a high degree of directiveness within the context of a particular activity to show a child that the challenging activity is possible not only to achieve, but also to enjoy.

Related to inner drive is another key feature of sensory integration treatment—the valuing of *active participation*, rather than passive participation, on the part of the child. Because the brain responds differently and learns more effectively when an individual is actively involved in a task rather than merely receiving passive stimulation, it is considered optimal for a child to be an active participant to the greatest degree possible. For example, sensory integration theory posits that a child experiences a greater degree of integration from pumping a swing or pulling on a rope to make it go than from being swung passively.

Maximal active involvement generally takes place when therapeutic activities are at just the right level of complexity, wherein the child not only feels comfortable and nonthreatened but also experiences some challenge that requires effort. The course of therapy usually begins with activities in which the child feels comfortable and competent and then moves toward increasing challenges. For example, for children with gravitational insecurity, therapy usually begins with activities close to the ground and with close physical support from the therapist to help the child feel secure. Gradually, over weeks of therapy, activities that require stepping up on different surfaces and moving away from the floor are introduced as the therapist subtly withdraws physical support. Introducing just the right level of challenge, while respecting the child's need to feel secure and in control, is a key to maximizing the child's active involvement in therapy (Figure 11-14).

However, there are situations in which passive stimulation is needed to help prepare a child for more complex or challenging activities. For example, the child with autism may show improved sensory registration after receiving passive linear vestibular stimulation (Slavik et al., 1984). The improved registration means that the child has greater awareness of the environment, and thus the passive stimulation is a stepping stone toward active involvement in an activity. Another example is the use of passive tactile stimulation as a means for reducing tactile

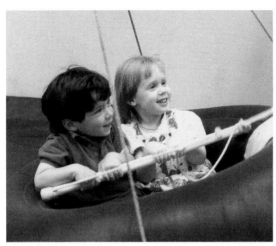

FIGURE 11-14 Rather than passively imposing vestibular input on the child, classical sensory integration treatment emphasizes active participation and self-direction of the child. (Courtesy of Shay McAtee.)

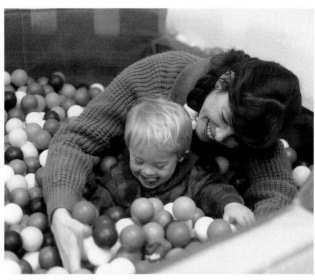

FIGURE 11-15 The setting in which classical sensory integration treatment takes place provides a variety of sensory experiences. Immersion in a pool of balls presents challenges to sensory modulation. (Courtesy of Shay McAtee.)

defensiveness (Ayres, 1972b; Wilbarger & Wilbarger, 1991). However, this aspect of therapy is seen as only a limited component of a sensory integrative treatment program and then only as a step toward facilitating more active participation.

Another key characteristic of sensory integrative treatment is the *setting* in which it takes place. The provision of a special therapeutic environment is an important aspect of this kind of intervention and has been described in detail by other authors (Slavik & Chew, 1990; Walker, 1991). Based on the research that shows that brain structure and function are enhanced when animals are permitted to actively explore an interesting environment (Jacobs & Schneider, 2001), a sensory-enriched environment is designed to evoke active exploration on the part of the child. The clinic that is designed for classical sensory integrative treatment contains large activity areas with an array of specialized equipment. The availability of suspended equipment is a hallmark of this treatment approach (Clark et al., 1989; Koomar & Bundy, 2002). Suspended equipment provides rich opportunities for stimulating and challenging the vestibular system. In addition, equipment and materials are available that provide a variety of somatosensory stimuli, including tactile, vibratory, and proprioceptive. Mats and large pillows are used for safety. Overall, this special environment provides the child with a safe and interesting place in which to explore his or her capabilities. At the same time it provides the therapist with a tool kit for creating sensory experiences that are enticing and for gently guiding the child toward activities that challenge perception, dynamic postural control, and motor planning (Figure 11-15).

Because of the prominence of vestibular stimulation in the classical sensory integration treatment environment, a few cautionary words are in order regarding this

powerful tool. Vestibular stimulation, most often in the form of linear movement, is commonly introduced early in the course of treatment for many children because it is believed to have an organizing effect on other sensory systems (Ayres, 1972b, 1979, 1981). However, it can have a highly disturbing and disorganizing effect on the child if used carelessly. Vestibular stimulation may produce strong autonomic responses, such as blanching and nausea. It directly influences the arousal level and, if not regulated carefully, may produce hyperactive, distractible states or lethargic, drowsy states. Used in classical sensory integration treatment, vestibular stimulation is not passively imposed on the child. Rather, the child is allowed to initiate and actively control vestibular input as much as possible, with the therapist stepping in to help modulate it when indicated. For example, if a child is actively rotating while sitting in a tire swing and begins to exhibit mild signs of autonomic activation, the therapist may intervene. The therapist may reduce the intensity of the swinging by guiding the child to shift to slow linear swinging or by offering the child a trapeze to pull to increase the amount of proprioceptive input. Proprioceptive input is believed to have an inhibiting effect on vestibular input, based on results of animal research (Fredrickson, Schwartz, & Kornhuber, 1966). Therefore knowledge of the effects of vestibular stimulation and its interactions with other sensory systems is critical in this treatment approach. Responsible use of vestibular stimulation as a treatment modality absolutely requires advanced training in sensory integration.

To summarize the key features of classical sensory integrative treatment, therapeutic activities are neither predetermined nor are they simply free play. The flow of the treatment session results from a collaboration between the therapist and child in which the therapist encourages and supports the child in a way that moves the child toward therapeutic goals. This all takes place within a special environment that is safe yet challenging. The use of special equipment and powerful sensory modalities requires that the therapist have special training well beyond the entry level of practice in occupational therapy.

Classical sensory integration treatment is an intensive, long-term intervention. Although treatment schedules vary, a typical schedule involves two sessions per week, each lasting 45 minutes to 1 hour. A typical course of therapy lasts for about 2 years. Most experts agree that at least 6 months of therapy are needed to detect results.

After Ayres (1972b, 1979) developed the classical sensory integrative treatment approach, her colleagues and students continued to further develop and expand on her intervention concepts. Koomar and Bundy (2002) provided a particularly thorough description of the application of sensory integration procedures for specific types of sensory integrative disorders. Holloway (1998) has imported classical sensory integration treatment concepts into the neonatal intensive care unit (NICU), where the treatment principles are used to help young infants when their developing nervous systems are most plastic. Others have adapted classical sensory integration intervention to address the needs of infants and toddlers who are developmentally at risk (Schaaf & Anzalone, 2001), and children with visual impairments (Roley, 2001), cerebral palsy (Blanche & Schaaf, 2001), environmental deprivation (Cermak, 2001), and fragile X syndrome (Hickman, 2001).

Use of the classical sensory integration treatment approach requires advanced study and training. Koomar and Bundy (2002) advocated a mentorship process as the best preparation for learning how to clinically apply sensory integration principles. Ayres also advocated this and established a 4-month course in which therapists receive both didactic instruction and intensive hands-on experience treating children under close supervision. Ayres believed that this level of intensity was required to master the classical sensory integration approach. Because of the highly specialized and complex nature of the classical sensory integration approach, it is important that occupational therapists gain mentored experience in this area before independently engaging in this form of practice.

In addition, ongoing study and discussion with peers is highly recommended to hone one's clinical expertise in this area, after acquiring advanced training. One technique that is useful in this regard is systematic analysis of cases using structures such as the STEP-SI model for clinical reasoning (Miller & Summers, 2001; Miller, Wilbarger, Stackhouse, & Trunnell, 2002). STEP-SI is an acronym for six dimensions to consider when reviewing an intervention session: sensation, task, environment, predictability, self-monitoring, and interactions. Systematic analysis of each of these dimensions can be used to organize assessment data, plan goals and priorities for intervention, and evaluate how well intervention is moving toward desired goals. We have found it to be particularly helpful for analyzing videotaped individual intervention sessions in order to identify therapeutic strategies that seem to be especially effective with a particular child.

While the traditional application of the classical sensory integrative approach as described here occurs within specialized therapy centers, many of the concepts can be applied in other settings as well. Many school-based occupational therapists have found ways to incorporate the central principles of the sensory integrative approach into the educational setting, including bringing specialized equipment into classrooms and playgrounds in ways that help to organize and prepare a child for learning. Successful therapy programs frequently involve helping families to understand and use the sensory integrative concepts that support and facilitate their children's success by developing activities at home and identifying resources within the community that reinforce the experiences emphasized during therapy (Pediatric Therapy Network, 2003).

Compensatory Skill Development

In contrast to the classical sensory integrative treatment approach, the compensatory skill development approach does not attempt to remediate an underlying sensory integrative disorder. Instead it aims to help the child and family develop specific skills or coping strategies in the face of a sensory integrative disorder. This approach may be used to supplement or to replace classical sensory integrative treatment.

The compensatory approach may be appropriate when a therapist trained in classical sensory integrative treatment is not available. It may also be selected as the treatment of choice for a child who urgently needs to accomplish specific tasks or skills and cannot wait for the longer-range but more widely generalizable outcomes of classical sensory integrative treatment. It may also be a desirable alternative for the child who has reached an age at which expected gains from the classical treatment are minimal. The compensatory approach may also be introduced to a child who has been involved with classical sensory integrative treatment. Such cases include children who (1) have responded well to a classical sensory integrative treatment for some time but have reached a plateau in gains, (2) are approaching or have reached ages at which expected gains from the classical treatment are minimal, (3) do not appear motivated to participate or show waning interest in the classical approach, (4) do not demonstrate improvement in response to the classical sensory integrative approach after a reasonable amount of time (usually a 6-month trial), or (5) urgently need to accomplish specific tasks or skills that could be trained as a supplement or replacement for classical sensory integrative treatment.

When the compensatory skill approach is selected, therapy is aimed at training specific skills or using techniques that permit better performance on a given task. For example, a child with poor proprioceptive feedback may need to keep up with handwriting exercises assigned in his or her second-grade class. The child is involved with classical sensory integrative treatment, which aims to help him or her develop better body awareness that eventually will help him or her not only with writing, but also with catching, throwing, cutting, buttoning, and many other proprioception-related difficulties. However, because of the everyday stress of the demands of handwriting, the child may not be able to afford to wait for these generalized capabilities to develop through sensory integrative treatment. For this child, specific handwriting training may be used to help him or her develop better handwriting skills, despite poor proprioceptive feedback. Adaptations may also be introduced to help the child compensate for the problem. For instance, a weighted pencil may provide augmented proprioceptive feedback regarding the position of the child's hand. Additionally, arrangements may be made with the child's teacher for the child to enter part of his or her schoolwork on a computer or to dictate it into a tape recorder to prevent poor writing skills from impeding other aspects of academic performance.

The therapist who chooses to use the compensatory skill development approach to individual therapy can do so while being mindful of the guiding principles of sensory integration theory (see Box 11-2). For example, it is optimal to involve self-direction and active participation as much as possible. This might be accomplished with the example child by having the child write his or her own stories related to his or her interests and experiences. Handwriting exercises that require active movement are expected to accomplish much more than any that are dependent on passive guidance of the child's hand. The therapist's ability to read the child's responses to writing activities helps ensure that the activities remain motivating and appropriately challenging. However, this approach generally tends to be much more therapist directed than the child-centered classical sensory integration approach.

Use of a compensatory skill approach for children with sensory integrative disorders requires that the therapist know enough about sensory integration to make sound judgments regarding when this approach is appropriate. Understanding the underlying sensory integrative disorder adequately is also essential so that the therapist does not interpret sensory-based problems as behavioral or neuromuscular in origin. Continuing education courses in specific training methods, such as the handwriting, are available and should be actively pursued by therapists desiring to use this approach.

Group Therapy Programs

Group rather than individual occupational therapy is sometimes recommended for children experiencing sensory integrative disorders. Sometimes *group therapy programs* are used as a transition from individual therapy so that the child can apply newly developed skills in a social peer context with less intensive support from a therapist (Figure 11-16). The need to help a child learn to function in the context of school- and community-based groups, such as in classrooms or on sports teams, is another important reason to consider placing the child in a therapeutic group setting. Furthermore, sensory integrative disorders often create social problems for children, and treatment in groups can provide an opportunity to help the child develop important peer interaction skills.

The occupational therapist working with a group of children cannot provide the same level of vigilance to individual responses that takes place during individual therapy. Therefore, some of the more intense applications of sensory stimulation or risk-taking behaviors that might be encouraged during classical sensory integrative treatment cannot be used within a group, nor can the therapist give the close guidance that is finely tuned to the individual child's needs every moment of the treatment session. Again, however, the principles of sensory integration theory outlined in Box 11-3 are important concepts to incorporate into the group format as much as possible.

Working with children in a group provides the opportunity to observe some of the ways in which sensory integrative disorders interrupt functional behavior in a social context. Some problematic child behaviors emerge only in a group situation and may not be evident during individual therapy. For example, tactile defensiveness may not be apparent in the safe constraints of individual

---

BOX 11-3 Expected Outcomes of Occupational Therapy Using Sensory Integration Principles

1 Increase in the frequency or duration of adaptive responses
2 Development of increasingly more complex adaptive responses
3 Improvement in gross and fine motor skills
4 Improvement in cognitive, language, and academic performance
5 Increase in self-confidence and self-esteem
6 Enhancement of occupational engagement and social participation
7 Enhancement of family life

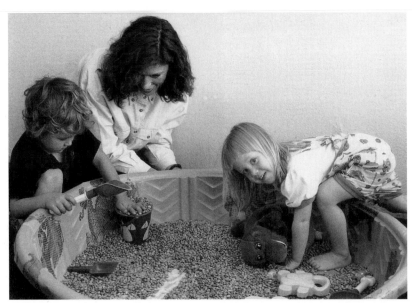

FIGURE 11-16 Group programs provide opportunities for children with sensory integrative disorders to develop coping skills that help them function in social context with peers. (Courtesy of Shay McAtee.)

therapy but may become obvious as a child tries to participate within a group of people who are brushing by in an unpredictable manner. Observing how the group dynamic affects the child can help the therapist know what aspects of the classroom, playground, park, or after-school activities are likely to pose a threat or challenge.

In some situations, external variables such as funding limitations, availability of staff, or organizational policies create the need for children to receive therapy in a group setting. It is important that occupational therapists make recommendations based primarily on the needs of the children being served, taking into consideration such outside factors, rather than allowing the external factors to dictate the type of intervention that is provided. It is also important to differentiate between what can be accomplished within a group versus an individual therapy session. Because group programs do not permit the same degree of intensive therapy as the classical sensory integration approach, they are not expected to lead to the same outcomes. Moreover, group programs usually resemble the compensatory skill approach more closely than classical sensory integrative treatment in aim and process, although some aim to facilitate and maintain sensory integrative functions.

Several resources are available to the therapist interested in developing group programs based on sensory integration concepts. Examples include group programs described by Bissell, Fisher, Owens, and Polcyn (1998), Inamura (1998), and Scheerer (1996). An especially innovative application of sensory integration concepts to groups is reflected in the work of Williams and Shellenberger (1994). Through a group format, their Alert Program helps children learn to recognize how alert they are feeling, to identify the sensorimotor experiences that they can use to change their level of alertness, and to monitor their arousal levels in a variety of settings.

To apply sensory integration principles to a group program, an occupational therapist should be familiar enough with sensory integration theory to understand precautions and general effects of various sensory and motor activities. Experience and training in working with groups, including how to maintain the attention of children in a group, how to address varying skill and interest levels, and how to deal with behavioral issues, are also recommended for occupational therapists applying sensory integration in group programs.

Consultation

Sensory integrative disorders are complex and are often misinterpreted as behavioral, psychologic, or emotional in origin. Helping family members, teachers, and others who come into contact with the child to understand the nature of the problem can be a powerful means toward helping the child. The provision of information to those who are in ongoing contact with the child and the development of strategies through collaboration with them are important ways that the therapist can indirectly intervene to influence the child's life positively across a variety of settings. The term *consultation* broadly refers to this indirect form of intervention.

Although many of the concepts that make up sensory integration theory and practice are not usually familiar to family members, teachers, or other professionals, once they are explained in everyday terms, a newfound understanding of the child often ensues. Cermak (1991) aptly referred to this process as *demystification*. Parents commonly express relief at finally having a name for behaviors that they have observed, and they may experience release from feeling that they have caused these problems through a maladaptive parenting style. Teachers also may appreciate having an alternative way to view child behaviors, especially when this new perspective is coupled with the application of strategies that promote responses from the child that are more productive.

Helping those around the child understand their own sensory integrative processes is sometimes a good way to make these new concepts more meaningful. Williams and Shellenberger (1994) use this tactic when introducing their Alert Program to promote optimal arousal states. They encourage the adults who are involved with the program to develop awareness and insight into their own sensorimotor preferences. This first step of the consultation process, increasing an understanding of sensory integration, can be achieved through several avenues, including parent conferences, experiential sessions, lecture and discussion groups, professional in-services, and ongoing education programs. Whatever format is used, it is likely that the greater the understanding of the basic concepts of sensory integration, the greater the openness and willingness to address these problems (Figure 11-17).

Perhaps the most important component of any consultation program is providing guidance for how to cope with the problems that stem from the sensory integrative dysfunction. Sometimes specific activities can be suggested that will help a child to prepare for a challenging task. For example, a child who has tactile defensiveness may be better able to tolerate activities such as finger painting or sand play if some desensitization techniques, such as applying firm touch-pressure to the skin, are used just before the activity. Promoting success in activities

can also be accomplished by suggesting individualized ways to help a child through difficult tasks. For example, some children with dyspraxia are likely to be more successful in completing a novel task when they receive verbal directions, whereas others respond optimally to visual demonstrations, and still others need physical assistance with the motion. Determining which method or combination of methods is most likely to help the individual child can assist adults in facilitating success.

Making adjustments in the environment can also be an important component of a consultation program for sensory integrative disorders. For example, children with autism often are highly affected by the sensory characteristics of their environments. Finding ways to manage sound, lighting, contact with other people, environmental odors, and visual distractions can make an important difference in attention, behavior, and, ultimately, performance. Dunn's work (1997, 2001) has led to a deeper understanding of how the sensory aspects of ordinary environments affect individuals who have the various sensory modulation styles that are depicted in her model (see Figure 11-9). Because individual differences in sensory processing tend to be lifelong tendencies, Dunn (2001) emphasizes how important it is for the person to learn to construct daily routines and manipulate sensory aspects of work and play environments in order to live as comfortably and successfully as possible. Consultation to develop the family's insight into a child's sensory characteristics, or to foster the child's own insight, may be a critical intervention.

Consultation services may be provided before, during, or after direct occupational therapy intervention, or they may be recommended as the intervention of choice instead of direct individual or group therapy. Whichever the case, the consultation should not be used to take the place of direct intervention if this would be most beneficial to the child. As previously mentioned, external pressures should not influence the form of therapy that is provided to the child with sensory integrative disorders, nor should procedures or techniques that require advanced training of an occupational therapist be recommended for parents and other professionals to do. For example, an appropriate consultation program never attempts to train a parent or teacher to provide individual therapy using the classical sensory integration approach. Therapists should also be familiar enough with the child to be aware of any precautions that might apply before they make any suggestions. For example, some children display delayed responses to vestibular stimulation and can become overstimulated or lethargic hours after receiving such stimulation. Many aspects of sensory integrative techniques can lead to adverse reactions and must be used with care.

At its best, consultation as a form of intervention for sensory integrative disorders requires training and experience. However, therapists with lesser degrees of

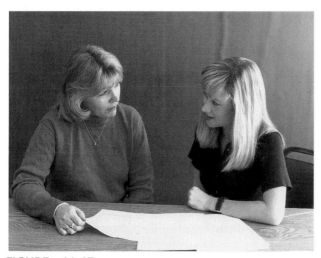

FIGURE 11-17 Consultation in school involves joint problem solving between the occupational therapist and the teacher. (Courtesy of Shay McAtee.)

experience and training can use this approach successfully, albeit to a more limited extent, as long as they do not overstep the bounds of their knowledge. The same background and training that are needed to provide individual therapy for sensory integrative dysfunction are desirable for this approach because the therapist needs to be able to predict what the child's likely responses will be to various activities and situations, given the characteristics of the child's sensory integrative disorder. In addition, the therapist should be well enough versed in sensory integration concepts to be able to explain them in simple yet meaningful terms. Also, it is imperative that the therapist have excellent communication skills and respect for the various people and environments that are involved. Bundy (2002) provided an excellent description of the communication process involved in a good consultation program.

Expected Outcomes of Occupational Therapy

As discussed previously, occupational therapy is not expected to "cure" sensory integrative disorders. Rather, occupational therapy aims to improve health and quality of life by engaging the child in meaningful and important occupations. To accomplish this with a child who has sensory integrative problems, the occupational therapist may aim to improve sensory integrative functions through direct remediation or to minimize the effects of the problems by teaching compensatory skills and coping strategies to the child, parents, and teachers. Often, remediation and compensatory approaches are thoughtfully combined in an intervention plan that is tailored to the particular needs of the child and family.

The goals and objectives that are formulated as part of a child's treatment plan target specific occupations in which positive changes are expected. These goals and objectives can be conceptualized as falling under the traditional occupational categories of work, rest, play, and self-care. For example, a toddler who tends to be overstimulated much of the time due to severe sensory modulation problems may consequently have difficulty falling asleep and staying asleep. One result of this situation is sleep deprivation, which aggravates defensiveness and behavior problems. A goal addressing the occupational domain of rest may be for the child to acquire more predictable sleep patterns with adequate amounts of sleep. A corresponding behavioral objective might be that the child will take a midday nap of at least 1 hour for 3 days per week. The intervention could involve both direct remediation to reduce the sensory defensiveness generally and parent consultation to teach strategies such as calming activities, a very predictable activity schedule including a specific rest time ritual, and creation of an arousal-reducing environment after lunch (e.g., lights dimmed and noise reduced and screened with rhythmic sounds or "white noise").

Sometimes specific behavioral objectives that address performance components are appropriate as a way to monitor progress toward the desired changes in daily occupations. Goals can be conceptualized as falling into seven general categories of expected outcomes that address component and occupational performance. These are summarized in Box 11-3 and discussed further in the following sections.

Increase in the Frequency or Duration of Adaptive Responses

As discussed in the introduction of this chapter, adaptive responses occur when an individual responds to environmental challenges with success. Application of sensory integration principles helps the therapist envision how to create opportunities for the child to make adaptive responses. This may be accomplished through systematic use of sensory input to promote organization within the child's nervous system. Ensuring that the sensory inputs inherent in activities are organizing rather than disorganizing and integrating rather than overwhelming requires careful monitoring on the part of the therapist, who must be sensitive to the child's response to each aspect of an activity and to each type of sensory input involved. The classical sensory integrative treatment approach intensively focuses on the child's demonstration of higher-level adaptive responses. However, compensatory skill approaches, group programs, and consultation services may also boost the frequency and duration of adaptive responses by changing the child's everyday environments in ways that enable the child to make adaptive responses more easily.

Increasing the duration and frequency of adaptive responses is an important outcome of sensory integration because it is on simple adaptive responses that functional behavior and skills are developed. For example, a child who has difficulty staying with an activity for more than a few seconds tends to shift from one activity to another. A desirable outcome for that child might be to stay for a longer time with a simple activity, such as swinging, in a therapy environment. Achievement of this simple adaptive response may eventually contribute to the functional behavior of staying with the reading circle in the school classroom for the required amount of time, despite the many distractions and cognitive challenges imposed by this occupation.

Development of Increasingly More Complex Adaptive Responses

Adaptive responses can vary in complexity, quality, and effectiveness (Ayres, 1981). A simple adaptive response might be simply holding onto a moving swing. A more complex adaptive response involving timing of action might be releasing grasp on a trapeze at just the right moment to land on a pillow. Over time, effective intervention is expected to enable the child to make adaptive responses that are more complex. This outcome is based on the assumption that sensory integrative procedures promote more efficient organization of multisensory input at primitive levels of functioning, which in turn is expected to enhance functions that are more complex. The result is an improvement in the child's ability to make judgments about the environment, what can be done with objects, and what specific actions need to be taken to accomplish a goal (Ayres, 1981).

Although repetition of a familiar activity may be important while a child is assimilating a new skill and may be useful in helping a child get ready for another more challenging activity, development of increasingly more complex abilities occurs only when tasks become slightly more challenging than the child's prior accomplishments. This is one of the main tenets of classical sensory integrative treatment. Because of the high degree of personal attention continuously given to the child during this kind of therapy, a fine gradient of complexity can be built into therapeutic activities while simultaneously ensuring that the child experiences success and a growing sense of "I can do it!"

Group program activities, compared with individual therapy, tend to place greater demands on children for several reasons, including limited opportunity for individualization of activities, the presence of other children with their unpredictable behaviors, and reduced opportunity for direct assistance from the therapist. Thus, a limitation posed by group programs is that challenges imposed on the group may at times be too great for an individual child, leading to frustration and failure. The therapist who provides a group program needs to be alert to the potential for this undesirable effect and strive to avoid it as much as possible. Whatever format for intervention is used, the therapist uses activity analysis, assessment information, ongoing observations, and knowledge of child development to ensure that the program engages the child's inner drive as much as possible to draw forth increasingly more complex interactions within the clinical, home, or community environments.

Improvement in Gross and Fine Motor Skills

The child who makes consistent and more complex adaptive responses shows evidence of improved sensory integration. Moreover, this child meets new challenges with greater self-confidence. A net result of these gains frequently is greater mastery in the motor domain. An example is the child with a vestibular processing disor-

der who exhibits greater competency and interest in playground activities and sports after classical sensory integrative treatment, even though these activities were not practiced during therapy. Motor skills may be among the earliest complex skills to show measurable change in response to a classical sensory integrative approach, probably because of the extent of the motor activity that is inherent in this treatment approach. Compensatory skill treatment, group intervention, or consultation for children with sensory integrative disorders should result in improvement of specific motor skills if these are targeted by the intervention. For example, if a compensatory approach to handwriting is used to help a child with poor somatosensory perception, specific gains in handwriting performance should follow if the intervention is successful.

Improvement in Cognitive, Language, or Academic Performance

Although cognitive, language, and academic skills are not specific objectives of occupational therapy for sensory integrative disorders, improvement in these domains has been detected in some intervention studies involving the provision of classical sensory integration treatment (Ayres, 1972a, 1976, 1978; Ayres & Mailloux, 1981; Cabay, 1988; Magrun, Ottenbacher, McCue, & Keefe, 1981; Ray, King, & Grandin, 1988; White, 1979). Application of classical sensory integration procedures is thought to generate broad-based changes in these areas secondary to enhancement of sensory modulation, perception, postural control, or praxis (Ayres, 1979, 1981; Cabay & King, 1989). For example, a child with autism may be helped through a sensory integrative approach to respond in a more adaptive way to sights, sounds, touch, and movement experiences that initially were disturbing. This improvement in sensory modulation may lead to a better ability to attend to language and academic tasks; thus, improvement in these areas may follow. A child who has a vestibular processing disorder may improve in postural control and equilibrium, freeing the child to more efficiently concentrate on academic material without the distraction of frequent loss of sitting balance or loss of place while copying from the blackboard. This child's vestibular-related improvements are also likely to have a positive effect on playground and sports activities because effects of classical sensory integration treatment are expected to generalize to a wide range of outcome areas.

Occupational therapy aimed at developing compensatory skills such as improved handwriting also may free the child to focus on the conceptual aspects of academic tasks rather than the perceptual-motor details of how to write letters on a page or how to keep a sentence on a printed line. In such compensatory programs, effects on outcome skills tend to be limited to the specific task of concern. Similarly, consultation programs may enhance language, cognitive, or academic skills by providing strategies for reducing the effect of sensory integrative disorders on these functions. For instance, helping a teacher understand how best to seat a child in class (such as in a beanbag chair versus a firm wooden chair or in the front corner of the room near the teacher's desk) may assist in reducing the effects of a sensory integrative disorder by making it easier for the child to attend to instruction in the classroom.

Increase in Self-Confidence and Self-Esteem

Ayres (1979) asserted that enhanced ability to make adaptive responses promotes self-actualization by allowing the child to experience the joy of accomplishing a task that previously could not be done. The outcome of therapy that encourages successful, self-directed experiences is a child who perceives the self as a competent actor in the world. Individual and group programs and direct and indirect services all can be geared to helping the child master the activities that are personally meaningful and essential to success in the world of everyday occupations. Mastery of such activities is expected to result in feelings of personal control that, in turn, lead to increased willingness to take risks and to try new things (Ayres, 1979). For example, a child with gravitational insecurity may experience not only fear responses to climbing and movement activities, but also feelings of failure and frustration at not being able to participate in the play of peers. In such a case, an increase in self-confidence and comfort in one's physical body is often accompanied by a general boost in feelings of self-efficacy and worth. Cohn, Miller, and Tickle-Degnen (2000) noted that parents' perceptions of the benefits of occupational therapy using a sensory integrative approach included a reconstruction of self-worth, in addition to improvement in abilities and activities. Parents in this study perceived that this intervention enabled their children to take more risks and to try new things, thus opening the door to greater possibilities.

Enhanced Occupational Engagement and Social Participation

Occupational therapy programs that address sensory integrative dysfunction encourage the child to organize his or her own activity, particularly in the classical sensory integration approach. As the child develops general sensory integrative capabilities and improved strategies for planning action, gains are seen in relation to the ability to master self-care tasks, to cope with daily routines, and to organize behavior more generally (Ayres, 1979). As a result, the child often is able to participate more fully in the occupations that are typical for his or her peers, a broad but critically important outcome of social participation. For example, intervention may help the child who is overly sensitive to touch or movement to deal with sensations in a more adaptive manner. As a result, the child approaches and engages in the challenges of everyday occupations, such as getting himself or herself ready for school in the morning, sharing a table with others in the school cafeteria, behaving appropriately in the classroom, and playing with friends on the playground with greater security and confidence. As noted previously, Cohn et al. (2000) reported that parents viewed their children as more willing to try new experiences following intervention, thus enhancing their opportunities for social participation. Not only is participation in daily occupations performed with greater competency and satisfaction, but also relationships with others are likely to become more comfortable and less threatening. Group therapy programs are ideal arenas in which the increases in self-confidence made in individual therapy can be tried out in the more challenging context of a social setting. Gains in occupational engagement and social participation are among the most significant of intervention outcomes.

Enhanced Family Life

When children with sensory integrative problems experience positive changes during intervention, their lives and the lives of other family members may be enhanced. One possible by-product of intervention based on sensory integrative principles is that parents gain a better understanding of their children's behavior and begin to generate their own strategies for organizing family routines in a way that is supportive of the entire family system. This kind of change can be particularly powerful for parents of children with autism, whose perceptions of child behaviors may be reframed as the parents become familiar with the sensory integrative perspective. For example, behavior that is interpreted as bizarre, such as insisting on wearing rubber bands on the arms, may be reframed as a meaningful strategy that the child uses to obtain deep pressure input for self-calming (Anderson, 1993). Instead of viewing the behavior as a frustrating, pathological sign that should be eliminated, reframing may lead the parents to explore other ways that they could provide the child with the deep pressure experiences that he or she seeks. Thus, an important outcome of sensory integrative intervention may include changes in parents' understanding of the child, leading to new coping strategies and alleviation of parental stress (Cohn & Cermak, 1998). In her studies of parental perspectives, Cohn (2001a, 2001b) has found that an important outcome of the sensory integrative approach is that parents tend to "reframe" their view and expectations of their children in a positive manner.

Measuring Outcomes

Because every child who demonstrates signs of sensory integrative dysfunction is unique, the expected outcomes of occupational therapy using a sensory integrative approach are individualized and diverse. Outcomes are sometimes measured using standardized tests. In fact, some of the SIPT tests are good measures of change due to strong test-retest reliability in addition to being relevant to concerns that are commonly voiced by parents and teachers (e.g., Design copying, Praxis on Verbal Command, Standing and Walking Balance, and others). However, standardized tests often do not address key occupational issues.

An alternative to standardized tests that addresses the individual nature of expected outcomes is a technique called *goal attainment scaling* (GAS). GAS is a method that was developed in the mental health arena as a program evaluation tool that facilitated patient participation in the goal-setting process (Kiresuk, Smith, & Cardillo, 1994). GAS provides a means to prioritize goals that are specifically relevant to individuals and their families, and to quantify the results using a standard metric that allows comparison of achievement across different types of goals. This process also captures functional and meaningful aspects of an individual's progress that are often challenging to assess using available standardized measures. For this reason, GAS is an attractive methodology for measuring change during occupational therapy, and it has now been successfully applied in occupational therapy effectiveness research in a variety of settings including rehabilitation (Joyce, Rockwood, & Mate-Kole, 1994; Mitchell & Cusick, 1998), school systems (Dreiling & Bundy, 2003; King et al., 1999), and mental health programs (Lloyd, 1986; Scott & Haggarty, 1984). This approach seems promising for capturing the diverse changes that are reported following sensory integration intervention programs. Case examples demonstrating how GAS has been applied to measure outcomes of sensory integration-based occupational therapy are described by Miller and Summers (2001).

Research on Effectiveness of Intervention

Therapists who wish to use a sensory integration approach in practice need to keep themselves up to date on research in this field to ensure that intervention is informed by the growing knowledge base. Research on the effectiveness of sensory integration-based interventions is particularly critical to evidence-based practice.

With respect to effectiveness research, more exists in the area of sensory integration than in any other practice area of occupational therapy. In one compendium of published research in sensory integration (Daems, 1994), a total of 57 efficacy and effectiveness studies were reviewed. Nearly a decade later, Miller (2003) reported finding more than 80 articles that addressed sensory integration effectiveness. However, the vast majority of these studies were poorly designed, addressed populations for which sensory integration interventions were not intended, or employed intervention methods that did not appear to be consistent with sensory integration theoretical principles.

Mulligan (2003) conducted a search to identify effectiveness studies published after 1980 that specifically evaluated treatment that was consistent with the general principles of sensory integration intervention and was implemented by occupational therapists working with children with sensory integrative dysfunction. She included studies that combined classical sensory integration with compensatory approaches, as well as meta-analyses that evaluated effect sizes of sensory integration-based intervention across multiple studies. Only studies published in peer-reviewed journals were considered. Using these criteria, Mulligan identified 21 articles that presented effectiveness studies or systematic reviews of effectiveness studies. These included meta-analyses, true experiments, quasi-experimental studies, single system studies, a qualitative study, a survey, and a case study.

In general, Mulligan (2003) found that the studies with the strongest research designs (the meta-analytic and experimental studies) reported mixed results. Four out of five true experimental studies reported that children receiving sensory integration treatment made significant gains on some outcome measures after intervention, compared to a control group. However, in studies that included an alternative treatment (including some quasi-experimental studies), the children who received sensory integration treatment did not significantly outperform the children who received an alternative treatment such as tutoring (Wilson, Kaplan, Fellowes, Gruchy, & Faris, 1992) or perceptual-motor training (Humphries, Wright, Snider, & McDougall, 1992; Polatajko, Law, Miller, Schaffer, & Macnab, 1991).

In a recent meta-analysis of experimental research on sensory integrative treatment, Vargas and Camilli (1999) analyzed 16 studies comparing sensory integrative treatment with no treatment and 16 studies comparing sensory integrative treatment with alternative treatments. These included studies of adults as well as studies with interventions that were inconsistent with sensory integration principles. A significant overall average effect size of 0.29 was found for sensory integrative treatment compared with no treatment, indicating an advantage for children receiving the treatment. The largest effect sizes were found for psychoeducational and motor outcome measures. However, older studies had a significantly higher effect size than more recent studies, which did not have a significant effect size when considered by themselves. The average effect size for sensory integrative treatment compared with alternative treatments was 0.09, a quite small effect, and the sensory integrative treatments did not differ significantly from alternative treatments in effect size. This latter finding indicates that sensory integrative treatment methods are as effective as other treatment methods, such as tutoring or perceptual-motor training.

The decline in effect size of sensory integrative treatment studies over the years is puzzling. The authors of the meta-analysis (Vargas & Camilli, 1999) suggest that the reason for this finding may lie in some unidentified difference in treatment implementation, or with selection and assignment of participants to experimental and control groups in the older studies versus the more recent ones. They point out that, in general, the studies examined sensory integration intervention in isolation and therefore do not represent the ways that sensory integration is implemented clinically, which usually involve incorporation of other treatment methods in addition to those that adhere to classical sensory integration principles.

After examining the effectiveness research on sensory integration, both Miller (2003) and Mulligan (2003) concluded that the effectiveness of sensory integration-based occupational therapy is neither proven nor unproven. This is because all of the existing studies that support the effectiveness of sensory integration intervention, as well as those that do not support its effectiveness, are flawed. Randomized, controlled clinical trials are considered to yield valid results only if they adhere to four standards: replicable intervention, homogeneous sample, sensitive and relevant outcome measures, and rigorous methodology (Boruch, 1997).

No published studies of sensory integration-based intervention to date meet all four of these criteria. For example, many studies use unclear or unsound methods to identify who is to receive sensory integration treatment; this creates the possibility that some children who do not have sensory integrative dysfunction are assigned to this treatment inappropriately. Another common flaw is that the intervention delivered in the study does not actually resemble the intervention that the researchers claim to be evaluating. Sometimes investigators use a rigid or very constrained treatment protocol in an effort to ensure that the sensory integration treatment is well defined and adheres to strict criteria. Although the purpose of this strategy is laudable (i.e., to ensure that the treatment is replicable), it may result in an intervention that lacks fidelity to the underlying treatment philosophy and principles. This is because a rigid treatment protocol is incompatible with the highly individualized, child-centered, fluid nature of classical sensory integration treatment, leading to results that do not represent the effects of the classical treatment. On the other hand, if treatment guidelines are too vague, or are not checked systematically during the delivery of the intervention, one cannot trust that the intervention was delivered in a consistent manner across the participants and across the intervention period of the study.

Another common problem is related to selection of outcome measures. Often children's responses to classical sensory integration treatment are as individualized as the methods used with them in intervention, making it difficult, perhaps impossible, for the researcher to select tests and other measurements that target the precise areas of gain for individual children. Moreover, it is likely that children with different types of sensory integrative dysfunction respond to this treatment with different kinds of gains. For example, children with tactile defensiveness are likely to show gains in different outcome domains than children with vestibular processing disorders; yet almost all of the research studies lump children together with sensory integrative dysfunction as if they should have similar responses to a standard treatment. This certainly was not Ayres's view, because she spent considerable effort attempting to identify subgroups of children with sensory integrative dysfunction who might differ from one another with respect to degree and type of responsiveness to intervention (Ayres, 1972a, 1978; Ayres & Tickle, 1980). It is hoped that researchers who conduct future effectiveness studies will become more sensitive to this important issue.

Another important issue that is rarely addressed is the maintenance of gains after a period of sensory integration-based occupational therapy is completed. An encouraging finding reported by Wilson and Kaplan (1994) suggests that children who receive sensory integration intervention may obtain long-term benefits that are not shared by children who receive other interventions. These researchers retested children who had participated in an earlier randomized, controlled clinical trial comparing sensory integration intervention with tutoring. Although no significant differences in outcomes were found between the two intervention groups in the original study (Wilson, Kaplan, Fellowes, Gruchy, & Faris, 1992), at follow-up 2 years later, only the children who had received the sensory integration treatment maintained the gross motor gains that they had made after intervention. Maintenance of intervention gains is a critical issue that has an influence on cost-effectiveness questions. Replication of Wilson and Kaplan's findings (1994) would make an important contribution to understanding the extent to which gains after sensory integration treatment can be maintained.

Although group experimental treatment designs are considered to be the gold standard of effectiveness studies, other research designs examining treatment outcomes also make valuable contributions to an understanding of the potential effects of sensory integration intervention. Single system research has been particularly useful in revealing individual differences in responses to sensory integrative treatment. In this kind of research, a child serves as his or her own control and is monitored repeatedly before intervention (the baseline phase) and during intervention. An advantage to this approach is that treatment and behavioral outcomes can be highly individualized. A recent example of this type of research is the study conducted by Linderman and Stewart (1999) on two preschoolers with pervasive developmental disorders. The researchers measured three behavioral outcomes for each child. Each outcome was observed in the child's home and was tailored to address functional issues for each child (e.g., response to holding and hugging for one child and functional communication during mealtime for the other). Results indicate significant improvements between baseline and intervention phases for five of the six outcomes measured.

A great deal of investigation remains to be done to explore questions regarding effectiveness of sensory integration treatment. It would be particularly beneficial to be able to better predict who will best respond to the classical sensory integration approach and who may be better served by other interventions. The effectiveness of combining classical sensory integration treatment with compensatory skill treatment, group programs, consultation, or other intervention methods is another area in need of research, particularly because such intervention combinations are what is typically done in clinical practice. The kinds of outcomes likely to proceed from various treatment approaches and the time frames in which those outcomes can be expected to emerge deserve close examination in effectiveness studies. Long-term maintenance of gains, particularly of those related to outcomes that are more global, such as social participation, is a particularly important question that should be addressed in research. Finally, studies need to explore which intervention outcomes are most meaningful to the families of children with sensory integrative dysfunction to ensure that intervention programs are responsive to the needs of the people served.

Case Study 1
History

Drew was diagnosed with autism (high functioning) when he was 7 years of age. His mother is Korean, and his father is American. All of Drew's early developmental milestones were attained within normal limits, except for language acquisition. He did not speak any words until 2 years of age, and by 3 years of age his family was concerned about his development because of delayed language skills. Drew attended an English-language preschool at 3 years of age and then a Korean language preschool. (His family speaks both Korean and English at home.) He was asked to leave the second preschool because of aggressive behavior. At 4 years of age, Drew attended a private special-education school where he received speech therapy and participated in a language-intensive playgroup. When Drew reached kindergarten age, he was enrolled in public special-education programs where he attended specialized classrooms for speech and language disorders, autism, and multiple handicaps.

Reason for Referral

Drew initially was referred by the state regional center for developmental disabilities to an occupational therapy private practice for evaluation when he was nearly 8 years of age. His regional center counselor thought that Drew had signs of a sensory integrative disorder, and he believed that Drew might benefit from occupational therapy. Drew's mother reported that her main concerns for Drew were related to his poor socialization skills, his limited ability to play with games and toys, and his tendency to become easily frustrated.

Evaluation Procedure

Although the Sensory Integration and Praxis Tests (SIPT) were attempted during the initial occupational therapy assessment, Drew was unable to follow the directions or attend to the tests sufficiently to obtain reliable scores. Therefore his occupational therapy evaluation consisted of a parent interview, including completion of a developmental and sensory history, and observation of Drew in a clinical therapy setting. At the time of assessment it was not possible to interview Drew's teacher. However, Drew's mother, who often observed him in the classroom, provided information about his performance at school.

Evaluation Results

Drew demonstrated inefficiencies in sensory processing in a number of sensory systems. During the assessment, signs of inconsistent responses to tactile input were evident. For example, Drew demonstrated a complete lack of response to some stimuli such as a puff of air on the back of his neck or the light touch of a cotton ball applied to his feet when he was not visually attending. However, he withdrew in an agitated fashion when the therapist attempted to position him. His mother reported that he showed extreme dislike for certain textures of food and clothing and that he disliked being touched. She also stated that he seemed to become irritated by being near other children at school and sometimes pinched or pushed peers who came close to him. Drew also appeared easily overstimulated by extraneous visual and auditory stimuli. His mother stated that he often covered his ears at home when loud noises were present and that at school he sometimes seemed confused as to the direction of sounds. He was observed to pick up objects and look at them very closely, and he appeared to rely on his vision a great deal to complete tasks. In response to movement, he enjoyed swinging slowly but became fearful with an increase in velocity. His mother stated that he often became fearful at the park when climbing.

Drew's balance was observed to be poor, and his equilibrium reactions were inconsistent. He also had trouble positioning himself on various pieces of equipment, showing poor body awareness. During the assessment he appeared to seek touch-pressure stimuli, including total body compression. He was reported to jump a great deal at home and at school. These types of proprioception-generating actions appeared to have a calming effect on Drew.

In the areas of praxis, Drew was able to imitate positions and follow verbal directions to complete motor actions, but he had a great deal of difficulty initiating activities on his own or attempting something that was unfamiliar to him. He also had difficulty timing and sequencing his actions. His mother reported that he tended not to participate in sports or in park activities and that he had trouble throwing, catching, and kicking balls. Drew was able to complete puzzles, string beads, and write his name; however, bilateral activities such as cutting and pasting were difficult for him.

Socially, Drew demonstrated poor eye contact and tended to use repetitive phrases that he had heard in the past. His mother stated that he wanted to play with peers but found it hard to make friends. Drew was independent in all self-care skills, except for tying shoes and managing some fasteners.

Based on an interview and questionnaire with Drew's mother, as well as observation of Drew in a clinical therapy setting, it was determined that he displayed irregularities in sensory processing, including hypersensitivity to some aspects of touch, movement, visual, and auditory stimuli. He also demonstrated difficulty with position sense, balance, bilateral integration, and the ideation, timing, and sequencing aspects of praxis. These difficulties were thought to interfere with Drew's ability to play purposefully with toys and to participate in age-appropriate games and sports. These problems, in combination with his language delays, were interfering significantly with his social skills and his ability to make friends, and they were increasing his tendency to become frustrated, all of which were the major concerns of his parents.

Recommendation

Individual occupational therapy was recommended to address Drew's sensory integrative dysfunction and the development of specific fine and gross motor skills. Because socialization issues were such a major concern for Drew's family and were interfering with his

performance at school, the evaluating therapist also recommended that Drew participate in an after-school group occupational therapy program to facilitate the acquisition of social skills.

Occupational Therapy Program

Drew received individual occupational therapy in a therapy clinic for 1 year. This individual therapy involved a combination of classical sensory integration and a compensatory skill development approach. During this time, Drew demonstrated significant gains in sensory processing with no further significant signs of tactile defensiveness or fear of movement activities. Motor planning of novel actions improved but continued to be of some concern for Drew. He did make notable gains in being able to catch and throw a ball and in writing and scissors skills. Through the group occupational therapy program, Drew became able to initiate and maintain interaction with peers, share objects, and play cooperatively with some assistance and structure from adults.

After this year of clinically based individual and group occupational therapy, it was recommended that individual therapy be continued at school. The focus of this occupational therapy program was to help Drew apply his improved sensorimotor and social skills in the natural context of school. Through a combination of direct service and consultation, several activities and adaptations were made to facilitate his performance at school. Because the initial year of intensive therapy using a classical sensory integrative approach had helped Drew tolerate and respond appropriately to sensory information and because he had developed many of the specific skills that he needed in the classroom during individual therapy, he was much better able to focus on the demands expected of him at school at that time. By the end of the school year, Drew's occupational therapist recommended that occupational therapy be discontinued because she believed that his teacher would be able to continue to help him in the areas that had been addressed through the consultation program.

However, when the individualized educational program (IEP) team met to discuss Drew's transition to a new school, there was significant concern about the possibility of Drew regressing in a new setting where he would need to adjust to many different routines. The IEP team requested that occupational therapy continue to ensure a smooth transition for Drew and to put in place a plan that would continue to help him develop socially.

When school resumed in the fall, the occupational therapist had arranged a "big buddy" program with a local high school. Two high school seniors worked with Drew as part of a social service assignment during recess for the fall semester. The occupational therapist trained the high school students to carry out a socialization program aimed at helping Drew feel comfortable with a new set of peers. Drew seemed to look up to the high school students and responded well to the "big buddy" program.

By the end of the fall semester in the new school, Drew played cooperatively with peers, interacting independently and communicating appropriately. His occupational therapy program was formally discontinued at this time, although the occupational therapist continued to check in with Drew's teacher when at his school site to work with other children. No additional intervention has been needed, but the option for further consultation or direct intervention is available should the need arise.

Case Study 2
History

Karen was born after a full-term pregnancy complicated by gestational diabetes. Labor, which was induced at 40 weeks, was long, and it was believed that Karen broke her right collarbone during delivery. Karen achieved her early motor and language milestones within average age ranges. However, she was described as an irritable baby who had difficulty breast feeding, startled easily, and could only be calmed by swinging. Karen attended a parent cooperative child development program as a toddler, and at 4 years of age she was eligible for a special-education preschool program through her school district. She has not been given any specific medical or educational diagnosis.

Reason for Referral

Karen's mother expressed concern about Karen's fine and gross motor skills to a neurologist, who referred Karen for an occupational therapy assessment when she was 4 years of age. When asked why she was seeking an evaluation for Karen, her mother wrote, "Up until recently I had been very patiently waiting for normal development to occur (for example, handedness, fine motor). The school psychologist feels that this still may occur, but I am convinced that something isn't right. Karen's increasing frustration and decreasing belief in herself prompted me to seek evaluations. While a part of me wishes to have a 'normal child,' the other part will be relieved to find that the child I have had so many doubts about since infancy does indeed have some behaviors and actions that are unusual."

Evaluation Procedure

The Sensory Integration and Praxis Tests (SIPT) were administered in one testing session. Karen was also observed in a clinical therapy setting and at home. In addition, Karen's mother was interviewed, and she com-

pleted a developmental and sensory history on which she provided detailed accounts of Karen's early and current sensorimotor, language, cognitive, social, and self-care development.

Evaluation Results

On the SIPT, Karen scored below average for age expectations on 7 of 17 tests. This profile was generated through computer scoring by the test publisher. The unit of measure represented by the scores is a statistic measure called a *standard deviation*, which represents how different the child's score is from that of an average child of the same age. The closer a child's score is to 0 on the horizontal axis, the closer to average is the child's performance on that test. Karen's scores are plotted as solid squares that are connected by a dark line on the computer-generated profile. Scores falling below −1.0 on the horizontal axis are considered to be possibly indicative of dysfunction.

One of Karen's scores was low on a motor-free visual perception test (space visualization), and it was noted that she had difficulty fitting a geometric form into a puzzle board during this test. Her mother reported that Karen knew colors at 18 months of age but had trouble learning shapes. However, she was reported to have a strong visual memory for roads, signs, and faces. These findings suggested difficulty with spatial orientation of objects but relative strengths in visual memory.

Karen had several low scores and showed signs of difficulty performing on several of the tests of somatosensory and vestibular processing. A low score on finger identification suggested inefficient tactile feedback involving the hands. This was corroborated by observations of poor manipulative skills during activities such as buttoning and using utensils. She was also observed to have signs of tactile defensiveness, also corroborated by her mother's report. Her low score on kinesthesia, as well as her difficulty in exerting the appropriate amount of pressure on a pencil and in positioning her body for dressing, suggested problems with proprioceptive feedback. Karen's lowest score on the SIPT was on the postrotary nystagmus test (−2.2 standard deviations). This low score, as well as below-average scores on standing and walking balance, observations of poor functional balance in dressing and playground activities, a tendency not to cross her body midline, poor bilateral coordination in activities such as cutting, and reports that she never appeared to get dizzy, pointed to the probability of vestibular processing problems.

Karen showed above-average performance on a praxis test on which she could rely on verbal directions. However, tests of motor planning that were more somatosensory dependent (oral praxis and postural praxis) were substantially more difficult for her. Karen was unable to ride a tricycle, pump a swing, or skip. She had extreme difficulty planning her movements to dress herself or even to let someone else dress her. She also had a great deal of difficulty using utensils during eating and often choked on food and drinks. Writing skills have been particularly difficult for Karen, and her lack of hand preference, immature grasp, and hesitancy to cross her midline have hampered her attempts at drawing or writing.

Karen was reported to be a social child who was liked by adults and younger peers. However, her mother worried that she did not seem able to "pick up on the hints and unwritten rules of her peers" and was "definitely starting to march to her own beat." She noticed increasing signs of frustration that she thought were beginning to impinge on Karen's willingness to participate with peers.

Overall, the evaluation results suggested deficits in sensory processing of some aspects of visual, tactile, proprioceptive, and vestibular sensory information. These difficulties were seen as related to somatodyspraxia, poor balance and bilateral integration, difficulties with specific gross and fine motor skills, and emerging concerns around socialization. Karen's strengths included age-appropriate cognitive and language skills, good ability to motor plan actions using verbal directions, and an exceptionally supportive and involved family.

Recommendation

Based on the evaluation results and a meeting of Karen's IEP team, who met shortly after the assessment, it was recommended that Karen receive individual occupational therapy using a sensory integration approach to enhance foundational sensory and motor processes. This program was funded by the school district as part of her special-education program, but because of her significant sensory integrative problems and need for a specialized approach, the therapy was recommended to initially occur in a therapy clinic equipped for classical sensory integrative treatment.

Occupational Therapy Program

In the first 6 months of individual occupational therapy a classical sensory integration approach was used that included individualized, carefully selected therapeutic activities aimed at enhancing visual, tactile, proprioceptive, and vestibular sensory processing. As part of her intervention program, Karen's therapist provided her with graded challenges to praxis, bilateral coordination, and balance.

After 6 months of therapy, Karen has shown decreasing tactile defensiveness, a reduced tendency to choke on food, acquisition of the ability to ride a tricycle, and an improved ability to plan new or unusual motor actions.

Although these are significant gains for Karen, she continues to exhibit substantial difficulties with many aspects of sensory processing, general motor planning ability, and many age-appropriate fine and gross motor skills. If she continues to respond to occupational therapy using a classical sensory integration approach, it is expected that by the beginning of the next school year (in about 6 months) she will have improved in basic sensory and motor functions to the extent that some specific skill training will become more appropriate. It is likely that at that time some therapy will occur at school with the introduction of a consultation program for her teacher. Her parents have already begun a home program, which appears to support the gains she is making through direct services. Karen's young age and initial positive response to therapy make her an optimal candidate for application of the sensory integration approach, and her long-term outlook is excellent.

STUDY QUESTIONS

1 How did A. Jean Ayres use the term *sensory integration*?

2 Describe how sensory integration plays a role in typical development. Provide specific examples of behaviors seen in infancy and early childhood, and explain how they relate to the development of sensory integration.

3 Identify the four main types of sensory integration problems, and describe some of the ways that each can influence daily function.

4 Imagine that you are explaining sensory modulation to a teacher who has never heard of this concept. How would you communicate that sensory modulation disorders affect classroom functioning?

5 What types of analyses did Ayres conduct to develop sensory integrative theory? What were some of the main tenets of sensory integration theory that emanated from these research studies?

6 Discuss the different methods that can be used as part of an occupational therapy assessment using a sensory integration approach.

7 Describe the Sensory Integration and Praxis Tests and the general domains that they assess.

8 Contrast the application of the classical sensory integration treatment approach with the compensatory skill approach. What would be the rationale for using one versus the other?

9 Under what circumstances would a group occupational therapy program or a consultation program be the intervention of choice for a child with a sensory integrative disorder?

10 How might expected outcomes of treatment differ for classical sensory integrative treatment versus compensatory skill, group, or consultation approaches?

REFERENCES

American Occupational Therapy Association (2002). Occupational therapy practice framework: Domain and process. *American Journal of Occupational Therapy, 56,* 609-639.

Anderson, E.L. (1993). *Parental perceptions of the influence of occupational therapy utilizing sensory integrative techniques on the daily living skills of children with autism.* Unpublished master's thesis. Los Angeles: University of Southern California.

Ayres, A.J. (1963). The Eleanor Clark Slagle Lecture. The development of perceptual-motor abilities: A theoretical basis for treatment of dysfunction. *American Journal of Occupational Therapy, 17* (6), 221-225.

Ayres, A.J. (1964). Tactile functions: Their relation to hyperactive and perceptual motor behavior. *American Journal of Occupational Therapy, 18* (1), 6-11.

Ayres, A.J. (1965). Patterns of perceptual-motor dysfunction in children: A factor analytic study. *Perceptual and Motor Skills, 20,* 335-368.

Ayres, A.J. (1966a). Interrelations among perceptual-motor abilities in a group of normal children. *American Journal of Occupational Therapy, 20* (6), 288-292.

Ayres, A.J. (1966b). Interrelationships among perceptual-motor functions in children. *American Journal of Occupational Therapy, 20* (2), 68-71.

Ayres, A.J. (1969). Deficits in sensory integration in educationally handicapped children. *Journal of Learning Disabilities, 2* (3), 44-52.

Ayres, A.J. (1971). Characteristics of types of sensory integrative dysfunction. *American Journal of Occupational Therapy, 25* (7), 329-334.

Ayres, A.J. (1972a). Improving academic scores through sensory integration. *Journal of Learning Disabilities, 5,* 338-343.

Ayres, A.J. (1972b). *Sensory integration and learning disorders.* Los Angeles: Western Psychological Services.

Ayres, A.J. (1972c). *Southern California Sensory Integration Tests.* Los Angeles: Western Psychological Services.

Ayres, A.J. (1972d). Types of sensory integrative dysfunction among disabled learners. *American Journal of Occupational Therapy, 26* (1), 13-18.

Ayres, A.J. (1975). *Southern California Postrotary Nystagmus Test.* Los Angeles: Western Psychological Services.

Ayres, A.J. (1976). *The effect of sensory integrative therapy on learning disabled children: The final report of a research project.* Los Angeles: Center for the Study of Sensory Integrative Dysfunction.

Ayres, A.J. (1977). Cluster analyses of measures of sensory integration. *American Journal of Occupational Therapy, 31* (6), 362-366.

Ayres, A.J. (1978). Learning disabilities and the vestibular system. *Journal of Learning Disabilities, 11* (1), 30-41.

Ayres, A.J. (1979). *Sensory integration and the child.* Los Angeles: Western Psychological Services.

Ayres, A.J. (1981). *Aspects of the somatomotor adaptive response and praxis.* (Audiotape). Pasadena, CA: Center for the Study of Sensory Integrative Dysfunction.

Ayres, A.J. (1985). *Developmental dyspraxia and adult-onset apraxia.* Torrance, CA: Sensory Integration International.

Ayres, A.J. (1989). *Sensory Integration and Praxis Tests manual.* Los Angeles: Western Psychological Services.

Ayres, A.J. (2004). *Sensory integration and the child* (2nd ed.). Los Angeles: Western Psychological Services.

Ayres, A.J., & Mailloux, Z. (1981). Influence of sensory integration procedures on language development. *American Journal of Occupational Therapy, 35* (6), 383.

Ayres, A.J., Mailloux, Z., & Wendler, C.L.W. (1987). Developmental apraxia: Is it a unitary function? *Occupational Therapy Journal of Research, 7* (2), 93-110.

Ayres, A.J., & Marr, D. (1991). Sensory Integration and Praxis Tests. In A.G. Fisher, E.A. Murray, & A.C. Bundy (Eds.), *Sensory integration: Theory and practice* (pp. 203-250). Philadelphia: F.A. Davis.

Ayres, A.J., & Tickle, L. (1980). Hyperresponsivity to touch and vestibular stimuli as a predictor of positive response to sensory integration procedures in autistic children. *American Journal of Occupational Therapy, 34,* 375-381.

Bach-Y-Rita, P. (1981). Brain plasticity. In J. Goodgold (Ed.), *Brain plasticity.* St. Louis: Mosby.

Baranek, G.T., Foster, L.G., & Berkson, G. (1997). Sensory defensiveness in persons with developmental disabilities. *Occupational Therapy Journal of Research, 17,* 173-185

Beery, K.E. (1997). *The Developmental Test of Visual-Motor Integration* (4th ed.). San Antonio, TX: Psychological Corporation.

Bennett, E.L., Diamond, M.C., Krech, D., & Rosenzweig, M.R. (1964). Chemical and anatomical plasticity of brain. *Science, 146,* 610-619.

Bissell, J., Fisher, J., Owen, C., & Polcyn, P. (1998). *Sensory motor handbook: A guide for implementing and modifying activities in the classroom.* San Antonio, TX: Therapy Skill Builders.

Blanche, E.I. (2002). *Observations based on sensory integration theory.* Torrance, CA: Pediatric Therapy Network.

Blanche, E., & Schaaf, R. (2001). Proprioception: A cornerstone of sensory integrative intervention. In S.S. Roley, E.I. Blanche, & R.C. Schaaf (Eds.), *Understanding the nature of sensory integration with diverse populations* (pp. 385-408). San Antonio, TX: Therapy Skill Builders.

Boruch, R.F. (1997). *Randomized experiments for planning and evaluation: A practical guide.* Thousand Oaks, CA: Sage.

Bretherton, I., Bates, E., McNew, S., Shore, C., Williamson, C., & Beeghly-Smith, M. (1981). Comprehension and production of symbols in infancy: An experimental study. *Developmental Psychology, 17,* 728-736.

Brown, C., & Dunn, W. (2002). *Adolescent/Adult Sensory Profile.* San Antonio, TX: The Psychological Corporation.

Bruininks, R.H. (1978). *Bruininks-Oseretsky Test of Motor Proficiency examiner's manual.* Circle Pines, MN: American Guidance Service.

Bundy, A.C. (2002). Using sensory integration theory in schools: Sensory integration and consultation. In A.C. Bundy, S.J. Lane, & E.A. Murray (Eds.), *Sensory integration:*

Theory and practice (2nd ed., pp. 309-332). Philadelphia: F.A. Davis.

Bundy, A.C., & Murray, E.A. (2002). Sensory integration: A. Jean Ayres' theory revisited. In A.C. Bundy, S.J. Lane, & E.A. Murray (Eds.), *Sensory integration: Theory and practice* (2nd ed., pp. 141-165). Philadelphia: F.A. Davis.

Burke, J. (2001). Clinical reasoning and the use of narrative in sensory integration assessment and intervention. In S.S. Roley, E.I. Blanche, & R.C. Schaaf (Eds.), *Understanding the nature of sensory integration with diverse populations* (pp. 385-408). San Antonio, TX: Therapy Skill Builders.

Burleigh, J.M., McIntosh, K.W., & Thompson, M.W. (2002) Central auditory processing disorders. In A.C. Bundy, S.J. Lane, & E.A. Murray (Eds.), *Sensory integration: Theory and practice* (2nd ed., pp. 141-165). Philadelphia: F.A. Davis.

Cabay, M. (1988). *The effect of sensory integration–based treatment on academic readiness of young, "at risk" school children.* Annual conference of the American Occupational Therapy Association, Phoenix, AZ.

Cabay, M., & King, L.J. (1989). Sensory integration and perception: The foundation for concept formation. *Occupational Therapy in Practice, 1,* 18-27.

Carrasco, R.C., & Lee, C.E. (1993). Development of a teacher questionnaire on sensorimotor behavior. *Sensory Integration Special Interest Section Newsletter, 16* (3), 5-6.

Case-Smith, J. (1991). The effects of tactile defensiveness and tactile discrimination on in-hand manipulation. *American Journal of Occupational Therapy, 45,* 811-818.

Cermak, S.A. (1988). The relationship between attention deficits and sensory integration disorders (Part I). *Sensory Integration Special Interest Section Newsletter, 11* (2), 1-4.

Cermak, S.A. (1991). Somatodyspraxia. In A.G. Fisher, E.A. Murray, & A.C. Bundy (Eds.), *Sensory integration: Theory and practice* (pp. 137-170). Philadelphia: F.A. Davis.

Cermak, S.A. (2001). The effects of deprivation on processing, play and praxis. In S.S. Roley, E.I. Blanche, & R.C. Schaaf (Eds.), *Understanding the nature of sensory integration with diverse populations* (pp. 385-408). San Antonio, TX: Therapy Skill Builders.

Chugani, H.T., & Phelps, M.E. (1986). Maturational changes in cerebral function in infants determined by 18FDG positron emission tomography. *Science, 231,* 840-843.

Clark, F.A., Mailloux, Z., & Parham, D. (1989). Sensory integration and children with learning disorders. In P.N. Pratt & A.S. Allen (Eds.), *Occupational therapy for children* (2nd ed., pp. 457-509). St. Louis: Mosby.

Cohn, E.S., Miller, L.J., & Tickle-Degnen, L.(2000). Parental hopes for therapy outcomes: Children with sensory modulation disorders. *American Journal of Occupational Therapy, 54,* 36-43.

Cohn, E.S. (2001a). Parent perspectives of occupational therapy using a sensory integration approach. *American Journal of Occupational Therapy, 55,* 285-294.

Cohn, E.S. (2001b). From waiting to relating: Parents' experiences in the waiting room of an occupational therapy clinic. *American Journal of Occupational Therapy, 55,* 168-175.

Cohn, E.S., & Cermak, S.A. (1998). Including the family perspective in sensory integration outcomes research. *American Journal of Occupational Therapy, 52,* 540-546.

Coster, W. (1998a). Occupation-centered assessment of children. *American Journal of Occupational Therapy, 52,* 337-344.

Coster, W., Deeney, T., Haltwanger, J., & Haley, S. (1998). *School Function Assessment.* San Antonio, TX: Therapy Skill Builders.

Daems, J. (Ed.). (1994). *Reviews of research in sensory integration.* Torrance, CA: Sensory Integration International.

Dreiling, D.S., & Bundy, A.C. (2003). A comparison of consultative model and direct-indirect intervention with preschoolers. *American Journal of Occupational Therapy, 57,* 566-569.

Dru, D., Walker, J.P., & Walker, J.B. (1975). Self-produced locomotion restores visual capacity after striate lesion. *Science, 187,* 265-266.

Dunn, W.W. (1981). *A guide to testing clinical observations in kindergartners.* Rockville, MD: American Occupational Therapy Association.

Dunn, W.W. (1997). The impact of sensory processing abilities on the daily lives of young children and families: A conceptual model. *Infants and Young Children, 9* (4), 23-25.

Dunn, W.W. (1999). *Sensory Profile: User's manual.* San Antonio, TX: Psychological Corporation.

Dunn, W. W. (2001). The sensations of everyday life: Empirical, theoretical, and pragmatic considerations. *American Journal of Occupational Therapy, 55,* 608-620.

Dunn, W. (2002). *The Infant/Toddler Sensory Profile manual.* San Antonio, TX: The Psychological Corporation.

Dunn, W., & Fisher, A.G. (1983). Sensory registration, autism, and tactile defensiveness. In J. Melvin (Ed.), *Occupational therapy in practice* (Vol. 1, pp. 181-182). Rockville, MD: American Occupational Therapy Association.

Dunn, W., Myles, B.S., & Orr, S. (2002). Sensory processing issues associated with Asperger syndrome: A preliminary investigation. *American Journal of Occupational Therapy, 56,* 97-102.

Fisher, A.G. (1991). Vestibular-proprioceptive processing and bilateral integration and sequencing deficits. In A.G. Fisher, E.A. Murray, & A.C. Bundy (Eds.), *Sensory integration: Theory and practice* (pp. 69-107). Philadelphia: F.A. Davis.

Fisher, A.G., & Murray, E.A. (1991). Introduction to sensory integration theory. In A.G. Fisher, E.A. Murray, & A.C. Bundy (Eds.), *Sensory integration: Theory and practice* (pp. 3-26). Philadelphia: F.A. Davis.

Fisher, A.G., Murray, E.A., & Bundy, A.C. (Eds.). (1991). *Sensory integration: Theory and practice.* Philadelphia: F.A. Davis.

Fredrickson, J.M., Schwartz, D.W., & Kornhuber, H.H. (1966). Convergence and interaction of vestibular and deep somatic afferents upon neurons in the vestibular nuclei of the cat. *Acta Otolaryngologica, 61,* 168-188.

Gregg, C.L., Hafner, M.E., & Korner, A. (1976). The relative efficacy of vestibular-proprioceptive stimulation and the upright position in enhancing visual pursuit in neonates. *Child Development, 47,* 309-314.

Gregory-Flock, J.L., & Yerxa, E.J. (1984). Standardization of the prone extension postural test on children ages 4 through 8. *American Journal of Occupational Therapy, 38,* 187-194.

Gunnar, M.R., & Barr, R.G. (1998). Stress, early brain development, and behavior. *Infants and Young Children, 11* (1), 1-14.

Henderson, A., Pehoski, C., & Murray, E. (2002) Visual-spatial abilities. In A.C. Bundy, S.J. Lane, & E.A. Murray (Eds.), *Sensory integration: Theory and practice* (pp. 123-140). Philadelphia: F.A. Davis.

Hickman, L. (2001). Sensory integration and fragile X syndrome. In S.S. Roley, E.I. Blanche, & R.C. Schaaf (Eds.), *Understanding the nature of sensory integration with diverse populations* (pp. 385-408). San Antonio, TX: Therapy Skill Builders.

Holloway, E. (1998). Early emotional development and sensory processing. In J. Case-Smith (Ed.), *Pediatric occupational therapy and early intervention* (pp. 163-197). Boston: Andover Medical.

Hubel, D.H., & Wiesel, T.N. (1963). Receptive fields of cells in striate cortex of very young, visually inexperienced kittens. *Journal of Neurophysiology, 26*, 994-1002.

Humphrey, T. (1969). Postnatal repetition of human prenatal activity sequences with some suggestions of their neuroanatomical basis. In R.J. Robinson (Ed.), *Brain and early behavior.* New York: Academic Press.

Humphries, T., Wright, M., Snider, L., & McDougall, B. (1992). A comparison of the effectiveness of sensory integrative therapy and perceptual-motor training in treating children with learning disabilities. *Journal of Developmental and Behavioral Pediatrics, 13*, 31-40.

Inamura, K.N. (1998). *Sensory integration for early intervention: A team approach.* San Antonio, TX: Therapy Skill Builders.

Jacobs, S.E., & Schenider, M. L. (2001). Neuroplasticity and the environment. In S.S. Roley, E.I. Blanche, & R.C. Schaaf (Eds.), *Understanding the nature of sensory integration with diverse populations* (pp. 29-42) San Antonio, TX: Therapy Skill Builders.

Joyce, B.M., Rockwood, K.J., & Mate-Kole, C.C. (1994). Use of goal attainment scaling in brain injury in a rehabilitation hospital. *American Journal of Physical Medicine and Rehabilitation 73*, 1, 10-14.

Kimball, J.G. (1999). Sensory integrative frame of reference. In P. Kramer & J. Hinojosa (Eds.), *Frames of reference for pediatric occupational therapy.* Baltimore: Williams & Wilkins.

King, G.A., McDougall, J., Tucker, M.A., Gritzan, J., Malloy-Miller, T., Alambets, P., et al. (1999). An evaluation of functional, school-based therapy services for children with special needs. *Physical & Occupational Therapy in Pediatrics, 19* (2), 5-29.

Kiresuk, T.J., Smith, A., & Cardillo, J.E. (1994). *Goal attainment scaling: Applications, theory, and measurement.* Hillsdale, NJ: Erlbaum Associates.

Knickerbocker, B.M. (1980). *A holistic approach to learning disabilities.* Thorofare, NJ: C.B. Slack.

Kolb, B., & Whishaw, I.Q. (1985). *Fundamentals of human neuropsychology* (2nd ed.). New York: W.H. Freeman.

Koomar, J.A., & Bundy, A.C. (2002). Creating direct intervention from theory. In A.C. Bundy, S.J. Lane, & E.A. Murray (Eds.), *Sensory integration: Theory and practice* (2nd ed., pp. 261-308). Philadelphia: F.A. Davis.

Lai, J.-S., Parham, L.D., & Johnson-Ecker, C. (1999). Sensory dormancy and sensory defensiveness: Two sides of the same coin? *Sensory Integration Special Interest Section Quarterly, 22*, 1-4.

Lee, J.R.V. (1999). *Parent ratings of children with autism on the Evaluation of Sensory Processing (ESP).* Unpublished Master's thesis, University of Southern California, Los Angeles.

Linderman, T.M., & Stewart, K.B. (1999). Sensory integrative-based occupational therapy and functional outcomes in young children with pervasive developmental disorders: A single-subject study. *American Journal of Occupational Therapy, 53*, 207-213.

Lloyd, C. (1986). The process of goal setting using goal attainment scaling in a therapeutic community. *Occupational Therapy in Mental Health, 6* (3), 19-30.

Magalhaes, L.C., Koomar, J., & Cermak, S.A. (1989). Bilateral motor coordination in 5- to 9-year-old children. *American Journal of Occupational Therapy, 43*, 437-443.

Magrun, W.M., Ottenbacher, K., McCue, S., & Keefe, R. (1981). Effects of vestibular stimulation on spontaneous use of verbal language in developmentally delayed children. *American Journal of Occupational Therapy, 35*, 101-104.

Mailloux, Z. (2001). Sensory integrative principles in intervention with children with autistic disorder. In S.S. Roley, E.I. Blanche, & R.C. Schaaf (Eds.), *Understanding the nature of sensory integration with diverse populations* (pp. 385-408). San Antonio, TX: Therapy Skill Builders.

Mailloux, Z., & Roley, S.S. (2002). Sensory integration. In H. Miller-Kuhaneck (Ed.), *Autism: A comprehensive occupational therapy approach.* Rockville, MD: AOTA Press.

Maurer, D., & Maurer, C. (1988). *The world of the newborn.* New York: Basic Books.

May-Benson, T. (2001) A theoretical model of ideation in praxis. In E. Blanche, S. Roley, & R. Schaaf (Eds.), *Sensory integration and developmental disabilities* (pp. 163-181). San Antonio, TX: Therapy Skill Builders.

McCune-Nicolich, L. (1981). Toward symbolic functioning: Structure of early pretend games and potential parallels with language. *Child Development, 52*, 785-797.

Miller, L.J. (1988). *Miller Assessment for Preschoolers manual* (Rev. ed). San Antonio, TX: Psychological Corporation.

Miller, L.J. (2003, February). Empirical evidence related to therapies for sensory processing impairments. *National Association of School Psychologist Communique, 31* (5), 34-37.

Miller, L.J., & Lane, S.J. (2000). Toward a consensus in terminology in sensory integration theory and practice: Part I: Taxonomy of neurophysiological processes. *Sensory Integration Special Interest Section Quarterly, 23* (1), 1-4.

Miller, L.J., Reisman, J., McIntosh, D.N., & Simon, J. (2001). An ecological model of sensory modulation: Performance of children with Fragile X Syndrome. In E. Blanche, S. Roley, & R. Schaaf (Eds.), *Sensory integration and developmental disabilities* (pp. 57-82). San Antonio, TX: Therapy Skill Builders.

Miller, L.J., & Summers, C. (2001). Clinical applications in sensory modulation dysfunction: Assessment and intervention considerations. In E. Blanche, S. Roley, & R. Schaaf (Eds.), *Sensory integration and developmental disabilities* (pp. 247-274). San Antonio, TX: Therapy Skill Builders.

Miller, L.J., Wilbarger, J., Stackhouse, T., & Trunnell, S. (2002). Use of clinical reasoning in occupational therapy: The STEP-SI model of intervention of sensory modulation dysfunction. In A.C. Bundy, S.J. Lane, & E.A. Murray

(Eds.), *Sensory integration: Theory and practice* (2nd ed., pp. 435-451). Philadelphia: F.A. Davis.

Mitchell, T., & Cusick, A. (1998). Evaluation of a client-centered pediatric rehabilitation programme using goal attainment scaling. *Australian Occupational Therapy Journal, 45,* 7-17.

Mulligan, S. (1998). Patterns of sensory integration dysfunction: A confirmatory factor analysis. *American Journal of Occupational Therapy, 52,* 819-828.

Mulligan, S. (2003). Examination of the evidence for occupational therapy using a sensory integration framework with children: Part two. *Sensory Integration Special Interest Section Quarterly, 26* (2), 1-5.

Parham, L.D. (1987). Evaluation of praxis in preschoolers. *Occupational Therapy in Health Care, 4* (2), 23-36.

Parham, L.D. (2002). Sensory integration and occupation. In A.C. Bundy, S.J. Lane, & E.A. Murray (Eds.), *Sensory integration: Theory and practice* (2nd ed., pp. 413-434). Philadelphia: F.A. Davis.

Parham, L.D., & Ecker, C.J. (2002). Evaluation of sensory processing. In A.C. Bundy, S.J. Lane, & E.A. Murray (Eds.), *Sensory integration: Theory and practice* (2nd ed., pp. 194-196). Philadelphia: F.A. Davis.

Parham, D., & Mailloux, Z. (2002). Sensory integration. In J. Case-Smith (Ed.) *Occupational therapy for children* (4th ed.) (pp. 329-381). St. Louis: Mosby.

Parush, S., Sohmer, H., Steinberg, A., & Kaitz, M. (1997). Somatosensory functioning in children with attention deficit hyperactivity disorder. *Developmental Medicine and Child Neurology, 39,* 464-468.

Pediatric Therapy Network (producer). (2003). *Applying sensory integration principles where children live, learn and play* (motion picture). Available from Pediatric Therapy Network, 1815 West 213th Street, Suite 100, Torrance, CA 90501.

Polatajko, H.J. (1985). A critical look at vestibular dysfunction in learning-disabled children. *Developmental Medicine and Child Neurology, 27,* 283-291.

Polatajko, H.J., Law, M., Miller, J., Schaffer, R., & Macnab, J. (1991). The effect of a sensory integration program on academic achievement, motor performance, and self-esteem in children identified as learning disabled: Results of a clinical trial. *Occupational Therapy Journal of Research, 11,* 155-176.

Provence, S., & Lipton, R. (1962). *Infants in institutions.* New York: International Universities Press.

Provost, E.M. (1991). *Measurement of sensory behaviors in infants and young children.* Doctoral dissertation. Albuquerque, NM: University of New Mexico.

Ray, T., King, L.J., & Grandin, T. (1988). The effectiveness of self-initiated vestibular stimulation in producing speech sounds in an autistic child. *Occupational Therapy Journal of Research, 8,* 186-190.

Reeves, G.D. (2001). From neurons to behavior: Regulation, arousal, and attention as important substrates for the process of sensory integration. In S.S. Roley, E.I. Blanche, & R.C. Schaaf (Eds.), *Understanding the nature of sensory integration in diverse populations* (pp. 89-108). San Antonio, TX: Therapy Skill Builders.

Reeves, G.D., & Cermak, S.A. (2002). Disorders of praxis. In A.C. Bundy, S.J. Lane, & E.A. Murray (Eds.), *Sensory integration: Theory and practice* (2nd ed., pp. 71-100). Philadelphia: F.A. Davis.

Roley, S.S. & Schenck, C. (2001). Sensory integration and visual deficits, including blindness. In S.S. Roley, E.I. Blanche, & R.C. Schaaf (Eds.), *Understanding the nature of sensory integration with diverse populations* (pp. 385-408). San Antonio, TX: Therapy Skill Builders.

Roley, S.S. (2002). Application of sensory integration using the Occupational Therapy Practice Framework. *Sensory Integration Special Interest Section Quarterly, 25* (4), 1-4.

Royeen, C.B. (1989). Commentary on "Tactile functions in learning-disabled and normal children: Reliability and validity considerations." *Occupational Therapy Journal of Research, 9,* 16-23.

Royeen, C.B., & Fortune, J.C. (1990). TIE: Touch Inventory for Elementary School-Aged Children. *American Journal of Occupational Therapy, 44,* 165-170.

Royeen, C.B., & Fortune, J.C. (2002). TIE: Touch Inventory for Elementary School-Aged Children. In A.C. Bundy, S.J. Lane, & E.A. Murray (Eds.), *Sensory integration: Theory and practice* (2nd ed., pp. 196-198). Philadelphia: F.A. Davis.

Royeen, C.B., & Lane, S.J. (1991). Tactile processing and sensory defensiveness. In A.G. Fisher, E.A. Murray, & A.C. Bundy (Eds.), *Sensory integration: Theory and practice* (pp. 108-136). Philadelphia: F.A. Davis.

Salthe, S.N. (1985). *Evolving hierarchical systems.* New York: Columbia University.

Schaaf, R. (1994). Neuroplasticity and sensory integration. Part 2. *Sensory Integration Quarterly, 22* (2), 1-7.

Schaaf, R., & Anzalone, M. (2001). Sensory integration with high risk infants and young children. In S.S. Roley, E.I. Blanche, & R.C. Schaaf (Eds.), *Understanding the nature of sensory integration with diverse populations* (pp. 385-408). San Antonio, TX: Therapy Skill Builders.

Scheerer, C. (1996). *Sensorimotor groups: Activities for school and home.* San Antonio, TX: Therapy Skill Builders.

Schneider, M.L. (1992). The effect of mild stress during pregnancy on birth weight and neuromotor maturation in rhesus monkey infants (*Macaca mulatta*). *Infant Behavior and Development, 15,* 389-403.

Schneider, M.L., Clarke, A.S., Kraemer, G.W., Roughton, E.C., Lubach, G., Rimm-Kaufman, S, Schmidt, D., & Ebert, M. (1998). Prenatal stress alters brain biogenic amine levels in primates. *Development and Psychopathology, 10,* 427-440.

Scott, A.H., & Haggarty, E.J. (1984). Structuring goals via goal attainment scaling in occupational therapy groups in a partial hospitalization setting. *Occupational Therapy in Mental Health, 4* (2), 39-58.

Shumway-Cook, A., Horak, F., & Black, F.O. (1987). A critical examination of vestibular function in motor-impaired learning-disabled children. *International Journal of Pediatric Otolaryngology, 14,* 21-30.

Slavik, B.A., & Chew, T. (1990). The design of a sensory integration treatment facility: The Ayres Clinic as a model. In S.C. Merrill (Ed.), *Environment: Implications for occupational therapy practice* (pp. 85-101). Rockville, MD: American Occupational Therapy Association.

Slavik, B.A., Kitsuwa-Lowe, J., Danner, P.T., Green, J., & Ayres, A.J. (1984). Vestibular stimulation and eye contact in autistic children. *Neuropediatrics, 15,* 333-336.

Solomon, P., Kubzansky, P.E., Leiderman, P.H., Mendelson, J.H., Trumball, R., & Wexler, D. (Eds.). (1961). *Sensory deprivation.* Cambridge: Harvard University.

Spitzer, S., & Roley, S.S. (2001) Sensory integration revisited: A philosophy of practice. In S.S. Roley, E.I. Blanche, & R.C. Schaaf (Eds.), *Understanding the nature of sensory integration with diverse populations* (pp. 3-27). San Antonio, TX, Therapy Skill Builders.

Stern, D.N. (1985). *The interpersonal world of the infant.* New York: Basic Books.

Vargas, S., & Camilli, G. (1999). A meta-analysis of research on sensory integration treatment. *American Journal of Occupational Therapy, 53,* 189-198.

Walker, K.F. (1991). Sensory integrative therapy in a limited space: An adaptation of the Ayres Clinic design. *Sensory Integration Special Interest Section Newsletter, 14* (3), 1, 2, 4.

White, M. (1979). A first-grade intervention program for children at risk for reading failure. *Journal of Learning Disabilities, 12,* 26-32.

Wilbarger, P. (1984). Planning an adequate "sensory diet": Application of sensory processing theory during the first year of life. *Zero to Three,* pp. 7-12.

Wilbarger, P., & Wilbarger, J.L. (1991). *Sensory defensiveness in children aged 2-12.* Denver, CO: Avanti Educational Programs.

Williams, M.S., & Shellenberger, S. (1994). *"How does your engine run?" A leader's guide to the Alert Program for Self-regulation.* Albuquerque, NM: TherapyWorks.

Wilson, B.N., & Kaplan, B.J. (1994). Follow-up assessment of children receiving sensory integration treatment. *Occupational Therapy Journal of Research, 14,* 244-266.

Wilson, B.N., Kaplan, B.J., Fellowes, S., Gruchy, C., & Faris, P. (1992). The efficacy of sensory integration treatment compared to tutoring. *Physical and Occupational Therapy in Pediatrics, 12,* 1-36.

Wilson, B.N., Pollock, N., Kaplan, B.J., & Law, M. (2000). *Clinical Observations of Motor and Postural Skills (COMPS)* (2nd ed.). Framingham, MA: Therapro.

Wiss, T. (1989). Vestibular dysfunction in learning disabilities: Differences in definitions lead to different conclusions. *Journal of Learning Disabilities, 22,* 100-101.

Adaptive response. A successful response to an environmental challenge (Ayres, 1979). The adaptive response is an important mechanism of sensory integrative development and is a central concept in classical sensory integration treatment.

Bilateral coordination. The ability of the two sides of the body to work together motorically.

Bilateral integration. The brain functions that enable coordination of functions of the two sides of the body.

Body scheme. An internal representation of the body; the brain's map of body parts and how they interrelate.

Dyspraxia. A condition in which the individual has difficulty with praxis. In children, this term is usually used to refer to praxis problems that cannot be accounted for by a medical condition, developmental disability, or lack of environmental opportunity.

Gravitational insecurity. A sensory modulation condition in which there is a tendency to react negatively and fearfully to movement experiences, particularly those involving a change in head position and movement backward or upward through space.

Hyperresponsivity. A disorder of sensory modulation in which the individual is disturbed by ordinary sensory input and reacts defensively to it, often with strong negative emotion, avoidance, and activation of the sympathetic nervous system. Often used interchangeably with the terms *overresponsivity* and *defensiveness*.

Hyporesponsivity. A disorder of sensory modulation in which the individual tends to ignore or be relatively unaffected by sensory stimuli to which most people respond. In some cases, the person may have an excessive craving for intense stimuli. Used interchangeably with the term *underresponsiveness*.

Ideation. The ability to conceptualize a new action to be performed in a given situation (Ayres, 1981, 1985). This aspect of praxis involves generating an idea of what to do. It precedes motor planning, which addresses the plan for how to perform the action.

Motor planning. The process of organizing a plan for action. This aspect of praxis is a cognitive process that precedes the performance of a new action.

Overresponsiveness. A disorder of sensory modulation in which the individual is disturbed by ordinary sensory input and reacts defensively to it, often with strong negative emotion, avoidance, and activation of

the sympathetic nervous system. Often used interchangeably with the terms *hyperresponsivity* and *defensiveness*.

Perception. The organization of sensory data into meaningful units. For example, stereognosis, a type of tactile perception, involves the organization of tactile details so that an object can be recognized by touch.

Praxis. The ability to conceptualize, organize, and execute nonhabitual motor tasks (Ayres, 1979, 1981).

Sensation seeking. A sensory modulation condition in which the individual actively seeks out particular kinds of sensations at higher frequencies or intensities than is typical. This condition often is considered to be a type of underresponsiveness.

Sensory defensiveness. A condition characterized by overresponsivity in one or more sensory systems.

Sensory discrimination. The ability to distinguish between different sensory stimuli. This term is usually used to refer to the ability to make fine distinctions between stimuli of one sensory modality, such as discriminating between two points of tactile contact or differentiating between similar sounds. It is sometimes also used to include the central process of organizing temporal and spatial characteristics of sensory stimuli (Miller & Lane, 2000).

Sensory integration. The organization of sensation for use (Ayres, 1979); a complex set of processes in the central nervous system that include modulation, perceptual, and praxic functions. This term is also used to refer to a frame of reference for treatment of children who have difficulty with these neural functions.

Sensory modulation. A complex central nervous system process by which neural messages that convey information about the intensity, frequency, duration, complexity, and novelty of sensory stimuli are adjusted (Miller & Lane, 2000). Behaviorally, this is manifested in the tendency to generate responses that are appropriately graded in relation to incoming sensations, neither underreacting nor overreacting to them.

Sensory processing. A term referring generally to the handling of sensory information by neural systems, including the functions of receptor organs and peripheral and central nervous systems. This includes the processes of reception, modulation, integration, and organization of sensory stimuli, including behavioral responses to stimuli (Miller & Lane, 2000.)

Sensory registration. The process by which the central nervous system attends to stimuli; this usually involves an orienting response. Sensory registration problems are characterized by failure to notice stimuli that ordinarily are salient to most people.

Sequencing. The ability to appropriately order a series of actions, an important element of motor planning. This term also is sometimes used to refer to the ability to replicate a series of sensory stimuli in the correct order.

Somatopraxis. An aspect of praxis that is heavily dependent on somatosensory processing (Ayres, 1989). An impairment of this aspect of praxis is termed *somatodyspraxia* (Cermak, 1991) and is characterized by poor tactile and proprioceptive processing as well as poor praxis.

Somatosensory. Pertaining to the tactile and proprioceptive systems.

Tactile defensiveness. A sensory modulation condition in which there is a tendency to react negatively and emotionally to touch sensations (Ayres, 1979).

Underresponsiveness. A disorder of sensory modulation in which the individual tends to ignore or be relatively unaffected by sensory stimuli to which most people respond. In some cases, the person may have an excessive craving for intense stimuli (see *sensation seeking*). Used interchangeably with the term hyporesponsivity.

Vestibular. Pertaining to the inner ear receptors, the semicircular canals, and the otolith organs that detect head position and movement as well as gravity.

Visuopraxis. An aspect of praxis that is heavily dependent on visual perception (Ayres, 1989). An impairment of visuopraxis is indicated by poor visual perception tests, along with difficulty replicating two-dimensional designs with paper and pencil, or difficulty with three-dimensional constructions such as building with blocks.

12 Visual Perception

Colleen M. Schneck

Visual perception
Visual-receptive component
Visual-cognitive component
Visual attention
Visual memory
Visual discrimination
Object (form) perception
Spatial perception

CHAPTER OBJECTIVES

1 Define visual perception.
2 Describe the typical development of visual-perceptual skills.
3 Identify factors that contribute to typical or atypical development of visual perception.
4 Explain the effects of visual-perceptual problems on occupations and life activities such as activities of daily living, education, work, play, leisure, and social participation.
5 Describe models and theories that may be used in structuring intervention plans for children who have problems with visual-perceptual skills.
6 Identify assessments and methods useful in the evaluation of visual-perceptual skills in children.
7 Describe intervention strategies for assisting children in improving or compensating for problems with visual-perceptual skills.
8 Give case examples, including principles of evaluation and intervention.

Some consider vision to be the most influential sense in humans (Bouska, Kauffman, & Marcus, 1990; Hellerstein & Fishman, 1987; Nolte, 1988). There is little argument that vision is the dominant sense in human perception of the external world; it helps the individual to monitor what is happening in the environment outside the body. Because of the complexity of the visual system, it is difficult to imagine the impact of a visual-perceptual deficit on daily living. Functional problems that may result include difficulties with eating, dressing, reading, writing, locating objects, driving, and many other activities necessary for engagement in occupation.

Given that occupational therapists focus on individuals' participation in activities of daily living, education, work, play, leisure, and social activities, the focus on the client factor of visual perception and its effects on performance skills can be critical. Although visual perception is a major intervention emphasis of occupational therapists working with children, it is one of the least understood areas of evaluation and treatment (Warren, 1993a). The information presented in this chapter describes current knowledge of visual perception that relates to evaluation of and intervention for children. The information in this area continues to evolve as research confirms or disproves explanatory models of the visual-perceptual system.

DEFINITIONS

Visual perception is defined as the total process responsible for the reception (sensory functions) and cognition (specific mental functions) of visual stimuli (Zaba, 1984). The sensory function, or visual-receptive component, is the process of extracting and organizing information from the environment (Solan & Ciner, 1986), and the specific mental functions, which constitute the visual-cognitive component, provide the ability to interpret and use what is seen. Together these two components enable a person to understand what he or she sees, and both are necessary for functional vision. Visual-perceptual skills include the recognition and identification of shapes, objects, colors, and other qualities. Visual perception allows a person to make accurate judgments on the size, configuration, and spatial relationships of objects.

Kwatney and Bouska (1980) defined the functions of the mature visual system, which demonstrate the interaction of the sensory (visual-receptive) component and the specific mental function (visual-cognitive) component. These functions are to:

1 Respond and adjust to retinal stimuli (anatomic and physiologic integrity)
2 Move both the head and eyes to collect raw data (oculomotor and vestibulo-ocular control)
3 Effectively interpret visual information (visuoperceptual ability)

4 Respond to visual cues through efficient limb movements (visuomotor ability)

5 Integrate the above functions

The term *visual information analysis* has come into use to define this ability to extract and organize information from the visual environment and to integrate it with other sensory information, previous experience, and higher cognitive functions (Tsurumi & Todd, 1998). Therefore integration of the visual-receptive (sensory functions and pain) and visual-cognitive (specific mental functions) systems is essential for functional vision. The visual-receptive components are described in the Occupational Therapy Practice Framework under client factors of sensory functions and pain, and the visual-cognitive components are described under specific mental functions (American Occupational Therapy Association [AOTA], 2002).

THE VISUAL SYSTEM

Hearing and vision are the distant senses that allow a person to understand what is happening in the environment outside his or her body or in extrapersonal space. These sense organs transmit information to the brain, the primary function of which is to receive information from the world for processing and coding. The visual sensory stimuli are then integrated with other sensory input and associated with past experiences. Approximately 70% of the sensory receptors in humans are allocated to vision. The eye, oculomotor muscles and pathways, optic nerve, optic tract, occipital cortex, and associative areas of the cerebral cortex (parietal and temporal lobes) are all included in this process. It is imperative that occupational therapists gain an understanding of the neurophysiologic interactions in the central nervous system (CNS) so that they can effectively evaluate and treat children with problems in the visual system. This discussion begins with the sensory receptor, the eye.

Anatomy of the Eye

A basic understanding of the anatomy and physiology of the eye aids comprehension of its influence on perception (Figure 12-1). The eye functions to transmit light to the retina, on which it focuses images of the environment. The eye is shaped to refract light rays such that the most sensitive part of the retina receives rays at a convergent point. The *cornea* covers the front of the eye and is part of the outermost layer of the eyeball. It plays a significant part in the focusing or bending of light rays that enter the eye. Behind the cornea is the *aqueous humor,* a clear fluid; the pressure of this fluid helps both to maintain the shape of the cornea and to focus light rays. The colored part of the eye, the *iris,* with its center hole, the *pupil,* is directly behind the cornea. The iris controls the amount of light entering the eye by increasing or decreasing the size of the pupil. The light then progresses through the crystalline *lens,* which does the fine focusing for near or far vision, and through a jelly-like substance called the *vitreous humor.*

The eye has three layers, the sclera, the choroid, and the retina. The *sclera,* which is fibrous and elastic, helps hold the rest of the eye structure in place; the *choroid* is composed primarily of blood vessels that nourish the eye; and the *retina* is the innermost layer. The retinal layer is composed of receptor nerve cells that contain a chemical activated by light. The retina has three types of receptor cells: *cones,* which are used for color perception and visual acuity; *rods,* which are used for night and peripheral vision; and *pupillary cells,* which control opening (dilation) and closing (constriction) of the pupil.

The *fovea centralis,* which is located in the retina, is the point of sharpest and clearest vision. It is most responsive to daylight and must receive a certain amount of light before it transmits the signal to the optic nerve. The retina responds to spatial differences in the intensity of light stimulation, especially at contrasting border areas, and provides basic information about light and dark areas. Light stimulates the visual receptor cells in the retina, causing electrochemical changes that trigger an electrical impulse to flow to the optic nerve. The *optic nerve* (cranial nerve II) transmits the visual sensory messages to the brain for processing. This information travels to the brain in a special way. Fibers from the nasal half of each retina divide, and half of the fibers cross to the contralateral side of the brain. Fibers from the outer half of each retina do not divide, therefore they carry visual information ipsilaterally. Thus visual information from either the left or right visual field enters the opposite portion of each retina and then travels to the same hemisphere of the brain. This organization means that even with the loss of vision in one eye, information is transmitted to both hemispheres of the brain. It also means that damage in the region of the left or right occipital cortex can cause a loss of vision, referred to as a *field cut,* in the opposite visual field (Hyvarinen, 1995a).

The optic nerve leads from the back of the eye to the lateral geniculate nucleus in the optic thalamus. It is here that binocular information is received and integrated at a basic level, which may contribute to crude depth perception. Information then passes from the two lateral geniculate bodies of the thalamus to the visual cortex in the occipital lobe (area 17). From the occipital cortex the refined visual information is sent in two directions via visual area 18 or 19 (Rafal & Posner, 1987; Ratcliff, 1987). Some impulses flow upward to the posterior parietal lobe, where visual-spatial processing occurs, focusing on the location of objects and their relationships to objects in space. This pathway is referred to as the *dorsal stream.* The magnocellular channel is dominant in the dorsal stream; this channel is associated with motion and depth detection, stereoscopic vision,

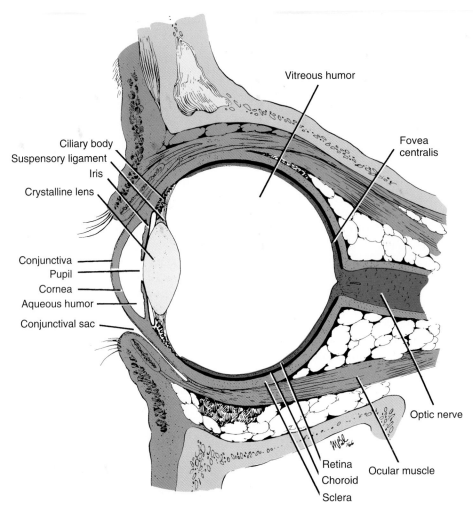

FIGURE 12-1 Cross-section of the eye. (From Ingalls, A.J., & Salerno, M.C. [1983]. *Maternal and child health nursing* [5th ed.]. St. Louis: Mosby.)

and interpretation of spatial organization (Hendry & Calkins, 1998). Other impulses flow downward to the inferior temporal lobe, where visual object processing takes place. Information sent here is analyzed for the specific details of color, form, and size needed for accurate object identification; the focus is on pattern recognition and detail and on remembrance of the qualities of objects. This is referred to as the *ventral stream*. The parvocellular channel is dominant in the ventral stream; this channel is thought to be important for color perception and for detailed analysis of the shape and surface properties of objects (Kandel, Schwartz, & Jessell, 1991).

Visual-Receptive Functions

The oculomotor system enables the reception of visual stimuli (visual-receptive process). The visual-receptive components include visual fixation, pursuit and saccadic eye movements, acuity, accommodation, binocular fusion and stereopsis, and convergence and divergence.

Visual fixation on a stationary object is a prerequisite skill for other oculomotor responses, such as shifting the gaze between objects (scanning) or tracking. Each eye is moved by the coordinated actions of the six extraocular muscles. These are innervated by cranial nerves III, IV, and VI (oculomotor, trochlear, and abducens). The oculomotor nuclei are responsible for automatic conjugate eye movements (lateral, vertical, and convergence). They also help regulate the position of the eyes in relation to the position of the head. The nuclei receive most of their information from the superior colliculus.

Two types of eye movements are used to gather information from the environment: pursuit eye movements, or tracking, and saccadic eye movements, or scanning. *Visual pursuit*, or *tracking*, involves continued fixation on a moving object so that the image is maintained continuously on the fovea. The smooth pursuit system is characterized by slow, smooth movements. Tracking may occur with the eyes and head moving together or with the eyes moving independently of the head. *Saccadic eye movements,* or *scanning,* are defined as a rapid change of fixation from one point in the visual field to another. A saccade may be voluntary, as when localizing a quickly displaced stimulus or when reading, or it may be involuntary, as during the fast phases of vestibular nystagmus. A saccadic movement is precise, although the presence of a slight overshoot or undershoot is normal.

In addition to voluntary control of eye movements, the vestibulo-ocular pathways control conjugate eye movements reflexively in response to head movement and position in space. These pathways enable the eyes to remain fixed on a stationary object while the head and body move.

In addition to the tasks of visual fixation, pursuit movements, and saccadic movements, other visual-receptive components include the following:

- *Acuity:* The capacity to discriminate the fine details of objects in the visual field. A vision measurement of 20/20 means that a person can perceive as small an object as an average person can perceive at 20 feet.
- *Accommodation:* The ability of each eye to compensate for a blurred image. Accommodation refers to the process used to obtain clear vision (i.e., to focus on an object at varying distances). This occurs when the internal ocular muscle (the ciliary muscle) contracts and causes a change in the crystalline lens of the eye to adjust for objects at different distances. Focusing must take place efficiently at all distances, and the eyes must be able to make the transition from focusing at near point (a book or a piece of paper) to far point (the teacher and the blackboard) and vice versa. It should take only a split second for this process of accommodation to occur.
- *Binocular fusion:* The ability mentally to combine the images from the two eyes into a single percept. There are two prerequisites for binocular fusion. First, the two eyes must be aligned on the object of regard; this is called *motor fusion,* and it requires coordination of the six extraocular muscles of each eye and precision between the two eyes. Second, the size and clarity of the two images must be compatible; this is known as *sensory fusion.* Only when these two prerequisites have been met can the brain combine what the two eyes see into a single percept.
- *Stereopsis:* Binocular depth perception or three-dimensional vision.
- *Convergence and divergence:* The ability of both eyes to turn inward toward the medial plane and outward from the medial plane.

For a more detailed description of the function of these components, see Gentile (1997).

Visual-Cognitive Functions

Interpretation of the visual stimulus is a mental process involving cognition, which gives meaning to the visual stimulus (visual-cognitive process). The visual-cognitive components are visual attention, visual memory, visual discrimination, and visual imagery.

Visual Attention

Visual attention involves the selection of visual input. It also provides an appropriate time frame through which visual information is passed by the eye to the primary visual cortex of the brain, where visual-perceptual processing can occur. Voluntary eye movements of localization, fixation, ocular pursuit, and gaze shift lay the foundation for optimal functioning of visual attention (Hyvarinen, 1994). The following are the four components of visual attention:

- *Alertness:* Reflects the natural state of arousal. *Alerting* is the transition from an awake to the attentive and ready state needed for active learning and adaptive behavior.
- *Selective attention:* The ability to choose relevant visual information while ignoring less relevant information; it is conscious, focused attention.
- *Visual vigilance:* The conscious mental effort to concentrate and persist at a visual task. This skill is exhibited when a child plays diligently with a toy or writes a letter.
- *Divided,* or *shared, attention:* The ability to respond to two or more simultaneous tasks. This skill is exhibited when a child is engaged in one task that is automatic while visually monitoring another task.

Visual Memory

Visual memory involves the integration of visual information with previous experiences. Long-term memory, the permanent storehouse, has expansive capacity. In contrast, short-term memory can hold a limited number of unrelated bits of information for approximately 30 seconds.

Visual Discrimination

Visual discrimination is the ability to detect features of stimuli for recognition, matching, and categorization. *Recognition* is the ability to note key features of a stimulus and relate them to memory; *matching* is the ability to note the similarities among visual stimuli; and *categorization* is the ability mentally to determine a quality or category by which similarities or differences can be noted. These three abilities require the capability both to note similarities and differences among forms and symbols with increasing complexity and to relate these findings to information previously stored in long-term memory.

Visual-perceptual abilities aid the manipulation of a visual stimulus for visual discrimination (Todd, 1999). Because visual perception has not been consistently defined, resources on visual perception use different terms and categories to define the same visual-perceptual skills. At times this contributes to confusion, because different disciplines may define the same terms differently.

It is also important to note that a distinction exists between object (form) vision (ventral stream) and spatial vision (dorsal stream) (Mishkin, Ungerleider, & Macko, 1983). Object vision is implicated in the visual identification of objects by color, texture, shape, and size (i.e., what things are). Spatial vision, which is concerned with the visual location of objects in space (i.e., where things are), responds to motor information and seems to be integral to egocentric localization during visuomotor tasks (Hyvarinen, 1995a). As discussed earlier, these two classes of function are mediated by separate neural systems. The cortical tracts for both object vision and spatial vision are projected to the primary visual cortex, but the object vision pathway goes to the temporal lobe and the spatial vision pathway goes to the inferior parietal lobe. These anatomic divisions have been verified repeatedly. However, researchers have emphasized differences in how these two areas use visual information (Goodale, 2000; Goodale & Milner, 1992). Visual information about object characteristics permits the formation of long-term perceptual representations that support object identification and visual learning. Spatial vision provides information about the location of object qualities that are needed to guide action, such as adjusting the hand during reach to the size and orientation of an object.

Based on studies done with individuals who had suffered brain damage, these two functions have been shown to be independent (Milner & Goodale, 1993; Necombe & Ratcliff, 1989). That is, disturbances of object recognition can occur without spatial disability, and spatial disability can occur with normal object perception (Dutton, 2002). The following are definitions of the object (form) and spatial-perceptual skills. Although they may not be separate entities, these groups of abilities or skills are labeled as follows:

1 Object (form) perception

a *Form constancy:* The recognition of forms and objects as the same in various environments, positions, and sizes. Form constancy helps a person develop stability and consistency in the visual world. It enables the person to recognize objects despite differences in orientation or detail. Form constancy enables a person to make assumptions regarding the size of an object even though visual stimuli may vary under different circumstances. The visual image of an object in the distance is much smaller than the image of the same object at close range, yet the person knows that the actual sizes are equivalent. For example, a school-age child can identify the letter *A* whether it is typed, written in manuscript, written in cursive, written in upper or lower case letters, or italicized.

b *Visual closure:* The identification of forms or objects from incomplete presentations. This enables the person quickly to recognize objects, shapes, and forms by mentally completing the image or by matching it to information previously stored in memory. This allows the person to make assumptions regarding what the object is without having to see the complete presentation. For example, a child working at his or her desk is able to distinguish a pencil from a pen, even when both are partly hidden under some papers.

c *Figure-ground:* The differentiation between foreground or background forms and objects. It is the ability to separate essential data from distracting surrounding information and the ability to attend to one aspect of a visual field while perceiving it in relation to the rest of the field. It is the ability to visually attend to what is important. For example, a child is able visually to find a favorite toy in a box filled with toys.

2 Spatial perception

a *Position in space:* The determination of the spatial relationship of figures and objects to oneself or other forms and objects. This provides the awareness of an object's position in relation to the observer or the perception of the direction in which it is turned. This perceptual ability is important to understanding directional language concepts such as in, out, up, down, in front of, behind, between, left, and right. In addition, position in space perception provides the ability to differentiate among letters and sequences of letters in a word or in a sentence (Frostig, Lefever, & Whittlesey, 1966). For example, the child knows how to place letters equal spaces apart and touching the line; he or she is able to recognize letters that extend below the line, such as *p*, *g*, *q*, or *y*. Another aspect of spatial perception, now referred to as *object-focused spatial abilities*, focuses on the spatial relations of objects irrespective of the individual (Voyer, Voyer, & Bryden, 1995). This includes skills evaluated by many formal assessments; however, poor performance on a formal test may or may not be linked to functional behavior.

b *Depth perception:* The determination of the relative distance between objects, figures, or landmarks and the observer and changes in planes of surfaces. This perceptual ability provides an awareness of how far away something is, and it also helps people move in space (e.g., walk down stairs).

c *Topographic orientation:* The determination of the location of objects and settings and the route to the location. *Wayfinding* depends on a cognitive map of the environment. These maps include information about the destination, spatial information, instructions for execution of travel plans, recognition of places, keeping track of where one is while moving about, and anticipation of features. These are important means of monitoring one's movement from place to place (Dutton, 2002; Garling, Book, & Lindberg, 1984). In addition, the images a person sees must be recognized if he or she is to make sense of what is viewed and if the individual is to find his or her way around (Dutton, 2002). For example, the child is able to leave the classroom for a drink of water from the water fountain down the hall and then return to his or her desk.

Visual Imagery

Another important component in visual cognition is visual imagery, or *visualization.* Visual imagery refers to the ability to "picture" people, ideas, and objects in the mind's eye even when the objects are not physically present. Developmentally, the child is first able to picture objects that make certain sounds and those that are familiar by taste or smell. The ability to picture what words say is the next step. This level of visual-verbal matching provides the foundation for reading comprehension and spelling.

Motor and Process Skills

Client factors may affect performance skills that in turn may affect activities and occupations. Motor skills of posture, mobility, and coordination may be affected by poor visual skills. For example in the area of mobility, research has shown the importance of vision in the development of proprioception of the hand prior to the onset of reaching in newborn infants (Clifton, Muir, Ashmead, & Clarkson, 1993). By 5 to 7 months, infants, in preparation for reaching, may use the current sight of the object's orientation, or the memory of it, to orient the hand for grasping; sight of the hand has no effect on hand orientation (McCarty, Clifton, Ashmead, Lee, & Goubet, 2001). If problems occur in visual memory, the hand may not be properly oriented during reach, and this affects coordination.

Process skills of knowledge, temporal organization, organization of space and objects, and adaptation all can be affected by visual perception. Children who have suffered damage to the white matter around the lateral ventricles or damage to the posterior parietal lobes can find it difficult to use vision to guide their body movements (Dutton et al., 1996). For example, a floor boundary between carpet and linoleum can be difficult to cross because it looks the same as a step. Black-and-white tiled floors can be frightening to walk across. At a curb, the foot may be lifted to the wrong height, too early, or too late, and walking down stairs without a banister is difficult.

Developmental Framework for Intervention

Warren (1993a) presented a developmental framework based on a bottom-up approach to evaluation and treatment. Using the work of Moore (Gilfoyle, Grady, & Moore, 1990), Warren suggested that with knowledge of where the deficit is located in the visual system, the therapist could design appropriate evaluation and treatment strategies to remediate basic problems and improve perceptual function. To apply this approach, the occupational therapist must have an understanding of the visual system, including both the visual-receptive and visual-cognitive components. Although Warren's model was presented as a developmental framework for evaluation and treatment of visual-perceptual dysfunction in adults with acquired brain injuries, it is useful as a model for children with visual-perceptual deficits. A hierarchy of visual-perceptual skill development in the central nervous system is presented in Figure 12-2. The definitions of components of each level are provided in the following list and are used in later descriptions of intervention.

1 *Primary visual skills* form the foundation of all visual functions.

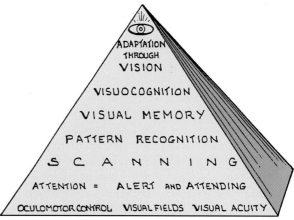

FIGURE 12-2 Hierarchy of visual-perceptual skills development. (Warren, M. [1993]. A hierarchical model for evaluation and treatment of visual perceptual dysfunction in adult acquired brain injury. I. *American Journal of Occupational Therapy, 47,* 42-54.)

a *Oculomotor control* provides efficient eye movements that ensure that the scan path is accomplished.

b *Visual fields* register the complete visual scene.

c *Visual acuity* ensures that the visual information sent to the CNS is accurate.

2 *Visual attention.* The thoroughness of the scan path depends on visual attention.

3 *Scanning.* Pattern recognition depends on organized, thorough scanning of the visual environment. The retina must record all the detail of the scene systematically through the use of a scan path.

4 *Pattern recognition.* The ability to store information in memory requires pattern detection and recognition. This is the identification of the salient features of an object.

a Configural aspects (shape, contour, and general features)

b Specific features of an object (details of color, shading, and texture)

5 *Visual memory.* Mental manipulation of visual information needed for visual cognition requires the ability either to retain the information in memory for immediate recall or to store for later retrieval.

6 *Visual cognition.* This is the ability to mentally manipulate visual information and integrate it with other sensory information to solve problems, formulate plans, and make decisions.

Warren's model provides a framework for assessing vision alone, without consideration of the other sensory systems. When visual-perceptual problems relate to sensory integration (SI) dysfunction, models based on SI theories guide evaluation and intervention (Burpee, 1997). These models consider organization of multisensory systems and the influence of vision as it integrates with other sensory systems.

Skeffington (1963) recognized that vision was more than light coming from the physical environment, entering the eye, and being transformed into an external phenomenon. He believed that vision cannot be separated from the total individual nor from any of the sensory systems because it is integrated into all human performance. He proposed a model that describes the visual process as the meshing of audition, proprioception, kinesthesia, and body sense with vision. This interaction is represented by four connecting circles, each denoting an important subsystem (Figure 12-3). The core, where each circle connects with the others, is vision. It should be clear from the model that visual perception is not obtained by vision alone. It comes from combining visual skills with all other sensory modalities, including the proprioceptive and vestibular systems.

Through extension of Skeffington's model, vision can be viewed as a dynamic blending of sensory information in which new visual and motor input are combined with previously stored data and then used to guide a reaction.

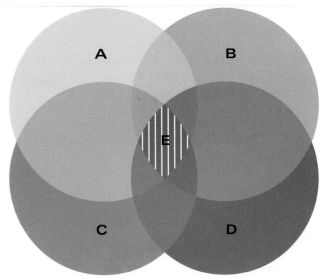

FIGURE 12-3 Skeffington's model of vision. **A,** Antigravity: Coming to terms with gravity to move. **B,** Centering: Ability to locate objects in space. **C,** Identification: Ability to focus on information, to refine and discriminate detail, and to save that information in the brain. **D,** Speech audition: Ability to communicate through speech and gesture and to use hearing. **E,** Vision: Interweaving of all these modalities. (Skeffington, A.N. [1963]. The Skeffington Papers [Series 36, No. 2, p. 11]. Santa Ana, CA: Optometric Extension Program.)

Research demonstrates an expansive interconnectivity of sensory systems (Damasio, 1989; Thelen & Smith, 1994). Studies of brain activity confirm that when an individual is using the visual system, many areas of the brain are activated. Evidence of full brain activity during visualization supports the concept that vision should be viewed in the totality of all sensory systems.

DEVELOPMENTAL SEQUENCE

Visual-Receptive Functions

As with other areas of development, the development of visual-receptive process and abilities takes place according to a prescribed timetable, which begins in the womb. By gestational week 24, gross anatomic structures are in place, and the visual pathway is complete. Between gestational weeks 24 and 40, the visual system, particularly the retina and visual cortex, undergoes extensive maturation, differentiation, and remodeling (Glass, 1993). As early as the fifth gestational month, eye movements are produced by vestibular influences (DeQuiros & Schranger, 1979). At birth the infant has rudimentary visual fixation ability and brief reflexive tracking ability. The visual system at this age is relatively immature compared with other sensory systems, and considerable development occurs over the next 6 months (Glass, 1993).

Toward the end of the second month, accommodation, convergence, and oculomotor subsystems are established (Bouska et al., 1990). Maximum accommodation is reached at 5 years of age, and the child should be able to sustain this skill effort for protracted periods at a fixed distance.

Controlled tracking skills progress in a developmental pattern from horizontal eye movements to eye movements in vertical, diagonal, and circular directions. By kindergarten a child should be able to move his or her eyes with smooth control and coordination in all directions. This can be demonstrated by asking the child to follow with the eyes a moving object located 8 to 12 inches from the child's face. If the child moves his or her head as a unit along with the eyes, this skill is still developing. Visual acuity is best at 18 years of age and tends to decline thereafter.

Visual-Cognitive Functions

Some visual-cognitive capacities are present at birth, whereas other higher level visual-cognitive abilities are not fully developed until adolescence. This development occurs through perceptual learning, the process of extracting information from the environment. Perceptual learning increases with experience and practice and through stimulation from the environment.

Object (Form) Vision

Long before infants can manipulate objects or move around space, they have well-developed visual-perceptual abilities, including pattern recognition, form constancy, and depth perception. Infants as young as 1 week of age show a differential response to patterns, with complex designs and human faces receiving more attention than simple circles and triangles. The infant learns to attend to relevant aspects of visual stimuli, to make discriminations, and to interpret available cues according to experiences.

Visual perception develops as the child matures, with most developmental changes taking place by 9 years of age. However, children vary in the rate at which they acquire perceptual abilities, in their effective use of these capacities, and in the versatility and comfort with which they apply these functions (Levine, 1987).

The abilities to perceptually analyze and discriminate objects systematically increase throughout childhood. It is generally believed that visual perception develops in the following ways:

- General to specific
- Whole to parts
- Concrete to abstract
- Familiar to novel

However, these sequences have not been proven, and in certain instances the opposite may occur. For example, visual development may proceed specific to general. The child first learns to recognize an object based on its general appearance and not by specific details. As the child learns to classify objects into categories and types, it becomes apparent that he or she is able to extract the features that make the object part of that category (Mussen, Conger, & Kagan, 1979). For example, the child learns to categorize cars as certain types or to classify animals according to their species. Further study is needed in this area. Williams (1983) estimated the developmental ages when primary visual-perceptual skills develop (Table 12-1).

Bouska and colleagues (1990) described three areas in which a child demonstrates increasing ability to discriminate visually. These areas include (1) the ability to recognize and distinguish specific distinctive features (e.g., that *b* and *d* are different because of one feature); (2) the ability to observe invariant relationships in events that occur repeatedly over time (e.g., a favorite toy is the same even when distance makes it appear smaller); and (3) the ability to find a hierarchy of pattern or structure, allowing the processing of the largest unit possible for adaptive use during a particular task (e.g., a map is scanned globally for the shape of a country, but subordinate features are scanned for the route of a river) (Gibson & Levin, 1975). These skills are important for learning to read and write. Justice and Ezell (2001) described emergent literacy as comprising two broad yet highly interrelated domains of knowledge: written language awareness and phonologic awareness. Written language awareness, also referred to as *print awareness* (Snow, Burns, & Griffin, 1998), describes children's knowledge of the forms and functions of printed language (e.g., distinctive features of alphabet letters, storybook conventions, environmental signs).

TABLE 12-1 Developmental Ages for Emergence of Visual-Perceptual Skills

Perception	Developmental Age
OBJECT (FORM)	
Figure-ground perception	Improves between 3 and 5 years of age; growth stabilizes at 6 to 7 years of age
Form constancy	Dramatic improvement between 6 and 7 years of age; less improvement from 8 to 9 years of age
SPATIAL	
Position in space	Development complete at 7 to 9 years of age
Spatial relationships	Improves to approximately 10 years of age

Modified from Williams, H. (1983). *Perceptual and motor development.* Englewood Cliffs, NJ: Prentice Hall.

The child's first perceptions of the world develop primarily from tactile, kinesthetic, and vestibular input. As these three basic senses become integrated with the higher level senses, vision and audition gradually become dominant. Young children or beginning readers tend to prefer learning through their tactile and kinesthetic senses and have lower preferences for visual and auditory learning (Carbo, 1983, 1997, 1998). At 6 or 7 years of age, most children appear to prefer kinesthetic, tactile, visual, and auditory learning, in that order. They learn easily through their sense of touch and whole-body movement and have difficulty learning through listening activities. The predominant reading style of primary grade children and struggling readers is global, tactile, and kinesthetic (Carbo, 1997). Generally, boys are less auditory and verbal and remain kinesthetic longer than girls (Restak, 1979). Around third grade most children become highly visual, and not until fifth grade do many children learn well through their auditory sense (Carbo, 1983). However, it is important to remember that reading style strengths and preferences develop at different times and rates (Carbo, 1997).

In the young child, visual discrimination of forms precedes by years the visual-motor ability to copy forms. Throughout elementary school, the child is able to handle more internal detail of figures and to understand, recall, and recreate such configurations (Levine, 1987). Children begin to use simultaneous and sequential data to develop strategies, and cognitive or learning styles begin to emerge. In addition, children learn best through their dominant sensory input channel. About 40% of school-age children remember visually presented information, whereas only 20% to 30% recall what is heard (Carbo, 1984, 1995; Carbo, Dunn, & Dunn, 1986).

Information processing in the visual-perceptual–motor domain has been identified as one of the major factors that can predict readiness for the first grade. There is evidence that the child who enters school with delayed perceptual development may not catch up with his or her peers in academic achievement (Morency & Wepman, 1973). Of the children who have difficulty reading in first grade, 88% have difficult reading at the end of fourth grade (Juel, 1988). Adequate perceptual discrimination is considered necessary for the development of reading and writing skills (Moore, 1979).

Children gradually develop the abilities to attend to, integrate, sort, and retrieve increasingly larger chunks of visual data. These stimuli from the environment usually arrive for processing either in a simultaneous array or in a specific serial order (Levine, 1987). An example of simultaneous processing involves observing and later trying to recall what someone wore.

Sequential processing involves the integration of separate elements into groups, of which the essential nature is temporal and each element leads only to one another. Sequential processing enables the child to perceive an ordered series of events (Kirby & Das, 1978). An example of sequential processing is the visual information provided in the written instructions for assembling a plastic model. An effective learner in the classroom needs to be able to evaluate, retain, process, and produce both simultaneous and sequential packages of information or action. In addition, children must learn to analyze and synthesize material containing more detail at a faster rate.

In adolescence, perceptual skills are enhanced by their interrelationship with expanding cognitive skill. Thus the adolescent can imagine, create, and construct complex visual forms. The adolescent is able to manipulate visual information mentally to solve increasingly complex problems, formulate plans, and make decisions. Of the children who are poor readers at the end of third grade, 75% remain poor readers in high school (Shaywitz, 1997). Teen rites of passage such as obtaining a driver's license or independent dating may be challenging or unobtainable for an individual with severe visual-perceptual deficits (Faye et al., 1984).

Spatial Vision

In the developmental process of organizing space, the child first acquires a concept of vertical dimensions, followed by a concept of horizontal dimensions. Oblique and diagonal dimensions are more complex, and perception of these spatial coordinates matures later. A 3- to 4-year-old child can discriminate vertical lines from horizontal ones, but children are unable to distinguish oblique lines until about 6 years of age (Cratty, 1970). The ability to discriminate between mirror or reversed-imaged numbers and letters, such as *b* and *d*, and *p* and *q,* does not mature in some children until around 7 years of age (Ilg & Ames, 1981).

The child develops an understanding of left and right from the internal awareness that his or her body has two sides (Suchoff, 1987). This understanding of left and right is called *laterality* and, according to Cratty (1970), proceeds in stages. A child's awareness of his or her own body is generally established by 6 or 7 years of age. Before 7 years of age, a child is not yet ready to handle spatial concepts on a strictly visual basis. The child must relate them to his or her own body.

Around the eighth year the child begins to project laterality concepts outside himself or herself. The child then develops *directionality,* or the understanding of an external object's position in space in relation to himself or herself. This allows the child to handle spatial phenomena almost exclusively in a visual manner. By sensing a difference between body sides, the child becomes aware that figures and objects also have a right and a left. The child "feels" this visually.

Directionality is thought to be important in the visual discrimination of letters and numbers for both reading and writing. The child first learns these concepts in relation to himself or herself and then transfers them to symbols and words.

ROLE OF VISION IN SOCIAL DEVELOPMENT

The importance of vision in facilitating infants' participation in social interactions has been widely recognized (Bruner, 1977; Fraiberg, 1977). Vision enables infants to acquire information from multiple locations at a range of distances and is a means for infants to organize information received from their other senses (Teplin, 1995). By coordinating visual and auditory input, infants accumulate information as they explore places, events, and individuals in the physical and social environments (Spelke & Cortelyou, 1981). Infants respond to attentive, social initiations from their parents by visually focusing on their parents' eyes, smiling, and occasionally shifting gaze to scan their parents' faces and the environment. Mutual gaze between parents and infants facilitates emotional attachment.

VISUAL-PERCEPTUAL PROBLEMS

Visual-Receptive Functions

The importance of good vision for classroom work cannot be overemphasized. More than 50% of a student's time is spent working at near-point visual tasks, such as reading and writing. Another 20% is spent on tasks that require the student to shift focus from distance to near and near to distance, such as copying from the board. For more than 70% of the day, therefore, tremendous stress is put on the visual system (Ritty, Solan, & Cool, 1993). Many students with visual dysfunctions can have difficulty meeting the behavioral demands of sitting still, sustaining attention, and completing their work.

Figure 12-4 presents a sample list of behaviors noted in children with specific visual problems (Optometric Extension Program Foundation, 1985). In addition to the behaviors noted in the list, Seiderman (1984) suggested that individuals with functional vision problems might use or develop any of the following compensatory techniques:

- Avoidance of reading work
- Visual fatigue
- Adaptation of the visual system through the development of a refractive error to perform near-centered visual task demands.

Impairment of oculomotor control can occur through disruption of cranial nerve function or disruption of central neural control. The pattern of oculomotor dysfunction depends on the areas of the brain that have been injured and the nature of the injury (Leigh & Zee, 1983). Oculomotor problems can limit the ability to control and direct gaze. In addition, when large amounts of energy must be used on the motor components of vision, little energy may be left for visual-cognitive processing (Hyvarinen, 1988, 1995a). Warren (1993a) and Scheiman (1997) present detailed descriptions of oculomotor deficits and other deficits seen in visual-receptive components

Refractive Errors

A child who is nearsighted has blurred distant vision but generally experiences clarity at near point. The child who is farsighted frequently has clear distant and near vision but has to exert extra effort to maintain clear vision at near point. The child with astigmatism experiences blurred vision at distance and near, with the degree of loss of clarity depending on the severity of the astigmatism. Measures of visual acuity alone do not predict how well children interpret visual information (Hyvarinen, 1988, 1995a). Other determinants include the ability to see objects in low-contrast lighting conditions, the ability of the eye to adapt to different lighting conditions, visual field problems, accommodation, and other oculomotor functions (Hyvarinen, 1988, 1995a).

If accommodation takes longer than previously described, words appear blurry and the child tends to lose his or her place, missing important information and understanding. When accommodation for near objects is poor, presbyopia exists; this individual is described as farsighted.

If the conditions of motor fusion and sensory fusion have not been met, allowing binocular fusion to occur (this process was described previously), single binocular vision is at best difficult and at worst impossible. If one eye overtly turns in, out, up, or down because of muscular imbalance, the condition is known as *strabismus,* sometimes referred to as a *crossed* or *wandering eye.* This can result in double vision or mental suppression of one of the images. This, in turn, can affect the development of visual perception. Some children have surgery to correct an eye turn. Although this intervention can correct the eye cosmetically, it does not always result in binocular vision.

Another type of binocular dysfunction is called *phoria.* Phoria refers to a tendency for one eye to go slightly in, out, up, or down, but overt misalignment of the two eyes is absent. Phoria requires the child to expend additional mechanical effort to maintain motor fusion of the two eyes, whether focusing near or far. The extra effort frequently detracts from the child's ability to process and interpret the meaning of what he or she sees.

Visual-Cognitive Functions
Attention

To review, visual attention is composed of alertness, selective attention, vigilance, and shared attention. If the child's state of alertness or arousal is impaired, the child

CHECKLIST OF OBSERVABLE CLUES TO CLASSROOM VISION PROBLEMS

1. **Appearance of eyes**
   One eye turns in or out at any time _____
   Reddened eyes or lids _____
   Eyes tear excessively _____
   Encrusted eyelids _____
   Frequent styes on lids _____
2. **Complaints when using eyes at desk**
   Headaches in forehead or temples _____
   Burning or itching after reading or
      desk work _____
   Nausea or dizziness _____
   Print blurs after reading a short time _____
3. **Behavioral signs of visual problems**
   a. Eye movement abilities (ocular motility)
      Head turns as reads across pages _____
      Loses place often during reading _____
      Needs finger or marker to keep place _____
      Displays short attention span in
         reading or copying _____
      Too frequently omits words _____
      Repeatedly omits "small" words _____
      Writes up or down hill on paper _____
      Rereads or skips lines unknowingly _____
      Orients drawings poorly on page _____
   b. Eye teaming abilities (binocularity)
      Complains of seeing double (diplopia) _____
      Repeats letters within words _____
      Omits letters, numbers, or phrases _____
      Misaligns digits in number columns _____
      Squints, closes, or covers one eye _____
      Tilts head extremely while working
         at desk _____
      Consistently shows gross postural
         deviations at all desk activities _____
   c. Eye-hand coordination abilities
      Must feel things to assist in any
         interpretation required _____
      Eyes not used to "steer" hand
         movement (extreme lack of
         orientation, placement of words
         or drawings on page) _____
      Writes crookedly, poorly spaced:
         cannot stay on ruled lines _____
      Misaligns both horizontal and vertical
         series of numbers _____
      Uses hand or fingers to keep place
         on the page _____
      Uses other hand as "spacer" to control
         spacing and alignment on page _____
      Repeatedly confuses left-right directions _____

   d. Visual-form perception (visual compar-
      ison, visual imagery, visualization) _____
      Mistakes words with same or similar
         beginnings _____
      Fails to recognize same word in next
         sentence _____
      Reverses letters and/or words in
         writing and copying _____
      Confuses likenesses and minor
         differences _____
      Confuses same word in same sentence _____
      Repeatedly confuses similar beginnings
         and endings of words _____
      Fails to visualize what is read either
         silently or orally _____
      Whispers to self for reinforcement
         while reading silently _____
      Returns to "drawing with fingers" to
         decide likes and differences _____
   e. Refractive status (e.g., nearsightedness,
      farsightedness, focus problems) _____
      Comprehension reduces as reading
         continued; loses interest too quickly _____
      Mispronounces similar words as
         continues reading _____
      Blinks excessively at desk tasks and/or
         reading; not elsewhere _____
      Holds book too closely; face too close
         to desk surface _____
      Avoids all possible near-centered tasks _____
      Complains of discomfort in tasks that
         demand visual interpretation _____
      Closes or covers one eye when reading
         or doing desk work _____
      Makes errors in copying from chalk-
         board to paper on desk _____
      Makes errors in copying from reference
         book to notebook _____
      Squints to see chalkboard, or requests
         to move nearer _____
      Rubs eyes during or after short periods
         of visual activity _____
      Fatigues easily; blinks to make chalk-
         board clear up after desk task _____

   NOTE: Students found to have any of the visual or eye problems on the checklist should be referred to a behavioral optometrist. Referral lists of behavioral optometrists are available from Optometric Extension Program Foundation, 2912 S. Daimler, Santa Ana, CA 92705.

FIGURE 12-4 Checklist of observable clues to classroom vision problems.

may demonstrate behaviors of overattentiveness, under-attentiveness, or poor sustained attention (Todd, 1999). Children who are overattentive may be compelled to respond to visual stimuli around them rather than attend to the task at hand, may be easily distracted by visual stimuli, and may demonstrate continual visual searching behaviors. Children who are underattentive may have difficulty orienting to visual stimuli, may habituate quickly to a visual stimulus, and may fatigue easily. At this level a child may refrain from attending to a familiar stimulus. A child with poor sustained attention may demonstrate a high activity level and may be easily distracted.

Selective attention is the next level of visual attention, and a child with difficulty in this area demonstrates a reduced ability to focus on a visual target. The child may have difficulty screening out unimportant or irrelevant information and may focus on or may be distracted by irrelevant stimuli. A child with difficulty in selective attention is easily confused. The child may focus on unnecessary tasks or information and therefore not obtain the specific information needed for the task.

A child with reduced vigilance skills shows reduced persistence on a visual task and poor or cursory examination of visual stimuli. The child cannot maintain visual attention. The more complex the visual structure of an object, the lengthier the process of visual analysis and the greater the vigilance skills needed. A child with deficits in shared attention can focus well only on one task at a time. He may be easily confused or distracted if required to share visual attention between two tasks.

Enns and Cameron (1987) suggested that visual inattention is the result of an inability to select the features that differentiate objects in a visual array. The child cannot see, recognize, or isolate the salient features and therefore does not know where to focus visual attention. Luria (1966) suggested that problems of visual recognition represent a breakdown of the active feature by feature analysis necessary for interpretation of a visual image. The current psychological literature focuses on such constructs as mental resource, automaticity, and stimulus selection (Arguin, Cavanagh, & Joanette, 1994). The research focuses on the attention demands that numerous competing stimuli make on individuals with a limited capacity to process those stimuli and on the fact that these exteroceptive stimuli can be processed either with awareness (i.e., effortful processing) or automatically (i.e., effortless processing).

Memory

The child with visual memory deficits has poor or reduced ability to recognize or retrieve visual information and to store visual information in short- or long-term memory. The child may fail to attend adequately, may fail to allow for storage of visual information, or may show a prolonged response time. The child may demonstrate the inability to recognize or match visual stimuli presented previously because he or she has not stored this information in memory, or the child may be unable to retrieve it from memory (Todd, 1999). The child may have good memory for life experiences but not for factual material and may fail to relate information to prior knowledge. He or she may demonstrate inconsistent recall abilities and poor ability to use mnemonic strategies for storage.

Visual Discrimination

The child with poor discrimination abilities may demonstrate an inadequate ability to recognize, match, and categorize. Ulman (1986) proposed that a finite set of visual operations, or *routines,* are performed to extract shape properties and spatial relationships. Usually an individual recognizes an object by orienting to its top or bottom. A child with poor matching skills may demonstrate difficulty matching the same shape presented in a different spatial orientation or may confuse similar shapes. A child with poor matching skills may have difficulty recognizing form in a complex field.

Object (Form) Vision. Children with form constancy problems may have difficulty recognizing forms and objects when they are presented in different sizes or different orientations in space or when differences in detail exist. This interferes with the child's ability to organize and classify perceptual experiences for meaningful cognitive operations (Piaget, 1964). This may result in difficulty recognizing letters or words in different styles of print or in making the transition from printed to cursive letters.

A child with a visual closure deficit may be unable to identify a form or object if an incomplete presentation is made; the child therefore would always need to see the complete object to identify it. For example, a child would have difficulty reading a sign if the letters were partly occluded by tree branches.

The child with figure-ground problems may not be able to pick out a specific toy from a shelf. He or she also may have difficulty sorting and organizing personal belongings. The child may overattend to details and miss the big picture or may overlook details and miss the important information. Children with figure-ground problems may have difficulty attending to a word on a printed page because they cannot block out other words around it. The child with figure-ground difficulties may not have good visual search strategies. Marr (1982) suggested that control of the direction of gaze is a prerequisite for efficiency of visual search. Cohen (1981) described the following visual search strategies:

1 The viewer looks for specific visual information and makes crude distinctions between figure and ground by isolating one figure from another.

2 The viewer determines which figures are most meaningful (the process stops here when recognition is immediate).

3 When recognition is not immediate, the viewer makes a hypothesis about the visual information received and directs attention to selected items to test the hypothesis.

Rogow and Rathwill (1989) found that good readers more frequently proceeded from the left to the right and from the top down to find "hidden figures" than did poor readers. Good readers were also more flexible in their approach; they rotated the page as needed and were not content until they found as many hidden figures as possible. The good readers also were less distressed by ambiguity, and they understood that pictures could be viewed in different ways.

Spatial Vision. A child with position in space difficulty has trouble discriminating among objects because of their placement in space. These children also have difficulty planning their actions in relation to objects around them. They may show letter reversals past 8 years of age and may show confusion regarding the sequence of letters or numbers in a word or math problem (e.g., was/saw). Writing and spacing letters and words on paper may be a problem. The children may show difficulty understanding directional language such as in, out, on, under, next to, up, down, and in front of.

Decreased depth perception can affect the child's ability to walk through spaces and to catch a ball. The child may be unable to determine visually when the surface plane has changed and may have difficulty with steps and curbs. Transference of visual-spatial notations across two visual planes can make copying from the blackboard difficult. Faulty interpretation of the spatial relationships can contribute to a problem with sorting and organizing personal belongings.

A child who has diminished topographic orientation may be easily lost and unable to find his or her way from one location to the next. The child may also demonstrate difficulty determining the location of objects and settings and may not recognize the images that help people find their way around the environment (Dutton, 2002). The child may be unable to walk from home to school without getting lost.

Diagnoses with Problems in Visual Perception

When children with disabling conditions have visual problems, the effects of the visual impairments can be tremendous. Numerous studies have found a high frequency of vision problems among individuals with disabilities (Fanning, 1971; Duckman, 1979; Scheiman, 1984; Ciner, Macks, & Schanel-Klitsch, 1991). Severe refractive errors are common among children with developmental problems (Rogow, 1992), and impaired visual attention can have a pervasive negative influence on the functional behavior of these children. Often considered distractible, these children may be able to locate objects but have difficulty sustaining eye contact or recognizing objects visually (Rogow, 1992).

Retinopathy of prematurity (ROP) is the single most cited cause of blindness in preterm infants. However, the number of infants with ROP has declined in recent years because of changes in medical interventions for premature infants (Stiles & Knox, 1996). Cortical visual impairment also occurs in preterm infants and is generally associated with severe CNS damage, such as periventricular leukomalacia. Other visual disorders common in preterm children include lenses that are too thick, poor visual acuity, astigmatism, extreme myopia, strabismus, amblyopia, and anisometropia (unequal refraction of the eyes) (Batshaw & Perret, 1986; Fledelius, 1976). These children also have difficulty processing visual information. Scores for visual attention, pattern discrimination, visual recognition, memory, and visual-motor integration are lower than those for full-term infants (Caron & Caron, 1981; Rose, 1980; Sigman & Parmelee, 1974). Studies of older children suggest that these problems often persist (Rogow, 1992; Siegel, 1983).

Children with developmental disabilities commonly have a co-existing diagnosis of blindness or other visual impairment. These children also may have sensory integrative deficits that further complicate their functional abilities (Smith Roley & Schneck, 2001).

Children with cerebral palsy (CP) frequently have been identified as a group with visual-perceptual deficits (Abercrombie, 1963; Breakey, Wilson, & Wilson, 1994). Children with CP often have a strabismus, oculomotor problems, convergence insufficiencies, or nystagmus. These problems may also limit the ability to control and direct visual gaze (Rogow, 1992).

Early research indicated that the degree of perceptual impairment in individuals with CP was related to the type and severity of the motor impairment (Birch, 1964). Children with athetosis have been found to have fewer visual-perceptual disorders than children with spasticity (Abercrombie, 1963). In a comparison study, children with CP scored significantly lower on a motor-free test of visual perception than typical children (Menken, Cermak, & Fisher, 1987). These findings supported earlier studies that showed that a group with spastic quadriplegia demonstrated the greatest problems in visual perception.

In children with language delay, poorly developed visual perception may contribute to the language difficulties. For example, language moves from the general to the specific. Young children call every animal with four legs a dog. Eventually they are able to discriminate visually between dogs and lions, and the vocabulary follows the visual-perceptual lead. Next, they can tell Dalmatians from dachshunds, but they are unable to recognize that both are dogs. Finally, the ability to categorize and generalize emerges somewhere between 7 and 9 years of age. In addition, the child who has visual-spatial perception deficits may show difficulty understanding directional language, such as in, on, under, and next to.

Visual-perceptual problems are found more frequently in individuals who have significantly higher verbal scores than performance scores on intelligence testing. Not all children with learning disabilities have visual-perceptual problems (Hung, Fisher, & Cermak, 1987). A recent study suggests that early brain damage can give rise to specific visual-perceptual deficits, independent of, although occurring in association with, selective impairment in nonverbal intelligence (Stiers, De Cock & Vandenbussche, 1999).

Children with learning disabilities may have difficulty filtering out irrelevant environmental stimuli and therefore have erratic visual attention skills. Children who have difficulty interpreting and using visual information effectively are described as having visual-perceptual problems because they have not acquired adequate visual-perceptual skills despite having normal vision (Todd, 1999).

Daniels and Ryley (1991) studied the incidence of visual-perceptual and visual-motor deficits in children with psychiatric disorders. In their study, deficits in visual-motor skills occurred far more frequently than deficits in visual-perceptual skills. When visual-perceptual problems occurred, they did so in conjunction with visual-motor skill problems. Some children with autism have demonstrated poor oculomotor function (Rosenhall, Johansson, & Gilberg, 1988). Children with autism often do not appear to focus their vision directly on what they are doing (Osterling & Dawson, 1994). A possible explanation is that they are using peripheral vision to the exclusion of focal vision. Recent research suggests that children with autism spend the same amount of time inspecting socially oriented pictures, have the same total number of fixations, and have similar scan path lengths as typically developing children (Van der Geest, Kemner, Camfferman, Verbaten, & van Engeland, 2002). These results do not support the generally held notion that children with autism have a specific problem in processing socially loaded visual stimuli. The authors suggested that the often-reported abnormal use of gaze in everyday life is not related to the nature of the visual stimuli, but that other factors, such as social interaction, may play a role.

Effects of Visual-Perceptual Problems on Performance Skills and Occupations

The effects of visual-perceptual problems may be subtle in nature. However, when the child is asked to perform a visual-perceptual task, he or she may be slow or unable to perform the task. Because visual-perceptual dysfunction affects the child's ability to use tools and to relate materials to one another (Ayres, 1979), bilateral manipulative skills are affected to a greater degree than the child's basic prehension patterns indicate. The child with visual-perceptual deficits may show problems with cutting, coloring, constructing with blocks or other construction toys, doing puzzles, using fasteners, and tying shoes. Visual perception deficits also can influence children's areas of occupation, such as activities of daily living, education, work, play, leisure, and social participation.

Children with visual-perceptual problems may demonstrate difficulty with activities of daily living (ADLs). In grooming, the child may have difficulty obtaining the necessary supplies and using a brush and comb and mirror to comb and style the hair. Applying toothpaste to the toothbrush may be difficult for the child. Fasteners; donning and doffing clothing, prostheses, and orthoses; tying shoes; and matching clothes may present problems. Skilled use of handwriting, telephones, computers, and communication devices may all present difficulty for the child with visual-cognitive problems. Instrumental activities of daily living, such as home management, may present problems. For example, the child may have trouble sorting and folding clothes. Community mobility may be difficult because the child is unable to locate objects and find his or her way. In play, the child may demonstrate difficulty with playing games and sports, drawing and coloring, cutting with scissors, pasting, constructing, and doing puzzles.

Classroom assignments may present problems for the child with visual-perceptual problems. He or she may have difficulty with educational activities such as reading, spelling, handwriting, and math. The following section elaborates on the educational problems seen in the school-age child.

Problems in Reading

At least a subgroup of children with reading problems confuses orientation and visual recognition of letters (Willows & Terepocki, 1993). Gibson (1971) delineated different characteristics of printed (written) information necessary for reading. These include a word's graphic configuration, orthography (order of letters), phonology (sounds represented), and semantics (meaning). The child benefits from these multiple simultaneous clues in reading. If the child has difficulty with one characteristic, he or she can rely on his or her perception of the other characteristics to extract the meaning. In early reading, children first encounter the visual configuration (graphics) and orthographics in a printed word. The child then must break the written word into its component phonemes (phonology), hold them in active working memory, and synthesize and blend the phonemes to form recognizable words (semantics). Visual word recognition seems to involve a subphonemic level of processing (Lukatela, Eaton, Lee, & Turvey, 2001). After practice, this step is accomplished and the word then can be dealt with as a gestalt or in its entirety rather than letter by letter and added to the child's growing sight vocabulary. Sight vocabulary consists of words that are instantly recognized as gestalts. As a child's reliance on sight vocabulary increases, decoding takes less time and the child develops automaticity, which allows the child to begin to concentrate on comprehension and retention.

Understanding sentences requires adding two more variables, context (word order) and syntax (grammatic construction), to the skills previously discussed (Levine, 1987). For reading paragraphs, chapters, and texts, it is assumed that decoding is automatic. A hierarchy can be assumed in that any developmental dysfunctions that impair decoding or sentence comprehension impede text reading.

The segmenting of written words in early reading calls for a variety of skills. First, children must be able to recognize individual letter symbols. This requires visual attention, visual memory, and visual discrimination. With severe dysfunction, recognition of words may be impaired (Levine, 1987), which interferes with the acquisition of sight vocabulary. Problems with visual perception might be suspected in a child who appears to be better at understanding what was read than at actually decoding the words. This child has good language abilities but some trouble processing written words.

Visual-perceptual attributes are different from the capacity to assimilate visual detail. The child may be diagnosed as having visual-perceptual problems when he or she is limited in attending to or extracting data presented simultaneously. In this instance the child does not have difficulty with the specific perceptual content but with the amount of information that must be simultaneously perceived to understand the whole.

Memory deficiencies also present reading problems (Levine, 1987). Children with visual memory problems may be unable to remember the visual shape of letters and words. Such children may also demonstrate an inability to associate these shapes with letters, sounds, and words (Greene, 1987). Children with weaknesses of visual-verbal associative memory have difficulty establishing easily retrievable or recognizable sound-symbol associations. They are unable to associate the sound, visual configuration, or meaning of the word with what is seen or heard.

Children who have difficulty with active working memory cannot hold one aspect of the reading process in suspension while pursuing another component. This ability is closely related to perceptual span, or the ability to recall the beginning of the sentence while reading the end of it. The child must take a second look at the beginning of a sentence after reading the end of it.

Children with visual discrimination deficits may not be able to recognize symbols and therefore may be slow to master the alphabet and numbers. Their relatively weak grasp of constancy of forms may make visual discrimination an inefficient process. Some children, therefore, cannot readily discern the differences between visually similar symbols. Confusion between the letters *p*, *q*, and *g* and between *a* and *o*, as well as letter reversals, may result, such as the notorious differentiation between *b* and *d*. A meta-analysis was conducted using 161 studies to examine the relationship between visual-perceptual skills and reading achievement (Kavale, 1982). The findings suggest that visual perception is an important correlate of reading achievement and should be included in the complex of factors predicting reading achievement. Visual discrimination abilities (form perception and spatial perception) are somewhat less important at advanced stages of the learning-to-read process than they are during the initial stages of reading acquisition (de Hirsch, Jansky, & Lanford, 1966; Jansky & de Hirsch, 1972; Lyle, 1969).

Confusion over the directionality and other spatial characteristics of a word may result in weak registration in visual memory, again possibly causing significant delays in the consolidation of a sight vocabulary. Even frequently encountered words need to be analyzed anew each time they appear. A child with visual-spatial deficits has difficulty with map reading and interpretation of instructional graphics such as charts and diagrams. Graphic representations require the child to integrate, extract the most salient elements from, condense, and organize the large amount of stimuli presented at once. Again, the child may not have difficulty with the perceptual content, but the amount of information to be assimilated simultaneously is more than the child can integrate and remember (Levine, 1987).

According to Raymond and Sorensen (1998), children with dyslexia have been shown to have normal detection but abnormal integration of visual-motion perception. The authors suggest that perhaps a collection of inefficient information-processing mechanisms produces the characteristic symptoms of dyslexia.

Problems in Spelling

Children with impaired processing of simultaneous visual stimuli may have difficulty with spelling (Boder, 1973). Their inability to visualize words may result from indistinct or distorted initial visual registration. Such children who have a strong sense of sound-symbol association may make what Boder calls *dyseidetic errors;* that is, they may spell words phonetically (e.g., lite for light) yet incorrectly. Their attempts at spelling reflect good phonetic approximations but are inaccurate. Visual sequential memory is necessary for remembering the sequence of letters in a word. Such children may exhibit poor spelling and may be unaware of letters omitted.

Problems in Handwriting

Pilot studies have begun to explore the relationship between visual-cognitive skills and handwriting (Chapman & Wedell, 1972; Yost & Lesiak, 1980; Ziviani, Hayes, & Chant, 1990). Tseng and Cermak (1993) suggested that visual perception shows little relationship to handwriting, whereas kinesthesia, visual-motor integration, and motor planning appear to be more closely related to handwriting. However, further research is necessary to provide information concerning the role of visual perception in handwriting.

Visual-cognitive abilities may affect writing in any one or any combination of the following situations. Children with problems in attention may have difficulty with the correct letter formation, spelling, and the mechanics of grammar, punctuation, and capitalization. They also have difficulty formulating a sequential flow of ideas necessary for written communication. For a child to write spontaneously, he or she must be able to revisualize letters and words without visual cues. Therefore if the child has visual memory problems, he or she may have difficulty recalling the shape and formation of letters and numbers. Other problems seen in the child with poor visual memory would be the mixing of small and capital letters in a sentence, the same letter written many ways on the same page, and an inability to print the alphabet from memory. In addition, legibility may be poor, and the child may need a model to write.

Visual discrimination problems may affect the child's handwriting. The child with poor form constancy does not recognize errors in his or her own handwriting. The child may be unable to recognize letters or words in different prints and therefore may have difficulty copying from a different type of print to handwriting. The child may also show poor recognition of letters or numbers in different environments, positions, or sizes. If the child is unable to discriminate a letter, he or she may show poor letter formation. A child with visual-closure difficulty always needs to see the complete presentation of what he or she is to copy. A child with figure-ground problems may have difficulty copying because he or she is unable to determine what is to be written; the child therefore may omit important segments or may be slower in producing written products compared with peers.

Visual-spatial problems can affect a child's handwriting in many ways. The child may reverse letters such as *m, w, b, d, s, c,* and *z* and numbers such as *2, 3, 5, 6, 7,* and *9*. If the child is unable to discriminate left from right, he or she may have difficulty with left to right progression in writing words and sentences. The child may demonstrate overspacing or underspacing and may have trouble keeping within the margins. The most common spatial errors in handwriting involve incorrect and inconsistent spacing between writing units (Ziviani & Elkins, 1984). When a child has a spatial disability, he or she may be unable to relate one part of a letter to another part and may demonstrate poor shaping or closure of individual letters or a lack of uniformity in orientation and letter size (Ziviani, 1995). The child may have difficulty with the placement of letters on a line and the ability to adapt the letter sizes to the space provided on the paper or worksheet.

Problems in Visual-Motor Integration

The results of a study by Parush, Yochman, Cohen, and Gerson (1998) suggest that clumsy children perform more poorly than typically developing children on visual-perceptual skills in motor and motor-free tasks. These findings suggest that visual perception and visual-motor integration are probably separate functions in typically developing children. When children who are clumsy are tested, a significant relationship is seen between these functions. Of the seven subtests of the Test of Visual-Perceptual Skills (TVPS), deficits on the subtests Visual Memory and Visual-Spatial Relationship seem the most likely related to visual-motor delays. These findings (Parush et al.) support previous findings by O'Brien, Cermak & Murray (1988).

Handwriting requires the ability to integrate the visual image of letters or shapes with the appropriate motor response. Visual-motor integration is not well understood because it is not a unitary process and consequently can be disrupted for a variety of reasons. Failure on visual-motor tests may be caused by underlying visual-cognitive deficits, including visual discrimination, poor fine motor ability, or inability to integrate visual-cognitive and motor processes, or by a combination of these disabilities. Therefore careful analysis is necessary to determine the underlying problem. Tseng and Murray (1994) examined the relationship of perceptual-motor measures to legibility of handwriting in Chinese school-age children. They found visual-motor integration to be the best predictor of handwriting. Weil and Cunningham-Amundson (1994) studied the relationship between visual-motor integration skills and the ability to copy letters legibly in kindergarten students. A moderate correlation was found between students' visual-motor skills and their ability to copy letters legibly. The researchers found that as students' scores on the Developmental Test of Visual-Motor Integration (VMI) increased, so did scores on the Scale of Children's Readiness in PrinTing (SCRIPT). Also, students who were able to copy the first nine forms on the VMI were found to perform better on the SCRIPT. Daly, Kelley, and Krauss (2003) partly replicated the Weil and Cunningham-Amundson study and found a strong positive relationship between kindergarten students' performance on the VMI and their ability to copy letter forms legibly. They suggest that students are ready for formal handwriting instruction once they have the ability to copy the first nine forms on the VMI.

Problems in Mathematics

The child with visual-perceptual problems has difficulty correctly aligning columns for calculation, and answers therefore are incorrect because of alignment and not because of calculation skills. Worksheets with many rows and columns of math problems may be disorganizing to children with figure-ground problems. Children with poor visual memory may have difficulty using a calculator. Visual memory difficulties also may present problems when addition and subtraction problems require multiple steps. Geometry, because of its spatial characteristics, is very difficult for the child with visual-spatial perception problems. Recognition, discrimination, and comparison of object form and space are part of the foundation of higher level mathematic skills. The visual imagery required to match and compare forms and shapes is difficult for students with visual-perceptual problems, which interfere with the learning of these underlying skills.

A longitudinal investigation that studied the relationship of sensory integrative development to achievement found that sensory integrative factors, particularly praxis, were strongly related to arithmetic achievement (Parham, 1998). This relationship was found at younger ages (6 to 8 years), and the strength of the association declined with age (10 to 12 years).

EVALUATION METHODS

Evaluation of visual-perceptual functions requires the therapist to consider the entire process of vision and examines the relationship of visual function to behavior and performance (Seiderman, 1984). Visual-receptive and visual-cognitive components may represent different issues in a child's school performance. Problems can and do exist in either area, with differing effects on the learning process. However, visual-receptive components can influence the information obtained for visual-cognitive analysis. Because receptive and cognitive components are important in the visual processing of information, individual assessment of the child should be conducted using an interdisciplinary approach, recognizing that the interplay of visual-receptive abilities, visual-cognitive skills, and school success is different for each child (Flax, 1984).

Reports generated by other educational or medical specialists often provide standardized measures of performance. Securing this information often eliminates the need for the occupational therapist to spend time administering additional visual-motor or visual-perceptual tests that yield the same information. This information also may assist the occupational therapist in selecting alternative measures that yield different data that could further help in understanding a child's problem. An interview with the teacher or classroom observation should be a major component of the assessment process. For example, information on visual stimulation in the classroom, which could affect the child's attention and focus, should be determined. The therapist might also determine whether most visual work for copying is done at near point or far point. The child's parents also should be interviewed, and they should be included as part of the team in the diagnosis and treatment of the child.

Through the interdisciplinary approach, the occupational therapist's findings can be integrated with those of the reading specialist, psychologist, speech-language pathologist, parent, and classroom teacher. By combining test results and analysis of the child's performance, the team members ascertain the nature of the interaction of the disability with the activity. A vision specialist, such as an ophthalmologist or an optometrist, may be needed to assess visual-receptive dysfunction and to remediate the condition.

Evaluation of Visual-Receptive Functions

Evaluation should begin by focusing on the integrity of the visual-receptive processes, including visual fields, visual acuity, and oculomotor control (Warren, 1993b). If deficits occur in these foundational skills, insufficient or inaccurate information about the location and features of objects is sent to the CNS, and the quality of learning through the visual sense is severely affected. Warren (1990) suggested that what sometimes appear to be visual-cognitive deficits are actually visual-receptive problems, which may include oculomotor disturbances. Therefore visual-receptive and visual-cognitive deficits may be misdiagnosed. The occupational therapist should be familiar with visual screening, because evaluation of vision and oculomotor skills assists in the assessment and analysis of their influence on visual perception and functional performance (Todd, 1999).

Visual screening consists of basic tests administered to determine which children are at risk for inadequate visual functions (Bouska et al., 1990; Hyvarinen, 1995a). The purpose of the screening is to determine which children should be referred for a complete diagnostic visual evaluation. Therefore the purpose of screening the visual-receptive system is to determine how efficient the eyes are in acquiring visual information for further visual-cognitive interpretation. The checklist presented in Figure 12-4 can help alert the therapist to visual symptoms commonly found in children who demonstrate poor visual performance.

Perimetry (computerized measurement of visual field by systematically showing lights of differing brightness and size in the peripheral visual field), confrontation, and careful observation of the child as he or she performs daily activities provide useful information about field integrity (Warren, 1993a). For example, missing or misreading the beginning or end of words or numbers may indicate a central field deficit.

The child's refractive status, which is the clinical measurement of the eye, should be determined. A school nurse or vision specialist usually performs this test. The refractive status reflects whether the student is nearsighted (myopic), farsighted (hyperopic), or has astigmatism. Several methods can be used to determine a child's refractive status. One method, the Snellen test, is used to screen children at school or in the physician's office. However, it measures only eyesight (visual acuity) at 20 feet. This figure, expressed commonly as 20/20 for normal vision, has little predictive value for how well a child uses his or her vision. It is estimated that the Snellen Test detects fewer than 5% of visual problems (Seiderman & Marcus, 1990). When a child passes this screening, he or she may be told that the existing vision is fine. However, it is only the eyesight at 20 feet that is fine.

Some schools and clinics use a Telebinocular or other similar instrument in vision screening. This device provides information on clarity or visual acuity at both near and far distances, as well as information on depth perception and binocularity (two-eyed coordination). Warren (1993b) suggested that the Contrast Sensitivity Test is best for measuring acuity. A pediatric version of this test is available (Vistech Consultants, Dayton, Ohio).

The occupational therapist may observe oculomotor dysfunction in the child. The screening test should answer several questions, including the following (Warren, 1993b; Hyvarinen, 1995b):

1 Do the eyes work together? How well?
2 Where is visual control most efficient? Least efficient?
3 What types of eye movements are most efficient? Least efficient?

Screening tools that can be used by occupational therapists are presented in Table 12-2.

In addition, the child's ocular health should be evaluated. The presence of a disease or other pathologic condition, such as glaucoma, cataracts, or deterioration of the nerves or any part of the eye, must be ruled out. An interview with the family regarding significant visual history helps identify any conditions that may be associated with visual limitations. This information can also be obtained from a review of the child's records and from

consultation with other professionals involved in direct care of the child (e.g., teacher or physician).

When visual problems are detected in screening, the child may be referred to a vision specialist such as an optometrist. The specialist can help determine whether the child has a visual problem that might be causing or contributing to school difficulties. The therapist then will be able to understand the effect those deficits have on function and can devise intervention strategies by designing and selecting appropriate activities that are within the child's visual capacity (Bouska et al., 1990).

Evaluation of Visual-Cognitive Functions

Clinical evaluation and observation may be the occupational therapist's most useful assessment methods. The therapist should observe the child for difficulty selecting, storing, retrieving, or classifying visual information. Observations could include visual search strategies used during visual-perceptual tasks (e.g., outside borders to inside), how the child approaches the task, how the child processes and interprets visual information, the child's flexibility in analyzing visual information, methods used for storage and retrieval of visual information, the amount of stress associated with visual activities, and whether the child fatigues easily during visual tasks. The therapist should analyze the tasks observed carefully to determine what visual skills are needed and to identify the areas in which the child has difficulty.

Visual-cognitive assessments typically administered by occupational therapists and those typically administered by other professionals are presented in Tables 12-3 to 12-6. Tsurumi and Todd (1998) have applied task analysis to the nonmotor tests of visual perception. This information greatly assists the therapist in analyzing the results of these tests. Currently, the best method for evaluating visual attention in children is informal observation during occupational performance tasks. Other assessments that may be used include the following:

- *Bruininks-Oseretsky Test of Motor Proficiency* (Bruininks, 1978)
- *Reversals Frequency Test* (Gardner, 1978): A norm-referenced test for children 5 to 15 years of age. This test measures reversals in a recognition and execution mode and includes a questionnaire for the teacher to complete that indicates the type and frequency of a child's reversals in both reading and writing.
- *Test of Pictures, Forms, Letters, Numbers, Spatial Orientation, and Sequencing Skills* (Gardner, 1992): A norm-referenced test for children 5 to 9 years of age that can be administered individually or to a group. The test, which has seven subtests, measures the ability visually to perceive forms, letters, and numbers in the correct direction and visually to perceive words with letters in the correct sequence.

TABLE 12-2 Vision Screening Tests

Test	Author	Description
Functional Visual Screening	Langley (1980)	Screening test developed for the severely or profoundly handicapped; it consists of 12 items, including pupillary reactions, blinking, peripheral orientation, fixation, gaze shift, tracking, and convergence.
Visual Screening	Bouska, Kauffman, & Marcus (1990)	Comprehensive screening test of distance and near vision, convergence near point, horizontal pursuits, distant and near fixations, and stereoscopic visual skills to identify children who should be referred to a qualified vision specialist for a complete diagnostic visual evaluation.
Erhardt Developmental Vision Assessment	Erhardt (1989)	Assessment that measures motor components of vision from fetal and natal periods to 6 months of age; the 6-month age level is considered a significant stage of maturity. The motor components of vision measured include both reflexive visual patterns and voluntary eye movements of localization, fixation, ocular pursuit, and gaze shift.
Sensorimotor Performance Analysis	Richter & Montgomery (1991)	Assessment of visual tracking, visual avoidance, visual processing, and hand-eye coordination during gross and fine motor tasks.
Crane-Wick Test	Crane & Wick (1987)	A norm-referenced test that can be administered individually or to a group, for children in kindergarten through grade 12; a sustained near-point visual skills test used to identify children with vision problems that interfere with learning and work activities. Subtests included are accommodation, saccadic eye movement, near point of convergence, eye teaming, pursuit of movement, visual processing, and functional hearing.
Visual Skills Appraisal	Richards & Oppenheim (1984)	An individually administered, norm-referenced test for children 5 to 9 years of age. Six subtests include pursuit, scanning, alignment, locating movements, hand-eye coordination, and fixation unity. Resulting subtest scores are converted to a scale, and a specialist provides cutoff points to indicate whether a student requires further examination.
OK Vision Kit	Williamson (1994)	A test that measures visual acuity using observable reflexive optokinetic nystagmus.
Pediatric Clinical Vision Screening for Occupational Therapists	Scheiman (1991)	A test that screens accommodation, binocular vision, and ocular motility.
Clinical Observations of Infants	Ciner, Macks, & Schanel-Klitsch (1991)	Description methods for testing vision in early intervention programs.
Clinical Observation for Adults	Warren (1993b)	A detailed description of visual screening is outlined for adults, but many items may be applied to children.

TABLE 12-3 Assessments of Visual Attention

Description	Test	Author
SCANNING		
Saccadic eye movements: rapid change of fixation from one point in the visual field to another.	Line Bisection* Letter Cancellation*	Warren (1993a)
VISUAL VIGILANCE		
Ability to handle substantial simultaneous detail; the task requires the child to sustain attention and emphasizes visual attention to detail by having the child find a particular, rarely occurring design embedded in many others.	Matching Familiar Figures Test* Visual Vigilance task on the Pediatric Early Elementary Examination (PEEX) Visual Vigilance task on the Pediatric Examination of Educational Readiness at Middle Childhood (PEERAMID)	Cairns & Cammock (1978) Levine & Rapport (1983) Levine (1985)
VISUAL SEQUENCING		
Registration and immediate recall of visual sequences.	Picture Arrangement subtest of the Wechsler Intelligence Scale for Children (WISC-III) Visual Sequential Memory subtest of the Test of Visual-Perceptual Skills (Non-Motor)*	Wechsler (1991) Gardner (1997)

*Test administered by occupational therapists.

TABLE 12-4   Assessments of Visual Memory

Description	Test	Author
VISUAL RETRIEVAL MEMORY TESTS		
Visualization and recall of entire configurations; the child studies a geometric form and then is asked to reproduce it from memory.	Benton Visual Retention Test* Visual Memory Scale* Spatial Memory subtest from the Kaufman Assessment Battery for Children (ABC)	Benton (1974) Carroll (1975) Kaufman & Kaufman (1983)
VISUAL RECOGNITION MEMORY		
Short-term visual memory; the child is shown a design and later is asked to select it from among similar sets of stimuli.	Visual Recognition subtests of the Pediatric Early Elementary Examination (PEEX)	Levine & Rapport (1983)
	Visual Recognition subtests of the Pediatric Examination of Education Readiness at Middle Childhood (PEERAMID)	Levine (1985)
	Visual Memory subtest of the Test of Visual Perception Skills (Non-Motor)*	Gardner (1997)

*Test administered by occupational therapists.

TABLE 12-5   Assessments of Visual Discrimination

Description	Test	Author
OBJECT (FORM) PERCEPTION		
The child is asked to match one design with another or to find a specific stimulus embedded within a complex background (usually administered as a motor-free assessment).	Motor-Free Visual Perception Test (revised)* Test of Pictures, Forms, Letters, Numbers, and Spatial Orientation* Developmental Test of Visual Perception (revised) (DTVP-II)* Subtests of the Test of Visual-Perceptual Skills (Non-Motor)*	Colarusso & Hammill (1996) Gardner (1997) Hammill, Pearson, & Voress (1993) Gardner (1997)
SPATIAL PERCEPTION		
The child is asked to match a design to one that has undergone some transformation but that retains its identity (e.g., mirror image or rotation).	Visual Form Constancy subtest of the Test of Visual-Perceptual Skills (Non-Motor)*	Gardner (1997)
	Matrix Analogies subtest of the Kaufman Assessment Battery for Children (ABC)	Kaufman & Kaufman (1983)
	Reversals Frequency Test* Jordon Left-Right Reversal Test (revised)* Concepts of Left and Right Test* Block Design and Object Assembly subtest of the Wechsler Intelligence Scale for Children (WISC-III)	Gardner (1978) Jordon (1980) Laurendau & Pinard (1970) Wechsler (1991)

*Test administered by occupational therapists.

TABLE 12-6   Assessment of Visual Motor Integration

Description	Test	Author
Integration of spatial input with fine motor production; the child is shown a geometric form and asked to copy it.	Bender Visual Motor Gestalt*	Bender (1963); see Koppitz scoring, 5 to 10 years of age (Koppitz, 1963)
	Benton Visual Retention Test Developmental Test of Visual-Motor Integration (VMI)*	Benton (1974) Beery (1997)

*Test administered by occupational therapists.

- *Concepts of Left and Right Test* (Laurendau & Pinard, 1970): A test that evaluates the child's understanding of left and right, from total lack of understanding to full internalization.
- *Test of Visual-Perceptual Skills (Non-Motor), revised (TVPS)* (Gardner, 1997).
- *Test of Visual Analysis Skills:* An untimed, individually administered, criterion-referenced test for children 5 to 8 years of age. The child is asked to copy simple to complex geometric patterns. The purpose of the assessment is to determine if the child is competent at or in need of remediation for perception of the visual relationships necessary for integrating letter and word shapes.
- *Developmental Test of Visual Perception, second edition (DTVP-2)* (Hammill et al., 1993): A norm-referenced test for children 4 to 10 years of age that is unbiased relative to race, gender, and handedness. The eight subtests include hand-eye coordination, copying, spatial relationships, position in space, figure-ground competence, visual closure, visual-motor speed, and form constancy.
- *Jordon Left-Right Reversal Test, revised* (Jordon, 1980): An untimed, standardized test for children 5 to 12 years of age that can be administered individually or to a group. It is used to detect visual reversals of letters, numbers, and words, and the test manual includes remediation exercises for reversal problems. The test takes about 20 minutes to administer and score.
- *Componential Assessment of Visual Perception (CAVP)* (Reid & Jutai, 1994): A computer-assisted evaluation tool that was designed as a process-based approach to the evaluation of visual-perceptual functioning in children and adults with neurologic disorders. Promising clinical usefulness has been reported in terms of utility, ease of use, format, and appeal (Reid & Jutai, 1997).

These tests can be used to evaluate how the child is processing, organizing, and using visual-cognitive information. Care should be taken in interpreting and reporting test results because it is not always clear what visual-perceptual tests are measuring. Because of the complexity of the tests, it is certain that they tap different kinds and levels of function, including language abilities. The effectiveness of any treatment method is largely determined by how the child is diagnosed, therefore careful analysis of test results and observations is important. Burtner et al. (1997) provide a critical review of seven norm-referenced, standardized tests of visual-perceptual skills frequently administered by pediatric therapists. Each assessment tool is critically appraised for its purpose, clinical utility, test construction, standardization reliability and validity. Discussion focuses on the usefulness of these assessment tools for describing, evaluating, and predicting visual-perceptual functioning in children.

INTERVENTION

Theoretic Approaches

The theoretic approaches that guide evaluation and treatment of visual-perceptual skills can be categorized as *developmental, neurophysiologic* or *compensatory.* The developmental model devised by Warren (1993a, 1993b), described in a previous section, is based on the concept that higher level skills evolve from integration of lower level skills and are subsequently affected by disruption of lower level skills. Skill levels in the hierarchy function as a single entity and provide a unified structure for visual perception. As pictured in Figure 12-2, oculomotor control, visual field, and acuity form the foundational skills, followed by visual attention, scanning, pattern recognition or detection, memory, and visual cognition. Identification and remediation of deficits in lower level skills permit integration of higher level skills. Occupational therapists who follow this model need to evaluate lower level skills before proceeding to higher level skills to determine where the deficit is in the visual hierarchy and to design appropriate evaluation and intervention strategies.

The *neurophysiologic* approaches aim to address the maturation of the human nervous system and the link to human performance. These approaches help create environmental accommodations to sensory hypersensitivity and visual distractibility. They also promote organization of movement around a goal, reinforcing the sensory feedback from that movement. Neurophysiologic approaches emphasize the importance of postural stability for oculomotor efficiency. The role of visual perception as part of sensory integration and the way the child perceives his or her environment are discussed in Chapter 11. The neurophysiologic approaches focus on improving visual-receptive and visual-cognitive components to enhance a child's occupational performance. Learning theories and behavioral approaches emphasize a child's development of visual analysis skills. The therapist provides the child with a systematic method for identifying the pertinent, concrete features of spatially organized patterns, thereby enabling the child to recognize how new information relates to previously acquired knowledge on the basis of similar and different attributes. The child learns to generalize to dissimilar tasks so that improvement in visual-perceptual skills leads to increased levels of occupational performance.

In *compensatory approaches,* classroom materials or instructional methods are modified to accommodate the child's limitations. The environment can also be altered or adapted. Adaptation and compensation techniques can include reducing classroom visual distractions, providing visual stimuli to direct attention and guide response, and modifying the input and output of computer programs. In daily living skills, adaptations to increase grooming,

BOX 12-1 Compensatory Instruction Guidelines

1 Limit the amount of new material presented in any single lesson.
2 Present new information in a simple, organized way that highlights what is especially pertinent.
3 Ensure that the child has factual knowledge.
4 Link new information with the information the child already knows.
5 Use all senses.
6 Provide repeated experiences to establish the information securely in long-term memory; practice until the child knows it and does not need to figure it out.
7 Group children with similar learning styles together.

dressing, eating, and communication skills can be made. In play situations, toys can be made more accessible, and in work activities, adaptations can be made to promote copying, writing, and organizational skills. Box 12-1 outlines compensatory instruction guidelines.

Perceptual training programs use learning theories to remediate deficits or prerequisite skills and have been implemented in the public schools for more than two decades. Occupational therapists generally use activities from these approaches in combination with neurophysiologic and compensatory approaches.

Optometry and occupational therapy have common goals related to the effects of vision on performance (Hellerstein & Fishman, 1987; Hyvarinen, 1995a; Kalb & Warshowsky, 1991; Scheiman, 1997). Collaboration is common and has been successful (Downing-Baum & Maino, 1996). When a visual dysfunction is identified, sometimes only environmental modifications (e.g., changes in lighting, desk height, or surface tilt) are needed to alleviate the problem. In many cases, glasses (lens therapy) are prescribed to reduce the stress of close work or to correct refractive errors. In other cases, optometric vision therapy may be prescribed by an optometrist and carried out collaboratively with an occupational therapist (Downing-Baum, 1995). Through vision therapy, optometrists provide structured visual experiences to enhance basic skills and perception.

Intervention Strategies

For a child of any age, an important treatment strategy is education (Tsurumi & Todd, 1998). The occupational therapist can help interpret the functional implications of the vision problem for the child and his or her parents, caregivers, and teachers. At times this can be the most helpful intervention for the child. The following sections present intervention suggestions according to age groups. However, activities should be analyzed and then selected according to the child's needs rather than according to his or her age group.

These activities illustrate both the developmental and compensatory approaches. Often activities combine approaches. For example, when classroom materials are adapted so that the print is larger and less visual information is presented (compensatory approach), the child might be better able to use visual-perceptual skills, with resulting improvement in those skills (developmental approach). For each age group, the focus of intervention is occupation in natural environments. The aim of occupational therapy intervention is to reduce activity limitations and enhance participation in everyday activities (Toglia, 2003).

Infants

Glass (1993) presented a protocol for working with preterm infants in a neonatal intensive care unit (NICU). Dim lighting allows the newborn to spontaneously open his or her eyes. Stimulation of the body senses (i.e., tactile-vestibular stimulation) can influence the development of distance sense (e.g., visual), which matures later (Rose, 1980; Turkewitz & Kenny, 1985). Based on research of neonatal vision, Glass suggested ways to use the human face as the infant's first source of visual stimulation. The intensity, amplitude, and distance of the stimulus depend on whether the intent is to arouse or quiet the infant. Glass also recommended beginning with softer, simpler forms and three-dimensional objects and to vary the stimuli on the intent to soothe or arouse the infant. Mobiles hung over cribs should be placed approximately 2 feet above the infant and slightly to one side. This allows for selective attention by the infant. In addition, Glass suggested that black and white patterns be reserved for full-term infants who are visually impaired and unable to attend to a face or toy. Once a visual response is elicited with the high-contrast pattern, a shift to a pattern with less contrast should be made. At $4\frac{1}{2}$ months of age, the preference for the familiar precedes the preference for novel as infants examine visual stimuli (Roder, Bushnell, & Sasseville, 2001). This presentation of stimuli is important in the formation of memory representations.

Preschool and Kindergarten

Occupational therapists can help preschool and kindergarten teachers organize the classroom activities to help children develop the readiness skills needed for visual perception. Teachers should understand the increased need for a multisensory approach with young children who are struggling with shape, letter, and number recognition. For example, the child might benefit from tactile input to help learn shapes, letters, and numbers. By using letters with textures, the child has additional sensory experiences on which he or she can rely when visual skills are diminished. Children should be encouraged to feel shapes, letters, and words through their hands and bodies. Letters can be formed with clay, sandpaper, beads, or chocolate pudding (Figure 12-5).

All preschool, kindergarten, and primary classes should include frequent activities that develop body-in-space concepts. Even with a range of levels of understanding among young students, group activities, such as Statue, shadow dancing, and Simon Says, can reinforce body-in-space comprehension. Children benefit from watching and imitating one another. The therapist may pair children so that one can model for the other in an obstacle course or other gross motor activity. In the occupational therapy literature, several publications detail activities for both classroom teachers and therapists (see Appendix 12-A).

Shared storybook reading has been found to provide a particularly useful context within which to promote at-risk preschoolers' emergent literacy knowledge (Justice & Ezell, 2002). Further study has shown that emphasis on the print concepts by talking about the print and by pointing to the print increases visual attention to the print. Children attended to print significantly more often when being read a storybook with large narrative print, relatively few words per page, and multiple instances of print embedded within the illustrations (Justice & Lankford, 2002).

Studies of handwriting suggest that no significant difference in letter writing legibility exists between kindergartners who use paper with lines and those who use paper without lines (Daly et al., 2003; Weil & Cunningham-Amundson, 1994). The authors suggest that kindergarten children be allowed to experiment with various types of writing paper when initially learning proper letter formation.

Elementary School

Therapy should begin at the level of the visual hierarchy where the child is experiencing difficulty. If the child is experiencing difficulty with visual-receptive skills, cooperative efforts between the occupational therapist and the optometrist may be helpful. The school-based occupational therapist's objectives for improving visual-receptive skills (as these appear on students' Individualized Education Program) are to support the child's academic goals and appropriate curricular outcomes.

Organizing the Environment. Visual perception affects a child's view of the entire learning environment. Visually distracting and competing information can be problematic to the child who has not yet fully developed his or her skills. The child may require that the classroom be less "busy" visually to allow him or her to focus on learning. Limiting a distractible child's peripheral vision by using a carrel is often helpful (Figure 12-6). In addition, the level of illumination needs to be monitored, and glare must be controlled.

The child needs a stable postural base that allows his or her eyes to work together. Children often sit at ill-fitting furniture, which can compound their problems. The occupational therapist can assist the teacher in properly positioning children. The therapist could add bolsters to seat backs, put blocks under a child's feet, or provide the child with a slant board if any of these

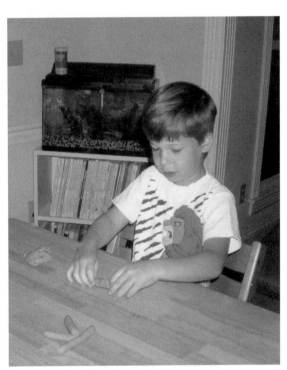

FIGURE 12-5 Kyle making letters with clay.

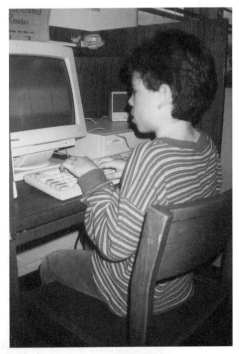

FIGURE 12-6 Todd in a study carrel.

materials will help the child use vision more efficiently or increase productivity. The therapist could also stress the importance of encouraging different positions for visual activity. Figure 12-7 shows such alternative positions as prone, "television position" for sitting, and side-lying for visual-perceptual activities such as reading. Each position should place the child in good alignment and should offer adequate postural support.

Children may benefit from color-coded worksheets to assist them in attending to what visually goes together. However, children with color vision problems may have difficulty with educational materials that are color coded, particularly when the colors are pastel or muddy. Therefore it is important to differentiate an actual visual color deficit from a problem either with color naming or with color identification (Ciner et al., 1991).

Christenson and Rascho (1989) proposed strategies to assist the elderly in topographic orientation, and these can be adapted for children. The authors found that use of landmarks and signage can enhance wayfinding skills and topographic orientation. They recommend the use of pictures or signs that are realistic and simple and that have high color contrast. For example, a simple, graphic depiction of a lunch tray with food could be used for the cafeteria door.

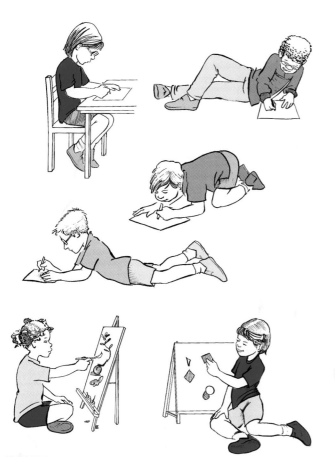

FIGURE 12-7 Alternate positions for visual-perceptual activities.

Visual Attention. With a sensory processing approach, general sensory stimulation or inhibition may be provided during or before visually oriented activities to improve visual attending skills. If the child is over-aroused, the therapist can diminish sensory input to calm him or her; if the child is underaroused, the therapist selects alerting activities to increase the level of arousal.

For the child with impaired visual attention, the therapist addresses goals using varied activities and time segments that are achievable. The therapist identifies activities that are intrinsically motivating to the child, because these help maintain the child's attention. The therapist should plan activities together with the child and use as many novel activities as possible. Most challenging to the therapist is adapting or modifying task activities while maintaining a playful learning environment for the child. For example, a therapist may have many activities focusing on the same visual-perceptual problem, and he or she changes activities frequently, depending on the child's sustained attention to the task. The therapist would gradually increase the amount of sustained attention needed to complete the task. Elimination of extraneous environmental stimuli is helpful at each level of visual attention. The occupational therapist can be a consultant to the classroom teacher and can suggest ways to improve the child's attention to learning in the classroom. For instance, using an inclusion model, the therapist could provide activities during a classroom session and then leave further suggestions for activities that the teacher can include during the week. Specific components of attention could be addressed in a hierarchical manner so that intervention tasks gradually place greater demands on attention (e.g., sustained attention to divided attention).

Visual attention skills are enhanced by activities that are developmentally appropriate and visually and tactilely stimulating. Manual activities such as drawing or manipulating clay encourage the eyes to view the movements involved (Rogow, 1992). In addition, the hand helps educate the eye about object qualities such as weight, volume, and texture and helps direct the eye to the object (Rogow, 1987). Simultaneous hand and eye movements construct internal representations of objects and serve the function of object recognition.

Activities to compensate for limitations in attention include (1) placing a black mat that is larger than the worksheet underneath it to increase high contrast, thereby assisting visual attention to the worksheet; (2) drawing lines to group materials; and (3) reorganizing worksheets (Todd, 1999). Visual stimuli on a worksheet or in a book can be reduced by covering the entire page except the activity on which the student is working or by using a mask that uncovers one line at a time (Figure 12-8). Reducing competing sensory input in both the auditory and visual modalities can be helpful for some students with poor visual attention. For example,

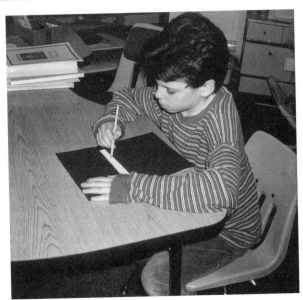

FIGURE 12-8 Todd's mask uncovers one line at a time.

headphones can be worn when working on a visual task. Good lighting and use of pastel-colored paper helps reduce glare. Encouraging children to search for high-interest photographs or pictures can help increase visual attention skills (Rogow, 1992). *Where's Waldo?* and similar books are highly motivating and encourage children to develop search strategies and visual attention.

Other suggestions include cueing the child to important visual information by using a finger to point, a marker to underline, or therapist verbalization to help the child maintain visual attention. Cooper (1975) found that subjects tended to look at a picture when it was named. The therapist can use large, colorful pictures combined with rhyming chants to encourage attention to the pictures (Rogow, 1992). Visual work should be presented when the student's energy is highest and not when he or she is fatigued (Rogow). Strategy training can be used to control distractibility, impulsivity, or a tendency to lose track or to overfocus (Toglia, 2003). Intervention strategies could include the following:

- Attending to the whole situation before attending to parts
- Taking timeouts from a task
- Monitoring the tendency to become distracted
- Searching the whole scene before responding
- Teaching self-instruction (Webster & Scott, 1983)
- Devising time-pressure management strategies (Fasotti, Kovacs, Eling, & Brouwer, 2000)

Visual Memory. Children with visual memory problems need consistent experiences; the therapist therefore should consult with the parents and teachers so that this consistency can be maintained at home and in the classroom. There is no evidence that repetitive practice of word lists or objects generalizes to other material (Cicerone, 2000). Instead, memory strategies may help with encoding or with the retrieval of memory. Grouping information in ways that provide retrieval cues can help a child remember interrelated data (Schneck, 1998). Several strategies may be helpful. *Chunking* is organizing information into smaller units, or chunks. This can be done by cutting up worksheets and presenting one unit or task at a time. *Maintenance rehearsal* (repetition) helps the child hold information in his or her short-term memory but seems to have no effect on long-term storage. An example of this strategy would be repeating a phone number until the number is dialed. *Elaborative rehearsal* is a strategy by which new information is consciously related to knowledge already stored in long-term memory. By the time a child is 8 years of age, he or she can rehearse more than one item at a time and can rehearse information together as a set to remember. Children can also relate ideas to more than one other idea. Mnemonic devices are memory-directed tactics that help transform or organize information to enhance its retrievability through use of language cues such as songs, rhymes, and acronyms. Gibson (1971) suggested that memory is composed primarily of distinctive features (what makes something different). If the child has good visualization, this can be used as a memory strategy for encoding information. Occupational therapists can help the child determine differences in visual stimuli to promote storage in memory. Games such as Concentration, copying a sequence after viewing it for a few seconds, or remembering what was removed from a tray of several items can be enjoyable ways to increase visual memory. The therapist first provides the student with short, simple tasks that he or she can complete quickly and successfully; gradually, as the student accomplishes tasks, the therapist increases their length and complexity.

External strategies and aids can also be used, such as notebooks, hand-held computers, and tape recorders, to name a few. These are easily available at a variety of stores. Also, tasks and environments can be rearranged so that they are less demanding on memory (Toglia, 2003). Examples include labeling drawers with the contents inside them, making cue cards with directions for tasks, and posting signs to help the child find his or her classroom.

Visual Discrimination. The therapist must use task analysis to design an intervention program. By analyzing the continuum of a task, the therapist can grade the activity from simple to complex to allow success while challenging the child's visual abilities (Blanksby, 1992). Remediation therefore should follow an orderly design (Bouska et al., 1990) so that the child can make sense of each performance. Intervention strategies should aim to help children recognize and attend to the identifying features by teaching them to use their vision to locate objects and then to use object features as well as other cues to form identification hypotheses (Schneck, 1998). Teaching children to scan or search pictures visually instructs the child in the value of looking and finding meaning. With high-interest materials the therapist can teach the child to look from top to bottom and left to right (Rogow, 1992). Using pictures from magazines, the therapist removes an important part of a picture and asks the student to identify what part is missing. Drawing, painting, and other art and craft activities encourage exploration and manipulation of visual forms. As the child moves from awareness to attention and then to selection, he or she becomes better able to discriminate between the important and unimportant features of the environment.

Occupational therapists can assist teachers in reorganizing the child's worksheets. Color-coding different problems may assist the child in visually attending to the correct section. Worksheets can also be cut up and reorganized to match the child's visual needs. It is important gradually to phase out the restructuring of the worksheets so the child can eventually use the sheets as they are presented in the workbooks.

When a child has problems copying from the chalkboard, an occupational therapist might recommend that the chalkboard be regularly cleaned in an effort to reduce clutter and provide high contrast for chalk marks. Notations on chalkboards, bulletin boards, or overhead transparencies should be color coded, well spaced, and uncluttered. These practices may reduce figure-ground problems. The therapist may also suggest that a teacher reduce use of the chalkboard by having the children copy from one paper to another with both papers in the same plane. A teacher may be encouraged to try bean bag games in which the targets are placed at approximately the same distance from the child's eyes as the chalkboard so that a student can practice focusing and fixating the eyes near and far in play.

Reducing the amount of print on a page (less print, fewer math problems) and providing mathematical problems on graph paper with numbers in columns in the ones, tens, and hundreds places help students with figure-ground difficulties. Masking the part of the worksheet that is not being worked on can help the child focus on one problem at a time. Cooper (1985) proposed a theoretic model for the implementation of color contrast to enhance visual ability in the older adult. Principles of color contrast and the ways in which color contrast can be achieved by varying hue, brightness, or color saturation of an object in relation to its environment are the foundation of the method of intervention. This helps a child identify the relevant information, such as the classroom materials and supplies.

Decoding Problems in Reading.

Children who have difficulty distinguishing between similar visual symbols may benefit from a multisensory approach. This includes tracing the shapes and letters, hearing them, saying them, and then feeling them, allowing a number of routes of processing to help supplement weak visual-perceptual processing. Thus the child sees it, hears it, traces it, and writes it. Eating letters is an activity children love; alphabet cereal, gelatin jigglers, cookies, and french fries in the shape of letters can be served for snacks. Children can trace the letters with frosting from tubes onto cookies and with catsup from packets for french fries.

For children with word recognition difficulty, the initial emphasis should be on recognition rather than retrieval. The child can be given a choice of visually similar words to complete sentences that have single words missing. In addition, using word families (ball, call, and tall) to increase sight vocabulary enhances word recognition skills. Phonic approaches may also be the best reading instruction method for children with poor word recognition. Textbooks recorded on audiotape cassettes can be ordered from local and state libraries from the American Printing House for the Blind (1839 Frankfurt Ave., P.O. Box 6085, Frankfurt, Kentucky 40206). The student can hear and read the textbook at the same time, which provides input through two sensory modalities.

If the child has strong verbal skills, verbal mediation (talking through printed words) should be stressed, and the child could be encouraged to describe what he or she sees to retain the information. A strategy that may assist a child who reverses letters in words is to follow along the printed lines with a finger. This technique helps stress reading of the letters in the correct sequence. Reading material rich in pictorial content (e.g., comic books), pictures with captions and cartoons, and computer software designed to enhance sight vocabulary can strengthen these associations.

Some support the use of colored filters to improve reading skills (O'Conner, Sofo, Kendall, & Olson, 1990). Blaskey et al. (2001) investigated the effectiveness of Irlen (colored) filters for improving comfort and reading performance and for determining whether traditional optometric intervention would be effective in relieving the symptoms commonly reported by people seeking help through the use of Irlen filters. Results revealed that subjects in both treatment groups showed improvement in vision functioning. The subjects in the Irlen filter group did not show any significant gains in reading rate, work recognition in context, or comprehension. However, they did report increased comfort in vision when reading.

Visualization.

The development of visualization techniques, or visual imagery, may be delayed. Like all skills, this proceeds from the concrete to the abstract. Therapists can start by helping students picture something that they can touch or feel. Using a grab bag with toys or objects inside that the child identifies without vision is a good way to do this.

As material becomes less concrete, more visual skills are drawn into play. A student might be asked to visualize something that he or she has done. The occupational therapist can facilitate the child's thinking by reminding him or her to consider various factors, such as color, brightness, size, sounds, temperature, space, movement, smells, and tastes. Hopefully, once the child practices orally, he or she will generalize the visualization process to reading (Bell, 1991).

Children with poor visualization may have difficulty spelling and may need to learn spelling rules thoroughly. They may also demonstrate reading comprehension problems. In addition, they may have difficulty forming letters because they are unable to visualize them. This would become evident when the child writes from dictation. Sometimes the child can visualize a letter from the sound, but it is reversed or missing parts.

Learning Styles. All students have a preferred learning style (Carbo, 1984, 1995; Carbo et al., 1986). When a student is taught through his or her preferred style, the child can learn with less effort and remember better (Dunn, Griggs, Olson, Gorman, & Beasley, 1995). Figure 12-9 shows diagnostic learning styles. All students need to be taught through their strongest senses and then reinforced through their next strongest sense.

Auditory learners are those who recall at least 75% of what is discussed or heard in a normal 40- to 45-minute period (Carbo et al., 1986). Visual learners remember what they see and can retrieve details and events by concentrating on the things that they have seen. Tactual and kinesthetic learners assimilate best by touching, manipulating, and handling objects. They remember more easily when they write, doodle, draw, or move their fingers. It is best to introduce material to them through art activities, baking, cooking, building, making, interviewing, and acting experiences. If a child has weaknesses in visual processing, it is more difficult for him or her to learn through the visual sense. This child may learn more effectively through the kinesthetic and tactile senses. Box 12-2 presents suggestions for kinesthetic learning.

Occupational therapists can greatly assist teachers by helping to determine a child's perceptual strengths and weaknesses so that an appropriate reading program can be matched to the child's preferred perceptual modality. Once the child is in first grade, it is important to determine what reading program the teacher is using. Table 12-7 matches reading methods to perceptual strengths and weaknesses and global and analytic styles.

In addition to perceptual strengths, the therapist must keep in mind the child's preferred manner of approaching new material. For instance, global learners require an overall comprehension first and then can attend to the details. Analytic learners piece details together to form an understanding.

Visual-Motor Integration. To review, the therapist should first focus on the underlying visual-receptive

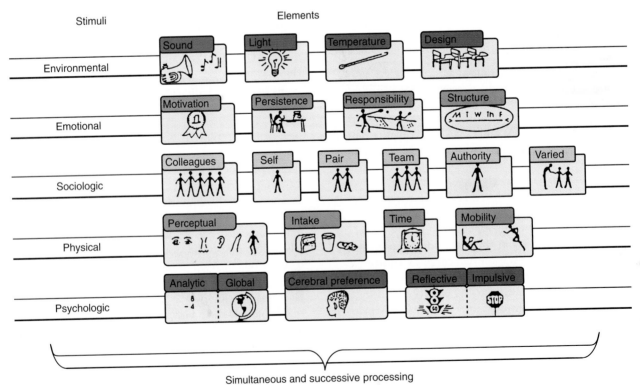

FIGURE 12-9 Diagnostic learning styles. (Courtesy Rita Dunn, Ed.D., St. John's University, Jamaica, NY.)

TABLE 12-7 Matching Reading Methods to Perceptual Strengths

Reading Method	Description	Reading Style Requirements
Phonics	Isolated letter sounds or letter clusters are taught sequentially and blended to form words.	Auditory and analytic strengths
Linguistic	Patterns of letters are taught and combined to form words.	Auditory and analytic strengths
Orton-Gillingham	Consists of phonics and tactile stimulation in the form of writing and tracing activities.	Auditory and analytic strengths combined with visual weaknesses
Whole word	Before reading a story, new words are presented on flash cards and in sentences, with accompanying pictures.	Visual and global strengths
Language-experience	Students read stories that they have written.	Visual, tactile, and global strengths
Fernald	Language-experience method, plus student traces over new words with index finger of writing hand.	Tactile and global strengths combined with visual weaknesses
Choral reading	Groups read a text in unison.	Visual and global strengths
Recorded book	Students listen two or three times to brief recordings of books, visually track the words, then read the selection aloud.	Visual and global strengths

From Carbo, M. (1987). Deprogramming reading failure: Giving unequal learners an equal chance. *Phi Delta Kappan, 69(3),*197-202.

BOX 12-2 **Suggestions for Tactile and Kinesthetic Learners**

- At story time, give the child a prop that relates to the story. The child can act out something that he or she just heard using the prop.
- Provide letter cubes for making words.
- To enable the student to build models and complete projects, provide simple written and recorded directions (the child sees and hears written directions simultaneously, which increases understanding and retention).
- Use games such as bingo, dominoes, or card games to teach or review reading skills. These activities allow movement and peer and adult interaction.
- Use writing activity cards. Paste colorful, high-interest pictures on index cards and add stimulating questions. (Carbo, Dunn, & Dunn, et al., 1986)
- Encourage the child to participate actively while he or she reads. For example, children can write while they read, underline or circle key words or place an asterisk in the margin next to an important section as they read, and inscribe comments when appropriate.
- Use glue letters.
- Use blocks from a Boggle game.
- Play Scrabble.

functions and then focus on the visual-cognitive functions. This should proceed in the sequence of visual attention, visual memory, visual discrimination, and specific visual discrimination skills. A multisensory approach to handwriting may be helpful to a child with visual-cognitive problems. Working with the eyes closed can be effective in reducing the influence of increased effort that vision can create and in lessening the visual distractions. Keeping the eyes closed can also improve the awareness of the kinesthetic feedback from letter formation.

The therapist should be aware of which handwriting approach is used in the classroom. The child whose preferred learning style is through the auditory system can be assisted in learning handwriting through use of a talking pen. Handwriting programs that are easier for

children with visual-cognitive problems include Loops and Other Groups (Benbow, 1990) and Handwriting without Tears (Olsen, 2003). Olsen described strategies to help children correct or avoid reversals. During handwriting lessons, the child should proofread his or her own work and circle the best-formed letters. Chapter 17 has comprehensive information on developing handwriting skills.

Children with visual-spatial problems often choose random starting points, which can confuse the writing task from the onset. Concrete cues must be used to teach abstract handwriting concepts. For example, colored lines on the paper or paper with raised lines can be helpful for the child who has trouble knowing where to place the letters on the page. In addition, green lines drawn to symbolize *go* on the left side of the paper and red lines to symbolize *stop* on the right side may help a child know which direction to write his or her letters and words. Upright orientation of the writing surface may also lessen directional confusion of letter formation (*up* means up and *down* means down) versus orientation at a desk on a horizontal surface, where *up* means away from oneself and *down* means toward oneself (Schneck, 1998).

Directional cues can be paired with verbal cues for the child who commonly reverses letters and numbers. These cognitive cues rely on visual images for distinguishing letters and include the following:

1 With palms facing the chest and thumbs up, the student makes two fists. The left hand will form a *b* and the right hand will form a *d*.
2 Lower case *b* is like *B*, only without the top loop.
3 To make a lower case *d*, remember that *c* comes first, then add a line to make a *d*.

The therapist can develop cue cards for the student to keep at his or her desk with common reversals.

Children with visual-cognitive problems often over-space or underspace words. The correct space should be slightly more than the width of a single lower case letter. When a child has handwriting spacing problems, the occupational therapist may recommend using a decorated tongue depressor to space words, using a pencil, or simply having the child use his or her finger as a guide. The child can also imagine a letter in the space to aid in judging the distance.

When students need additional help to stop at lines, templates with windows can be used in teaching handwriting. These templates can be made out of cardboard with three windows; one for one-line letters (*a, c, e, i, m,* and *n*), one for two-line letters (*b, d, k, l,* and *t*), and the third for three-line letters (*f, g, j, p, q, z,* and *y*). It is important to consider that visual memory is used to recognize the letters or words to be written, and motor memory starts the engram for producing the written product. Therefore it may be that motor memory, not visual memory, is the basis for the problem.

Dankert, Davies, and Gavin (2003) evaluated whether preschool children with developmental delays who received occupational therapy would demonstrate improvement in visual-motor skills. The children received occupational therapy, at minimum, of one individual 30-minute session and one group 30-minute session per week for one school year. Their performance was compared with that of two control groups: typically developing peers who received occupational therapy and typically developing peers who did not receive occupational therapy. The results showed that the students with developmental delays demonstrated statistically significant improvement in visual-motor skills and developed skills at a rate faster than expected compared to typically developing peers.

Computers. Many excellent educational computer programs for young children that the occupational therapist can use are already on the market. Software programs that are highly motivating for children of all ages are available. Living books on the computer reinforce the written word with the spoken word and assist in developing a sight-word vocabulary.

The computer can be used as a motivational device to help increase the child's attention to the task. It also provides a means to practice skills in an independent manner. Drill and practice software record data on accuracy and the time taken to complete the drills, allowing the therapist to record the child's progress. The therapist can adapt the computer program by changing the background colors to those that enhance the child's visual-perceptual skills. The therapist can also enlarge the written information so that less information is present on the screen. Sands and Buchholz (1997) provide a discussion on the use of computers in reading instruction. Appendix 12-A includes a list of computer software and hardware companies that provide current information on technologic and educational resources available for children with a variety of special needs.

Studies on the treatment effectiveness of computer use in fields other than the occupational therapy profession are varied and could help guide effective treatment. For example, a single-subject reversal design study was done to examine the effectiveness of using a computer to increase attention to developmentally appropriate visual analysis activities of five children 3 to 5 years of age who had developmental disabilities (Cardona, Martinez, & Hinojosa, 2000). The results suggested that each child's attention to task performance improved during the computer-based activities as measured by the number of off-task distractions. Sitting tolerance and visual attention to the task did not change. All participants seemed to be interested in and motivated to engage in the computer-based activities.

More research is needed to examine a longer intervention phase and the effectiveness of computer-based intervention in natural settings, such as a classroom. Authors who have studied the effects of computer games in kindergarten-age children recommend their use in improving visual-perceptual skills (Perov & Kozminsky, 1989). Their findings indicate that, on the basis of required time and motivation level, computer games are more efficient than other educational programs.

Currently a considerable body of literature supports the use of virtual environment technology to train spatial behavior in the real world (Durlach et al., 2000). Occupational therapists should incorporate this information into treatment.

SUMMARY

Children with visual-perceptual problems often receive the services of occupational therapists. This chapter described a developmental approach that emphasizes methods of identifying the underlying client factors of visual-receptive and visual-cognitive skills. The relationship of these components to various performance skills was described. Using the developmental approach, the occupational therapist helps the child increase his or her visual-perceptual skills by improving the skill problems that appear to be limiting function. By adapting classroom materials and instruction methods, the therapist also helps the child compensate for visual-perceptual problems. Intervention often includes a combination of developmental and compensatory activities. This holistic approach enables the child with visual-perceptual problems to achieve optimal function and learning.

Little evidence exists in the occupational therapy literature regarding treatment effectiveness for visual-perceptual problems in children. As a profession, occupational therapy has defined its domain of practice and frames of reference used in the treatment of children with visual-perceptual problems. The next step is to test the effectiveness of these treatment programs systematically.

CASE STUDY

When Todd was a 9-year-old student in the third grade, most of his day was spent in the regular third grade classroom, where he functioned at grade level in all areas of academics except reading. Todd received daily resource room instruction in this area. This instruction consisted of copying, worksheet completion, and drill and repetition techniques and did not include opportunities for manipulative activities.

An occupational therapy evaluation indicated that Todd's perceptual skills were delayed about 2 years, with weaknesses noted in visual-spatial relations, figure-ground perception, and visual sequential memory. From interviewing the teacher, the therapist learned that Todd was not moving from learning to read to reading to learn. His decoding was not automatic, therefore he was spending considerable time figuring out what the words were rather than comprehending what he was reading. He also reported that his eyes tired easily while reading. Good eye movements were needed to sustain reading for longer periods. Because of poor spatial abilities, Todd had difficulty discerning differences in visually similar symbols and had difficulty with words that only differed by sequence (*three* and *there*) or spatial orientation (*dad* and *bad*). The third grade reading books had more print per page and fewer illustrations to give cues. Too many words on the page made it difficult for Todd because of his poor figure-ground abilities. He demonstrated an inability to recall the exact order of words, poor sight vocabulary, and poor spelling caused by poor visual sequential memory.

The therapist referred Todd for optometric evaluation because of his reported visual fatigue during reading tasks. Planning together with Todd, the therapist and teacher developed strategies to assist him in increasing his visual memory. Initially, short visual memory tasks were used, and gradually the length of tasks was increased. This was done using visual memory games and activities on the computer. In addition, visual discrimination tasks were started, beginning with simple forms and moving to forms that were more complex.

In consultation with the teacher, the therapist recommended reducing the amount of print per page and masking what was not immediately needed when this could not be done. Phonics approaches to word recognition were recommended (see Table 12-7), as were using verbal mediation to decode words.

STUDY QUESTIONS

1 Describe the relationship of the sensory functions/visual-receptive and the specific mental functions/visual-cognitive components.

2 What are the differences between object (form) vision and spatial vision? Describe different forms of each.

3 Define three occupational therapy recommendations for a second grade teacher who has a child with difficulties in visual attention.

REFERENCES

Abercrombie, M.L.J. (1963). Eye movements, perception, and learning. In *Visual Disorders and Cerebral Palsy*. London: Heinemann.

American Occupational Therapy Association (AOTA). (2002). Occupational Therapy Practice Framework: Domain and process. *American Journal of Occupational Therapy, 56,* 609-639.

Arguin, M., Cavanagh, P., & Joanette, Y. (1994). Visual feature integration with an attention deficit. *Brain and Cognition, 24,* 44-56.

Ayres, A.J. (1979). *Sensory Integration and the Child.* Los Angeles: Western Psychological Services.

Batshaw, M.L., & Perret, Y.M. (1986). *Children with handicaps: A medical primer* (2nd ed.). Baltimore: Brookes.

Beery, K.E. (1997). *Developmental Test of Visual-Motor Integration* (4th ed.). Los Angeles: Western Psychological Services.

Bell, N. (1991). *Visualizing and verbalizing for language comprehension and thinking.* Paso Robles, CA: Academy of Reading Publishers.

Benbow, M. (1990). *Loops and other groups.* Tucson: Therapy Skill Builders.

Bender, C.L. (1963). *Bender Visual-Motor Gestalt Test.* Cleveland: Psychological Corporation.

Benton, A.L. (1974). *Benton Visual Retention Test.* Chicago: Psychological Corporation.

Birch, H.G. (1964). *Brain damage in children: The biological and social aspects.* New York: Williams & Wilkins.

Blanksby, B.S. (1992). Visual therapy: A theoretically based intervention program. *Journal of Visual Impairment and Blindness, 86,* 291-294.

Blaskey, P., Scheimen, M., Parisi, M. Ciner, E.B., Gallaway, M., & Sleznick R. (1990). The effectiveness of Irlen Filters for improving reading performance: A pilot study. *Journal of Learning Disabilities, 23,* 604-612.

Boder, E. (1973). Developmental dyslexia: A diagnostic approach based on three atypical reading-spelling patterns. *Developmental Medicine and Child Neurology, 15,* 661.

Bouska, M.J., Kauffman, N.A., & Marcus, S.E. (1990). Disorders of the visual perception system. In D. Umphred (Ed.), *Neurological rehabilitation* (2nd ed., pp. 522-585). St. Louis: Mosby.

Breakey, A.S., Wilson, J.J., & Wilson, B.C. (1994). Sensory and perceptual functions in the cerebral palsied. *Journal of Nervous and Mental Diseases, 158,* 70-77.

Bruininks, R.H. (1978). *Bruininks-Oseretsky Test of Motor Proficiency.* Circle Pines, MN: American Guidance Service.

Bruner, J.S. (1977). Early social interaction and language acquisition. In H.R. Schaffer (Ed.), *Studies in mother-infant interaction* (pp. 271-290). New York: Academic Press.

Burpee, J.D. (1997). Sensory integration and visual functions. In M. Gentile (Ed.), *Functional visual behavior: A therapist's guide to evaluation and treatment options.* Bethesda, MD: American Occupational Therapy Association.

Burtner, P.A., Wilhite, C., Bordegaray, J., Moedl, D., Roe, R.J., & Savage, A.R. (1997). Critical review of visual perceptual tests frequently administered by pediatric therapists. *Physical and Occupational Therapy in Pediatrics, 17,* 39-61.

Cairns, E., & Cammock, T. (1978). Development of a more reliable version of the matching familiar figures test. *Developmental Psychology, 14,* 555.

Carbo, M. (1983). Reading styles change from second to eighth grade. *Education Leadership, 40,* 56-59.

Carbo, M. (1984, 1995). *Reading Style Inventory.* Roslyn, NY: National Reading Styles Institute.

Carbo, M. (1987). Deprogramming reading failure: Giving unequal learners an equal chance. *Phi Delta Kappan, 69* (3), 197-202.

Carbo, M. (1997). Reading styles times twenty. *Educational Leadership, 54,* 38-42.

Carbo, M. (1998). The power of reading styles: Accommodating students' strengths. In *Perspectives on Reading Instruction.* Alexandria, VA: Association for Supervision and Curriculum Development.

Carbo, M., Dunn, R., & Dunn, K. (1986). *Teaching students to read through their individual learning styles.* Englewood Cliffs, NJ: Prentice-Hall.

Cardona, M., Martinez, A.L., & Hinojosa, J. (2000). Effectiveness of using a computer to improve attention to visual analysis activities of five preschool children with disabilities. *Occupational Therapy International, 7,* 42-56.

Caron, A., & Caron, R. (1981). Processing of relational information as an index of infant risk. In S. Friedman & M. Sigman (Eds.), *Preterm birth and psychological development.* New York: Academic Press.

Carroll, J.L. (1975). *Visual memory scale.* Mt. Pleasant, MI: Carroll Publications.

Chapman, L.J., & Wedell, K. (1972). Perceptual-motor abilities and reversal errors in children's handwriting. *Journal of Learning Disabilities, 5,* 321-325.

Christenson, M.A., & Rascho, B. (1989). Environmental cognition and age-related sensory change. *Occupational Therapy Practice, 1,* 28-35.

Cicerone, K.D. (2000). Evidence-based cognitive rehabilitation: Recommendations for clinical practice. *Archives of Physical Medicine and Rehabilitation, 81* (12), 1596-1615.

Ciner, E.B., Macks, B., & Schanel-Klitsch, E. (1991). A cooperative demonstration project for early intervention vision services. *Occupational Therapy Practice, 3,* 42-56.

Clifton, R.K., Muir, D.W., Ashmead, D.H., & Clarkson, M.G. (1993). Is visually guided reaching in early infancy a myth? *Child Development, 64,* 1099-1110.

Cohen, K.M. (1981). The development of strategies of visual search. In D.F. Fisher, R.A. Monty, & J.W. Senders (Eds.), *Eye movements: Cognition and visual perception.* Hillsdale, NJ: Erlbaum.

Colarusso, R.P., & Hammill, D.D. (1996). *Motor-Free Visual Perception Test, revised.* Novato, CA: Academic Therapy Publications.

Cooper, B.A. (1985). A model for implementing color contrast in the environment of the elderly, *American Journal of Occupational Therapy, 39,* 253-258.

Cooper, L.A. (1975). Mental rotation of random two-dimensional shapes. *Cognitive Psychology, 7* (2), 20-43.

Crane, A., & Wick, B. (1987). *Crane-Wick Test.* Houston: Rapid Research Corporation.

Cratty, B.J. (1970). *Perceptual and motor development in infants and children,* New York: Macmillan.

Daly, C.J., Kelley, G.T., & Krauss, A. (2003). Relationship between visual-motor integration and handwriting skills of children in kindergarten: A modified replication study. *American Journal of Occupational Therapy, 57,* 459-462.

Damasio, A.R. (1989). Time-locked multiregional retroactivation: A systems level proposal for the neural substrates of recall and recognition. *Cognition, 33,* 25-62.

Daniels, L.E., & Ryley, C. (1991). Visual-perceptual and visual-motor performance in children with psychiatric disorders. *Canadian Journal of Occupational Therapy, 58* (30), 137-141.

Dankert, H.L., Davies, P.L. & Gavin, W.J. (2003). Occupational therapy effects on visual-motor skills in preschool children. *American Journal of Occupational Therapy, 57,* 542-549.

de Hirsch, K., Jansky, J., & Lanford, W. (1966). *Predicting reading failure.* New York: Harper & Row.

DeQuiros, J.B., & Schranger, O.L. (1979). *Neuropsychological fundamentals in learning disabilities.* Novato, CA: Academic Therapy Publications.

Downing-Baum, S. (1995). Exercises in pediatric vision therapy. *OT Week, 9,* 20-22.

Downing-Baum, S., & Maino, D. (1996). Case studies show success in OT-OD treatment plans. *ADVANCE for Occupational Therapists, 18.*

Duckman, R. (1979). The incidence of anomalies in a population of cerebral palsied children. *Journal of the American Optometric Association, 50,* 1013.

Dunn, R., Griggs, S.A., Olson, J., Gorman, B., & Beasley, M. (1995). A meta-analytic validation of the Dunn and Dunn learning styles model. *Journal of Educational Research, 88,* 353-363.

Durlach, N., Allen, G., Dorken, R., Garnett, R., Loomis, J., & Templeman, J., et al. (2000). Virtual environments and the enhancement of spatial behavior. *Presence: Teleoperators and Virtual Environments, 9,* 593-616.

Dutton, G. (2002). Visual problems in children with damage to the brain. *Visual Impairment Research–2002, 4,* 113-121.

Dutton, G., Ballantyne, J., Boyd, G., Bradnam, M., Day, R., & McCulloch, D., et al. (1996). Cortical visual dysfunction in children: A clinical study. *Eye, 10,* 302-309.

Enns, J.T., & Cameron, S. (1987). Selective attention in young children: The relation between visual search, filtering, and priming. *Journal of Experimental Child Psychology, 44,* 38-63.

Erhardt, R.P. (1989). *Erhardt Developmental Vision Assessment (EDVA)* (Rev. ed.). Tucson: Therapy Skill Builders.

Fanning, G.S. (1971). Vision in children with Down's syndrome. *Australian Journal of Optometry, 54,* 74.

Fasotti, L., Kovacs, F., Eling, P., & Brouwer, W.H. (2000). Time pressure management as a compensatory strategy training after closed head injury. *Neuropsychological Rehabilitation, 10,* 47-65.

Faye, E.E., Padula, W.V., Padula, J.B., Gurland, J.E., Greenberg, M.L., & Hood, C.M. (1984). The low vision child. In E.E. Faye (Ed.), *Clinical low vision* (2nd ed., pp. 437-475). Boston: Little, Brown.

Flax, N. (1984). Visual perception versus visual function. *Journal of Learning Disabilities, 17,* 182-185.

Fledelius, T. (1976). Prematurity and the eye. *Acta Ophthalmology Supplement, 128,* 3-245.

Fraibery, S. (1977). Insights from the blind: Comparative studies of blind and sighted infants. New York: Basic Books.

Frostig, M., Lefever, W., & Whittlesey, J.R.B. (1966). *Administration and scoring manual for the Marianne Frostig Developmental Test of Visual Perception.* Palo Alto, CA: Consulting Psychologists Press.

Gardner, M.F. (1992). *Test of Pictures-Forms-Letters-Numbers-Spatial Orientation & Sequencing Skills.* Burlington, CA: Psychological and Educational Publications.

Gardner, M.F. (1997). *Test of Visual-Perceptual Skills (Non-Motor), revised (TVPS).* Burlington, CA: Psychological and Educational Publications.

Gardner, R.A. (1978). *Reversals frequency test.* Cresskill, NJ: Creative Therapeutics.

Garling, R., Book, A., & Lindberg, E. (1984). Cognitive mapping of large-scale environments: The interrelationship of action plans, acquisition and orientation. *Environment and Behavior, 16,* 3-34.

Gentile, M. (1997). *Functional visual behavior: A therapist's guide to evaluation and treatment options.* Bethesda, MD: American Occupational Therapy Association.

Gibson, E.J. (1971). Perceptual learning and the theory of word perception. *Cognitive Psychology, 2,* 351.

Gibson, E.J., & Levin, H. (1975). *The psychology of reading.* Cambridge, MA: MIT Press.

Gilfoyle, E., Grady, A., & Moore, J. (1990). *Children adapt* (2nd ed.). Thorofare, NJ: Slack.

Glass, P. (1993). Development of visual function in preterm infants: Implications for early intervention. *Infants and Young Children, 6* (1), 11-20.

Goodale, M. (2000). Perception and action in the human visual system. In M.S. Gazzaniga (Ed.), *The new cognitive neurosciences* (2nd ed., pp. 365-377). Cambridge, MA: MIT Press.

Goodale, M., & Milner, L.S. (1992). Separate visual pathways for perception and action. *Trends in Neuroscience, 15,* 20-25.

Greene, L.J. (1987). *Learning disabled and your child: a survival handbook.* New York: Ballantine Books.

Hammill, D.D., Pearson, N.A., & Voress, J.K. (1993). *Developmental Test of Visual Perception* (2nd ed.). Austin, TX: Pro-Ed.

Hellerstein, L., & Fishman, B. (1987). Vision therapy and occupational therapy: An integrated approach. *AOTA Sensory Integration Special Interest Section Newsletter, 10* (3), 4-5.

Hendry, S.H.C., & Calkins, D.J. (1998). Neuronal chemistry and functional organization in the primate visual system. *Trends in Neurosciences, 21,* 244-349.

Hung, S.S., Fisher, A.G., & Cermak, S.A. (1987). The performance of learning-disabled and normal young men on the test of visual-perceptual skills. *American Journal of Occupational Therapy, 41,* 790-797.

Hyvarinen, L. (1988). *Vision in children: Normal and abnormal.* Medford, Ontario: Canadian Deaf, Blind and Rubella Association.

Hyvarinen, L. (1994). Assessment of visually impaired infants. *Ophthalmology Clinics of North America, 7,* 219-225.

Hyvarinen, L. (1995a). Considerations in evaluation and treatment of the child with low vision. *American Journal of Occupational Therapy, 49,* 891-897.

Hyvarinen, L. (1995b). *Vision testing manual.* La Salle, IL: Precision Vision.

Ilg, F.L., & Ames, L.B. (1981). *School readiness.* New York: Harper & Row.

Jansky, J., & de Hirsch, K. (1972). *Preventing reading failure: Prediction, diagnosis, and intervention.* New York: Harper & Row.

Jordon, B.A. (1980). *Jordon Left-Right Reversal Test* (2nd ed.). Los Angeles: Western Psychological Services.

Juel, C. (1988). Learning to read and write: A longitudinal study of 54 children from first through fourth grades. *Journal of Educational Psychology, 80,* 437-447.

Justice, L.M., & Ezell, H.K. (2001). Descriptive analysis of written language awareness in children from low income households. *Communication Disorders Quarterly, 22,* 123-134.

Justice, L.M., & Ezell, H.K. (2002). Use of storybook reading to increase print awareness in at-risk children. *American Journal of Speech-Language Pathology, 11,* 17-29.

Justice, L.M., & Lankford, C. (2002). Preschool children's visual attention to print during storybook reading: Pilot findings. *Communication Disorders Quarterly, 24* (1), 11-21.

Kalb, L., & Warshowsky, J.H. (1991). Occupational therapy and optometry: Principles of diagnosis and collaborative treatment of learning disabilities in children. *Occupational Therapy Practice, 3* (1), 77-87.

Kandel, E.R., Schwartz, J.H., & Jessell, T.M. (1991). *Principles of neural science,* New York: Elsevier Science.

Kaufman, A.S., & Kaufman, N.L. (1983). *Kaufman Assessment Battery for Children.* Circle Pines, MN: American Guidance Service.

Kavale, K. (1982). Meta-analysis of the relationship between visual perceptual skills and reading achievement. *Journal of Learning Disabilities, 15,* 42-51.

Kirby, J., & Das, J.P. (1978). Information processing and human abilities. *Journal of Educational Psychology, 70,* 58-66.

Koppitz, E.M. (1963). *The Bender Visual-Motor Gestalt Test for Young Children.* New York: Grune & Stratton.

Kwatney, E., & Bouska, M.J. (1980). *Visual system disorders and functional correlates: Final report.* Philadelphia: Temple University Rehabilitation and Training Center No. 8.

Langley, M.B. (1980). *Functional vision inventory for the severely/profoundly handicapped.* Chicago: Stoelting.

Laurendau, M., & Pinard, A. (1970). *Development of the concept of space in the child.* New York: International University Press.

Leigh, R.J., & Zee, D.S. (1983). *Neurology of eye movements.* Philadelphia: F.A. Davis.

Levine, M. (1985). *The ANSER system.* Cambridge, MA: Educators Publishing Service.

Levine, M. (1987). *Developmental variation and learning disorders.* Cambridge, MA: Educators Publishing Service.

Levine, M., & Rapport, L. (1983). *The ANSER system.* Cambridge, MA: Educators Publishing Service.

Lukatela, G., Eaton, T., Lee, C., & Turvey, M.T. (2001). Does visual word identification involve a sub-phonemic level? *Cognition, 78,* B41-B52.

Luria, A. (1966). *Higher cortical functions in man.* New York: Basic Books.

Lyle, J.G. (1969). Reading retardation and reversal tendency: A factorial study. *Child Development, 40,* 833-843.

Marr, D. (1982). *Vision.* San Francisco: Freeman.

McCarty, M.E., Clifton, R.K., Ashmead, P.L., Lee, P., & Goubet, N. (2001). How infants use vision for grasping objects. *Child Development, 72,* 973-987.

Menken, C., Cermak, S.A., & Fisher, A.G. (1987). Evaluating the visual-perceptual skills of children with cerebral palsy. *American Journal of Occupational Therapy, 41* (10), 646-651.

Milner, A.D., & Goodale, M.A. (1993). Visual pathways to perception and action. In T.P. Hicks, S. Molotchnikoff, & T. Ono (Eds.), *The visually responsive neuron: From basic neurophysiology to behavior* (pp. 317-337). New York: Elsevier Science.

Mishkin, M., Ungerleider, L., & Macko, K. (1983). Object vision and spatial vision: Two cortical pathways. *Trends in Neuroscience, 6,* 414-417.

Moore, R.S. (1979). *School can wait.* Provo, UT: Brigham Young University Press.

Morency, A., & Wepman, J. (1973). Early perceptual ability and later school achievement. *Elementary School Journal, 73,* 323.

Mussen, P.H., Conger, J.J., & Kagan, J. (1979). *Child development and personality* (5th ed.). New York: Harper & Row.

Necombe, F., & Ratcliff, G. (1989). Disorders of spatial analysis. In E. Boller & J. Grafman (Eds.), *Handbook of neuropsychology* (Vol. 2). New York: Elsevier Science.

Nolte, J. (1988). *The human brain* (2nd ed.). St. Louis: Mosby.

O'Brien, V., Cermak, S.A., & Murray, E. (1988). The relationship between visual-perceptual motor abilites and clumsiness in children with and without learning disabilities. *American Journal of Occupational Therapy, 42,* 359-363.

O'Conner, P., Sofo, F., Kendall, L., & Olsen, G. (1990). Reading disabilities and the effects of colored filters. *Journal of Learning Disabilities, 23* (10), 597-620.

Olsen, J.Z. (2003). *Handwriting without tears: Teacher's Guide. Cabin John,* MD: Olsen.

Optometric Extension Program Foundation. (1985). Santa Ana, CA: The Foundation.

Osterling, J., & Dawson, G. (1994). Early recognition of children with autism: A study of first birthday videotapes. *Journal of Autism and Developmental Disorders, 24,* 247-257.

Parham, L.D. (1998). The relationship of sensory integrative development to achievement in elementary students: Four-year longitudinal patterns. *Occupational Therapy Journal of Research, 18,* 105-127.

Parush, S., Yochman, A., Cohen, D., & Gershon, E. (1998). Relation of visual perception and visual-motor integration for clumsy children. *Perceptual and Motor Skills, 86,* 291-295.

Perov, A., & Kozminsky, E. (1989). The effect of computer games practice on the development of visual perception skills in kindergarten children. *Computers in the Schools, 6* (3/4), 113-122.

Piaget, J. (1964). *Development and learning.* Ithaca, NY: Cornell University Press.

Rafal, R.D., & Posner, M.I. (1987). Cognitive theories of attention and the rehabilitation of attentional deficits. In M.J. Meier, A.L. Benton, & L. Diller (Eds.), *Neuropsychological rehabilitation.* New York: Guilford.

Ratcliff, G. (1987). Perception and complex visual processes. In M.J. Meier, A.L. Benton, & L. Diller (Eds.), *Neuropsychological rehabilitation* (pp. 182-201). New York: Guilford.

Raymond, J.E., & Sorensen, R.E. (1998). Visual motion perception in children with dyslexia: Normal detection but abnormal integration. *Visual Cognition, 5,* 389-404.

Reid, D.T., & Jutai, J. (1994). *The Componential Assessment of Visual Perception manual.* Toronto, ON: University of Toronto, Department of Occupational Therapy.

Reid, D.T., & Jutai, J. (1997). A pilot study of perceived clinical usefulness of a new computer-based tool for assessment of visual perception in occupational therapy practice. *Occupational Therapy International, 4,* 81-98.

Restak, R. (1979). *The brain: The last frontier.* New York: Doubleday.

Richards, R.G., & Oppenheim, G.S. (1984). *Visual skills appraisal.* Novato, CA: Academic Therapy Publications.

Richter, E., & Montgomery, P. (1991). *The sensorimotor performance analysis.* Hugo, MN: PDP Products.

Ritty, J.M., Solan, H., & Cool, S.J. (1993). Visual and sensory-motor functioning in the classroom: A preliminary report of ergonomic demands. *Journal of the American Optometric Association, 64* (4), 238-244.

Roder, B.J., Bushnell, E.W., & Sasseville, A.M. (2001). Infant preferences for familiarity and novelty during the course of visual processing. *Infancy, 1* (4), 491-507.

Rogow, S.M. (1987). The ways of the hand: hand function in blind, visually impaired, and visually impaired multiple handicapped children. *British Journal of Visual Impairment, 5* (2), 58-63.

Rogow, S.M. (1992). Visual perceptual problems of visually impaired children with developmental disabilities. *Re:View, 24* (2), 57-64.

Rogow, S.M., & Rathwill, D. (1989). Seeing and knowing: An investigation of visual perception among children with severe visual impairments. *Journal of Vision Rehabilitation, 3* (3), 55-66.

Rose, S.A. (1980). Enhancing visual recognition memory in preterm infants. *Developmental Psychology, 16,* 85.

Rosenhall, J., Johansson, E., & Gilberg, C. (1988). Oculomotor findings in autistic children. *Journal of Laryngeal Otology, 102,* 435-439.

Sands, S., & Buchholz, E.S. (1997). The underutilization of computers to assist in the remediation of dyslexia. *International Journal of Instructional Media, 24* (2), 153-175.

Scheiman, M. (1984). Optometric findings in children with cerebral palsy. *American Journal of Optometric Physiology, 61,* 321-323.

Scheiman, M. (1991). *Pediatric clinical vision screening for occupational therapists.* Philadelphia: Pennsylvania College of Optometry.

Scheiman, M. (1997). *Understanding and managing vision deficits: A guide for occupational therapists.* Thorofare, NJ: Slack.

Schneck, C.M. (1998). Intervention for visual perceptual problems. In J. Case-Smith (Ed.), *Occupational therapy: Making a difference in the school system.* Bethesda, MD: American Occupational Therapy Association.

Seiderman, A.S. (1984). Visual perception versus visual function. *Journal of Learning Disabilities, 17,* 182-185.

Seiderman, A.S., & Marcus, S.E. (1990). *20/20 is not enough: The new world of vision.* New York: Alfred B. Knopf.

Shaywitz, B.A. (1997). The Yale Center for the study of learning and attention: Longitudinal and neuro-biological studies. *Learning Disabilities: A Multidisciplinary Journal, 8,* 21-30.

Siegel, L. (1983). The prediction of possible learning disabilities in preterm and full-term children. In T. Field & A. Sostek (Eds.), *Infants born at risk: Physiological, perceptual, and cognitive processes.* New York: Grune & Stratton.

Sigman, M., & Parmelee, A. (1974). Visual preferences of four-month-old premature and full-term infants. *Child Development, 45,* 969-965.

Skeffington, A.N. (1963). *The Skeffington Papers* (Series 36, No. 2, p. 11). Santa Ana, CA: Optometric Extension Program.

Smith Roley, S., & Schneck, C. (2001). Sensory integration and the child with visual impairment and blindness. In S. Smith Roley, E. Blanche, & R. Schaff (Eds.), *Sensory integration and developmental disabilities.* Tucson: Therapy Skill Builders.

Snow, C., Burns, M.S., & Griffin, P. (Eds.) (1998). *Preventing reading difficulties in young children.* Washington, DC: National Academy Press.

Solan, H.A., & Ciner, E.B. (1986). *Visual perception and learning: Issues and answers.* New York: SUNY College of Optometry.

Spelke, E.S., & Cortelyou, A. (1981). Perceptual aspects of social knowing: Looking and listening in infancy. In M.E. Lamb & L.R. Sherrod (Eds.), *Infant social cognition: Empirical and theoretical considerations* (pp. 61-83). Hillsdale, NJ: Erlbaum.

Stiers, P., De Cock, P., & Vandenbussche, E. (1999). Separating visual perception and non-verbal intelligence in children with early brain injury. *Brain and Development, 21,* 397-406.

Stiles, S., & Knox, R. (1996). Medical issues, treatments, and professionals. In M.C. Holbrook (Ed.), *Children with visual impairments: A parent's guide* (pp. 21-48). Bethesda, MD: Woodbine House.

Suchoff, I.B. (1987). *Visual-spatial development in the child* (2nd ed.). New York: State University of New York, State College of Optometry.

Teplin, S.W. (1995). Visual impairment in infants and young children. *Infants and Young Children, 8,* 18-51.

Thelan, D., & Smith, L.B. (1994). *A dynamic systems approach to the development of cognitions and action.* Cambridge, MA: MIT Press.

Todd, V.R. (1999). Visual perceptual frame of reference: An information processing approach. In P. Kramer & J. Hinojosa (Eds.), *Frames of reference for pediatric occupational therapy* (2nd ed.). Baltimore: Williams & Wilkins.

Toglia, J.P. (2003). Cognitive-perceptual retraining and rehabilitation. In E.B. Crepeau, E.S. Cohen, & B.A.B. Schell (Eds.), *Willard and Spackman's Occupational Therapy* (10th ed., pp. 607-629). Philadelphia: Lippincott Williams & Wilkins.

Tseng, M.H., & Cermak, S.A. (1993). The influence of ergonomic factors and perceptual-motor abilities on handwriting performance. *American Journal of Occupational Therapy, 47* (10), 919-926.

Tseng, M.H., & Murray, E.A. (1994). Differences in perceptual-motor measures in children with good and poor handwriting. *Occupational Therapy Journal of Research, 14* (1), 19-36.

Tsurumi, K., & Todd, V. (1998). Tests of visual perception: What do they tell us? *School System Special Interest Section Quarterly, 5* (4), 1-4.

Turkewitz, G., & Kenny, P.A. (1985). The role of developmental limitations of sensory input on sensory/perceptual organization. *Developmental and Behavioral Pediatrics, 6,* 302.

Ulman, S. (1986). Visual routines. In S. Pinker (Ed.), *Visual cognition.* Cambridge: MIT Press.

Van der Geest, J.N., Kemner, C., Camfferman, G., Verbaten, M.N., & van Engeland, H. (2002). Looking at images with human figures: Comparison between autistic and normal children. *Journal of Autism and Developmental Disorders, 32,* (2), 69-75.

Voyer, D., Voyer, S., & Bryden, M.P. (1995). Magnitude of sex differences in spatial abilities: A meta-analysis and consideration of critical variables. *Psychological Bulletin, 117,* 250-270.

Warren, M. (1990). Identification of visual scanning deficits in adults after CVA. *American Journal of Occupational Therapy, 44,* 391-399.

Warren, M. (1993a). A hierarchical model for evaluation and treatment of visual perceptual dysfunction in adult acquired brain injury. I. *American Journal of Occupational Therapy, 47* (1), 42-54.

Warren, M. (1993b). A hierarchical model for evaluation and treatment of visual perceptual dysfunction in adult acquired brain injury. II. *American Journal of Occupational Therapy, 47* (1), 55-66.

Webster, J.S., & Scott, R.R. (1983). The effects of self-instructional training on attentional deficits following head injury. *Clinical Neuropsychology, 5,* 9-74.

Wechsler, D. (1991). *Wechsler Intelligence Scale for Children–III.* New York: Psychological Corporation.

Weil, M.J., & Cunningham-Amundson, S.J. (1994). Relationship between visuomotor and handwriting skills of children in kindergarten. *American Journal of Occupational Therapy, 48,* 982-988.

Williams, H. (1983). *Perceptual and motor development.* Englewood Cliffs, NJ: Prentice-Hall.

Williamson, T. (1994). *OK Vision Test.* Farmersville, OH: Vision Lyceum.

Willows, D.M., & Terepocki, M. (1993). The relation of reversal errors to reading disabilities. In D.M. Willows, R.S. Kruk, & E. Corcois (Eds.), *Visual processes in reading and reading disabilities* (pp. 265-286). Hillsdale, NJ: Erlbaum.

Yost, L.W., & Lesiak, J. (1980). The relationship between performance on the developmental test of visual perception and handwriting ability. *Education, 101,* 75-77.

Zaba, J. (1984). Visual perception versus visual function. *Journal of Learning Disabilities, 17,* 182-185.

Ziviani, J. (1995). The development of graphmotor skills. In A. Henderson & C. Pehoski (Eds.), *Hand function in the child: Foundations for remediation* (pp. 184-193). St. Louis: Mosby.

Ziviani, J., & Elkins, J. (1984). An evaluation of handwriting performance. *Educational Review, 36,* 251-261.

Ziviani, J., Hayes, A., & Chant, D. (1990). Handwriting: A perceptual motor disturbance in children with myelomeningocele. *Occupational Therapy Journal of Research, 10,* 12-26.

WEB SITES

Visual Perception

The Joy of Visual Perception: A Web Book: http://www.yorku.ca/eye/thejoy.htm

Assessments

The 14th Mental Measurement Yearbook: Buro's Institute Test Reviews Online: http://www.unl.edu/buros

Visual Perception tests: http://www.lea-test.sgic.fi/en/vistests/pediatric/percepti/percepts.html

Reading Styles

Carbo Reading Styles Institutes: http://www.nrsi.com/previoustips/tip101397.html

Computer Programs

Virtual School (freeware and shareware programs): http://www.en.eun.org/eun.org2/eun/en/vs-primary/content.cfm?lang = encov = 7951

Optometry

Optometrists Network: http://www.children-special-needs.org/questions.html

Optometric Extension Program: http://healthy.net/oep/vision.htm

Publications for Classroom Activities

- *Sensory Motor Handbook* (J. Bissell, J. Fisher, C., Owens, & P. Polcyn; Sensory Integration International, 1988, Torrance, CA). A wonderful guide for implementing and modifying activities in the classroom. Both visual-perceptual and spatial concerns are addressed. Exercises are indexed according to the skill they are designed to remediate.
- *Little Kim's Left and Right Book* (C.W. McMonnies; Superior Educational Publications, 1992, Sydney, Australia).* A very appealing picture book for preschoolers.
- *A Practical Guide for Remedial Approaches to Left/Right Confusion and Reversals* (C.W. McMonnies; Superior Educational Publications, 1991, Sydney, Australia).
- *Overcoming Left/Right Confusion and Reversals: A Classroom Approach* (C.W. McMonnies; Superior Educational Publications, 1992, Sydney, Australia). Group and individual remediation exercises for older children. The 18 remedial procedures follow a developmental sequence, starting with body awareness of oneself, which is used as a basis for acquiring the ability to project that internal awareness into space (directionality). The aim is to provide variety to activities that will establish an internal/automatic/reflex/somatesthetic awareness of right and left that does not depend on external cues such as identifying the writing hand, watch-wearing hand, or ring-wearing hand. Specific activities are used to help children overcome difficulty with left-to-right reading.
- *Reversal Errors: Theories and Therapy Procedures* (K.A. Lane; Vision Extension, 1988, Santa Ana, CA) and *Developing Your Child for Success* (K.A. Lane; Vision Extension, 1991, Santa Ana, CA). For use by school-based practitioners, teachers, and parents.
- *Classroom Visual Activities* (CVA) (R.G. Richards; Academic Therapy Publications, 1988, Novato, CA). More than two dozen exercises are provided to remediate underlying laterality, directionality, and midline problems, as well as activities focused on the underlying visual skills necessary to achieve efficient visual perception. The exercises are categorized by the areas addressed, which include muscle movement, oculomotor skills, accommodation, and visualization.
- *Songs for Sensory Integration: The Calming Tape and the Vision Tape* (L. Hickman; Belle Curve Records, 1992, Boulder, CO). Auditory tapes. Optometrist Lynn Hellerstein is the narrator of the vision tape. Included is a clear, simple explanation of vision and exercises that can be used to supplement optometric vision therapy.
- *Classroom Activities for Correcting Specific Reading Problems* (S.A. Pavlak; Parker Publishing, 1985, West Nyack, NY). For children who are having trouble remembering letters and their sounds. Presents 41 letter- and letter-sound recognition activities and 52 consonant- and vowel-recognition activities.

Computer Programs

- Many computer programs that work on visual-perceptual skills are available commercially. Only a few are listed. Others can be found through http://search.epnet.com/direct.asp?an=0705304988&db=aph
- *Xerox Imaging Systems* (800-248-6550): Makers of the Kurzweil Reading Machine that is used in the BookWise PC computer-based tutoring system. BookWise converts the text into synthesized speech, integrating the child's auditory processing and visual tracking skills by simultaneously highlighting the work.
- *Lexia Learning Systems* (800-435-3942): Offers interactive reading programs designed to facilitate the acquisition of decoding skills.
- *The Learning Company* (800-852-2255): Publishes the Reader Rabbit Series, which helps students to strengthen visual-perception, eye-hand coordination, spatial awareness, and visual-memory.
- *Don Johnson, Inc.* (800-999-4660): Provides a wide array of both adaptive computer hardware and computer software programs to strengthen areas of computer access, communication, productivity, and literacy for people with special needs.

---

*All McMonnies' materials are distributed in the United States through the Optometric Extension Program (OEP), Santa Ana, CA.

- *Hartley Courseware* (800-247-1380): Offers visual tracking software and more than 200 computer programs.
- *DLM* (800-843-8855): Provides programs that break down decoding for early readers.

- *Great Wave Software* (800-423-1144): Provides software for early readers.
- *International Society for Technology in Education* (800-336-5191): Offers a wide array of resources and support materials for education.

Psychosocial Issues Affecting Social Participation

Debora A. Davidson

CHAPTER OBJECTIVES

1 Understand the dynamic interaction of emotional, cognitive, neurobehavioral, and environmental factors as they influence aspects of occupational performance through the course of typical development during infancy, childhood, and adolescence.

2 Explain means of promoting the psychosocial wellness of infants, children, and adolescents in natural contexts.

3 Identify the diagnostic hallmarks and contributing factors of common mental health conditions and relate these to the occupational performance of children and adolescents.

4 Understand the continuum of services available to children and adolescents with psychosocial disorders.

5 Explain the variety of service delivery models and frames of reference used by occupational therapists in psychosocial settings.

6 Define the roles of occupational therapists who provide services to children and adolescents with psychosocial disorders, as well as the roles of other team members.

7 Understand evaluation and intervention processes related to the special needs of children and adolescents whose occupational performance has been affected by psychosocial problems.

Promotion of a child's social participation in the contexts of family, friendships, classmates, caregivers, and teachers is an essential domain of occupational therapy in all practice settings (Davidson & LaVessar, 1998; Florey, 1989; Peloquin, 1993; Williamson, 1993). Achievement of developmental milestones and occupational goals is the result of continuously evolving interactions between aspects of the child and the environmental contexts that envelop him or her. Social relationships are a critical part of that environment; the mutual influences of the individual and his or her social contexts combine to largely determine the child's quality of life and participation in those social contexts.

The purposes of this chapter are to (1) describe dynamic aspects of healthy psychosocial development in the child and the family, (2) outline common causes of psychosocial problems in children and adolescents and their implications for occupational performance, (3) describe the roles of occupational therapy practitioners and other team members in a variety of intervention settings, and (4) introduce selected evaluation and intervention methods, including intervention goals for common psychosocial needs.

The unifying frame of reference for this chapter is the person-environment-occupation (PEO) model (Law et al., 1996). This frame of reference emphasizes the dynamic interaction between elements of the individual and elements of the various aspects of the environments, as well as the ways these interactions influence occupational performance. *Person factors* include qualities of the individual such as gender, age, developmental levels, skills, preferences, and values. *Environment factors* encompass the social and physical contexts within which the child functions. Person and environment factors are viewed as reciprocally influential and as directly relevant to the child's occupational performance. Appreciating and understanding these elements and their potential for dynamic interaction enable the occupational therapist to approach intervention flexibly and effectively.

TEMPERAMENT AS IT INFLUENCES AND IS INFLUENCED BY THE ENVIRONMENT

Children vary in their development of interests, habits, talents, and social competence. Standardized pediatric tests reveal variations among children in the rate and sequence of their acquisition of motor, language, and cognitive skills. Curiosity about these differences among children has inspired more than 30 years of research. Chess and Thomas were among the first scholars to study children's styles of responding to various experiences and of carrying out activities such as sleeping, eating, and exploring objects (Thomas, Chess, & Birch, 1968). Their work developed the concept of temperament. Temperament refers to a collection of inborn, relatively stable traits that influence the ways in which individuals process and respond to the environment.

Chess and Thomas identified nine basic characteristics of temperament, which remain useful today (Chess, 1997). These are (1) activity level, (2) rhythmicity (i.e., the degree to which the child's patterns of sleeping, eating, and play are predictable), (3) approach to or withdrawal from novel situations, (4) intensity of emotional responses, (5) sensory threshold, (6) mood (general emotional state), (7) adaptability, (8) distractibility, and (9) attention span and persistence. Temperament characteristics are not considered to be inherently good or bad, and they are not under the control of the child or the parents. However, behaviors arising from temperament traits may be more or less adaptive or pleasing, depending on the context. Children whose temperament style approaches extremes on any of the nine parameters may have more difficulty negotiating the social and emotional demands of childhood (Cronin, 2001). Environmental demands and expectations must always be considered whenever an attempt is made to predict the effects of temperament on occupational performance. Recent research indicates that the assessment of each child's temperament is influenced by the observer's point of view and that the determination of function or dysfunction has much to do with the situational compatibility with the family and other social environments (Vaughn & Bost, 1999).

Chess and Thomas (1987) were interested in learning about the influence of personality characteristics on the parent-child relationship and the child's development. They took the statistical concept, *goodness of fit*, and applied it to interpersonal relationships. They found that when the expectations of individuals important to the child are compatible with the child's temperament, there is a good fit. When the child's temperament is at odds with parental expectations, mutual distress may result (see Box 13-1). Although Chess and Thomas focused on parent-child fit, other research has supported these findings in teacher-child and peer-child relationships (Keogh, 1986; Keogh & Burstein, 1988).

Chess and Thomas (1983) identified three common patterns of temperament from the nine temperament traits described above. They gave these combinations the labels *easy child, difficult child,* and *slow-to-warm-up child* (Figure 13-1). The easy child is positive in mood and approach to new stimuli. This child is calm, expressive, and malleable and has a generally low to moderate activity level. Children characterized as easy tend to adapt effectively to changing situations and demands. The difficult child is at the opposite end of the temperament spectrum. Characteristics that characterize this style are a negative mood and approach, slow adaptability, a high activity level, and high emotional intensity. Extremes of sensory threshold often occur among children with a difficult temperament pattern. A slow-to-warm-up child demonstrates mildly intense negative reactions to new stimuli and is slow to adapt to changing situations and demands. This child requires repeated exposure to new environments before he or she feels comfortable. Once a slow-to-warm-up child has established a routine, he or she usually functions well, but transitions are often problematic for children of this temperament type (Cronin, 2001).

BOX 13-1   Case Example: Goodness of Fit

Theresa is a highly active, inquisitive 8-year-old. She likes to move around and interact with others and dislikes sedentary activities. Although her mood is generally happy, Theresa's emotional responses are intense, and she expresses her feelings loudly. Theresa's temperament is a good fit with running with her friends on the playground, and her peers regard her as someone who is exciting and fun to be with. Theresa's temperament is not such a good fit when she attends church services with her family; her parents often scold and correct her for looking around, moving, and talking.

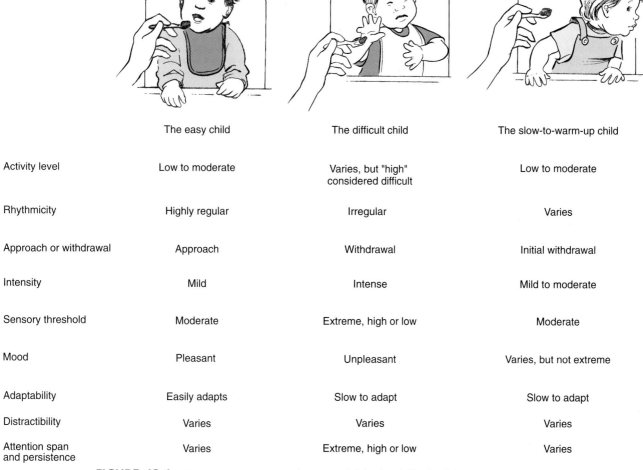

	The easy child	The difficult child	The slow-to-warm-up child
Activity level	Low to moderate	Varies, but "high" considered difficult	Low to moderate
Rhythmicity	Highly regular	Irregular	Varies
Approach or withdrawal	Approach	Withdrawal	Initial withdrawal
Intensity	Mild	Intense	Mild to moderate
Sensory threshold	Moderate	Extreme, high or low	Moderate
Mood	Pleasant	Unpleasant	Varies, but not extreme
Adaptability	Easily adapts	Slow to adapt	Slow to adapt
Distractibility	Varies	Varies	Varies
Attention span and persistence	Varies	Extreme, high or low	Varies

FIGURE 13-1 Temperament types: the easy child, the difficult child, and the slow-to-warm-up child.

Research has linked various temperament characteristics to parental **stress** in child rearing (Honjo et al., 1998), certain psychiatric disorders in adulthood (Kagan & Zentner, 1996; Nigg & Goldsmith, 1998), adolescent substance abuse (Weinberg, Rahdert, Colliver, & Glantz, 1998), and disruptive behavioral disorders (Harden & Zoccolillo, 1997). A growing body of research supports the notion that temperament, although inborn, is not unchanging across a child's life span. Experiences and environmental circumstances, such as the interpersonal styles of the primary caregivers, have been shown to have a potentially significant influence on the developing child's temperament style (Belsky, Fish, & Isabella, 1991). These findings suggest that therapeutic intervention can be helpful if goodness of fit is lacking between a child and his or her caregiver.

Occupational therapists often see children who are in distress and whose behavior is disruptive or upsetting to the family. Practitioners can help parents, caregivers, teachers, and children explore and understand their temperaments and learn to predict when behavior may not match environmental demands (e.g., a very active child at the theater, the effect of beginning a new school year on a slow to warm up child). This perspective may reduce frustration and increase the possibility of organizing environments and activity demands to promote goodness of fit and successful occupational engagement.

ATTACHMENT: A DYNAMIC INTERACTION OF BIOLOGY AND ENVIRONMENT

A child's neuromaturational progress greatly influences social participation. The healthy, full-term infant is biologically prepared to participate in interactions with a nurturing and consistent caregiver, resulting in a loving attachment that is essential for healthy development. As the infant nurses, cuddles, gazes with fascination at his or her mother's face, and responds to comforting, emotions are elicited that become the foundation of the baby's self-concept and a safe base from which to explore the world (Thompson, 2002). Simultaneously, the mother experiences hormonal and neurochemical effects from interacting with her infant that promote feelings of well-being, protectiveness, and love for her baby (Hofer, 1994). Healthy attachment occurs when a caregiver and an infant consistently interrelate in such a way that the infant develops confidence that his or her needs will be met, and that he or she is safe and cared for (Belsky & Cassidy, 1994; Main, 1996). Many experts contend that the quality of early attachment influences the capacity to form relationships later in life (Feeny, 1996; Hazan & Zeifman, 1999; Waters & Stroufe, 1983). Some researchers are studying the influence of early attachment experience on neurodevelopment itself, at the biochemical and cellular levels (Ebert, Seale, & McMahon, 2001; Kraemer, 1992; Main, 1995). Thompson asserts that the quality of early relationships "is far more significant on early learning than are educational toys, preschool curricula, or Mozart CDs." (p. 11)

Traits and behaviors of the parent and child interact dynamically in environmental contexts to determine the quality of attachment that develops; each party is simultaneously influencing and influenced by the other and by other features of the environment. Researchers have identified four patterns of attachment behavior between parents and infants: secure, avoidant, resistant or ambivalent, and disorganized/disoriented (Table 13-1) (Ainsworth, Blehar, Waters, & Wall, 1978; Main & Soloman, 1990).

Parent-child attachment relationships continuously change in relation to the child's and parent's stages of development and changing environmental circumstances (Rothbart, 1991). As the infant becomes mobile, then develops language and self-care skills, the caregiving style of the parent adjusts accordingly, and the attachment relationship is altered. Attachment patterns may also be influenced by environmental factors, such as the loss or addition of family members. Adjustments in attachment continue throughout the child's developmental course, and in the best circumstances the positive reciprocity initiated early in infancy is maintained throughout.

Understanding that patterns of attachment between children and their parents are mutable implies that attachment is a process that can be influenced. This notion is supported by research with high-risk infants and mothers who received intervention to promote healthy attachment through three home visits focused on teaching mothers how to observe and respond effectively to their infants' behaviors (van den Boom, 1990). The group of 50 receiving the training developed significantly more secure attachments than did those in the control group. These effects from interventions to promote attachment have been found in other studies as well (van Ijzendoorn, Juffer, & Duyvesteyn, 1995).

Many infants, children, and adolescents served by occupational therapists have neurodevelopmental problems. The social experience of children who have intrinsic difficulty with receptive and/or expressive communication, sensory processing, or motor performance is different from that of typically developing children (Richardson, 2002). Difficulty with feeding, an inability to establish regular patterns of activity and sleep throughout the day and night, resistance to cuddling, and other behaviors common to infants with neurologic dysfunction are incompatible with easy attachment and may put the process at risk. Environmental factors, such as a parent's long hours of work, can limit the time available for child-focused interaction, potentially interfering with the attachment process. Likewise, a parent whose

TABLE 13-1 Patterns of Attachment in Infants and Parents

Attachment Style	Characteristic Caregiver Behavior	Characteristic Infant Behavior
Secure	Emotionally available, responds to infant's emotional and physical needs in a timely, consistent, and effective manner	Seeks proximity to parent, but as mobility develops, explores the immediate environment; demonstrates mastery motivation and self-confidence; misses parent upon separation, but is easily comforted upon parent's return
Avoidant	Emotionally unavailable, typically not adequately responsive to infant's communications of need	Avoids parent; emotionally blunted; interacts with objects in the environment rather than with the parent
Resistant or ambivalent	Inconsistently available and responsive to infant's communications of need; caregiving style is determined by parent's moods and is an unpredictable combination of adequate and inadequate responses	Clingy and preoccupied with the parent; does not actively explore the environment; difficult to comfort after separation; mood may be angry or passive
Disorganized/disoriented	Highly anxious or threatening toward the child; does not respond effectively or appropriately to infant's communications; may be abusive or psychotic	Disorganized or disoriented when interacting with the parent; displays approach-avoidance behaviors, including staring and "freezing," clinging, or huddling on the floor

behavior is anxious, irritable, or emotionally disengaged or who has difficulty interpreting and responding to the child's communications cannot fully participate in reciprocal interaction. When such behaviors are frequent, attachment is at risk. Occupational therapists can support healthy interaction between caregivers and children by understanding this essential process, educating parents about their child's development and communication style, and helping them to generate solutions for problems that inhibit the formation of a strong attachment.

CHILD ABUSE AND NEGLECT: PROBLEMS WITH THE PARENT-CHILD RELATIONSHIP AND ENVIRONMENT

At its most extreme, inadequate attachment formation between a parent and child can be a factor in the physical abuse or neglect of the child. This is a common problem for children and families, one that affected at least 903,000 American families in 2001 (U.S. Department of Health and Human Services, Administration on Children, Youth and Families, 2003). Experts assert that epidemiologic figures consistently underrepresent the number of true cases because of underreporting (Sedlak & Broadhurst, 1996; Starr, Dubowitz, & Bush, 1990). Child abuse has been defined as neglect, physical abuse, sexual abuse, or emotional maltreatment, all of which may occur alone or in combination.

Neglect is defined as the withholding of nutrition, shelter, clothing, and medical care such that the child's health is endangered. Undersupervision and abandonment are included in this category. This is the most common form of child abuse, accounting for about 60% of reported cases.

Physical abuse, which affects about 19% of child abuse victims, includes punching, shaking, kicking, biting, throwing, burning, and other forms of injurious punishment.

Sexual abuse, found in about 12% of cases, includes any seduction, coercion, or forcing of a child to observe or participate in sexual activity for the sexual gratification of a more powerful individual.

Emotional maltreatment is marked by withholding of affection, criticism, chronic humiliation, or threats of harm to the child or to people, animals, or items important to him or her. This type of child abuse is the most difficult to measure, and the estimated figure of 6% likely grossly underrepresents the true incidence (U.S. Department of Health and Human Services, Administration on Children, Youth and Families, 2003).

Developmental and psychological outcomes that have been associated with childhood abuse include traumatic brain injury, depression, substance abuse, learning disorders, conduct disorders, and personality disorders

(Bagley & Mallick, 2000; Egeland, Sroufe, & Erickson, 1983; Hoffman-Plotkin & Twentyman, 1984; Jasinski, Williams, & Siegel, 2000). These problems often carry lifelong consequences, including the increased risk of such individuals eventually behaving abusively toward their own children (Wolfner & Gelles, 1993). Most tragically, approximately 1,300 children died of the effects of abuse or neglect in 2001 (U.S. Department of Health and Human Services, Administration on Children, Youth and Families, 2003). Clearly, such pathologic behavior is incompatible with healthy family functioning.

Attachment patterns between parents and children are the result of a dynamic interaction of factors related to the child, the parent, and the environment. Risk factors for child abuse and neglect have been identified in these three spheres (Box 13-2). No single factor is consistently associated with child abuse. The more risk factors present

---

BOX 13-2 Risk Factors for Child Abuse

PHYSICAL AND EMOTIONAL ABUSE
Parent Factors
- Youth/immaturity
- Substance abuse
- Low empathy
- Difficulty interpreting child's communications
- Impulsiveness
- Limited coping skills
- Lack of knowledge about child development
- Unrealistic expectations
- Emotionally needy
- History of abuse
- Disappointment in child's gender or appearance

Child Factors
- Prolonged dependency for developmental or medical reasons
- "Difficult" temperament
- High activity level
- Limited skill at interpreting parent's nonverbal communications
- Appearance displeasing to parent

Environmental Factors
- Social isolation, lack of support
- Culture that condones or encourages aggression or abuse
- Poverty

CHILD NEGLECT
Parent Factors
- Depression or other mental disorders
- Cognitive limitations
- Substance abuse
- History of extreme deprivation

Child Factors
- Prolonged dependency for developmental or medical reasons

Environmental Factors
- Social isolation, lack of support
- Poverty
- Family disorganization

and the more severe each one is, the higher the risk of abuse and neglect in a family.

A child's disability increases the risk of maltreatment. The incidence of abuse and neglect may be as high as 3.4 times greater for children with disabilities than for those without (Sullivan & Knutson, 2000). Disabilities that have been associated with an increased risk of maltreatment include behavior disorders, communication disorders, cognitive disabilities, physical impairments, and craniofacial anomalies (Jaudes & Diamond, 1985; Sullivan & Knutson, 2000; Verdugo, Bermejo, & Fuertes, 1995; Wald & Knutson, 2000). Any condition that prolongs a child's dependency or stimulates parental rejection adds to the risk of abuse or neglect. For example, having a difficult temperament or being born prematurely increases the risk (Frodi, 1981). Most of the young clients seen by occupational therapy practitioners have delayed development in one or more areas and, as a group, are at increased risk of abuse and neglect.

Environmental factors interact dynamically with child factors, affecting the level of risk of abuse and neglect. Certain qualities of the parents (particularly the mother, who usually is the primary caretaker) have been identified as risk factors. These include having a personal history of receiving inadequate parenting; a personality characterized by immaturity, egocentrism, and impulsivity; and alcohol or drug abuse (Main & Goldwyn, 1984; Ogata et al., 1990; Steele, 1997; Wolfner & Gelles, 1993).

Characteristics of the larger community may further contribute to environmental risk factors. Poverty has been shown to correlate positively with increased rates of child abuse and neglect (Coulton, Korbin, Su, & Chow, 1995; Sedlak & Broadhurst, 1996). Social isolation is a powerful risk factor, one that puts single-parent families at significantly higher risk of abuse than two-parent families (Sedlak & Broadhurst). Communities with high crime rates present a high risk of child abuse due to a combination of a cultural acceptance of aggressive behavior, high levels of economic distress, and the social isolation that results when residents are fearful to step out onto the street.

Although poverty and a parent's troubled background may increase the likelihood of child abuse, high levels of social integration and community morale appear to be mediating factors that can reduce the incidence of child abuse (Gabarino & Kostelny, 1992). Successful intervention and prevention programs address family and community needs for safe and enjoyable places to gather and engage in meaningful occupation (Daly et al., 1998, Steele, 1999; Vondra, 1990). A meta-analysis of abuse prevention and family wellness programs indicated that the most effective programs supported parents using a strengths-based, empowerment approach. Successful programs continued over 6 months and provided at least two sessions per month (MacLeod & Nelson, 2000).

Occupational therapists have opportunities to intervene with individuals and families through direct service, program development, consultation, and administrative roles.

Children who are physically abused and/or neglected may bear outward signs of this, and therapists should always observe for bruises, cuts, or other injuries or for behaviors that may reflect pain. The appropriateness of the child's clothing for fit and for weather conditions should be noted over time. This is not an assessment of fashionability but of adequacy. Therapists should ask the child about his or her eating and sleeping habits and activities throughout the day when at home. They should also ask how the adults at home respond to children's misbehavior (e.g., "What kinds of things do you do that get you in trouble sometimes?" "What happens then?"). Some children will describe inadequate or unsafe situations, given gentle encouragement. Teachers and therapists should observe what has been brought to school for lunch, or how the child responds to food that is offered; a child with too little to eat at home may hoard food or eat more than is typical.

Socially, children from abusive homes may behave in a variety of ways that reflect individual temperaments and coping styles. Behaviors may range from being withdrawn and guarded to acting intrusive and demanding. Often children who have been abused are themselves aggressive, but this is not universal (Kolko, 2002). Many abused children are socially immature and emotionally needy. The description of resistant/ambivalent and disorganized/disoriented attachment styles also fits many of these children.

Occupational therapy practitioners are required by federal law to report suspected cases of abuse and neglect to state child protective service agencies (National Clearinghouse on Child Abuse and Neglect Information, 2000). Reports of suspected child abuse or neglect may be made by telephone and should be followed with a letter documenting the child's demographic information, the specific observations that led to the report, and the practitioner's contact information. Referrals to child protective services are held in confidence, and individuals who submit referrals in good faith are protected by law from prosecution. Discovery of a failure to report suspected cases of abuse or neglect may result in prosecution and/or disciplinary action by the practitioner's licensing board. Referrals to child protective services are reviewed and classified according to the situational risk. Families that are evaluated often receive a variety of intervention services, including respite care, parenting education, assistance with housing, day care, home visits, individual and family counseling, substance abuse treatment, and transportation. In 2001 approximately 19% of children who were found to be victims of abuse or neglect were removed from their homes and placed in temporary or long-term foster care (U.S. Department of

Health and Human Services, Administration on Children, Youth and Families, 2003).

ENVIRONMENTAL FACTORS AND SOCIAL PARTICIPATION

Social participation can be fully experienced only when children and families live in supportive environments that provide opportunities for self-expression and connection with others. When these conditions go unmet, even for a limited time, occupational performance suffers. When conditions are less than adequate for prolonged periods, the child's very course of development may be altered, with lifelong effects. Assessing the nature of a child's environment is a critical stage of clinical reasoning in the attempt to determine the psychosocial contributors to occupational dysfunction.

Environmental factors that relate to psychosocial performance may be roughly divided into those that are time limited and relatively brief and those that are more long-term (Table 13-2). Time-limited environmental stress factors are personal and family stressors that are keenly experienced and then resolved over a period of weeks or months. Long-term environmental stress factors are events and situations in which the stressors are pervasive and continue for months or years. Although they are useful for general conceptual purposes, these categorizations should be used with caution. Whether an event or circumstance falls into one category or the other partly depends on the coping style and circumstances of the individual affected. For example, the death of a grandparent may be an event about which a child feels acutely sad for several weeks and then to which he or she adjusts, especially if the relationship was limited by distance or other factors. For a very sensitive child or for

TABLE 13-2 Environmental Stress and Its Effects on Children

Time-Limited Environmental Stress Factors*	Long-term Environmental Stress Factors*
▪ Changing schools or childcare providers	▪ Violence in the home or neighborhood
▪ Illness of an immediate family member	▪ Chronic illness of a parent
▪ Death of a family member or friend	▪ Death of a parent
▪ Temporary financial crisis	▪ Chronic poverty
▪ Family relocation	▪ Long-term homelessness
▪ Temporary marital distress of parents	▪ Chronic parental conflict
▪ Divorce with closure	▪ Societal discrimination/ prejudice

*These categorizations are general examples. Whether a stress is experienced in a time-limited or chronic fashion ultimately depends on a number of individual and environmental factors.

one for whom the grandparent was a primary caregiver, such a loss could result in months of grief. If the child did not know the grandparent at all, the loss may be irrelevant.

Time-Limited Environmental Stress and Its Impact on Occupational Performance

Short-acting environmental conditions, such as the death of a member of the extended family or of a friend, a temporary marital crisis, a change of school or day care, or a family relocation, can have significant effects on the child's social participation. Children's reactions to such events often include decreased performance in play or academic activities. The child may act preoccupied, fatigued, or disinterested in his or her usual pastimes. Sometimes children temporarily "lose" their self-care skills and revert to more dependent, infantile ways. These reactions are normal and healthy ways for children to focus their internal resources on dealing with distress, and they may also stimulate the emotional support needed from caregivers to help the child cope with increased levels of stress. The occupational therapist can reassure parents and teachers of this and can encourage them to find ways to meet the child's need for extra nurturing while supporting a return to more age-appropriate behavior.

Case Example: Brooke

Brooke is a 3-year-old girl who has been receiving occupational therapy services for developmental dyspraxia. A month ago Brooke's mother gave birth to Ryan. Initially Brooke responded to this event with positive excitement and continuously begged to hold and help care for her brother. However, during the past week, she has been talking "baby talk" and resisting bedtime and has even wet her pants on two occasions, with no visible embarrassment or remorse. Brooke's parents are understandably concerned, and they are wondering what to do. They tried telling her to "talk like a big girl" and ignored her when she used infantile language. They have been irritable and exasperated at bedtime, because both parents are exhausted from getting up at night with the baby. Now that she has wet her pants, they are fearful that Brooke may have a "major psychological problem." The occupational therapist, who has been working with Brooke and her family for several months, responds, "You all have your hands full, with the changes and demands of a new baby in the family! I can see that everyone is working to capacity to cope, including Brooke. She is showing her stress the way 3-year-olds do. She has regressed in her development in some ways; the way she talks, needing lots of extra support at bedtime, and not using the potty all the time. The good news is that these behaviors are very normal for preschoolers who are stressed, and they are temporary. As the family finds its new routines, so should Brooke. The challenging news is that Brooke probably really does need extra attention right now, just when time and energy are so stretched. Can her aunt or grandfather arrange an outing with Brooke, to give her some extra attention? Also, if someone can take over Ryan's care for short periods, you will be able to give Brooke the special time with you that she so needs. There are some wonderful children's books that explore how it feels to become an older sister or brother; reading one of these with Brooke may give her some emotional support. Looking at videos or photos of Brooke's infant years and reminiscing with her about what a cute and cared-for baby she was (and what an adorable 3-year-old she is now) may also provide her some reassurance as to her position in the family. Taking a nap cuddled up together might be restorative for both of you. You will know what methods work for her when she asks to repeat them! I think that by meeting some of her extra needs now, you can hasten Brooke's return to her 3-year-old self. What are your thoughts?"

Chronic Environmental Stress and Its Impact on Occupational Performance

Long-term sources of social stress are circumstances and events that do not resolve over the course of weeks or months (see Table 13-2). Examples of these include poverty, social discrimination, and severe family dysfunction that may occur when one or both parents suffer from substance abuse or other mental disorders. These kinds of environmental conditions may have long-term effects on children's development and social participation through the life span, especially if combined with other complications such as the child's own neurodevelopmental problems.

More than 20% of the children in the United States live in poverty. Poverty affects 16.3% of all white children, 39.9% of all African American children, and 40.3% of all Hispanic children (Economic Report of the President, 1998). Long-term poverty has been associated with a number of serious problems for children and adolescents and for the adults who care for them (Chafel & Hadley, 2001). The home environments of families with few resources may offer limited access to items considered necessities by the majority of the culture, such as books, toys, a telephone, television, or computer. Language opportunities in low-income homes are often different and reduced compared with those found in middle-class homes (Locke, Ginsborg, & Peers, 2003). Due to a combination of health and environmental factors, children who live in chronic economic deprivation are at increased risk of having lower cognitive abilities and more behavioral problems (Bendersky & Lewis,

1994). Parents who experience the stress of chronically worrying about meeting basic needs for food, shelter, and safety are more prone to discipline their children harshly, have marital conflicts, experience depression, and have substance abuse problems (Belle, 1990; Jones-Webb, Snowden, Herd, Short, & Hannan, 1997; McLoyd, 1990). They may be too overwhelmed, discouraged, or disorganized to become involved in their children's schooling. These conditions place many low-income students at a disadvantage and diminish their future opportunities. Some children who have experienced lifetimes of severe family and community dysfunction reach adolescence feeling hopeless about their future. Their occupational performance is clearly affected by this as they struggle with society's expectations to further their education in order to prepare for a productive adulthood, whereas from the adolescent's perspective, this is impossible to achieve.

Case Study: Marcus

Marcus is a 15-year-old boy who is a ninth grade student in a large public high school. Marcus's family has struggled with poverty for six generations. He lives in a neighborhood where he has observed drug-related activities, fighting, and adults' sexual behavior on a regular basis. His favorite uncle was killed in a knife fight last year. Marcus's cousin, a rising star in basketball, was permanently disabled in a shooting. Last week one of his teachers quit her job after being mugged in her classroom. Marcus's mother has a tenth grade education and four children, whom she is raising independently. She has a day job as a hotel maid and a night job as a cashier in a convenience store. She is chronically exhausted and irritable. She encourages all of her children to work hard in school so that they can have a better life than hers. Marcus is also exhausted. He tries to go to school and to do what he can to help his mother, but he sees no real way out of their current situation. The bills are always greater than the family's resources. To Marcus it seems that no matter how hard people try, they never seem to get ahead, and often they do not even survive. The teachers at school seem critical and uncaring, and their questions and reprimands make Marcus anxious. Schoolwork is difficult, boring, and unrelated to his real concerns. When he was a child, Marcus wanted to be a professional football player or a doctor when he grew up. Now he is convinced that these are childish, impossible dreams, but he has no new plans with which to replace them. He is on the verge of quitting school and has no job skills. The likelihood that he eventually will achieve a satisfying career and contribute positively to the community is extremely small.

This case shows how poverty and other chronic stress factors can affect a child's occupational performance, both in terms of preparation for and the availability of opportunities to achieve social participation. Although these environmental factors are clearly influential in determining a child's occupational performance, the PEO model reflects a balance of emphasis among its three components (Law et al., 1996). The following section provides information about the role mental functioning plays in the enact-ment and development of children's occupational performance.

Relationship of Mental Health to Social Participation

A child's developmental progress and occupational performance are as dependent on the extent to which psychosocial needs are met as they are on the adequacy of nutrition and shelter. In 1999, Surgeon General David Satcher of the U.S. Public Health Service, supervised the publication of the results of a multiagency study sharing the expertise of hundreds of service providers, researchers, and consumers. In *Mental Health: A Report of the Surgeon General,* Dr. Satcher said, "From early childhood until death, mental health is the springboard of thinking and communication skills, learning, emotional growth, resilience, and self-esteem. These are the ingredients of each individual's successful contribution to community and society" (U.S. Public Health Service, 1999).

A fixed definition of mental health is difficult to formulate; behaviors and beliefs construed as healthy by one individual or in a particular context may be considered inappropriate or unhealthy by someone else or in another context. For example, American parents of Northern European descent often value independence and achievement. Such parents might be concerned about the behavior of their 5-year-old son, who wants his mother to help him with dressing and bathing even though he can do these things for himself. This behavior might cause the parents to wonder if their child is immature or spoiled. Parents from a cultural background that promotes a climate of interdependence, such as that found in Japan, might find such behavior to be expected and quite acceptable.

It is clear that practitioners must be competent in assuming a multicultural approach to evaluate social and emotional behavior effectively. Despite differences with regard to specific indicators of mental wellness, it is possible to consider the issue from a more occupational perspective. *Mental Health: A Report of the Surgeon General* states that "Mental health is a state of successful performance of mental function, resulting in productive activities, fulfilling relationships with other people, and the ability to adapt to change and to cope with adversity. Mental health is indispensable to personal well-being, family and interpersonal relationships, and contribution to community or society" (U.S. Public Health Service, 1999). This description of mental health

is one that occupational therapists can apply across cultures and developmental stages.

The ability of children and adolescents to participate socially and academically may be severely impaired by poor mental health. It is estimated that 15% to 22% of children have a mental disorder, and only 2% receive evaluation and intervention (National Advisory Mental Health Council, 1990; U.S. Public Health Service, 1999). As a result of contributing social pressures and problems, as well as increased awareness of the signs of such disorders, increasing numbers of children are being diagnosed with mental disorders (Constantino, 1993; Prothro-Stith, 1991; Wolfner & Gelles, 1993). Effective interventions for these types of conditions often require a combination of family education, special services at school, various therapies for the child and family, and medication.

Occupational therapists approach their work from a client-centered, occupational performance approach rather than from a medical or pathology-focused perspective (Burke, 2003; Law et al., 1996). However, client-centered approaches do not preclude an understanding of the nature and course of a client's illness or disability. To develop and implement client-centered, contextually appropriate interventions, the therapist must understand the child's symptoms, the effects and side effects of any medications the child is taking, and the prognosis. In addition, practitioners who recognize the diagnostic hallmarks of mental disorders that occur in childhood and adolescence can play an important role in referring children and adolescents in need of a diagnostic evaluation to specialists such as psychologists or psychiatrists. In many settings the occupational therapist may be the only team member who understands the symptoms and various interventions for mental disorders and their implications for occupational performance in school, child care, and at home. The following is an overview of hallmark symptoms of the more common mental disorders experienced by children and adolescents and their implications for occupational performance. The *Diagnostic and Statistical Manual of Mental Disorders,* Fourth Edition–Text Revised (DSM-IV-TR) (APA, 2000) is used to classify clinical problems into diagnostic categories.

MENTAL DISORDERS COMMONLY AFFECTING CHILDREN AND ADOLESCENTS

Mood Disorders

Mood disorders involve long-term changes in the child's prevailing emotions. The presence of symptoms may be cyclic in nature, increasing and decreasing periodically, but symptoms typically endure for months or years if left untreated (Kovacs, Feinberg, Crouse-

Novak, Paulauskas & Finkelstein, 1984a). The diagnostic criteria for *major depression* stipulate that symptoms must have reached a level of severity that results in changes in occupational performance (APA, 2000). Depression manifests as persistent or repeated episodes of a combination of irritability, a loss of interest in and enjoyment of usual activities, increased or decreased activity level, sadness, periods of crying, decreased energy, inability to concentrate and learn, agitation, sleep and/or appetite disturbance, anxiety, guilt, and/or thoughts of death or suicide. Depression is estimated to occur in 3% of children and 8% of teenagers (APA, 2000; Milling, 2001). Children and adolescents who have experienced clinical depression are likely to have repeated episodes into adulthood (Kovacs, Feinberg, & Crouse-Novak, 1984b; Harrington, Fudge, Rutter, Paulauskas, Finkelstein, Pickles, & Hill, 1990). The diagnostic evaluation of depression should be made by a psychologist or psychiatrist through structured interviews with the child and parents (Milling, 2001; Sabatino, Webster, & Vance, 2001). Determining a diagnosis in children may be complicated because the outward symptoms may appear inconsistently (i.e., the child may play and seem happy some of the time). Intervention often includes a combination of medications, psychotherapy, and counseling of the parents (Milling, 2001; Sabatino, Webster et al., 2001). Brief hospitalization may be required if the risk of suicide exists.

Occupational performance and satisfaction are adversely affected by the symptoms of depression. The loss of enjoyment and interest, as well as the difficulty with thinking, reduces a child's motivation to play and diminishes his or her ability to attend and learn in school. Children with depression may sleep during the day, even in classes. They often complain of being tired or bored during previously preferred activities. Activity levels may be decreased or increased, and the child may be chastised for being lazy or "out of control," depending on the situation. Unexpected tearfulness or displays of temper place the child in social jeopardy with adults and peers. Changes in appetite may affect social interactions during meals, because the child may be scolded for eating too little or too much. There may be resistance to attending family, church, and other social activities. Probably the most occupationally debilitating aspects of depression are the child's feelings of incompetence, hopelessness, and helplessness. These emotions, however irrational, are symptoms of depression that can prevent children and adolescents from participating in activities that involve any risk of humiliation, such as deciding which answer to choose on a test, raising one's hand in class, inviting a peer to play, or joining in a game. Adolescents with depression experience the anxiety and self-doubt of depression in addition to the feelings of self-consciousness typically experienced during this phase of life. Depression in adolescence increases the risk of alcohol and drug use, as teens seek relief from emotions that are overwhelmingly painful (U.S. Department of Health and Human Services, 1997).

Bipolar disorder, or manic-depressive illness, is diagnosed when individuals experience periods of extreme overactivity and agitation, irritability, rapid ("pressured") speech, and sleep disturbance. Less often children and adolescents may display elation and grandiosity (Biederman, 1997; Katic & Steingard, 2001). Episodes of mania alternate with periods of typical or depressed mood and may fluctuate through the course of a day or over a period of weeks or months. Sometimes changes in mood may be difficult to distinguish from behavioral problems of a learned nature (Katic & Steingard, 2001). Mania in children may be confused with attention deficit disorder, although the cyclic nature of mania and the cognitive symptoms constitute points of difference. During manic phases some people have confused and bizarre thinking that may involve feelings of omnipotence and euphoria and/or hallucinations. A diagnostic evaluation should be completed by a psychologist or psychiatrist specializing in the care of children and adolescents, using structured interviews with the child and parents, and direct behavioral observation. Intervention often includes medication, psychotherapy or counseling, and client and family education (Katic & Steingard, 2001; Sabatino et al., 2001).

Children and adolescents who have bipolar disorder may have periods when their behavior is noticeably out of character or socially inappropriate, or they may seem consistently irritable and active (Biederman, 1997). Behaviors that are commonly experienced during low levels of mania include talking continuously, attention seeking, disregard for others' feelings or social norms, sudden changes in emotions, and impulsiveness. The child may resist adults' attempts to guide or correct him or her and may act "bossy" toward adults. He or she may act aggressively toward property, other children, or adults. These behaviors are not compatible with performance as a student and may occur sometimes even if the child is taking medication. It is important that the adults who regularly interact with a child with recurring symptoms of bipolar disorder know that these behaviors may not always be under the child's control, and the adults should have plans in place for responding effectively, avoiding behavioral outbursts that are disruptive or dangerous.

Anxiety Disorders

Anxiety disorders are characterized by pervasive, long-standing feelings of uneasiness, fearfulness, or dread that are not founded on realistic concerns. Estimated to occur in 4% to 13% of children, anxiety is a relatively common problem (APA, 2000; U.S. Public Health Service, 1999). The diagnosis of a clinical disorder is made by a psychiatrist or psychologist through observation, interviews with the child and family, and self-report questionnaires (Rothe & Castellanos, 2001). Symptoms of anxiety and depression often occur together, and medications may be combined to address both problems (Katic & Steingard, 2001). Subclinical levels of anxiety may also have a negative impact on children's occupational performance and social participation and should receive attention from occupational therapists and others who work with children in schools and other settings.

Anxiety disorders often appear during childhood or adolescence. Characteristic symptoms include excessive worrying about others' evaluations of oneself or about one's past and future behavior. These children also show considerable self-consciousness and a high need for reassurance by others (APA, 2000; Leary & Kowalski, 1995). Children and adolescents who have social anxiety may be unable to participate in many of the activities in which they would like or are expected to engage (Beidel, Turner, & Morris, 1995; Silverman & Ginsburg, 1998). Whenever the child feels placed at risk of criticism or embarrassment, he or she may become overwhelmed by automatic reactions, such as a racing heart, difficulty breathing effectively, and perspiring. Thinking is derailed by emotions of fear or even panic. This reaction may occur in any situation, such as when a teacher is calling on students to perform in class, during a piano lesson, when meeting the new minister at church, or when learning to drive a car. Such experiences are subjectively unpleasant and may cause embarrassment because of others' real or imagined reactions. Children and adolescents who have social anxiety may avoid participating in many cherished and expected activities and sometimes even avoid going places where unfamiliar people are present, such as school, church, and shops (Crick & Ladd, 1993). Social participation is extremely compromised.

Obsessive-compulsive disorder is a subset of the anxiety disorders that is characterized by engagement in repetitive thoughts and behaviors that have little or no functional purpose beyond reducing anxiety. Obsessive-compulsive disorder affects relatively few children and adolescents (fewer than 1%) but is thought by some experts to be underreported (Gilbert, Greening, & Dollinger, 2001). Symptoms of obsessive-compulsive disorder may occur consistently or episodically but tend to be durable over many years (Thomsen & Mikkelsen, 1995). Children and adolescents with this disorder may spend many hours a day engaging in behaviors such as washing the hands, counting objects, arranging objects in a particular way, checking on the status of something (e.g., whether an appliance is unplugged), or cleaning. These behaviors may be visible to the casual observer or may be performed surreptitiously. In either case, if the repetitive activity is interrupted or prevented, the affected individual experiences anxiety. Intervention often includes medication, client and family education, and cognitive behavioral therapy (Gilbert, Greening, & Dollinger, 2001). Children and adolescents with obsessive-compulsive disorder often are also diagnosed with neurologic impairments such as Tourette's syndrome (Gilbert, Greening, & Dollinger, 2001; Rothe & Castellanos, 2001).

A child's balance of activity is negatively affected by the amount of time spent on obsessive-compulsive rituals. Tasks that ordinarily would take minutes may require hours as the child restarts the process again and again. Task interruption may occur as the adolescent stops to readjust unrelated objects or to wash his or her hands. Schoolwork, cleaning one's bedroom, packing for a sleepover, grooming oneself, and dressing are just some activities that could be severely affected by obsessive-compulsive symptoms. The child with obsessive-compulsive behavior also suffers socially, because even though the child may know that the repetitive actions are irrational and, by others' standards, "weird," he or she feels compelled to continue doing them. It becomes easier to spend time alone and at home, rather than to cope with others' reactions and misunderstanding.

Attention Deficit Disorder

Attention deficit disorder is characterized by significant difficulty with selective and/or sustained attention to tasks. It is estimated to affect 3% to 5% of children and adolescents, with more boys than girls represented (APA, 2000). A diagnosis is made through structured observations in a variety of settings and across time. Intervention often includes a combination of medication, behavior management, client education, support, and environmental adaptation (Zametin & Ernst, 1999).

Children and adolescents with attention deficit disorder may have difficulty performing tasks in environments that are moderately or highly stimulating, such as the typical classroom or household. When trying to engage in activities, the child may have to work at continuously redirecting his or her attention from extraneous sounds and sights and back to the targeted task. Reading comprehension and listening skills are often affected. Impulsiveness may result in acting before thinking, producing errors on schoolwork, or in inappropriate social behavior. Adolescents with attention deficit may have difficulty following through on commitments as a result of disorganization and "forgetfulness." They are less able to organize their time and materials than most of their peers. They may have difficulty sustaining effort on tasks, quickly become bored, and leave tasks unfinished.

Pervasive Developmental Disorders

Pervasive developmental disorders constitute a grouping of neurobehavioral disorders that manifest within the first 3 years of life. They are characterized by (1) abnormal relating to people, objects, and events; (2) delayed or missing speech, language, and nonverbal communication skills; (3) abnormal sensory processing; and (4) restricted, repetitive, and stereotyped patterns of behavior, interests, and activities (APA, 1994). Diagnoses included in this category are *Asperger's syndrome* and *autism*. There exists a wide range of ability and variation in severity of symptoms within this population. At one extreme, children have functional language and cognitive skills at levels that allow their participation in typical classrooms; children at the other end of the spectrum are functionally nonverbal and require continuous assistance and accommodation. Approximately 60% to 70% of individuals with autism require moderate to high levels of support throughout life; about 5% to 15% are able to work and live independently (Nordin & Gillberg, 1998). The diagnosis of pervasive developmental disorders has increased over the past 20 years, with current estimates indicating a prevalence of approximately 6 per 1000 population for autism, and much higher rates for Asperger's syndrome (Wing & Potter, 2002). This apparent increase has been attributed variously to a broadening of the diagnostic criteria, the advent of assessments that allow earlier diagnosis, and a possible increase in mistaking other language and cognitive disorders for autism (Sabatino et al., 2001). Intervention for problems associated with pervasive developmental disorders often include behavioral methods, psychoeducational approaches, language therapy, social skills training, and a variety of medications to address specific symptoms (Osterling, Dawson, & McPartland, 2001; Sabatino et al.). Occupational therapy may include sensory integration therapy and life skills training (Hickman & Orentlicher, 2001; Mailloux & Roley, 2001). A variety of alternative interventions with limited or no empirical support are available, including modified diets, auditory training, and holding therapy. As with all interventions, families should be encouraged and supported in making a critical evaluation of the evidence to date before engaging in a course of action (Sabatino et al.).

Role of the Occupational Therapist With Regard to Medication

All the mental disorders previously described include medications as a central or adjunctive treatment. The use of psychotropic medications with children and adolescents has increased significantly over the past 10 years despite concerns about the lack of research (Jensen et al., 1999; Katic & Steingard, 2001). Research evidence to date indicates that, just as for adults, a combination of medication and therapy is more effective than either approach alone for anxiety and attention deficit disorders (Kolko, Bukstein, & Barron, 1999; Pfefferbaum, 1997).

Many children who receive occupational therapy services take psychotropic medications. The medical management of such drugs is made challenging by the child's continuous growth and development and by the lack of research to guide decision making (Katic & Steingard). Occupational therapists should stay apprised of their clients' medications and should consult the prescribing physician to learn about the expected effects, possible side effects, and precautions. As a general guideline, therapists should consistently observe their clients for positive changes and possible unwanted drug effects; these should be reported to the prescribing physician and noted in the client's official record. Any time a child displays an abrupt or marked change in the state of arousal (i.e., acts unusually drowsy or agitated), demonstrates signs of neurologic change (e.g., previously unobserved motor or cognitive difficulties), or complains of discomfort (e.g., nausea or headaches), the possibility of medication side effects should be considered. If the observed symptoms are severe or of sudden onset, the situation should be treated as an emergency, requiring immediate notification of the child's parents and evaluation by a physician. All such observations and referrals should be documented by the occupational therapy practitioner in a timely manner.

Children and adolescents with psychological and behavioral problems live, work, and play in all kinds of environments. Their problems and needs may be viewed in a variety of ways, depending on the context. The following section explores the wide range of possible settings in which occupational therapists work with children whose occupational performance is affected by psychosocial dysfunction and the ways occupational therapy may be practiced in each.

PRACTICE ENVIRONMENTS

The purpose of this section is to describe ways in which occupational therapists provide psychosocial intervention in a variety of settings and to show how occupational therapists apply holistic, client-centered approaches. A variety of treatment settings that represent a continuum from less to more psychiatrically oriented and from less to more intensive and restrictive are described. The mission, clientele, services, frames of reference, and staffing patterns for each type of facility are outlined, as are the traditional or potential roles for occupational therapists in each setting. Case studies synthesized from the author's clinical experiences illustrate psychosocial intervention in a variety of traditional and nontraditional settings.

Therapeutic environments to be discussed include early childhood intervention programs, public schools, outpatient mental health centers, day treatment programs, residential treatment centers, correctional facilities, and inpatient acute care hospitals. Some of these programs are designed specifically to assist children and adolescents who have identified mental health problems; other programs are oriented toward meeting more general educational or developmental needs. Occupational therapists are well established in some of these settings and pioneers in others. In any case, pediatric occupational therapists have the knowledge base, the skills, and the opportunities to provide psychosocial intervention to children and adolescents with mental health and social problems in all service settings.

Early Childhood Intervention Programs

The primary mission of early childhood intervention (ECI) programs is the prevention and amelioration of developmental disabilities in children from birth to 3 years of age. Clients include infants and toddlers who have been diagnosed as having developmental delay and those who are considered at risk for developmental problems, as well as their families (Individuals with Disabilities Act [IDEA], 1990, 1997). Although infants and toddlers are referred to early intervention programs primarily for evaluation and treatment of neurologic and physical conditions, they also may be referred when their development is at risk because of parental mental health problems, such as chemical dependency, domestic violence, parental depression, or other psychiatric disorders. Occasionally the infant may have a diagnosed mental health disorder, such as failure to thrive or pervasive developmental disorder (APA, 2000; Hunter & Powell, 1990).

Professionals working in ECI programs are likely to use developmental, neurodevelopmental, rehabilitative, behavioral, interactional, and family systems frames of reference (Table 13-3). Occupational therapists, educated to recognize and treat persons with mental illness, contribute significantly to the ECI team's effectiveness with high-risk families. For example, parents experiencing depression are often unable to meet their infant's needs for responsive interaction (Pickens & Field, 1993). Parents who are addicted to drugs are at increased risk of neglecting or abusing their children (Wolfner & Gelles, 1993). Occupational therapists can screen clients for problems such as depression and substance abuse and can aid their efforts to obtain evaluation and treatment by a qualified care provider. Environmental stressors such as poverty, social isolation, and community violence also need to be evaluated and addressed, because they play a major part in a family's ability to meet the needs of infants and children (Coulton, Korbin, Su, & Chow, 1995; Humphry, 1995; Vondra, 1990). If the parent of a child with medical complications reports that the family is having difficulty following through with the child's

care because of unemployment and marital stress, the ECI team can refer the parents for financial assistance, work placement, and counseling services. Once these concerns have been resolved, parents have more energy available for childcare. If the danger of child abuse or neglect appears to exist, the occupational therapist is required by law to report these concerns to that state's child protection agency (National Clearinghouse on Child Abuse and Neglect Information, 2000). The following case study presents an example of family-centered early intervention.

Case Study: Vanessa

Part A

Vanessa, who is 16 years old, and her 4-month-old daughter, Emily, live independently in a subsidized housing development in a large city. Emily was referred to an ECI program by her pediatrician, who was concerned about the possibility of developmental delay related to her low birth weight and probable fetal alcohol effects. Emily was evaluated by the center's interdisciplinary team. She was found to be a passive baby who rarely interacted with people or the environment, had low muscle tone, and was slow to drink from a bottle. Because of transportation problems, Vanessa decided that she would prefer home-based intervention. The team agreed that the occupational therapist would provide therapeutic and case management services.

1 What are key personal, environmental, and occupational issues for this mother and child?

2 If you were the therapist, how could you find the answers to these questions?

3 As a direct service provider, what assessments would you use? What information would these tools or methods provide?

4 What is the role of a service coordinator? How would you fulfill this role with Vanessa and her baby?

Part B

The therapist worked with Emily and Vanessa individually and together. To coordinate care, she established communication with two other agencies that were also providing services to the family: the state's Department of Children and Family Services and the Public Health Department. Intervention for Emily focused on increasing her arousal level and responsiveness to the environment, developing motor control, and improving her efficiency at eating. Neurodevelopmental and sensory integrative therapy and feeding techniques were applied to reach these goals. The therapist provided a selection of toys each week and encouraged Vanessa to give Emily opportunities to move and explore the environment.

Vanessa initially was shy and guarded with the therapist but became increasingly comfortable as the weeks passed. The therapeutic relationship was forged when the

TABLE 13-3 Settings for Psychosocial Treatment of Children and Adolescents

	Early Childhood Intervention Programs	School Systems	Outpatient and Day Treatment Programs	Residential Treatment Centers	Correctional Facilities	Inpatient Hospitals
Frames of reference	▪ Developmental ▪ Neurodevelopmental ▪ Rehabilitative ▪ Behavioral ▪ Family systems	▪ Educational ▪ Developmental ▪ Behavioral	▪ Behavioral ▪ Cognitive ▪ Developmental ▪ Psychodynamic ▪ Family systems ▪ Neurobehavioral	▪ Behavioral ▪ Developmental ▪ Milieu	▪ Behavioral ▪ Educational	▪ Developmental ▪ Neurobehavioral ▪ Cognitive ▪ Psychodynamic ▪ Family systems
Clientele	▪ Families of children from birth to 3 years of age who are diagnosed with developmental delay or are at risk for delay	▪ Children and adolescents 2 to 18 years of age	▪ Children and adolescents 5 to 18 years of age and their families	▪ Children and adolescents 5 to 10 years of age, sometimes families	▪ Children and adolescents 10 to 18 years of age	▪ Children and adolescents 3 to 18 years of age
Staffing*	▪ Dominant team style: 2 and 3 ▪ Special educators ▪ Speech-language pathologists ▪ Audiologists ▪ Occupational therapists ▪ Physical therapists ▪ Social workers ▪ Psychologists ▪ Nurses ▪ Nutritionists	▪ Dominant team style: 1 and 2 ▪ Educators ▪ Special educators ▪ Speech-language pathologists ▪ Occupational therapists ▪ Physical therapists ▪ Counselors ▪ Psychologists ▪ Administrators	▪ Dominant team style: 1, 2, and 3 ▪ Psychiatrists ▪ Psychologists ▪ Social workers ▪ Nurses ▪ Counselors ▪ Occupational therapists ▪ Art therapists ▪ Recreational therapists ▪ Music therapists	▪ Dominant team style: 2 and 3 ▪ House parents ▪ Psychologists ▪ Social workers ▪ Educators	▪ Dominant team style: 1 and 2 ▪ Guards ▪ Police officers ▪ Parole officers ▪ Lawyers ▪ Psychologists ▪ Psychiatrists ▪ Social workers ▪ Educators ▪ Counselors ▪ Occupational therapists	▪ Dominant team style: 1 and 2 ▪ Psychiatrists ▪ Nurses ▪ Unit staff ▪ Psychologists ▪ Social workers ▪ Occupational therapists ▪ Recreational therapists ▪ Music therapists ▪ Art therapists

*Dominant team style: 1, multidisciplinary; 2, interdisciplinary; 3, transdisciplinary.

occupational therapist and Vanessa worked together to assemble a colorful mobile for the baby's crib. During that session, Vanessa confided that she was living in fear of Emily's father, who had beaten Vanessa repeatedly during her pregnancy and was threatening her life if she did not agree to let him move into the apartment.

1 What are the therapist's legal and ethical responsibilities at this point?

2 What resources are available for this family?

The occupational therapist assisted Vanessa in contacting a battered women's service organization, which offered support groups, crisis shelter, legal services, and adult education programs. She also helped Vanessa identify family members who might be able to assist with childcare and help with occasional transportation needs. During the course of their relationship, the occupational therapist continued to listen to Vanessa's concerns and encouraged her to pursue the resources available to her. She also monitored the home situation for potential violence toward Emily in case a referral to Child Protective Services was needed. In addition, she maintained regular communication with the referring pediatrician, who assisted with monitoring of Emily's health and the family's progress.

Although Vanessa consistently expressed strong feelings of affection for her daughter and the desire to be a good mother to her, the therapist observed that mother-infant interactions were often poorly synchronized, resulting in frustration for both.

1 What risk factors for child neglect or abuse are present in this case?

2 What are appropriate short-term and long-term therapy goals for this family?

The occupational therapist taught Vanessa to recognize Emily's changing states of arousal and to time her attempts to engage the baby in social play when Emily was calm and alert. Vanessa learned to involve Emily in developmentally appropriate interactive activities such as peek-a-boo, gentle tickling, and "so big." She also learned the importance of providing Emily with a variety of sensory, motor, and language experiences.

After 6 months of therapy, Vanessa was regularly attending educational and support activities sponsored by the women's shelter. She planned to enroll in her school's vocational training program. Emily had become appropriately active and sociable, and both she and her mother interacted warmly in a manner that bespoke their mutual emotional development and attachment. The therapist in this example helped the family address key psychosocial needs through direct intervention and community referral. The ECI team carried out its mission by providing direct assistance and coordinating the provision of services among various agencies. As with most young families, the psychosocial and physical needs of the infant could be met fully only when those of the primary caregiver were met as well.

Public School Systems

Prevalence studies have indicated that 10.5% of secondary special education students have a primary classification of emotional disturbance, making this the second largest group after learning disabilities (Blackorby & Wagner, 1996). Beyond this group, many other students also have behavioral problems that disrupt their performance in school. The primary mission of public education is academic and social preparation for future education and work roles. Research shows that this goal has been largely unreached for students who have emotional and behavioral problems (Blackorby & Wagner; Carson, Sitlington, & Frank, 1995; Maag & Katsiyannis, 1996; Walker & Bunsen, 1995). Students with moderate to severe behavioral problems are unable to take full advantage of education and experience repeated academic and social failure. As many as 40% of students with emotional or behavioral disorders drop out of high school (U.S. Department of Education, 1993). These students have a significantly increased risk of economic dependency and crime (Blackorby & Wagner). The public schools are an arena in which occupational therapists have an unrealized opportunity to have a tremendous effect on the lives of children with psychosocial problems.

Students whose special needs are primarily of a psychosocial nature are classified by the school system as *seriously emotionally disturbed (SED)*. The Individuals with Disabilities Education Act (IDEA) defines this special education classification in the following way:

> A condition exhibiting one or more of the following characteristics over a long period of time and to a marked degree, which adversely affects educational performance: (A) An inability to learn that cannot be explained by intellectual, sensory, or health factors; (B) An inability to build or maintain satisfactory interpersonal relationships with peers or teachers; (C) Inappropriate types of behavior or feelings under normal circumstances; (D) A general pervasive mood of unhappiness or depression; or (E) A tendency to develop physical symptoms or fears associated with personal or school problems (IDEA, 1997, Section 300. 7[c][4])

Children who exhibit psychosocial disorders are included in the SED classification. This category does not include children who demonstrate socially maladjusted behavior (e.g., delinquency, school truancy, conduct disorder) in the absence of the problems previously listed. Other categories in which psychosocial problems and behavioral disorders are often present include pervasive developmental disorders, mental retardation, and traumatic brain injuries (IDEA, 1990).

A variety of school settings serves special education students with behavioral problems, depending on the school district's and individual school's philosophies and resources, the individual student's needs, and the parents' preferences. Self-contained classroom arrangements allow students whose behavior is frequently disruptive or otherwise inappropriate to receive intensive behavioral intervention while being educated in a small group setting. However, students in such classrooms are segregated from peers and role models and suffer the stigma of being identified as "different." The current trend is toward inclusion of special education students in regular education settings as much as possible. In this model, students attend regular education classrooms with support services that may include a resource room for specific subjects, classroom aides, crisis intervention, and counseling services. The benefits of this approach include regular exposure to a normal school environment, opportunities to interact with typically developing peers, and positive experiences that reinforce learning of social skills. However, problems can arise when teachers have a large number of students and little training in preventing or managing disruptive behaviors. Teachers and students then feel inadequate and frustrated.

Many schools incorporate social skills training programs into the regular curricula taught by classroom teachers. These programs, which are suitable for all children, address areas such as communication skills (Gresham & Elliot, 1993), social problem solving (Shure & Spivack, 1982; Weissburg, 1985; Weissberg, Caplan, & Bennetto, 1988), and drug abuse prevention (Cohen, Brennan, & Sexton, 1984). Such educational programs can provide an excellent means of developing positive social thinking and behavior in typically developing children. However, these programs do not provide the intensive guidance required by children and adolescents whose psychosocial dysfunction affects performance in these areas (Robinson & Rapport, 2002).

School-based therapeutic intervention is directed toward enhancing students' academic and future vocational performance, with an emphasis on both scholastic and social development. Traditionally the school psychologist, counselor, or social worker assumes responsibility for evaluating psychosocial needs and may work with students in individual or small group sessions. These professionals serve the needs of all students, not just those in special education, and they may not have an extensive clinical background in psychopathology (Maag & Katsiyannis, 1996). They apply behavioral, cognitive, and developmental approaches (see Table 13-3).

Many leaders in education and occupational therapy believe that the services provided to students with behavioral disorders are inadequate in quantity and quality (Florey, 1989; Maag & Katsiyannis, 1996; Martin, Lloyd, Kauffman, & Coyne, 1995; Schultz, 2003). Teachers express despair as they sacrifice creative educational methods to address behavioral crises. Parents of students with behavioral disorders are frustrated by the paucity of services to address their children's particular needs. All parents are concerned about their children's safety and education at school.

Occupational therapy activity groups have been described as effective for elementary students who have social and behavioral difficulties (Agrin, 1987; Davidson & LaVessar, 1998; Schultz, 1992; Schultz, 2003). Motivating activities such as planning and preparing meals, creating craft projects, producing a newspaper, performing skits and plays, and refinishing furniture help students develop competencies in daily living skills while practicing adaptive responses to interpersonal challenges and developing self-confidence. The goals of this type of approach support improved occupational functioning in the classroom and other school settings. Students' behavioral improvements in occupational therapy task groups have been shown to generalize to the classroom and other contexts, thus winning the support of educators and administrators in the school (Agrin & Schultz, 2003). Agrin speculated that the students' future success in less restrictive settings could be predicted by the development of their social skills in the activity groups.

Students who are referred for occupational therapy services to address fine motor, perceptual, or orthopedic problems may also have social and emotional needs that impair academic performance. The case study for Dylan exemplifies how one student's multiple needs were addressed. With the advent of inclusion, general education teachers are working with increasing numbers of special needs children, including those who have educational diagnoses of SED. Their classrooms also include children who are not enrolled in special education but who are troubled and preoccupied with acute and/or chronic life stressors, such as poverty, community violence, and family turmoil. In some schools the majority of students are trying to learn despite a climate of constant crisis. Behavioral disruptions are frequent, and educators feel endangered and unsupported. Occupational therapists are positioned to provide consultation to teachers who need ideas regarding environmental adaptation and group management and to assist with determining which students should be referred for evaluation. By educating and supporting teachers, therapists can have a positive influence on the school experiences of hundreds of children.

The School to Work Opportunities Act (1994) and IDEA (1997) both reflect the high priority placed on preparing students for gainful employment. Middle and high school students who have emotional and behavioral problems are considered by many to be among the most difficult to transition successfully into independent living and satisfying, economically sustaining work (Carson, Sitlington, & Frank, 1995; Maag & Katsiyannis, 1998). Although no universally successful means have been identified, research to date indicates that the most promising interventions include individualized planning that involves the student and parents. The intervention should also include social skills training and support, classroom education regarding work values and life skills, and actual work experience in positions in which the fit between student and job is optimal (Maag & Katsiyannis, 1998). Age- and situational-appropriate occupations should be emphasized over performance components training, and environments should be structured to facilitate students' success (Brollier, Shepherd, & Markley, 1994). Occupational therapists are able to provide any and all of these interventions, and they can serve educational teams, as well as transitional planning specialists.

School-based occupational therapists do not always embrace psychosocially oriented intervention. Based on a review of the special education literature, Schultz (1992) concluded that teachers would welcome the kind of assistance occupational therapists can provide in improving students' social skills. School administrators who are concerned about occupational therapists meeting the needs of the traditional referrals may initially be less encouraging. School-based therapists who are committed to providing holistic services need to educate and persuade colleagues regarding the potential effectiveness of occupational therapy approaches to help students meet central academic goals by developing the essential skills needed for social participation. This may be approached directly through discussions with key administrators, in-service sessions for teachers and related services professionals, and program development. Concurrently, psychosocial goals may be gradually incorporated into students' individual education programs. Trends in inclusionary and transitional education have created an atmosphere in which occupational therapy leadership in comprehensive holistic intervention approaches is needed and welcomed.

Case Study: Dylan

Part A

Dylan, an 8-year-old second grader, was referred for an occupational therapy evaluation because his handwriting was slow and illegible. The teacher completed a Pre-Assessment Checklist for Teachers (Figure 13-2), which indicated that Dylan often showed problems with incomplete and careless work, disorganized work habits, and peer relations characterized by teasing and rejection, as well as the handwriting difficulty that precipitated the referral.

1 What assessment tools and methods would you choose to use with Dylan? What information would you want to obtain from these?
2 Does your assessment battery provide information about the student as a person, his environment, and his occupational performance?

Part B

During the evaluation session Dylan was polite and compliant. His affect was generally sad, and he made frequent self-disparaging comments, such as, "I'm not good at this." After motor testing had been completed, the occupational therapist asked Dylan about his feelings about school this year and whether there was anyone in his class with whom he played on a regular basis. He reported feeling "okay" about school in general but said, "I don't have any friends at school. They all say I'm fat and dumb." Dylan's fine motor skills were significantly below average.

1 What are this student's key strengths and limitations?
2 What kinds of short-term and long-term treatment goals would you formulate? How can these goals be written to relate directly to Dylan's academic performance?
3 What intervention approach do you recommend?

Part C

Dylan was enrolled in 30 minutes per week of occupational therapy with two other second graders. The group worked on developing writing and cutting skills by making group collages with themes, such as, "I can be a friend by . . ." and "The five best things about me are . . ."; by drawing pictures of what they would like to be doing 20 years in the future; and by writing and illustrating collective stories. Group members discussed their ideas and, with guidance and encouragement from the therapist, began to listen to one another, express their ideas, and give and accept positive feedback. The boys shared ideas about how to make friends and cope with teasing and rejection. Dylan and another boy developed a friendship that continued outside of the sessions. The group members voted to name themselves "The Tuesday Club," adding to their sense of belonging. In addition, the therapist worked with Dylan's teacher on adaptations that would facilitate improved organization, handwriting performance, and social interactions. Together they designed a chart to reward desirable behaviors. Finally, the occupational therapist advised the parents regarding recreational opportunities, such as YMCA day camp and the Boy Scouts, that would further enhance Dylan's social and motor skills.

After one semester of occupational therapy, Dylan's grades had improved significantly. His mother reported that he no longer resisted attending school on most days, and Dylan reported satisfaction with his school performance and social life. The teacher was pleased both with Dylan's progress and with her success in using a behavior charting system. At that point the occupational therapist reduced intervention to biweekly monitoring and occasional consultation with the teacher.

The therapist in this example met the concerns of the referring teacher, who could not read the student's writing, and the concerns of the student, who felt

Please rate the student's performance as it compares with that of most of the other children in his or her class	Usually	Sometimes	Never
Works independently on written assignments			
Writing is legible			
Writing is efficient/speed is adequate			
Writing is accurate for copied work			
Writing is accurate for spontaneous work			
Completes all parts of worksheets			
Written work is neat			
Approach to work is logical, organized			
Independently identifies errors in work			
Independently corrects errors in work			
Persists when tasks are challenging			
Seeks help as needed			
Works at a reasonable pace			
Reads at a level close to his/her cognitive level			
Follows instructions and rules			
Cooperates with peers			
Cooperates with teachers			
Expresses emotions appropriately			
Focuses on tasks despite typical distractions			
Stays seated, refrains from excessive fidgeting			
Appears uncoordinated			
Bumps into people or things			
Trips or falls			
Knocks things over			
Holds objects in an unusual manner			
Has trouble cutting with scissors			
Acts before thinking			

FIGURE 13-2 Pre-Assessment Checklist for Teachers (Revised).

isolated and anxious at school. Both problems significantly impaired the student's academic progress and were effectively and efficiently addressed through a combination of direct service and consultation.

Outpatient Mental Health Services

Children and adolescents who seek outpatient mental health services usually have significant behavioral disturbances. Typically, the young person's problems have caused moderate to severe levels of disturbance for family, school, or community members by the time mental health care commences. The primary goals of outpatient mental health services are the diagnosis and management of mental health problems to improve functioning in the community and the prevention of crises necessitating hospitalization.

The child's initial contact with an outpatient mental health facility usually consists of an intake interview, which explores the nature and severity of the child's and

Is under- or over-active (circle one)			
Has difficulty learning new motor tasks			
Seeks unusual sensations (smelling, twirling, rubbing)			
Over-reacts to: movement, heights, touch, sounds, smells (Circle any that apply)			
Under-reacts to: movement, heights, touch, sounds, smells (Circle any that apply)			
Engages in body-rocking			
Scratches, pinches, strikes, or bites self			
Chews or mouths non-food objects			
Disregards or over-reacts to pain (circle one)			
Appears anxious			
Harms or destroys property			
Is verbally aggressive (threatens, curses)			
Is physically aggressive toward peers or adults			

FIGURE 13-2—Cont'd.

the family's problems. The responses given in the interview form the basis for decisions regarding appropriate evaluation and intervention. In many cases, the intake interviewer is a social worker or paraprofessional trained in mental health screening. Possible dispositions include outpatient evaluation at a later date or crisis evaluation with immediate short-term intervention.

Outpatient mental health services may be provided through freestanding clinics, hospital-based programs, community mental health centers, health maintenance organizations, and private practice offices. Funding sources may include the clients' families, private insurance, Medicaid, federal grants, and state assistance (Manderscheid & Sonnenschein, 1992). The agency's sources of funding influence the types of clientele served and the types of services provided. For example, private for-profit services generally are affordable only for upper-income families with generous insurance plans. These programs may offer special services such as yoga or academic tutoring in addition to the traditional interventions. Middle- and lower-income families usually seek services that are partly publicly funded and therefore more basic (Tuma, 1989).

Parents seek services from community and outpatient mental health services for their children and adolescents for problems ranging from attention deficit disorder to depression. Service provision often begins with screening and crisis intervention. Comprehensive evaluation of the child and family may consist of interviews, play sessions, and standardized psychological or developmental testing. Therapy may be provided for the individual child or parent, couples, groups, and families. Parent education groups, pharmacotherapy, and case management

may also be available. Some mental health centers offer primary prevention services, such as public education, wellness programs, and consultation with public schools. Other services include vocational training, respite care, and day care services (Homonoff & Maltz, 1991).

The frames of reference used in outpatient programs vary with the philosophies of the specific facilities, but they commonly draw from cognitive, behavioral, family systems, neurobiologic, and psychodynamic theories (see Table 13-3). Treatment approaches are most commonly goal focused and time limited and involve the family and school. Clients generally attend one or two 1-hour sessions per week for a specified period. In publicly funded mental health centers, payment for services is based on the individual's income. Third-party payers have varied levels of coverage for mental health care. Therapeutic modalities commonly include play therapy (for young children), talking, expressive art, therapeutic board games, group discussions, and family discussions. These programs may be staffed by a combination of psychologists, social workers, and psychiatrists, with some combination of psychiatric nurses, licensed counselors, and trained paraprofessionals (Manderscheid & Sonnenschein, 1992).

The number of occupational therapy practitioners who currently work with children and adolescents in community-based mental health practice is relatively small. Only 5% of occupational therapy practitioners specialize in mental health, and an even smaller percentage of this group works primarily with children or adolescents (AOTA, 2000). However, most children and adolescents with behavioral and social problems are not seen in mental health settings. Many children with social participation needs are encountered in public schools and early intervention programs, which employ 29% of all occupational therapists and 26% of occupational therapy assistants (AOTA, 2000). Work with children and adolescents who have significant emotional and behavioral problems is extremely challenging. A thorough understanding of child development and the frames of reference used by other members of the mental health team is needed, as are ways to relate these other frames of reference to occupational therapy. Excellent communication and behavioral management skills, personal maturity, and comfort with role sharing are also required. Empathy and the ability to relate to troubled children and their families must co-exist with the knowledge that often the clients' values and behaviors run counter to those of the therapist. Many communities lacking in economic resources such as work training and social activities may not be able to provide comprehensive programs for these children and families, which limits what the mental health team can help their clients achieve.

Community-based mental health practice allows a focus on occupations in the child's natural environment. The crafts, games, and daily living activities that are so much a part of occupational therapy are extremely motivating and developmentally appropriate for most young people. The therapeutic relationships formed with many young clients can be powerful in their capacity to facilitate positive change. Working with clients in the context of their families, schools, and communities affords the greatest opportunities for generalizing therapeutic effects into everyday living. In addition, occupational therapists have a unique combination of skills (e.g., expertise in developmental evaluation, sensory integration evaluation and therapy, and activities-based therapy) that is highly valued by intervention teams (Case-Smith, 1994). Client and public education regarding issues such as parenting, stress reduction, and child development are needed services that occupational therapists can provide. Teaching childcare workers, educators, and vocational trainers ways of promoting effective social and work-related behavior is a valuable consultation service. Service coordination and interfacing with other service agencies are also important roles well suited to occupational therapists (Adams, 1990). Program planning and administration are areas of mental health practice in which occupational therapists can excel (Nielson, 1993). Such services may be provided in clinical or community settings, including the public schools or clients' homes.

In 1992, Congress authorized the Comprehensive Community Mental Health Services for Children and their Families Program. This program provides federal funding through demonstration grants to states and communities and is designed to promote effective ways to organize, coordinate, and deliver mental health services and supports for individual children and their families. Cultural competence is a critical goal of the program, and each grant must document that the policies and practices of each agency address the impact of and show respect for the race, culture, and ethnicity of the children and families they serve. The agencies that have been receiving funding provide a broad array of services, including occupational therapy, and are designed to meet the multiple and changing needs of children and adolescents with serious emotional disturbances and their families. The projects place emphasis on family involvement and support and linkage between home and school. Many of these projects involve day treatment services for culturally diverse children and adolescents (U.S. Department of Health and Human Services, 2004).

Day treatment programs are offered in a variety of settings, including psychiatric hospitals, community mental health facilities, and schools for students with special needs (Pruitt & Kiser, 1991). Such programs provide a middle step between outpatient intervention and hospitalization and are becoming popular for clinical and economic reasons (Erker, Searight, Amant, & White, 1993). Clients attend programs from 4 to 6 hours a day, 5 days a week, and are at home during the evenings and on weekends (Block & Lefkovitz, 1992). Interventions often include a variety of therapies and academic classes.

Day treatment may facilitate a child's transition from the hospital back to the home and community, provide crisis stabilization, allow comprehensive evaluation, or serve as an intensive therapeutic alternative to outpatient or inpatient treatment (Pruitt & Kiser, 1991). Programs often follow a psychoeducational model and may include vocational evaluation and training for adolescents (Nelson & Condrin, 1987). A psychiatrist or psychologist who specializes in child and adolescent mental health typically leads the intervention team. Other team members, which often include occupational therapists, are listed in Table 13-3.

Occupational therapy activities are designed to motivate and facilitate self-awareness and communication skills, to develop grooming and etiquette habits, and to teach life skills such as cooking and community mobility. Crafts, role-playing exercises, cooperative action games, and therapeutic board games are popular modalities in such occupational therapy programs. Working with the client's parents, childcare providers, teachers, or job coach, the occupational therapist can facilitate the transition from intensive day treatment programs to the community and public school and enhance the carryover of interventions and goals. The family may also benefit from assistance with locating and securing social and leisure activity resources. The following case study describes how a consultative model of intervention may be used to assist with the transition of a client from day treatment back to full community involvement. The focus in this example is on educating and problem solving with personnel from another agency.

Case Study: Mario

Part A

Mario is 17 years old and has been diagnosed with mild mental retardation, anxiety disorder, and impulse control disorder. He has a lifelong history of poor socialization with people other than his family, separation anxiety, and occasional temper tantrums. He also takes medications for a seizure disorder and asthma. Mario was admitted to day treatment after a series of explosive episodes during which he broke furniture and a window.

Mario, his family, and the treatment team decided that Mario would begin a job training program as part of his day treatment. It was determined that the occupational therapist would arrange and implement this. The supervisor at the job training site expressed both interest and a little trepidation at the notion of working with a client who had a history of psychiatric disturbance with aggressive behavior. The occupational therapist's task included helping Mario to develop and use new interpersonal and practical skills needed for success in his training, such as meeting new people, asking questions, maintaining acceptable standards of dress and grooming, and reading a clock. This was accomplished through group and individual sessions in the day treatment program. Another part of the intervention involved preparing the job training site to work effectively with Mario.

To facilitate the transition, the occupational therapist visited the job training site to evaluate its appropriateness for Mario and to establish a working relationship with the people there. The occupational therapist then accompanied Mario to his interview at the job training program. As the job trainer and Mario discussed the program's operations, the therapist made suggestions to increase Mario's chances of success.

One suggestion was for Mario to write the program schedule into his pocket calendar and to negotiate with the job trainer the times needed for regular psychiatric or medical appointments. Another suggestion was for the job trainer to provide Mario with a written list of basic expectations for participation in the program, such as arriving on time, wearing appropriate clothing, and bringing a sack lunch. Mario's need for a high degree of structure and routine was discussed, and the supervisor provided him with a detailed schedule of activities for the upcoming week. The occupational therapist also helped Mario ask the supervisor questions about issues she knew he was concerned about, such as what would happen if he made mistakes and what he should do if he was confused or had questions. The occupational therapist also helped Mario answer the job training supervisor's questions, such as how the supervisor should respond if Mario became agitated. (Mario suggested that he could take a break in the break room if he felt overwhelmed, and the therapist gave the supervisor her cell phone number.) The occupational therapist, Mario, and the job training supervisor left the interview feeling prepared and excited about working together.

1 In what other ways could Mario's transition into this new environment be facilitated?

Part B

Once Mario began the job training program, he experienced periods of intense anxiety and agitation, causing concern for his supervisor and co-workers. The supervisor called the occupational therapist, who visited the job training facility. Through discussion with Mario, the occupational therapist was able to establish that he had become upset when he was given conflicting or inconsistent directives from different supervisors. It was also observed that Mario did not interact with co-workers, even if they greeted him.

1 How could these problems be addressed?

The therapist met with Mario and the supervisor to negotiate a plan. It was decided to (1) as much as possible, assign Mario routine tasks that needed to be performed the same way each time; (2) limit Mario's supervision to one person at a time; and (3) encourage Mario to verbalize his feelings of confusion, anxiety, and frustration to his supervisor before he felt overwhelmed. The therapist assisted Mario and his supervisor in writing and signing a behavioral contract that outlined consequences for behavioral outbursts: a 30-minute break after the first outburst and suspension without pay for the remainder of the day if there was a second outburst. Finally, the occupational therapist spent some time in the company lunchroom helping Mario meet and get to know his co-workers. Once Mario was integrated with his colleagues and supervisor, he was able to demonstrate his full potential as a reliable and capable worker.

Residential Treatment Centers

Residential treatment centers present an environment that is more restrictive and intensive than a day treatment program but less restrictive than an acute care hospital setting. Although only 8% of children receiving mental health services use residential treatment, this form of intervention accounts for nearly 25% of the total cost of children's mental health care (Burns, Hoagwood, & Maultsby, 1998). The length of stay in residential treatment centers varies considerably and is influenced by funding constraints, the facility's philosophy, and the needs of the client and family (Spreat & Jampol, 1997). Placement may last from weeks to years (Durrant, 1993). Facilities often serve children who are unable to function in home and community settings because of behavioral problems that have grown out of chronic neglect and abuse (Spreat & Jampol). Program philosophies range from highly structured and intensively therapeutic to more naturalistic and homelike environments. Facilities vary in size from a few to hundreds of residents. Children and adolescents who require residential treatment are usually troubled by combinations of psychologic, social, behavioral, and family problems that are severe and chronic enough to warrant extended periods of care and respite.

The immediate mission of residential care programs is to provide a safe and therapeutic environment for children and adolescents whose behavioral, emotional, and social problems preclude their safety and competence in the community (Stein, 1995). The intended outcome of residential care is for children and adolescents to function as full participants in the community and family, foster family, transitional living, or independent living settings. Experts in the area of residential care assert that treatment is not limited to formal individual, group, and family therapy sessions. To be meaningful, therapeutic intervention must continue in the everyday experiences of children as they interact with childcare staff and their peers (Beker & Feurstein, 1991; Durrant, 1993; Stein). The effectiveness of intervention is determined by the skills of the therapeutic, educational, and childcare staff in building relationships, managing children's behavior, and structuring leisure and work activities (Daly et al., 1998).

Staffing reflects each residential care facility's philosophy and target populations. Frames of reference often used in residential care include behavioral, psychodynamic, and activities-based approaches (Kennedy et al., 1990; Stein, 1995). Most programs are largely staffed by trained paraprofessionals (sometimes called "house parents" or "childcare workers") who provide around-the-clock care. Psychotherapists and administrators, who may be social workers, psychologists, or psychiatrists, provide supervision. Educational services for the children may be provided on site or through the local public school system. Traditionally, occupational therapists are not full-time staff members. Some residential treatment facilities may contract for services that include consultation to the house staff regarding the residents' developmental needs and limitations, ways to organize and guide household responsibilities to include the residents, and ways to teach self-care and community living skills. Other occupational therapists provide services as part of the child's school programs, addressing goals related to academic and social performance.

Children who live in even the most deluxe institutional settings do not have access to many occupational experiences that are part of the daily cultures of others. Occupational therapy can have a tremendous impact on the quality of life and therapeutic effectiveness of residential treatment. Direct intervention with children and adolescents could include many of the goals and approaches outlined in the discussion of occupational therapy in day treatment programs. Often the therapist intervenes to facilitate the resident's participation in community activities such as shopping, playing sports, participating in activity clubs, and attending church. Opportunities for as much family interaction as possible during such activities increase the benefits of such experiences (Spreat & Jampol, 1997).

A small but growing area of occupational therapy psychosocial practice is the juvenile justice system. Many incarcerated young people have serious emotional disturbances that have not been addressed therapeutically (Atkins et al., 1999). Children and adolescents who steal, vandalize property, or assault others may enter either the mental health or the correctional system, depending on whether the behavior is interpreted as a symptom of a conduct disorder or a violation of the law (Tuma, 1989). Occupational therapists are increasingly involved in the comprehensive psychiatric evaluation of children and adolescents who are either under consideration for psychiatric commitment or who are to be tried as adults. Youth offenders who are enrolled in diversional programs or are treated in state or other psychiatric facilities may also receive occupational therapy.

Inpatient Psychiatric Hospitals

Inpatient psychiatric hospitals provide the most restrictive, intensive, and costly therapeutic intervention (U.S. Public Health Service, 1999). It is generally reserved for children and adolescents who pose a serious safety risk to themselves or others, who have complicating medical conditions, or who are considered to have poor prognoses if treated as outpatients (Mabe, Riley, & Sunde, 1989). Inpatient psychiatric units may be found in general hospitals, state psychiatric hospitals, and private psychiatric hospitals. There was a burgeoning of inpatient facilities from the middle 1970s through the 1980s, when reimbursement for such care was abundant. This trend ended and reversed with the advent of managed mental health care and the increased control by third-party payers on admissions and length of stay (Dalton & Forman, 1992). Despite such shifts in service availability, there will always be a need for the rapid diagnosis and stabilization that such specialized facilities provide.

Child and adolescent inpatient psychiatric units are usually locked facilities directed by a psychiatrist and staffed by nurses and paraprofessionals trained in the care and management of severely impaired patients (Dalton & Forman, 1992). Very often patients are hospitalized when in crisis, such as after a suicide attempt, an assault, or a psychotic episode. Sometimes patients are admitted for comprehensive psychological and medical evaluation of complex chronic problems. In most cases the length of stay is limited to days or weeks, with the goal being rapid discharge to less costly and restrictive treatment alternatives.

The treatment team is interdisciplinary and may include psychiatrists, nurses, paraprofessional direct care staff, social workers, recreational therapists, psychologists, special educators, and music therapists, as well as occupational therapists (see Table 13-3). Interns and trainees representing these professions may also circulate through the team. The professional staff applies a variety of psychosocial theories, with behavioral and neurobiologic approaches among those most commonly used (Dalton & Forman, 1992).

Occupational therapists who work with children and adolescents experiencing acute psychiatric problems play an important role by contributing to diagnosis, stabilization, and discharge planning. Activities in a locked hospital unit typically are quite structured, which limits opportunities for individual choices and participation in many occupational roles. Often the occupational therapist's evaluation of hospitalized children includes observation of the patient performing activities that are motivating and require the cognitive, social, and adaptive skills needed at home and school. In addition, occupational therapists evaluate the child's performance levels as they compare with those of typical children. This information allows the team to predict more reasonably how the child performs when coping with the demands of community settings.

It is essential for members of any interdisciplinary team to combine their unique perspectives on each patient's needs into a cohesive, coherent plan that is mutually agreeable. This cohesion is especially important when working with patients who are challenging and often volatile. The following case study illustrates how an occupational therapist recognized a program need and worked with an administrator and interdisciplinary team to implement changes.

Case Study: Assertiveness Group

Part A

A common goal of psychiatric treatment with adolescents is to facilitate the client's identification with the peer group. This developmentally appropriate goal may be met counterproductively, such as when the patients group together to perform antisocial activities, such as smuggling alcohol into the unit or assisting a peer in running away from the hospital. This type of dynamic occurred in a long-term psychiatric care facility about twice a year, usually soon after a large influx of new patients entered the adolescent unit. The traditional manner of response to such group behavior was unit restriction, during which time the regular schedule of therapies, school, and passes was suspended. During unit restriction the patients, nurses, and therapists gathered several times daily to try to facilitate the adolescents'

understanding of the group process and their individual roles in contributing to the negative behaviors. Often this was a lengthy and painful process because of the adolescents' limited comfort and skills in communicating their feelings and concerns. Meetings were characterized by periods of silence and blaming, and they often ended in frustration on all sides.

The occupational therapist hypothesized that the group meetings would be more productive if the patients had basic communication skills and a better sense of their own values and feelings. The therapist met with the program director and proposed incorporating daily self-awareness and assertiveness groups into the unit restriction protocol in an effort to catalyze the unit restriction process. The director approved the idea and suggested presenting it to the rest of the team for feedback. Other team members were less enthusiastic because they viewed occupational therapy as fun and rewarding to the patients. They thought that this would undermine the punitive aspects of unit restriction.

1 How could you gain the team's support for trying a new approach?

2 What kinds of activities would you want to do with the clients? How could these be structured to maintain discipline and the spirit of "restriction"?

Part B

The occupational therapist explained that the highly structured activities would develop the basic communication skills that were needed. Inappropriate behavior would lead to suspension from the session. The team agreed to a trial of occupational therapy during unit restriction with the provision that if the misbehavior increased, the sessions would be discontinued. Unit nurses and staff were invited to observe or join the sessions at their discretion.

The adolescents, many of whom felt bored, isolated, and confused by the unit restriction, immediately welcomed the occupational therapy sessions. Initial sessions incorporated games and art activities to facilitate identification and expression of feelings about being hospitalized, being a part of the patient group, and the causes and effects of unit restriction. Subsequent sessions were devoted to teaching concepts and practicing skills related to assertive communication. Discussions, worksheets, and role playing games were used for this.

The incidence of inappropriate and antisocial behavior declined significantly, and as a result the nurses had to cope with fewer disciplinary problems. Most important, the patients discussed pertinent issues during the group process meetings. They were able to explore and understand the group's responsibility to the progress of each member and each individual's responsibility to the betterment of the group. The ensuing maturation led to the development of a positive peer group culture in which the majority discouraged individual antisocial behaviors.

Staff members were pleasantly surprised to observe that the occupational therapy sessions were clearly related to the goals of the unit restriction, and they expressed their support by direct feedback and by helping to prepare the room and gather the patients for sessions. The occupational therapist also believed that her treatment philosophy and skills were better understood by the rest of the team, resulting in greater job satisfaction.

The case examples found throughout this chapter depict a number of ways to intervene with children and adolescents who have psychosocial problems. The following section outlines occupational therapy evaluation and intervention options more specifically and in more detail.

EVALUATION

The evaluation process is foundational to the intervention process and largely determines its success. Evaluating children who exhibit behavioral problems can be challenging, both because of the complex nature of the task and because the child may be unable to cooperate with traditional assessment approaches. As much information as possible should be gleaned indirectly from past and current school or medical records; evaluating therapists need to learn about teacher and parent checklists; and naturalistic observations should be made in typical contexts, such as various settings in the school, home, and community.

The evaluation process begins with an occupational profile that includes an occupational history, the client's perceptions of current functioning, the client's concerns about performance, and priorities for intervention (AOTA, 2002). A thorough occupational profile adds to the therapist's knowledge of the person, environment, and occupations. The profile may be obtained through an informal interview or with the assistance of a structured interview, such as the *Canadian Occupational Performance Measure* (Law et al., 1994). An interview or a paper and pencil activity may be used to gain an understanding of the child's habits and balance of activity. Some children are better able to express their concerns and hopes for the future in pictures. For them, a large piece of paper and some colorful markers or crayons, along with an invitation to "draw a picture of yourself doing something" or "make a picture of some things you want to be doing next month" may give the therapist and child a way to begin their dialog. The purpose of beginning the evaluation process with an occupational profile is to obtain a sense of the scope and immediacy of issues concerning the client. When working with children, the "client" includes the referring adult, who could be the parent, a teacher, a foster parent, or some other closely involved person. When the child is very young, has limited functional communication, or is being seen in the context of school, the occupational profile should include information from the involved adults. This information guides decisions about subsequent steps in the evaluation process and helps with the formulation of intervention goals and methods.

In school settings, completion of the Pre-Assessment Checklist for Teachers before the child is evaluated can help define issues of concern and inform teachers about the scope of occupational therapy (see Figure 13-2). This tool is designed with items related to the production of written schoolwork listed first and is cast with a positive slant (e.g., "Works independently on written assignments"). The second section relates more to cognitive and social performance, and the items are cast from a more problem-oriented perspective (e.g., "Has difficulty learning new motor tasks"). Teachers respond to these items using a Likert scale and can write in specific concerns.

One of the most valuable assessment methods for children and adolescents who have social participation problems is to observe them interacting with peers or family members during motivating activities such as crafts, board games, or preparing and enjoying food. During such sessions the therapist can see the child in action as he or she responds to opportunities to initiate interactions, make choices, share opinions, request help, try something new, cope with competition or conflict, and other typical demands of social participation. The activity-focused session can also allow observation of other types of skills, such as reading ability, planning and organization, safety awareness, concentration, problem solving, postural control, and small tool use. If the session includes classmates, family members, or others with whom the child relates at home or school, information about the child's social environment is also obtained.

An evaluation of play can provide invaluable, multifaceted information about a child's social, emotional, cognitive, and motor development and addresses a critical area of occupational performance. Assessments for this purpose include structured observational measures, such as the Knox Preschool Play Scale (Knox, 1974, 1997), or the Test of Playfulness (Bundy, 1997). Florey and Greene (1997) outlined an activity observation guide to facilitate practitioners' evaluation of play in children 6 to 12 years of age.

The Social Skills Rating System (Gresham & Elliott, 1990) was developed by psychologists to evaluate and classify social behavior in students from kindergarten through 12th grade. There are three versions of the protocols, each for a different grade range. Through a combination of teacher, parent, and student (self) rating scales, this tool measures perceived performance in the domains of social skills, academic competence, and problem behaviors. The 30 social skills items are stated in positive terms (e.g., "Initiates conversation with peers") and include items indicative of cooperation, assertion, responsibility, empathy, and self-control. Respondents are asked to rate the items in terms of frequency and importance. The problem behavior items, which are answered only by parents and teachers, classify behaviors as externalizing (behaviors that are intrusive or disruptive), internalizing (behaviors reflecting anxiety or sadness), and hyperactivity. The results of the Social Skills Rating System are easily translated into intervention and Individualized Education Program (IEP) goals and objectives.

The School Function Assessment (SFA) is an observational assessment that assists with the evaluation of the performance in school of students with disabilities (Coster, Deeney, Haltiwanger, & Haley, 1998). It is administered as a paper and pencil form that can be completed by the occupational therapist, the child's teacher, and others who know his or her school behavior well. It is followed by a structured interview that elaborates on the written responses. More than 100 items on the SFA pertain to social participation in categories of Functional Communication, Memory and Understanding, Following Social Conventions, Compliance with Adult Directives and School Rules, Task Behavior/Completion, Positive Interaction, Behavior Regulation, and Safety.

The Occupational Therapy Psychosocial Assessment of Learning (OTPAL) uses a combination of observation and interviewing to evaluate a student's psychosocial abilities as they relate to his or her specific school environment (Townsend et al., 2001). This assessment is designed for children in elementary school who have been identified as having social participation difficulties.

Standardized assessments of skills, such as measures of the child's fine and gross motor abilities, developmental levels, handwriting, sensory integration, and cognitive-perceptual abilities, should be done as needed for intervention planning. The following are some general guidelines for structured evaluation of students who may resist following directions.

1 Remember that the main goal is to measure the student's best performance on assessment items and to form a therapeutic alliance.
2 Allow extra time for relationship building and breaks during the assessment sessions. Take several brief sessions to complete the battery, if that is needed to ensure a valid measure. Do not be afraid to stop a session early if the child becomes agitated or intractable; crisis prevention is always preferable to crisis intervention.
3 Ask the teacher beforehand for tips about the child's preferences and dislikes. Find out what behavior

management techniques work well in the classroom and what interaction styles to avoid. Ask if there is any history of aggressive behavior, and if so, what forms it takes.
4 Be prepared to use rewards to help the child persevere. Favored items include stickers, small candies, or an enjoyed activity at the end of the session.
5 Involve the student as a partner in the evaluation process; explain the nature and purpose of the assessments, conduct a personable interview, ask for feedback, and make responsive adjustments as often as possible.

INTERVENTION

If it is to be meaningful and effective, intervention with children and adolescents who have social performance problems must include goals that directly address these concerns. These goals should relate directly to the contexts and activities in which the child needs and wants to participate. The following are examples of such goals:

- *Long-term goal I:* James will participate successfully in physical education classes, requiring 0 to 1 verbal correction per class session by (date).
- *Short-term goal Ia:* Given verbal reminders and adult support, James will consistently take turns with peers during a 20-minute ball game by (date).
- *Short-term goal Ib:* James will independently locate his "square" upon entering the gym and, given occasional verbal cues, will sit or stand on his square as directed by the teacher on 4 of 5 days by (date).
- *Short-term goal Ic:* James will refrain from leaving the gym without permission 100% of the time by (date).
- *Short-term goal Id:* Given opportunities to take brief "breaks" as needed, James's behavior will be age appropriate and polite during sports and games in physical education classes on 4 of 5 opportunities by (date).

Contemporary models of occupational therapy emphasize interventions using activities in their natural contexts (AOTA, 2002; Law et al., 1996; Schkade & Schultz, 1992; Schultz & Schkade, 1992). Schultz (2003) has described such an approach with boys who were classified with behavior disorders in school, using the model of Occupational Adaptation. The boys attended small groups, in which they participated in craft activities that were motivating and appropriately challenging. The therapist's role was to arrange and maintain an environment that supported the participants' efforts toward learning ways of adapting to new and familiar challenges, both social and otherwise. The participants were supported in evaluating their own performance, with minimal and carefully chosen direction from the therapist. If a participant was aggressive toward another person or property, he was instructed to leave that session and allowed to try again the next. As the students progressed, they began to give one another corrective and positive feedback. Once the group achieved sufficient progress during parallel craft activities, the challenge was increased to focus on cooperative group projects, such as the development and creation of a hallway display depicting social studies concepts. Positive changes in the boys' social participation were attributed to a combination of improvement in the boys' adaptive capacities and changes in the social environment at school. During her 2 years of intervention with the boys, Schultz observed that the adults and students in the school had developed negative expectations of them, such that inappropriate and maladaptive behavior was inadvertently encouraged. When the group members behaved appropriately in the school context, expectations and opinions about them began to shift, resulting in improved environmental support for future successes.

In contrast with the environmentally focused approach of Occupational Adaptation, other interventions generally are more therapist structured and may be more removed from the everyday environments of children. For example, behavioral methods such as point- or token-reward systems may be incorporated into activities-based therapy. This type of operant behaviorism is well researched and has been found to be effective for many children as they build new skills (Powers, 2001). However, operant behavioral approaches have been criticized by some because they take power away from the naturalistic environmental influences and the child's learning and place it more on the artificial rewards and the therapist (Schultz, 2003; VanderVen, 1995). Ideally, operant behavioral methods, if used at all, are temporary facilitators for children who have learned to get their needs met through unacceptable behaviors and who can quickly learn adaptive behaviors when given a temporary reward, which is phased out as the naturally occurring social rewards become available.

Case Study: Max

Max typically shouts and knocks over board games when he fears he will lose, resulting in broken games and disrupted friendships. The therapist initially talked with Max about his behavior, and they discussed better ways of coping. However, although he can describe alternative ways to handle his distress, Max continues to act inappropriately when playing competitive games. Max is enrolled in small activity group sessions during which the children play board games. The players are intermittently rewarded with praise and small treats for "being patient" and "good sportsmanship." As Max becomes more capable, the natural rewards of enjoying a game with

friends become available to him, and he requires less structure and fewer artificial rewards to maintain his role as a player in the games. Soon he will be able to engage in this type of play as well as other children his age.

A more socially based behavioral approach is that of Rational Intervention (RI), a cross-disciplinary, decision-making system that assists those interacting with children and adolescents with the clinical reasoning needed to make immediate responses that facilitate social participation (Table 13-4) (Davidson, 2001). The primary goal of RI is to help children attain and maintain behaviors that are adaptive and appropriate for participation in natural contexts and to create a consistent approach that

TABLE 13-4 Levels of Social Appropriateness and Rational Intervention

Level	Child's Behavior	Rational Interventions
5	Within a functional range for acceptable performance in the community	Facilitate
4	Approximates behavior that is acceptable, with minor errors	Facilitate, monitor, or gently correct: ■ Alter the environment ■ Redirect ■ Model ■ Cue ■ Discuss alternatives
3	Not positive but not disruptive or dangerous (may be withdrawn, passive, quietly off task)	Monitor or gently correct: ■ Alter the environment ■ Redirect ■ Model ■ Cue ■ Discuss alternatives
2	Disruptive but not dangerous (noncompliant with rules and directives, makes rude sounds or gestures, curses)	Gently correct: ■ Alter the environment ■ Redirect ■ Model ■ Cue ■ Discuss alternatives and/or moderately correct: ■ Time-out
1	May escalate to dangerous level (shouting, verbal or physical threats of violence, spitting, pinching or hitting self, harming expendable property)	Gently correct: ■ Alter the environment ■ Cue verbally ■ Explain outcomes/alternatives and/or moderately correct: ■ Time-out
0	Imminently harmful to self or others (striking, kicking, biting, head banging, cutting, running away, destroying valuable property)	Strongly correct: ■ Time-out ■ Physically manage ■ Seclusion room ■ Physically restrain

supports this for all staff members and adult family members who interact with the child. The general principles of RI are:

- Every interaction between a child and an adult is a learning session.
- Intervention begins with the adult's consistent enactment of respectfulness and caring toward the child.
- The main goals of intervention are all persons' immediate safety and the continuous improvement of the child's ability to make decisions that support successful participation in life at home and in the community.
- Opportunities for making choices and decisions are built into daily activities as often as possible. Children should have regular, frequent opportunities to practice skills needed for community living through educational and leisure experiences in the community.
- To promote children's opportunities for decision making, adults should impose the least amount of external control needed to maintain safety and promote positive, functional behavior.

In using the RI approach, the therapist initially observes and assesses the child's behavior, and classifies it as belonging in one of three color-coded zones. Green zone behaviors are adaptive and would be acceptable in most community and home settings. Yellow zone behaviors are mildly to moderately problematic, and require monitoring, environmental modification, or cueing to facilitate adaptive social behavior. Red zone behaviors present the threat or actuality of danger to the child or others and require direct and immediate verbal or physical management. Therapeutic responses include facilitation, monitoring, gentle correction, moderate correction, and strong correction and may be incorporated into therapy sessions and all social participation contexts (Box 13-3).

Case Study: Brenda

Brenda is an occupational therapist who works at a therapeutic school for children with behavioral and emotional problems. Today she is helping to care for the children during recess. As Brenda walks around the busy playground area, she encounters many scenes, each of which requires Rational Intervention.

- Three children have acquired a basketball. They are discussing what to play, and seem to be making headway toward consensus. This is functional, safe, level 5 behavior; Brenda leaves them to their game.
- A girl keeps running into the midst of a kickball game that is in progress, and the players are shouting angrily at her. It appears to Brenda that the girl wants to play the game but does not have the skills to ask to join. This is level 4 behavior; that is, generally positive but not well executed. Brenda gives the child a verbal cue, calling out to her, "Ask Tom if you can be on his

---

BOX 13-3 Response Options in Rational Intervention

FACILITATION
- Observe unobtrusively.
- Improve environmental supports (i.e., provide comfortable seating and a quiet work area for children who want to play a board game together).

MONITORING
- Observe visibly so that children are aware of adult presence.
- Express encouragement as needed.
- Facilitate problem solving by asking guiding questions.

GENTLE CORRECTION
- Alter environment as needed (i.e., change the seating arrangement to reduce conflict between participants).
- Remind children of rules, expectations, or new skills that may be used.
- Join in activity and model adaptive behavior.
- Redirect child to alternative activity.
- Discuss alternatives to current behavior.

MODERATE CORRECTION
- Give child a break from activity through redirection.

STRONG CORRECTION
- Impose formal time-out (child is seated away from activity for 1 to 5 minutes, until calm).
- Use physical management of the child and remove him or her from activity and/or activity area.

---

team!" She watches to make sure the intervention is successful, then moves on.

- Brenda notices a boy who has tied a garden hose into a series of knots. She approaches and asks him to take the knots out of the hose. The boy responds, "Get lost, Bozo!" and keeps making knots in the hose. Although this behavior is inappropriate and rude, it is not dangerous. It is level 2, yellow zone behavior. Brenda says, "Tying up the hose can damage it. Please take out the knots now. I will help, if you like." The boy abruptly stands and swings the hose at Brenda, missing her by several feet. His behavior has declined to level 2, red zone, and could potentially be dangerous. Brenda responds in a calm, firm voice, "Please put the hose down right now, or you will have to go inside for the rest of recess." The boy drops the hose and says, "You're mean! You took away my recess!" Brenda recognizes this as an improvement, and responds supportively, "I'm glad you decided to put down the hose. Let's hurry and fix it, so you'll have more time to play outside."

SUMMARY

Children and adolescents with emotional, cognitive, and behavioral problems are unable to participate satisfactorily in home, school, and community life. Social problems such as poverty, family sociopathic conditions, and cultural violence have been linked with an increased incidence of psychosocial dysfunction in young people (Constantino, 1993; Prothro-Stith, 1991; Wolfner & Gelles, 1993). Such social problems are steadily increasing in the United States, whereas mental health services for young people continue to be inadequate in amount and quality. Occupational therapists who work with children and adolescents have the knowledge and skills to help improve their clients' occupational functioning by addressing key psychosocial needs. This may be accomplished through individual and group therapy, program development, and consultation. Pediatric occupational therapists in all settings need to become psychosocial practitioners to meet the mental health and behavioral needs of young people and their families effectively.

STUDY QUESTIONS

1 Review the characteristics of temperament. How would you characterize your temperament? How does your temperament affect your choice of leisure activity, friendships, study style, or behavior when you are ill? Answer these questions again with regard to a brother or sister or a friend. How does the "fit" between you work or not work?

2 What are the characteristics of bipolar disorder in young children? What kinds of problems might a child with this disorder have in school and at home? Would the symptoms or occupational problems be the same for a 16-year-old? If so, in what way? How would you explain this disorder to a child's teacher?

3 Review the case study for Dylan (p. 465). In designing a behavioral charting program for Dylan, what three behaviors would you like to reinforce? What adaptive techniques or interventions might help with organization, handwriting, and social interaction?

4 What kinds of interventions could an occupational therapist provide to children and adolescents living in a residential treatment environment that would most help ameliorate the occupational restrictions inherent to such a setting?

REFERENCES

Adams, R. (1990). The role of occupational therapists in community mental health. *Mental Health Special Interest Newsletter, 13* (1), 1-2.

Agrin, A. (1987). Occupational therapy with emotionally disturbed children in a public school. *American Journal of Occupational Therapy, 7,* 105-114.

Ainsworth, M.D., Blehar, M.C., Waters, E., & Wall, S. (1978). *Patterns of attachment: A psychological study of the strange situation.* Hillsdale, NJ: Earlbaum.

American Occupational Therapy Association (AOTA). (2000). *The AOTA Membership Composition Survey.* Bethesda, MD: The Association.

American Occupational Therapy Association. (2002). The Occupational Therapy Practice Framework. *American Journal of Occupational Therapy, 56,* 609-639.

American Psychiatric Association (APA). (1994). *Diagnostic and statistical manual of mental disorders* (4th ed., pp. 65-78). Washington, DC: The Association.

American Psychiatric Association (APA). (2000). *Diagnostic and statistical manual of mental disorders* (4th ed., revised). Washington, DC: The Association.

Atkins, D., Pumariega, A., Rogers, K., Montgomery, L., Nybro, C., & Jeffers, G., et al. (1999). Mental health and incarcerated youth: II. Prevalence and nature of psychopathology. *Journal of Child and Family Studies, 8* (2), 193-204.

Bagley, C., & Mallick, K. (2000). Prediction of sexual, emotional and physical maltreatment and mental health outcomes in a longitudinal cohort of 290 adolescent women. *Child Maltreatment, 5,* 218-226.

Beidel, D.C., Turner, S.M., & Morris, T.L. (1995). A new inventory to assess childhood social anxiety and phobia: The Social Phobia and Anxiety Inventory for Children. *Psychological Assessment, 8,* 235-240.

Beker, J., & Feuerstein, R. (1991). The modifying environment and other environmental perspectives in group care: A conceptual contrast and integration. *Residential Treatment for Children and Youth, 8* (3), 21-36.

Belle, D. (1990). Poverty and women's mental health. *American Psychologist, 45,* 385-389.

Belsky, J. & Cassidy, J. Attachment: Theory and evidence. In M. Rutter & D.F. Hayes (Eds.) *Development through life: A handbook for clinicians* (pp. 373-402). Oxford: Blackwell.

Belsky, J., Fish, M., & Isabella, R. (1991). Continuity and incontinuity in infant negative and positive emotionality: Family antecedent and attachment consequences. *Developmental Psychology, 27,* 421-431.

Bendersky, M., & Lewis, M. (1994). Environmental risk, biological risk, and developmental outcome. *Developmental Psychology, 30,* 484-494.

Biederman, J. (1997). Is there a childhood form of bipolar disorder? *Harvard Mental Health Letter, 13,* 8.

Blackorby, J., & Wagner, M. (1996). Longitudinal post school outcomes of youth with disabilities: Findings from the National Longitudinal Transition Study. *Exceptional Children, 62,* 399-413.

Block, B., & Lefkovitz, P. (1992). *Standards and guidelines for partial hospitalization.* Alexandria, VA: American Association for Partial Hospitalization.

Brollier, C., Shepherd, J., & Markley, K. (1994). Transition from school to community living. *American Journal of Occupational Therapy, 48,* 346-353.

Bundy, A. (1997). Play and playfulness: What to look for. In L.D. Parham & L.S. Fazio (Eds.), *Play in occupational therapy for children* (pp. 52-66). St. Louis: Mosby.

Burke, J.P. (2003). Philosophical basis of human occupation. In P. Kramer, J. Hinojosa, & C.B. Royeen (Eds.), *Perspec-*

tives in human occupation: Participation in life (pp. 32-44). New York: Lippincott Williams & Wilkins.

Burns, B., Hoagwood, K., & Maultsby, K. (1998). Improving outcomes for children and adolescents with serious emotional and behavioral disorders: Current and future directions. In M.H. Epstein, K. Kutash, & A.J. Duchnowski (Eds.), *Outcomes for children and youth with emotional and behavioral disorders and their families: Programs and evaluation best practices* (pp. 686-707). Austin, TX: Pro-Ed.

Carson, R.R., Sitlington, P.L., & Frank, A.R. (1995). Young adulthood for individuals with behavioral disorders: What does it hold? *Behavioral Disorders, 20,* 127-135.

Case-Smith, J. (1994). Defining the specialization of pediatric occupational therapy. *American Journal of Occupational Therapy, 48,* 791-802.

Chafel, J.A., & Hadley, K.G. (2001). Poverty and the well-being of children and families. In C.E. Walker & M.C. Roberts (Eds.), *Handbook of clinical psychology* (pp. 48-71). New York: John Wiley & Sons.

Chess, S. (1997). Temperament: Theory and clinical practice. *Harvard Mental Health Letter, 14,* (5), 5-7.

Chess, S., & Thomas, A. (1983). Dynamics of individual behavioral development. In M.D. Levine, W.B. Carey, A.C. Crocker, & R.T. Gross (Eds.), *Developmental-behavioral pediatrics* (pp. 158-175). Philadelphia: WB Saunders.

Chess, S., & Thomas, A. (1987). *Know your child.* New York: Basic Books.

Cohen, J., Brennan, C., & Sexton, B. (1984). *A social cognitive approach to the prevention of adolescent substance abuse. Intervention I: Sixth grade.* New Haven, CT: Yale University School of Medicine, The Consultation Center.

Constantino, J. (1993). Parents, mental illness, and primary health care of infants and young children. *Zero to Three, 13* (5), 1-10.

Coster, W., Deeney, T., Haltiwanger, J., & Haley, S. (1998). *School Function Assessment.* San Antonio, TX: Psychological Corporation.

Coulton, C., Korbin, J., Su, M., & Chow, J. (1995). Community level factors and child maltreatment rates. *Child Development, 66,* 1262-1276.

Crick, N.R., & Ladd, G.W. (1993). Children's perceptions of their peer experiences: Attributions, loneliness, social anxiety and social avoidance. *Developmental Psychology, 29,* 244-254.

Cronin, A. (2001). Psychosocial and emotional domains. In J. Case-Smith (Ed.). *Occupational therapy for children (4th ed).* (pp. 413-452). St. Louis: Mosby.

Dalton, R., & Forman, M. (1992). *Psychiatric hospitalization of school-age children.* Washington, DC: American Psychiatric Press.

Daly, D., Schmidt, M., Spellman, D., Criste, T., Dinges, K., & Teare, J. (1998). The Boys' Town Residential Treatment Center: Treatment implications and preliminary outcomes. Child and Youth Care Forum, 27 (4), 267-279.

Davidson, D. (2001). Measuring the outcome of Rational Intervention: A behavior management approach for children and adolescents in residential care. Unpublished manuscript.

Davidson, D., & LaVessar, P. (1998). Facilitating adaptive behaviors in school-aged children with psychosocial problems. In J. Case-Smith (Ed.), *AOTA self-study series: Occupational therapy: Making a difference in school-based practice.* Bethesda, MD: American Occupational Therapy Association.

Durrant, M. (1993). *Residential treatment: A cooperative, competency-based approach to therapy and program design.* New York: W.W. Norton.

Ebert, J., Seale, T. & McMahon, E. (2001). Genetic influences on behavior and development. In C.E. Walker & M.C. Roberts (Eds.) Handbook of clinical psychology (3rd ed., pp. 207-244) New York: John Wiley & Sons.

Economic Report of the President. (1998). Washington, DC: U.S. Government Printing Office.

Egeland, B., Sroufe, L., & Erickson, M. (1983). The developmental consequences of different patterns of maltreatment. *Child Abuse and Neglect, 7,* 459-469.

Erker, G., Searight, H.R., Amant, E., & White, P. (1993). Residential versus day treatment for children: A long-term follow-up study. *Child Psychiatry and Human Development, 24,* 31-39.

Feeny, J.A. (1996). Attachment, caregiving, and marital satisfaction. *Personal Relationships, 3,* 401-416.

Florey, L. (1989). Nationally speaking: Treating the whole child: Rhetoric or reality? *American Journal of Occupational Therapy, 43,* 365-368.

Florey, L., & Greene, S. (1997). Play in middle childhood: A focus on children with behavioral and emotional disorders. In L.D. Parham & L.S. Fazio (Eds.), *Play in occupational therapy for children* (pp. 126-143). St. Louis: Mosby.

Frodi, A. (1981). Contribution of child characteristics to child abuse. *American Journal of Mental Deficiency, 85,* 341-345.

Gabarino, J., & Kostelny, K. (1992). Child maltreatment as a community problem. *Child Abuse and Neglect, 16,* 455-464.

Gilbert, B.O., Greening, L., & Dollinger, S.J. (2001). Neurotic disorders in children: Obsessive-compulsive, somatoform, dissociative, and post-traumatic stress disorders. In C.E. Walker & M.C. Roberts (Eds.), *Handbook of clinical psychology* (3rd ed., pp. 414-431). New York: John Wiley & Sons.

Gresham, F., & Elliot, S. (1993). Social skills intervention guide: Systematic approaches to social skills training. *Special Services in the Schools, 8,* 137-158.

Harden, P.W., & Zoccolillo, M. (1997). Disruptive behavior disorders. *Current Opinions in Pediatrics, 9* (4), 339-45.

Harrington, R., Fudge, H., Rutter, M., Pickles, A., & Hill, J. (1990). Adult outcomes of childhood and adolescent depression I. *Archives of General Psychiatry, 47,* 465-473.

Hazan, C., & Zeifman, D. (1999). Pair bonds as attachments. In J. Cassidy & P. Shaver (Eds.), *Handbook of attachment: Theory, research, and clinical applications* (pp. 336-354). New York: Guilford Press.

Hickman, L., & Orentlicher, M. (2001). Transition from school to adult life for students with autism. In H. Miller-Kuhaneck (Ed.), *Autism: A comprehensive occupational therapy approach* (pp. 237-268). Bethesda, MD: American Occupational Therapy Association.

Hofer, M. (1994). Hidden regulators in attachment, separation, and loss. *Monographs for the Society for Research in Child Development, 59,* 192-207, 250-283.

Hoffman-Plotkin, D., & Twentyman, C. (1984). A multimodal assessment of behavioral and cognitive deficits in abused and neglected preschoolers. *Child Development, 55,* 794-802.

Homonoff, E., & Maltz, P. (1991). Developing and maintaining a coordinated system of community-based services to children. *Community Mental Health Journal, 27,* 347-358.

Honjo, S., Mizuno, R., Ajiki, M., Suzuki, A., Nagata, M., & Goto, Y., et al. (1998). Infant temperament and child-rearing stress: Birth order influences. *Early Human Development, 51* (2), 123-135.

Humphry, R. (1995). Families who live in chronic poverty: Meeting the challenge of family-centered services. *American Journal of Occupational Therapy, 49,* 687-693.

Hunter, J., & Powell, G. (1990). Failure to thrive. In C. Semmler & J. Hunter (Eds.), *Early occupational therapy intervention.* Gaithersburg, MD: Aspen Publications.

Individuals with Disabilities Education Act. (1990). Amendments (P.L. 102-119), 20 USC et seq., 1400-1485.

Individuals with Disabilities Education Act. (1997). Amendments (P.L. 105-17), 20 U.S.C. et seq.

Jasinski, J.L., Williams, L.M., & Siegel, J. (2000). Childhood physical and sexual abuse as a risk factor for heavy drinking among African-American women: A prospective study. *Child Abuse and Neglect, 24,* 1061-1071.

Jaudes, P.K., & Diamond, L.J. (1985). The handicapped child and child abuse. *Child Abuse and Neglect, 9,* 341-347.

Jensen, P., Bhatara, V., Vitiello, B., Hoagwood, K., Feil, M., & Burke, L. (1999). Psychoactive medication prescribing practices for U.S. children: Gaps between research and clinical practice. *Journal of the American Academy of Child and Adolescent Psychiatry, 38,* 557-565.

Jones-Webb, R.J., Snowden, L., Herd, D., Short, B., & Hannan, P. (1997). Alcohol-related problems among black, Hispanic, and white men: The contributions of neighborhood poverty. *Journal of Studies on Alcohol, 58,* 539-545.

Kagan, J., & Zentner, M. (1996). Early childhood predictors of adult psychopathology. *Harvard Review of Psychiatry, 3* (6), 341-350.

Katic, A., & Steingard, R.J. (2001). Pharmacotherapy. In C.E. Walker & M.C. Roberts (Eds.), *Handbook of clinical psychology* (3rd ed., pp. 928-951). New York: John Wiley & Sons.

Kennedy, P., Kupst, M., Westman, G., Zaar, C., Pines, R., & Schulman, J. (1990). Use of timeout procedures in a child psychiatry inpatient milieu: Combining dynamic and behavioral approaches. *Child Psychiatry and Human Development, 20* (3), 207-216.

Keogh, B.K. (1986). Temperament and schooling: Meaning of "goodness of fit"? *New Directions in Child Development, 31,* 89-108.

Keogh, B.K., & Burstein, N.D. (1988). Relationship of temperament to preschoolers' interactions with peers and teachers. *Exceptional Child, 54* (5), 456-461.

Knox, S. (1974). A play scale. In M. Reilly (Ed.), *Play as exploratory learning: Studies in curiosity behavior.* Beverly Hills, CA: Sage Publications.

Knox, S. (1997). Development and current use of the Knox Preschool Play Scale. In L.D. Parham & L.S. Fazio (Eds.), *Play in occupational therapy for children* (pp. 35-51). St. Louis: Mosby.

Kolko, D., Bukstein, O., & Barron, J. (1999). Methylphenidate and behavior modification in children with ADHD and co-morbid ODD or CD: Main and incremental effects across settings. *Journal of the American Academy of Child and Adolescent Psychiatry, 38,* 578-586.

Kolko, D.J. (2002). Child physical abuse. In J.E.B. Myers, L. Berliner, J. Briere, C.T. Hendrix, C. Jenny, & T.A. Reid (Eds.), *The APSAC handbook on child maltreatment* (2nd ed.). Beverly Hills, CA: Sage Publications.

Kovacs, M., Feinberg, T.L., Crouse-Novak, M.A., Paulauskas, S.L., & Finkelstein, R. (1984a). Depressive disorders in childhood I. *Archives of General Psychiatry, 41,* 229-237.

Kovacs, M., Feinberg, T.L., Crouse-Novak, M.A., Paulauskas, S.L., & Finkelstein, R. (1984b). Depressive disorders in childhood II. *Archives of General Psychiatry, 41,* 643-649.

Kraemer, G. (1992). A psychobiological theory of attachment. *Behavioral and Brain Sciences, 15,* 493-541.

Law, M., Baptiste, S., Carswell, A., McColl, M., Polatajko, H., & Pollack, N. (1994). *The Canadian Occupational Performance Measure* (2nd ed.). Ottawa, ON: Canadian Association of Occupational Therapy.

Law, M., Cooper, B., Strong, S., Stewart, D., Rigby, P., & Letts, L. (1996). The person-environment-occupation model: A transactive approach to occupational performance. *Canadian Journal of Occupational Therapy, 63,* 9-23.

Leary, M.R., & Kowalski, R.M. (1995). *Social anxiety.* New York: Guilford Press.

Locke, A., Ginsborg, J., & Peers, I. (2003). Development and disadvantage: Implications for the early years and beyond. *International Journal of Language and Communication Disorders, 37,* 3-15.

Maag, J.W., & Katsiyannis, A. (1996). Counseling as a related service for students with emotional or behavioral disorders: Issues and recommendations. *Behavioral Disorders, 21,* 293-305.

Maag, J., & Katsiyannis, A. (1998). Challenges facing successful transition for youths with E/BD. *Behavioral Disorders, 23,* 209-221.

Mabe, P., Riley, W., & Sunde, E. (1989). Survey of admission policies for child and adolescent inpatient services: A national sample. *Child Psychiatry and Human Development, 20,* 99-111.

MacLeod, J., & Nelson, G. (2000). Programs for the promotion of family wellness and the prevention of child maltreatment: A meta-analytic review. *Child Abuse and Neglect, 24,* 1127-1149.

Mailloux, Z., & Roley, S.S. (2001). Sensory integration. In H. Miller-Kuhaneck (Ed.), Autism: A comprehensive occupational therapy approach. (pp. 101-132) Bethesda, MD: American Occupational Therapy Association.

Main, M. (1995). Attachment: Overview, with implications for clinical work. In S. Goldberg, R. Muir, & J. Kerr (Eds.), *Attachment theory: Social, developmental, and clinical perspectives* (pp. 407-474). Hillsdale, NJ: Analytic Press.

Main, M. (1996). Overview of the field of attachment. *Journal of Consulting and Clinical Psychology, 64,* 237-243.

Main, M., & Goldwyn, R. (1984). Predicting rejection of her infant from mother's representation of her own experience: Implications for the abused-abusing intergenerational cycle. *Child Abuse and Neglect, 8,* 203-217.

Main, M., & Soloman, J. (1990). Procedures for identifying infants as disorganized/disoriented during the Ainsworth Strange Situation. In M.T. Greenberg, D. Cicchetti, & E.M. Cummings (Eds.), *Attachment in the preschool years: Theory, research, and intervention* (pp. 121-160). Chicago: University of Chicago Press.

Mandersheid, R., & Sonnenschein, M. (Eds.) (1992). Mental health, United States, 1992. Rockville, MD: U.S. Department of Health and Human Services.

Martin, K., Lloyd, J., Kauffman, J., & Coyne, M. (1995). Teachers' perceptions of educational placement decisions for pupils with emotional and behavioral disorders. *Behavioral Disorders, 20,* 106-117.

McLoyd, V.C. (1990). The impact of economic hardship on black families and children: Psychological distress, parenting, and socioemotional development. *Child Development, 61,* 311-346.

Milling, L.S. (2001). Depression in preadolescents. In C.E. Walker & M.C. Roberts (Eds.)., *Handbook of clinical psychology* (3rd ed., pp. 373-392). New York: John Wiley & Sons.

National Advisory Mental Health Council. (1990). *National plan for research on child and adolescent mental disorders.* Washington, DC: National Institute of Mental Health.

National Clearinghouse on Child Abuse and Neglect Information. (2003). Guidelines and laws for reporting child abuse and neglect: Mandatory reporters of child abuse and neglect. http://www.nccanch.acf.hhs.gov

Nelson, R., & Condrin, J. (1987). A vocational readiness and independent living skills program for psychiatrically impaired adolescents. *Occupational Therapy in Mental Health, 7,* 105-113.

Nielson, C. (1993). Occupational therapy and community mental health: A new and unprecedented turn. *Mental Health Special Interest Newsletter, 16* (3), 1-2.

Nigg, J., & Goldsmith, H. (1998). Developmental psychopathology, personality, and temperament: Reflections on recent behavioral genetics research. *Human Biology, 70* (2), 387-412.

Nordin, V., & Gillberg, C. (1998). The long-term course of autistic disorders: Update on follow-up studies. *Acta Psychiatrica Scandinavica, 97,* 99-108.

Ogata, S., Silk, K., Goodrich, S., Lohr, N., Westen, D., & Hill, E. (1990). Childhood sexual and physical abuse in adult patients with borderline personality disorder. *American Journal of Psychiatry, 147,* 1008-1013.

Osterling, J., Dawson, G., & McPartland, J. (2001). Autism. In C.E. Walker & M.C. Roberts (Eds.), *Handbook of clinical psychology* (3rd ed., pp. 188, 432-452). New York: John Wiley & Sons.

Peloquin, S. (1993). The patient-therapist relationship: Beliefs that shape care. *American Journal of Occupational Therapy, 47,* 935-942.

Pfefferbaum, B. (1997). Posttraumatic stress disorder in children: A review of the past 10 years. *Journal of the American Academy of Child and Adolescent Psychiatry, 36,* 1503-1511.

Pickens, J., & Field, T. (1993). Facial expressivity in infants of depressed mothers. *Developmental Psychology, 29,* 986-988.

Powers, S.W. (2001). Behavior therapy with children. In C.E. Walker & M.C. Roberts (Eds.), *Handbook of clinical psychology* (3rd ed., pp. 825-839). New York: John Wiley & Sons.

Prothro-Stith, D. (1991). *Deadly consequences: How violence is destroying our teenage population and a plan to begin solving the problem.* New York: Harper Collins.

Pruitt, D., & Kiser, L. (1991). Day treatment: Past, present, and future. In M. Lewis (Ed.), *Child and adolescent psychiatry: A comprehensive textbook.* Baltimore: Williams & Wilkins.

Richardson, P. (2002). The school as social context: Social interaction patterns of children with physical disabilities. *American Journal of Occupational Therapy, 56,* 296-304.

Robinson, K., & Rapport, L. (2002). Outcomes of a school-based mental health program for youth with serious emotional disorders. *Psychology in the Schools, 3,* 661-676.

Rothbart, M.K. (1991). Temperament: A developmental framework. In J. Strelau & A. Angleitner (Eds.), *Explorations in temperament: International perspectives on theory and measurement* (pp. 2235-2260). London: Plenum Press.

Rothe, E.M., & Castellanos, D. (2001). Anxiety disorders in children and adolescents. In H.B. Vance & A.J. Pumariega (Eds.), *Clinical assessment of child and adolescent behavior* (pp. 383-412). New York: John Wiley & Sons.

Sabatino, D.A., Vance, H.B., & Fuller, G. (2001). Pervasive developmental disorders. In H.B. Vance & A.J. Pumariega (Eds.), *Clinical assessment of child and adolescent behavior* (pp. 188-230). New York: John Wiley & Sons.

Sabatino, D.A., Webster, B., & Vance, H.B. (2001). Childhood mood disorders: History, characteristics, diagnosis, and treatment. In H.B. Vance & A.J. Pumariega (Eds.), *Clinical assessment of child and adolescent behavior* (pp. 413-449). New York: John Wiley & Sons.

Schkade, J., & Schultz, S. (1992). Occupational adaptation: Toward a holistic approach for contemporary practice. I. *American Journal of Occupational Therapy, 46,* 829-837.

Schultz, S. (1992). School-based occupational therapy for students with behavioral disorders. *Occupational Therapy in Health Care, 8,* 173-196.

Schultz, S. (2003 Sept 8). AOTA continuing education article: Psychosocial occupational therapy in schools. *OT Practice, 8* (16), CE-1-CE-8.

Schultz, S., & Schkade, J. (1992). Occupational adaptation: Toward a holistic approach for contemporary practice. II. *American Journal of Occupational Therapy, 46,* 917-925.

Sedlak, A.J., & Broadhurst, D.D. (1996). *Executive summary of the Third National Incidence Study of Child Abuse and Neglect.* Washington, DC: U.S. Department of Health and Human Services, National Center on Child Abuse and Neglect.

Shure, M., & Spivack, G. (1982). Interpersonal problem-solving in young children: A cognitive approach to prevention. *American Journal of Community Psychology, 10,* 341-356.

Silverman, W.K., & Ginsberg, G.S. (1998). Anxiety disorders. In T.H. Ollendick & M. Hersen (Eds.), *Handbook of child psychopathology* (3rd ed., pp. 239-268). New York: Plenum Press.

Spreat, S., & Jampol, R. (1997). Residential services for children and adolescents. In R.T. Ammerman & M. Hersen (Eds.), *Intervention in the real world context: Handbook of prevention and treatment with children and adolescents* (pp. 106-133). New York: John Wiley & Sons.

Starr, R.H. Jr., Dubowitz, H., & Bush, B.A. (1990). The epidemiology of child maltreatment. In R.T. Ammerman & M. Hersen (Eds.), *Children at risk: An evaluation of factors contributing to child abuse and neglect* (pp. 149-165). New York: Plenum Press.

Steele, B. (1997). Psychodynamic factors in child abuse. In R.E. Helfer & R.S. Kempe (Eds.), *The battered child* (5th ed., pp. 73-106). Chicago: University of Chicago Press.

Stein, F. (1995). *Residential treatment of adolescents and children: Issues, principles, and techniques.* Chicago: Nelson-Hall Publishers.

Sullivan, P.M., & Knutson, J.F. (2000). Maltreatment and disabilities: A population-based epidemiological study. *Child Abuse and Neglect, 24,* 1257-1273.

Thomas, A., Chess, S., & Birch, H. (1968). *Temperament and behavior disorders in children.* New York: New York University Press.

Thompson, R. (2002). The view from research: The roots of school readiness in social and emotional development. *Kauffman Early Education Exchange, 1* (1), 8-29.

Thomsen, P., & Mikkelsen, H. (1995). Course of OCD in children and adolescents. *Journal of the American Academy of Child and Adolescent Psychiatry, 34,* 1432-1440.

Townsend, S., Carey, P., Hollins, N., Helfrich, C., Blondis, M., & Hoffman, A., et al. (2001). *Occupational Therapy Psychosocial Assessment of Learning.* Chicago: Model of Occupational Therapy Products.

Tuma, J. (1989). Mental health services for children: The state of the art. *American Psychologist, 44,* 188-199.

U.S. Department of Education. (1993). Fifteenth annual report to Congress on the implementation of the Individuals with Disabilities Education Act. Washington, DC: U.S. Department of Education.

U.S. Department of Health and Human Services, Administration on Children, Youth, and Families (1997). *Annual report to Congress on the evaluation of the comprehensive community mental health services for children and their families program.* Washington, DC Retrieved on June 15, 2004 at http://www.mentalhealth.samhsa.gov/cmhs/surgeongeneral/

U.S. Department of Health and Human Services, Administration on Children, Youth and Families (2003). *Child maltreatment 2001.* Washington, DC: U.S. Government Printing Office.

U.S. Department of Health and Human Services. (2004). Comprehensive community mental health services program for children and their families. Washington, DC: Substance Abuse and Mental Health Services Administration.

U.S. Public Health Service (1999). *Mental health: A report of the Surgeon General.* Washington, DC: U.S. Public Health Service. Web site: www.surgeongeneral.gov/library/mentalhealth/home.html

van den Boom, D. (1990). Preventive intervention and the quality of mother-infant interaction and infant exploration in irritable infants. In W. Koops, H. Soppe, J.L. van der Linden, P.C.M. Molenaar, & J.J.F. Schroots (Eds.), *Developmental psychology behind the dikes* (pp. 249-270). Amsterdam: Eburon.

van Ijzendoorn, M., Juffer, F., & Duyvesteyn, M. (1995). Breaking the intergenerational cycle of insecure attachment: A review of the effects of attachment-based interventions on maternal sensitivity and infant security. *Journal of Child Psychology and Psychiatry, 36,* 225-248.

VanderVen, K. (1995). "Point and level systems": Another way to fail children and youth. *Child and Youth Care Forum, 24,* 345-367.

Vaughn, B.R., & Bost, K.K. (1999). Attachment and temperament: redundant, independent, or interactive influences on interpersonal adaptation and personality development? In J. Cassidy & P. Shaver (Eds.), *Handbook of attachment: Theory, research, and clinical applications* (pp. 198-225). New York: Guilford Press.

Verdugo, M.A., Bermejo, B.G., & Fuertes, J. (1995). The maltreatment of intellectually handicapped children and adolescents. *Child Abuse and Neglect, 19,* 205-215.

Vondra, J.I. (1990). Sociological and ecological factors. In R.T. Ammerman & M. Hersen (Eds.), *Children at risk: An evaluation of factors contributing to child abuse and neglect* (pp. 149-165). New York: Plenum Press.

Wald, R.L., & Knutson, J.F. (2000). Childhood disciplinary experiences reported by adults with craniofacial anomalies. *Child Abuse and Neglect, 24,* 1623-1627.

Walker, R., & Bunsen, T. (1995). After high school: The status of youth with emotional and behavioral disorders. *Career Development of Exceptional Individuals, 18,* 97-107.

Waters, E., & Stroufe, A. (1983). Social competence as a developmental construct. *Developmental Review, 3,* 79-97.

Weinberg, N., Rahdert, E., Colliver, J., & Glantz, M. (1998). Adolescent substance abuse: A review of the past 10 years. *Journal of the American Academy of Child and Adolescent Psychiatry, 37* (3), 252-261.

Weissberg, R. (1985). Developing effective social problem-solving programs for the classroom. In B. Schneider, K.H. Rubin, & J. Ledingham (Eds.), *Peer relationships and social skills in childhood* (Vol. 2). New York: Springer-Verlag.

Weissberg, R., Caplan, M., & Bennetto, L. (1988). *The Yale–New Haven problem solving (SPS) program for young adolescents.* New Haven, CT: Yale University.

Williamson, G. (1993). Enhancing the social competence of children with learning disabilities. *Sensory Integration Special Interest Section Newsletter, 16,* 1-2.

Wing, L., & Potter, D. (2002). The epidemiology of autistic spectrum disorders: Is the prevalence rising? *Mental Retardation and Developmental Disabilities Research Reviews. 8* (3), 151-161.

Wolfner, G., & Gelles, R. (1993). A profile of violence toward children: A national study. *Child Abuse and Neglect, 17,* 197-212.

Zametin, A.J., & Ernst, M. (1999). Review article: Problems in the management of attention deficit–hyperactivity disorder. *New England Journal of Medicine, 340* (1), 40-46.

Feeding Intervention

Jane Case-Smith ▪ Ruth Humphry

CHAPTER OBJECTIVES

1 Describe children's participation in mealtimes.
2 Define factors that influence feeding, eating, and mealtime occupations.
3 Understand the sequence of typical feeding and self-feeding skills.
4 Describe how feeding contributes to and reflects the parent-child relationship.
5 Analyze how a disability can interfere with feeding interactions.
6 Explain the evaluation of and intervention for oral sensory and motor impairments as they affect feeding skills of children.
7 Define and describe swallowing disorders and intervention for swallowing problems.
8 Describe common oral structural problems, and explain interventions to promote early feeding in children with these problems.
9 Describe interventions that enhance the child's ability to self-feed and to drink from a cup.
10 Identify and explain the nutritional aspects of feeding and the nature of collaboration with nutritionists.
11 Explain the behavioral issues that interfere with feeding and intervention strategies to improve mealtime behaviors.

Eating meals is an essential occupation that occurs several times a day and provides children with nutritional intake and learning and interactional experiences that affect every aspect of the young child's life. Mealtimes create a temporal organization to the day and give the child opportunities to practice object manipulation, experience new sensations, and learn how to communicate needs and desires. The interaction during feeding helps the parent bond with the child and helps the child trust in and rely on the parent to meet his or her needs. For young children, eating food occurs as a co-occupation with caregiving adults who select the types of food, amount presented, time of eating, and method of feeding. The caregiver bases these carefully made selections on what he or she believes is age-appropriate performance, what is nutritionally sound, and what he or she values as cultural tradition.

Children experience problems in feeding for various reasons. Premature infants and those born with congenital problems such as heart defects may lack the ability to organize behavior or the energy to suck effectively. Other children born with oral anomalies, such as cleft palate, require parents and health care professionals to implement compensation strategies so that the child can ingest food. Children who have underlying problems with motor control (e.g., cerebral palsy) or difficulty learning everyday skills (e.g., mental retardation) can experience associated problems with eating or mastering utensil use. Other children have delayed feeding skills secondary to problems that the parent experiences in presenting food or understanding what to expect of young children at mealtime. To plan effective interventions for a child's problem in feeding, the therapist synthesizes information about the mealtime environment, performance of the child and caregivers, and relationship of the child's performance to an eating task. Given the complexity of performing this occupation and the interactive effects of the occupation, person, and environment described in Chapters 3 and 4, the occupational therapist works at many levels to help a child with feeding problems.

The first section of this chapter describes developmental changes in the acquisition of eating and feeding skills. Occupational performance of eating and feeding for typically developing children goes through major transformations in the first 3 years, starting with total dependency to independence in using spoons and forks and consuming various foods. The first section also presents a general framework for the evaluation of feeding and eating problems. The next section describes evaluation and intervention for specific sensory, motor, and structural problems that delay or interfere with the development of eating skills. The third section presents interventions to promote self-feeding. Nutritional and interactional issues are discussed.

PARTICIPATION IN MEALTIME

Mealtime is typically a family time that provides a context for physical, cognitive, and emotional nourishment of all members. Meals provide a temporal organization to the day, dividing it into periods where certain activities end and new activities begin. They are an important part of everyone's routines and generally afford a time for rest, communication, and socialization. When parents feed their children, they communicate symbolic and emotional meanings while meeting a need for nourishment (DeVault, 1991). Many adults believe that to nourish the child is to nurture. Mealtimes constitute an essential aspect of family life, where members bond, learn to communicate and share, and practice their cultural routines.

Caregivers and children have both shared and individual roles during mealtime. Expectations for the child at mealtime are that he or she remains seated, attends to the caregiver, participates in self-feeding and eating, communicates with the caregivers and others, and follows the family's routines. The caregiver is expected to provide nourishing food in sufficient quantities to satisfy, to assist in feeding young children, to communicate and interact with other family members present, and to establish mealtime norms and routines.

A child's mealtime participation changes from infancy to adulthood. Initially, during infancy, the parents are occupied in feeding and holding tasks, and later, during preschool/school age years, in communicating or disciplining. Almost all parents make efforts to create a pleasant and relaxing family time during meals. These efforts are not always successful when a child has a disability affecting eating performance. The child's temperament, health, disposition and the parent's health and mood are among the factors that contribute to mealtime social interactions.

Contextual Influences on Mealtime

Family composition can determine who is present at mealtime. The child may be fed in an isolated setting alone with his mother or may sit with all family members around the dinner table. Large families may have chaotic or noisy mealtimes. Such an environment creates difficulties for a child with hypersensitivities or high sensory arousal. Caregivers may not notice that a child has poor intake when many are present at the dinner table. A positive aspect of a large family is that extra hands are available to feed a child who needs assistance. Sometimes children who need a quieter environment or who need

maximal assistance are fed separately before or after other family members. Sometimes only one family member can feed the child successfully. When a child only has one feeder, the responsibility for feeding around the clock can be stressful and exhausting over time.

Cultural beliefs and values also influence the role of children during mealtime. In some cultures, children are fed by a caregiver through the preschool years, while in others infants are encouraged to self-feed despite the mess that results. For example, Puerto Rican mothers continue to feed their children to significantly later ages than Anglo mothers (Schulze, Harwood, & Schoelmerich, 2001). The Puerto Rican mothers who feed their children as toddlers emphasize maintaining respectful relations and appropriate interpersonal relationships during the meal. In contrast, the Anglo mothers who allow self-feeding at 12 months of age emphasize the young child's independence and autonomy (Schulze et al.). Cultural beliefs also affect the amounts and types of food that parents believe their children should eat. In another example, southern African American children are fed sweetened tea to supplement their diet, because parents believe that physical and cognitive ability are enhanced by the tea (Lee, Murry, Brody, & Parker, 2002). The tea may replace other drinks (e.g., milk) that have more vitamins and nutrients.

A *family's socioeconomic status* also influences mealtime. Families in poverty may not have sufficient food or may eat less expensive foods that tend to be high in carbohydrates and fat. Parents who are not educated may not know about nutrition and nutritionally balanced diets. Although chronic undernutrition is rare in the United States, it has been estimated that as many as 8% of 12-year-olds experience food inadequacy (Kleinman et al., 1998), almost all of whom can be categorized as having low socioeconomic status.

Single mothers are particularly at risk for falling into a low socioeconomic status. A single mother may experience more stress and have less structure/routine, such that mealtime routines with her child are not established. The child may graze throughout the day when hungry, eating whatever happens to be available. Single mothers may not have access to information on child development and feeding. These mothers may feed their young children inappropriate foods or foods with poor nutritional value.

All parents make decisions about how to feed their children and the appropriate amount of flexibility based on what they believe the child should learn from the situation. In a descriptive study, Humphry and Thigpen-Beck (1997) asked parents whether they approve of flexibility with a child when he or she refuses to eat a dish. *Social contexts* were important in understanding how different parents respond. Older, more educated parents were more inclined to be flexible and change what they fed the child. Parents who believed that good behavior and obedience are important were less likely to accept flexibility. A larger agenda often influences the type of feeding strategy that the parents use and how parents interpret the child's behaviors at mealtime (Humphry & Thigpen-Beck, 1998).

Personal Influences on Mealtime

Personal factors of the child that influence mealtime include health, eating skills, and communication/interaction skills. This chapter describes how health problems and delayed or deficit oral motor skills affect feeding. Occupational therapists often provide intervention when feeding problems are caused by a child's health problems, sensory processing difficulties, or neurodevelopmental delays/deficits.

The caregiver's personal factors may also influence mealtime and the child's ability to feed. Initially mealtime is like a dance between the caregiver and child. It begins when the child signals a cue that he or she is hungry or ready to eat. The caregiver responds to the child's cues of hunger, readiness to take a bite, and indications of distress and satiation. The child responds to the parent's gestures and verbalizations with eye contact, smiles, and verbalizations indicating what he wants and how he feels. When the caregiver does not take pleasure in feeding a child, the task can lose much of its meaning and becomes a job (Brazelton, 1993), changing the mealtime experience for the adult and child. For example, some caregivers are anxious about feeding, and tend to be controlling when the child is a poor eater. The caregiver may have preset ideas about how much the child should eat and therefore force food on the child or become disappointed with the child's input. A controlling parent may find that the child desires control of what she eats, and a battle of wills may result.

TYPICAL DEVELOPMENTAL SEQUENCE OF MEALTIME PARTICIPATION, FEEDING, AND EATING

Progression of Mealtime Participation

In the first months of life (e.g., birth to 6 months), parents feed their infant in their arms. Feeding is generally a time for bonding, characterized by close holding and warmth, eye contact, and nonverbal communication between parents and child. The parent strokes and touches the child who often grasps the mother's breast or hair or father's shirt. Although the parent decides what the infant eats, the infant typically controls the pace of the meal and when feeding ends. When this interaction is less than positive, the parent may compensate by

trying to control more of the interaction. When first mealtimes are positive, the interactions contribute to bonding and development of the parent-child relationship.

Feeding and eating become more independent between 7 and 24 months. The 7-month-old infant can finger-feed and by 18 months is attempting to use a spoon and cup. With this emerging independence, mealtimes become messier and more chaotic. Although the parent selects the foods to give the child, the child can choose to eat those foods or not. During this age range, the toddler is offered a greater variety of foods. The parent no longer holds the child who is now in a high chair or booster chair. The toddler explores his or her foods and enjoys making a mess. Most toddlers explore the sensory qualities of foods with their hands and tongues. Parents encourage their child's efforts at self-feeding and allow him or her to try different foods. They also limit foods that are difficult to chew and digest. Eating remains a time for communication, which is now both verbal and nonverbal. Parents verbally describe the child's foods to provide a rich source of new vocabulary; food names are often some of the first words toddlers speak.

Once the child is 2 and is feeding relatively independently, he or she usually becomes a full participant in family mealtime. The child sits at the table where she or he can model the actions and behaviors of other members. The preschooler begins to eat some or all of the foods that other family members are eating. Family members model appropriate feeding behaviors and instruct the child in self-feeding rules. For most preschool children, mealtimes are enjoyable, social times, where parents attempt to create a positive, relaxing environment and emphasis is placed on communication and togetherness. Disability can have a negative effect on mealtime and accomplishing these outcomes. Pressure on preschoolers to eat more, eat neatly, or eat certain foods may create anxiety about eating and may be harmful in the long run by preventing the child from enjoying eating and viewing mealtime as a positive social event.

Development of Eating and Self-Feeding Skills

As with other developing occupations, a child's eating and self-feeding skills emerge from physical maturation, changing performance components, new challenging tasks that the caregiver presents, and feedback about success in performance. When helping children develop eating skills, the occupational therapist considers maturity of the child's underlying skills, such as motor control of the tongue, but the relationship of motor performance to quality of feeding is not hierarchic (i.e., the maturation of the specific skill does not always come first with a subsequent change in occupational performance). Rather there is an interaction between eating occupations and specific process and motor skills. For example, underlying control of the lips to remove food from the spoon depends to some extent on maturation of nerves controlling oral motor actions (Wolf & Glass, 1992). Understanding a spoon's function in self-feeding requires cognitive abilities in recognition and classification of objects. The child's motivation to self-feed may improve the quality of oral motor control and promote learning of form and space. Practice with a spoon enables discovery of new patterns of lip movement, which contributes to the child's self-feeding skills. Concurrently, through manipulation of the spoon into the mouth, the child alters his or her understanding of the nature of tools. A child challenged to change patterns of feeding before he or she is ready to apply new motor or cognitive abilities will become distressed and uncooperative with meals. Thus, therapists must consider the child's readiness to learn new eating skills before introducing new tasks.

The occupation of feeding consists of different phases as the child progresses from breast-feeding to self-feeding a complete meal of table foods with utensils. During early infancy, changes occur in the method of the infant's sucking from a nipple. Typically, changes in eating and self-feeding demonstrate a sequence of new behaviors as parents present new feeding challenges. Because the timing to introduce new eating experiences varies from one family to the next and typically developing children mature at varying rates, the range in the ages when new skills in feeding are demonstrated is great.

The child's occupational performance in feeding depends on his or her dynamical integration of motor, cognitive, and social/interactive skills, which are also developing. Although this chapter focuses on intervention to promote oral motor skill development, consuming food in the context of a social experience *organizes behavior and motivates the child.* In designing intervention, the occupational therapist considers occupational performance (feeding) and underlying systems that contribute to performance (oral motor, sensory, neuromotor, cognitive, and social/interactive abilities).

TYPICAL DEVELOPMENT OF ORAL STRUCTURES

Intact oral structures and cranial nerves are prerequisites for eating and drinking. Different actions of the mouth develop concurrently as the child gains control of jaw, tongue, cheek, and lip movement. The anatomic structures of the mouth and throat change significantly in the first 12 months. The growth and maturation of the oral structures allow for development of more mature feeding patterns. Table 14-1 lists the oral structures involved in feeding.

The newborn has a small oral cavity filled with fatty cheeks and the tongue. When the nipple is placed inside the mouth, the tight fit enables the infant to easily compress the nipple and achieve automatic suction. The negative pressure that automatically occurs during sucking movements of the jaw expresses liquid from the nipple (Morris & Klein, 2000). Therefore the full-term, healthy newborn is successful in sucking from a breast or bottle nipple.

The structures in the infant's throat are also in close proximity to one another. The infant's epiglottis and soft palate are in direct approximation. As a result, the liquid from the nipple safely passes from the base of the tongue to the esophagus. During swallowing, the larynx elevates and the epiglottis falls over it to protect the trachea. Therefore aspiration is unlikely before 4 months of age, and the infant can safely feed in a reclined position.

As the infant grows, the neck elongates and the relationship of the oral and throat structures changes. The oral cavity becomes larger and more open. The fatty tongue becomes thin and muscular, and the cheeks lose much of their fatty padding. With the increase in oral

TABLE 14-1　Functions of Oral Structures in Feeding

Structure	Parts	Function During Feeding
Oral cavity	Hard and soft palate, tongue, fat pads of cheeks, upper and lower jaws, and teeth	Contains the food during drinking and chewing and provides for initial mastication before swallowing
Pharynx	Base of tongue, buccinator, oropharynx, tendons, and hyoid bone	Funnels food into the esophagus and allows food and air to share space; the pharynx is a space common to both functions
Larynx	Epiglottis and false and true vocal folds	Valve to the trachea that closes during swallowing
Trachea	Tube below the larynx and cartilaginous rings	Allows air to flow into bronchi and lungs
Esophagus	Thin and muscular esophagus	Carries food from the pharynx, through the diaphragm, and into the stomach; at rest, it is collapsed and distends as food passes through it

Modified from Wolf, L.S., & Glass, R.P. (1992). *Feeding and swallowing disorders in infancy: Assessment and management.* Tucson, AZ: Therapy Skill Builders.

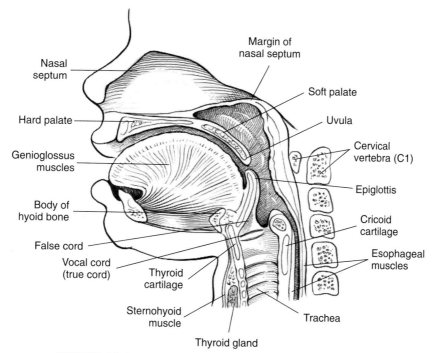

FIGURE 14-1 Anatomic structures of the mouth and throat.

cavity space, the tongue, lips, and cheeks must provide greater control of liquid or food within the mouth. New sucking patterns emerge to enable the infant to handle liquid without the structural advantages of early infancy. These include up-and-down movements of the tongue to express liquids from the nipple. The increasing oral space also provides room to masticate food and to move the tongue in the rolling pattern required during chewing (Wolf & Glass, 1992).

As the infant approaches 12 months of age, the hyoid, epiglottis, and larynx descend, creating space between these structures and the base of the tongue. The hyoid and larynx become more mobile during swallowing, elevating with each swallow. The infant requires greater coordination of these structures during the suck-swallow-breathe sequence. With the elongation of the pharynx, feeding in a reclined position creates a greater possibility of aspiration. The pull of gravity in a reclined position can interfere with the control an infant needs to move the liquid to the entrance of the esophagus. Figure 14-1 shows the structures of the mouth and pharynx of the infant.

TYPICAL ORAL MOTOR DEVELOPMENT ASSOCIATED WITH EATING SKILLS

The development of sucking, drinking, biting, and chewing is highly related to the overall motor development of the child. The development of more mature oral patterns occurs as the child has changing nutritional needs, demonstrates interest in self-feedings, and expands communication efforts. The changes in jaw, tongue, lip, and cheek movements are associated with the development of skills in (1) sucking and drinking; (2) coordinating sucking, swallowing, and breathing; and (3) biting and chewing. Table 14-2 summarizes the sequence of eating skill development.

Sucking and Drinking Skills

The sucking reflex is present in the fetus and predominates as the method of oral feeding through the first 8 to 10 months of life. Sucking patterns differ when the child is sucking on a pacifier (nonnutritive) compared with sucking on a bottle nipple (nutritive). The nonnutritive pattern is rapid and rhythmic, usually about two sucks per second. The nutritive pattern is rhythmic but is characterized by a burst-and-pause pattern. This pattern allows the infant to breathe and rest between sucking bursts.

Premature infants typically are fed by nonoral means through 33 weeks' gestational age. Before this age, the infant demonstrates a rhythmic nonnutritive sucking pattern, but sucking strength and endurance limit oral feeding. In a healthy premature infant of 35 weeks' gestational age, the jaw and tongue movements are sufficiently strong to allow for oral feeding at least part of the time. The rate of sucking, the force of suction or compression, and the length of time that the infant eats determines the amount of liquid taken in. Two characteristics that are important to feeding efficiency are the

TABLE 14-2 Developmental Sequence of Eating Skills

Age	Type of Food	Sucking/Drinking Skills	Swallowing	Biting and Chewing
1 month	Liquids only.	Uses a suckling or sucking pattern.	Tongue moves in extension-retraction to swallow.	Does not bite or chew.
3 months	Liquids or pureed.	Uses a suckling or sucking pattern. Tongue moves in extension/retraction.	Uses a primitive suckle-swallow pattern. Sequences 20 or more sucks from bottle/breast.	Rarely exhibited, may demonstrate reflexive biting.
5 months	Eats pureed foods. Formula or breast milk remain primary source of nutrition.	Continues to use sucking pattern. Tongue moves up and down. One sip at a time taken from cup.	Choking on breast or bottle is rare. Takes pureed food well.	Uses a primitive phasic bite-and-release pattern. Biting is not yet controlled or sustained. Jaw moves up and down in munching and biting.
6 months	Liquids and pureed foods.	No longer loses liquids during sucking. Uses a suckling or sucking pattern for cup drinking. Tongue moves up and down on bottle but in extension-retraction with cup. Has difficulty drinking from a cup and loses liquids.	Swallows thicker pureed foods and some lumpy foods. Uses long sequences of sucking, swallowing, and breathing with breast or bottle. May cough or choke when using a cup.	The up and down jaw movements are more variable and less automatic. Uses diagonal rotary movement when moving the tongue to the side. Some tongue lateralization when food is placed to the side. Lips help to hold the food in place for chewing.
9 months	Soft foods, mashed table foods.	Strong sucking pattern, no liquid loss.	Uses long sequences of sucking during cup drinking. Takes one to three sucks before stopping to swallow or breathe.	Munches with diagonal movements as food is transferred from center to sides. Voluntary biting on food and objects. Lips are active with jaw during chewing. Uses lateral movements to transfer food from the center to sides of mouth.
12 months	Easily chewed foods including meats, coarsely chopped foods.	Most of liquid is now from a cup. Uses a sucking pattern (up and down tongue movement). May lose liquid when using a cup.	Swallows liquids and semisolid foods with tongue tip elevation. At times exhibits tongue protrusion. Lips are closed during swallow.	Controlled, sustained bite with soft cookie. Begins rotary chewing movements. Lips are active during chewing. Easily transfers food from the center to both sides.
18 months	Coarsely chopped table foods, including most meats and raw vegetables.	Mature sucking patterns. Jaw is stable when drinking from the cup.	Uses tongue-tip elevation with swallowing. Swallows solid foods with easy lip closure. No loss of food.	Uses a controlled sustained bite on a hard cookie. Chews with lips closed. Demonstrates rotary chewing.
24 months	All table foods, all foods except those with skins, very tough meats, or foods that break into large pieces.	Adult-like sucking patterns: up-and-down tongue movements.	No liquid loss. Swallows solid foods with easy lip closure. Tongue-tip elevation used for swallowing.	During chewing, can transfer food from both sides of the mouth. Lips are closed during chewing. Uses circular rotary movements when transferring food across the midline from one side to the other.

Ages are approximate and may vary among infants.
Adapted from Glass, R., & Wolf, L. (1998). Feeding and oral motor skills. In J. Case-Smith (Ed.), *Pediatric occupational therapy and early intervention*. Boston, MA: Butterworth Heinemann; Morris, S.E., & Klein, M. (2000). *Prefeeding skills* (2nd ed.). San Antonio, TX: Therapy Skill Builders.

rhythm of sucking and the type of suction (i.e., negative pressure for expression of liquid) that the infant is able to achieve and sustain over time (Daniels, Devlieger, Casaer, & Eggermount, 1986). Wolf and Glass (1992) explained that both compression and suction are needed to express liquid. The infant achieves these aspects of feeding through sucking patterns that include sealing the lips around the nipple and moving the tongue in simultaneous extension and retraction and up-and-down movements. By 36 weeks' gestational age, the typical premature infant takes all food by mouth and uses a sucking pattern similar to that of the full-term infant.

The full-term infant (born at 40 weeks' gestation) has strong oral reflexes that enable him or her to take in liquid nutrition without difficulty. Given tactile stimulation near the mouth, the hungry infant's rooting reflex induces the infant to turn his or her head, thereby allowing him or her to latch onto any potential nutritional source. The infant also exhibits a gag and cough reflex to protect the airway from the intake of liquid.

The sucking pattern of the full-term infant is rhythmic, sustained, and efficient, diminishing appropriately with satiation. The pattern of each infant is unique and varies in efficiency of sucking according to the infant's level of fatigue and hunger. Most infants complete an oral feeding in 20 to 25 minutes.

The infant's first sucking pattern is termed *suckling* (Morris & Klein, 2000). A forward-backward movement of the tongue characterizes this pattern. Jaw opening and closing accompany this rhythmic back-and-forth tongue movement (Yokochi, 1997). The tongue typically extends but not beyond the border of the lips.

Suckling predominates in the first 4 months. The pattern may cause slight liquid loss and intake of air and is primarily observed in the second and third months of life, after the infant's physiologic flexion has disappeared and before the infant has established mature oral motor control. At 4 months of age, the tongue begins to move in an up-and-down direction that characterizes a true sucking pattern. The wide jaw excursions of the young infant are reduced. Less liquid is lost, and suction on the nipple increases.

The 6-month-old infant demonstrates strong up-and-down tongue movement with minimal jaw excursion during sucking. Jaw stability increases and allows for better control of tongue movement. The lip seal is good, such that the infant does not lose liquid during sucking on a nipple. Many cultures in the United States introduce the cup to the infant at 6 months of age (usually a sipper cup with a spout). When first presented a cup, the infant will try to continue to use a suckling pattern so the jaw continues to move up and down and the tongue moves forward and backward in the mouth. The wide jaw excursions result in liquid loss. Some coughing may occur as the infant first attempts this skill.

By 9 months of age, the infant continues to feed from the bottle using strong sucking patterns. Long sequences of continuous sucks occur when the infant drinks from the cup. The jaw is not consistently stable on the rim of the cup, so the infant is messy drinking from a cup.

At 12 months of age, many infants make the transition from the bottle to the cup for drinking during mealtime but continue to bottle-feed at other times. Jaw stability for supporting the cup's rim remains incomplete. The tongue may protrude slightly beneath the cup to provide additional stability (Morris & Klein, 2000). For the first time, tongue tip elevation occurs during swallowing.

With practice the infant uses an up-and-down sucking pattern to obtain liquids from a cup. He or she bites on the rim of the cup to obtain external jaw stabilization. The upper lip closes on the edge of the cup to provide a seal for drinking. The tongue elevates to bring the liquid into the mouth.

At 24 months of age, the child can efficiently drink from a cup. He or she uses up-and-down tongue movements and tip elevation. Internal jaw stabilization emerges so that the jaw appears still. Therefore, the rim of the cup rests on the stable jaw, and biting on the cup's rim is no longer necessary. The child swallows with easy lip closure and does not lose liquids from the cup. Lengthy suck-swallow sequences occur.

Coordination of Sucking, Swallowing, and Breathing

As the infant demonstrates increasing control of jaw, tongue, and lip movement, he or she also learns to coordinate and sequence oral movements into rhythmic patterns of sucking, swallowing, and breathing. The coordination of the oral structures as they work together to prepare and swallow food is perhaps more important to the feeding process than development of control of any one oral structure.

The 1-month-old infant demonstrates one suck to one swallow at the beginning of the feeding. He or she can sequence two to three sucks per swallow after his or her initial hunger has been satiated. By 3 or 4 months of age, the infant sequences 20 or more sucks from the breast or bottle before pausing. Swallowing occurs intermittently (after four to five sucks) and without pausing. Breathing slows during sucking and occurs within and between sucking sequences. Occasionally the infant may cough or choke when he or she momentarily loses coordination of sucking, swallowing, and breathing.

As the infant approaches 12 months of age, these long sequences continue in bottle-feeding or breast-feeding. When the infant begins to drink from the cup, he or she loses this coordination. At 9 months of age, the infant stops to swallow or breathe after one to three sucks from the cup. By 12 months of age, swallowing follows sucking without pausing and the infant takes three continuous swallows before pausing. Swallowing is efficient (without coughing) when liquid flow presents at an appropriate rate.

By 15 to 18 months of age, the infant has excellent coordination of sucking, swallowing, and breathing. When drinking from a cup, the infant's swallowing follows sucking without pauses. The infant performs at least three suck-swallow sequences before pausing, and the amount of liquid swallowed each time increases to at least 1 ounce. Coughing or choking rarely occurs.

Biting and Chewing

The first *biting* or *chewing* movements of the infant are reflexive. At 4 to 5 months of age, the infant uses a rhythmic, stereotypic, phasic bite-and-release pattern on almost any substance placed in the mouth (e.g., a soft cookie, cracker, or toy). Jaw movements are up and down rather than diagonal. When the phasic bite-and-release pattern is used in a repeated rhythm, it is termed a *munching pattern*. A munching pattern is characterized by jaw movement in the vertical direction and tongue movement in extension and retraction (lateralization has not yet developed). Therefore, the munching pattern appears as an effective solution when the infant receives pureed foods or soft foods that quickly dissolve.

By 7 to 8 months of age, the infant demonstrates some variability in the up-and-down munching pattern. He or she begins to use some diagonal jaw movement when the texture of the food requires variation in jaw movement. The infant continues to use the phasic bite-and-release pattern when he or she bites a cookie, thus the jaw closes abruptly on the cookie and then the infant sucks on it. The jaw holds the cookie, but the infant cannot yet successfully bite through it. A bite is obtained by breaking off the piece while the jaw is held closed on the cookie. When the infant receives food on a spoon, the upper lip actively cleans it from the spoon. The lips become more active during sucking and maintaining the food within the mouth.

By 9 months of age, the infant handles pureed and soft food well. He or she continues to use a munching pattern; however, the vertical up-and-down jaw movements now include diagonal movements. The infant transfers the food from the center of the mouth to the side using lateral tongue movements. These same lateral movements keep the food on the side during munching, making that process effective in mastication of soft or mashed table food. The lips are active during chewing, so they make contact as the jaw moves up and down.

Rotary chewing movements begin at approximately 12 months of age, made possible as the child gains jaw stability and controlled mobility. This control is also exhibited when the child demonstrates sustained, well-graded bite on soft cookies. The tongue is active in chewing by moving food from the center of the mouth to the sides, licking food from the lips, and demonstrating tip elevation on occasion. The infant is able to retrieve food on the lower lip by drawing it inward into the mouth.

The infant at 18 months of age demonstrates well-coordinated rotary chewing. He or she is able to chew soft meat and various table foods. The child can control and sustain bite and can bite off a piece of a hard cookie or pretzel. The tongue becomes increasingly mobile and efficiently moves food within the mouth.

At 24 months of age, the child can eat most meats and raw vegetables. The child can grade and sustain the bite and can bite on hard foods with ease. Circular rotary jaw movements that characterize mature chewing are present. The tongue transfers food from one side of the mouth to the other using a rolling movement. The tongue moves skillfully to clear the lips and gums. Lip closure during chewing prevents food loss.

Self-Feeding Skills

Motivation to eat and the social meaning of eating can be equally important for the therapist to develop interventions for *self-feeding skills*. To consider cognitive and psychosocial development relative to activities of daily living (ADLs), Humphry and Morrow (1998) have provided insights into how children play with and master toys to suggest how these components influence performance of occupations. The caregiver can introduce new challenges in mealtimes even before the child shows full mastery in an earlier area of performance. Table 14-3 outlines the developmental sequence of self-feeding. The ages are approximate and overlapping.

The infant displays his or her active nature of "discovering" new forms of feeding when given baby cereal for the first time on a spoon. Initially, the infant tries to use a suckling action, so the tongue pushes forward and pushes the food out of the mouth. With repeated challenge across several meals, the child applies alternative motor patterns of the lips and tongue to manage the new food texture. Learning to move the baby cereal to the back of the mouth takes time, sometimes several weeks. The infant elicits active learning by experience, and regardless of whether baby food is introduced at 5 or 7 months of age, the infant's first response is to repeat the original suckling pattern used with the nipple. Older infants master the action quicker than younger ones.

Children are often eager to feed themselves. As early as 6 months of age, the infant may bring his or her hands up to the bottle and try to hold it. The caregiver should not prop the bottle because the infant lacks motor skills necessary to remove the bottle if choking occurs. Also the infant typically lacks the cognitive

TABLE 14-3 Developmental Continuum in Self-Feeding and Associated Component Areas

Age (mo)	Eating and Feeding Performance	Concurrent Changes in Performance Components		
		Sensorimotor	Cognition	Psychosocial
5-7	Takes cereal or pureed baby food from spoon.	Has good head stability and emerging sitting abilities; reaches and grasps toys; explores and tolerates various textures (e.g., fingers, rattles); puts objects in mouth.	Attends to effect produced by actions, such as hitting or shaking.	Plays with caregiver during meals and engages in interactive routines.
6-8	Attempts to hold bottle but may not retrieve it if it falls; needs to be monitored for safety reasons.		Object permanence is emerging and infant anticipates spoon or bottle.	Is easily distracted by stimuli (especially siblings) in the environment.
6-9	Holds and tries to eat cracker but sucks on it more than bites it; consumes soft foods that dissolve in the mouth; grabs at spoon but bangs it or sucks on either end of it.	Good sitting stability emerges; able to use hands to manipulate smaller parts of rattle; guided reach and palmar grasp applied to hand-to-mouth actions with objects.	Uses familiar actions initially with haphazard variations; seeks novelty and is anxious to explore objects (may grab at food on adult's plate).	Recognizes strangers; emerging sense of self.
9-13	Finger-feeds self a portion of meals consisting of soft table foods (e.g., macaroni, peas, dry cereal) and objects if fed by an adult.	Uses various grasps on objects of different sizes; able to isolate radial fingers on smaller objects.	Has increased organization and sequencing of schemas to do desired activity; may have difficulty attending to events outside visual space (e.g., position of spoon close to mouth).	Prefers to act on objects than be passive observer.
12-14	Dips spoon in food, brings spoonful of food to mouth, but spills food by inverting spoon before it goes into mouth.	Begins to place and release objects; likely to use pronated grasp on objects like crayon or spoon.	Recognizes that objects have function and uses tools appropriately; relates objects together, shifting attention among them.	Has interest in watching family routines.
15-18	Scoops food with spoon and brings it to mouth.	Shoulder and wrist stability demonstrate precise movements.	Experiments to learn rules of how objects work; actively solves problems by creating new action solutions.	Internalizes standards imposed by others for how to play with objects.
24-30	Demonstrates interest in using fork; may stab at food such as pieces of canned fruit; proficient at spoon use and eats cereal with milk or rice with gravy with utensil.	Tolerates various food textures in mouth; adjusts movements to be efficient (e.g., forearm supinated to scoop and lift spoon).	Expresses wants verbally; demonstrates imitation of short sequence of occupation (e.g., putting food on plate and eating it).	Has increasing desire to copy peers; looks to adults to see if they appreciate success in an occupation; interested in household routines.

understanding that a dropped bottle can be retrieved and put back into the mouth. Infants older than 8 months of age actively hold the bottle, but the caregiver should monitor their self-feeding to ensure adequate intake because infants are easily distracted once they satisfy their initial hunger.

Typically, finger-feeding develops quickly and naturally as the infant receives soft cookies or crackers to hold by about 8 months of age. At this age, infants typically exhibit a radial digital grasp, which positions the cookie well for entry into the mouth. From 9 to 13 months of age, the infant develops several skills that contribute to his or her ability to self-feed. Control of sitting posture and improved sitting balance, development of refined pincer grasp with controlled release, and refinement of isolated forearm and wrist movements result in efficient finger-feeding. By 12 months of age, finger-feeding is generally a preferred and enjoyed activity and matches changes in psychosocial components as the infant wishes to have increased independence and may refuse to be fed.

The selection of finger foods should match the child's oral motor skills (e.g., cooked vegetables are easily grasped and mashed with the tongue and gums). The infant should not be given nuts, hard candy, chunks of hot dog, or grapes because these can occlude the airway if they are aspirated.

Infants younger than 1 year of age will grasp, wave, and bang spoons when being fed. At around 12 months of age, the infant demonstrates an understanding of the spoon by poking at a bowl of food with a spoon and bringing it to the mouth. The infant is easily frustrated as visual monitoring of the spoon's position is poor and he or she has difficulty sequencing movements to scoop or adjusting the forearm and wrist. The food frequently slips from the spoon before it reaches the mouth. Attending to the whole activity and recognizing when the spoon is empty (sufficient cognitive changes to use feedback) is necessary before the infant starts to control the wrist and forearm sufficiently for spoon-feeding. Infants, despite marginal ability, will frequently insist on self-feeding even though independence means less success at satisfying hunger.

Proficiency in spoon-feeding emerges between 15 and 18 months of age when the infant brings the spoon with sticky food, such as yogurt, into the mouth with minimal spillage. The infant holds the spoon in a pronated gross grasp and uses primarily shoulder movement to bring it to the mouth. By 24 months of age, the child spoon-feeds without spillage (with more solid foods). He or she holds the spoon in the radial fingers with the forearm supinated and is able to obtain the food and efficiently place the spoon into the mouth. Between 30 and 36 months of age, the child may begin to prefer a fork for stabbing foods and may learn to eat foods that are more difficult to maintain on a spoon (e.g., cold cereal and rice with gravy).

Drinking

The infant may demonstrate interest in drinking from a cup as early as 6 months of age. However, skills in drinking from a cup do not emerge until about 12 months of age. At that time the infant is better able to correctly orient the cup to the mouth and to tip it to a degree that spillage is not inevitable. Several types of cups are available that make learning to drink from a cup an easy transition for the child. The first cup that the infant uses has a lid and a spout. It may have handles or may be a small cup that the infant can hold in one hand. Initially, the parent places only a small amount in the cup to decrease spillage and promote the child's success in directing the flow of liquid. The child may begin to use a small (4- to 6-ounce) cup without a lid at 24 months of age; however, spillage is inevitable at that time. The child continues to use a small cup.

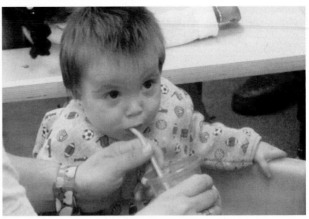

FIGURE 14-2   Using a straw to drink requires lip pursing and active lip seal. (Courtesy of Jayne Shepherd.)

Straw drinking emerges at about 2 years of age. It may become a skill before that time if the caregiver exposes the child to straw drinking. Use of a straw requires good lip seal and strong suction to bring the liquid into the mouth (Figure 14-2). In addition to the oral motor skills required to draw the liquid into the mouth, cognitive skills are needed to problem-solve how to use the straw. The infant often bites or blows on the straw before learning how to suck through it. This framework of typical development helps the therapist identify problems and establish realistic intervention goals and expected outcomes.

EVALUATION

Overview of Feeding Issues

Evaluation begins by assessing mealtime participation and appreciating the issues from the caregiver's point of view. The child's developmental and health history is also important to understanding the feeding problem and making decisions about further evaluation and potential intervention approaches. This information may be gathered from written reports. The child and family priorities, relevant history, and level of mealtime participation provide an overall picture of the feeding problem. This information is gained through parent interview, informal observation, and written reports about the child. The therapist obtains information about the current feeding methods by asking the parents to describe feeding over the course of a typical day. This open-ended request allows the parents to bring forward their concerns. After this, the therapist can guide the discussion to obtain comprehensive information (Box 14-1).

A discussion regarding the feeding problem from the perspective of the parents is critical to determine their primary concerns. Are the parents most concerned about

BOX 14-1 Questions Regarding Feeding at Home

1 Who feeds your child at home?
   a Do different caregivers feed your child in different ways (e.g., different positions)?
   b Does your child seem to respond differently to various feeders?
   c If only one caregiver feeds your child, what is the effect of this total responsibility on this caregiver?
2 Describe your child's problems with feeding.
   a Does your child have difficulty sucking or drinking?
   b Does your child have problems biting or chewing?
   c Does your child cough or choke? When? How often?
   d What do you think is causing your child's problems with eating?
3 How much help does your child need with feeding?
   a Do you manually assist your child in chewing and drinking?
   b Does your child self-feed, or do you assist him or her in self-feeding?
   c Is your child independent in using a cup, or do you have to assist him or her?
4 How do you know when your child is hungry?
5 How do you know when your child has had enough to eat or drink?
   a Does your child stop eating when satiated?
   b Can your child's endurance cause him or her to stop eating before he or she is full?
6 When and how often is your child fed, and how long does a meal take?
7 How much formula, milk, baby food, or other food does your child consume? Each meal? Each day?
8 If your child gets something other than formula, milk, and baby food, do you do anything special to prepare the food (e.g., mash it or cut it into small bites)?
9 When your child is fed at home, where does he or she sit (e.g., in a regular chair at the table, in a high chair, or in a wheelchair)?
   a How do you position your child?
   b Do you do anything special to adapt the seating?
10 What bottles, nipples, or spoons are used in feeding? (Explore specific types or shapes.)
   a If adapted equipment is used for feeding, what is it and how is it used?
   b Have you tried special equipment before and decided that it was not working for you and your child?
11 Describe your child's response to feeding. When does your child most enjoy feeding?
12 How does your child react to foods that are new or that have different textures, tastes, or temperatures?
13 Does your child's performance and behavior during feeding differ in the morning, midday, or night?
14 Who is around during most meals, and what else is going on in the room?
15 Has anyone given you suggestions on how to feed your child? How did these work for you?
16 What routines and behaviors reflect cultural beliefs?

weight gain? Is the length of time required for feeding dominating the parent's daily activities? Does the child seem to lose most of the food consumed during feeding (e.g., through vomiting or reflux)? Is the child's behavior during feeding creating havoc for the entire family during mealtime? Although the parents' expressed concerns become the focus of intervention, the therapist should consider concerns of the professionals in developing the feeding plan when they differ from the concerns of the parents.

The parents also provide the team with information about the child's developmental history and feeding history. Obtaining this history helps the therapist identify the basis of the feeding problem (e.g., if longstanding sensory or behavioral issues have influenced feeding performance). By asking about the feeding history, the therapist also obtains a sense of the parents' frustration and ability to cope with the child's feeding issues. The techniques that the parents use and their experiences in feeding the infant are helpful in identifying appropriate intervention strategies. Parents whose children have received therapy services in the past probably have important information to share regarding interventions that worked and those that did not. The parent's interview can also provide guidance regarding who may implement intervention recommendations and which adults need to receive communication about an oral-motor or feeding program or the child's progress in developing eating/feeding skills.

Recorded developmental histories supplement the parents' report. The written reports of other occupational and physical therapists, early childhood specialists, and teachers provide foundational knowledge about the child. For example, a child with sustained hospitalization for another condition may not have been given the same opportunities to progress, or an early history of restricted upper extremity movement may lead to restricted oral play, influencing sensory system and secondarily the ability to eat. Understanding the child's developmental course and rate of change in other occupational performance areas such as object play and social interactions is important for the therapist to make realistic goals for what will change in the next few months, prioritize objectives, and select appropriate intervention strategies.

Eating and Feeding Performance

The child is observed in feeding and eating to assess level of performance and to analyze how motor, sensory, cognitive, and communication skills contribute to performance. It is important that the observation is as naturalistic as possible, using foods that the child typically eats. Ideally the therapist has an opportunity to play with the child before feeding. During play, the therapist can observe overall exploration and play performance and can analyze which systems (e.g., cognitive, motor) constrain performance. The therapist should focus on cognitive ability and interest in imitation, response to sensory input, communication style, postural control, ability to manipulate objects, and if age appropriate, use toys in a functional manner. This information helps the therapist plan the feeding evaluation (e.g., how to position the child, whether to offer opportunities to use a utensil, and how to communicate with the child during the feeding observation). This play session also helps build rapport between the therapist and the child. The relaxed and positive interaction can influence the nature of the interaction during feeding, given that feeding experiences may have a history of being stressful and uncomfortable for the child.

If the evaluation takes place in a clinic or school, the child should receive foods that he or she typically eats. Parents can help the team select the menu, or the team may ask them to bring preferred foods from home. The therapist places the child in his or her typical feeding position and provides feeding utensils and methods familiar to the child. The therapist initially asks one parent to feed the child a portion of the meal.

The observation of the parent-child interaction helps the therapist to understand factors that may promote or inhibit the child's intake. During this time, the therapist reflects on the potential meaning of the occupation to the child and his or her interest in participating. Observations of parent-child interaction also give the therapist insights into the everyday context for feeding from which to make recommendations. Does the parent talk to the child? Does the child send clear cues regarding readiness to eat, satiation, or preferences in foods? Does the parent respond to his or her nonverbal cues?

Further Analysis of Feeding: Identifying Underlying Factors

After observing feeding by the caregiver, the therapist should also feed the child. This gives the therapist additional information about the child's responses to new positions and different foods. This part of the evaluation helps the therapist determine the potential effectiveness of intervention techniques that will improve the child's ability to eat or self-feed. Therefore, the therapist obtains assessment information regarding what intervention strategies seem to promote skills and the child's responsiveness to different intervention methods.

The focus of the observational assessment is to explore hypothesized impairments that may relate to the health, safety, endurance, and interactional issues identified through the initial interview and record review. Throughout the evaluation, the therapist considers the child's ability to communicate, respond, and interact during eating. Component level analysis includes the child's oral sensitivity; postural control; jaw, lip, cheek,

and tongue movements; coordination of those movements; and overall strength and endurance during feeding. A speech pathologist may assist in analysis of oral motor skills.

To further analyze the child's feeding and eating issues, the therapist may return to the child's medical record for additional information. Does the child have a medical condition that leads to feeding problems or poor weight gain? Reports of metabolic or neurologic evaluations, including results of computerized tomography (CT) scans or brain imaging scans, may help the therapist understand systemic problems. Instances of pneumonia and frequent and prolonged upper-respiratory infection suggest a problem with swallowing. When swallowing problems are suspected, a videofluoroscopic swallow study may be completed.

Videofluoroscopic Swallow Study

VFSS is used to analyze the swallow mechanism and is particularly important for children who aspirate or are at high risk for aspiration because of severe motor problems (Gisel, Applegate-Ferrante, Benson, & Bosma, 1995). Factors that suggest swallowing problems include gagging or choking, repeated ineffective swallows, and reflux. Many times the aspiration may be silent, so the only indications are wet, noisy respiration after feeding and the occurrence of repeated respiratory infections (Benson & Lefton-Greif, 1994). The therapist should distinguish aspiration from penetration. Laryngeal penetration occurs when food or liquid enters the vestibule to any extent down to the level of the true vocal cords, but not into the airway. Aspiration involves entry of the food into the airway, below the vocal folds (Arvedson & Lefton-Greif, 1998; Freidman & Frazier, 2000; Logemann, 1993). The feeding team can identify and distinguish these problems with a VFSS.

The VFSS is also referred to as a *modified barium swallow*. The therapist or technician saturates a food substance with barium and videotapes ingestion of the barium to show how the food passes from the mouth through the pharynx. The occupational therapist consults with the radiologist so that he or she can place the infant or child in typical feeding positions or potentially therapeutic positions. The therapist also selects the types of food textures based on knowledge of the child's current diet and feeding goals (Schuberth, 1994).

In a typical VFSS, the therapist mixes liquid barium with other liquids or pureed foods and spreads barium paste on crackers or cookies. The therapist can give the food using a bottle, cup, or spoon. The purpose of the VFSS is to identify whether the child aspirates and how the child swallows liquids and different textures in different positions. Because the video record shows how the food travels through the mouth and pharynx, the therapist receives detailed information about the swallowing problem (Schwarz, 2003; Wolf & Glass, 1992).

The results of the VFSS indicate the safety and appropriateness of oral feeding and guide the therapist's recommendations (Zerilli, Stefans, & DiPietro, 1990). For example, the therapist may recommend positions and textures for the parents to use during feeding that seem to result in optimal swallowing patterns without aspiration. Although the VFSS gives the therapist important information and insight regarding the swallowing problem, it may not be representative of the child's typical feeding in a more natural environment.

Other Medical Procedures

Children with gastroesophageal reflux (GER) or suspected GER may require additional medical tests to determine the frequency and duration of the reflux. A pH probe reveals the amount of acid that penetrates the esophagus as an indicator of the frequency of GER. The probe is inserted into the esophagus through the nose to monitor acid levels (usually for 24 hours). A pH probe is advantageous because it examines the frequency of GER over 24 hours, which other tests (e.g., a barium swallow) cannot accomplish. Another procedure that uses nuclear medicine technology to diagnose severity of GER and problems in gastric emptying is gastroesophageal scintigraphy. In this procedure, the infant or child ingests a radionuclide isotope, and its movement through the esophagus, stomach, and intestines is recorded by a camera. The extensive filming (recording generally continues for one hour) provides accurate evidence of GER, if present, and records the time required for stomach emptying. This information is used by physicians when considering fundoplication (surgery that tightens the gastroesophageal sphincter).

Contextual Factors

Evaluation of the context for feeding is essential to development of intervention goals and plans. In some cases, feeding problems are primarily based on contextual issues. Important contextual issues to consider are physical, social, temporal, and cultural. Box 14-2 lists some of the contextual factors that should be considered when assessing feeding.

Understanding the contextual factors that influence mealtimes and feeding performance helps to determine the basis for the problem and possible solutions. Certain contextual factors can easily be changed (e.g., a child can be positioned in a chair that is more upright and has straps that maintain good alignment). Other contextual factors that cannot be expected to change (e.g., cultural beliefs and family routines) should be accommodated in the intervention plan. Contextual factors may determine

---

BOX 14-2   Guiding Questions to Evaluate the Contexts for Feeding

PHYSICAL
- Is seating and positioning adequate? Supportive? Does it provide stability?
- Are head, neck, shoulders, and pelvis well aligned?
- Is space adequate for eating activities?
- Are noise and activity levels conducive to eating?

SOCIAL
- Who feeds the child?
- Who is present during the meal?
- What is the nature of the social interaction among family members during the meal?
- What communication/interaction occurs between caregiver and child during feeding?

TEMPORAL
- Is sufficient time allotted and available for a relaxing meal?
- How often is the child fed?
- How long does feeding take?

CULTURAL
- How do cultural beliefs and values influence mealtime?
- What foods does the family eat?

---

the success of the intervention (i.e., which recommended strategies the family will implement). For example, if the caregivers do not value or prioritize the child's independence in feeding, then they are unlikely to follow through with suggestions to increase feeding independence.

The assessment findings are discussed and interpreted by team members, including the family, to develop a cohesive intervention plan. Intervention for feeding problems considers the whole child, involves the family, and requires collaboration with professionals of other disciplines (Schwarz, 2003; Tarbell & Allaire, 2002).

The following sections identify key issues that affect feeding and eating in infants and children. Although the issues are discussed separately, feeding problems are seldom attributable to a singular cause and usually are the result of delays or impairment in multiple performance areas. For example, children with severe sensory problems generally have oral motor skill delays, and children with swallowing disorders often have motor deficits.

INTERVENTION FOR SENSORY ISSUES

Young children with feeding problems often exhibit hypersensitivity in and around the mouth. Diagnoses in which oral hypersensitivies are common include autism (Baranek, 1999), pervasive developmental disorders, cerebral palsy, multiple disabilities (Schwarz, 2003), and sensory integration dysfunction (Tarbell & Allaire, 2002). These children demonstrate aversive responses to touch in the mouth and demonstrate extreme responses to textured food within the mouth. Behaviors observed when pureed food on a spoon is placed in the mouth include spitting, coughing, or gagging. These behaviors are typical when a new texture is introduced to most children. However, the child with oral hypersensitivities persists beyond the time usually required to develop tolerance. Infants with sensory problems may hold the food in their mouths to avoid moving it through the mouth. Sensory defensiveness is a critical problem for the child because it often limits the amount of nutritional intake, restricts variety of foods, and creates a negative interaction that is disruptive to the co-occupation of feeding. Adding textured food to the infant's meal is important to facilitating higher levels of oral motor skill (i.e., chewing and diagonal tongue movements are elicited when the texture of the food requires those movements). Knowing the basis of the child's defensiveness is important for the therapist to plan an intervention program that helps resolve the problem. Oral hypersensitivity can relate to any one of three causative factors (Wolf & Glass, 1992):

1 Oral hypersensitivity is often associated with the early experiences of the child (i.e., as a newborn and young infant) (Bazyk, 1990). Newborns with medical problems at birth often endure procedures that are noxious to the oropharyngeal area. Examples of nursing and medical procedures associated with oral tactile defensiveness are mouth and lung suctioning, intubation, and nasal gastric feeding. In each of these procedures, hard plastic tubes are entered into the mouth and throat, almost always causing gagging and coughing. Over time, when such experiences are repeated, the infant develops defensive responses to all oral-sensory input, perhaps in an attempt to protect that highly sensitive area.

2 Hypersensitivity also may result in the child who is not fed by mouth for an extended period (Tarbell & Allaire, 2002). When the child does not receive oral feedings and compensatory oral stimulation, he or she develops hypersensitivity of the oral area. Oral stimulation is critical at certain developmental periods for establishing sensory processing around and inside the mouth. Lack of oral experiences may be the easiest type of sensory defensiveness to overcome.

3 A neurologic impairment that directly affects the sensory tracts can also cause oral-sensory defensiveness. Infants with neurologic immaturity often have difficulty with sensory modulation and are hypersensitive to tactile input. Children with cerebral palsy or other disorders may demonstrate oral

defensiveness as a manifestation of neurologic impairment. Children with autism may exhibit generalized hypersensitivity and may require a program emphasizing sensory integration (SI).

Oral hypersensitivity often is the result of a combination of these three causative factors. Infants who have neurologic impairment with associated hypersensitivity often are recipients of nonoral feedings and invasive oral procedures. Feeding intervention is particularly challenging for children whose defensiveness seems to be related to both offensive oral experiences and general sensory impairment. In many children, sensory problems evolve into behavioral problems, where sensory issues resolve, but behaviors (e.g., picky eating, food refusal) remain because they become habits or are rewarded by caregivers. For these children, a multipronged approach using sensory and behavior techniques is indicated.

Evaluation
Mealtime Participation

To understand how the child participates in family and school mealtimes, the therapist interviews the parent or teacher. The goal of the interview is to assess the level of the child's participation in mealtime and specifically his or her acceptance of various sensory stimuli in his or her mouth. In the interview the therapist explores the questions outlined in Box 14-1. The child with hypersensitivity may accept only one or two food textures, may swallow food without mastication or preparation, may spit out foods on a regular basis, or may exhibit a hyperactive gag that seems unrelated to the amount of food placed into the mouth.

Feeding and Eating Performance

The therapist also needs to observe the child's eating using a variety of textures. When possible, the therapist precedes a trial of different textures with relaxed play with the child so that he or she becomes comfortable. Nonintrusive play can also help to establish rapport. To observe the child's sensory responses, the therapist should use various textures and attempt placement of food in different parts of the mouth. When the child exhibits aversive responses to food inside the mouth, the therapist asks the parent if the responses are typical or exaggerated because of discomfort with an unfamiliar feeder.

Intervention

Hypersensitivity can seriously interfere with the nutritional intake and oral motor skills of the child. It is often a problem that can improve significantly with intervention. At first the therapist should implement intervention activities at times other than during meals. Because intervention activities are often uncomfortable and challenging for the child, the therapist may best perform them between feedings to avoid disruption of mealtimes and the child's nutritional intake (Morris & Klein, 2000; Tarbell & Allaire, 2002).

Activities in Between Mealtimes

The occupational therapist first focuses on establishing a relationship of trust with the child. The child may distrust anyone who attempts to place food in his or her mouth; therefore good rapport and positive interactions are critical. The therapist can playfully embed activities to desensitize into the child's play activities. When possible, the activities are self-guided, and the therapist introduces the sensory stimulating activities gradually. Once the therapist begins oral desensitization, he or she can maintain the trusting relationship if he or she always acknowledges the child's physical cues of discomfort (by at least a verbal response and when appropriate by withdrawal of the oral stimulus). The therapist should also allow turn taking, decision making, and as much active participation by the child as possible. Children will tolerate greater sensory input if the activity is under the child's control and provided in the context of a motivating, developmentally appropriate activity (Bundy & Koomar, 2002).

The therapist can begin oral desensitization by encouraging the infant to explore his or her mouth with his or her own hands. The infant can begin to suck on his or her hands and fingers with the guidance of the therapist's hand. The therapist can introduce rubber toys into the oral play. The therapist may use the NUK toothbrush or a regular toothbrush to brush and massage the gums (Morris & Klein, 2000). The therapist can engage in turn-taking games with the infant using a rubber toy or toothbrush in a hide-and-seek game to stimulate different areas of the mouth using different degrees of pressure. The parent can rub the infant's gums with a warm washcloth, applying firm sustained pressure and allowing the child to chew or suck on the cloth. The texture of the washcloth is easily accepted by children and is helpful in improving sensory tolerance of other textures. For older children with higher-level oral motor skills, the therapist can use blow toys to desensitize the oral area. Blowing bubbles and making sounds are particularly motivating activities that help the child become more aware of his or her mouth and oral movements.

Desensitization activities between meals should include small amounts of food. The therapist can dip rubber toys in pureed food and toothbrushes in fruit juice before entry into the infant's mouth. The therapist should introduce the taste and texture of different foods into the oral play as much as possible. Once the child is in preschool, snack time is an excellent time to focus on oral desensitization because it may not be as important to eat a certain amount of food. Turn-taking games and sharing with peers can encourage oral intake and improve the child's willingness to try new textures.

Activities to Prepare for Eating

Application of oral desensitization immediately before the child's mealtime can be beneficial. The therapist should develop a program that prepares the child for oral intake and requires only a brief amount of time and energy by the caregiver and child (Figure 14-3). Using a warm washcloth around and inside of the mouth can desensitize this area before feeding. The infant may tolerate the washcloth better than the parent's finger. The therapist may instruct the parent to place his or her finger inside a nipple or inside an Infa-Dent toothbrush, then to rub the baby's gums, tongue, and palate (Klein & Delaney, 1994). When demonstrating to the parent or applying any method of direct oral stimulation, the therapist should wear gloves and follow Occupational Safety and Health Administration (OSHA) guidelines for exposure to body fluids such as saliva (Federal Register, 1991). These regulations require that "gloves be worn when it can be reasonably anticipated that the employee may have hand contact with blood, other potentially infectious materials, mucous membranes, and nonintact skin" (pp. 64133-64134).

Sometimes the infant benefits from overall application of deep pressure. In this case, the therapist can systematically apply sensory preparation, beginning with stroking in body areas where it is tolerated. Firm rubbing and deep pressure (e.g., infant massage) are stimuli that desensitize and increase tolerance to touch (Klein & Delaney, 1994). Gradually, and based on the child's

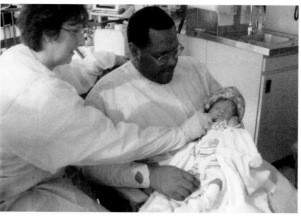

FIGURE 14-3 The occupational therapist coaches the father in application of touch pressure prior to feeding. (Courtesy of Jayne Shepherd.)

response, the therapist applies the tactile stimulation to the cheeks, outer lips, inside of the mouth, gums, and tongue (Glass & Wolf, 1998). Sustained firm pressure to the upper palate can desensitize the entire mouth, enabling the child to accept touch in other parts of his or her mouth. This pressure can produce calming and more organized responses. Certain older children (e.g., those with autism) seem to benefit from vibration applied to the lower jaw and around the mouth. The therapist should allow the child to guide this strong proprioceptive input, and the child may request vibration to the gums and inside the mouth. The therapist should monitor responses to vibration; the proximity to the vestibular receptor may cause vestibular system reactions. If tolerated by the child, vibration can decrease sensitivity and increase oral motor responses.

In addition to these preparatory activities, the therapist should consider adaptations to the child's position. The therapist should support the child's trunk and head so that the child feels secure and stable but not overly confined. Children who have generalized sensory defensiveness may be more comfortable in a chair than in the arms of the caregiver because human touch is a very powerful and potentially distracting stimulus. The therapist should place children with concomitant respiratory problems in upright positions that allow for maximum thoracic expansion and optimal respiration during feeding.

Mealtime Interventions

Modifying the texture of the child's food is perhaps the most important intervention that the therapist can offer to the child with hypersensitivity. Box 14-3 provides guidelines for adapting food texture to accommodate and decrease the child's hypersensitivity.

The therapist encourages the parent to introduce new textures gradually and in a way that makes them palatable to the child and easily consumed. For example, the parent can mix mashed potatoes with other vegetables and soft meats to help hold those foods together. The child may accept this sensory experience better than the new food alone, which may become a collection of discrete bits after chewing. The therapist should encourage parents to add the right amount of moisture to food to make it easily manageable in the mouth. Thickening foods becomes important for the child with poor oral motor control because the thicker substance moves more slowly within the mouth and provides more sensory input, making it easy for the child to control.

When the therapist recommends changes in the types of food (e.g., more fruits and vegetables), consultation with a nutritionist regarding the effect of the dietary change is important. Children with disabilities often need high-caloric and high-protein intake, making the balance of nutrients more difficult to achieve.

BOX 14-3 **Guidelines for Adapting Food Texture for Children with Hypersensitivity**

1 The therapist should ensure adequate nutritional intake by attending to the nutrient value and amount of food intake when changing the texture of foods consumed.
2 Pureed, smooth foods are the first solid foods that the therapist should attempt with a child with severe oral-sensory defensiveness. The therapist can gradually increase the texture of pureed foods by adding food with lumps or of more coarse texture.
3 The therapist should vary the textures within any one meal from those least tolerated to those most tolerated. When the child successfully eats a food with strong sensory input, the therapist can reward him or her with a spoonful of a favorite food.
4 Soft foods that have cohesion when masticated offer increased sensory experiences. When placed between the teeth, cheese, chicken, and well-cooked vegetables (with no skins) increase chewing.
5 Graham crackers, butter cookies, and some cereals (e.g., Cheerios) provide discrete bits of food in the mouth that promote desensitization. Soft crackers and cookies promote chewing and dissolve quickly once inside the mouth, presenting less danger of choking.
6 For children who need altered food texture over time, a food grinder to puree the child's food is a useful tool. The therapist can progressively alter the food texture by changing the food grinder setting.
7 Grainy breads provide more texture than soft white breads, which tend to form a ball and adhere to the upper palate.
8 It may be helpful to introduce textured foods that require some chewing by mixing them in with foods that are familiar to the child and that add cohesion to the food bolus.
9 The therapist should maintain a pleasant, fun atmosphere during feeding and, when appropriate, use play and verbal interaction to distract the child from focusing attention on the food within his or her mouth. Verbal encouragement and looks of delight are rewarding to the child who has eaten a new food. Offering another bite can be frustrating rather than rewarding.

Modified from Case-Smith, J. (1999). Self care strategies for children with developmental deficits. In C. Christiansen (Ed.), *Ways of living: Self-care strategies for special needs* (pp. 83-122). Bethesda, MD: AOTA.

In addition to adjusting the food texture, the therapist should assess the utensils used and the placement of the spoon in the child's mouth relative to the child's tolerance. A child often better tolerates food placed in the anterior part of the mouth as opposed to food placed on the posterior tongue. He or she may better tolerate food on the center of the tongue than on the sides. However, food placement on the side is often desirable for increasing chewing and tongue lateralization.

Table 14-4 is a chart of food progression from smooth, pureed foods to coarse and chewy foods. The chart lists foods in different nutrient groups in the sequence that a typical child learns to tolerate and handle

TABLE 14-4 Food Progression Based on Texture Consistency

	Pureed	Mashed, Coarse Pureed	Ground/ Mashed/ Well cooked	Soft	Soft/Some regular	Full diet
Meats and meat substitutes	Strained meats and egg yolk	Commercial junior foods; soft meats ground fine in food grinder with liquids added; mashed egg yolk	Ground meats with gravy; soft cooked eggs	Ground meats; scrambled eggs; smooth peanut butter	Well-cooked, soft meats, hard-cooked eggs	Cut-up meats (all types except very tough, e.g. roast beef, ham)
Dairy products	Thinned puddings, plain yogurt; strained cottage cheese	Fork-mashed cottage cheese; pudding; custard; thickened cream soups	Cottage cheese	Yogurt with soft fruits; ice cream; some soft cheeses	Cheeses of medium hardness (cheddar)	
Breads and cereals	Infant cereals thinned with milk	Thicker infant cereals; Cream of Wheat	Cooked cereals such as oatmeal; crackers; toast; plain cookies; bread without crust	Cooked cereals with soft fruits added; bread with crust; well-cooked pasta	Dry cereals with milk; sandwiches with smooth filling cut into small pieces; rice; firmer texture pasta	Sandwiches with various fillings
Fruits and vegetables	Strained fruits and vegetables	Junior fruits, applesauce, ripe mashed bananas; junior vegetables; mashed potatoes	Fork-mashed, soft canned fruits without skins; soft ripe mashed fresh fruits; fork-mashed, well-cooked vegetables	Canned fruits (peaches, pears); soft, ripe fresh fruits (peeled); well-cooked vegetables cut into small pieces	Canned fruits of increased texture (fruit cocktail); vegetables of increased texture (cooked carrots); soups with well-cooked vegetables	Raw fruits; dried fruits; raw vegetables with skins (corn, peas, lima beans); chunky soup

solid foods. The food groups also follow the progression of oral motor skills achievement.

INTERVENTION TO IMPROVE ORAL MOTOR PERFORMANCE

Children with significant motor impairments often exhibit oral motor delays. Examples of children with motor dysfunctions that can affect feeding are those with cerebral palsy, traumatic brain injury, prematurity, or genetic syndromes such as trisomy 21. Children with moderate to severe cerebral palsy often exhibit significant oral motor impairment and feeding dysfunction. Dahl, Thommessen, Rasmussen, and Selberg (1996) found that 60% of their sample of children with cerebral palsy had daily feeding problems that included difficulty chewing and swallowing. Schwarz (2003) reported that up to 90% of nonambulatory children with cerebral palsy exhibited evidence of malnutrition. Using a sample of 49 children with cerebral palsy from the United Kingdom, Reilly, Skuse, and Poblete (1996) found that 91% had some degree of oral motor impairment, with 33% of these categorized as severe.

Often the muscle tone of children with cerebral palsy in the proximal areas of the face, neck, and trunk is hypotonic, resulting in poor head and trunk stability. The child's jaw tends to move in wide excursions, completely open or clamped shut. The child often demonstrates inability to grade the jaw's movement in the midranges typically observed in sucking and chewing. When the child has low facial muscle tone, the mouth is often open, resulting in excessive drooling and loss of food from the mouth during feeding. An open mouth during feeding also makes swallowing difficult. In a descriptive study of 58 children with severe physical disabilities, more than half exhibited an up-and-down pattern of jaw movement to take in food. In more than a third of the children, their mouths were open some or all of the time during feeding (Yokochi, 1997).

In the child with hypotonia, the tongue may be inactive, moving primarily with the lower jaw. The tongue may move only in extension and retraction, or it may move into extreme ranges (e.g., completely retracted into the back of the mouth) (Yokochi, 1997). The tongue's extreme ranges or lack of movement may be associated with poor jaw stability such that the jaw does not function as a base for tongue movement. The lips of children with cerebral palsy are often inactive and hypotonic. Lip seal on the bottle's nipple, the cup rim, or a spoon is inadequate and results in food loss or air intake. Hypotonic cheeks result in less suction of the nipple and difficulty maintaining food in the tongue's center.

Children with hypotonic oral musculature often have overall postural instability. Postural instability results in poor postural alignment and increased difficulty with oral motor skills. When upright, the child may fall into trunk and cervical flexion. When slightly reclined, his or her head may fall into extension. When the child's neck is in hyperextension, neck alignment is not appropriate for safe and efficient swallow.

Sometimes a child who initially exhibits low tone may exhibit spasticity as he or she matures and attempts to assume positions more upright against gravity. Children with hypertonicity tend to exhibit hyperextension of the trunk and neck without reciprocal flexion. They may exhibit tonic oral reflexes or abnormal oral motor patterns that are never observed in a typically developing child. Children with hypertonicity differ from children with low muscle tone who exhibit delayed oral motor patterns that are observed in children who are younger. The following are examples of oral motor patterns observed in children with hypertonicity:

- *Tonic bite.* The gums or teeth close or clamp together in a forceful motion. Once closed, the jaw remains clamped and the therapist may need to reposition the child to open the mouth. The tonic bite occurs more often when the child is inappropriately positioned in some neck extension or when he or she has extreme tactile defensiveness.
- *Tongue thrust.* In tongue thrust the child completely extends his or her tongue outside the border of the lips. The tongue's movement is forceful and is often maintained in the extended position. Tongue thrust also occurs more often when the child is positioned in trunk and neck extension. This forceful tongue movement results in loss of food or liquid from the mouth and does not initiate a swallow. Children with severe tongue thrust may lose much of the food presented to them. The therapist may observe jaw thrust (a strong, forceful, downward movement of the lower jaw) with tongue thrust.

- *Lip retraction and lip pursing.* Some children with high muscle tone associated with cerebral palsy exhibit lip retraction. The lips pull away from the midline and stay fixed in the retracted position when utensils and food or a cup and drink are entered into the mouth. This stiffening replaces the soft seal of the lips typically observed. Lip pursing is a response in which the lips draw tightly together at midline. Both movement patterns result in food loss and difficulty obtaining the food from the spoon or the drink from the cup. These movement patterns occur most frequently when the neck is extended and appropriate head and trunk alignment is not achieved. They also occur when the child experiences an emotional reaction to a situation.

Evaluation
Mealtime Participation

Children with severe cerebral palsy almost always require physical assistance during the meal, although this may be limited to cutting the food into bite-size pieces. Children with significant oral motor problems are often fed before or after the family's mealtime. They may have a special seat or may sit in their wheelchair during the meal. Guiding questions to include in the assessment are as follows:

- Does the child eat with the family or eat at a separate time?
- Does the child sit with the family at mealtime (whether or not he or she eats)?
- What special food preparations are necessary?
- How much does he or she participate in the mealtime conversation and interaction?

Feeding and Eating Performance

Specific assessment of the child's eating skills focuses on oral motor factors. Overall motor patterns, strength, and muscle tone are evaluated:

- Postural alignment and postural control, including asymmetries, with a focus on head and trunk stability
- Jaw, tongue, cheek, and lip movement patterns
- Coordination and sequencing of jaw, tongue, and lip movements during feeding (i.e., coordination of suck-swallow-breathe)
- How oral movement patterns are affected by the child's posture using different external sources of postural support (e.g., in the caregiver's lap versus in a feeder chair or small child's chair)
- How oral motor patterns change when the jaw or cheeks are supported and the child's response to handling around the mouth before and during feeding

The goal of the evaluation is to assess oral motor skills with the child in typical positioning, with optimal positioning and environmental conditions, and during application of intervention strategies. The resulting information provides the therapist with guidance as to the nature of the child's oral motor strengths and problems and the types of intervention that seem to promote improved oral motor control.

Intervention
Postural Alignment

Improving the child's postural alignment and stability through good positioning is often helpful in promoting oral motor function. Some oral motor problems immediately resolve when the child is well positioned in good postural alignment. Appropriate alignment for feeding consists of the following:

- Neutral pelvic alignment of the trunk. Pelvic alignment is promoted when the child sits well supported against a flat back, on a flat seat, and square on the buttocks with 90° of hip flexion and 90° of knee flexion
- Good head, neck, and shoulder alignment with the head in slight flexion or at neutral
- Chin tuck with the back of the neck in an elongated position

The child can achieve correct postural alignment in various positions, depending on the size of the child and his or her postural stability. One guideline for the therapist is to provide the child with more external postural stability than he or she actually needs. The therapist positions the child with oral motor deficits associated with a motor delay in a slightly reclined position with head and trunk fully supported. Feeding requires high-level, intricate oral movement and focused concentration; therefore complete postural stability, excellent alignment, and comfort are critical to successful eating.

Characteristics of Feeding Positions and Positioning Devices

- *Infant held sideways in the caregiver's arms.* This position allows for full body contact. It is appropriate for infants; however, it may be difficult for the caregiver to maintain optimal head and shoulder alignment. This position is fatiguing and is inappropriate for the older infant or the infant who has poor postural control.
- *Infant held on caregiver's thighs facing caregiver* (Figure 14-4). This position provides excellent stability and good alignment and promotes midline. It frees both of the caregiver's hands. This intimate position allows for eye contact and therefore promotes communication. It does not work with older, larger children.
- *Infant placed in an infant seat.* The infant seat works well for infants with fair head control who

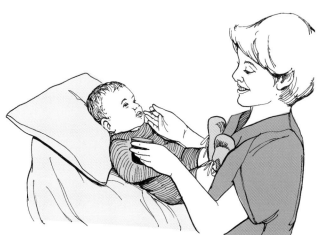

FIGURE 14-4 Face-to-face position for feeding.

are not yet independent in sitting. The caregiver can adapt the infant seat with small rolls on the side to maintain a symmetric posture. When the infant is placed in the infant seat, the caregiver can free his or her hands and use them for support at the chin or chest during feeding. Straps are available with this seat, and the cost is low. The infant seat is not an appropriate device for an infant with established sitting balance or for the infant who weighs more than 25 pounds.

- *Infant placed in a cradle bouncer.* This seat is similar to an infant seat. It holds the infant in more extension and is inappropriate for an infant with increased extensor muscle tone. The bouncing motion of the seat can promote rhythmic movement during feeding but is a distraction to the infant who has difficulty tolerating vestibular system input.
- *Infant placed in a foam-filled (Tumble Forms2) feeder seat.* This positioner offers full head and trunk support and promotes good alignment. The feeder seat comes with a strapping system, and the caregiver can order different chest straps. The curved sides of the chair promote midline and decrease shoulder retraction. The caregiver can recline the infant seat to the angle desired for feeding (i.e., the angle at which the head is in an optimal position). The Tumble Forms2 chair is available in different sizes and is easily cleaned, easily transported, and safe when used with its wedge or mobile base. It is more expensive than an infant seat and is inappropriate for infants who sit independently (Figure 14-5).
- *Infant placed in a regular car seat.* Most car seats provide good alignment and postural stability for the infant. Usually adjusting the seat's degree of tilt is more difficult and small adjustments are not possible.

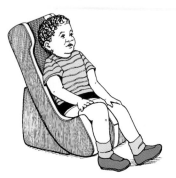

FIGURE 14-5 Tumble Forms Feeder Chair offers support and an adjustable feeding angle.

■ *Child placed in a transport chair or wheelchair.* A transport chair or pediatric wheelchair may be the optimal seating device for feeding a child with severe motor limitations. It is typically the most supportive seating arrangement for the child. Transport chairs offer individualized seating with customized head support, lateral supports, and trunk straps. Therefore the chair offers optimal external stability of the child's posture. The tray provides an additional truncal support and a surface for weight bearing on arms. A key feature beneficial to children with poor head control is that the chair tilts into various positions while maintaining optimal postural alignment for feeding (neutral pelvis and 90° hip and knee flexion). This tilt-in-space feature allows the child to recline in small increments. The transport chair places the child at a height that makes feeding convenient for the adult. A disadvantage of feeding in the transport chair is that its height can create a barrier to peer interaction, as in a preschool setting where the children eat snacks seated in small chairs at a low-level table.

■ *Child placed in a beanbag chair.* The beanbag chair is a comfortable seating option for the child who otherwise may be in a wheelchair or on the floor. It brings the child into a semi-upright position for visualization of the environment and for eye contact with peer or adults. The beanbag chair is not the best option for feeding because postural alignment is difficult to control and the infant tends to be primarily in extension. The beanbag is particularly inappropriate for children with extensor posturing because it does not successfully inhibit these postures.

■ *Infant placed in a high chair.* A high chair is standard furniture for many families with infants learning to eat solid foods. It is the positioner of choice if the infant has adequate postural stability and motor control. Minimally, the infant should be able to independently maintain a propped sitting position for several seconds. The high chair provides back support, side supports, pelvic strapping, and a tray. The caregiver can easily adapt it to give additional foot support and lateral support. The high chair places the infant at a height that allows him or her to participate in the family's mealtime. This height is convenient for the caregiver who is feeding. The high chair is desirable because it is readily available and economical; it is particularly appropriate for the infant who will soon be sitting independently.

Summary. Caregivers should have a range of options for positions; however, the therapist should discourage certain positioning choices. For example, although holding the infant in the caregiver's lap is a comforting position, it does not give the caregiver optimal control when the infant has poor control of movement. Infants with postural instability benefit from placement in a stable seating device that helps the infant focus on oral movements and frees the caregiver's hands for providing manual assistance to the infant's oral movements.

Handling Techniques in Support of Oral Movement

After positioning the child in good postural alignment with optimal postural stability, the therapist can apply handling techniques to support oral movements. The techniques involve touch in and around the mouth; therefore desensitization of the oral area is often a required prerequisite to handling.

Occupational therapists often collaborate with speech pathologists in developing an intervention program to address oral motor issues. Occupational and speech therapists have described handling techniques to either compensate for motor impairments or support the development of oral motor abilities associated with eating (Klein & Delaney, 1994; Morris & Klein, 2000; Wolf & Glass, 1992). These handling techniques have evolved over years of applied experience, but therapists have only recently subjected them to systematic study. The reflective clinician recognizes that certain handling techniques are more effective with some types of oral movement problems than with other conditions affecting children's oral motor abilities. The therapist also needs to consider pragmatic issues, such as the immediate need to help families incorporate safe and effective feeding methods and the frequency and duration of direct therapy services, in selecting treatment techniques and describing expected outcomes.

Some handling techniques can provide mechanical assistance when the child does not have the muscle strength or oral motor control to do the occupation independently. Compensation strategies, such as good positioning, immediately influence quality of occupational performance. Researchers have investigated the effectiveness of oral support using the therapist's fingers on the infant's cheeks and under the chin in a study of premature infants (Einarsson-Backes, Deitz, Price, Glass, & Hays, 1994). Preterm infants have the potential but lack the neurologic maturation to perform sucking movements in an organized manner. The caregiver's hands support jaw stability and control the bridge until the infant matures sufficiently to acquire his or her own control.

Handling before Feeding. The therapist and caregiver can best address certain neuromotor problems both before and during feeding. Children with hypotonicity of the oral musculature often benefit from techniques to at least temporarily improve muscle tone. Glass and Wolf (1998) described techniques that improve muscle tone and therefore muscle responsivity during feeding. Tapping or quick stretch of cheeks and lips provides sensory input that increases muscle tone around the mouth. The therapist should apply the tapping or stretch symmetrically and rhythmically, repeating the stimulation several times within a brief period immediately before feeding. Vibration is a stronger stimulus that can increase tone and ready muscles for movement. Children with low muscle tone and hypersensitivity may benefit from vibration around the mouth. Vibration should be used with caution to avoid overstimulating the child.

Preparation for Children with Hypertonicity. When the child has high muscle tone of the lips, cheeks, and tongue, the therapist can recommend that the parent apply deep and firm pressure using a downward stroking motion symmetrically to the cheeks and around the lips. The therapist or parent can apply firm rhythmic sustained pressure through the lower jaw (chin), facilitating a chin tuck position. He or she can also apply touch pressure to the child's cheeks to inhibit or decrease lip retraction.

In the child with oral hypertonicity, often the tongue retracts to the back of the mouth or extends beyond the lips. Good postural alignment often helps inhibit these extreme tongue positions. Facilitation techniques can temporarily change movements of the tongue. The therapist can place his or her finger (or the bowl of the spoon) in the middle of the tongue and apply rhythmic, downward pressure. The pressure should be forward for the retracted tongue and backward for the extended tongue. Rhythmic pressure using a downward motion of one beat per second can promote a sucking pattern (Morris & Klein, 2000). Jiggling or lateral movement of the spoon or finger on the tongue can be inhibitory and should be used based on the child's response. Once feeding begins, the parent should continue downward pressure with the use of the bowl of the spoon.

Techniques during Feeding. The therapist's or parent's fingers can provide external support of the jaw under and around the lower jaw. The therapist can apply his or her hand to the child's chin either from the front or from the side (Figure 14-6). One finger places pres-

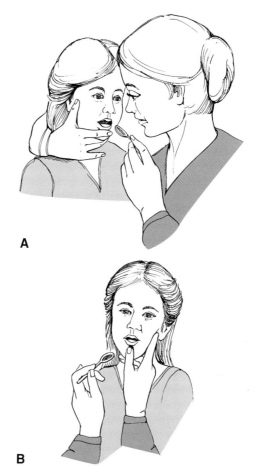

FIGURE 14-6 Jaw control and oral support. **A,** From the side. **B,** From the front.

sure through the front of the chin to promote chin tuck, and another provides support under the jaw. The finger under the jaw provides a source of stability, inhibits wide jaw excursions, and provides a support base for tongue movement. Important aspects of successfully using jaw support include use of the flat side of the finger (rather than the fingertip) and use of the finger as a source of support to the child's jaw movement, not to direct the child's movement. Forcefully moving the child's jaw is inappropriate. The therapist places the finger under the chin midway between the tip of the jaw and the throat and is careful not to move the hand's pressure into the throat. The therapist or parent should maintain his or her hand under and around the jaw during the entire feeding rather than removing and reapplying it with each bite. This support to the jaw may be particularly critical when the child is drinking from a cup, at which time the jaw's movement may increase. The goal of this activity is for the child to gain adequate internal jaw and tongue stability to eat and drink without physical assistance.

Cheek Support. In infants the therapist may apply touch pressure to the cheeks using the thumb and index finger (with the third finger under the jaw). This pressure is appropriate only during bottle-feeding as a

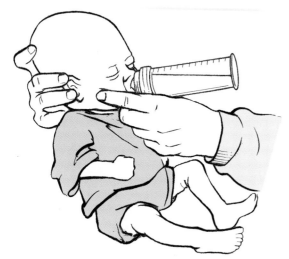

FIGURE 14-7   Jaw and cheek support of the infant during bottle-feeding.

method to increase negative pressure within the mouth and therefore improve suction on the nipple (Einarsson-Backes et al., 1994). The pressure to the cheeks can improve the lip's seal and sucking patterns (Figure 14-7).

Spoon Placement.   A small spoon with a swallow bowl allows for easy food removal. The placement of the spoon can influence the child's oral motor responses. Downward pressure of the spoon on the center of the tongue can facilitate a sucking response. This can be effective for moving the food to the back of the tongue for swallowing.

Downward and inward pressure with the spoon (or nipple) can promote the up-and-down tongue movement observed in mature sucking. This pressure can also inhibit tongue thrust during feeding. Central placement of the spoon is appropriate when the child has only a sucking pattern and the tongue moves in extension and retraction. To encourage tongue lateralization and the beginning of chewing patterns, the therapist recommends to the parent placing the spoon to the side. Food placement between the gums and teeth directly promotes chewing. The therapist instructs the parent to place food on alternating sides and to place food in the central to anterior part of the mouth. Inserting the spoon or food to the posterior portion of the tongue results in gagging and does not allow the child to move, chew, and control the food before swallowing.

Head Position.   A chin tuck position with the head well aligned on the shoulders is generally best for feeding. This head position may require the support of the caregiver or therapist's arm in the back of the neck or under the occipital lobe.

Although complete upright posture allows for correct swallowing and helps reduce the possibility of aspiration, certain children may need a position of slight neck flexion to help them swallow. Positioning the head slightly forward in neck flexion reduces the possibility of aspiration because it reduces the distance that the larynx must move upward to initiate the swallow.

The therapist should use a position of neck flexion with caution because it may interfere with breathing. Some children posture in neck hyperextension despite efforts to hold them in a position of neutral neck alignment. This is the case with children who have difficulty breathing and are seeking a completely open air passageway. A VFSS may help elucidate if aspiration occurs in this position, giving guidance to the therapist as to how important neutral neck alignment is to the child's feeding. The therapist should avoid pushing the neck into extension during feeding by handling the neck at key points to improve neck alignment (e.g., manual pressure on the upper chest).

Altering the Sensory Quality of Foods.   The progression of the food textures listed in Table 14-4 provides examples of food consistencies that require progressively higher-level oral motor skills. Although the therapist and parent use strategies to help the child develop improved oral motor skills, foods selected for the child's diet should accommodate the child's current skill level and should challenge the child to develop higher-level skills. Thin liquids are the most difficult consistency to control in the mouth and should be thickened when the child has poor tongue control and an inefficient suck-swallow pattern.

Eating pureed foods requires no more than a suck-swallow response; therefore giving the child pureed foods elicits sucking. To elicit munching and chewing patterns, the child must receive soft foods with greater texture. Increasing the sensory input using highly textured foods facilitates tongue lateralization and tip elevation, active lip movements, and increased chewing responses.

The therapist can hold a long piece of vegetable or soft meat between the child's side teeth to promote graded biting. He or she may initially use strips of soft cheese, chicken, or a long green bean. Soft cookies and crackers placed to the side can also promote controlled biting. Pretzels, French fries, and apple slices require more jaw strength and can be tried as a next step in promoting biting skills.

Certain foods can increase muscle tone and chewing. Cheese and apples can promote rotary chewing and graded jaw movements. Some dried fruits (e.g., raisins, apricots, and apples) can help increase chewing. Tough or fibrous meats are contraindicated. Box 14-4 provides a list of foods that are indicated and contraindicated for children with immature oral motor skills.

Efficacy of Techniques.   Therapists have guided traditional treatment for children with cerebral palsy through handling techniques designed to provide sensory and motor experiences that replicated normal

BOX 14-4   Foods Indicated and Contraindicated for Children with Immature Oral Motor Skills

PROPERTIES OF INDICATED FOODS
Even consistency
Increased density and volume
Thick (liquids)
Uniform texture
Stays together (will not break up in the mouth)
Easy to remove and suck

PROPERTIES OF CONTRAINDICATED FOODS
Multiple textures and consistencies (tacos, vegetable soup, stews, and salads)
Sticky (peanut butter)
Greasy (fried foods)
Tough (red meat, processed meats, and diced fruit)
Fibrous and stringy (celery, citrus fruits, and raw vegetables)
Skins (raw fruits and peanuts)
Spicy (pepper and horseradish)
Seeds and nuts (plain or in breads and cakes)
Thin (liquids such as water, carbonated drinks, broth, coffee, tea, and apple juice)
Quickly liquefying (Jell-O and watermelon)
Foods that break up in the mouth (some cookies and flaky pastries)
Crunchy (chips and carrots)

movements (Adams & Snyder, 1998). Therapists, over time, found that higher parts of the motor system would learn and be able to replicate the experienced movement as part of an action during an occupation. Therapists have questioned the effectiveness of techniques that emphasize practicing movements if there is significant motor impairment (Heriza, 1991; Mathiowetz & Haugen, 1994). Gisel et al. (1995) examined the efficacy of intervention to enhance sensory and motor oral functions for 27 children with cerebral palsy over 10- to 20-week periods. They individualized treatment to the child, which lasted 5 to 7 minutes, 5 days a week. The children practiced components of oral motor skills, including tongue lateralization, lip control, and vigor of chewing. The researchers used food to elicit specific oral movements. Treatment included monitoring progress to introduce more food texture during snack or lunch as new oral motor skills were observed. The researchers found some significant changes in the children's ability to eat. After intervention, the researchers decreased the duration of meals slightly and the children progressed to eating increased texture. These gains were modest but suggested that the intervention may produce greater change if implemented over a longer period of time.

In selecting handling techniques to promote oral motor skills, therapists continually monitor the effects of their strategies on the child's eating skill. Working at the level of client factors (e.g., lip closure or increased tongue lateralization) is likely to be a long-term process and can be worthwhile if the functional goal is kept in mind (Rogers & Holms, 1998). The therapist should maintain eating food and drinking liquids as the source of motivation and the goal that organizes movement (Humphry & Morrow, 1998). Handling techniques will be most effective if the strategy feels natural and can be incorporated into daily routines by caregivers and parents.

INTERVENTION FOR SWALLOWING PROBLEMS

Children with swallowing disorders tend to have severe neuromotor impairments or physiologic immaturity that interferes with the coordination of the *suck-swallow-breathe sequence*. These children may not be oral feeders. If the child is at risk for aspiration or is known to aspirate, he or she may feed through a gastrostomy or jejunostomy tube. Children who do not feed by mouth have limited ability to participate in mealtime. A child with a gastrostomy may be limited to tasting small bites of food during the mealtime. Sometimes the child eats the same foods as the family with them pureed to a consistency that allows their flow through the gastrostomy tube. The child's participation may be limited to sitting and interacting with the family during mealtime without eating.

Other children with swallowing problems may continue to eat by mouth and benefit from intervention to improve the suck, swallow, and breathe sequence. To understand swallowing disorders related to neuromotor dysfunction or physiologic immaturity, this section briefly describes the normal phases of swallowing.

Swallowing and Coordinating the Suck-Swallow-Breathe Sequence
Oral Phase

In the first phase of swallowing, the oral phase, the food enters into the mouth, where it is processed. This phase consists of biting, sucking, chewing, or munching. The food is moved side to side for chewing and comes to the center as a bolus for transit to the back of the tongue. In the oral transit phase, the masticated food or liquid is moved to the back of the tongue, where swallowing is initiated. Therefore swallowing is essentially a reflexive response to the sensory input of the food on the posterior portion of the tongue (Morris & Klein, 2000). The oral and oral transit phases are the only swallow phases that the child controls. These phases establish the timing and coordination of the swallow and are therefore critical to efficient swallowing. Therapeutic input to influence swallowing improves the child's control of the initial oral phases.

Pharyngeal Phase

In the pharyngeal phase the bolus moves from the back of the tongue through the pharynx to the opening of the esophagus. The propulsion of the bolus is based on negative pressure; therefore closure of the nasal, laryngeal, and oral openings is important for efficient bolus transit. The larynx is protected by the closure of the epiglottis over the trachea and the contraction of the true and false vocal cords. At the same time that the esophagus opens, the negative pressure propels the bolus through the pharynx to the esophagus opening.

Esophageal Phase

In the esophageal phase the food or liquid moves through the esophagus using peristalsis. The swallow itself and the sensation of the food involuntarily initiate peristalsis (Tuchman, 1994). The upper esophageal sphincter closes immediately after a bolus enters the esophagus. A combination of gravity and peristaltic action moves the food into the stomach. After the bolus enters the stomach, the lower sphincter closes to prevent upward movement of the food (Morris & Klein, 2000).

Problems

The following problems can affect the child's ability to coordinate sequential swallows without aspiration. When neuromotor problems are severe, the tongue moves primarily in extension or demonstrates minimal movement and tone. Children with severe oral motor dysfunction are often unable to gather the food into a bolus for swallowing. The food may trickle over the sides of the tongue and the pharynx without eliciting a swallow. Foods that break apart can scatter in the mouth, and bits may fall into the pharynx. When a swallow is not triggered, the protective closure of the epiglottis does not occur, leaving the trachea open, and aspiration becomes highly probable. When liquids and food pool in the pharynx, the child is at high risk for aspiration. When the oral transit phase is slow or is without a rhythmic sequence, the swallow either appears delayed or seems to occur at random. The primary problem created by delayed swallowing is that food enters the pharynx before or after the swallow, where it pools or where it may enter the larynx.

The child with a respiratory disorder is also at high risk for swallow dysfunction. Although the child typically demonstrates adequate oral motor skills and swallowing, the suck-swallow-breathe sequence is poorly coordinated. Typically the infant with respiratory distress syndrome demonstrates rapid and shallow breathing patterns. The infant's oxygen level may plummet when breathing momentarily pauses to allow for swallowing. Rapid breathing in an irregular pattern prevents development of a regular, rhythmic pattern of swallowing.

The infant who struggles to breathe has increased respiratory difficulty when feeding. He or she may attempt to breathe and swallow at the same time.

Evaluation

Assessment of swallowing disorders or the possibility of a swallowing disorder includes all of the strategies described previously in the chapter, including obtaining the following:

- History of feeding and description of mealtime participation from the caregiver
- Medical history by written or parental report
- Clinical observation of feeding
- VFSS

Parental Report

As described previously, the therapist requests a detailed description of typical feeding from the parent. Guiding questions are as follows:

1 How does the child participate in mealtime?
2 Where and when is the child fed?
3 What kinds of foods are given to the child?
4 How does the child respond during feeding? Does he or she demonstrate aversive responses and, if so, to what types of food?
5 Does the child choke, gag, or cough? Is food lost during feeding?
6 Does the child sound raspy during feeding? Does his or her breathing sound noisy (wet) during or after feeding?
7 Does the child have frequent upper respiratory infections?

For the child who is underweight or is eating a restricted diet because of problems swallowing some types of food, a detailed record of the amount of food eaten over a 3-day period is important for the therapist to identify nutritional intake (Crist, Napier-Phillips, McDonnel, Dedwidge, & Beck, 1998). The nutritionist analyzes this record to develop a comprehensive intervention plan for increased nutritional intake and a balanced diet.

Medical History

The therapist should obtain all medical records, including records of neurologic examination and results of CT scans and brain imaging scans. Frequently occurring pneumonia and upper respiratory infections are typical in the child who regularly aspirates. The therapist should carefully read past records of the results of VFSS and consider them in the intervention plan. Consultation with a speech pathologist that has completed an evaluation of the child can also help the therapist gain understanding of the child's oral motor function.

Clinical Observation

The therapist should observe feeding in the child's natural environment. If the evaluation takes place in a clinic or school, the therapist should use foods that the child typically eats. The therapist should place the child in his or her typical feeding position and use feeding utensils and methods familiar to the child. After observing typical feeding, the therapist should attempt new positions and different foods as appropriate. The foods and methods tried during the evaluation are techniques that the therapist postulates will improve oral motor skill and swallow. Therefore the therapist obtains assessment information regarding what intervention strategies seem to promote skills and the child's responsiveness to different intervention methods. As discussed previously, the therapist should ask the parent if the child's behaviors are typical or unique to the stress of the evaluation situation (e.g., interacting with strangers in an unfamiliar setting).

Videofluoroscopic Swallow Study

The VFSS is an essential component of the evaluation process when a child exhibits the clinical signs of swallow dysfunction. Often the VFSS provides the most conclusive evidence of the swallowing problem and results in specific recommendations for food consistencies and feeding positions that seem to promote oral motor skill and reduce the possibility of aspiration (Zerilli, Stefans, & DiPietro, 1990).

Intervention

Intervention for swallowing dysfunction relates specifically to the child's unique strengths and limitations as shown in the evaluation. The following techniques were outlined by Glass and Wolf (1998) and address components of eating. At all times the first concern of the therapist is safety, so his or her first consideration is compensation strategies to ensure safe intake of nutrition.

Increase Initiation of Swallowing

For young infants, the therapist can activate the muscles involved in swallowing by applying cold stimulation to the tongue and soft palate using a frozen pacifier. When the muscles are readied for action, the swallow reflex is initiated more quickly. Wolf and Glass (1992) also recommend the use of chilled formula to quicken the swallow reflex. In an older child, the therapist can use a popsicle or piece of ice before feeding or intermittently during feeding. Logemann (2000) recommended giving the child a cold or sour (e.g., lemon juice) bolus to elicit a swallow reflex. As with any technique, the therapist should carefully evaluate and adjust the effect of using cold stimulation as needed.

Improve Oral Transit

Many children have swallowing dysfunction associated with poor oral motor control. The food is not efficiently masticated, gathered into a bolus, and moved to the back of the tongue, where the swallow reflex is triggered. This child may benefit from head and jaw support. The jaw support should include facilitation of mouth closure and tongue movement. Jaw support allows the child to focus on moving the tongue within the mouth. Improving mouth closure can increase pressure gradients in the mouth, thereby improving the efficiency of swallowing. Thickening liquids is often extremely helpful in improving swallowing. The thickened liquid moves more slowly within the mouth, allowing the child to better control it; it also has greater adhesion and therefore tends to remain a bolus. Thickened liquid also is heavier and therefore gives more proprioceptive input to the tongue during oral transit.

Position can improve the child's ability to swallow. When the child is positioned in extension, he or she has less control of the food's movement because of the effects of gravity. With the neck extended, the child has difficulty with mouth closure and efficient tongue movements. Positioning the child's head in neck flexion can improve closure of the larynx during swallowing, therefore decreasing the possibility of aspiration. Good neck alignment increases the child's ability to control the food's movement.

Handling and Intervention during Feeding

When children have respiratory disorders, swallowing is problematic as it relates to breathing and the child's coordination of the suck-swallow-breathe sequence. In therapy with the infant who remains on some oxygen support, use of a nasal cannula or another source of oxygen during feeding is important. With oxygen support, rapid breathing is slowed to a pace that better allows for intermittent swallowing. Slowing of respiration encourages better control of the suck-swallow-breathe sequence.

Placing the child in a full upright position can also improve respiration during feeding and can facilitate coordination of swallowing. Often the infant with a respiratory disorder struggles during feeding because he or she initiates a rapid sequence of sucking and is unable to establish an appropriate suck-swallow-breathe sequence. As a result, the infant coughs or chokes when the breathing becomes an absolute, immediate necessity. Glass and Wolf (1998) recommended a technique termed *external pacing*. To pace the infant's sucking pattern, the therapist breaks the infant's sucking sequence by gently removing the nipple from the mouth. By interrupting an otherwise long sucking sequence, the therapist gives the child an opportunity to breathe and relax. This method gives the child an externally imposed pace and suck-swallow-breathe sequence.

With older children who are spoon feeding, helping the child to self-feed can slow the pace of the feeding and cue the child to swallow (Logemann, 2000). Also, encouraging the child to dry swallow in between swallows of food can help to clear the pharynx of liquid.

Modify the Infant's Food

Children with respiratory or cardiac disorders typically have poor endurance and less oral intake than other children. One way to improve their nutrient and caloric intake is to increase the caloric density of their food. Formula is available in different caloric densities, and Karo syrup can be added. For older children, the caregiver can add peanut butter, butter, gravies, and powdered milk to foods. These diet changes require consultation and direction by a nutritionist. The therapist should discuss any diet change with a nutritionist or the physician to ensure that the child's overall nutritional intake is positively affected.

Mealtime Participation

Often a child who has difficulty swallowing needs one-on-one attention during a meal. The therapist encourages the family to allow the child to participate in family mealtime by tasting and exploring foods at the table. Therapists need to appreciate that children who have significant swallow problems require extensive time to feed. When recommendations are given, the therapist considers the caregivers' time investment and attempts to give solutions that do not increase the time needed to feed.

Nonoral Feeding

Several methods of nonoral feeding are available to infants with persistent swallowing disorders that result in aspiration, with poor feeding endurance that results in failure to thrive, or with limitations in oral motor function that prevent adequate food intake. Nonoral methods include nasogastric, oral gastric, gastrostomy, and jejunostomy tubes. In any infant or child whose food intake is inadequate for growth or whose lack of oral motor skills and swallow efficiency make feeding unsafe, the feeding team should consider nonoral feedings. The therapist helps the parent view nonoral feeding as a method to improve the health and developmental status of the child. It should not result in complete removal of oral stimulation or complete removal of

the feeding interaction. In many instances, the placement of a gastrostomy or the use of other nonoral feeding methods is a temporary measure to promote the child's nutritional status and growth (Tarbell & Allaire, 2002).

Hyperalimentation, also termed *parenteral nutrition*, involves a medical procedure in which a central line introduces highly nutritional solutions directly into the bloodstream. It provides protein and calorie intake sufficient to sustain life and to promote growth in the absence of adequate gastrointestinal tract function. Hyperalimentation is used for children with congenital bowel anomalies or in severe medical crises (Batshaw & Perret, 1992). It requires a surgical procedure to insert the catheter into a large vein, typically a vein near the heart. The surgeon may use the brachial artery. The surgeon pumps the fluid into the bloodstream, requiring that the child be connected to an intravenous pump at all times (Wong, 1997). A complication of this form of nutritional intake is yeast and bacterial infection, which can result in death. Although long-term use of hyperalimentation is possible, generally children who cannot make the transition to another form of nutritional intake do not survive beyond infancy.

Use of nonoral feeding should not end the child's oral experiences and the enjoyment of interaction during feeding. When the caregiver administers bolus feedings, he or she can also give the child oral stimulation. The parent or caregiver can give the child small amounts of food before the nonoral feeding or during the feeding. If the child has routine aspiration, sucking on a pacifier during gastrostomy feeding may be safest. The goal is to link a pleasurable oral experience with the satiation of hunger. This type of oral stimulation during nonoral feeding is particularly critical for the child who is expected to return to oral feeding.

Transition from Nonoral Feeding to Oral Feeding

The feeding team initiates the transition from nonoral to oral feeding with a physician's recommendation, based on the child's medical status and an evaluation of the child's oral motor skills by an occupational or speech therapist. After considering the health care team's recommendations, the family decides whether a transition to oral feeding is desirable and, if so, when and how they would like to approach this process. Occupational therapists often are instrumental in each phase of the transition.

The first step in a program to transition a child from nonoral to oral feeding is *oral motor intervention*. The child must demonstrate that he or she is capable of oral feeding. The therapist works with the child to desensitize the areas around the mouth and the structures within the mouth. The therapist facilitates specific oral motor skills during sensory play. Activities to desensitize include chewing and sucking of rubber toys, a NUK toothbrush, and a textured cloth (described in the section on hypersensitivities). The therapist gradually offers small amounts of food textures to the child, usually while feeding the child through the gastrostomy tube (Schauster & Dwyer, 1996).

Other activities that encourage oral motor skill development are making sounds, blowing bubbles, and giving kisses. The therapist emphasizes brushing teeth and oral play with toys. The therapist can point out the small successes that the child makes and can help the parent and child maintain an appropriate perspective on the goals (e.g., enjoyment of oral-sensory experiences). The therapist praises and encourages whatever the child chooses to do with food.

Often the child vies for control of the oral sensory experiences, perhaps because of the discomfort involved and the associated lack of meaning of the occupations around meals. The parent, who has anxiety about the child's achieving oral feeding and successfully making the transition without weight loss or health problems, often awards the child's avoidance or manipulative behaviors during feeding with increased attention. Approaches to behavior issues are described in later sections of this chapter.

Another component of the transition from nonoral to oral feeding is *manipulation of the gastrostomy feedings* so that bolus feedings are given rather than continuous feeding (e.g., feeding overnight). The physician instructs the parents to give bolus feedings four to five times per day to emulate a meal schedule. Once the child's digestive tract adjusts to the bolus feedings, health and weight are evaluated to determine if feedings can be reduced. If the child is expected to accept food by mouth, he or she needs to experience hunger; therefore the child must receive a reduced amount of food. Schauster and Dwyer (1996) suggested that a reduction of 25% of the tube feeding is necessary to stimulate hunger. Often children who require gastrostomy feedings are not medically and nutritionally stable enough to reduce their caloric intake; therefore, the transition to oral feeding requires a lengthy time. Some weight loss almost always results from this process; therefore, children who cannot tolerate any weight loss are not candidates for making the transition.

The therapist's support and encouragement are important to the child's and the parents' success in this process. The longer the child has been on nonoral feeding, the more difficult the transition. *Continual support* to the family is needed, and regular communication with the family is critical. The parents need encouragement for the small increments of progress and the loss of progress that occurs at times. The therapist's encouragement helps the parents maintain the energy and positive attitude needed to successfully reach the goal of oral feeding. Parents who experience feeding problems with their child can provide mutual support and assist each other in problem solving. Parent-to-parent support can strengthen their abilities to cope with stressful problems on a day-to-day basis (Chamberlin, Henry, Roberts, Sapsford, & Courtney, 1991). Parent groups are particularly appropriate when children have difficult feeding problems that include behavioral issues that need to be managed over lengthy periods.

INTERVENTION FOR ORAL STRUCTURAL PROBLEMS

Children with oral structural problems at birth may have feeding problems that directly relate to the structural deficits, and a compensation strategy is indicated. Two structural problems that can occur are *cleft lip and palate* and *micrognathia*. Cleft lip and palate is the fourth most common disability in children, affecting almost 1 in 700 children in the United States. These problems often create feeding difficulties, particularly in the perinatal period (Emondson & Reinhartsen, 1998). The role of the occupational therapist is to make recommendations for feeding equipment, adapted methods, and positions to be used until the child undergoes plastic surgery or outgrows the structural problem. Because oral structural problems rarely occur with neurologic impairment, the child with cleft lip and palate or micrognathia typically demonstrates intact oral movement and effective suck-swallow coordination once the structural problems are resolved.

A cleft lip and palate is a separation of parts of the mouth usually joined together during the early weeks of fetal development. A cleft lip is separation of the upper lip and often the upper dental ridge. A cleft palate is a separation of the hard or soft palate and occurs with or without a cleft lip. Because of the lack of closure between the oral and nasal cavities, newborns have difficulty maintaining sufficient negative pressure to express liquid from a nipple (Glass & Wolf, 1999). The infant's tongue does not have an upper surface to express milk from the breast or bottle.

Cleft lips and palates are closed through surgery. Surgeons can repair cleft lips in the first few months of life. Repair of a cleft palate is more extensive, and the surgeon generally waits until the infant reaches a certain weight, usually by 12 months of age. Generally, surgeons perform multiple procedures to correct the abnormalities. These surgeries include bone grafting, orthodontic repair, and placement of ear tubes.

Micrognathia refers to a small, receded lower jaw. The mouth and tongue may be of normal size but are posteriorly positioned in relation to the upper jaw and the airway. Children with Pierre Robin syndrome have both micrognathia and cleft palate.

Evaluation

Evaluation involves inspection of the oral structures and assessment of how the defects limit the feeding process. Evaluation should include observation of feeding to assess how the food travels through the mouth and how well the infant can express liquids from the nipple.

During the evaluation process, the therapist should try several different feeding devices, methods, and positions to identify methods that overcome the structural defects and allow safe oral intake. The infant may need a VFSS to identify if aspiration occurs or if liquids move into the nasal passageway.

Intervention

The therapist sometimes recommends that the parent use squeeze bottles to express liquids into the infant's mouth when suction is limited. Because the parent rather than the infant controls the flow of liquid, it is more difficult for the infant to predict and time an effective swallow. A variety of nipples are designed for use with children who have structural problems. These nipples compensate for lack of negative pressure and for limitations in tongue position and movement. The Habermann nipple was developed specifically for infants with cleft palate to deliver flow without requiring suction (Figure 14-8). It has a one-way valve that allows the infant to express fluid by compression alone, compensating for lack of suction (Glass & Wolf, 1999). This nipple allows the infant to independently control milk flow.

Some nipples adjust the flow of the liquid during feeding by turning the nipple's rim. The therapist can use long thin nipples to carry the liquid to the back of the mouth past the cleft palate to avoid liquid flow into the nasal passageway. The physician sometimes recommends a prosthetic device (i.e., an obturator) to lengthen

the palate to prevent liquid from escaping into the nasal cavity (Edmondson & Reinhartsen, 1998).

Glass and Wolf (1999) suggested that therapists avoid cross-cut nipples because they create an uneven flow that is more difficult for the infant to control. The therapist must work carefully with the parent so that the liquid flows easily from the bottle but is not excessive, resulting in a flow that the child cannot control. The therapist should consider the nipple characteristics in Table 14-5 when making recommendations to parents or nurses.

The infant with cleft lip and palate or micrognathia benefits from upright positioning. By holding the infant in a vertical position, the risk of aspiration is reduced. Upright positioning can promote forward movement of a recessed jaw and can prevent nasal and pharyngeal aspiration in the infant with cleft palate.

When micrognathia is severe, the tongue may occlude the airway. When the condition compromises respiration, the child may need placement of tracheostomy and

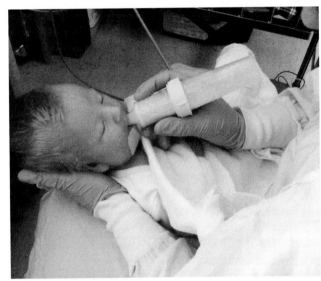

FIGURE 14-8 Infant uses Habermann feeder. (Courtesy of Jayne Shepherd.)

TABLE 14-5 Nipple Characteristics Related to Use with Children Who Have Oral Structural Defects

Nipple Type	Characteristics
Long, thin nipples	Work well when the tongue is recessed; can bring the tongue forward
Single nipple hole	Results in a steady liquid stream, which can be easier to handle than bursts of liquid
Wide nipple	Can be compressed for liquid expression for the child with a cleft palate
Broad-based nipple	Can help the infant with a cleft lip gain suction
Nipple with cross-cut hole	Can create an uneven liquid flow or a burst of fluid that is difficult for the infant to control
Nipple with enlarged hole	Should be used with great care; when the caregiver enlarges the hole, it is difficult to predict what type of liquid flow will result
Soft, pliable nipple	Appropriate for infants with cleft palates who are unable to achieve suction
NUK nipple	Has the hole on top of the nipple and should not be used with children with cleft palates; this nipple may be functional if its position on the tongue is reversed

gastrostomy tubes. These procedures provide temporary support of respiration and nutrition until the surgeon can repair the structural problems. Use of a long, firm nipple can assist with tongue position and movement. Downward pressure on the tongue can promote a sucking response. The therapist helps to control and slow the flow of liquid by selecting a low flow nipple and by periodically removing the nipple to allow the infant to take extra breaths without swallowing (Glass & Wolf, 1999).

The following example illustrates the role of the occupational therapist with the infant who has Pierre Robin syndrome.

Case Study

Sarah was born with Pierre Robin syndrome and presented with a small recessed chin and retracted tongue. She also had a deep cleft in her hard and soft palates. She struggled with her first feedings. On the third day of life, her retracted tongue fell into her airway, completely occluding it. Because Sarah was connected to a monitor, the medical team immediately intubated her. She then received a tracheostomy and gastrostomy to avoid further complications caused by the position of her tongue. She was discharged home on continuous feedings and moist air to her tracheostomy. She required respiratory treatment and frequent suctioning to keep her lungs clear. In the first few months she had frequent pneumonia, but she became healthy by 3 months of age. Her growth was adequate, although she remained in the fifth percentile of weight for height.

An occupational therapist initiated home-based therapy to develop an oral motor program that would promote development of her oral motor skills while she received gastrostomy feedings and awaited surgery, which was anticipated to occur at 18 months. The therapist initiated and recommended that the family implement a program of graded oral input. Because Sarah did not exhibit mouthing of her hands or objects, the therapist's first efforts were to initiate a hand-to-mouth movement pattern and to rub her gums with the pacifier. Sarah used the pacifier for brief periods, but she was unable to maintain suction on it to independently hold it in her mouth. Her preferred oral stimulus was her mother's finger.

The therapist applied slow, rhythmic stroking to Sarah's tongue to bring it forward. By 5 months of age, Sarah could hold the pacifier in her mouth. At that time the therapist dipped her pacifier in fruit juice to introduce tastes. She frequently mouthed her fingers. Sarah's mother began using the NUK toothbrush for additional stimulation, and Sarah enjoyed chewing on it. Sarah demonstrated increased tolerance of a warm washcloth on her face.

By 7 months of age, Sarah learned to sit upright when supported at the pelvis and to sit at midline in an infant seat. Her increased stability of neck and trunk allowed for more oral motor experiences. The therapist introduced pureed foods, first on the nipple and NUK toothbrush. The therapist applied desensitization, using stroking with a washcloth to increase her sensory tolerance. She then began to take two to five spoonfuls of pureed fruits. The therapist applied downward and forward pressure with the bowl of the spoon. Sarah tolerated this procedure and seemed to enjoy it after several weeks. She developed good suction on the pacifier. The physician recommended that the parent give feedings in boluses to emulate oral feedings. When the parent began bolus feedings, she performed oral stimulation immediately before the gastrostomy feeding with the hope that Sarah would be hungry and more receptive to oral stimulation. She was receptive but did not consume more than five spoonfuls. She was not hungry because she received total nutrition through the gastrostomy. At that time, her suck-swallow sequence was well coordinated, and her tongue was in a forward position.

At 9 months of age, Sarah tolerated various food textures in her mouth. Oral motor skills rapidly progressed and were only slightly behind those of her typically developing peers. Her tongue and mandible had moved into a forward position, and the physician recommended that she transition to oral feedings without waiting for repair of the cleft palate, which was 9 months in the future. The therapist and nutritionist met with Sarah's mother to design a diet that would increase oral intake and simultaneously reduce gastrostomy feedings. Because oral sensory issues had been addressed in the occupational therapy program and because Sarah's oral motor skills were almost age appropriate, the team thought that the transition would proceed quickly. As the therapist reduced gastrostomy feedings, she carefully monitored Sarah's weight to ensure that her oral intake maintained the nutritional intake required for growth. Although children almost always lose weight in the transition from nonoral to oral feedings, Sarah did not. She and her mother were ready for oral feedings to begin, and Sarah successfully made the transition in 2 weeks.

INTERACTIONAL ASPECTS OF THE CO-OCCUPATION OF FEEDING

As described in Chapter 5, a parent and child form a subsystem within the dynamic family system. Because early feeding is always a shared interaction between the caregiver and infant, any intervention that targets how the child eats affects the parent who is responsible for feeding. When therapeutic activities occur without participation of the child's usual feeders and out of the context of mealtimes, the meaning of the occupation for the child is diminished. When intervention targets impairments or subskills (e.g., practice of lip closure or tolerance of textures by sucking on a toy), the therapist should make a plan for incorporating the newly emerging skills into mealtime activities. Naturally, this generalization of skills needs to involve the child's feeders.

A systems model of the feeding process suggests that one cannot isolate the cause from the consequences of feeding dysfunction in understanding the parent's and child's behaviors around meals (Humphry, 1995). Except in situations where structural oral problems such as cleft lip make immediate identification possible, frequently the therapist does not identify feeding dysfunction until after the parent and child have had weeks, sometimes months, of frustrating experiences in feeding. Understanding factors that influence interactional and social issues during feeding is important as these issues during childhood influence the individual's lifelong eating patterns. Using a systems model enables the occupational therapist to understand the complex issues that affect feeding and to focus on more than one part of the system at a time. Using this model helps the therapist understand how a busy, overstimulating environment and a mother pressed for time can negatively influence the child's ability to use lip closure in taking food from the spoon. Conversely, a child who has difficulty feeding and requires continual caregiver assistance may be disruptive to the family's mealtime, and the therapist can recognize that the family's first priority is social aspects of dinner. In this situation, it may be necessary to address nutritional needs in another context. A focus on parent-child interaction is important when working with children who are diagnosed with failure to thrive. In the past when children did not gain weight, therapists categorized failure to thrive as either organic (a medical problem that led to poor nutrition) or nonorganic (a problem related to parenting and factors in the environment). The interactive systems model offers a more complete picture of feeding (Humphry, 1995). Children that are diagnosed with nonorganic failure to thrive, where parental neglect and inappropriate feeding practices are identified problems, may also demonstrate oral motor delays that affect their nutritional intake and compound the other issues, such as limited time allotted by the parent for the meal. Regardless of the source of feeding problems, the multilevel systems model helps the therapist consider the quality of fit between the parent and child and suggests intervention that will enhance feeding skill acquisition in the child, parenting practices, and interaction of the feeding dyad. The following sections present the caregiver and child's perspectives when feeding is a challenge.

Caregiver's Perspective When a Child Has Feeding Problems

Parents of children with feeding problems frequently report that their difficulties began when the child was 6 months of age (Ramsay, Gisel, & Boutry, 1993). Some parents show great perseverance and creativity in trying to accommodate their child's special needs (Bakker & Woody, 1995). However, these early experiences can have a negative effect on parents and subsequent caregiving behaviors. Mothers of infants with eating problems feed their infants more frequently, feed them for longer periods, worry more about the infant's health, and experience more isolation from social support systems than mothers of infants with no feeding problems (Hagekull & Dahl, 1987). Among infants and preschool-age children with a history of mealtime problems, the parent is more likely to be coercive and have behaviors that can contribute to or sustain feeding problems in the child (Sanders, Patel, LeGrice, & Shepherd, 1993).

Statements made by parents about their choices at mealtimes help the therapist understand what importance and meaning the caregiver derives from feeding. In a qualitative study, Bakker and Woody (1995) interviewed parents of children with developmental disabilities who had feeding problems. They found one common theme—*the importance of nutrition*—suggesting that parents understand the implications of the child's problems for general health. However, sometimes the importance of nutrition is in conflict with another theme—*what is best for the child*. Parents' ideas about what their children experienced during meals helps them define what is best. At times the parent has to decide which theme will guide caregiving decisions. The following is an example of a parent who determines what will guide her decisions.

Joan, the mother of a 5-year-old with athetoid cerebral palsy, worried that her son would not feel that he was part of the family if he sat in his chair and used a tray rather than sitting at the table to eat. In spite of the fact he had better control of the spoon in supported seating with a tray and dropped food onto himself and the floor when he was sitting at the table, Joan wanted the family to be together.

As described previously, part of parenting is integrating advice with what the parent thinks about that child and the meaning of the occupation. In the Bakker and Woody interviews (1995), Sarah said the following while looking at her daughter:

> In the chair there she'll do all this stuff, but in my lap, she relaxes. Of course, now she sees people at the evaluation center, and they all have hissy fits that I do this. Honest. It's more relaxing just to feed her like this than to put her in that chair or to fight her, and it's just me as a mom.

This parent understands the desired therapeutic actions for feeding her daughter with severe motor problems. However, the occupational therapist needs to address how positioning alters the meaning of the occupation for the parent before the parent can expect any substantial changes in the child's seating during meals.

Occupational therapy intervention for feeding problems facilitates behavioral change in both the child and the parent or other adult caregiver. The therapist first considers how to establish a working relationship with the parent and communicate intervention strategies in a way that supports adaptive and effective strategies that the parent already uses, and respects the feelings that the parent expresses about what is important about feeding the child. The therapist recognizes that the parent may experience a sense of failure as a caregiver if nutritional status and growth are poor. Acknowledging the legitimate basis for the parent's stress is a first step in the parent being able to articulate his or her needs. As adults who think about their occupations, parents also have their own theories about why the child is not eating well (Humphry, 1995). Once the therapist and parent establish a collaborative relationship, the therapist can suggest alternative strategies to achieve a feeding goal and ask the parent to select those that he or she feels comfortable implementing. Two important strategies to promote success are to recommend ways that feeding techniques can be incorporated into daily routines and to allow the parent to decide when and how frequently he or she will implement the techniques. A parent may determine that working on drinking from a cup is only realistic at night, just before he or she changes the child's clothes for bed. Another parent may decide that giving the child time to practice self-feeding is only possible on weekends.

Child's Perspective When Feeding Is a Problem

Because children eat several times a day, meals represent frequent learning opportunities that can influence motor, cognitive, and psychosocial functions. The perception of hunger, signaling need, and receiving adult response are the first contingency-response experiences of many infants. Children, especially infants, create opportunities to interact with adults. Once the immediate feelings of hunger are satiated, infants use feeding time to engage and interact with their caregivers (Brazelton, 1993). The reciprocity developed during feeding experiences may be a foundation for subsequent communication. The close physical contact during breast-feeding or bottle-feeding also provides various sensory and motor experiences. As the infant gets older, self-feeding is one of the first experiences to negotiate the issue of autonomy between the child and parent. For preschool- and school-age children, verbal interactions of families during meals provide learning experiences that promote language and concepts about the world (Beals, 1993).

When a child has feeding problems, his behaviors may be negative or oppositional because he or she is fearful of choking or sensory discomfort. The child may experience anxiety about the eating, and behaviors may be negative because of past experiences and his or her memories of discomfort. Sometimes negative or controlling behaviors learned as a protective mechanism during eating become habits and are demonstrated long after feeding or swallowing problems have resolved. The occupational therapist and other team members need to consider how to help parents work through negative behaviors and compensate for the secondary effects on parent-child interaction. Clinicians, teachers, and parents can work together to understand the child's typical communicative acts. If the child signals preferences by making faces or looking toward a desired drink, caregivers should recognize and honor these communications. The following is an example of an interaction between a teacher and a child.

Megan is a 3-year-old girl with spastic cerebral palsy. When feeding Megan, the teacher implemented the occupational therapist's suggestions to promote jaw stabilization by placing her fingers under Megan's jaw as she offered a bite of ground food. The teacher noted that Megan looked at the chocolate pudding on the side of the tray. The teacher could acknowledge Megan's interest in the pudding by naming it and talking about how she could have the pudding after her meal. If Megan's feeders only concentrated on head position and jaw stability, Megan would learn that her efforts at making her needs known were not worth the effort.

IMPLICATIONS OF SOCIAL CONTEXTS IN FEEDING

All aspects of the environment—cultural, physical, and interpersonal—influence feeding. Meals also have a temporal context in other life routines, so feeding must occur within the demands of time for other family or classroom occupations. Direct observation is an ideal strategy for the therapist to understand contextual factors in feeding. When this is unrealistic, the therapist should ask the parent to describe a typical meal and request specific details of the child's behaviors and the environment to appreciate variations in the elements of the social context.

As discussed at the beginning of the chapter, the family's cultural background can determine selection and preparation of food and the interactive rituals during mealtimes. One component of social context is ethnicity and its implications for feeding practices. For example, despite common recommendation that children not be given products with cow's milk, a mother from the Middle East may feel that yogurt, a common food in a family's diet, is an ideal first food for an infant. Asking parents about the different foods in their culture helps build rapport because it shows the therapist's interest in the family's traditions.

The family's interactive routines may also determine physical features of mealtime. For example, some families strive to always eat together watching a television show or sitting in a special dining area. In addition, the family's background may determine how the child is seated during feeding; therefore, therapists must consider whether changing positions is essential.

Another component of the social context of feeding is the generally shared assumptions about good parenting and feeding. Confusion exists about the amount of food that children typically eat at different ages, even among parents of typically developing children. Occupational therapists are just one of many sources of information on feeding. Caregivers acquire information about how and what to feed an infant from family members, neighbors, texts on child development, and other health professionals. The occupational therapist who asks about the feeding techniques that the parent has tried should specifically explore suggestions that have come from relatives and neighbors (see Box 14-1). If the family structure is hierarchic, the therapist may need to discuss feeding alternatives with the family member who has the authority to make decisions rather than the primary caregiver who is feeding the child. The therapist often needs to meet with several family members to come to a consensus. The occupational therapist may see the child in a clinic or special part of the classroom where the social and physical context of feeding cannot be directly observed. Questions about meals (see Box 14-1) are important for the therapist to make effective suggestions.

Intervention for Self-Feeding Issues

Delays in self-feeding skills result when the child's performance in cognitive, behavioral, sensory, or motor skills is delayed or deficit. The respondents of a survey of occupational therapists who were interested in developmental disability reported that the largest proportion of children with feeding delays were experiencing problems primarily associated with motor deficits (41%). The second most common issues influencing feeding were sensory problems (30%) and general developmental delays or behavioral problems (22%) (Thigpen-Beck & Dovenitz, 1995). In planning intervention, the first consideration of the therapist is to determine that the child can safely eat daily and with reasonable efficiency for his or her parents and teachers. After ensuring that safety and daily nutritional needs are met, the therapist will work to promote self-feeding independence.

Evaluation

To design interventions to assist a child in learning to self-feed, a complete assessment of the child's motor, sensory, cognitive, and communication skills is needed. The child must indicate an interest in self-feeding and an interest in exploring food. Postural stability and alignment is assessed to determine how much and what types of external support are needed. Specific skills in grasping a utensil and moving hand to mouth are assessed to determine strategies for promoting independence in spoon and fork feeding.

Intervention

Occupational therapists may propose compensation or remedial strategies to improve a child's self-feeding. Strategies during mealtime include position of the child, handling techniques, adaptation of the tasks, and use of adapted equipment. Behavior issues in self-feeding require a comprehensive team approach. Many general issues about behaviors are discussed in Chapter 13. Interventions at the impairment level to improve arm and hand strength and control are described in Chapter 10.

Positioning

Correct postural alignment and stability are critical to the child's success in self-feeding. Control of the arm in space while bringing the spoon to the mouth requires a stable postural base. Children with cerebral palsy often lack adequate postural stability for a base of arm control, moving the arm toward midline. The child must feel secure and relaxed during self-feeding so that his or her endurance is adequate to feed the entire meal. Various seating arrangements are available to stabilize the child for self-feeding.

Wheelchair. The child's wheelchair may offer ideal positioning and comfort for feeding and often has a tray to support the plate and cup. Positioning with the head, neck, and trunk in upright alignment is similar to the positioning described previously for feeding the child. Correct posture for self-feeding includes a tucked chin, depressed shoulders, and a neutral pelvis. The child can maintain an upright position for feeding if the wheelchair has a firm seat and is an appropriate size. Pelvic and hip abductor straps and lateral trunk support help support the position of a neutral pelvis and a symmetric, upright trunk. When the child tends to retract his or her shoulders, padded humeral "wings" on the back of the chair or on the wheelchair tray can maintain the arms in a forward protracted position. These "wings" help increase arm stability and maintain the child's hands at midline for self-feeding.

Rifton Child's Chair. Once the child has fair to good sitting stability, the Rifton chair is an excellent choice for feeding. The Rifton chair places the child in a completely upright position and requires good head control. This chair has a firm seat and back, adjustable foot rests, arm supports, and pelvic strapping. A pelvic abductor pad can be added to the system. A tray is desirable for weight bearing on arms during feeding and for additional sitting stability. The tray provides a surface for play with food or for self-feeding if the child has those skills.

Child's High Chair. The advantages of using a high chair are discussed in the previous section and apply to self-feeding as well.

Tray Adaptations. Regardless of the chair selected, the tray fitted for the chair offers opportunities for modification of positioning. A tray adaptation that helps increase arm stability and improve the arm's position for feeding is a small (short) bolster that can be placed under the arm. By separating the elbow from the trunk, the shoulder is abducted and the elbow is stabilized at a height that enables the child to scoop food onto the spoon and reach the mouth using a pattern of elbow flexion. The bolster serves as a lever from which the child can efficiently reach the tray (and food) and his or her mouth.

Another effective compensation strategy to improve control of the hand-to-mouth pattern is to raise the tray or feeding surface. Raising the tray brings it higher on the child's trunk, thereby assisting with trunk stability. A higher tray also holds the arms in greater humeral abduction, which decreases the distance that the hand travels to reach the mouth and can improve control of the hand-to-mouth movement. By stabilizing the elbow on the tray, the child can move in a simple pattern of elbow flexion and extension to self-feed.

Handling Strategies during Self-Feeding

Self-feeding is a particular challenge for children with poor arm and hand control, such as those with athetoid cerebral palsy. These individuals may benefit from handling during feeding to improve control and to enhance the movement patterns used during feeding. The techniques that therapists use often involve facilitation of shoulder depression and protraction and scapular stability to increase the child's control of distal arm movement. The therapist may place his or her hand on top of the child's shoulders or scapula. Support or guidance of the humerus may be necessary to establish a smooth hand-to-mouth pattern. The therapist helps stabilize and support the arm with his or her arm underneath the child's arm. By supporting underneath, the child controls the arm's movement. Arm support should be intermittent and as needed based on the responses of the child.

Other children have poor control of free movement in space and rely on vision to guide movements. This is especially challenging since self-feeding involves moving the hand through space toward a target that the child cannot visualize (the mouth). The child lacks feedback about wrist position and when the food spills, and he or she has difficulty understanding what to change. In one recommended technique, the therapist holds the spoon handle between the extended index and third fingers. The therapist slips these fingers into the child's palm with a thumb on the dorsum of the child's hand. The child holds onto the fingers and spoon using a palmar grasp, and the therapist facilitates a self-feeding pattern using subtle and natural facilitation from within the child's hand. Klein and Delaney (1994) recommended that the therapist hold the spoon in the child's palm by placing one finger in the palm and the thumb on the back of the wrist. Using this handling technique, the therapist can facilitate wrist extension and apply pressure in the palm to encourage sustained grasp. These techniques are particularly successful with a child who has developed a basic hand-to-mouth pattern but has difficulty placing the spoon into his or her mouth. One disadvantage of these handling techniques is that they require the therapist, teacher, or parent to be seated behind or to the side of the child. This positioning limits eye-to-eye interaction with the child during feeding and can create a barrier to communication. This limitation is not as important in a group situation, such as the family mealtime or the school's snack time. Practice of self-feeding using these techniques on an intermittent basis can improve the movement pattern when the caregiver provides consistent feedback and reinforcement to the child regarding his or her self-feeding efforts. In applying these techniques, the therapist's goal is to facilitate the child's success and gradually decrease the amount of physical assistance and adaptive equipment required in self-feeding.

Adaptive Equipment. A variety of adaptive equipment has been specifically designed to accommodate the needs of children who experience difficulty in self-feeding. Often the equipment provides simple, yet critical, adaptations to the feeding experience that enable the child to be independent in self-feeding. Examples of adapted feeding equipment include utensils, plates, bowls, cups, and straws. Utensils with built-up handles that are easier to grasp or straps on the handle to secure it to the hand can compensate for limited grasp. Children with orthopedic impairments that influence the upper extremity may be more successful with spoon handles that are longer or shorter or that are curved or bent. Children need sturdy spoons with short handles and small, shallow bowls. Various spoons are available for children and may cost less than special equipment ordered through catalogs. To scoop food onto the spoon, the child may need a dish with a raised edge. These "scoop dishes" often have suction cups underneath to stabilize them on the tray or table. The high curved side of the dish makes scooping the food easier when the child is unable to use an assisting hand to obtain the food. The fork is generally introduced after the spoon. A short fork with blunt prongs can work well even when the child uses a palmar grasp. Cups with lids reduce spillage by controlling the flow of liquid into the mouth. Lids without spouts are recommended when the child exhibits suckling tongue movement. Straws can promote the child's ability to suck and can allow the child to drink without lifting the cup from the table surface. Straw drinking can also promote a chin tuck position because the child must move forward using active neck flexion to obtain the straw. More sophisticated adapted equipment, such as the electric feeder, may enable a child to self-feed without using the arms. Criteria for selecting adaptive equipment to improve the child's independence in self-feeding include durability, ease of cleaning and use, and developmental appropriateness.

Task Modifications. Children who have problems controlling the spoon because of abnormal muscle tone can also benefit from modification of the self-feeding activity itself. For example, children with ataxic cerebral palsy who exhibit tremor in the upper extremity during purposeful activities often have difficulty having enough control to self-feed. Without the experience needed for feedback, the child does not learn more refined modifications of the arm and wrist. If children struggle when attempting to eat spillable foods on a spoon, stabbing food with a blunt fork may be a more effective self-feeding method.

In addition to learning how to control the utensil, the child learns to perform self-feeding occupations in a manner consistent with his or her social context. The adult usually sets the performance criteria and provides feedback regarding what is or is not finger food. Another powerful force in providing information about adequate self-feeding is observations of peers. Siblings and classmates eating the meal at the same time act as models for adequate occupational performance or will challenge the child to learn a new skill. Therefore, part of intervention planning includes strategies to ensure that the child engages in self-feeding as a part of the social context of the family or classroom.

NUTRITION

Adequate nutrition is necessary for a healthy life. Malnutrition and nutritional issues are of particular concern for children with development disabilities who demonstrate the feeding problems described in this chapter. This compromised feeding and nutritional status results from a combination of factors, including exceptional nutritive requirements, limited feeding skills, and drug- or disease-induced food intolerance. In addition, the parent's emotional, physical, and social stresses associated with caring for a child with special health care needs can disrupt the feeding interaction (Baroni & Sondel, 1995; Brizee, Sophos, & McLaughlin, 1990).

Malnutrition or a failure-to-thrive condition can exacerbate or worsen the developmental condition. Accordingly, the therapist needs to adjust diets with higher or lower daily requirements of certain nutrients to provide optimal nutrition and prevent detrimental side effects of the medications. Unfortunately, early interventionists, including occupational therapists, often do not make appropriate referrals to nutritionists (Clark, Oakland, & Brotherson, 1998). Clinicians sometimes assume that if the family receives assistance through programs such as Women, Infants, and Children (WIC), a nutritionist is involved with the family and will provide sufficient guidance. Because children with special needs have exceptionally complex problems the WIC nutritionist does not have sufficient time or knowledge to address these issues.

The occupational therapist can perform nutritional screening with guidance by the nutritionist. Therapists will also see children for eating problems. The following require a referral to a nutritionist and incorporation of recommendations (Clark, Wood, & Lawson, 1998):

- An infant consumes less than the desired 16 to 32 ounces of milk or formula.
- The child has constipation.
- The parent expresses concerns.
- The child's diet is not consistent with his or her chronologic age.
- The child has problems with eating and self-feeding.
  A nutritional screening consists of the following:
1 Interviewing the caregivers regarding amounts and types of foods consumed daily
2 Collecting data on height, weight, and weight for height
3 Observing general appearance of skin, hair, and gums
4 Reviewing medical records

The following are problems identified in the screening that indicate the need for a more in-depth nutritional assessment and services (Brizee et al., 1990):

- Weight for height below the tenth percentile
- Weight for height above the nineteenth percentile
- Height and weight below the fifth percentile
- Parents' concern about nutrition
- Behavioral or oral motor problems that result in severe limitations in the types or amounts of food ingested

The following is an example of a child who required in-depth nutritional assessment:

> When Joey was 5 years old, the preschool interdisciplinary team followed his development. His home-based teacher asked for additional input from the rest of the team because she suspected that Joey had autism. His parents wanted Joey to start in a kindergarten program but were worried about meals. Although he fed himself, Joey refused to eat anything but Cheerios with milk. His weight was at the twentieth percentile. The preschool interdisciplinary team referred Joey to the nutritionist because of his restricted diet. His analysis revealed adequate caloric intake but a diet that was missing many

nutrients typically found in fruits and vegetables. The team began vitamin supplements immediately and agreed that one of the first priorities was for the occupational therapist to work with the teacher on expanding Joey's tolerance of different types of foods.

With the close link between nutrition and health, priorities in intervention are to promote nutrition by adjusting occupational therapy strategies. The following principles apply to the occupational therapist's intervention and its potential effect on the child's nutritional status.

When oral intervention for sensory or motor problems is stressful for the child, the intervention activities should occur at times other than mealtime. Mealtime should be the time for the child to receive an optimal amount of nutrition and experience the satisfaction of satiation. Challenging oral interventions, particularly those that strongly influence the sensory system, may upset or frustrate the child and result in food refusal. Mealtime can then evolve into a battle of the child who exerts control of a situation that creates discomfort or stress by refusing food. When the therapist addresses oral desensitization and new oral motor skills at times other than mealtime, the child and the parent or therapist can approach these activities in a more relaxed, playful manner.

The therapist should always consider the consequences of food intake and nutrition when developing therapeutic strategies to improve oral motor abilities. Strategies that prolong a meal beyond 40 minutes may make unreasonable demands on the caregivers' time or may exhaust the child before he or she has consumed a sufficient amount of food (Gisel et al., 1995).

Often therapists recommend changes in food texture. To overcome an aversive response to sensory challenges, they may select sweet food, like cookies or pudding, to increase motivation. When the therapist attempts new textures, he or she should consider the nutritional value. Acceptance does not translate into good nutrition, especially if the snack for therapy translates into less hunger for the next meal. When attempting new textures of food, the therapist should reinforce the importance of nutrition by selecting foods with high nutritional value. The therapist should use cheese and fruits to work on chewing rather than cookies and monitor intake at other meals.

A nutritionist should assess all major changes in the child's diet. For example, blanket recommendations to use high-caloric foods can be inappropriate, even when the goal for the child is weight gain. Sometimes high-caloric food supplements actually decrease the child's overall appetite and food intake. The therapist needs to balance increases in the caloric density of foods with increases in fluid intake. The therapist should consider the long-term effects of artificially increasing caloric density.

Collaboration with the nutritionist is essential for children who are underweight, and frequent consultation with the nutritionist is critical for the therapist to avoid malnutrition and improve the child's overall health and development. Often the therapist interacts with the failure-to-thrive child and his or her family more frequently than the nutritionist and is privy to information regarding the child's eating. Food refusal and loss of appetite can be particularly detrimental to these children. The therapist can share insight into the interactional components of the problem. Issues other than failure to thrive warrant referral to the nutritionist. The therapist may recommend that the family consult with a nutritionist in the following instances:

- When a child begins a new medication that is known to have a food and medication interaction
- When changes in the child's health suggest concern for drug and nutrient interaction
- When the child gains or loses weight suddenly
- When major changes in diet occur
- When conditions such as constipation are longstanding problems

Although these problems do not always require direct intervention and changes in diet, it is important that the nutritionist monitor them and follow recommendations to improve the child's nutrition.

SUMMARY

Intervention to promote a child's feeding and eating skills is an important role of the occupational therapist. For the child, the ability to participate in mealtime is influenced by oral sensory and motor function, physiologic parameters, cognitive underpinnings, and social abilities to interact with family members while eating. For the parent or caregiver, other factors influence how she or he feeds the child, including informal ideas about feeding a child, anxiety that the child eat a sufficient amount or specific foods, and the family's cultural tradition and eating routines.

Given these influences, feeding interventions require a holistic approach in which multiple aspects of the child's behaviors and the environment are considered. Because of the complexity and critical importance of feeding interaction and nutritional intake, a collaborative interdisciplinary approach is recommended, with the family's concerns and priorities central to the intervention plan. This chapter provides a foundation for occupational therapists to help children develop eating skills that allow for good nutritional intake and thus for growth and development. The occupational therapist emphasizes interventions that support positive interactions during feeding and helps caregivers gain confidence, skills, and enjoyment in feeding their children.

Case Study 1

Carol was born prematurely at 30 weeks' estimated gestational age and had hyperbilirubinemia, respiratory distress, and a grade III intraventricular hemorrhage. A developmental assessment at 12 months of age indicated mild delays in gross and fine motor skills. Her parents fondly called her their "lazy baby." She was alert and pleasant and had recently begun to babble in long sequences. She learned to sit independently at 11 months of age. She rolled from place to place and did not creep or cruise. She could hold two objects, one in each hand, waving and banging them. She did not yet combine objects and had limited control of release.

The therapist interviewed Carol's mother at the 12-month assessment. She reported that Carol fed completely from the bottle. Her mother had tried pureed foods on several occasions; however, Carol spit them from her mouth and became upset. These behaviors prevented Carol's mother from continuing to try pureed foods and cereals. Carol demonstrated a strong sucking pattern, but she did not demonstrate tongue lateralization or graded bite. Her jaw was unstable when she attempted cup drinking. Although her weight was appropriate for her age, her mother wanted to introduce new foods and progress to feeding with a spoon and cup.

Feeding Evaluation

The therapist's evaluation indicated that Carol was hypersensitive in and around her mouth. Although she exhibited an effective sucking pattern, her tongue and jaw movement were unorganized when she was introduced to pureed foods. She coughed and choked on pureed food, losing most of the food placed on her tongue. Carol's parents were anxious to progress to a variety of foods and a more balanced diet. The failed attempts to introduce new foods into Carol's diet discouraged her parents.

Intervention

The therapist first addressed Carol's oral hypersensitivity at times other than feeding. Using a warm, wet washcloth, the therapist began by stroking her face around the mouth and then in the mouth, rubbing the gums and palate. The therapist used the NUK toothbrush to rub her gums. Carol seemed to like this; therefore the therapist used the NUK toothbrush to introduce food tastes and textures. The therapist dipped the toothbrush into fruit baby food before oral stimulation. The therapist then dipped a nipple with her finger inside into the baby food and pressed it onto the anterior tongue, lateral tongue, and gums.

As Carol's tolerance of the baby food presented on the nipple and toothbrush increased, the therapist introduced a latex-covered spoon with pureed food. The therapist asked the parent to use smooth pureed food at first, and then introduced foods with greater texture. The therapist and parent provided jaw support to inhibit her jaw's excessive movement and to promote the tongue's movements. The parent removed this support as Carol's suck-swallow sequence of pureed foods became efficient.

By 15 months of age, Carol's diet included a variety of pureed foods. At this time, the therapist introduced coarse foods, and the therapist and parent initiated placement of the food on the side of her tongue and between her gums. The therapist reintroduced jaw support as a support of tongue lateralization. The therapist initiated cup drinking at this time because Carol's jaw stability had increased. The therapist used a small, transparent plastic cup. Its transparency helped the parents and therapist regulate the flow of liquid into Carol's mouth. The therapist gave small, single sips at first and then facilitated a sequence of suck-swallow movements.

By 18 months of age, Carol was eating soft foods. Because she was unable and unsuccessful in self-feeding with a spoon, she preferred finger foods, such as strips of soft cheese or processed meats such as turkey. Cup drinking remained difficult, although she was learning to bite on the cup for stability. Her mother used thickened liquids, such as milk with yogurt and juice with baby food, to slow the movement of the liquid and to give her a better opportunity to control its flow. At that time, oral sensitivity was no longer a primary issue, although Carol exhibited mild discomfort when new foods were introduced. Carol's mother was pleased with the variety of foods that Carol consumed and with her continued weight gain and growth.

Case Study 2

Jonathan was diagnosed with spastic quadriparesis when he was 6 months old. His lower extremities exhibited high muscle tone, particularly in hip adductors and hamstrings. As a result, he demonstrated a scissoring pattern when standing or when held in his mother's arms. At $2\frac{1}{2}$ years of age, he had many assets: a ready smile, good social skills and responsivity to social interaction, beginning language (about 20 words), and a pleasant affect. He sat with minimal assistance, had begun to crawl on his belly, and rolled segmentally about the room. He required external postural support to play with toys; however, once he had postural stability, he brought his hands to midline, grasped using a radial palmar grasp, released toys in a container, transferred objects, and began to fit an object into a precise space. Although hand-eye coordination was emerging, he continued to have difficulty with integrating visual skills with arm and hand movements.

Evaluation

Parent Interview. Jonathan ate soft foods and had begun to try some harder foods such as pretzels, ham, and apples. He took the food from a cup or spoon using active lip movements. Lip closure while chewing was fair, but not perfect, as he continued to have some food loss. He used both a munching pattern and some rotary chewing. He reverted to a vertical up-and-down munching pattern with more difficult foods (e.g., those that were hard or tough). He used a sucking pattern with pureed foods and a diagonal rotary pattern with soft foods. Jonathan demonstrated a variety of patterns of tongue movement, including tip elevation, lateralization, and beginning rolling. Jaw control was emerging; he exhibited a sustained bite pattern, and jaw stabilization increased on the cup rim. He continued to bite on the cup during drinking. The occupational therapist and Jonathan's parent implemented a program to upgrade the texture of his foods, and he made continual progress in feeding skills. Drinking thin liquids remained difficult, and his mother managed his drinking by providing some manual head and jaw support and by thickening his liquids to a nectar quality. Jonathan handled liquids better when using a straw and when taking small sips of liquid at a time. As his appetite increased and he continued to demonstrate improvements in oral skills, he showed increasing interest in self-feeding. He began to finger feed bites of sandwiches, crackers, cheese, and strips of ham or chicken.

Jonathan's mother gave him a spoon on several occasions; his first attempts at self-feeding resulted in much more food going on his face and clothes than in his mouth. His mother tried to have Jonathan self-feed in his high chair using an adult spoon and a bowl of yogurt. In spite of his lack of success, Jonathan seemed eager to try to use the spoon and often grabbed it from his mouth during feeding. The occupational therapist evaluated his feeding to help his mother develop a system for self-feeding that was efficient and began to address self-feeding as a goal in the intervention program.

Feeding Observation. In the high chair, Jonathan was without foot support and had minimal trunk support. He frequently fell to one side. The therapist evaluated the self-feeding movements; he successfully scooped the yogurt, then fully abducted his shoulder and flexed his elbow to bring the spoon to his mouth. Although this motion brought the food to his mouth, Jonathan was unable to turn the spoon for entry into his mouth. His efforts to get the food resulted in spillage. Although he failed to get food into his mouth, he remained highly motivated and seemed to enjoy the activity.

Intervention

The therapist adjusted Jonathan's position for self-feeding and recommended simple equipment to enhance the quality of fit between Jonathan and the desired occupation, self-feeding. Instead of feeding in the high chair, the occupational therapist suggested that he sit in the Rifton chair for self-feeding. He was stable in the Rifton chair, which had lateral supports, foot supports, and a tray that could be positioned close to his body at a height that enabled solid weight-bearing on elbows. He demonstrated his best hand and arm control in this chair (Figure 14-9). The therapist used a scoop dish with suction cups on the bottom. This bowl allowed him to obtain food without holding the bowl with his other hand. The therapist also used a small child's adapted spoon. The spoon selected was short; had a bent angle at the bowl; and had a flat, small bowl and a thick handle. Jonathan could easily handle the spoon with a radial palmar grasp and could enter it into his mouth without wrist rotation or radial deviation. Initially the therapist provided some support at his hand by entering her index finger into his hand and placing her thumb on the hand's dorsum as he grasped the spoon. The therapist's hand supported his arm and wrist movements, and she only exerted pressure when his arm movement appeared inadequate for entry into his mouth (Figure 14-10). The therapist soon eliminated this assistance. The therapist used a small padded block under his elbow, which proved to be helpful as an extra source of stability. Jonathan maintained his elbow on the pad and used elbow flexion to bring food to his mouth.

The therapist suggested that pudding be the first food used in feeding practice because of its cohesive, sticky

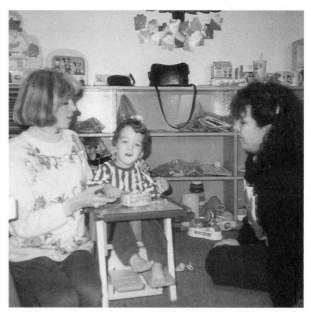

FIGURE 14-9 Rifton chair provides a firm base of support to trunk and feet during self-feeding.

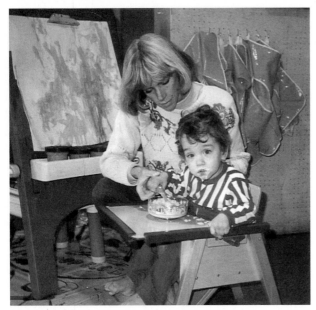

FIGURE 14-10 The therapist supports and guides the child's hand during self-feeding using the thumb on hand dorsum and finger in his palm.

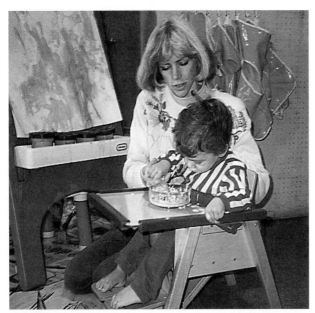

FIGURE 14-11 Foods that are successful when first attempting self-feeding are those that stick together, are easily scooped, hold to the spoon, and taste good.

texture. The therapist soon added yogurt and ice cream, which quickly became Jonathan's favorite treats (Figure 14-11).

The therapist and Jonathan's mother developed a plan to increase the fine motor skills that Jonathan needed to improve self-feeding. Activities to enhance self-feeding with the spoon included games that required forearm supination with objects held in a radial digital grasp. Examples included placing pegs vertically into a

pegboard, placing peg people into a school bus or airplane, and using a toy accordion with vertically oriented handles. Jonathan performed these activities in the Rifton chair or corner chair with a tray, where he was well supported and posturally stable with feet flat. With this equipment and position, Jonathan regularly practiced self-feeding.

STUDY QUESTIONS

1 You receive a referral for a 9-month-old infant who refuses all attempts to be fed pureed baby foods. She currently takes six bottles of formula per day. Your initial evaluation indicates that she has significant hypersensitivity of the oral area. Describe the first three activities that you would implement in intervention. Identify two recommendations that you would give to her parents.

2 You are working with a 12-year-old child who has severe motor delays and difficulty feeding. He has fair head control and poor trunk control, and he is not a candidate for self-feeding at this time. He demonstrates primitive oral movements; his jaw is unstable and moves in wide excursions, and his tongue moves in extension and retraction. He often loses food from his mouth and frequently chokes and coughs during feeding. Coughing is most frequent during drinking. Describe in detail how you would position him for feeding and what positioning devices you may use. What types of food and drink would you recommend?

3 You are the occupational therapist for a 6-year-old child with feeding difficulties. When you feed her at school, you suspect that she is aspirating some of her food and drink. List two ways that you would pursue investigating this possibility. What two questions would you ask her parents? What may you ask of the physician to further investigate the possibility of aspiration?

4 One of the children with whom you are working on oral feeding is demonstrating a keen interest in feeding himself. He has poor control of his upper extremities. His shoulder stability is poor, and he exhibits only a gross grasp and involuntary release. He does not yet have the ability to maintain grasp of a utensil while guiding it to his mouth. What activities may you implement to improve his ability to self-feed? What would be the first foods and eating activities that would allow him to succeed in self-feeding?

5 When a child has significant oral motor problems, often drinking is a more difficult skill to achieve than eating solid foods. Given the importance of

maintaining hydration, what three recommendations would you make for children whose oral motor skills suggest the possibility of aspiration when drinking liquids?

REFERENCES

Adams, R.C., & Snyder, P. (1998). Treatments of cerebral palsy: Making choices of intervention from an expanding menu of options. *Infants and Young Children, 10* (4), 1-22.

Arvedson, J.C., & Lefton-Greif, M.A. (1998). *Pediatric Videofluorographic Swallow Studies*. San Antonio: Communication Skill Builders.

Bakker, T., & Woody, A. (1995). *Primary caregivers' experiences with children with feeding issues*. Unpublished research project, University of North Carolina at Chapel Hill.

Baranek, G.T. (1999). Autism during infancy: A retrospective video analysis of sensory-motor and social behaviors at 9-12 months of age. *Journal of Autism and Developmental Disorders, 29*, 213-224.

Baroni, M., & Sondel, S. (1995). A collaborative model for identifying feeding and nutrition needs in early intervention. *Infants and Young Children, 8* (2), 26-36.

Batshaw, M.L., & Perret, Y.M. (1992). *Children with disabilities: A medical primer*. Baltimore: Brookes Publishing.

Bazyk, S. (1990). Factors associated with the transition to oral feeding in infants fed by nasogastric tubes. *American Journal of Occupational Therapy, 44*, 1070-1078.

Beals, D.E. (1993). Explanatory talk in low-income families' mealtime conversations. *Applied Psycholinguistics, 14*, 489-513.

Benson, J.E., & Lefton-Greif, M.A. (1994). Videofluoroscopy of swallowing in pediatric patients: A component of the total feeding evaluation. In D.N. Tuchman & R. Walter (Eds.), *Disorders of feeding and swallowing in infants and children* (pp. 187-200). San Diego: Singular Publishing Group.

Brazelton, T.B. (1993). Why children and parents must play while they eat: An interview with T. Berry Brazelton. *Journal of the American Dietetic Association, 93*, 1485-1487.

Brizee, L.S., Sophos, C.M., & McLaughlin, J.F. (1990). Nutrition issues in developmental disabilities. *Infants and Young Children, 2* (3), 10-21.

Bundy, A.C., & Koomar, J.A. (2002). Orchestrating intervention: The art of practice. In A.C. Bundy, S.J. Lane, & E.A. Murray (Eds.), *Sensory integration: Theory and practice* (2nd ed.). Philadelphia: F.A. Davis.

Chamberlin, J., Henry, M.M., Roberts, J.D., Sapsford, A.L., & Courtney, S.E. (1991). An infant and toddler feeding group program. *The American Journal of Occupational Therapy, 45*, 907-911.

Clark, F., Wood, W., & Lawson, E.A. (1998). Occupational science: Occupational therapy's legacy for the 21st century. In M.E. Neisdtadt & E.B. Crepeau (Eds.), *Willard & Spackman's occupational therapy* (pp. 13-21). Philadelphia: J.B. Lippincott.

Clark, M.P., Oakland, M.J., & Brotherson, M.J. (1998). Nutrition screening for children with special health care needs. *Children's Health Care, 27*, 231-245.

Crist, W., Napier-Phyillips, A., McDonnell, P., Ledwidge, J., & Beck, M. (1998). Assessing restricted diet in young children. *Children's Health Care, 27* (4), 247-257.

Dahl, M., Thommessen, M., Rasmussen, M., & Selberg, T. (1996). Feeding and nutritional characteristics in children with moderate or severe cerebral palsy. *Acta Paediatrics 85*, 697-701.

Daniels, H., Devlieger, H., Casaer, P., & Eggermont, E. (1986). Nutritive and non-nutritive sucking in preterm infants. *Journal of Developmental Physiology, 8*, 117-121.

DeVault, M.L. (1991). *Feeding the family: The social organization of caring as gendered work*. Chicago: Chicago Press.

Edmondson, R., & Reinhartsen, D. (1998). The young child with cleft lip and palate: Intervention needs in the first three years. *Infants and Young Children, 11* (2), 12-20.

Einarsson-Backes, L., Deitz, J., Price, R., Glass, R., & Hays, R. (1994). The effect of oral support on sucking efficiency in preterm infants. *The American Journal of Occupational Therapy, 48*, 490-498.

Federal Register, 56 (235), December 6, 1991.

Friedman, B., & Frazier, J.B. (2000). Deep Laryngeal Penetration as a Predictor of Aspiration. *Dysphagia, 15*, 153-158.

Gisel, E.G., Applegate-Ferrante, T., Benson, J.E., & Bosma, J.F. (1995). Effect of oral sensorimotor treatment on measures of growth, eating efficiency and aspiration in the dysphagic child with cerebral palsy. *Developmental Medicine and Child Neurology, 37*, 528-543.

Glass, R., & Wolf, L. (1998). Feeding and oral motor skills. In J. Case-Smith (Ed.), *Pediatric occupational therapy and early intervention* (pp. 225-288). Boston: Butterworth-Heinemann.

Glass, R.P., & Wolf, L.S. (1999). Feeding management of infants with cleft lip and palate and micrognathia. *Infants and Young Children, 12*, 70-81.

Hagekull, B., & Dahl, M. (1987). Infants with and without feeding difficulties: Maternal experiences. *International Journal of Eating Disorders, 6*, 83-98.

Heriza, C. (1991). Motor development: Traditional and contemporary theories. In *Contemporary management of motor control problems*. Fredericksburg, VA: APTA.

Humphry, R. (1995). The nature and diversity of problems leading to failure to thrive. *Occupational Therapy in Health Care, 9*, 73-90.

Humphry, R., & Morrow, J. (1998). *Developmental processes behind the acquisition of occupations in self care*. Unpublished manuscript. University of North Carolina at Chapel Hill.

Humphry, R., & Thigpen-Beck, B. (1997). Caregiver role: Ideas about feeding infants and toddlers. *Occupational Therapy Journal of Research, 17*, 237-263.

Humphry, R., & Thigpen-Beck, B. (1998). Parenting values and attitudes: Views of therapists and parents. *The American Journal of Occupational Therapy, 52*, 835-843.

Klein, M.D., & Delaney, T.A. (1994). *Feeding and nutrition for the child with special needs*. Tucson, AZ: Therapy Skill Builders.

Kleinman, R., Murphy, J., Little, M., Pagano, M., Wheler, C., Regal, K., & Jellinek, M. (1998). Hunger in children in the United States: Potential behavioral and emotional correlates. *Pediatrics, 101*, 101-103.

Lee, E.J., Murry, V.M., Brody, G., & Parker, V. (2002). Maternal resources, parenting, and dietary patterns among rural African American children in single-parent families. *Public Health Nursing, 19*, 104-111.

Logemann, J.A. (1993). *Manual for the Videofluorographic Study of Swallowing*, Second Edition. Austin: Pro-Ed.

Logemann, J.A. (2000). Therapy for children with swallowing disorders in the educational setting. *Language, Speech, and Hearing Services in Schools, 31,* 50-55.

Mathiowetz, V., & Haugen, J.B. (1994). Motor behavior research: Implications for therapeutic approaches to central nervous system dysfunction. *The American Journal of Occupational Therapy, 48,* 733-745.

Morris, S.E., & Klein, M.D. (2000). *Pre-feeding skills* (2nd ed.). Tucson, AZ: Therapy Skill Builders.

Papousek, H., & Papousek, M. (1995). Intuitive parenting. In M.H. Bornsteing (Ed.), *Handbook of parenting* (Vol. 2, pp. 117-136). Mahwah, NJ: Lawrence Erlbaum Associates.

Ramsay, M., Gisel, E.G., & Boutry, M. (1993). Non-organic failure to thrive: Growth failure secondary to feeding-skills disorder. *Developmental Medicine and Child Neurology, 35,* 285-297.

Reily, S., Skuse, D., & Poblete, X. (1996). Prevalence of feeding problems and oral motor dysfunction in children with cerebral palsy: A community survey. *The Journal of Pediatrics, 128,* 877-882.

Rogers, J.C., & Holm, M.B. (1998). Evaluation of occupational performance areas. In M.E. Neistadt & E.B. Crepeau (Eds.), *Willard & Spackman's occupational therapy* (9th ed., pp. 185-208). Philadelphia: J.B. Lippincott.

Sanders, M.R., Patel, R.K., LeGrice, B., & Shepherd, R.W. (1993). Children with persistent feeding difficulties: An observational analysis of the feeding interactions of problem and non-problem eaters. *Health Psychology, 12,* 64-73.

Schauster, H., & Dwyer, J. (1996). Transition for tube feedings to feedings by mouth in children: Preventing eating dysfunction. *The Journal of the American Dietetic Association, 96* (3), 277-281.

Schuberth, L.M. (1994). The role of occupational therapy in diagnosis and management. In D.N. Tuchman & R. Walter (Eds.), *Disorders of feeding and swallowing in infants and children* (pp. 115-130). San Diego: Singular Publishing Group.

Schulze, P.A., Harwood, R.L., & Schoelmerich, A. (2001). Feeding practices and expectations among middle-class Anglo and Puerto Rican mothers of 12-month-old infants. *Journal of Cross-Cultural Psychology, 32,* 397-406.

Schwarz, S.M. (2003). Feeding disorders in children with developmental disabilities. *Infants and Young Children, 16,* 317-330.

Tarbell, M.C., & Allaire, J.H. (2002). Children with feeding tube dependency: Treating the whole child. *Infants and Young Children, 15,* 29-41.

Thigpen-Beck, B., & Dovenitz, S. (1995). *The values, beliefs, and attitudes of occupational therapists regarding selected baby behaviors associated with eating.* Unpublished research project. University of North Carolina at Chapel Hill.

Tuchman, D.B. (1994). Physiology of the swallowing apparatus. In D.N. Tuchman & R. Walter (Eds.), *Disorders of feeding and swallowing in infants and children* (pp. 1-25). San Diego: Singular Publishing Group.

Wolf, L.S., & Glass, R.P. (1992). *Feeding and swallowing disorders in infancy: Assessment and management.* Tucson: Therapy Skill Builders.

Wong, D.L. (1997). *Whaley & Wong's essentials of pediatric nursing.* St. Louis: Mosby.

Yokochi, K. (1997). Oral motor patterns during feeding in severely physically disabled children. *Brain & Development, 19* (8), 552-555.

Zerilli, K.S., Stefans, V.A., & DiPietro, M.A. (1990). Protocol for the use of videofluoroscopy in pediatric swallowing dysfunction. *The American Journal of Occupational Therapy, 44* (5), 441-446.

Activities of Daily Living and Adaptations for Independent Living

Jayne Shepherd

KEY TERMS

Activities of daily living (ADL)
Instrumental activities of daily living (IADLs)
Performance context
Adaptation approach
Grading techniques

Backward chaining
Forward chaining
Cues
Prompts
Assistive devices
Environmental adaptations
Adaptive positioning

CHAPTER OBJECTIVES

1 Describe the effects of context on a child's performance and parental expectations for activities of daily living (ADLs) and instrumental activities of daily living (IADLs) occupations.
2 Identify the body structures and functions, performance skills, performance patterns, and activity demands that may affect a child's ADL and IADL performance.
3 Identify evaluation procedures and methods in ADL and IADL occupations that target child and family preferences for intervention.
4 Describe intervention strategies and approaches, both general and specific.
5 Describe the selection and modification of equipment, techniques, and environments for certain ADL and IADL occupations.

Activities of daily living and instrumental activities of daily living encompass some of the most important occupations children learn as they mature. Self-care or basic activities of daily living (ADLs) include learning how to take care of one's body, such as toilet hygiene, bowel and bladder management, bathing and showering, personal hygiene and grooming, eating and feeding, dressing,

functional mobility, and sleep and rest (American Occupational Therapy Association [AOTA], 2002). Other ADL tasks may be assumed, such as care of a personal device and learning to express sexual needs (AOTA). As the child matures, he or she learns to perform ADLs and IADLs in socially appropriate ways so that he or she can engage in the other occupations of education, play, leisure, social participation, and work in the family and the community.

Instrumental activities of daily living (IADLs) are more complex ADLs that may be delegated to others but that generally are needed to participate independently in home, school, community, and work environments (AOTA, 2002; Brown et al., 1991; Spencer, Murphy, Bean, & Shelley, 1991). These IADL occupations include use of a communication device, community mobility, shopping, home management (e.g., clothing care, cleaning, and household maintenance), meal preparation and cleanup, health maintenance (e.g., taking medications, exercise, and nutrition), care of pets and care of others, and safety procedures and emergency responses. Children and young people learn these occupations to prepare them for independent living as adults.

This chapter discusses the dynamic interaction of child factors, contexts, activity demands, and performance skills and patterns, which allows a child to engage in ADL and IADL occupations. Evaluation methods, intervention approaches, and strategies for improving outcomes in ADL and IADL activities are described. Typical development, problems, and adaptations for toileting, dressing, bathing, grooming, and performing other related ADL tasks are given (feeding is discussed in Chapter 14). IADL occupations are discussed in relation to performance in the home, hospital, community, and school environment. Examples of adaptations to physical and social environments are provided, with consideration given to cultural, temporal, and personal influences.

IMPORTANCE OF DEVELOPING ADL AND IADL OCCUPATIONS

The foundations for ADLs begin in infancy and are refined throughout the various stages of development. As unique individuals living in certain contexts, children learn these activities at varying rates and have occasional regression and unpredictable behaviors. Cultural values, social routines, and the physical environment influence the timing of when children assume ADLs and IADLs. Overall, society and families assume that children develop increasing levels of competence and self-reliance to meet their own ADL and IADL needs. Growth and maturity allow the child to participate in various roles and environments with decreasing levels of adult supervision.

When a child is born with or acquires a disability, parental and child expectations for ADL and daily living independence are modified. Occupational therapists are instrumental in helping parents and children learn how to modify activity demands and routines so that children use ADL and IADL occupations. Active participation in ADLs has several benefits for the child, including maintaining and improving body functions (e.g., strength, endurance, range of motion [ROM], coordination, memory, sequencing, concept formation, and body image) and mastering tasks meaningful and purposeful to the child. For example, when children dress themselves, they choose their own clothing, participate in dress-up during playtime, put on a coat when going outside, change clothes for gym class, or dress in a uniform to work at a restaurant. As the child learns new ADL and IADL tasks, he or she develops a sense of accomplishment and pride in his or her abilities. The child becomes responsible for developing and maintaining routines or patterns that prevent further illness (e.g., checking skin conditions, maintaining cleanliness of himself or herself and the environment, and cooking nutritious meals), as well as for meeting role expectations for community living. This increasing independence also gives parents, teachers, and other caregivers more time and energy for other tasks.

FACTORS AFFECTING PERFORMANCE

Child factors, the performance context, and the specific demands of the self-care activity affect the child's performance patterns and performance skills (i.e., motor, process, and communication/interaction), as well as his or her ability to participate successfully in ADL and IADL occupations. According to the Occupational Therapy Practice Framework (AOTA, 2002), child factors include body functions and body structures that may be affected by the disability. ADLs and IADLs are performed in a context of interwoven internal and external conditions, some from within the child (personal, spiritual, and temporal contexts) and others around the child (social, cultural, and physical contexts). During ADL occupations, the context influences the activity demands, which vary in object use, space and social demands, sequencing and timing, and required actions, body functions, and body structures. As therapists consider these factors, they determine the knowledge and performance skills (goal-directed actions) and patterns the child needs in order to learn how to care for himself or herself and to live independently.

Child Factors and Performance Skills

Occupational therapy intervention to increase ADL and IADL function considers what the child and family value and the context in which the tasks occur. The levels of independence, safety, and adequacy of occupational performance of the child and family determine the child's motor, process, and communication ADL occupations in various contexts.

The child has specific functional issues (body structures and functions), interaction skills, and performance patterns that affect ADL and IADL performance. For example, children with tactile hypersensitivity may cry during dressing and refuse to dress despite having the motor and process skills to dress themselves. Children with visual impairments may use their sense of touch when brushing their hair. A child with cerebral palsy may not have the postural control to sit up during dressing but may have the perceptual functions (e.g., body functions of right-left discrimination and figure-ground) to dress in a side-lying position. A child with an attention deficit disorder may be able to do all the steps in a self-care task, but his or her organization, sequencing, and memory may interfere with adequate, safe performance (Stein, Szumowski, Blondis, & Roizen, 1995).

Interest level, self-confidence, and motivation are strong forces that help children attain levels of performance that are either above or below expectations. Children with mental retardation, traumatic brain injury, or multiple disabilities experience difficulties in coordination, initiative, attention span, sequencing, memory, safety, and ability to learn and generalize activities across environments. However, with instruction and opportunity, ADLs and IADLs sometimes become the tasks these children perform most competently (Kellegrew, 1998; Orelove & Sobsey, 1996).

The child's disability or health status may affect his or her ability to perform ADL and IADL tasks. The therapist considers the child's capacity for learning and ability to complete difficult tasks safely. Pain, fatigue, the amount of time the child needs to complete the task, and the child's satisfaction with his or her performance influence the choice of ADL occupations (Holm, Rogers, & James, 2003).

Children who are acutely ill or who have multiple disabilities that require numerous procedures throughout the day (e.g., tube feeding, tracheostomy care, and bowel and bladder care) may not have the time or energy to work on ADL and IADL tasks. For example: Jenna, a 10-year-old child with a C_6 spinal cord injury and quadriplegia, can dress herself independently within a 45-minute period, but she and her family prefer that someone else dress her so that she has more energy for school tasks. Children with multiple disabilities may physically be unable to do all or any part of ADL tasks, but they can partially participate or direct others on how to care for them. When children are hospitalized for long periods, they often need to have some control over their participation in self-care routines. Figure 15-1 shows how doing a small part of self-care routines is possible and meaningful for children in the hospital with acute illnesses.

Performance Context

The initiation and completion of ADL tasks are influenced by the context of the tasks, including interwoven conditions, both internal and external to the child (e.g., personal and temporal contexts) and around the child (social, cultural, physical, and virtual contexts). Children in early and middle childhood often perform ADLs and IADLs in different settings. The four primary settings that children experience are the home, school, community, and work. Once the occupational therapist understands the contexts in which occupation occurs, he or she can choose intervention strategies that are congruent with the demands of the activity or can change aspects of the environment that are barriers to the child's

performance of ADL and IADL tasks. Although this section has divided the contexts into various areas, all the areas are interrelated.

Personal and Temporal Contexts: Family Life Cycle and Developmental Stage

Age, gender, education, and socioeconomic status define the personal context for ADL and IADL occupations. Children typically develop ADLs and IADLs in a sequence, achieving specific tasks as overall competency increases. The sequence of ADL development helps therapists and families form realistic expectations for children at different ages and helps determine the appropriate timing for teaching these occupations. By considering the child's age, therapists determine when it is time to stop working on specific preparatory or therapeutic activities. For example, 6-year-old Tilly had occupational therapy for 5 years to enhance eating by trying to increase lip closure and to develop a more efficient suck-swallow pattern. If she had not learned this over the past 5 years, what are her chances of learning it this year? It may be time for the therapist to work on self-feeding strategies or on an IADL activity, such as operating an appliance with a switch for meal preparation.

Families vary in their ability and availability to assist and encourage the child to perform ADLs and IADLs. This ability often depends on where the family and child are in the family life cycle and their ability to be flexible in everyday routines (Turnbull & Turnbull, 2001). During infancy, parents often seek instruction on feeding, dressing, and bathing. By 3 years of age, the child's self-feeding, dressing, and toileting skills may become issues for parents. For example, if Mary is the

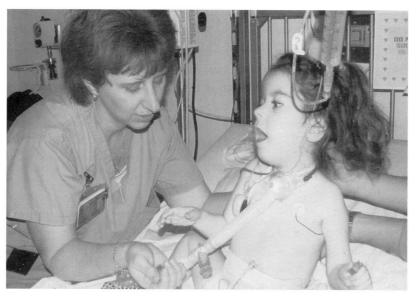

FIGURE 15-1 Partial participation. This child partially participates in hair combing and picks out her barrettes while therapists support her in her hospital bed.

last of nine children, ADL independence may not have priority because the older siblings love to feed and dress Mary.

When the child enters school, by 6 years of age, functional mobility in the school environment, dressing (especially outerwear), toileting, socialization with peers, grooming (e.g., washing the hands and face), and IADL functional communication (e.g., writing, drawing, and expressing needs) become increasingly important. Simple household activities, such as taking out the trash, setting and clearing the table, making a simple sandwich, washing or dusting countertops, and following safety precautions, are appropriate goals. Older siblings may become more aware of and sensitive to their brother's or sister's disability, and the therapist may ask them to help their sibling learn ADL tasks and perform household tasks.

During adolescence (13 to 21 years of age), increasing independence in ADL and IADL tasks often determines whether a child will fit in with peers or be successful in obtaining a job outside the school environment. The child takes on increased responsibility for care of personal devices, medication routines, and health maintenance routines. During this stage, families further investigate current community resources as they think about future living arrangements, vocational opportunities, and the availability of other recreational activities for their child (Turnbull & Turnbull, 2001). Parent issues may focus on the child's ability to express sexual needs, to be safe in many environments, and to respond to emergency situations appropriately. The therapist may address additional IADL tasks to promote independence during this stage, including caring for clothing, preparing meals, shopping, managing money, and maintaining a household (Healy & Rigby, 1999).

During adolescence, concerns and goals for therapy may differ between parents and child. Both may be concerned about the adolescent's independence in ADLs and IADLs; however, adolescents may have more concerns about fitting in with a social group (McGavin, 1998). Children with severe disabilities who require maximum physical assistance in ADLs become a great concern to parents as they get older and their children approach adulthood. For the first time, parents may not have the physical strength to handle the daily care needs of their child.

Social Context

The social environment, family, other caregivers, and peers provide encouragement and support ADL independence. They also hold certain expectations regarding the child's ADL occupations, based on the family structure (e.g., the number of family members). In large families, different members may be assigned to perform or to help with specific ADL tasks for a child with a disability; in other families, the parent may be the sole person responsible for the daily living needs of the child. Family expectations, roles, and routines for managing daily living needs also influence the child's development of ADLs and IADLs and performance patterns (Turnbull & Turnbull, 2001). For example, parents living on a farm may expect their child to get up at dawn, put on overalls and boots, do chores such as feeding the animals, receive home schooling, and help sell eggs to augment the family income.

The therapist considers personal characteristics of family members, such as temperament, coping abilities, flexibility, and health status, when planning treatment (Turnbull & Turnbull, 2001) (see Chapter 5). For example, the mother may put her child in the "mothering" role if she is depressed and unable to get out of bed to cook dinner. Another child may not learn how to do yard chores if the father is disorganized and has not structured the tasks for the child. Parents with mental retardation or mental health problems may need to see a therapist modeling a behavior to learn how to cue and structure a task for their children (Turnbull & Turnbull). Parents with physical problems may need instructions and practice in using specific techniques and assistive devices safely.

An analysis of social routines helps determine when and how ADLs and IADLs are taught. Routines may differ significantly in home, school, community, and recreational environments, and children need to adapt to these differences. The variation in routine may confuse or disorganize children with mental retardation, autism, or attention deficit disorders but may be motivating to children without attention, sensory, or cognitive problems. School-based and early intervention therapists need to be aware of the social routines so that they can choose appropriate times to teach tasks. When tasks are taught or practiced at times and places where they naturally occur, they more quickly become part of the child's behavior repertoire (Brown et al., 1991). For example, school-based therapists may meet children at the bus to work on functional mobility and may be present as the child removes his or her coat to work on dressing. When tasks are embedded throughout all environments, children have multiple opportunities to practice activities and learn how to use the natural cues in the environment to modify their behavior. Social interactions and networks of peer buddies are extremely powerful in motivating children (Hughes & Carter, 2000) and helping them succeed in self-care.

Cultural Context

As therapists work with children and families in an array of service provision models, they must be aware of their own and others' cultural beliefs, customs, activity patterns, and expectations for performance in ADLs and IADLs (Lynch & Hanson, 1998). Occupational therapists may become involved with a family because someone else believes that their services are needed, and the family may not welcome the therapists' personal questions about the child's and family's self-maintenance occupations and routines. Cultural expectations of the family, caregivers, and social group as a whole may determine behavior standards. Family beliefs, values, and attitudes about child rearing, autonomy, and self-reliance influence how parents perceive ADLs and IADLs. In Anglo-European cultures, parents usually are concerned about children meeting developmental milestones (Hanson, 1998), yet other cultures (e.g., Hispanic) may be more relaxed about milestone attainment (Zuniga, 1998). In some adult-centered Indian cultures, parents expect children to be independent at an early age. In some cultures, parents and society generally reward children for taking the initiative to do chores around the house or in the community. In other cultures, parents may give children more time to be childlike and may not push them to do adult-type chores until a later age (Willis, 1998).

Social role expectations and routines are influenced by culture. Many Anglo-European parents encourage children to become independent and self-reliant (Hanson, 1998). In contrast, many Hispanic families (Zuniga, 1998) and Asian families (Chan, 1998) may encourage dependency or interdependency in the family. Routines for dressing, feeding, bathing, going to bed, and carrying out household tasks vary among cultural groups.

Culture also influences the type and availability of the tools, equipment, and materials a child uses to perform ADLs or IADLs. Customs and beliefs may determine how parents dress their children, what they feed them, what utensils the parents use in the kitchen, how they prepare and store food, what type of bed they use, and how they meet health care needs. Economic conditions, geographic location, and opportunities for education and employment can help determine the types of resources and supports that are available to families.

Physical Context

Barriers in the physical environment, including terrain and furniture and other objects, can hinder the child's development of ADLs and IADLs. Inaccessible buildings and rooms crowded with furniture limit how children in wheelchairs move throughout the environment. On the other hand, a large, open space may be too much room to allow a preschooler to contain his or her excitement and complete ADL tasks. Differences in surfaces also affect mobility; for example, rugs can make use of a walker or wheelchair more difficult. Other physical characteristics that the therapist assesses relate to the type of furniture, objects, or assistive devices in the environment and whether they are usable and accessible. What is usable in one environment (e.g., a particular type of phone at home) may not be usable in other environments, such as a hospital or job site. Sensory aspects of the physical environment often influence performance (e.g., the type of lighting, noise level, temperature, visual stimulation, and tactile or vestibular input of tasks). In particular, children with autism or attention deficit hyperactivity disorder (ADHD) can be overly sensitive to and distracted by the sensory aspects of an environment.

Virtual Context

In today's world, the virtual context is considered for ADL and IADL evaluation and intervention. Numerous checklists, assessments, and schedulers, and a wealth of information about ADLs and IADLs, can be found online. Parents, teachers, children, and therapists can collaborate in the use of these resources to enhance performance. Box 15-1 lists Internet resources for ADLs, and Box 15-2 lists such resources for IADLs.

Children and adolescents communicate with friends using Internet chat rooms or e-mail. Assistive technology may help children with disabilities access the Internet, communicate, or set up reminders to perform ADL and IADL occupations (see Chapter 18). Shopping, banking, meal planning, access to public transportation schedules, health information, home improvement businesses, and even information about pet care are all available on the Internet. Mentors and support groups for individuals learning how to care for their own needs and live in the community are also available. An exceptional web site is Blackboards and Bandaides (http:// www.faculty.fairfield.edu/fleitas), which was developed by a nurse to offer a forum for children and adolescents with chronic health care needs. Here children talk about themselves, allowing other professionals, families, siblings, and friends to understand their dilemmas and celebrations while living with a health care problem. Discussion of their disease and how they fit into the social context are common themes, and participants also share poetry, art, and other information.

Activity Demands

The activity demands in certain contexts can facilitate or impede the quality of ADL and IADL performance. A task analysis helps the therapist understand the complexity and various aspects of the activity. This evaluation involves analyzing the objects used, space and social demands, sequencing and timing, and required actions and skills (AOTA, 2002). Activity demands vary in the clinic, home, school, and community. For example, when a child with a traumatic brain injury is making a sandwich in an outpatient clinic, the child's performance skills

BOX 15-1   Online Resources for Help with Activities of Daily Living (ADLs)

All Areas

- Children's Hemiplegia and Stroke Association
  Site has a variety of resources on research, adaptive techniques for activities of daily living (ADLs) and instrumental activities of daily living (IADLs), and forums for children with these disabilities and their families.
  http://www.chasa.org/
- Family Village
  Site has numerous links and resources for all types of disabilities.
  http://www.familyvillage.wisc.edu/at/adaptive-devices.html
- Guide for ADLs for children who are visually impaired
  http://www.viguide.com/vsnadl.htm
  Neuromuscular Diseases: 101 Hints to "Help-with-Ease" for Patients with Neuromuscular Disease: A Do-It-Yourself Owner's Guide published by the Muscular Dystrophy Association
  http://www.mdausa.org/publications/101hints/index.html

Products for Daily and Independent Living

- AbleNet, Inc.
  Site offers assistive technology products.
  http://www.ablenetinc.com/Product.htm
- The Equipment Shop
  http://www.equipmentshop.com
- Handy Gadgets for One Handers
  Site demonstrates a variety of devices for ADLs and instrumental activities of daily living (IADLs).
  http://www.usinter.net/wasa/handy.html
- Independent Living Aids, Inc.
  www.independent-living.co.uk
- Maddak, Inc.
  http://www.maddak.com
- Sammons/Preston, Inc.
  http://www.sammonspreston.com/pedCat.htm
- Maxi-Aids, Inc.

Site offers aids for children who are blind or visually impaired.
http://www.maxiaids.com

Dressing and Clothing Solutions

- Adaptive bras
  http://www.wearease.com/bra.html
- Clothing Solutions
  http://www.caringconcepts.com/index.html
- Easy Access Clothing for Children
  http://www.easyaccessclothing.com/
- Latex-free, waterproof underwear (Netti Supersoft)
  http://www.llmedico.com/home/
- Vinyl wear
  http://www.vinylwear.com/

Sexuality

- Anatomically correct dolls
  http://www.feelingscompany.com
- Curriculums and other video resources for teaching adolescents with disabilities about sexuality
  http://www.sexualhealth.com/resources/library.cfm?list=curr
- Through the Looking Glass
  Site provides supports, resources, and services for parents with disabilities
  www.lookingglass.org
- Information on sexuality and individuals with Down syndrome
  http://www.ndss.org
- *Table Manners and Beyond: The Gynecological Exam for Women with Developmental Disabilities and Other Functional Limitations*
  http://www.bhawd.org/sitefiles/TblMrs/cover.html
- *You Deserve to Be Safe: A Guide for Girls With Disabilities* (2002)
  http://dawn.thot.net/safe.html

---

may vary significantly in the occupational therapy kitchen compared with his or her home kitchen. The child's unfamiliarity with the kitchen appliances or utensils may disrupt the flow of motor skills, and the spatial arrangements, lighting, and surface availability may cause process skill problems. For the activity, specific steps are followed and sequenced according to time requirements (e.g., the bread is put into the toaster, before the sandwich is made, and is toasted for 90 seconds so that it doesn't burn). If the child is making a sandwich for another person or with another person in the kitchen, the increased number of tasks or steps and the social demands to share supplies and to converse have increased the demand on performance skills during completion of the activity. In summary, ADL and IADL performance may be graded by adapting the environment, the type of activity or interactions required, the sequence of the activity, and whether an activity is new or familiar to the child. Occupations are viewed according to the context

in which they occur, the demands of the activity, and the child's abilities.

EVALUATION OF ADL AND IADL OCCUPATIONS

Families and their children play key roles in the determination of which evaluation procedures should be used. By working collaboratively with families, therapists learn about the child, the various environments in which ADLs and IADLs occur, the demands of the activities, and the expectations and concerns of the family. When children get older and are able to communicate, the therapist includes them in the determination of what areas of ADLs and IADLs are important to them. The parents and child often become more vested in the results if the therapist gives them a chance to select or refuse evaluations and to choose where and when the evaluation is completed (Giangreco, Cloninger, & Iverson, 1998).

BOX 15-2   Online Resources for Help with Instrumental Activities of Daily Living (IADLs)

Community Mobility
- Child Passenger Safety
  http://www.nhtsa.dot.gov/people/injury/childps/ChildSS/DocumentList.cfm
- National Center of Accessibility
  Site provides information on travel, recreation, parks, and tourism.
  http://ncaonline.org/research/
- National Highway Traffic Safety Administration (NHTSA)
  http://www.nhtsa.dot.gov/
- National Safety Belt Coalition
  http://www.nsc.org/traf/SBC/sbcchild.htm
- *Ride Safe*
  Brochure that provides information and pictorial cues on how to secure wheelchair tiedowns and occupant restraints.
  www.travelsafer.org
- U.S. Access Board
  Site gives accessibility requirements for built environments, transit vehicles, telecommunications equipment, and electronic and information technology.
  http://www.access-board.gov/

Health Management and Maintenance
- Blackboards and Bandaides
  Web site at which children and adolescents can talk about their chronic illness.
  http://www.faculty.fairfield.edu/fleitas/
- Porter, S., Freeman, L., & Griffin, L. (2000). *Transition planning for adolescents with special health care needs and disabilities: Information for families and teens.* Boston: Institute for Community Inclusion, Children's Hospital UAP.
  http://www.communityinclusion.org/transition/pdf/familyguide.pdf

Household Maintenance and Management
- *Ansell-Casey Life Skills Assessment and Guidebook* (2nd revision) (Seattle: Casey Family Programs)
  http://www.caseylifeskills.org/lsm/guidebook/full.pdf
- Ansell-Casey Life Skills Inventory
  Free online assessment of life skills that is completed online and then automatically scored. Inventory has 92 items.
  http://www.caseylifeskills.org

- *Ready, Set, Fly: A Parent's Guide to Teaching Life Skills* (Seattle: Casey Family Programs)
  http://www.caseylifeskills.org/lsg/resources/RSF.pdf

Use of Communication Devices
- Assistive Technology Training OnLine
  Great ideas for the use of communication devices and adaptations for writing.
  http://atto.buffalo.edu/
- Making talking books (for ADL and IADL intervention)
  These books can be done in Powerpoint, Hyperstudio, and Clicker 4 software programs.
  http://atto.buffalo.edu/registered/Tutorials/talkingBooks/

Financial Management
- Consumer Jungle
  http://www.consumerjungle.org

Meal Preparation
- Glossary of cooking terms
  http://www.goodstuffonline.com/glossary.html
- Meal planning
  http://www.my-meals.com

Safety and Emergency Response
- Easter Seals Easy Access Housing and Safety
  http://www.easter-seals.org/site/PageServer?pagename=ntl_resources_home
- National Children's Center for Rural and Agricultural Health and Safety (NCCRAHS)
  Marshfield Clinic
  http://research.marshfieldclinic.org/children
- National Program for Playground Safety
  University of Northern Iowa
  http://www.uni.edu/playground/
- National SAFE KIDS Campaign
  http://www.safekids.org
- S.A.F.E.T.Y. First
  Site explains preplanning of evacuation procedures.
  http://www.easter-seals.org/site/PageServer?pagename=ntl_safety_first
- *You Deserve to Be Safe: A Guide for Girls With Disabilities* (2002)
  http://dawn.thot.net/safe.html

This approach also gives therapists a better understanding of the contexts in which the child performs occupations and of current performance patterns that may be valued by the family.

Evaluation Methods

Evaluation of ADLs and IADLs begins with an analysis of occupational performance, which may collect data from numerous sources. Interviews, inventories, and structured and naturalistic observations are evaluation methods typically used to measure ADL and IADL performance in occupational therapy. The therapist uses these methods alone or in combination to analyze occupational performance (abilities and limitations), develop

intervention strategies, and/or measure outcomes of treatment. The choice of instrument depends on the reason for the evaluation. Table 15-1 lists instruments that assess children's ADL and IADL performance for different purposes.

For ADL and IADL independence, the child must be able to obtain and use supplies to complete a particular task. The therapist generally rates performance according to the child's ability to set up and complete a task and may assess performance by grading the child's level of independence. Table 15-2 presents one example of how the therapist may rate a child's independence in bathing. The therapist may use a system for grading the child's level of independence with any of the methods or purposes discussed in the following section.

TABLE 15-1 Instruments for Assessing ADL and IADL Performance in Children and Adolescents

Instrument and Publisher	Interview/ Inventory	Observation	Age Range	Description
ABS-S: 2 AAMR Adaptive Behavior Scale–School (2nd ed.) (Lambert, Nihira, & Leland, 1993) Pro-Ed 8700 Shoal Creek Boulevard Austin, TX 78757-6897 http://www.proedinc.com	X	X	3-8.11 yr	■ ABS is a standardized, criterion-referenced measure for adaptive behaviors in nine domains related to instrumental activities of daily living (IADLs): independent functioning, physical development, economic activity, language development, numbers and time, prevocational/ vocational activity, self-direction, responsibility, and socialization. ■ Maladaptive behaviors are measured in seven behavior domains. ■ ABS is useful for children with mental retardation (MR), autism, and behavior disorders.
AMPS Assessment of Motor and Process Skills (5th ed.) (Fisher, 2003a, 2003b) AMPS Project International P.O. Box 42 Hampton Falls, NH 03844 http://www.ampsintl.com	X	X	3 yr-adult	■ AMPS is a criterion-referenced test for activities of daily living (ADL) and IADL tasks that assesses the underlying motor and process performance skills used to perform the task. ■ Clients choose two or three ADL tasks they want to do (the test has 83 possible tasks, graded easy to hard). ■ Examiners need to be trained at a course, observe and rate at least 10 clients, and then have their scores calibrated according to rater severity through AMPS International. before using the assessment. ■ AMPS is useful for individuals ages 3 yr or older and with most disabilities. ■ Test's reliability and validity have been established, and normative data for typical individuals are available.
BDI Battelle Developmental Inventory (Newborg, Stock, Wnek, Guidubaldi, & Svinicki et al., 1988) BDI-II (expected release in Fall 2004) Riverside Publishing 425 Spring Lake Drive Itasca, IL 60143-2079 http://www.riverpub.com/ contact/index.html	X	X	6 mo-8 yr	■ ADL domain includes grooming, toilet hygiene, dressing, and eating. ■ The evaluator can use an in-depth assessment or a screening format.
CCITSN Carolina Curriculum for Infants and Toddlers with Special Needs (3rd ed.) (Johnson-Martin, Attermeier, & Hacker, 2004)	X	X	0–2 yr	Both CCITSN & CCPSN: ■ Include self-care as one of the five domains measured (self-care skills assessed in the CCITSN are eating, dressing, and grooming; the CCPSN assesses these three plus toileting) ■ Include sequences in responsibility, self-concept, and interpersonal skills ■ Provide an assessment log for collecting information
CCPSN Carolina Curriculum for Preschoolers with Special Needs (2nd ed.) (Johnson-Martin, Hacker, & Attermeier, 2004) Paul Brookes Publishing P.O. Box 10624 Baltimore, MD 21285 http://www. brookespublishing.com	X	X	2-5 yr	■ Give teaching suggestions for routines and modifications ■ Can be used with children with visual, motor, and hearing impairments ■ Have been field tested in more than 32 locations ■ Have high reliability and validity

TABLE 15-1   Instruments for Assessing ADL and IADL Performance in Children and Adolescents—*cont'd*

Instrument and Publisher	Interview/ Inventory	Observation	Age Range	Description
COACH Choosing Options and Accommodations for Children (2nd ed.) (Giangreco, Cloninger, & Iverson, 1998) Paul Brookes Publishing P.O. Box 10624 Baltimore, MD 21285 http://www. brookespublishing.com	X	X	3-21 yr	■ COACH is a curriculum-referenced, transdisciplinary team assessment and curriculum with four domains: personal management, community, home, and vocational. ■ The instrument is used as a team planning tool in the domains and does not assess specific skills. ■ Tasks are scored and given a potential priority and rank by each evaluator. ■ COACH is intended for children with moderate, severe, or profound disabilities but has been used with children with mild disabilities.
FIM Functional Independence Measure FIMware user guide and self-guided training manual, Version 5.20 (1997, 1999) Buffalo, NY 14214: State University of New York at Buffalo. http://www.udsmr.org/	X	X	8 yr-adult	■ FIM is a functional outcome measure for clients with physical disabilities. ■ Scores predict the intensity and extent of the assistance needed. ■ Six domains are assessed: self-care, mobility, locomotion, sphincter control, communication, and social cognition; there are 18 subdomains. ■ FIM uses a seven-point ordinal scale to measure the level of independence. ■ The test is norm referenced and part of the Uniform Data System for Medical Rehabilitation.
HELP Hawaii Early Learning Profile–Revised (Furuno, O'Reilly, Hosaka, Zeisloft, & Allman 1997) *Inside HELP: An Administration Manual* (Parks, 1999) VORT P.O. Box 11132 Palo Alto, CA 94306 http://www.vort.com/	X	X	Birth-3 yr	■ HELP is a curriculum-referenced assessment. ■ Self-care is one of six domains that cover 622 skills. ■ The instrument includes an inventory of developmental skills, an activity guide, and other materials intended for parents with disabilities. ■ Psychometric testing is not included.
PEDI Pediatric Evaluation of Disability Inventory (Haley, Coster, Ludlow, Haltiwanger, & Andrellos, 1992) Psychological Corporation Therapy Skill Builders 555 Academic Court San Antonio, TX 78204-2498 http://marketplace. psychcorp.com/ http://www.bu.edu/cre/pedi/ about-pedi.html	X	X	6 mo-7 yr (and older if skills below those of a 7-year-old)	■ PEDI is a normative, judgment-based outcome measurement (i.e., caregiver interview and/or observation). ■ Three domains are measured: self-care, mobility, and social function. ■ Some of the self-care skills assessed are drinking, utensil use, dressing, brushing the hair, and washing the face. ■ Functional skills (197 tasks), caregiver assistance (20 tasks), and modifications of adaptive equipment are rated.

Continued

TABLE 15-1 Instruments for Assessing ADL and IADL Performance in Children and Adolescents—*cont'd*

Instrument and Publisher	Interview/ Inventory	Observation	Age Range	Description
SFA School Function Assessment (Coster, Deeney, Haltiwanger, & Haley, 1998) Psychological Corporation Therapy Skill Builders 555 Academic Court San Antonio, TX 78204-2498 http://marketplace.psychcorp.com/	X	X	5-12 yr	■ SFA is a criterion-referenced assessment. ■ The test measures student function in the school setting according to participation in regular class, special education class, playground/recess, transportation, bathroom/toileting, transitions, and mealtime/snack time. ■ Task supports and activity performance are rated. ■ SFA produces a functional profile in comparison to peers. ■ The test is reliable and valid.
VINELAND Vineland Adaptive Behavior Scales (Sparrow, Balla, & Cicchetti), 1984) Vineland-II (expected release in 2005) American Guidance Service Circle Pines, MN 55014 (http://www.agsnet.com)	X		Birth-18.11 yr (and low-functioning adults)	■ The instrument is a norm-referenced evaluation. ■ Social competency is assessed, with behavioral observations in daily living skills (personal, domestic, community), communication, socialization, and motor domains. ■ An optional maladaptive behavior domain is provided for children 5 yr or older. ■ Three versions are available: interview/survey form; interview/expanded form; and classroom/teacher form (3-12.11 yr); online scoring is available. ■ The scales are appropriate for students with or without disabilities. ■ The instrument is reliable and valid for children with mental retardation. (Balboni, Pedrabissi, Moltoni, et al., 2001)
WeeFIM Functional Independence Measure for Children (Hamilton & Granger, 2000) *WeeFIM system^{SM} clinical guide: Version 5.01.* (1998, 2000). Buffalo, NY 14214: University at Buffalo.	X	X	6 mo-6 yr	■ WeeFIM® is a functional outcome evaluation for children with physical disabilities. ■ The instrument determines the amount of caregiver assistance needed. ■ Three domains are assessed: (1) self-care (eating, grooming, bathing, dressing [upper body and lower body], toileting, bladder management, and bowel management); (2) mobility, and (3) cognitive skills; 18 items are assessed. ■ This instrument is a direct adaptation of the Functional Independence Measure (FIM™) for adults. ■ WeeFIM® has interrater reliability and stability.

TABLE 15-2 Rating of Self-Care Skill Independence during Task Analysis

Level of Independence	Definition	Bathing Example
Independent	Child does 100% of the task, including setup.	Child gets out needed supplies and equipment and bathes, rinses, and dries himself or herself without assistance.
Independent with setup	After another person sets up the task, child does 100% of the task.	Caregiver places bathtub seat in tub and organizes bath supplies; child bathes, rinses, and dries himself or herself without assistance.
Supervision	Child performs task by himself or herself but cannot be safely left alone; he or she may need verbal cueing or physical prompts for 1% to 24% of task.	Child bathes, rinses, and dries himself or herself without assistance but needs monitoring when getting into and out of tub and when washing lower extremities because of poor balance and judgment.
Minimal assistance or skillful	Child does 51% to 75% of task independently but needs physical assistance or other cueing for at least 25% of task	Child bathes and rinses body parts independently but needs physical assistance getting into and out of tub; he or she is cued to monitor water temperature and to dry body parts.
Moderate assistance (26% to 50% partial participation)	Child does 26% to 50% of task independently but needs physical assistance or other cueing for at least 50% of task.	Child adjusts water temperature and washes and rinses face, torso, and upper extremities independently; he or she needs physical assistance getting into and out of tub and for washing and rinsing lower extremities and back.
Maximal assistance (1% to 25% partial participation)	Child does 1% to 25% of task independently but needs physical assistance or other cueing for 75% of task.	Child independently washes, rinses, and dries face but needs verbal cues to wash torso; he or she needs physical assistance getting into and out of tub and for washing other body parts.
Dependent	Child is unable to do any of the task.	Caregiver physically picks up child, places him or her in tub, and washes, rinses, and dries child's body parts; child does not lift body parts to be washed or dried.

Modified from Trombly, C.A., & Quintana, L.A. (1989). Activities of daily living. In C.A. Trombly (Ed.), *Occupational therapy for physical dysfunction* (3rd ed., p. 387). Baltimore: Williams & Wilkins.

An occupational analysis is done both during evaluation procedures and after they have been completed. Rogers, Holm and Stone (1997) suggested that therapists collect four types of data when evaluating ADL and IADL performance: (1) precise identification of limitations in the task, (2) causes of limitations, (3) capacity for change, and (4) possible interventions needed. For example, when a child puts on his socks, the therapist identifies that pulling the sock up over the ankle is difficult because of problems with upper extremity weakness and the tightness of the sock. Because the child has a neuromuscular disease with progressive weakness, he does not have the capacity to get stronger; therefore changes in the activity demands or compensatory techniques (e.g., loose fitting socks or a sock aid) will be needed to enable him to complete this activity independently. These data help therapists identify appropriate strategies and outcomes in intervention.

Interviews may be informal and unstructured. For example, the therapist may ask the interviewee (e.g., parent, child, teacher, and other significant caregiver) about the child's abilities, performance patterns (habits, routines, and roles), environmental characteristics, goals, and dreams. Sometimes simply asking the child, "What do you want to be able to do?" gives the therapist a place to start for further evaluation. The therapist may use interviewing techniques and inventory methods together to obtain useful information about how the child performs in different contexts.

Therapists also commonly use two types of observation. With *structured observation*, the therapist gives the child a task to do and then rates the child's performance in completing the task. Structured observation of ADL performance provides information about how well the child performs the task in a structured situation; however, it does not determine whether the child will begin the task at the appropriate time or perform the task in different contexts (e.g., whether the child will dress himself or herself when left alone).

With *naturalistic* or *ecologic observation*, the therapist gathers information in the typical or natural setting in which the activity occurs. Usually the therapist completes a task analysis to identify the activity demands. This includes looking at the steps of the activity, the sequence of these steps, and how the child adapts to the demands of the environment. In a naturalistic task analysis, the therapist evaluates the child's ability to do the task itself and the physical, social, and cultural characteristics of the environment. For example, when observing a child's ability to use the toilet at school, the therapist notes accessibility barriers, the sensory characteristics of the environment, typical classroom routines and expectations for toileting, and any cultural aspects of the toileting process (e.g., type of clothing the child is wearing), as well as how the child adapts to these factors. By understanding these contexts and the steps and sequence needed to complete the task, the therapist can choose appropriate intervention strategies according to the demands of the activity in the school context. Environmental observation is time-consuming, but it provides an abundance of information when used in a team effort (Rempfer, Hildenbrand, Parker, Brown, 2003). In addition to evaluating the performance skills and patterns used, the therapist identifies the level of assistance and the number of modifications needed to improve the child's independence.

Ecologic or environmentally referenced assessments are appropriate for all children and are particularly useful for children with moderate to severe disabilities who have difficulty generalizing tasks from one environment to another (Orelove & Sobsey, 1996; Sailor et al., 1986; York-Barr, Rainforth, & Locke, 1996). A *top-down approach* considers the contexts in which the child performs valued occupations in addition to what the child can or cannot perform (Bryze & Curtin, 1993; Coster, 1998; Trombly, 1995). With this approach, the therapist (1) asks the parent and child what they want or need to do; (2) identifies the environments or context in which the task occurs, the steps of the task, and the child's capabilities; (3) compares the demands of an identified task with the child's actual performance skills while completing the task; and (4) identifies and prioritizes the discrepancies to develop an intervention plan.

Team Evaluations

Curriculum-referenced or -guided assessments are often used by interdisciplinary teams in settings such as early intervention or school system practice. Self-care is often an area of assessment. The Carolina Curriculum for Infants and Toddlers with Special Needs (CCITSN) (Johnson-Martin, Attermeier, & Hacker, 2004), the Carolina Curriculum for Preschoolers with Special Needs (CCPSN) (Johnson-Martin et al., 2004) and the Hawaii Early Learning Profile (Furuno, O'Reilly, Hosaka, Zeisloft, & Allman, 1997) are typical curriculum-referenced assessments used in early intervention. Others are listed in Table 15-1.

Giangreco et al., (1998) developed a useful transdisciplinary, curriculum-based assessment and guide, Choosing Options and Accommodations for Children (COACH). Therapists use COACH to identify areas of concern (not specific skills) for school-age children with moderate to severe disabilities and to help plan inclusive educational goals with a family prioritization interview and environmental observations. The team identifies priorities, outcomes, and needed supports for specific environments and across environments in the areas of communication, socialization, personal management, leisure and recreation, and applied academics. Team members plan goals together, write interdisciplinary goals, and then decide which services the child needs. The team may decide that an occupational therapist is needed only as a consultant if the special education teacher is able to address the ADL task adequately.

Measurement of Outcomes

The health care and educational systems are demanding evidence-based practice and cost-effectiveness for therapy intervention. Within the past decade, professionals in the fields of rehabilitation and occupational therapy have developed universal assessments to measure the outcomes of ADLs and IADLs (see Table 15-1). Outcomes may include occupational performance, adaptation, client satisfaction, and/or role competence (AOTA, 2002). In addition to providing a means to evaluate children individually, the collection of aggregated ADL assessment results or outcome measures may help justify program expansion or changes in intervention strategies.

In rehabilitation, four primary assessments, which are valid and reliable, are used to measure occupational performance and adaptation to ADL tasks in children and adolescents. The Functional Independence Measure (FIM) is a universal assessment tool developed for adults but also used for children as young as 8 years old. The FIM assesses the severity of a disability and outcome progress after rehabilitation. For children 7 years of age or younger, therapists use the Functional Independence Measure-II for Children (WeeFIM-IISM) (Hamilton & Granger, 2000; Tsuji et al., 1999). The Pediatric Evaluation of Disabilities Inventory (PEDI) (Haley, Coster, Ludlow, & Haltiwanger, & Andrellos, 1992) is used for children from birth to 7 years of age. Numerous studies have used these assessment tools to demonstrate positive outcomes in ADL performance for children with brain injuries and other physical disabilities (Bedell, Haley, Coster, & Smith, 2002a & 2002b; Dumas, Haley, Fragala, & Steva, 2001; Knox & Usen, 2000; Kothari, Haley, Gill-Body, & Dumas, 2003). However, the question arises of whether a change in an assessment score really means that the child has made significant functional gains in self-care. Iyer, Haley, Watkins, & Dumas. (2003) found that occupational therapists, physical therapists, and speech therapists who were blinded to PEDI scores rated the magnitude of functional change in those scores as meaningful when an 11% change had occurred. In a recent study by Ziviani et al. (2001), the WeeFIM and the PEDI appeared to measure the same construct of self-care. The choice of which assessment to use depends on the characteristics of the child and the context for intervention.

The Assessment of Motor and Process Skills (AMPS) (Fisher, 2003a, 2003b) assesses ADL performance skills in various environments, both familiar (home or school) and unfamiliar (occupational therapy clinic). It has been used with children over 3 years of age from different cultural backgrounds and with an array of disabilities. The AMPS has been used widely in outcome studies, mostly with adolescents and adults; however, it also is appropriate for children (Fisher, 2003a; Pierce, Daly, Gallagher, Gershoff, & Schaumburg, 2002; Sellers, Fisher, & Duran, 2001). In the AMPS, the therapist assesses the dynamic interaction of process and motor skills while the child attempts to meet the demands of the activity in a certain environment. The therapist has a choice of 83 ADL tasks and gives the child or adolescent a list of approximately five to six familiar tasks, from which the child chooses two to complete. Because the AMPS has a task challenge hierarchy, from very easy to much harder than average, many of the activities are appropriate for children (e.g., putting on socks and shoes, brushing the teeth, folding laundry, setting a table, upper and lower body dressing, making a sandwich, vacuuming, baking brownies, or cooking an omelet). While the child performs the chosen ADL task according to the instructions given, the therapist rates the motor and process skills. The AMPS tasks use a top-down approach to evaluate skills and gives a comprehensive view of how efficiently, safely, and independently the child is functioning in performance contexts (Bryze & Curtin, 1993; Fisher, 2003a, 2003b). These results help the therapist predict what other ADLs the child may or may not be able to perform. The AMPS has potential for evaluating progress over time after clients have been taught adaptive patterns, organizational strategies, and environmental adaptations. A limitation of the AMPS is that the rater must be trained in a five-day course, then after observing and rating clients, his or her scoring is calibrated according to rater severity. This training and calibration must occur before he or she can perform the assessment.

School therapists may not find the PEDI, WeeFIM-II, or FIM as useful as an outcome assessment as it is in rehabilitation. As discussed in Chapter 22, the School Function Assessment (SFA) (Coster et al., 1998) assesses the child's participation in six different environments (transportation, transitions, classroom, cafeteria, bathroom, and playground). This assessment gives the therapist a profile of valuable information about self-care performance and role performance in the school environment, which the therapist can use to develop projected Individualized Education Plan (IEP) outcomes. For the School AMPS (Fisher & Bryze, 1997),

the therapist observes the child in the natural school environment while the child does typical school tasks. Currently the assessment includes 20 possible school tasks in five categories: pen/pencil writing tasks, drawing and coloring tasks, cutting and pasting tasks, computer writing tasks, and manipulative tasks (Fingerhut, Madill, Darrah, Hodge, & Warren, 2002; Fisher, Bryze, & Atchison, 2000). The School AMPS helps therapists assess motor and process skills during typical school graphic communication and communication device tasks. Because adaptations to ADL and IADL tasks often involve assistive technology (AT), it is important that the therapist consider the emerging outcome AT assessments in this area related to satisfaction and performance (see Chapter 18).

The Canadian Occupational Performance Measure (COPM) (Law et al., 1998) assesses a client's perception of his or her ADLs, productivity, and leisure occupations. The COPM provides an interview framework for children and families that helps the therapist identify how they are performing in everyday occupations and environments and how satisfied they are with their performance. Personal care, functional mobility, and community management are the areas covered in ADL performance. The child identifies his or her most important concern and rates his or her performance and satisfaction with that task; this helps the child prioritize intervention goals (McGavin, 1998).

INTERVENTION STRATEGIES AND APPROACHES

When planning intervention procedures, the therapist must consider the child's characteristics/factors and performance skills and patterns in relation to the context and the demands of the activity. Therapists need to be sensitive to parents' and other caregivers' needs and concerns. They must listen to and reassure these individuals, involve them in making observations, and engage them in problem solving. When planning treatment for children with performance problems in ADLs and IADLs, the therapist must ask himself or herself the following questions (Brollier, Shepherd, & Markley, 1994; Snell & Brown, 2000):

- What ADLs and IADLs are *useful* and *meaningful* in current and future contexts?
- What are the *preferences* of the child or the family?
- Are the activities *age appropriate* (i.e., used by peers without disabilities)?
- Is it *realistic* to expect the child to perform or master this task?
- What *alternative methods* can the child use to perform tasks (e.g., including the use of activity modifications or assistive technology)?
- Does learning this task *improve the child's health, safety, and social participation?*

- Do *cultural issues* influence how tasks are taught?
- Can the task be assessed, taught, and *practiced in a variety of environments?*

Therapists can use various approaches to improve ADLs and IADLs in children, including (1) establishing, restoring, and maintaining performance; (2) activity adaptations or compensatory methods; and (3) prevention/education. Therapists often use a combination of these approaches and various theoretic orientations to help children participate in ADL occupations. Table 15-3 gives examples of these approaches and possible theoretic orientations for the therapist to use when teaching a child to button his or her shirt. These approaches are discussed throughout each area of ADL tasks and IADL in later sections of the chapter.

Establishing, Restoring, and Maintaining Performance

The therapist may attempt to establish ADL or IADL performance and patterns using a developmental approach or, if this is not possible, he or she may try to restore or remediate the child's abilities that interfere with performance. To establish ADL and IADL patterns, the therapist uses the child's developmental and chronologic age and plans treatment according to a typical

TABLE 15-3	Approaches to Improving the Performance of Activities of Daily Living	
Approach	**Appropriate Frame of Reference**	**Problem: Buttoning Buttons without the Use of the Right Hand**
Establish, restore, and maintain	Developmental Biomechanical Neurodevelopmental treatment Sensory integration Person-environment-occupation (PEO)	Use specific activities to establish hand use and prehension patterns for buttoning. ■ Use coins in a piggy bank, board games with small, thin game pieces, craft activities (e.g., friendship bracelets, mosaics) to work on hand strength and coordination before beginning with buttons. ■ Provide tasks to develop, improve, or restore body functions (e.g., range of motion of hand, weight bearing to decrease tone; increase sensory input by playing with foam or Play-Doh); use dexterity activities to improve motor skills (coordinate, manipulate, flow, calibrate, grip). ■ Maintain performance patterns by using a dressing routine or other tasks that provide practice opportunities for buttoning on a regular basis (e.g., have a calendar on which the day of the week has to be buttoned to the calendar); maintain dexterity and strength through a daily exercise routine.
Modification/adaptation	PEO Human occupation Rehabilitation Biomechanical Sensory integration Neurodevelopmental treatment	Revise current activity demands or the context to compensate for body function and body structure limitations that affect performance skills and performance patterns. ■ *Adapt the task method:* Child uses one-handed buttoning technique, uses a pullover shirt so that buttoning is not an issue, or uses an extra large shirt with buttons already buttoned; he or she wears the button shirt over a pullover shirt like an open jacket. ■ *Adapt the object or use assistive technology:* Buttons are replaced with other buttons that have long shanks or that match the child's tactile preference; child uses a buttonhook, elastic sewn on buttons, or pressure-sensitive tape; child and devices are positioned for stability during activity (e.g., child sits in a chair with arms to button a shirt.) ■ *Adapt the task environment:* Child practices buttoning in the bedroom, away from distracting toys or siblings; parent, sibling, or peer is asked to button the shirt; shirt with buttons is used because it is culturally important to a teenager not to wear a pullover shirt.
Prevention/education	Human occupation Developmental Rehabilitation Biomechanical Sensory integration Coping	Educate and prevent failure at buttoning. ■ Therapist models and teaches the child and parent how to use the above approaches and lets them practice the approach while he or she watches. ■ Therapist provides home ideas for developing opportunities to practice games or tasks; he or she gives written/pictorial, verbal, or video instructions. ■ Therapist consults with day care provider or teacher to ensure carryover of the method used.

Modified from American Occupational Therapy Association (AOTA). (2002). Occupational therapy practice framework: Domain and process. *American Journal of Occupational Therapy, 56,* 609-639; and Dunn, W., Brown, C., & McGuigan, A. (1994). Ecology of human performance: A framework for considering the effect of context. *American Journal of Occupational Therapy, 48* (7), 595-607.

developmental sequence. In this approach the therapist examines underlying body structures and functions (e.g., strength, and tactile discrimination), selects age-appropriate tasks and habits to target in intervention, and gives parents some expectations for skill development (Kramer & Hinojosa, 1999).

In an establish or restore approach, therapists identify gaps in performance skills and intervene to teach or remediate the underlying problem that is interfering with a child's ADL performance. This approach focuses on the child's deficits in body function and structure. Therapists often use biomechanical, neurodevelopmental therapy (NDT), sensory integration (SI), behavioral, or motor control tasks to restore performance skills. For example, before dressing a child with spastic cerebral palsy and tight extensors, the therapist may use preparatory handling techniques (NDT) to inhibit the child's tone. In such a case the therapist would place the child in a supine position and slowly roll the child's hips from one side to the other to reduce the tone, increase range of motion, and encourage trunk rotation (Boehme, 1988). After this preparation the child's task performance will improve, and the therapist may then facilitate movement patterns by stabilizing the pelvis while the child pulls up his or her pants. When using this approach, therapists provide parents and children with suggestions on how to practice these movement patterns in various tasks.

Occupational therapists also use behavioral approaches. They may use backward or forward chaining to teach the tasks. In backward chaining, the therapist performs most of the task, and the child performs the last step of a sequence to receive positive reinforcement for completing the task. Practice continues, with the therapist performing fewer steps and the child completing additional steps. This method is particularly helpful for children with a low frustration tolerance or poor self-esteem because it gives immediate success. In forward chaining, the child begins with the first step of the task sequence, then the second step, and continues learning steps of the task in a sequential order until he or she can perform all steps in the task. Forward chaining can be helpful for children who have difficulty with sequencing and generalizing activities. The therapist can give varying amounts of cues, or prompts, before or during an activity. Therapist or person cues and environment or task cues can occur naturally or artificially in an environment. Therapists use verbal, gestural, or physical cues or a combination of all three (Biederman, Fairhall, Raven, & Davey, 1998; Snell & Vogtle, 2000). Environmental or task cues may include picture sequences or checklists, color coding, positioning, or adaptation of the sensory properties of the environment or materials used in a task. Figure 15-2 shows an example of a visual picture sequence for hand washing. Reese and

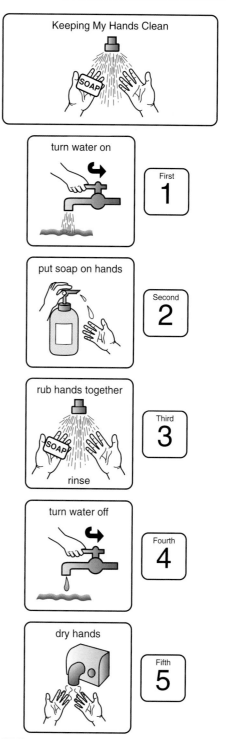

FIGURE 15-2 This simple picture sequence gives Adam the needed cues to wash his hands independently. (Courtesy Judith Schoonover, Loudoun County Public Schools, Virginia; Picture Communication Symbols from Mayer-Johnson, Inc, Solana Beach, CA.)

Snell (1991) described a hierarchic approach to presenting artificial cues from being least intrusive to most intrusive: verbal cues, verbal and gestural cues, and verbal and physical cues. Reese and Snell described a hierarchy of physical cues: shadowing the child's movements, using two fingers to guide the child, and using a hand-over-hand approach to guide movement. The therapist or parent uses the least amount of cues possible and fades cues to promote independence. Figure 15-3 presents

examples of these different types of cues, which can be used as a child performs various self-care occupations.

Once self-care routines and patterns have been developed, it is important to maintain them and any of the environmental supports that promote continued ADL success. Repetition and the development of habits and routines are essential organizers, particularly for children who take a long time to learn new skills, have poor memory, or thrive on routine or practice. Schedules for

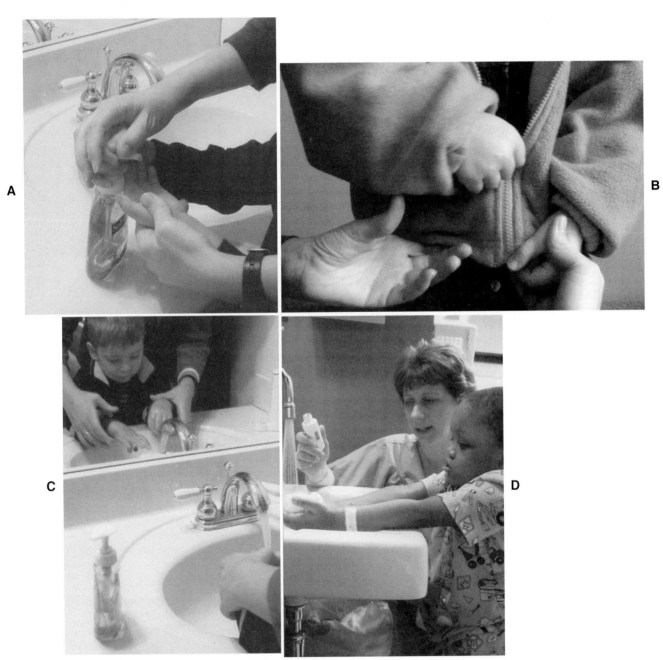

FIGURE 15-3 Hierarchy of cues, from most intrusive to least intrusive. **A,** A hand-over-hand approach is used for squirting soap on the child's hands. **B,** Two fingers are used to guide zipping of the child's coat. **C,** The therapist shadows her hand over the top of the child's hands to cue hand movements for hand washing. **D,** The therapist verbally cues the child on how to wash the hands.

toileting or dressing, visual prompts displayed on the wall, a set place for items when grooming, and a checklist for grocery shopping are all examples of contextual supports. Health maintenance activities (e.g., self-catheterization, wheelchair push-ups, ROM exercises, taking medication regularly, and eating nutritious meals) support task performance in all occupations.

Adaptation (Compensatory) Approach

In the adaptation approach (also called the compensatory approach), the therapist does not expect to establish or restore client factors; therefore he or she uses alternative physical techniques, substitute movement patterns, or other adaptive performance patterns to enable the child to complete a task. Compensatory strategies may include modification of the task or task method, use of assistive technology, or modification of the environment (Geyer, Kurtz, & Byram, 1998). Therapists often use a combination of these strategies to improve a child's performance, giving consideration to the performance context. Table 15-4 provides examples of typical adaptation approaches used with different functional problems.

Therapists practice adaptation or compensatory strategies in various contexts and modify them until they become functional. For example, a child with a bilateral upper extremity amputation may have several compensatory strategies to use for ADL tasks. As an adapted method, the child can use his or her feet or mouth to write or dress, or he or she can learn new movement patterns to operate a prosthetic arm (assistive device) for manipulating objects. Another compensatory strategy may include using personal assistance in the home or school environment. A child's mother can place clothes in drawers the child can reach while sitting in a wheelchair.

Adapting Task Methods

The therapist often modifies tasks by using grading techniques. Grading is the adaptation of a task or portions of a task to fit the child's capabilities. By using a task analysis, the therapist rates subtasks of the activity and varies them according to their degree of ease or difficulty for the child. The therapist may modify the activity demands to compensate for limited capacities and performance skills. He or she may grade the tasks according to qualities (e.g., simple to complex). Grading of a task may include gradually increasing the number of steps for which the child is responsible, fading the amount of personal assistance or cueing the child receives, or reducing the length of time the child takes to complete an activity.

Each ADL and IADL involves a series of steps that are performed together in a specific sequence. Through task analysis, the therapist gains an understanding of the sequence of steps involved in each ADL task. The therapist uses *personal assistance* when a child cannot complete a task independently or when completion of the task requires too much of the child's energy, which is needed for other, more important tasks (Smith, Benge, & Hall, 2000). The therapist uses *partial participation* when a child cannot complete a task independently; the child performs some steps of the task, and a caregiver completes the remainder. This helps the child to become part of the activity and to use his or her current abilities. Partial participation often is used when children are first learning a task or when their abilities are severely limited (Ferguson & Baumgart, 1991).

Adapting the Task Object or Using Assistive Technology

Several assistive devices are available through equipment vendors, catalogs, and specialty department stores. These devices are changing constantly, and they vary in complexity, price, and quality. Assistive devices are commercially available or are custom-made by the therapist or by skilled craftsmen, orthotists, or rehabilitation engineers. By using local and national databases, publications, and Internet searches on product comparison, therapists can keep informed of the availability of new assistive devices in order to find equipment for unique or specific problems (Smith et al., 2000).

The choice of an assistive device is a cooperative decision made by the child, the parents, therapists, and others who work with the child. Together these individuals systematically evaluate what the child needs to do, his or her performance contexts, the child's abilities and limitations, and the capabilities of the device itself. They choose the device that has the best "environmental fit." Adolescents who are striving to identify with their peers tend to reject devices that call attention to their disabilities. Children are easily frustrated if use of the device exceeds their coordination abilities or attention span. To be worthwhile, an assistive device should meet the following requirements:

- *Assist in the task* the child is trying to complete without being cumbersome
- Be *acceptable* to the child and family and in the contextual environments in which it will be used (e.g., appearance, functions, upkeep, and storage)
- Be *practical and flexible* for the environments in which it will be used (e.g., dimensions, portability, positioning, and use with other assistive devices)
- Be *durable* and easy to clean
- Be *expandable* (i.e., able to meet the child's needs now and when the child has grown and has more sophisticated abilities)
- Be *safe* for the child to use (e.g., cognitive, behavioral, or physical characteristics such as drooling, throwing,

TABLE 15-4 Typical Adaptation Principles Used with Children and Adolescents with Disabilities

Behavior/Disability	Adaptation Principles
Low vision or hearing (or both)	■ Use intact or residual senses ■ Amplify sensory characteristics of objects (e.g., color, size, tactile and auditory features) ■ Give cues consistently to determine whether activity is beginning or ending ■ Use tactile, verbal, visual, or object cues (e.g., put hand on washcloth or say, "It's time to wash your face.") ■ Use gestures (e.g., point to arm that is put in sleeve first) ■ Decrease auditory and visual distractions
Dislike of being touched (tactile defensive)	■ Prepare child for touch by giving deep pressure and organized, rhythmic touch ■ Give choices for tactile preferences (e.g., clothes, washcloths, brushes) ■ Let child perform touching on himself or herself (e.g., use toothbrush or wash face or body) ■ Allow child to wear snug clothing (e.g., turtleneck) or loose clothing per his or her preference
Inability to find clothes or to understand top, front, or bottom	■ Amplify characteristics ■ Reduce distracters (e.g., place only one utensil on countertop for cooking activity) ■ Use visual or gestural cues (e.g., mark medial border of shoes with happy faces to keep shoes on correct feet) ■ Use systematic scanning when searching for objects (e.g., clothes in closet)
Inability to sit up or maintain balance	■ Provide support externally (e.g., use positioning device) ■ Change position of child (e.g., have child sit to put on shoes or dress in side-lying position) ■ Change position of activity (e.g., keep grooming items together in a bucket on top of the sink)
Limited reach	■ Reduce amount of reach needed ■ Change position of activity ■ Lengthen handles (e.g., use long-handled bath sponge or reacher)
Difficulty grasping objects	■ Build up handles of objects (e.g., brushes and spoons) ■ Substitute assistive devices so that grasping is not necessary (e.g., use universal cuffs or straps) ■ Stabilize objects with other body parts (e.g., in teeth or between legs)
Weakness with little endurance	■ Eliminate gravity (e.g., prop elbow, or dress in side-lying position) ■ Use lightweight objects ■ Use power equipment
Difficulty controlling movement	■ Provide stable base of support (e.g., sit on floor with wide base) ■ Eliminate need for fine control (e.g., use an enlarged zipper pull) ■ Use weighted devices to give proprioceptive feedback (e.g., weighted toothbrushes and cups)
Poor memory; inability to remember sequences or directions	■ Establish and practice set routines and sequences ■ Use partial participation, grading techniques, and backward and forward chaining ■ Use visual cues (e.g., pictures, labels, checklists, color coding) ■ Substitute assistive technology (e.g., alarm on watch or timers) ■ Use verbal cues (e.g., "First, then second," jingles, rhymes, songs) ■ Use real life materials in the setting in which the occupation occurs
Tendency to become easily frustrated; outbursts	■ Identify purpose of "problem behavior" (e.g., escape, avoid, attention, obtain, transition, or stimulate) by analyzing antecedents and consequences ■ Limit exposure to context associated with misbehavior ■ Use preferred tasks and give choices ■ Reinforce, coach, and expand appropriate alternate behaviors ■ Avoid personal assistance and coaching (use partial participation) ■ Use grading, prompting, fading prompts, and generalization

Developed from Geyer, L.A., Kurtz, L.A., & Byram, L.E. (1998). Prompting function in daily living skills. In J.P. Dormans & L. Peliegrino (Eds.), *Caring for children with cerebral palsy: A team approach* (pp. 323-346). Baltimore: Brookes; and Koegel, L.K., Koegel, R.L., Kellegrew, D., & Mullen, K. (1996). Parent education for prevention and reduction of severe problem behaviors. In L.K. Koege, R.L. Koegel, & G. Dunlap (Eds.), *Positive behavioral support: Including people with difficult behavior in the community* (pp. 3-30). Baltimore: Brookes.

or difficulty with sequencing do not interfere with use of the device)
■ Have a *system of maintenance or replacement* with continued use
■ *Meet the cost constraints* of the family or purchasing agency
Overall, the child should complete tasks at a higher level of efficiency using the device than he or she could without it. Trial use of a device is highly recommended;

this helps determine the feasibility of its use and demonstrates its value to the child and primary caregivers.

Recently computers and cognitive prosthetic devices have come into use for purposes such as visual schedules, social stories, and to give children the visual and/or auditory prompts needed to initiate, sequence, sustain, and terminate ADL and IADL activities (Gentry, 2003; Gray, 2000). For example, a talking book from Microsoft's PowerPoint can help a child learn shoe tying, how to

Use your right hand to make a loop
close to the knot.
Hold it between your two fingers.

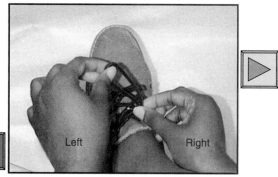

FIGURE 15-4 Sample talking book. This frame from *Talking Shoes* was created with Microsoft PowerPoint. (Courtesy Laura Pal and Kelly Showalter, Virginia Commonwealth University, Richmond.)

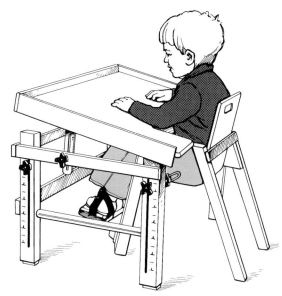

FIGURE 15-5 Commercially available chair with positioning components and a desk with an adjustable height and an adjustable inclined work surface.

dress himself or herself, and how to set a table if the technology is nearby. As shown in Figure 15-4, while tying his shoes, the child or adolescent uses the talking book as a visual and auditory prompt on his computer or his personal digital assistant device (PDA). Other cognitive prosthetic devices that can aid ADL and IADL tasks include portable memory aids (e.g., checklists, voice-activated tape recorders), medication alarm pill boxes, watches with specialized features (alarms, schedules, talking), alarm organizers, pagers, sound-activated key rings, and simple switches that program up to three steps.

Making Adaptations to the Context

In all the approaches discussed, the therapist uses the interaction between the child and the environmental contexts to improve performance. The therapist can adapt physical environments by recommending modifications of architectural and other physical barriers or sensory characteristics. To facilitate wheelchair access, the child's caregivers can install ramps or move furniture. For example, the family can place their computer on a more usable work surface in a more accessible location so that the child who is wheelchair dependent can use it for doing homework and communicating with a brother or sister at college. For some children, therapists minimize sensory stimuli and eliminate visual and auditory distractions. Other children may require increased environmental stimulation (e.g., color or music) to cue their performance. Table 15-5 presents examples of how the physical environment can be adapted.

Work Surface. The work surface supports the child, materials, tools, and assistive devices in an activity. The boundaries of the work space help children keep within usable or safe environments. For example, a cutout surface on a table or a lip on a wheelchair tray or

sink countertop makes boundaries for children. The therapist adds various textures, colors, and pictures to the work surface area to give sensory cues about boundaries or to structure the task. Even with these adaptations, some children (e.g., those with weakness in one side of the body) need assistance in stabilizing objects. Table 15-6 presents suggestions for stabilizing objects when they are placed on the work surface or held by the child.

Characteristics of the work surface that are amenable to adaptation include height, angle of incline (Figure 15-5), size, distance from the body, distance from other work areas, and general accessibility of a work surface. Changes in these characteristics enhance the child's function in various ways, including improving arm support, increasing the visual orientation of a task, adapting seat height for easier transfers, and improving table height for wheelchair access.

Positioning. Therapists consider the position of the child and the position of the materials or activity when planning intervention. Children who have problems with posture and movement often lack sufficient control to assume or maintain stable postures during activity performance and benefit from adaptive positioning. Adaptive positioning may include using different positions (e.g., sitting instead of standing), low technology devices (e.g., lapboards, pillows, towel rolls), or high technology (e.g., customized cushions or wheelchairs). When possible, the therapist uses the most typical position for a given activity with the fewest restrictions or adaptations to stabilize the body for function (Bergen, Presperin, & Tallman, 1990; Finnie, 1997).

Alternative body positions are extremely helpful to children with disabilities. These changes help compensate for physical limitations in body functions such as

TABLE 15-5 Environmental Adaptations for the Home When Accessibility is Limited

Architectural Barrier	Structural Changes	Possible Assistive Devices	Task Modification
Entrances and exits	Hand rails Hand stairs Ramp Built-up terrain to door height Stair lift In-home elevator Increased door width (33 to 36 inches minimum) Step-back hinges Door rehinged to open in or out Pocket or folding door Electric door openers	Straps or loop door handle Lever handles Portable doorknob Built-up key holders Combination locks Environmental control unit	Use different entrance Remove inside doors Use curtains for privacy Use hip or wheelchair to open doors
Bathroom	Increased door width (33 to 36 inches minimum); French doors or accordion door Enlarged room Sink mounted low Open space under cabinet Showers with built-in seat Placement of tub faucets changed Ramped shower stall Toilet bidet installed Linen closet shelves with no door	Safety rails Seat reducer Raised commode seat Step placed in front of commode Wheelchair commode Insulated pipes Single-lever faucets Tub seats Wheelchair shower chair Hydraulic lifts Toilet paper tongs Toilet paper mounting Angled mirror Wall-mounted hairdryer with switch Suction-cupped bucket to hold supplies	Freestanding commode in secluded area Urinal Bed bath Sponge bath Liquid soap Soap on a string Shampoo pump Dry shampoo
Bedroom	Downstairs bedroom Enlarged space Enlarged closet doors Low closet pole Closet storage system with shelves Built-in bookshelves at low and medium heights Cut holes in work surfaces for holding objects and electrical cords Built-in dressers or dressers bolted to the wall Special glides for wall drawers	Leg extenders Bed rails Firm mattress Straps or rope ladders Mounted shoe rack Environmental control units or switches for TV, radio, and light access Enlarged drawer handles or loop added Positioning devices Adaptive chairs	Place bed on floor Keep most-used clothes in accessible drawers Use shelves instead of dresser drawers for clothes Store toys in shoe bag
Kitchen	Enlarged space Lowered countertops Lowered cabinets No cabinets under sink Built-in rangetop Sliding drawers and organizers in cabinets Wall-mounted, side-by-side oven Dishwasher mounted higher or has front-opening Front-opening washing machine		Keep items most used in low cupboards or on accessible surfaces Hang bowls and pans on wall instead of storing in cabinets Eat on wheelchair lap tray instead of table Keep water in insulated pump bottle on table Use a stool for washing dishes

strength, joint movement, control, or endurance and provide relief to skin areas and bony prominences. A therapist considers positions that maximize independent task performance. Key points for stability that enable the child to use available voluntary movement are the pelvis and trunk, head, and extremities (Bergen & Colangelo, 1985; Finnie, 1997). The following questions guide decision making about positioning:

■ Is the child aligned properly? Are the hips, shoulders, and head in good alignment (Figure 15-6)?
■ What positions or devices increase trunk stability (e.g., using a hard seat insert or lateral supports, using a

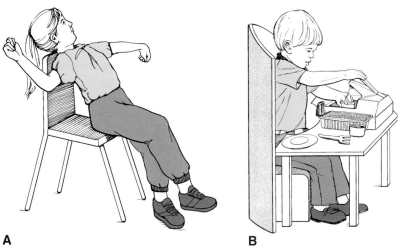

FIGURE 15-6 Sitting postures. **A,** Incorrect sitting resulting from a massive extension pattern and an asymmetric tonic reflex posture. **B,** Correct sitting posture. Weight is equally distributed on the sitting base, and the feet and elbows are supported.

TABLE 15-6 Stabilization Materials and Application Procedures

Materials	Application Procedures
Tape	Applies quickly but often is a temporary solution; includes masking, electrical, and duct tapes (duct tape is sturdy and has holding power).
Nonslip pressure-sensitive matting	Fits under objects or around them and can be glued to objects; friction between materials minimizes slipping and sliding of objects; available in rolls or pads.
Suction cup holders	Hold lightweight materials, maintaining suction between object and work surface; single-faced suction cups can be applied permanently to objects (e.g., with nails, screws, or glue); double-faced suction cups can be moved from object to object.
C-clamps	Secures flat objects to lap trays, table edges, and other surfaces.
Tacking putty	Sticks posters onto walls; holds lightweight objects on surfaces such as tables, lap trays, angle boards, and walls.
Pressure-sensitive hook-and-loop tapes (Velcro)	Sewn to cloth or glued to the base of objects and work surfaces; soft loop tape is used on areas that will contact the child's skin or clothing.
Wing nuts and bolts	Secure objects to a table surface or lapboard when holes are drilled through the object and holding surface; sturdy and more permanent.
Magnets	Affix to an object; stabilize objects on metallic surfaces such as refrigerator doors, metal tables, and magnetic message boards.
L-brackets	Hold objects in an upright plane; holes are drilled in both the work surface and the object to correspond with the L-bracket holes; objects are secured with nuts and bolts.
Soldering clamps	Hold small items for intricate work (e.g., mending a shirt, sewing on a button, or putting on a bracelet); mounted to freestanding base; bases are weighted, suction cupped, or held to the surface with a C-clamp.
Elastic or webbing straps	Attach to or around objects or positioning devices to hold them down; they also secure flat objects onto a work surface; straps are secured by tying, pressure-sensitive hook-and-loop table, D-rings and buckles, grommets, or screws.

surface to support the feet, or widening the sitting base by abducting the legs)?

■ Is support adequate to maintain upright posture with head in the midline?

■ Can the child use his or her hands and visually focus on the task?

Sitting and sometimes standing are the most appropriate positions for the child to perform ADL tasks. In addition to postural alignment, the therapist recommends positions that provide the child with (1) good orientation of his or her body to the work surface and the materials being used, (2) good body and visual orientation to the therapist (if instruction is being given), and (3) the ability independently to get to the place where the ADL occurs, maintain the necessary position, and leave. The therapist modifies chair heights so that the child's feet are touching the floor to support postural stability and facilitate transfers. If the therapist raises the seat height, he or she provides a footrest. The therapist shortens or lengthens chair legs with blocks or leg extenders.

Kangas (1998) advocates a "task-ready position" for children with moderate to severe motor disabilities. Instead of positioning the child's hips, knees, and ankles at 90-degree angles, Kangas positions them so that they are ready to move. In the task-ready position, the pelvis is secure, the trunk and head are slightly forward so that the shoulders are in front of the pelvis, the arms and hands are in front of the body, and the feet are flat on the floor or behind the knees. The therapist removes or loosens as many restraints or chair adaptations as safely possible so that the child has maximal potential for movement. The movement, even when subtle, provides visual, vestibular, proprioceptive, and kinesthetic feedback. A carved or molded seat and a seat belt across the thighs give additional sensory feedback and are used for positioning of the pelvis and safety.

Prevention/Education Approach

Child and caregiver education is essential in all therapy for children. By educating others, the therapist helps prevent injuries and possible failure in occupational performance. This education helps children perform ADL occupations in their environments and helps caregivers and children learn safety information, specific techniques, and coping strategies. When providing information, occupational therapy practitioners must consider the learning capacity and environmental contexts of children and their families, as well as the demands of the activity (Holm et al., 2003).

Because a young child or a child with moderate developmental delays may not be ready to assume health maintenance tasks independently, parents, caregivers, and occasionally siblings are responsible for learning appropriate methods and adaptations to perform ADLs and IADLs. Instructional methods depend on individual preferences, family life cycle needs, and the physical, learning, and psychosocial capacities of children, families, and caregivers.

Therapists present child or caregiver education in various ways. They often demonstrate, or model, how to do the task (e.g., tub transfers) when instructing. In addition the therapist may use visual aids, written instructions, audiotapes, videotapes, and checklists. The method chosen often depends on the comfort level and preferences of the parents and therapists and the contextual demands. In a study by Feldman (1999), videotaped instructions were used to teach parents with limited cognition about child care (including dressing skills) and child safety. The information was learned and was retained for longer than 65 months.

Children require multiple opportunities to practice new tasks, and families may need help assessing routines and identifying when children can practice ADL occupations (Koegel, Koegel, Kellegrew, & Mullen, 1996).

In a study by Kellegrew (1998), parents used self-monitoring forms to record the number of opportunities their child had to perform an ADL task and the amount of assistance they gave the child during the task. The parents did not receive specific instructional methods; rather, broad concepts were conveyed, for example, that ADL tasks were important, that their children were ready and able to learn, and that their children required many opportunities to practice the tasks. Families were creative in finding ways and opportunities to help their children practice tasks, and ADLs increased only when children were given multiple opportunities to engage in them. These results suggest that it is important for the therapist to assess a child's opportunities to practice tasks when developing home programs.

An educational approach provides parents and children the chance to make informed choices about the services, methods, assistive technology, and environmental adaptations they will use (Bayzak, 1989). Grading, forward and backward chaining, partial participation, and modeling help train caregivers. Unfortunately, parent education and the information provided may not receive adequate emphasis in some programs (King, Law, King, & Rosenbaum, 1998). In this chapter, education of caregivers and children is discussed as an integral part of the intervention approaches for ADLs and IADLs.

SPECIFIC INTERVENTION TECHNIQUES FOR SELECTED ADL TASKS

Specific intervention strategies for toilet hygiene and bowel and bladder management, dressing, bathing and showering, personal hygiene and grooming, and sexual activity are described in the following sections. Interrelationships among child factors, contexts, and activity demands are considered. A combination of the approaches and strategies described previously is used to help children become as independent as possible in ADL occupations. As with all treatment, the therapeutic use of self-purposeful and meaningful activities, consultation, and education are methods used to help others learn ADL occupations.

Toilet Hygiene and Bowel and Bladder Management
Typical Developmental Sequence

Independent toileting is an important self-maintenance milestone, and its achievement varies widely among children. It carries considerable sociologic and cultural significance. Self-sufficiency may determine participation in day care centers, school programs, recreational and community opportunities, and secondary school vocational choices. Like other ADL tasks, toileting is a complex task requiring a thorough analysis of the demands of the activity and the ways the context and the child's capabilities influence performance skills and patterns. To begin to learn this task, a child must be physically and psychologically ready. Also, parents or caregivers need to be ready to devote the time and effort to toilet training the child. A communication system between caregivers and the child is essential.

At birth a newborn voids reflexively and involuntarily. As the child matures, the spinal tract is myelinated to a level for bowel and bladder control at the lumbar and sacral areas, and the child learns to control sphincter reflexes for volitional holding of urine and feces. Children are often physiologically ready for toileting if they have a pattern of urine and feces elimination.

Bowel control precedes bladder control, and studies indicate that girls are trained an average of $2\frac{1}{2}$ months earlier than boys. Independence in toileting includes getting on and off the toilet, managing fasteners and clothing, cleansing after toileting, and washing and drying hands efficiently without supervision. Children progress in sequence, according to each child's unique pace of development. The typical developmental sequence for toileting is presented in Table 15-7.

TABLE 15-7   Typical Development Sequence for Toileting

Approximate Age (yr)	Toileting Skill
1	■ Indicates discomfort when wet or soiled ■ Has regular bowel movements
$1\frac{1}{2}$	■ Sits on toilet when placed there and supervised (short time)
2	■ Urinates regularly
$2\frac{1}{2}$	■ Achieves regulated toileting with occasional daytime accidents ■ Rarely has bowel accidents ■ Tells someone that he or she needs to go to the bathroom ■ May need reminders to go to the bathroom ■ May need help with getting on the toilet
3	■ Goes to the bathroom independently; seats himself or herself on toilet ■ May need help with wiping ■ May need help with fasteners or difficult clothing
4-5	■ Independent in toileting (e.g., tearing toilet paper, flushing, washing hands, managing clothing)

Modified from Coley, I. (1978). *Pediatric assessment of self care assessment* (p. 145, 149). St. Louis: Mosby; and Orelove, F., & Sobsey, D. (1996). Self-care skills. In F. Orelove & D. Sobsey (Eds.), *Educating children with multiple disabilities* (2nd ed., p. 342). Baltimore: Brookes.

Typical Problems That Interfere with Toileting Independence

Children with spinal cord injury, spina bifida, or other conditions that produce full or partial paralysis require special management for bowel and bladder activities. Loss of control over these bodily functions can produce embarrassment and decreased feelings of self-esteem. School-age children are characteristically modest about their bodies, and adolescents are struggling with identity issues and the need to be like their peers.

The type of bladder problem depends on the level and type of neurologic impairment. When the lesion is in the lumbar region or below, the reflex arc is no longer intact and the bladder is flaccid (lower motor neuron bladder). When the lesion is above the level of bladder innervation, the result is an automatic bladder (upper motor neuron bladder). The child undertakes training programs for the upper motor neuron bladder to develop an automatic response. Children with a flaccid bladder cannot be trained because the bladder has insufficient tone to empty and requires assistance in emptying.

The therapist works with physicians and nurses to determine bladder training and management programs after medical testing and collaborative discussions with children and their parents. Four main methods can be used to manage urine: (1) condom catheterization (for males), (2) indwelling catheters, (3) intermittent catheterization (every 4 to 6 hours), and (4) ileal conduits. Parents are asked to restrict the child's fluid intake to prevent bladder distention. When girls have partial control of bladder function, they wear disposable diapers or incontinence pads.

A basic principle for success in bowel reeducation is to have a regular, consistent evacuation of the bowel. The time for this is a matter of choice, but there should be a schedule that remains consistent. In some cases the child receives suppositories and a warm drink before evacuation. This stimulates contraction and relaxation of muscle fibers in the walls of the intestine, moving the contents onward. Other techniques include digital stimulation, massage around the anal sphincter, or manual pressure using the Credé method on the abdomen. Occasionally, removal of the stool by hand or by a colostomy is recommended. As with an ileostomy, colostomy collection bags are emptied and cleansed on a regular basis.

Children who perform catheterizations or bowel programs may have difficulty in any of the following areas: maintaining a stable yet practical position, hand dexterity, perceptual awareness, strength, range of motion, and stability and accuracy when emptying collection devices. Memory, safety, and sensory awareness are needed for any of these procedures. Although nurses are often the professionals who teach bowel and bladder control methods, the occupational therapist may be involved to establish the hand skills necessary, to adapt the context by providing assistive devices or adapted methods, or to establish a routine that becomes habitual and easy for the child and helps prevent future infections or embarrassment.

Closely associated with bowel and bladder care is care of the skin in the perineal area. The skin should be cleansed thoroughly to protect the tissue against the effects of contact with waste matter and to eliminate odor. All children with decreased sensation are susceptible to *decubiti*, which are pressure sores that occur fairly rapidly when blood vessels are compressed (e.g., around a bony prominence such as the ischial tuberosity).

Children with Limited Motor Skills and Body Functions

Diapering becomes a difficult task when infants or children have strong extensor and adduction (muscle and movement function) patterns in their legs. Therapists teach the mother restorative or remedial methods to decrease extensor patterns before diapering and to incorporate these methods into the diapering routine. For example, the mother may first place a pillow under the child's hips, flex the hips, and slowly rock the hips back and forth before she helps the child abduct the legs for diapering.

Toileting independence may be delayed in children with limitations in strength, endurance, range of motion, postural stability, and manipulation or dexterity. With an unstable sitting posture, the child has difficulty relaxing and maintaining a position for pressing down and emptying the bowels. With weakness and limited range of motion, the child may be unable to manage fastenings because of hand involvement or may have problems sitting down or getting up from the toilet seat because of hip-knee contractions or quadriceps weakness.

Cleansing after a bowel movement may be difficult if the child cannot supinate the hand, flex the wrist, or internally rotate and extend the arm. An anterior approach may work. The therapist must caution girls against contamination from feces, which can cause vaginitis. If at all possible, girls should wipe the anus from the rear. Solutions to cleansing problems are difficult and often discouraging. These children may require remediation strategies to improve body capacities (e.g., active range of motion), or adaptation strategies (e.g., assistive technology and environmental adaptations) to perform the toileting task.

Children with Cognitive Limitations

Children with mental retardation take longer to learn toileting, but they often become independent (Orelove & Sobsey, 1996). Problems with awareness, initiation,

sequencing, memory, and dexterity in managing their clothes are typical. As with all children, physiologic readiness for toileting is a prerequisite for training programs. The therapist uses task analysis to determine which steps of the process are problems, and he or she then determines what cues and prompts are needed to achieve the child's best performance. The therapist also evaluates which methods work as successful reinforcement (Snell & Vogtle, 2000).

Adaptation or Compensatory Strategies for Improving Toileting Independence

Compensatory strategies include remodeling or restructuring the environment, selecting assistive devices, or devising alternative methods to enhance independence. Adaptations to provide privacy are particularly important for the older child and adolescent. The therapist also addresses caregiver needs as the child becomes heavier and more difficult to assist with toileting.

Characteristics of physical and social environments at home or school influence how a child manages toileting hygiene. Assisting children in determining where to perform the procedure and how to manage it in their home, school, and recreational environments is often a challenge. Social routines and expectations are also important variables for the therapist to consider when making recommendations for managing toileting. These expectations depend on the child's age and abilities and how the family perceives the child's ability to manage this aspect of his or her ADLs.

Social Environment.   Of all ADL tasks, toileting requires the most sensitive approach on the part of those who work with the child on a self-maintenance program. Children may purposely restrict their fluid intake at school in an effort to avoid the need for elimination. Unfortunately, limited fluid intake promotes infections, which increases the difficulty of regulating the bowel and bladder. Families, teachers, nurses, and paraprofessionals work with therapists to evaluate the social environment and find the best place, time, and routine for the child. When self-catheterization is done in the school or community environment, the child can ensure privacy by using the health room, a private bathroom stall, or a time when children are usually not taking bathroom breaks. Carrying catheterization supplies in a fanny pack or a small nylon (nontransparent) bag also protects the child's privacy.

Therapists help children who lack bowel and bladder control develop routines and health habits that eliminate possible odors. By focusing on performance patterns, the therapist reinforces and incorporates regular cleaning and changing of appliances (collection bags for ileal conduits and colostomies) and urine collection bags into daily schedules. A good fluid intake also is recommended to prevent odors and bacterial growth.

Children with autism often have a difficult time learning toilet training. Maria Wheeler (1998) has written a practical guide to toilet training for children with autism and related disorders. Her discussion of support strategies such as modeling, social stories, and preteaching and her numerous examples of common problems and solutions associated with training individuals with autism are excellent. She uses the social context and many visual prompts to structure the steps for toileting. Table 15-8 provides suggestions for adapting toileting.

Physical Environment.   The bathroom often is the most inaccessible room in the house, yet it is essential that every family member have access to it. The floor space may be insufficient to allow the child to turn a wheelchair for a toilet transfer. The location and height of the sink, faucets, towels, soap, and toilet paper may make them inaccessible to young children. Sensory aspects of the objects in the environment may hinder performance. Children with hypersensitivity may have difficulty tolerating bathroom odors (e.g., air freshener, perfumed toilet paper or soap) or tactile sensations (e.g., a towel or a rug by the toilet). Therefore the bathroom's space, equipment, and objects may need to be adapted or modified.

TABLE 15-8   Analysis and Interventions for Toileting

Area	Analysis	Intervention Ideas
Required (task analysis)	■ Recognizes signal to go to the bathroom (visual or sensation) ■ Goes to bathroom and closes door ■ Pulls clothes down (only as much as needed) ■ Sits or stands at toilet ■ Urinates or defecates (or words child uses) ■ Gets toilet paper ■ Wipes, then throws toilet paper in toilet ■ Flushes once ■ Pulls clothes up ■ Washes and dries hands ■ Throws away trash ■ Leaves bathroom	■ Have visual routine on wall (objects, pictures, or action words). ■ Make tasks smaller or larger, depending on child's abilities (e.g., separate washing and drying of the hands). ■ Add task if child is omitting it or is having trouble (e.g., if child is smearing feces, use "WIPE" as one of the steps). ■ Child uses too much toilet paper: (1) remove toilet paper roll and use Kleenex, or pull off correct amount to be used and hand it to child, or (2) place a tape mark on the wall of how much paper to roll out. ■ Child does not sit: use timer and instruct child to stay "seated" until timer rings; use potty that is close to the floor.
Client factors (body functions and structures)	■ Sensations (bladder fullness, voluntary control, emptying bladder, wet or dry, toilet paper texture, noise of flushing) ■ Physiologic readiness ■ Strength, coordination, and endurance to manage clothing and fasteners ■ Balance to stand or sit on toilet ■ Emotional readiness: fears of flushing or disease, need for privacy, attitude toward toileting	■ Use habit training if no pattern is evident: go at the same times every day. ■ Have child dress in easy-to-manipulate clothing. ■ Use preparatory activities at other times to build strength and coordination for fasteners. ■ Support child's body (e.g., grab bars, foot support, ring reducer, or potty chair on floor). ■ Change toilet papers or use different material, such as wet wipes or cloth.
Contexts (cultural, social, physical, personal, temporal)	■ *Cultural:* Family and societal expectations of toileting; words used; whether child uses a public bathroom and sits on the toilet seat; institutional practices (e.g., co-toileting in preschool, language used) ■ *Social:* Acceptance of use of a diaper; how child indicates need to toilet (e.g., pee pee, gestures), others in bathroom, flushing, gender-specific public bathroom rules ■ *Physical:* Size, temperature, sounds; set up; way to flush, height of toilet, adaptations (toilet seat or potty chair; grab bars or safety frame around toilet); faucets and other fixtures ■ *Personal:* Chronologic age, grade in school, gender ■ *Temporal:* Previous experiences, fears of flushing or disease, need for privacy, attitude toward toileting	■ Spell out expectations in the beginning. ■ Dedicate a bathroom to toilet training, if possible. ■ Play soft music or toilet song on a tape player. ■ Public bathrooms: Boys need cueing for bathroom behavior and may need a social story: leave a space between yourself and someone else at a urinal; keep your pants up over your buttocks while urinating at a urinal; don't talk or look others in the eye while at the urinal; be quick and leave when you are finished; only you will touch your body while in the bathroom (unless catheterization training). ■ If child dawdles in bathroom, have him or her go with a peer buddy or go at a less busy time. ■ If child is fearful, have him or her open door for escape, then flush.

Continued

TABLE 15-8 Analysis and Interventions for Toileting—*cont'd*

Area	Analysis	Intervention Ideas
Performance skills (motor, process, communication/inter-action)	■ Posture, mobility coordination, strength, and effort needed ■ Temporality: initiate, sequence, and terminate ■ How child communicates need to go to bathroom (e.g., physically or by speaking)	■ Provide way to indicate a need to go: ○ Picture cues of entire sequence ○ Object cues or transitional object ■ Social story ■ Timer ■ Spoken cues ■ Physical, gestural cues
Performance patterns (habits, routines, roles)	■ Recognizes typical routines in the family for eating and drinking ■ Recognizes typical times and patterns when child urinates or defecates ■ Uses habit training to go at a certain time of the day, every day ■ Cleans up accidents by himself or herself without harsh reprimanding ■ Behavior challenge may be provoked by changes in routines.	■ Limit or increase liquids. ■ Use wet/dry chart to determine typical times for toileting. ■ Use visual schedule for toileting steps (including wiping) and times, as well as times for drinking fluids. ■ Use same routine and rituals for toileting (e.g., particular times or when waking, before trips, after meals). ■ Urge family, school, and day care all to follow the same routine and collect data.
Activity demands (objects, spatial, social, sequencing, timing)	■ Placement of potty chair or toilet seat; height of toilet, flushing mechanism, toilet paper dispenser ■ Space in bathroom, arrangement of items ■ Door shut or closed; whether child announces it's time to go ■ Steps to toileting, flushing after going potty; when to close door, get toilet paper or paper towel ■ Public bathroom social expectations	■ Change layout of objects or accessibility of environment. ■ Include "Shut door" as part of toileting sequence. ■ Discuss public bathroom expectations; have social story available to talk about them. ■ Public bathroom (boys): Use private stall first, then move to urinal.

Compiled from Wheeler, M. (1998). *Toilet training for individuals with autism and related disorders.* Arlington, TX: Future Horizons.

Toileting Adaptations. Numerous adaptations are available to assist the child in positioning and maintaining cleanliness after toileting. Urinals, catheters, leg bag clamps, long-handled mirrors, positioning devices to provide postural stability or to hold the legs open, and universal cuffs with a catheter or digital stimulator attached are some examples of assistive devices that therapists may provide. For children with good postural control but limited range of motion or grasp, simple, inexpensive aids include various types of toilet paper tongs and toilet paper holding devices.

A combined bidet and toilet offers a means of total independence. Several models are available that attach to a standard toilet bowl. A self-contained mechanism spray washes the perineal area with thermostatically controlled warm water and dries it with a flow of warm air. The child can operate controls with the hand or foot (Figure 15-7). Various special cushions designed to prevent tissue trauma are commercially available.

The type of clothing worn during toileting often hinders the child's independence or the caregiver's ability to promote independence. For children who wear diapers, a full-length crotch opening with a zipper or a hook-and-loop (e.g., Velcro) closure makes changes easier. When children are first learning toilet training, the use of elastic-waisted diapers that pull up gives them the

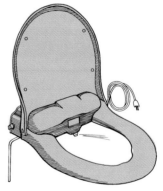

FIGURE 15-7 Electrically powered bidet makes it possible to clean the perineal area independently, without using hands or paper.

opportunity to practice this part of the toileting sequence yet also protects clothing from accidents. As children mature, they may be responsible for changing their own diapers or caring for their appliances and equipment. Girls may wear wraparound or full skirts because these are easy to put on and adjust for diaper changes or toileting. The child can reach and drain leg bags with greater ease when his or her pants have zippers or hook-and-loop closures along the seams. Flies with long zippers or hook-and-loop closures make it easier for boys to urinate or catheterize themselves when in wheelchairs.

Adaptations for Unstable Posture. When children sit on the toilet, they need to feel posturally secure. When toilet seats are low enough that the feet rest firmly on the floor, the abdominal muscles that normally aid in defecation can effectively fulfill their function.

Small children often need reducer rings to decrease the size of the toilet seat opening and thus improve sitting support. A step in front of the toilet helps small children get onto it. Safety rails that attach to the toilet or wall may assist with balance and allow the child to freely use his or her hands. The child who has outgrown small training potties can use freestanding commodes, which may be useful when wheelchair access to the bathroom is impossible. Units that roll into place over the toilet may be an option.

Families can purchase commodes that feature such modifications as adjustable legs, safety bars, angled legs for stability, and padded, upholstered, and adjustable backrests and headrests. Commodes are also available with seat reducer rings, seat belts, and adjustable footrests.

Dressing

Typical Development

Independence in dressing usually takes 4 years of practice. Characteristically, learning to undress comes before learning to dress. Caregivers introduce self-dressing in a natural way, at bedtime, by allowing the child to complete the final step in pulling off a garment. Similarly, when the child becomes more goal directed and motivated to be independent, he or she is ready to try the more difficult tasks of learning to put on clothing. Often the caregiver uses backward chaining by putting the garment on the child and allowing the child to complete the action. Gradually the child performs more of the task and the caregiver performs less. Table 15-9 presents the typical development of dressing.

Dressing requires children to use a variety of performance skills and patterns to meet the unique demands of the activity. They need to know where their bodies are in space and how body parts relate while they use visual and the kinesthetic systems to guide arm and leg movements. The visual and somatosensory systems enable the child to understand form and space and how clothing conforms to and fits on the body. Dynamic postural stability is important as the child reaches, bends, and shifts his or her center of gravity while getting dressed. If the child avoids crossing the midline and performs dressing tasks on the right side of the body with the right hand and those on the left with the left hand, he or she most likely will have difficulty with tasks that require both hands to work together, such as fastening clothing and tying shoelaces. How the child coordinates the two sides of the body, manipulates the clothing, grips fasteners,

Age (yr)	Self-Dressing Skills
	TABLE 15-9 Typical Developmental Sequence for Dressing
1	■ Cooperates with dressing (holds out arms and feet) ■ Pulls off shoes, removes socks ■ Pushes arms through sleeves and legs through pants
2	■ Removes unfastened coat ■ Removes shoes if laces are untied ■ Helps pull down pants ■ Finds armholes in pullover shirt
$2\frac{1}{2}$	■ Removes pull-down pants with elastic waist ■ Assists in pulling on socks ■ Puts on front-button coat or shirt ■ Unbuttons large buttons
3	■ Puts on pullover shirt with minimal assistance ■ Puts on shoes without fasteners (may be on wrong foot) ■ Puts on socks (may be with heel on top) ■ Independently pulls down pants ■ Zips and unzips jacket once on track ■ Needs assistance to remove pullover shirt ■ Buttons large front buttons
$3\frac{1}{2}$	■ Finds front of clothing ■ Snaps or hooks front fastener ■ Unzips zipper on jacket, separating zipper ■ Puts on mittens ■ Buttons series of three or four buttons ■ Unbuckles shoe or belt ■ Dresses with supervision (needs help with front and back)
4	■ Removes pullover garment independently ■ Buckles shoes or belt ■ Zips jacket zipper ■ Puts on socks correctly ■ Puts on shoes, needs assistance in tying laces ■ Laces shoes ■ Consistently identifies the front and back of garments
$4\frac{1}{2}$	■ Puts belt in loops
5	■ Ties and unties knots ■ Dresses unsupervised
6	■ Closes back zipper ■ Ties bows ■ Buttons back buttons ■ Snaps back snaps

Modified from Klein, M.D. (1983). *Pre-dressing skills.* Tucson, AZ: Communication Skill Builders.

and calibrates the amount of strength and effort determines how the activity is completed. Process skills such as choosing the appropriate clothing, temporally organizing the task, and adapting to contextual changes (e.g., new materials, noise in the environment, placement of clothing) also affect dressing outcomes.

Typical Problems and Intervention Strategies

Limitations in Cognition and Process Skills

Children who have underlying cognitive and perceptual deficits may also have problems in process performance skills. They may demonstrate problems with choosing, using, and handling clothing. This may include difficulty distinguishing right and left sides of the body, putting a shoe on the correct foot, turning the heel of a sock, or differentiating the front of clothing from the back or identifying the correct leg or sleeve. Applying concepts such as above, in front of, or behind may be difficult for these children. Temporal organization, especially initiating, continuing, sequencing, terminating, and organizing the dressing task, often is problematic for children with mental retardation or autism. The pacing may be too slow or too fast, and they may be unable to remember instructions or to use environmental cues to find their clothing or to notice or benefit from their mistakes. Instead, they may perseverate on using the same unsuccessful action to put on the clothing or to use fasteners. The therapist uses an establish or adaptive approach by modifying the demands of dressing in various environments.

Behaviorally the child may become frustrated with the complexity of certain dressing tasks. Language may be delayed, which restricts the child's verbal capacity to express frustration. This may increase when the child is faced with tasks that require fine manipulations if coordination is limited or if the child has sensory modulation problems. Often a behavioral approach is effective for acquiring independence. After making a baseline assessment, the therapist carefully analyzes the demands of each dressing task. Once the therapist determines the limitations and strengths in performance skills and

patterns, he or she uses partial participation and backward and forward chaining methods. Environmental and task adaptations include visual charts or pictures, social stories, checklists, and selection of clothing that is easy to manipulate (e.g., slightly larger clothing, stretchy materials, pullover shirts, and loafers). Simultaneous prompting in the dressing activity itself helps children learn the task (Sewell, Collins, Hemmeter, & Schuster, 1998). Figure 15-8 presents an example of a social story for a child who has sensory issues and who dislikes changes in routines or dressing for outside play. By giving repetitive positive statements, the child is more ready to follow the routine in the story and initiates the task.

Physical or Motor Limitations. Children with various conditions find dressing difficult because of the coordination and the range and strength required for pulling clothes on and off and connecting fasteners. Children with arthritis who have pain with finger movement frequently require assistance during a flare-up of their disease. They may be unable to move their arms freely or to reach certain areas of the body. Children with the use of only one hand find it difficult to zip trousers, tie shoelaces, and button shirts or blouses. The therapist may focus on improving the child's strength or coordination. In most cases the child learns adaptation techniques, often through his or her own experimentation or use of assistive technology. Children with cerebral palsy often have difficulty balancing and controlling arm and leg movement when donning and removing clothing. Limited dexterity may also interfere with dressing.

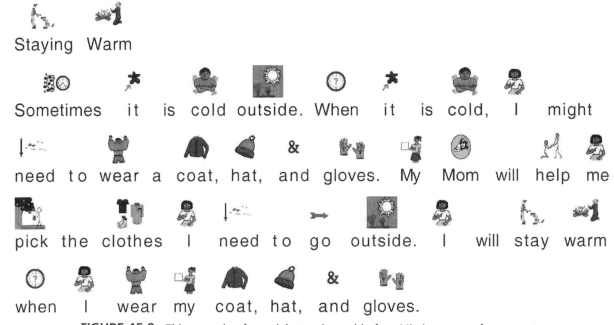

FIGURE 15-8 This example of a social story is used before Mimi goes out for recess to help her rehearse what she is going to do and to help her understand why. (Courtesy Rebecca E. Argabrite Grove, Loudoun County Public Schools, Virginia; story created with Pix Writer by Slater Software, Guffey, CO)

Therapists suggest methods to modify the demands of the activity; such as supportive positioning or the use of adaptive aids such as buttonhooks, rings on zippers, one-handed shoe fasteners, or hook-and-loop closures. Because clothing manufacturers recognize the value of universal design, many of these adaptations are available commercially (Schwarz, 2000).

Adaptive Methods for Dressing Children with Motor Limitations. Although it is common to dress an infant while he or she is lying in the supine position, this position frequently increases extensor tone in infants with neurologic impairment. For this reason some therapists advocate placing the infant prone across the knees with the infant's hips flexed and abducted, thereby inhibiting leg extensor and adduction tone. When the infant gains head and trunk control, the caregiver can dress him or her in a sitting position with the child's back resting against and supported by the caregiver's trunk. In this position the infant has an opportunity to observe his or her own body during dressing.

When dressing an infant with increased extensor tone, the caregiver carefully bends the infant's hips and knees before putting on shoes and socks (Figure 15-9) and brings the infant's shoulders forward before putting his or her arm through a sleeve. By flexing the child's hip and knee, postural tone is decreased and dressing becomes easier. When a child achieves sitting balance, a good way to proceed with dressing is to place the child on the floor and later on a low stool, continuing to provide support where needed from the back. Orientation to the child's body parts should remain a focus in the social interaction. The caregiver helps the child understand how his or her body relates to his or her clothes and to the various positions (e.g., "The arm goes through the sleeve" and "the head goes through the hole at the top of the shirt").

When the child is older and heavier, there may be no alternative but to dress the child while he or she is in the side-lying or supine position. Placing a hard pillow under the child's head, thus slightly raising his or her shoulders, makes it easier for the caregiver to bring the child's arms forward and to bend his or her hips and knees. If it is possible to maintain the child in a side-lying position, this posture may make it easier for the caregiver to manage the child's arms and legs and for the child to assist in the dressing task (Figure 15-10).

Adaptive Methods for Self-Dressing. The child who has hand coordination but poor balance may be able to take advantage of the function that he or she possesses when in a side-lying position with the effect of gravity lessened. For the child who can sit but is unstable, a corner of two adjoining walls or a corner seat on the floor may provide enough postural support for independent dressing. Sitting balance is more precarious as one reaches when donning overhead garments or pants and shoes, therefore the child needs additional external support. Sitting in chairs with arms or sitting on the floor against a wall may improve performance.

The occupational therapist helps improve the child's dressing by offering the parent and child various problem-solving strategies, from which the child and parents may choose. Table 15-10 offers choices in problem solving that can be used in putting on and taking off different garments. Clothing selections, assistive technology, and adaptations to the task are methods for improving a child's performance in self-dressing.

Increased attention to the needs of individuals with disabilities has been shown over the past decade, with some adaptive clothing becoming available through catalog supply companies. These companies generally offer attractive, fashionable clothing that meets functional requirements yet conforms in appearance to the child's peer group standards and fashion trends. Modifications should be inconspicuous, and the appearance of the clothing should not single out the wearer. When

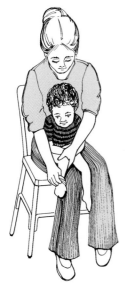

FIGURE 15-9 When dressing a child who is hypertonic, the caregiver should carefully flex the hip and knee before putting on socks and shoes.

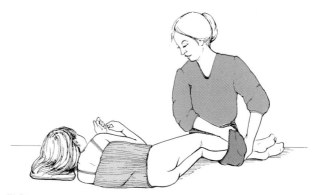

FIGURE 15-10 The side-lying position may reduce stiffness and make dressing easier.

TABLE 15-10 Adaptation Strategies for Dressing with Different Types of Garments

Garment	Design Features of Clothing or Assistive Technology Adaptations for Easier Dressing	Adaptations to Task Method
Pull-up garments	■ Large size ■ Stretchy material ■ Loops sewn into waistband ■ Elastic waistbands, but not too tight ■ Pressure-sensitive tape ■ Zipper pulls ■ Dressing sticks	■ Sit on chair ■ Lie on floor ■ Lie on side and roll side to side to pull up pants ■ Use chair or grab-bar to stabilize oneself while pulling up pants ■ Put weak or affected leg in first
Pullover garments	■ Large, easy opening for head ■ Flexible rib knit fabric ■ Large armholes and sleeve openings; raglan sleeves ■ Elastic cuffs and waistbands	■ Lay garment on lap, floor, or table, front side down; put arms in and flip over head ■ Pull garment over head, then put in arms ■ Put weak or affected leg in first
Front-opening garments	■ Loose style ■ Fullness in back of garment ■ On shirt or jacket, collar of different color than main garment ■ Short-sleeve garments first, proceeding to long-sleeve garments ■ Raglan sleeves ■ Garment with no closures or one or two buttons (e.g., sweater, jacket)	■ Lay garment on lap, floor, or table, with neck of garment toward child; put in arms, duck head, extend arms, and flip garment over head; shrug shoulders and use arms to help garment fall into place ■ Put weak or affected arm in first, pull up to shoulder; follow collar, then put in other arm
Buttons	■ Flat, large buttons ■ Buttons contrast in color with garment ■ Buttons with shanks (easier to grasp) ■ Buttons sewn on loosely ■ Buttons sewn on one side; hook-and-loop tape on both sides to close shirt or pants ■ Front buttons first, proceeding to side and back buttons	■ Use pullover styles instead of buttons ■ Button all but the first two or three buttons and put shirt on like a pullover ■ Begin buttoning with bottom button (easier to see and align) ■ Use a buttonhook ■ Use elastic thread to sew on sleeve buttons; put on sleeve without buttoning ■ Use backward chaining
Zippers	■ Nylon zippers (easier than metal) ■ Zipper tabs or rings ■ Zipper pulls ■ Hook-and-loop tape instead of zipper while pulling up zipper tab with other hand ■ Longer zippers (more space for donning and doffing clothes) ■ Front zippers first, proceeding to side and back zippers	■ Sit to gain stability ■ Stand to keep jacket zipper flat ■ Hold zipper taut with one hand at bottom of zipper ■ For side zipper, lean against wall to hold bottom of zipper
Socks	■ Soft, stretchy socks ■ Large size ■ Tube sock (no set place for heel) ■ Ankle socks first, proceeding to calf or over-the-calf socks ■ Loops sewn into socks ■ Sock aide or donner	■ Sit on stable surface (e.g., chair, floor) ■ Lie on back and prop foot on opposite knee ■ Fold or roll sock before putting it over the toes and pulling it up ■ Use backward chaining
Shoes	■ Long-opening shoes (many eyes) with loose laces ■ Broad shoe (not tight) ■ Slip-on shoes ■ Hook-and-loop tab closures ■ Elastic laces already tied ■ Elastic curly laces that do not need tying ■ Tabs at heels for pulling shoes on ■ Long-handled shoehorns	■ Sit on stable surface (e.g., chair, floor) ■ Prop up foot on stool or chair ■ Lie on back and prop foot on opposite knee ■ Flex legs and point toes downward ■ Use gravity to help push heel into shoe (e.g., child pushes down on a hard surface)

possible, clothing should conceal physical disabilities or at least should not attract attention to them. Clothing contributes to the wearer's sense of well-being. Functionally, the design of the clothing should enable the wearer to take care of personal needs, help maintain proper body temperature, and provide freedom of movement.

Most clothing is made for individuals in a standing position. For those who spend long hours in a wheelchair, the sitting position can cause pulling and straining on some areas of the garment and a surplus of fabric in others. The caregiver can make alterations to provide more comfort in sitting (e.g., pants that are cut higher in the back and lower in the front and cut larger to give additional room in the hips and thighs) (Kennedy, 1981; Kernaleguen, 1978; Schwarz, 2000). A longer inseam also allows the proper hem height for pants when sitting (rests on top of shoe). Pockets in the back may cause shearing or skin breakdown with prolonged sitting. Instead, pockets can be placed on the top of the thigh or on the side of the calf for easy access. Front and side seams can be sewn with hook-and-loop fasteners or zippers and wrist loops to assist in donning. Pullover tops with raglan and gusset sleeves allow more room when maneuvering a wheelchair. If the shirt is cut longer in the back and shorter in the front, it is easier to keep a neat appearance. Rain or winter capes are comfortable in a wheelchair. They are cut longer in the front to cover the child's legs and feet and shorter in the back so that they do not rub against the wheel of the chair (Schwarz).

For children who wear orthoses for spinal support, front openings that extend from the neck to the lower abdomen make self-dressing easier, whereas back openings are easier when others dress the child (Lawrence & Niemeyer, 1994; Schwarz, 2000). Caregivers should use larger clothing that fits over orthoses but should avoid loose sleeves for children who push wheelchairs because the sleeve may get caught in the spokes of the wheel. The child who wears an ankle-foot orthosis may need to have clothing reinforced to protect against rubbing. This can be done by sewing fabric patches inside the garment where friction and stress occur and by adapting the pants with side seams and hook-and-loop closures so that the pants go over the orthosis more easily.

When children require gastrostomy feedings, tracheostomy care, catheterization, or diapering, they need clothing that allows easy access. Caregivers can sew moisture-resistant fabric into the seat of pants, on collars, on attaching bibs, and on sleeve cuffs (if the child bites clothing) (Sweeney, 1989). Jumpsuits or shirts with hook-and-loop closures at the gastrostomy site, neckline, or shoulder, crotch, or pant leg allow caregivers to perform medical procedures without removing the child's clothing (Lawrence & Niemeyer, 1994; Schwarz, 2000; Sweeney).

Bathing or Showering
Typical Development

A child's interest in bathing begins before 2 years of age when he or she begins to wash while in the tub. By 4 years of age, children wash and dry themselves with supervision. It is not until children are 8 years of age that they can independently prepare the bath and shower water (e.g., the appropriate depth and temperature) and independently wash and dry themselves.

Good grooming habits are important for all children but take on added significance for children with disabilities. At an early age the caregiver needs to encourage and help the child with a disability to achieve cleanliness to maintain his or her health. Bathing should be a pleasurable activity, but for the parent of a child who lacks postural stability, it can be a tedious task that requires constant attention and alertness. The work involved multiplies as the child grows and becomes larger and heavier.

Cultural expectations and social routines for bathing vary, and the therapist should consider them when assessing a child's independence. The therapist must respect family preferences on how often a person bathes and with whom (e.g., parent and children bathing together).

Restore Approach

Therapists often use bathing therapeutically to restore body capacities that interfere with independence. A warm bath may calm a child who is distressed and may decrease tonicity and increase range of motion and independent movement (Case-Smith, 2000). When a child has hypersensitivity, rubbing with a washcloth, water play, and deep pressure or rubbing while drying the child may help reduce the child's sensitivity to touch. For children who have difficulty interacting with others or the environment, bath play may motivate the child to explore objects, engage in pretend play, and interact with a sibling or parent (Case-Smith).

For children with motor limitations, the therapist may use a restore approach to prepare the child for self-bathing. The therapist may use activities to improve range of motion, bilateral coordination, grasp, postural control, and motor planning before teaching bathing. Activities or games (e.g., Simon Says) that require a child to reach above or behind or down to the toes may give children the body awareness and necessary movement for self-bathing.

Adaptation Approach

The caregiver's positioning and handling are prime considerations in adapting bathing of children. Children with cerebral palsy may lose their balance when startled. Keeping the child's head and arms forward when lifting and lowering him or her into the tub can prevent a reaction of full extension. The caregiver should use slow, gentle movements with the child and provide simple verbal cues about the steps of bathing. Draining the tub and wrapping the child in a towel before lifting him or her from the tub can make the child feel more secure.

Parents often need suggestions for bathing a child who is hypersensitive to touch. This child may be avoiding bathing at all costs and is at risk of getting hurt while in the tub. Understanding the child's sensory needs and using adaptive techniques may help bathing become a positive experience for both parent and child. Preparatory activities that give the child deep pressure prior to bathing are sometimes helpful, especially deep pressure to the head prior to shampooing. The child may prefer washing the back and extremities first, and then the stomach and face, using rhythmic, organized, deep strokes. Some parents and children find a hand-held shower with an eye guard hat useful for removing soapsuds (especially during hair washing) and avoiding getting soap in the eyes. Adjusting the water flow of the hand-held shower and allowing the child to use it himself or herself gives the child more control over the direction of the water pressure on his or her body while holding it. Sometimes, with children who have tactile sensitivity, using a cup with water is a more relaxing way to rinse off than a shower spray. Wrapping the child in a tight towel after bathing and holding the child with deep pressure also can help.

Adaptive positioning or special equipment that gives support can help the child feel safe and secure. Bath hammocks fully hold the body and enable the parent to wash the child thoroughly (Figure 15-11, *A*). Commercially, a light, inconspicuous bath support offers good design features (Figure 15-11, *B*). The front half of the support ring swings open for easy entry and then locks securely, holding the child at the chest to give trunk stability. Various kinds of bath seats and shower benches (Figure 15-11, *C*) are available for the older child to aid bathtub seating and transfers. For the child with severe motor limitations who is lying supine in the tub in shallow water, a horseshoe-shaped inflatable bath collar (Figure 15-11, *D*) can support the neck and keep the child's head above water. A bath stretcher is constructed like a cot and fits inside the bathtub at rim or mid-tub level to minimize the caregiver's bending while transferring and bathing the child.

Prevention/Education for Bathing Safety

Parent and child education about bathing safety helps prevent injury. Constant monitoring until the child demonstrates safety in the tub is necessary. Sometimes parents do not teach independence in bathing because they worry that the child may injure himself or herself if they are not there. Following a safe routine for bathing,

teaching the child what he or she is and is not allowed to do in the tub or shower, and grading the amount of assistance and monitoring helps develop independence. Nonslip bath mats beside the tub and in the tub are essential for safety. Grab bars and their placement require careful thought and planning in each individual case. A rubber cover for the bathtub faucet can prevent injury if the child touches it or slips and hits his or her head. Faucets need to be marked for temperature, and children may begin running their own bathwater by first putting on the cold water, then slowly adding hot water.

Parents are taught to use good body mechanics during bathing to prevent back injury. To lessen strain, it is best for the adult to sit on a stool beside the tub or to kneel on a cushion. Lifting is done with the knees bent and the back straight, with the legs used for power. As children get older and heavier, a Hoyer lift or easily accessed shower stall arrangement may be necessary.

Personal Hygiene and Grooming
Skill Development

By 2 years of age, children imitate their parents when brushing their teeth. Supervision of tooth brushing continues until about 6 years of age. Tooth brushing is especially difficult for the child with oral sensitivity. The child should use his or her preferred brushing methods until tolerance improves and he or she can accomplish more thorough cleaning. A small, soft brush is easier to move around in the mouth, especially if the child has a tongue thrust or gag reflex. When the child's gums are tender, the caregiver may substitute a soft, sponge-tipped toothette for a brush. For the child who brushes independently, an electric toothbrush or oral irrigation device (e.g., Water-Pik) allows more thorough cleaning. This is a good solution for children with limited dexterity, although for children with weakness, an electric toothbrush may be too heavy to manage.

If a child has problems with a weak grasp, the caregiver may enlarge the toothbrush handle with sponge rubber or may add a hook-and-loop strap. One-handed flossing tools are available in large and small sizes and can be adapted by enlarging the size and length of the handle. A hand-over-hand technique helps a child learn how to direct the toothbrush in the mouth and to reach all teeth (Figure 15-12). As the child starts doing the movement, gestures or only verbal prompts may be needed. As always, a routine sequence for tooth brushing, gradual fading of cues, and visual pictures about the process assist the child with underlying memory or performance skill problems.

Face washing, hand washing, and hair care are typical grooming activities taught to preschoolers and young children. The child's culture, family values, and individual interests strongly influence the timing of the development of grooming independence. Adolescence begins

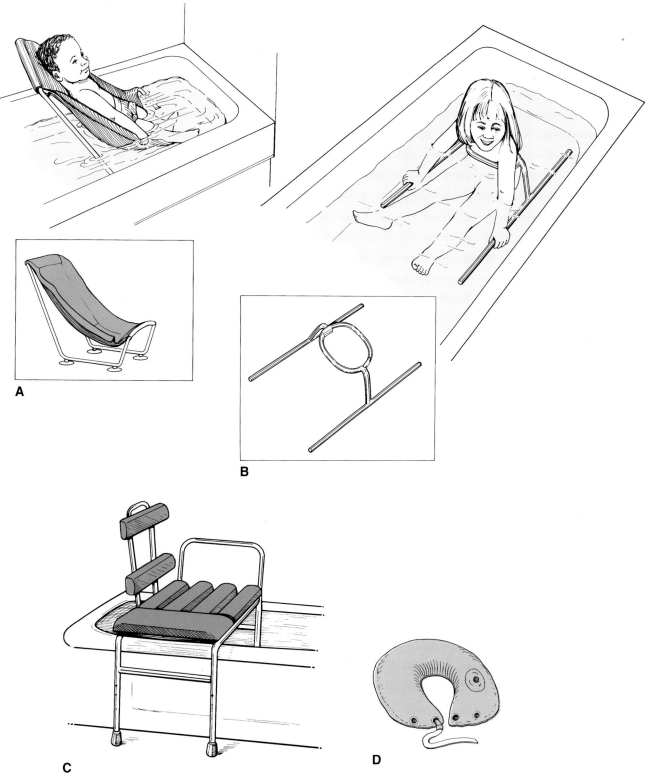

FIGURE 15-11 Adapted seating equipment for bathing. **A,** The hammock chair is adjustable and equipped with oversized suction feet. It fully supports the child who has no sitting balance and poor head control. **B,** Trunk support ring is lightweight and compact and fits all bathtubs. **C,** A shower bench aids seating and transfers. **D,** An inflatable bath collar can be used when the child is in either the supine or prone position.

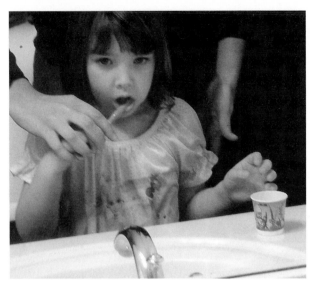

FIGURE 15-12 A hand-over-hand approach works well for Lydia, who is sensitive to tooth brushing, as she is participating in the activity and directing which part of the teeth she wants to brush first.

at the onset of puberty and is a period of remarkable growth toward physical, sexual, emotional, and social maturity. The physiologic changes that occur at puberty are partly attributable to the increased output of hormones by the pituitary gland. For example, body hair grows, and the sebaceous glands become more active, producing oily secretions. With these physical changes and different social expectations (depending on the culture), new self-maintenance tasks emerge, including skin care, hair styling, hair removal, and the application of cosmetics.

Intervention

Grooming is an aspect of ADLs that is highly influenced by cultural values. The therapist must respect the child's and family's preferences in hair style, cosmetics, and routines. The family and child or adolescent need to take the lead in identifying their concerns and priorities in this area. Problem solving follows the principles and approaches identified in the first sections of this chapter. The following is an example of an adolescent who desires independence in grooming.

Josie demonstrates incoordination, poor memory, and limited judgment, but she wants to be independent in her grooming. Restorative activities are somewhat helpful, but adaptation strategies are more essential to increasing her independence in grooming. The occupational therapist recommends that Josie use a brush with a built-up handle, rest her elbow on the table while brushing her hair to stabilize her ataxic movements, use a checklist and visual model, and ask a peer to help style her hair. Josie and her parents are educated about ways

to incorporate grooming tasks into everyday routines by placing visual and natural cues in the environment; for example, the deodorant can be kept on the dresser, and facial cleansing equipment can be left out on the sink as a visual cue to Josie to use it before applying makeup.

Sexual Activity

While the therapist is working with children on personal ADL tasks such as bathing or hygiene, sexuality questions may arise. Children and adolescents of all disabilities are sexual beings, and sexual activities need to be discussed to prevent social exploitation, abuse, sexually transmitted diseases, and pregnancy. Children with developmental disabilities are more prone to the risk of exploitation because often (1) they must depend on others for basic needs; (2) they frequently have multiple caregivers; (3) their connection with authority figures is one of learned helplessness or nondiscriminatory compliance; and (4) they have difficulty with social, reasoning, judgment, and problem-solving skills (O'Neill, 2002; Sullivan & Knutson, 2000). For therapists working with children on very personal daily living activities, it is important to help children differentiate between necessary touch (e.g., diaper changing, catheter instruction, menstrual care, hygiene) and intimate touch. Hinsburger (1993) suggested that therapists and parents always do the following:

- Ask permission before touching
- Describe what they are doing and why
- Facilitate participation when performing necessary touch activities
- Communicate with the child about what was done and why and about any feelings following intimate touch

Parents may be receptive to discussing their child's *sexuality,* or they may feel unprepared to address these issues. If parents and professionals begin talking about sexuality education in early childhood (e.g., body, gender, touching, privacy, expressing affection, and boundaries), the need to approach complex subjects such as refusal behavior, dating, birth control, and sexuality rights will not be as difficult a transition. Melberg-Schwier and Hingsburger (2000) have written an excellent book to guide parents as they embark on this topic. If the child is under 18 years of age, therapists must obtain parental permission to discuss sexuality issues. Therapists need to consider the contextual aspects of the child's family and social groups and determine whether it is appropriate to discuss sexuality and who should discuss it (receiver and informant). Therapists who decide to enter a discourse on sexuality must consider their own knowledge, beliefs, and attitudes so that they can give children and their families the correct information in a nonjudgmental way. Occupational therapists may refer the child to someone who is more knowledgeable about sexuality and more comfortable discussing it. Responsible therapists are careful to separate their personal values with regard to sexuality from those of the client and family.

Children and adolescents with cognitive problems related to mental retardation or a traumatic brain injury often need guidelines for expressing their sexuality appropriately in various contexts (Couwenhoven, 2001). Appropriate touch from others, dress and hygiene, masturbation, touching of others, and appropriate interactions with the opposite gender are areas in which education is required to prevent abuse and prosecution from the courts for sexual misconduct.

Older adolescents with chronic health conditions need specific answers and ideas for expressing sexuality in a healthy way (Shapland, 1999). An adolescent may question the physical and psychosocial aspects of sexuality and his or her ability to conceive. Information about contraceptive use and techniques for avoiding intercourse are essential for the adolescent to avoid unwanted pregnancies. As adolescents with disabilities consider conceiving and bearing children in the future, it may be helpful to talk to other parents with disabilities or become aware of online support groups and resources. Table 15-11 presents more of the information children need about sexual activity across the age span.

TABLE 15-11 Typical Sexuality Concepts Discussed with Children and Adolescents with Disabilities

Age (yr)	Typical Behaviors or Concepts to Learn
Birth-2	■ Touches genitals for sensory pleasure ■ Experiences affection and touch
3-5	■ Shows interest in genitals of the opposite sex ■ Learns proper names of genitals (social demands) ■ Plays "Show me" games with other children ■ Understands that others should not touch his or her genitals ■ Learns that some behaviors are acceptable in public, others are to be done in private (e.g., masturbation, undressing) ■ Begins to learn privacy rights (e.g., close doors, knock and wait to enter, close blinds) ■ Begins to learn rules for touch and affection boundaries and authority figures
6-8	■ Knows differences between boys and girls ■ Names body parts correctly ■ Learns basic elements and language of reproduction and pregnancy ■ Learns about relationships (e.g., friends, mutual respect) and decision making ■ Thinks about social responsibility ■ Understands appropriate and inappropriate social and sexual behaviors ■ Understands necessary (e.g., personal hygiene) and intimate touch ■ Avoids and reports sexual exploitation (understands necessary touch and intimate touch)
9-11	■ Shows interest in social relationships ■ Discusses body image ■ Discusses sexuality within family ■ Understands personal boundaries ■ Knows how to use refusal skills ■ Understands body changes that will occur during puberty (and, if able, the impact on his or her disease or disability) ■ Knows about reproduction and pregnancy ■ Learns about sexually transmitted diseases and the need to abstain from sexual intercourse ■ Avoids or reports sexual abuse (understands necessary touch and intimate touch)
12-18	■ Is sensitive and private about body ■ Compares body to others and may be critical ■ Asks questions about changes occurring (physical and emotional) ■ Shows more interest in caring for body (e.g., hair, face, exercise) ■ Discusses sexuality and sexual identity with friends ■ Uses preventive health care routinely (e.g., breast, gynecologic and testicular examinations) ■ Begins dating and learning about communication and love ■ Uses values to guide actions in intimacy ■ Expresses sexuality through dress, actions, or intercourse ■ Understands reproduction, pregnancy, and birth control ■ Knows how to use contraceptives and prevent diseases (safe sex) ■ Asks for or is given genetic counseling ■ Identifies and uses community sexual health services

Compiled from Couwenhoven, T. (2001). Sexuality education: Building a foundation of healthy attitudes. *Disability Solutions, 4,* (6), 1-8. http://www.disabilitysolutions.org/4-6.htm; Lawrence, K.E., & Niemeyer, S. (1994). Behavior management and psychosocial issues: Sexuality issues. In K.E. Lawrence & S. Niemeyer (Eds.), *Caregiver education guide for children with developmental disabilities: Aspen Reference Group* (pp. 236-245). Frederick, MD: Aspen; and National Information Center for Children and Youth with Disabilities (NICHCY). (1992). Sexuality education for children and youth with disabilities. *NICHCY News Digest, 1* (3), 1-6.

Annon (1976) developed the PLISSIT model to teach people with disabilities about sexuality. This model is based on four phases of information giving: (1) permission to ask about sexuality, (2) limited information given, (3) specific suggestions, and (4) intensive therapy (usually provided by a trained counselor or psychologist who understands sexuality in individuals with disabilities). This model teaches staff about sexuality issues and informs clients about who is willing to discuss sexuality with them. In some settings, staff wear a button saying, "I'm askable" to designate their comfort in talking about sexuality (Dawe & Shepherd, 1985). While practicing bed mobility, dressing, personal hygiene, positioning, and communication/interaction skills, the adolescent often asks sexuality questions. Depending on the situation and the therapy setting, therapists address these questions in the context in which the questions are asked. For example, while practicing bed mobility, 17-year-old Belinda, who recently suffered a spinal cord injury, asks, "How can I ever have sex with a guy? Can I have a baby?" With prior parental permission, this may be an opportune time to discuss contraceptives, positioning, use of intact senses, control of distracting environmental stimuli, and the medical need to empty her bladder before sexual activity (Friedman, 1997). Referral to her physician or to a gynecologist who is knowledgeable about women with disabilities is appropriate, as is referral to her psychologist or counselor. If the parents approve, therapists can give additional information in a written, oral, or video format and can provide the adolescent with the opportunity to talk to older adolescents or adults who have similar disabilities. Sexuality education needs a team approach, and therapists may work with physicians, nurses, or pharmacists to discuss the use of certain medicines and how they affect sexual function (Dunn, 1997). Memory aids for medicine schedules or contraceptive use may also be helpful (Friedman, 1997). If the therapist is uncomfortable talking about sexual activity, the client should be told this and referred to someone who has the comfort level and knowledge to answer questions.

INSTRUMENTAL ACTIVITIES OF DAILY LIVING

Health Maintenance

As children with disabilities mature, taking responsibility for their health maintenance becomes realistic. By adolescence, families and therapists encourage young people to be responsible for caring for personal devices (e.g., hearing aids, wheelchairs, or splints), taking medications, and general health maintenance. Initially, children or adolescents can partially participate in any of these tasks or can direct others in how to perform the task. As

children make decisions about their health routines, they learn first hand what happens if they do not follow bowel and bladder programs or develop routines for physical fitness or proper nutrition (Betz, 1998). Activities that promote the development of problem-solving skills and help children gain confidence in their abilities to be self-sufficient are critical to the child's development of ADL independence. Children and adolescents with chronic health care needs have numerous medical tasks to learn besides general health care maintenance. Age-specific tasks must be accomplished to aid the transition to the adult health care (Bloomquist, Brown, Peersen, & Presler, 1998; Luther, 2001; Peterson, Rauen, Brown, & Cole, 1994). Table 15-12 presents examples of health maintenance issues for children with chronic medical needs, and Box 15-2 lists many of the online sources available on this topic.

Use of a Communication Device

As children mature and begin to take more responsibility for their own health maintenance and sexuality, their need to communicate independently with others increases. Children learn how to send and receive messages to and from other people through verbal, nonverbal, and graphic communication systems. Children who are nonverbal may use gestures, writing, or assistive devices to communicate their needs. This section discusses emergency systems and telephones as forms of communication.

Emergency Alert and Call Systems

Children with serious medical problems or with life-support systems need more frequent monitoring day and night. This need is more critical for children who have impaired mobility, dexterity, or communication abilities. Intercom systems assist parents with this responsibility and give the child a way to initiate calls for help or social interaction. Call switches or buzzers that attach to the bed or wheelchair can provide an independent means of seeking assistance from individuals in other rooms. Various portable intercoms and inexpensive electronic aids for daily living (EADLs) are available at electronics supply stores and children's stores. Caregivers may position a wireless or cellular telephone near the child. The child can use this device as a telephone or as an intercom, depending on the model chosen.

Emergency alert systems, worn as pendants or stabilized on wheelchairs, are available for purchase with a service that places emergency calls when the system is activated. The child can use outside alarms that can be heard in the neighborhood to summon assistance. Caregivers must carefully plan arrangements and alternatives in advance. The ability to exit the house quickly is most

TABLE 15-12 Health Care Maintenance for Typically Developing Children and Children with Spina Bifida

Age (yr)	Additional Health Typical Development of Health Maintenance*	Maintenance Issues for Child with Spina Bifida
5-9	■ Follows safety rules at home and school ■ Informs others of emergencies ■ Uses basic first aid techniques for minor injuries ■ Tells other when he or she is sick ■ Cares for health care items with reminders (e.g., glasses and toothbrush) ■ Routinely washes hands, takes a bath, and washes hair with reminders ■ Assists in getting medicine ready	■ Does pressure reliefs and checks for skin breakdown (e.g., legs, buttocks, and feet) with reminders ■ Tells others when he or she is injured or feels sick (e.g., headache, pain, swelling, or change in bowel and bladder patterns) ■ Cares for personal adaptive devices (e.g., crutches, wheelchair, or catheters) with reminders ■ Catheterizes himself or herself at home and school ■ Carries a list of current medicines and doctors' names
10-14	■ Recognizes when he or she is getting sick or needs to see a doctor ■ Knows emergency procedures (e.g., phone numbers, who to call, what to do) ■ Cares for health care items (e.g., glasses, braces, retainers, facial scrubs) ■ Uses first aid procedures ■ Eats nutritious meals with supervision ■ Exercises with supervision ■ Takes medicine with supervision ■ Avoids cigarettes, drugs, and sexual abuse	■ Recognizes when he or she is injured or feels sick (e.g., headache, pain, swelling, or change in bowel and bladder pattern) ■ Knows dosage of medications ■ Knows names of doctors (e.g., primary care, urologist, neurologist, or orthopedist) ■ Cares for personal adaptive devices (e.g., wheelchair, walker, braces) or instructs others in how to maintain devices ■ Catheterizes himself or herself in community environments ■ Prevents further health care problems (e.g., drinks to avoid bladder infection, exercises [push-ups]; avoids latex; maintains good hygiene, eating, and exercise practices)
15-18	■ Recognizes when a change in medicine or health intervention is needed ■ Makes appointment to see doctors ■ Eats nutritious meals ■ Exercises regularly ■ Cares for personal hygiene and follows good health habits ■ Uses first aid procedures for major and minor injuries ■ Takes medicine when needed ■ Uses birth control as needed	■ Takes medications independently and knows side effects ■ Knows how to access therapy, doctors, and other health care services ■ Knows how to obtain and pay for medical supplies ■ Prevents secondary disabilities (e.g., manages weight, follows routine medical care, skin care, and equipment maintenance)

Modified from Ford, A., Schnorr, R., Meyer, L., Davern, L., Black, J., & Dempsey, P. (1989). *The Syracuse community-reference curriculum guide* (pp. 324-327). Baltimore: Brookes; and Peterson, P.M., Rauen, K.K., Brown, J., & Cole, J. (1994). Spina bifida: The transition into adulthood begins in infancy. *Rehabilitation Nursing, 19* (4), 229-238.
*Medicines, personal devices, health routines, and other such skills.

directly influenced by the child's ability to get to the door and open it, therefore the therapist may still practice these activities in intervention sessions.

Telephones

Universal designs in commercially available telephones have improved access for all individuals with disabilities. Telephones may have large numbers and many features, such as redial, preprogrammed telephone numbers, and built-in intercoms or amplifiers. These features are useful for children with limited dexterity and limited abilities to sequence or remember telephone numbers. Children with auditory limitations can use special telephones with visual indicators (e.g., flashing light or strobe light), vibration, or hearing aid compatibility, or a telecommunication device for the deaf (TDD)

(McInnes & Treffry, 1993). Telephones with remote control dialing, large, illuminated letters or Braille, talk-back features (e.g., repeats last telephone number dialed or caller identification information), and voice-activated answering machines can assist children with limited vision.

If coordination or endurance is problematic, the child can use a headset or a telephone mounted on a gooseneck or with an attached universal cuff. The child dials buttons with a T-bar or universal cuff with a pencil. Answering machines that record and save messages are helpful when writing is difficult. Some adolescents record a message asking the caller to "Stay on the line until I can get to the phone!" Voice-activated answering machines and remote control dialing assist children with limited physical capabilities. Car telephones, cellular telephones, and other portable telephones or pagers are also beneficial to children and adolescents with disabilities. These easily accessed devices are helpful for emergencies and can be equipped with the features described previously.

Parents may not have the financial resources or the desire to change telephone systems. Familial preferences and the environmental context often influence which telephone is selected. Sample questions for the therapist to ask include the following:

- What is the purpose of having the telephone (e.g., safety, socialization, work)?
- In which room or rooms will the child use the telephone?
- If a child uses a headset or an electronic aid to daily living to talk on the telephone, can other family members also access it easily?
- If the child uses a cellular telephone or a pager system, are these devices permitted at school?
- Can the child or will a family member be responsible for recharging the telephone or changing the batteries?

Household Management Tasks

During childhood, children learn home management tasks that help them contribute to family functioning. Performing these tasks gives children a feeling of self-worth and develops future abilities for independent living and work environments. Home management tasks include cleaning, caring for clothing, preparing and cleaning up after meals, shopping, managing money, and maintaining a household.

Typical Developmental Sequence

As early as 18 months of age, children begin to understand what it means to "help out" in performing household chores. As children observe their parents routinely dust, sweep, set tables, or do laundry, they often initiate simple household tasks without cues from a parent. "Me do it" or "I want to sweep" are typical comments. As children get older, they become more capable of performing household chores, and parents often wish that enthusiasm for helping around the house would continue! Instead, adolescents become more absorbed in personal grooming or social activities and participate less in household chores (Duckett, Raffaelli, & Richards, 1989). Table 15-13 shows the developmental sequence for learning to perform home management tasks.

Contextual Considerations

Participation in home management tasks depends on the child's age and capabilities and the temporal and environmental contexts. The size of the family and the accessibility of the environment can encourage or dis-

TABLE 15-13   Developmental Sequence for Household Management Tasks

Age	Task
13 mo	■ Imitates housework
2 yr	■ Picks up and puts toys away with parental reminders
	■ Copies parents' domestic activities
3 yr	■ Carries things without dropping them
	■ Dusts with help
	■ Dries dishes with help
	■ Gardens with help
	■ Puts toys away with reminders
	■ Wipes up spills
4 yr	■ Fixes dry cereal and snacks
	■ Helps with sorting laundry
5 yr	■ Puts toys away neatly
	■ Makes a sandwich
	■ Takes out trash
	■ Makes bed
	■ Puts dirty clothes in hamper
	■ Answers telephone correctly
6 yr	■ Runs simple errands
	■ Does household chores without redoing
	■ Cleans sink
	■ Washes dishes with help
	■ Crosses street safely
7-9 yr	■ Begins to cook simple meals
	■ Puts clean clothes away
	■ Hangs up clothes
	■ Manages small amounts of money
	■ Uses telephone correctly
10-12 yr	■ Cooks simple meals with supervision
	■ Does simple repairs with appropriate tools
	■ Begins doing laundry
	■ Sets table
	■ Washes dishes
	■ Cares for pet with reminders
13-14 yr	■ Does laundry
	■ Cooks meals

courage participation in household chores. Age, gender, socioeconomic status, geographic location (Light, Hertsgaard, & Martin, 1985), and customs and values about self-sufficiency (Lynch & Hanson, 1998) may influence when and how the child performs chores. Often girls participate in chores more than boys do (Seymour, 1988), and they may choose more cooperative indoor chores than boys, who choose more independent outdoor chores (e.g., washing the car and lawn care) (Duckett et al., 1989). Expectations often differ for children from low socioeconomic environments or rural versus urban areas. Families may encourage independence or they may promote interdependency among family members. Therapists need to consider these factors when working with children and their families.

The family's modeling behaviors, patience, routines, and expectations and the child's preferences influence which chores children do. This role modeling of chores by all family members is important in establishing household chores as routine and expected. If the parents do household chores inconsistently or rarely, the child may not be included in "helping out" roles and may not learn the typical routines or habits for completing household tasks.

When children with or without disabilities first begin to wash tables, dust, or vacuum, extra time and patience from the parent and modified expectations for performance are necessary. The parents repeat instructions, and the child often must redo the tasks, taking more time than if the parents had completed the task themselves. Parents give the child time to problem solve and ideally allow him or her to learn from mistakes.

Performance Problems in Household Tasks

The medical-physical or educational needs of a child with a disability often overshadow the development of IADL occupations. Occupational therapists collaborate with parents to set up routines and modify tasks and environments so that the child can perform all or part of a household task. Often independence in household tasks is not a goal; however, some level of participation allows the child to contribute to the family's daily functions.

Children with motor problems have difficulty obtaining materials, manipulating and using typical equipment, or completing the entire task. Children with process skill limitations have difficulty initiating and terminating the task, following and remembering the sequence, and generalizing the tasks to other environments (e.g., differences in cleaning kitchen and living room floors). When a child has a low frustration level and poor impulse control, parents are often fearful to give them tasks that could potentially be unsafe.

Intervention Strategies

Environmental modifications, assistive technology, task modification, and varying levels of help from others are often the approaches that therapists use to teach home management tasks. Home modifications may also include adding effective safety features to help prevent injuries (Lyons et al., 2003). Table 15-5 gives examples of how caregivers can adapt various environments in the home with structural changes and assistive devices to allow the child to participate in household tasks.

Natural cues in the physical or social environment assist in the development of a child's IADLs. If memory is a problem, the caregiver should keep all the needed supplies where the child will use them. For example, a sponge can be placed next to the bathroom sink to help the child find the object and remind him or her to clean the sink after tooth brushing or face washing. Artificial cues such as color coding or labeling shelves, cabinets, and bins with pictures or words also help children locate objects in the environment. Picture charts and checklists assist the child in remembering the sequence of tasks. Figure 15-13 gives an example of a visual cue to help the boy set the table correctly. Using natural teaching moments and embedding ADL routines into the school or home schedule help children learn new tasks and feel a sense of efficacy (Stowitschek, Laitinen, & Prather, 1999). For example, if Jake washes clothes and turns everyone's underwear pink because he did not sort the clothes properly, it becomes a teachable moment to remind him to sort the clothes before washing them.

Children with ROM, strength, coordination, or postural control problems may need modified equipment. For cleaning table surfaces, typical equipment may

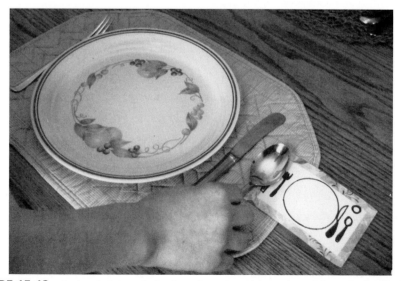

FIGURE 15-13   A visual picture helps Raoul set the table and participate in family chores.

include dusting or wiping mitts or adapted spray bottles for cleaning solutions. Long-handled dustpans, dusters, or buckets on wheels with a stick attached may help the child who cannot bend forward. Broom, mop, and vacuum handles can be enlarged or adapted with additional pieces to allow the child to hold them.

Children with limitations in mental capacities may encounter problems with sequencing, judging, and performing the tasks on a regular basis (Browder & Bambura, 2000). These children need pictorial cues in the form of a chart on the wall or a flip-card book. The charts list the steps of a task or a sequence of tasks (e.g., task analysis), and the child checks off each step or task when he or she completes it. The picture helps the child remember the sequence and helps him or her judge whether the task has been done correctly. For example, a pictorial recipe allows the child to see how many cups of cheese to use and whether he or she has put the cheese correctly on top of the pizza. If the measuring cup has an acetate or plastic covering, the parent can mark the correct level with a washable marker. The caregiver should fade the use of pictorial cues as the child learns the task. Figure 15-14 gives an example of how a child who cannot read can use pictures, words, and an aisle number on index cards to complete a grocery shopping task.

The caregivers use verbal, gestural, or physical cues when the child is first learning a task. For example, the caregiver uses verbal cues to tell the child how many times to squirt a solution when cleaning tables or mirrors. An example of a gestural cue is holding up three fingers (one at a time) to remind the child of how many times to spray; a physical cue would be tapping the child's hand or using a hand-over-hand approach to show him or her how to spray three times.

Most families are interdependent in performing household management tasks. Although independent performance is highly valued, complete self-reliance in a task may not be achievable or even desirable if the task requires too much time and energy or if it exacerbates abnormal behaviors or movement patterns. Dependence in some tasks is appropriate at times and may permit completion of other, more readily achieved independent living activities.

Children with disabilities participate in household management tasks at different levels. Some may never be independent in cooking, but the caregiver can include them in an activity through partial participation. For example, a child with athetoid cerebral palsy may not have the coordination to control stirring strokes, but he or she can participate in the task of making a cake or cutting vegetables by using an automated learning device (ALD) with an electric mixer (Levin & Scherfenberg, 1987). An ALD is essentially an electronic aid to daily living that has a switch that activates an appliance. The ALD reduces the voltage of the appliance to a lower voltage at the switch. It may have a timer that allows the appliance to remain on for a set amount of time without the child activating the switch during this time.

Prevention/Education in Household Safety. Many parents fear that their children with disabilities will be injured when performing household tasks. Safety while using appliances, utensils, and other equipment is of utmost importance. For example, children with myelomeningocele may not have sensation in their lower extremities. Education in safety precautions is needed to prevent burns from hot plates or pots carried on the lap or from touching a stove, dryer, or other hot item. Fire alarms, carbon monoxide detectors, gas detectors, and propane detectors can have amplified sound, flashing

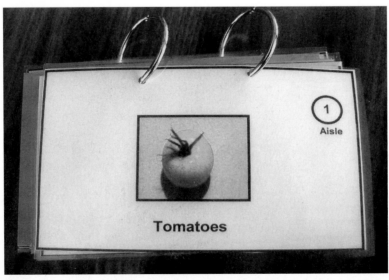

FIGURE 15-14 These cue cards attach to the grocery cart with rings and can be turned over as each item is purchased.

lights, and/or vibration to alert children and adolescents with sensory impairments. Children also need to be ready to respond if an emergency occurs. Access to the telephone and the correct telephone numbers and the ability to get in and out of the house are key tasks. A portable cell phone, a wireless phone, or an accessible telephone station, combined with knowledge of how to contact emergency services or a designated helper, is also important.

Therapists consider cultural characteristics in relation to safety issues. In some cultures, parents are expected to protect their children until they are married and leave the house; they may not want children (with or without disabilities) exposed to uncertain or potentially risky situations. In addition, safety knowledge may be lacking for some families and for some therapists. For example, recently immigrated families may not have experience with electricity or plumbing and may not be aware of safety issues with water and electricity (Lynch & Hanson, 1998). Therapists working in rural counties need to understand typical farm chores, a framework for tasks that are age appropriate, and the risks to children with disabilities (Castillo, Hard, Myers, Pizatella, & Stout, 1998; Clark, 1994).

Caring for Pets and Others

As children grow, they are given responsibility for caring for others. This responsibility typically begins with an animal and later may include caring for younger siblings. Table 15-13 presents the typical development of caregiving activities for children and adolescents. Children and adolescents with disabilities are often cared for by others and have few opportunities to reciprocate this caring to others. Others model caregiving in social and cultural environments. With grading, prompting, and guidance, some children with disabilities learn how to do errands or favors, clean up, share materials, baby-sit, and perform volunteer work (Ford et al., 1989). For example, children with significant delays in development can learn how to complete an errand or help their mother or a sibling feel better by rubbing her shoulders or bringing her a blanket. Visual, verbal, gestural, and physical cues may assist the child in learning caregiving occupations. Giving children these opportunities may help them feel more competent later at becoming caregivers or parents themselves. Adolescents may benefit from talking to and observing other parents with disabilities and accessing support networks (listed in Box 15-1 under sexuality).

Community Activities and Occupations

Shopping, eating in restaurants, banking, and attending sports and recreational events involve many similar activities, including achieving mobility, communicating with strangers, handling money and packages, reading and writing, and performing ADLs in various settings. The therapist performs an ecologic assessment to target the necessary tasks and performance skills, to identify areas where adaptation or skill development is needed, and to develop and analyze instructional strategies that fit the environmental demands. The therapist teaches children these tasks in the community setting (Falvey, 1986; York-Barr, Rainforth, & Locke, 1996). The use of assistive devices in public depends on their degree of portability and ease of use and the attitudes of the child and family.

Managing money during shopping tasks is often difficult for the child with physical or cognitive disabilities. Instead of wallets, these children can use small zippered purses (e.g., fanny packs) that go around the waist or are hooked to the wheelchair. These are adapted with a large zipper pull and can be attached with hook-and-loop fasteners to a lapboard for stability. The child can hand the fanny pack to the store clerk and ask him or her to get the money out or put the change in the fanny pack. When purchasing an item, children can also instruct clerks to put their change in the paper bag that is given to them. The child can use a calculator to help with arithmetic and carry cue cards to remind himself or herself of the value of money. For children with visual limitations, a money brailler, coin sorter, or specific folding technique or placement of money can help in identifying denominations of money.

As the child matures, learning how to purchase and pay for items online or through catalogs is essential. Some grocery stores have online or phone services; the customer orders selected items, the store puts the items together, and the customer picks up the goods at a designated time. Adolescents need to have practice planning and staying within a budget and using a checking account. The virtual world of online banking and record keeping for checking and savings accounts is useful for the adolescent limited in mobility or mathematical skills.

Community Mobility

Functional mobility in the community is critical to the child's development and to the family's ability to be active outside the home. Community participation ranges from the early stages, when the child accompanies his or her parents on errands, to the time when the child goes out on his or her own. When a child is in a wheelchair, skills such as street crossing, navigating a mall or store, or riding public transportation are essential mobility skills to learn. The therapist educates the family and child with disabilities about functional mobility and addresses transportation of the child from a safety standpoint. Furthermore, when the therapist selects new equipment for a child, he or she considers the methods used for home, school, and community mobility to ensure that the child can use and transport the device as necessary.

Family Vehicle

In the United States, all 50 states have safety laws requiring children to use car seats and restraint systems while traveling in cars; however, the requirements for using these seats vary across the country. Car seats and restraint systems protect children from injury and are one of the most used—and most improperly used—pieces of equipment on the market (Decina & Lococco, 2004). In a study by the National Highway Traffic Safety Administration (NHTSA) done in six states, 76% of the 5,527 children weighing less than 80 pounds were placed in car restraint systems that were misused (Decina & Lococco). This highly technical field requires that therapists become acquainted with the federal regulations, the variety of car seats and cars, and ways to choose, fit, and install child restraint systems.

In general, infants and children are always placed in the back seat until they weigh 80 pounds and are 4 feet, 9 inches tall, because passenger-side airbags can be deadly to small children who are restrained. Restraint systems or harness straps may be the five-point type (shoulders, hips, and pelvis) or the three-point type (shoulders and crotch) and should be adjusted to the shoulder level. If a retainer clip is available for harness straps, it should be used and should be kept at armpit level. As with wheelchairs, children should not travel with toys, mirrors, or special play trays attached to the seat, because these may interfere with the harness or may become missiles during a crash (Berres, 2003).

The NHTSA conducts research on car seats and updates its recommendations and standards as new findings emerge. The following are NHTSA recommendations for car seats:

- Infant seats should be backward facing and should be used for infants (up to 1 year) until the child reaches 20 to 22 pounds. The harness straps should be at the infant's shoulder level or below.
- Toddler or convertible seats are used first as backward-facing infant seats (5 to 35 pounds) and then as forward-facing toddler seats (20 to 40 pounds). The harness straps should be at shoulder level or above for forward-facing seats.
- Booster seats for children over 40 pounds should use lap belts that fit low and tight across the lap or upper thigh and shoulder belts that are tight across the chest.

Car seat designs change yearly and some are recalled for defects so therapists need to keep abreast of alerts and changes in standards. The NHTSA web site updates information on transporting children with disabilities based on their newest research.

Berres (2003), an occupational therapist and special needs transportation instructor, cautions therapists not to add any extra padding to the seat (under or behind) or to the straps without reading the manufacturer's labels or working with someone certified as a child passenger safety technician (CPS) through the NHTSA. If trunk or head support is needed, rolls for lateral supports may be added as long as the harness system is not disrupted. Any other adaptations could change how the crash forces are distributed over the body and could lead to injury or death (Berres).

Education and Prevention of Injury. A variety of commercial car seats available are useful for children with disabilities if the seat is chosen and installed correctly. Children who weigh more than 80 pounds and/or have skeletal deformities, poor head or trunk control, spica casts, or abduction braces often need specialized commercial seats to increase access, support, comfort, and protection. The type of car used, the child's age, size (weight and height) and physical capacities, and the ease of correct installation in the car determine which seat is the best fit for the child (Berres, 2003). Also, even if the correct-size car seat is purchased, it may not be installed properly. In a study by Lane, Liu, and Newlin (2000), modeling, direct hands-on practice, and written instructions for parents did not ensure proper installation of the car seat. With the proper knowledge, family instruction or community education on car seat safety is certainly an area in which occupational therapists can make a difference. The Task Force on Community Preventive Services (Zaza et al., 2001) found strong evidence for the effectiveness of using a combination of community education programs, loaner programs, walk-in safety check clinics, and publicity of laws and enforcement to improve the correct use of child safety seats.

Children who have outgrown standard commercial car seats but have not yet developed adequate sitting balance may use car seats designed specifically for larger children with disabilities. Transport/travel type wheelchairs (see Chapter 19) are also designed as car seats and are an option for some children. Restraint harnesses or vests, attached to the regular car or school bus seat, can help restrain children with postural or behavior problems. Older, heavier children who cannot manage car transfers may benefit from freestanding portable or special car lifters or power-assist seats.

Many children with physical disabilities ride vans and buses seated in their wheelchairs. These vehicles are especially helpful for children in power wheelchairs that do not dismantle or fold. Ramps or power van lifts help transfer the child into the vehicle. A voluntary wheelchair standard, American National Standards Institute/Rehabilitation Engineering Society of North America (ANSI/RESNA) WC/19, addresses the use of wheelchairs as seats in motor vehicles. These standards can guide parents in choosing safer, easier to use wheelchairs. Minimal crashworthiness tests have been performed with all the varieties of mobility devices (e.g., type, size, weight, and construction), and few states keep information on automobile accidents involving wheelchairs (Schneider, 2002).

If possible, the child should transfer out of the wheelchair and into a seat in the vehicle and use the already tested occupant restraint systems. As children are able, they need to know how to instruct others in ways to safely transport them in a wheelchair on a bus or in a car. If a child must be transported in a wheelchair, Bertocci, Hobson, and Digges (2000) and Schneider (1996, 2002), and van Roosmalen, Bertocci, Hobson, and Karg (2002) recommend the following with regard to wheelchair tiedown and occupant restraint systems (WTORS):

- All wheelchairs should be placed facing forward, *never* sideways. When chairs are placed sideways, they can fold and collapse on impact, potentially causing more injury;
- An occupant restraint system must be available and must be attached on the wheelchair itself. This restraint is separate from the wheelchair restraint system and is effective if it is a belt-type system. Restraints should be for the upper and lower torso and should be applied over skeletal regions such as the pelvis and shoulders rather than over the soft abdominal area.
- A wheelchair restraint system separate from the occupant restraint system should be in place. This tiedown system should secure the wheelchair frame to the floor of the vehicle and should be independent from the occupant restraint system. Four-point strap systems for manual docking or powered docking tiedowns are recommended. Securement points for the tiedowns are on the wheelchair, and anchored points are on the wheelchair and/or the vehicle. These securement points must be easily accessible.
- Items attached to the wheelchair need to be removed and strapped down onto the wall of the bus or under a seat. On impact in an accident, a lapboard or augmentative communication device could act as a missile and further injure the child or other occupants of the vehicle.

School Transportation

Rules and equipment for transporting children with disabilities and their equipment vary among school systems, although the standards set by the NHTSA are recommended. As with the family vehicle, it is first recommended that the child transfer to the bus seat whenever possible. The occupational therapist's role often involves working with school transportation officials in implementing the above safety guidelines and issues and helping to solve special problems for individual children. With the physical therapist, the occupational therapist may help assess and implement the safest way to ascend and descend the bus and transfer into the bus seat if possible. Therapists also make sure that the lockdown procedures for wheelchairs, lap trays, communication systems, and other devices meet the requirements of the individual school system and that restraining systems are maintained properly. Wheelchairs need sufficient positioning controls to maintain the child's posture throughout the bus ride, and a designated place for containing belongings safely should be available. Federal Head Start rules now require safety vests for children who weigh less than 50 pounds. These vests must be tethered to the lap belt or to the frame of the seat behind the child.

Public Transportation

The Architectural and Transportation Barriers Compliance Board and the Department of Transportation (1998) have developed guidelines for public transportation on buses, rapid transit trains, and planes. These guidelines and regulations increase the opportunities for children with disabilities to travel. Even though more communities have accessible rapid transit programs, many still have Dial-a-Ride type programs that provide door-to-door bus or van service. This is typically arranged in advance by telephone. Children who are able to board buses or rapid rail systems must learn important skills such as handling money and tickets, using transit schedules, and identifying the correct buses, trains, and stops. How to get on a lift, how to lock the wheelchair, and how to direct others in ways to secure items on the chair and the chair to the bus are responsibilities children should be taught as appropriate. For children with memory and sequencing problems, instructional strategies such as partial participation and graded cueing may assist them with sequencing the task. Shadowing the child the first time he or she takes the bus may also be an option.

Large major transportation systems accommodate passengers with disabilities by priority and special seating. With the new regulations, each rapid transit company must provide at least one car designated and accessible for persons with disabilities. Different companies and transportation modes have varying amenities, therefore it is necessary to compare policies in advance. Regulations for aircraft boarding chairs, transfer procedures, and the storage of wheelchairs and batteries are available from the U.S. Access Board (see Box 15-2). Airplane companies have boarding chairs that are accessible to the airplane's 17-inch aisles and are designed with locks, restraint systems, and removable arms for transfers into the airplane seat. In most cases, individuals with disabilities cannot sit in their wheelchair on planes and trains, which makes it difficult to use the restroom. If a child has respirator or other needs requiring electricity, pre-planning is essential. Advance checks on accessibility are advised before taking a trip.

Contextual Factors Affecting Mobility

Environmental factors that affect mobility include other people and crowds, street crossings, use of personal or public transportation and elevators, and architectural barriers. Occupational therapists often are involved with a team to select the most appropriate mobility device for a child. (Chapter 19 elaborates on devices available for children.) Once the therapist identifies problems in mobility, he or she may consult with or teach the child, parent, and other caregivers remedial and compensatory techniques for improving mobility in various community settings. The therapist can use his or her expertise to educate the child and caregivers on how to get in and out of doorways and elevators, get up and down curbs, and maneuver in tight spots. The therapist also uses his or her knowledge about sensory modifications, energy conservation, time management, and positive behavior supports to help children move in routine environments such as the school or home. The following example shows how an adolescent can be taught to overcome environmental barriers.

Geoff is a 16-year-old sophomore in high school who has spastic cerebral palsy. He wants to hang out with his friends at a fast-food restaurant but has mostly depended on his family to take him places and get his food. Geoff uses an augmentative communication device and a power wheelchair with a lap tray. As a consultant, the therapist visits the community site to perform an ecologic evaluation. After assessing Geoff in the fast-food restaurant, the therapist uses task analysis to determine six steps for Geoff to accomplish. She uses backwards chaining to get Geoff to be successful at this task. Table 15-14 summarizes the approaches and adaptations that Geoff used to improve his performance. Using systematic record keeping, the team determined the steps that Geoff did consistently and the strategies that needed modification. Graphing Geoff's progress also cued the certified occupational therapy assistant (COTA), his teacher, and his family to reduce prompting, eliminate unnecessary adaptive equipment, and increase the level of performance expected from Geoff. In addition to preplanning an activity and eating out, Geoff experienced getting on and off public transportation, crossing a street, asking for help, making transactions, manipulating money, choosing the most nutritious meal with the least amount of fat, and interacting with others without disabilities. Geoff's performance is influenced by a contextually based occupation that has meaning to him. In spite of Geoff's spastic cerebral palsy with quadriplegia, he independently manipulates money, puts his food on a lap tray, selects a napkin and straw, and brings his food to the table.

Independent Driving

Adolescents with or without disabilities are often excited about being able to drive, because this ability gives the child more independence from his or her parents. The therapist usually consults with adapted driving program specialists unless he or she has had specialized training in driving adaptations and instruction. In most states, as the adolescent prepares to drive, he or she must first pass a written test to receive a learner's permit. For some students with learning disabilities, this is the first hurdle to driving, because many written driving tests are given online, and students may have difficulty understanding testing procedures, symbols, and the wording of questions, especially if they have perceptual or reading difficulties. The adolescent may need to self-advocate for assessment accommodations if this proves difficult.

After passing the written test for driving, students complete the application process, which includes bringing the correct documents and passing the vision test. Therapists consider body functions and structures and performance skills when first evaluating driving capabilities. For example, therapists may examine the adolescent's body functions in relation to neuromotor (strength, ROM), perceptual, or sensory functions important for getting into a car, turning on the motor, and operating the car's controls. Evaluation of body structures (e.g., eyes, ears, skeletal structure, cardiac and respiratory systems) and of motor skills (e.g., posture, mobility, coordination, strength and effort, energy) and process skills (e.g., attends, shows temporal organization, navigates, notices and responds, adjusts, and benefits from or adapts to changes) is crucial before any teenager with a disability gets behind the wheel for further driving tests.

Automobile adaptations for the teenage driver with a disability range from simple add-on components to those that convert a car or van permanently. Add-on adaptations that do not affect others' use of the car are preferred when feasible. Access modifications, steering systems, brake accelerator systems, secondary backup systems, and driver access modifications are typical, and 8.9% of modifications are done for drivers under 21 years of age (Bureau of Transportation Statistics, 2002).

Steering knobs facilitate grasping and turning of the wheel, and for adolescents with quadriplegia or significant upper extremity weakness, zero-effort steering may be useful. Built-up brakes and accelerator pedals or left-footed accelerators are useful for adolescents with ROM, weakness, or coordination difficulties. Right- or left-hand controls or relocation of the horn and dimmer switches are examples of other adaptations for the family automobile. Each year, new technologies are making it

TABLE 15-14 Geoff: An Example of Instructional Procedures and Adaptations to Build Successful Occupational Performance in the Community*

Geoff is a 16-year-old sophomore in high school who has spastic cerebral palsy. He wants to hang out with his friends at a fast-food restaurant but has mostly depended on his family to take him places and get his food. Geoff uses an augmentative communication device and a power wheelchair with a lap tray. As a consultant, the therapist visits the community site to perform an ecologic evaluation. After assessing Geoff in the fast-food restaurant, the therapist uses task analysis to determine six steps for Geoff to accomplish. She uses backwards chaining to get Geoff to be successful at this task.

Instructional Goals and Procedures	Task Method and Materials/Assistive Technology	Environmental Adaptations	Time	Motivational Strategies
6. Throws away trash and exits fast-food restaurant, asking for help, if needed, in 5-min period (1 : 1; prompt; wait outside for him)	Power wheelchair, lapboard, augmentative communication device, watch	Wads up trash before moving to trash can; chooses trash container not in the main flow of restaurant traffic; pushes open doors and trash can" go in the next column exits through door closest to table area where people may be seated; has Epson programmed to say, "Please open the door for me" and "Thank you"; tries automatic and manual doors	5 min	Being able to socialize with others with preprogrammed message; working toward independence; "beat the clock"
5. Opens or requests help with opening packages and eats food independently (1 : 1; begin with drink, add one item each time)	Drink; french fries; finger foods	Eats at table on his lap tray; chooses items he can open (i.e., in paper sacks, not boxes) and grasp; has preprogrammed Epson to say, "Please help me open this."	Two or three items per visit	Eating; time to socialize one on one
4. Gets food, napkin, straw, and utensils and carries to table area on his lapboard without spilling items (1 : 1; verbal and gestural cues to maneuver wheelchair)	Power wheelchair, lapboard, possibly non-slip matting	Goes to restaurant at nonpeak hours; therapist or friend may put tray on lapboard; goes to table with removable chairs	Performs actions independently	Wants to perform actions independently
3. Independently manipulates money and pays for food (1 : 1; therapist stands behind Geoff; verbal or gestural cues)	Puts money in side pocket of wheelchair; places money on lapboard	Practices money skills in classroom; uses preprogrammed Epson message to ask clerk to put his change on tray	Practices money skills for 2 weeks before outing	Wants to be able to do this at other businesses
2. Uses augmentative communication device independently to order food (1 : 1; decides on what to eat before coming; preprograms Epson communication device; uses timer on watch as cue; peer added to eat with him)	Epson augmentative communication device; lapboard	Hands clerk card that says, "I use this machine to talk to you"; does not go to counter until ready, and goes to counter on "off times" when restaurant is not extremely busy	2 min	Wants to eat food different from that in cafeteria at school; wants to go with friends; can choose own food
1. Determines his order and if he has enough money (1 : 1; verbal prompting; counts money before going out and writes down amount; uses timer on watch as cue)	Lapboard, side pocket for wheelchair; watch; calculator	Practices rounding numbers and counting money in math class; talks about what he thinks items will cost before going to restaurant; uses calculator to add money	3 min	Receives a certain amount of money to spend; is allowed to keep the change

*Objective: Geoff will be able to purchase and eat a meal at a fast-food restaurant by completing each subskill and criterion as established.

possible for adolescents and adults with disabilities to drive, and therapists need to refer adolescents to facilities and clinics that are certified to teach driving to persons with disabilities and that are updated and may even have the newest technologies available.

Teenagers may learn to drive with adapted controls, but independence is limited if they cannot transfer themselves and their equipment (e.g., wheelchairs) into and out of the car. Therapists teach various transfer techniques, depending on the child's capabilities, especially strength and postural control. Car door openers, enlarged controls (e.g., door locks), transfer boards, webbing loops, modified dressing sticks (to close the door), or wooden jigs to guide wheelchairs into a specific space (i.e., trunk or backseat) are examples of assistive devices the adolescent may use. Teenagers who ambulate for short distances may be able to put a chair into the trunk or side door of a car. Other teenagers who are nonambulatory may also place the chair in the backseat of the car or may get in the front seat on the passenger side of the car and pull the wheelchair in with them. Vehicle access devices (e.g., power doors, a raised roof, a lowered floor, or raised door openings) and driver position modifications (e.g., removable seat or power-assist seat) are also helpful to students with weakness and other disabilities. Wheelchair carriers and lifts that go on the rear or top of the car may be another option.

SUMMARY

This chapter presented a wide range of options for enhancing ADLs and IADLs for children and adolescents with disabilities. Typical developmental sequences and special methods for evaluating ADLs and IADLs were presented. The environmental context in which ADLs and IADLs occur, the child's capacities, and the demands of the task, as well as parent and child preferences, were discussed in the planning of evaluation and intervention. Performance skills during an activity and performance patterns were noted as influences on the outcomes of intervention. Intervention strategies were illustrated, including task adaptation, assistive technology, and environmental modification. The importance of positioning and orienting the child to the work surface was stressed. As technology changes and outcome data become available, a responsibility of the occupational therapist is to remain knowledgeable about current methods and equipment that promote independent functioning in children with disabilities.

STUDY QUESTIONS

1   Linda is 2 years old and has high tone and spasms. Her mother has asked for suggestions for dressing and diapering. Linda's mother explains that her daughter is very tight when she undresses her in the evening. What approach and method would you suggest?

2   Mark is 7 months old and has Down syndrome. His mother has just returned to work, and his grandmother is taking care of him. She is having difficulty dressing Mark, who feels like a rag doll to her, and she complains of back pain. What adaptations to the task and environment would you suggest?

3   Hank is 16 years old and has diabetes. He is cognitively intact but has peripheral neuropathies, low endurance, and poor coordination. He is in a wheelchair and lives in a wheelchair-accessible home. Hank wants to be able to stay by himself when he comes home from school, but his mother is not sure this is a good idea. He needs to be able to take his medicine and fix himself a snack. As Hank's therapist, what factors do you need to consider? What adaptations may he need?

4   José is $2\frac{1}{2}$ years old and has begun toilet training. He is extremely distractible and sensitive to environmental smells, has below-average equilibrium reactions for his age, and has difficulty with fasteners. What suggestions do you have for his day care providers as they begin to address toilet training?

5   Colin is 5 years old and has been identified as having severe perceptual problems and low tone and endurance. What do you hypothesize will be his problems with dressing? What can you do to grade the dressing task so that it is easier?

6   Nine-year-old Nailah has poor postural control and tactile defensiveness. Bath time is difficult for her mother because Nailah particularly hates to have her hair washed. What suggestions do you have for Nailah's mother? (Think of preparatory activities as well as the consultation method you will use.)

7   Twelve-year-old Melinda has difficulty with balance, but she is motivated to dress herself. What positions could help facilitate her independent performance in putting on pants, shoes, or a shirt?

8   Mario is an 8-year-old with low muscle tone. He currently weighs 75 pounds, and he is outgrowing his booster seat. What other seating options would you consider for him and why?

9   Ahmad is 10 years old and was placed in traction for 4 months because of a severe break in his femur. He is modest and wants to be able to wash and dress himself. Are there any social or cultural considerations you should explore? What

suggestions would you give Ahmad and his caregivers?

REFERENCES

American National Standards Institute/Rehabilitation Engineering Society of North America (ANSI/RESNA). (2000). ANSI/RESNA WC/19: Wheelchairs used as seats in motor vehicles (Vol. 1). RESNA: Arlington, VA.

American Occupational Therapy Association (AOTA). (2002). Occupational therapy practice framework: Domain and process. *American Journal of Occupational Therapy, 56,* 609-639.

Annon, J. (1976). The PLISSIT model: A proposed conceptual scheme for the behavioral treatment of sexual problems. *Journal of Sex Education and Therapy,* 1-15.

Balboni, G., Pedrabissi, L., Molteni, M. & Villa, S. (2001). Discriminant validity of the Vineland Scales: Score profiles of individuals with mental retardation and a specific disorder. *American Journal of Mental Retardation, 106* (2), 162-172.

Bayzak, S. (1989). Changes in attitude beliefs regarding parent participation in home programs. *American Journal of Occupational Therapy, 43,* 723-728.

Bedell, G.M., Haley, S.M., Coster, W.J., & Smith, K.W. (2002a). Developing a responsive measure of change for paediatric brain injury inpatient rehabilitation. *Brain Injury, 16,* 659-671.

Bedell, G.M., Haley, S.M., Coster, W.J., & Smith, K.W. (2002b). Participation readiness at discharge from inpatient rehabilitation in children and adolescents with acquired brain injury. *Pediatric Rehabilitation, 5,* 107-116.

Bergen, A.F., & Colangelo, C. (1985). *Positioning the client with CNS deficits: The wheelchair and other adapted equipment* (2nd ed.). Valhalla, NY: Valhalla Rehabilitation Publications.

Bergen, A.F., Presperin, J., & Tallman, T. (1990). *Positioning for function: Wheelchairs and other assistive devices.* Valhalla, NY: Valhalla Rehabilitation Publications.

Berres, S. (2003). Keeping kids safe: Passenger restraint systems. *OT Practice, 8* (9), 13-19.

Bertocci, G.E., Hobson, D.A., & Digges, K.H. (2000). Development of a wheelchair occupant injury risk assessment method and its application in the investigation of wheelchair securement point influence on frontal crash safety. *IEEE Institute of Electrical and Electronic Engineers: Transportation Rehabilitation Engineer, 8* (1), 126-139.

Betz, C.L. (1998). Facilitating the transition of adolescents with chronic conditions from pediatric to adult health care and community settings. *Issues in Comprehensive Pediatric Nursing, 21,* 97-115.

Biederman, G.B., Fairhall, J.L., Raven, K.A., & Davey, V.A. (1998). Verbal prompting, hand-over-hand instruction, and passive observation in teaching children with developmental disabilities. *Exceptional Children, 64,* 503-511.

Bloomquist, K.B., Brown, G., Peersen, A., & Presler, E.P. (1998). Transition to independence: Challenges for young people with disabilities and their caregivers. *Orthopaedic Nursing, 17,* 27-35.

Boehme, R. (1988). *Improving upper body control: An approach to assessment and treatment of tonal dysfunction.* Tucson: Therapy Skill Builders.

Brollier, C., Shepherd, J., & Markley, K. (1994). Transition from school to community living. *American Journal of Occupational Therapy, 48* (4), 346-353.

Browder, M., & Bambara, B. (2000). Home and community. In M.E. Snell & P. Brown (Eds.), *Instruction of students with severe disabilities* (5th ed., pp. 543-589). New York: Macmillan.

Brown, L., Schwarz, P., Udvari-Solner, A., Kampschroer, E., Johnson, F., Jorgensen, J., et al. (1991). How much time should students with severe intellectual disabilities spend in regular education classrooms and elsewhere? *Journal of the Association for Persons with Severe Handicaps, 16,* 39-47.

Bryze, K., & Curtin, C. (1993). A top-down approach: Relationships to research and occupational performance. *Developmental Disabilities Special Interest Section Newsletter, 2,* 2-4.

Bureau of Transportation Statistics. (2002). Research Note: Common vehicle modifications for persons with disabilities. Retrieved at http://www.nhtsa.dot.gov/cars/rules/adaptive/BTSRN/ResearchNote0209.html Retrieved January 9, 2004.

Case-Smith, J. (2000). ADL strategies for children with developmental deficits. In C. Christiansen (Ed.), *Ways of living: ADL strategies for special needs* (pp. 83-121). Bethesda, MD: American Occupational Therapy Association.

Castillo, S., Hard, D.H., Myers, J.R., Pizatella, T., & Stout, N. (1998). A national childhood agricultural injury prevention initiative. *Journal of Agricultural Safety and Health Special Issue, 1,* 183-191.

Chan, S. (1998). Families with Asian roots. In E.W. Lynch & M.J. Hanson (Eds.), *Developing cross-cultural competence: A guide for working with children and their families* (2nd ed., pp. 251-354). Baltimore: Brookes.

Clark, R.W. (1994). Development characteristics of children: A framework for age appropriate tasks. National Institute for Farm Safety. Madison, WI: University of Wisconsin.

Coster, W.J. (1998). Occupation-centered assessment of children. *American Journal of Occupational Therapy, 52* (5), 337-344.

Coster, W., Deeney, T.A., Haltiwanger, J.T., & Haley, S.M. (1998). *School function assessment: User's manual.* San Antonio, TX: Therapy Skill Builders.

Couwenhoven, T. (2001). Sexuality education: Building a foundation of healthy attitudes. *Disability Solutions, 4* (6), 1-8. Web site: http://www.disabilitysolutions.org/4-6.htm

Dawe, N.J., & Shepherd, J.T. (1985). Occupational therapy in the sexuality program of a rehabilitation hospital. *American Occupational Therapy Association Physical Disabilities Special Interest Section Newsletter, 8,* 1-2.

Decina, L.E., & Lococco, K. (2004). Misuse of child restraints. Office of Research and Technology, National Highway Traffic Safety Administration. Retrieved January 31, 2004, from http://www.nhtsa.gov/people/injury/research

Duckett, E., Raffaelli, M., & Richards, M. (1989). Taking care: Maintaining the self and the home in early adolescence. *Journal of Youth and Adolescence, 18* (6), 549-565.

Dumas, H.M., Haley, S.M., Fragala, M.A., & Steva, B.J. (2001). Self-care recovery of children with brain injury:

Descriptive analysis using the Pediatric Evaluation of Disability Inventory (PEDI) functional classification levels. *Physical and Occupational Therapy in Pediatrics, 21* (2-3), 7-27.

Dunn, K.L. (1997). Sexuality education and the team approach. In M.L. Sipski & C.J. Alexander (Eds.), *Sexuality education function in people with disability and chronic illness: A professional's guide* (pp. 381-402). Baltimore, MD: Aspen.

Dunn, W., Brown, C., & McGuigan, A. (1994). Ecology of human performance: A framework for considering the effect of context. *American Journal of Occupational Therapy, 48* (7), 595-607.

Falvey, M. (1986). *Community-based curriculum: Instructional strategies for students with severe handicaps.* Baltimore: Brookes.

Feldman, M.A. (1999). Teaching child-care and safety skills to parents with intellectual disabilities through self learning. *Journal of Intellectual and Developmental Disability, 24* (1), 27-44.

Ferguson, D.L., & Baumgart, D. (1991). Partial participation revisited. *Journal of the Association for Persons with Severe Handicaps, 16,* 218-227.

Fingerhut, P., Madill, H., Darrah, J., Hodge, M., & Warren, S. (2002). Classroom-based assessment: Validation for the School AMPS. *American Journal of Occupational Therapy, 56,* 210-213.

Finnie, N. (1997). *Handling the young child with cerebral palsy at home* (3rd ed.). Woburn, MA: Butterworth-Heinemann.

Fisher, A.G. (2003a). *Assessment of Motor and Process Skills: Vol. 1. Development, standardization, and administration manual* (5th ed.). Fort Collins, CO: Three Star Press.

Fisher, A.G. (2003b). *Assessment of Motor and Process Skills: Vol. 2. User manual* (5th ed.). Fort Collins, CO: Three Star Press.

Fisher, A.G., & Bryze, K. (1997). *School AMPS: School version of the Assessment of Motor and Process Skills.* Fort Collins, CO: Three Star Press.

Fisher, A.G., Bryze, K., & Atchison, B.T. (2000). Naturalistic assessment of functional performance in school settings: Reliability and validity of the School AMPS scales. *Journal of Outcome Measurement, 4,* 504-522.

Ford, A., Schnorr, R., Meyer, L., Davern, L, Black, J., & Dempsey, P. (1989). *The Syracuse community-reference curriculum guide.* Baltimore: Brookes.

Friedman, J.D. (1997). Sexual expression: The forgotten component of ADL. *OT Practice, 2* (1), 20-25.

Functional Independence Measure FIMware User Guide and Self-Guided Training Manual, Version 5.20. WeeFIM System^SM Clinical Guide: Version 5.01. Buffalo, NY 14214: University at Buffalo; 1998, 2000.

Furuno, S., O'Reilly, K., Hosaka, C.M., Zeisloft, B., & Allman, T. (1997). *Hawaii Early Learning Profile–Revised.* Palo Alto, CA: Vort.

Gentry, A. (2003). Cognitive prosthetics: 21st century tools for the rehabilitation of thinking skills [online course]. Retrieved September 2, 2003, http://www.cerebreon.com/courses/cp/

Geyer, L.A., Kurtz, L.A., & Byram, L.E. (1998). Promoting function in daily living skills. In J.P. Dormans & L. Peliegrino (Eds.), *Caring for children with cerebral palsy: A team approach* (pp. 323-346). Baltimore: Brookes.

Giangreco, M., Cloninger, C., & Iverson, V. (1997). *Choosing options and accommodations for children (COACH)* (2nd ed.). Baltimore: Brookes.

Gray, C. (2000). *The new social story book: Illustrated edition.* Arlington, TX: Future Horizons.

Haley, S.M., Coster, W.J., Ludlow, L.H., Haltiwanger, J., & Andrellos, P. (1992). *Administration manual for the Pediatric Evaluation of Disability Inventory.* San Antonio, TX: Psychological Corporation.

Hamilton, B.B., & Granger, C.U. (2000). *Functional Independence Measure for Children (WeeFIM-II).* Buffalo, NY: Research Foundation of the State University of New York

Hanson, M. (1998). Families with Anglo-European roots. In E.W. Lynch & M.J. Hanson (Eds.), *Developing cross-cultural competence* (2nd ed., pp. 93-126). Baltimore: Brookes.

Healy, H., & Rigby, P. (1999). Promoting independence for teens and young adults with physical disabilities. *Canadian Journal of Occupational Therapy, 66* (5), 240-248.

Hingsburger, D. (1993). *I openers: Parents ask questions about sexuality and children with developmental disabilities.* Vancouver, BC: Family Support Institute Press.

Holm, M.B., Rogers, J.C., & James, A.B. (2003). Interventions for daily living. In E.B. Crepeau, E. Cohn, & B. Schell (Eds.), *Willard and Spackman's occupational therapy* (10th ed., pp. 491-554). Philadelphia: J.B. Lippincott.

Hughes, C., & Carter, E. W. (2000). *The transition handbook: Strategies high school teachers use that work!* Baltimore: Brookes.

Iyer, L.V., Haley, S.M., Watkins, M.P., & Dumas, H.M. (2003). Establishing minimal clinically important differences for scores on the Pediatric Evaluation of Disability Inventory for inpatient rehabilitation. *Physical Therapy, 83* (10), 888-898.

Johnson-Martin, N., Attermeier, S.M., & Hacker, B. (2004). *The Carolina curriculum for infants and toddlers with special needs* (3rd ed.). Baltimore: Brookes.

Johnson-Martin, N., Hacker, B., & Attermeier, S.M. (2004). *The Carolina curriculum for preschoolers with special needs.* (2nd ed.). Baltimore: Brookes.

Kangas, K. (1998). *Using your head: Access and integration of independent mobility and communication "Head First."* Presentation at TechKnowledgy '98 Conference, Children's Hospital, Richmond, VA October *28,* 1998.

Kellegrew, D. (1998). Creating opportunities for occupation: An intervention to promote the ADL independence of young children with special needs. *American Journal of Occupational Therapy, 52* (6), 457-465.

Kennedy, E. (1981). *Dressing with pride* (Vol. 1). Groton, CT: PRIDE Foundation.

Kernaleguen, A. (1978). *Clothing designs for the handicapped.* Edmonton, Canada: University of Alberta Press.

King, G., Law, M., King, S., & Rosenbaum, P. (1998). Parents' and service providers' perceptions of the family-centeredness of children's rehabilitation services. *Physical and Occupational Therapy, 18* (1), 21-40.

Knox, V., & Usen, Y. (2000). Clinical review of the Pediatric Evaluation of Disability Inventory. *British Journal of Occupational Therapy, 63* (1), 29-32.

Koegel, L.K., Koegel, R.L., Kellegrew, D., & Mullen, K. (1996). Parent education for prevention and reduction of severe problem behaviors. In L.K. Koegel, R.L. Koegel, & G. Dunlap (Eds.), *Positive behavioral support: Including people with difficult behavior in the community* (pp. 3-30). Baltimore: Brookes.

Kothari, D.H., Haley, S.M., Gill-Body, K.M., & Dumas, H.M. (2003). Measuring functional change in children with acquired brain injury (ABI): Comparison of generic and ABI-specific scale using the Pediatric Evaluation of Disability Inventory (PEDI). *Physical Therapy, 83* (9), 776-785.

Kramer, P., & Hinojosa, J. (1999). *Frames of reference for pediatric occupational therapy* (2nd ed.). Baltimore: Lippincott Williams & Wilkins.

Lambert, N.M., Nihira, K., & Leland, H. (1993). *AAMR Adaptive Behavior Scale–School-2.* Austin, TX: Pro-Ed.

Lane, W.G., Liu, G.C., & Newlin, E. (2000). The association between hands-on instruction and proper child safety seat installation. *Pediatrics, 106*(4 Suppl), 924-929.

Law, M., Baptiste, S., Carswell, A., McColl, M.A., Polotajiko, H., & Pollock, N. (1998). *Canadian Occupational Performance Measure* (3rd ed.). Toronto: Canadian Association of Occupational Therapists.

Lawrence, K.E., & Niemeyer, S. (Eds.). (1994). *Home care issues/activities of daily living: Caregiver education guide for children with developmental disabilities* (pp. 4:31-4:46). Gaithersburg, MD: Aspen.

Levin, J., & Scherfenberg, L. (1987). *Selection and use of simple technology in home, school, work, and community settings.* Minneapolis: Ablenet.

Light, H., Hertsgaard, D., & Martin, R. (1985). Farm children's work in the family. *Adolescence, 20* (7), 425-432.

Luther, B. (2001). Age-specific activities that support successful transition to adulthood for children with disabilities. *Orthopaedic Nursing, 20* (1), 23-39.

Lyons, R.A., Sander, L.V., Weightman, A.L., Patterson, J., Jones, S.A., & Lannon, S., et al., (2003). Modification of the home environment for the reduction of injuries (Cochrane Review). In *The Cochrane Library,* Issue 4, 2003. Chichester, UK: John Wiley & Sons.

Lynch, E., & Hanson, M. (1998). *Developing cross-cultural competence* (2nd ed.). Baltimore: Brookes.

McGavin, H. (1998). Planning rehabilitation: A comparison of issues for parents and adolescents. *Physical and Occupational Therapy, 18* (1), 69-82.

McInnes, J.M., & Treffry, J.A. (1993). *Deaf-blind infants and children: A developmental guide.* Toronto: University of Toronto Press.

Melberg-Schwier, K.M., & Hingsburger, D. (2000). *Sexuality: Your sons and daughters with intellectual disabilities.* Baltimore: Brookes.

Newborg, J., Stock, J.R., Wnek, L., Guidubaldi, J., & Svinicki, J. (1988). *Battelle Developmental Inventory.* Chicago: Riverside Publishers.

O'Neill, P. (2002). *Abuse and neglect of children with disabilities: A collaborative response.* Richmond, VA: Virginia Institute for Developmental Disabilities, Virginia Commonwealth University.

Orelove, F., & Sobsey, D. (1996). ADL skills. In F. Orelove & D. Sobsey (Eds.), *Educating children with multiple disabilities* (3rd ed., pp. 333-375). Baltimore: Brookes.

Parks, S. (1999). *Inside HELP: An administration manual.* Palo Alto, CA: Vort.

Peterson, P.M., Rauen, K.K., Brown, J., & Cole, J. (1994). Spina bifida: The transition into adulthood begins in infancy. *Rehabilitation Nursing, 19* (4), 229-238.

Pierce, S.R., Daly, K., Gallagher, K.G., Gershoff, A.M., & Schaumburg, S.W. (2002). Constraint-induced therapy for a child with hemiplegic cerebral palsy: A case report. *Archives of Physical Medicine and Rehabilitation, 83,* 1462-1463.

Porter, S., Freeman, L., & Griffin, L. (2000). *Transition planning for adolescents with special health care needs and disabilities: Information for families and teens.* Boston: Institute for Community Inclusion, Children's Hospital UAP. Retrieved October 1, 2003, at http://www.communityinclusion.org/transition/pdf/familyguide.pdf

Reese, G.M., & Snell, M.E. (1991). Putting on and removing coats and jackets: The acquisition and maintenance of skills by children with severe multiple disabilities. *Education and Training in Mental Retardation, 26,* 398-410.

Rempfer, M., Hildenbrand, W., Parker, K., & Brown, C. (2003). An interdisciplinary approach to environmental intervention: Ecology of human performance. In L. Letts, P. Rigby, & D. Stewart (Eds.), *Using environments to enable occupational performance* (pp. 119-136). Thorofare, NJ: Slack.

Rogers, J.C., Holm, M.B., & Stone, R.G. (1997). Assessment of daily living activities: The home care advantage. *American Journal of Occupational Therapy, 51,* 410-422.

Sailor, W., Halvorsen, A., Anderson, J., Goetz, L., Gee, K., & Doering, K., et al. (1986). Community intensive instruction. In R. Horner, L. Meyer, & B. Fredericks (Eds.), *Education of learners with severe handicaps* (pp. 251-288). Baltimore: Brookes.

Schneider, L.W. (1996). Working toward safer motor-vehicle transportation for people in wheelchairs. *Transportation Research Institute (UMTRI) Research Review, 27* (3), 1-16.

Schneider, L. (2002). *Providing safer transportation to children in wheelchairs* (lecture). Pediatric Assistive Technology and Rehab Symposium, Children's Hospital, Richmond, VA, (August 28, 2002).

Schwarz, S.P. (2000). *Attainment's dressing tips and clothing resources for making life easier.* Verona, WI: Attainment.

Sellers, S.W., Fisher, A.G., & Duran, L. (2001). Validity of the Assessment of Motor and Process Skills with students who are visually impaired. *Journal of Visual Impairment and Blindness, 95,* 164-167.

Sewell, T.J., Collins, B.C., Hemmeter, M.L., & Schuster, J.W. (1998). Using simultaneous prompting within an activity-based format to teach dressing skills to preschoolers with developmental delays. *Journal of Early Intervention, 21,* 132-142.

Seymour, S. (1988). Expressions of responsibility among Indian children: Some precursors of adult status and sex roles. *Ethos, 17* (4), 355-370.

Shapland, C. (1999). Sexuality issues for youth with disabilities and chronic health conditions: *Healthy and ready to work because everyone deserves a future:* An occasional policy brief of the Institute for Child Health Policy (pp. 1-24). Gainesville, FL: University of Florida. Retrieved August 1, 2003, at http://hctransitions.ichp.edu/policypapers/SexualityIssues.pdf

Smith, R., Benge, M., & Hall, M. (2000). Using assistive technologies to enable self-care and daily living. In C. Christiansen (Ed.), *Ways of living: ADL strategies for special needs* (2nd ed., pp. 57-81). Bethesda, MD: American Occupational Therapy Association.

Snell, M.E., & Brown, F. (2000). Development and implementation of educational programs. In M.E. Snell & F. Brown (Eds.), *Instruction of students with severe disabilities*

(5th ed., pp. 115-165). Upper Saddle River, NJ: Prentice-Hall.

Snell, M.E., & Vogtle, L.K. (2000). Methods for teaching self-care skills. In C. Christiansen (Ed.), *Ways of living: ADL strategies for special needs* (2nd ed., pp. 57-81). Bethesda, MD: American Occupational Therapy Association.

Sparrow, S., Balla, D., & Cicchetti, D. (1984). *Vineland Adaptive Behavior Scales.* Circle Pines, MN: American Guidance Services.

Spencer, K., Murphy, M., Bean, G., & Schelly, C. (1991). Vocational needs assessment: A functional, community referenced approach. In K. Spencer (Ed.), *From school to adult life: The role of occupational therapy in the transition process* (pp. 185-213). Fort Collins, CO: Department of Occupational Therapy, Colorado State University.

Stein, M.A., Szumowski, E., Blondis, T. & Roizen, N.J. (1995). Adaptive skills dysfunction in ADD and ADHD children. *Journal of Child Psychology & Psychiatry, 36* (4), 663-670.

Stowitschek, J.J., Laitinen, R., & Prather, T. (1999). Embedding early self-determination opportunities in curriculum for youth with developmental disabilities using natural teaching incidents. *Journal of Vocational Special Needs Education, 21,* 15-26.

Sullivan, P.M., & Knutson, J.F. (2000). Maltreatment and disabilities: A population-based epidemiological study. *Child Abuse and Neglect, 4* (10), 1257-1273.

Sweeney, J. (1989). *Clothing for children with severe disabilities: A guide to adaptive garments for use in the institutional setting.* Alexandria, VA: Special Clothes.

Trombly, C.A. (1995). Occupation: Purposefulness and meaningfulness as therapeutic mechanisms: 1995 Eleanor Clarke Slagle lecture. *American Journal of Occupational Therapy, 47,* 253-257.

Tsuji, T., Liu, M., Toikawa, H., Hanayama, K., Sonoda, S., & Chino, N. (1999). ADL structure for nondisabled Japanese children based on the Functional Independence Measure for Children (WeeFIM). *American Journal of Physical Medicine & Rehabilitation, 78* (3), 208-212.

Turnbull, A.P., & Turnbull, H.R. (2001). *Families, professionals, and exceptionality: Collaborating for empowerment* (4th ed.). Columbus, OH: Merrill/Prentice Hall.

WeeFIM II^{SM} system clinical guide: Version 5.01. (1998, 2000). Buffalo, NY: University at Buffalo.

Wheeler, M. (1998). *Toilet training for individuals with autism and related disorders.* Arlington, TX: Future Horizons.

Willis, W. (1998). Families with African-American roots. In E.W. Lynch & M.J. Hanson (Eds.), *Developing cross-cultural competence* (2nd ed., pp. 165-208). Baltimore: Brookes.

York-Barr, J., Rainforth, B., & Locke, P. (1996). Developing instructional adaptations. In F.P. Orelove & D. Sobsey (Eds.), *Educating children with multiple disabilities* (3rd ed., pp. 119-159). Baltimore: Brookes.

Zaza, S., Sleet, D.A., Thompson, R.S., Sosin, D.M., Bolen, J.C., & Task Force on Community Preventive Services. (2001). Reviews of evidence regarding interventions to increase use of child safety seats. *American Journal of Preventive Medicine, 21*(Suppl 4), 31-47.

Ziviani, J., Ottenbacher, K.J., Shephard, K., Foreman, S., Astbury, W., Ireland, P. (2001). Concurrent validity of the Functional Independence Measure for Children (WeeFIM) and the Pediatric Evaluation of Disabilities Inventory in children with developmental disabilities and acquired brain injuries. *Physical and Occupational Therapy in Pediatrics, 21* (2-3), 91-101.

Zuniga, M.E. (1998). Families with Latino roots. In E.W. Lynch & M.J. Hanson (Eds.), *Developing cross-cultural competence* (2nd ed., pp. 209-250). Baltimore: Brookes.

SUGGESTED READINGS

Epps, S., Stern, R.J., & Horner, R.H. (1990). Comparison of simulation training on self and using a doll for teaching generalized menstrual care to women with severe mental retardation. *Research in Developmental Disabilities, 11,* 37-66.

Jarus, T., & Ratzon, N.Z. (2000). Can you imagine? The effect of mental practice on the acquisition and retention of a motor skill as a function of age. *Occupational Therapy Journal of Research, 20* (3), 163-178.

National Research Council, Committee on the Health and Safety Implications of Child Labor (1998). *Protecting youth at work.* Washington, DC: National Academy Press.

Rheingold, H. (1982). Little children's participation in the work of adults: A nascent prosocial behavior. *Child Development, 53,* 114-125.

Schwier, K.M., & Hingsburger, D. (2000). *Sexuality: Your sons and daughters with intellectual disabilities.* Baltimore: Brookes.

Unruh, A.M., Fairchil, D.S., & Versnel, J. (1993). Parents' and therapists' ratings of self-care skills in children with spina bifida. *Canadian Journal of Occupational Therapy, 60* (3), 145-148.

van Roosmalen, L., Bertocci, G.E., Hobson, D.A., & Karg, P. (2002). Preliminary evaluation of wheelchair occupant restraint system usage in motor vehicles. *Journal of Rehabilitation Research and Development, 39* (1), 83-93.

Play

Susan H. Knox

CHAPTER OBJECTIVES

1 Describe the importance of and relationship of play to occupational therapy.
2 Describe play theories in terms of form, function, meaning, and context.
3 Describe play assessments and determine their usefulness for assessment and treatment planning.
4 Describe environmental and individual qualities that facilitate or constrain play.
5 Describe how play is used in treatment.

INTRODUCTION

"Play . . . is the way the child learns what no one can teach him. It is the way he explores and orients himself to the actual world of space and time, of things, animals, structures, and people. Through play he learns to live in our symbolic world of meanings and values, of progressive striving for deferred goals, at the same time exploring and experimenting and learning in his own individualized way. Through play the child practices and rehearses endlessly the complicated and subtle patterns of human living and communication, which he must master if he is to become a participating adult in our social life" (Franz, 1963, pp. v-vi)."

All children play, and it is through play that they learn about themselves and about the world around them. Watching children play is like looking through a window into their very being. Play has been identified as one of the primary occupations in which people engage, according to the American Occupational Therapy Association (AOTA) Practice Framework (AOTA, 2002). As defined by Parham and Fazio (1997), play is "any spontaneous or organized activity that provides enjoyment, entertainment, amusement or diversion" (p. 252) and is "an attitude or mode of experience that involves intrinsic motivation, emphasis on process rather than product and internal rather than external control; an 'as-if' or pretend element; takes place in a safe, unthreatening environment with social sanctions" (p. 252).

There are two sides of play: the science of play, where play is a critical aspect of human development that deserves serious study, and the art of play, where the therapist and the child are players, where there is joy, pleasure, and freedom. Occupational therapists need knowledge and skill in both aspects. This chapter describes play as the child's occupation from an historical perspective, discusses why play is important to occupational therapists, describes methods of assessing play, and discusses play in intervention.

PLAY THEORIES

Clark et al. (1991) defined occupations as "the chunks of culturally and personally meaningful activity in which humans engage" (p. 310). People create or orchestrate their daily experiences through planning and participating in occupations (Yerxa et al., 1989). Occupational therapy generally considers work, self care, leisure, play, and rest to be the major occupations of people. Occupations can be explained through the substrates of form, function, meaning, and context (Clark et al., 1991.)

Play can be viewed through these substrates of occupation:
1 As activities having certain characteristics (i.e., its form, including activities, characteristics, and products)
2 As a developmental phenomenon contributing to a child's development and enculturation (i.e., its function, including purposes, process, and experience)
3 As an experience or a state of mind (i.e., its meaning, including what motivates or satisfies the child).
Play, as any other activity, takes place within context, which denotes the individual's environments and the personal, physical, and social elements of each environment.

571

Form

Many play theorists (Bergen, 1988; Caillois, 1958; Cohen, 1987; Ellis, 1973) describe play as categories of activities in which children engage. These include such activities as games, building and construction, social play, pretend, sensorimotor play, and symbolic or dramatic play. Children's play activities change over time and reflect their development (Bergen, 1988; Neulinger, 1981).

Sensorimotor and exploratory play predominate in infancy (Figure 16-1) as infants develop mastery over their own bodies and learn the effect of their actions upon objects and people in the environment (Piaget, 1952; Rubin, Fein, & Vandenberg, 1983). Sensorimotor play peaks in the second year of life, then declines. Children continue to use sensory motor play when they learn new motor skills. Exploratory play begins in infancy, and by the end of the first year, infants actively explore their surroundings, demonstrate a beginning understanding of cause and effect, and are interested in how things work. In the second year, play centers around combining objects and learning their meaning. Children begin to classify objects and develop purpose in their actions. Exploratory play gradually declines through the preschool years, but it reappears when the child is learning new skills (Bergen, 1988).

Constructive play has identifiable outcomes and predominates during the preschool years as practice. Constructive play remains high during middle childhood and adolescence but becomes more abstract. It may develop into arts and crafts.

Symbolic play and pretense develop at the end of the first year and through the second, peaking at around 5 years of age and evolving into dramatic and sociodramatic play. During middle childhood, symbolic play and fantasy play are seen in mental games, secret clubs, and daydreaming, and in language play such as riddles or secret codes (Bergen, 1988). Television, computer games, and movies are also ways of indulging in fantasy play.

Social play begins very early with interaction between the infant and mother, and by age 3, children engage in complex social games. Children use role play to learn about social systems and cultural norms. Garvey (1977a) described four types of roles seen in group play: (1) functional roles, such as pretending to be a doctor; (2) relational roles, such as pretending to be mother and baby; (3) character roles, such as those from television and movies; and (4) roles with no identifiable identity. Social play combined with motor play develops into rough-and-tumble play (Bergen, 1988). Games with rules teach children to take turns and to initiate, maintain, and end social interactions (Johnson, Christie, & Yawkey, 1999). This type of play predominates during the school-age years (Bergen). Social play and games with rules are particularly influenced by the culture. The physical environments available for play, peer groups, and the types of play encouraged by parents have changed as our society has become more urbanized (Neulinger, 1981). Currently, time, places, and types of play are more planned and structured such as with organized sports and "play dates" (Knox, 1999) (Figure 16-2).

Adolescents are concerned with autonomy and being socialized into adult roles. This is a period of transition as obligations, time available for play, changes and refinements of interests, family and peer pressures all affect teen activity (Neulinger, 1981). In a study by Csikszentmihalyi and Larson (1984), the largest single activity of adolescents was socializing. Second was television, and third, sports, games, hobbies, reading, and music.

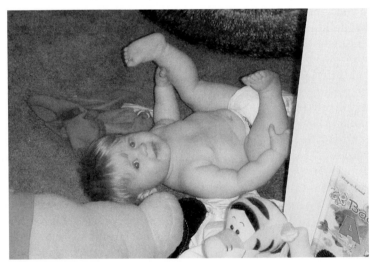

FIGURE 16-1 A first type of sensory motor-exploratory play is the infant's exploration of her own body. (Courtesy of Dianne Koontz Lowman.)

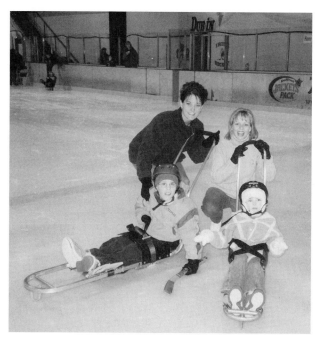

FIGURE 16-2 Play today is often highly structured; for example, this play date takes place at the ice-skating rink. (Courtesy of Jill McQuaid.)

Another way to look at the forms of play, or play forms, is through their characteristics. Scholars of play have not identified a single characteristic common to all kinds of play but have suggested many qualities or characteristics of play that differentiate play from nonplay. These characteristics include intrinsically motivated, suspension of reality, internal locus of control, spontaneous, fun, flexible, totally absorbing, vitalizing, an end in and of itself, nonliteral, and challenging (Cohen, 1987; Ellis, 1973; Huizinga, 1950; Levy, 1978, Neumann, 1971; Reilly, 1974). According to Rubin et al. (1983), play is characterized by the following traits: it (1) expresses intrinsic motivation and self-direction; (2) focuses on means rather than ends; (3) is organism centered rather than object centered; (4) is noninstrumental or symbolic; (5) shows freedom from externally imposed rules; and (6) reveals active engagement in the activity. Takata (1971) defined the following principles of play: (1) it is a complex set of behaviors characterized by "fun"; (2) it involves sensory, neuromuscular, or mental processes; (3) it involves repetition of experience, exploration, experimentation, and imitation; (4) it precedes within its own time and space boundaries; (5) it functions as an agent for integrating the internal and external worlds; and (6) it follows a sequential developmental progression.

Function

Another way of looking at play is in relation to function, or how play influences adaptation. Play functions include

processes, experiences, and purposes. Historically, play has been described as the way a child develops those skills necessary for life (Groos, 1976; Rubin et al., 1983), as a way of working off surplus energy (Schiller, 1957), or for recreation and relaxation (Rubin, Fein, Vandenberg, et al., 1983). Modern or contemporary theories emphasize the value of play in contributing to the child's development or to enculturation. They include using play to achieve optimal arousal (Berlyne, 1966; Ellis, 1973), to develop ego function (Erikson, 1963), and to develop cognitive skills (Bruner, 1972; Piaget, 1962; Vygotsky, 1966). Sociocultural explanations include the development of social abilities (Parten, 1933; Smilanski, 1968), role development (Reilly, 1974; Shannon, 1974), and play's contribution to culture (Huizinga, 1950; Schwartzman, 1978). Johnson et al. (1999) identified three ways to consider play and development: (1) play reflects development; (2) play reinforces development; and (3) play is an instrument of developmental change.

Meaning

Play meaning refers to the quality of the experience or *to a person's state of mind*. The attitude a person assumes during play is usually termed playfulness. Liebermann (1977) felt that a person had an internal disposition to play that could be described along five dimensions: physical spontaneity, cognitive spontaneity, social spontaneity, manifest joy, and sense of humor. Barnett (1990, 1991) and Barnett and Kleiber (1982, 1984) further related playfulness to the development of cognitive abilities. In the occupational therapy literature, Bundy (1991, 1993) defined the qualities of playfulness as a person's intrinsic motivation, internal control, and the ability to suspend reality. These three elements are best expressed as continua, and "it is the sum contribution of these three elements that tips the balance toward play or nonplay, playfulness on nonplayfulness" (Bundy, 1993, p. 219). In addition to these three elements, children give and receive social cues to denote that they are playing.

Knox (1996), in a qualitative study of preschool children's play, identified actions and behaviors that characterized playful children. The playful children showed flexibility and spontaneity in their play and in social interactions, curiosity, imagination, creativity, joy, the ability to take charge of situations, the ability to build on and change the flow of play, and total absorption. Nonplayful children were less flexible and had difficulty with transitions or changes, expressed negative or immature affect or speech, often withdrew either physically or emotionally from play sequences, did not have control over situations, and tended to prefer adults or younger children for play.

Context

Play also obtains meaning through context. Children's activities can never be isolated from the environment within which they are playing, nor from familial, social, and cultural influences. The presence or absence of other persons, animals, the physical setting, and the availability of toys and other objects upon which to interact all have a profound effect on children's play (Figure 16-3). Play context includes cultural and societal expectations of play. Yerxa et al. (1989) stated, "The environment provides physical, psychological, social, cultural, and spiritual demands and resources" (p. 7).

A number of authors (Barnett & Kleiber, 1984; Bergen, 1988; Howes & Stewart, 1987; Jacobs & White, 1994) have studied the effects of the environment, quality of care, and types of interactions between caregivers and children on play behavior. They found that higher socioeconomic status correlated with greater levels of imaginary play, that permissive home environments encouraged creativity, and that high program quality improved children's social interaction and level of play. The variety of materials and opportunities for children to explore and interact with and their ability to control their activities were associated with improved quality of play. In addition, caregivers and peers who were emotionally and verbally responsive helped to improve the child's quality of play. Cultural and ecological factors also influence the way children play (Johnson Charlie, & Yawkey, 1999; Rubin et al., 1983). The cultural factors include child-rearing and parental influences, peer experiences, the physical environment, the schools, and the media (Figure 16-4). Ecological influences on play include the effects of stimulus novelty on play, object and material influences, play space density, and indoor versus outdoor play space.

All environments offer affordances and constraints to an individual's behavior. Knox (1974) and Michelman (1974) described factors in the environment that either promote or inhibit play. Factors that promote play include the availability of objects and persons, freedom from stress, provision of novelty, and opportunities to make choices. Factors that might inhibit play include external constraints, self-consciousness, too much novelty or challenge, limited choices, and over competition.

Contextual components that appear to promote play include (1) familiar peers, toys, and other materials; (2) freedom of choice; (3) adults who are nonintrusive or directive; (4) safe and comfortable atmosphere; and (5) scheduling that avoids times of fatigue, hunger, or stress (Rubin et al., 1983). These elements appear to facilitate playfulness (i.e., the expression of internal motivation and internal control to explore or pretend).

PLAY IN OCCUPATIONAL THERAPY

Play has always been a part of the pediatric occupational therapist's repertoire although its importance has altered over the years. Adolph Meyer (1922) wrote of work, play, rest, and sleep as being the four rhythms that shaped

FIGURE 16-3 Books are an early play activity even before the child is able to read. (Courtesy of Dianne Koontz Lowman.)

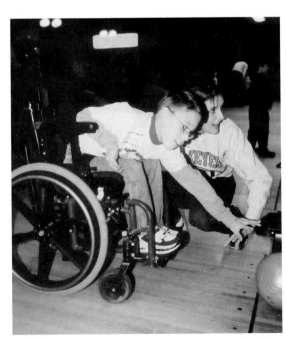

FIGURE 16-4 Mom's enthusiasm and encouragement add to the playfulness experienced in bowling. (Courtesy of Jill McQuaid.)

human organization. In one of the earliest articles on play in the occupational therapy literature, Alessandrini (1949) referred to play as a "serious undertaking, not to be confused with diversion or idle use of time. Play is not folly. It is purposeful activity, the result of mental and emotional experiences" (p. 9). Richmond (1960) spoke of play as the vehicle for communication and growth of the child. Play in the early years of occupational therapy was used for a variety of purposes such as diversion, development of skills, or for remedial purposes.

Mary Reilly was instrumental in bringing play into the forefront of occupational therapy in the late 1960s. She described play along a continuum that she called occupational behavior (Reilly, 1974). Through play, children learn skills and develop interests that later affect choices and success in work and leisure. Play is the arena for the development of sensory integration, physical abilities, cognitive and language skills, and interpersonal relationships. In their play, children practice adult and cultural roles and learn to become productive members of society (Bergen, 1988; Levy, 1978; Reilly, 1974). Reilly felt that play is a multidimensional system to adapt to the environment and that the exploratory drive of curiosity underlies play behavior. This drive has three hierarchical stages: exploration, competency, and achievement. Exploratory behavior is seen most in early childhood and is fueled by intrinsic motivation. Competency is fueled by effectance motivation, a term defined by White as an inborn urge toward competence (White, 1959). This stage is characterized by experimentation and practice in order to achieve mastery. Achievement is linked to goal expectancies and is fueled by a desire to achieve excellence. Using this frame of reference, other scholars studying under Reilly expanded the concepts of play. Florey (1971) offered a developmental framework of play and explored the concept of intrinsic motivation as being central to play. Takata (1969, 1974) developed a taxonomy of play and described play epochs based on Piagetian stages, and Knox (1974) examined play developmentally for the purposes of evaluation.

In researching the relationship between play and sensory integration, Clifford and Bundy (1989) found that children with sensory integration dysfunction differed in play scores on the Preschool Play Scale but that many of their play skills were within normal expectations. This led Bundy to conclude that there were other foundations for play than sensory integration or physical capabilities and that led into her studies on playfulness (Bundy, 1991, 1993, 1997).

Occupational science developed in the late 1980s as an academic discipline to study the nature of occupation and how it influences health. Because play is the primary occupation of children, a number of researchers have studied various aspects of play. Primeau (1995) studied parent-child routines and how play is orchestrated into daily routines. She proposed that parents use two types of play strategies: segregation and inclusion. In the segregated strategy, play times were separate from other daily routines; whereas in the inclusion strategy, play was incorporated into other daily routines. Parents use play routines to support their children's learning. Pierce (1991, 1997) studied object play of infants. She described three types of object rules learned by children: (1) object property rules (that is, the child's internal representation of the properties of objects); (2) object action rules (the repertoire of actions on the objects); and (3) object affect rules (those factors affecting object choice and keeping play enjoyable).

Knox (1999) expanded the concept of playfulness to study the play styles of preschool children. Four dimensions of play style were identified using grounded theory methods: preferences, attitudes, approach, and social reciprocity. Within these dimensions, elements of style were determined. Preferences included setting, toys, types of play, roles, and playmates. Attitudes included mood, consistency, and humor. Approach included direction, focus, and spontaneity. Social reciprocity included social orientation, responsivity, and flexibility. The children were described in terms of their unique play style and the elements of style were analyzed across the children. Knox found that play style differed among all the children and the way they approached play episodes was dependent on their play style.

PLAY ASSESSMENT

Even though play is considered the child's major occupation, and most occupational therapists would agree that it is important to the child, few therapists routinely evaluate it (Couch, 1996; Crowe, 1989; Lawlor & Henderson, 1989). Couch found that 62% of pediatric occupational therapists who responded to her questionnaire stated that they evaluated play, but less than 20% used criterion-referenced play assessments. Play was usually evaluated through clinical observations or as a part of developmental tests.

Play assessments are usually of four types: (1) those that assess skills in a particular area through play; (2) those that assess developmental competencies; (3) those that assess the way a child plays, including playfulness and play style; and (4) narratives.

Skills

Most of the play assessments described in the literature are designed to evaluate a particular skill area, such as cognition or social interaction. These assessments use structured play settings, materials, and activities or play observations. The assessments described here include those most often cited in the occupational therapy literature. Rosenblatt (1977) and Hulme and Lunzer (1966) assessed play in relation to language and reasoning. The

Piagetian stages of cognitive development have formed the basis of a number of play assessments (Rubin, Maioni, & Hornung, 1976; Smilanski, 1968). The classic assessment of the social aspects of play was developed by Parten (1933). She assessed social participation in play of preschool children by examining two dimensions: degree of participation and degree of leadership. Degree of participation included the social interaction during play and was rated as unoccupied, solitary, onlooker, parallel, associative, and organized supplementary play. Degree of leadership included how much the child depended on or directed others in play.

Development

A few assessments rate the developmental skills of the child through play. Linder (1993) developed a transdisciplinary play-based assessment that assesses the child in cognitive, social-emotional, language, physical, and motor development through naturalistic play.

Two assessments developed by occupational therapists explore play developmentally: the Play History (Takata, 1969, 1971, 1974) and the Knox Preschool Play Scale (Knox, 1968, 1974, 1997; Bledsoe & Shepherd, 1982). Takata described play developmentally within time and space and felt that play reflected the interaction between the individual and the external environment. The Play History is a semistructured interview and play observation, yielding information on the child's daily activity schedule. She identified two elements of play: form and content. Form parallels changes in development and includes the choice of play materials, amount and nature of playfulness, and organization in play. Content reflects life's situations and is the expression of the child's immediate needs, impulses, and physical and emotional state. Takata developed a taxonomy of play epochs based on the Piagetian stages in order to analyze the interview and play observation. Behaviors are classified as evident, not evident, encouraged, and not encouraged. As a result of the analysis, a play prescription can be developed. Behnke and Fetokovich (1984) conducted reliability and validity studies on the Play History and found it to be a reliable and valid instrument for assessing children's play behavior.

The Knox Preschool Play Scale (Knox, 1968, 1974, 1997) is an observational assessment designed to describe developmental skills as seen during play for children through 6 years of age. This assessment was revised by Bledsoe and Shepherd (1982) and more recently by Knox (1997). The scale describes play in terms of 6-month increments through age 3 and yearly increments through age 6. Four dimensions are examined: space management, material management, pretense/symbolic, and participation. Space management is the manner in which the child learns to manage his or her body and the space around him or her. Material management is the way in that the child manages material surroundings. The pretense/symbolic dimension is the way in which the child learns about the world through imitation and the development of the ability to understand and separate reality from make-believe. Participation is the amount and manner of social interaction. Children are observed indoors and outdoors and rated on all four dimensions. Bledsoe and Shepherd (1982) examined reliability and validity on the first revision with typically developing children. Harrison and Kielhofner (1986) did the same with children with disabilities. Both studies found the scale to be highly reliable and valid. Many studies have been conducted using the Knox Preschool Play Scale, and these have been summarized by Knox (1997).

Experience

The third way therapists assess play is to analyze the child's experience or state of mind when playing (i.e., playfulness and play style). Barnett (1990, 1991) devised a rating scale based on Liebermann's playfulness concepts. Children were rated on items representing the five playfulness traits: physical spontaneity, manifest joy, sense of humor, social spontaneity, and cognitive spontaneity.

Bundy (1993, 1997) developed the Test of Playfulness (ToP), designed to assess the individual's degree of playfulness. The scale contains 68 items representing four elements of playfulness, intrinsic motivation, internal control, ability to suspend reality, and framing; the child is rated on scales of extent, intensity, and skill. The ToP can be scored from direct observations or videotapes of children engaged in free play.

Advantages and Disadvantages of Evaluating Play

Observing children play is like looking through a window into their lives. An analysis of children's play is helpful in assessing their physical and cognitive abilities, social participation, imagination, independence, coping mechanisms and environment (Bergen, 1988; Brown & Gottfried, 1985, Garvey, 1977a). An evaluation of play and of the child's abilities as seen through play provides important information regarding the child's occupational performance as well as performance skills and patterns.

Play is most often evaluated in routine, self-chosen, familiar activities in naturalistic settings, providing the therapists with a picture of everyday competencies. Play assessments based on identifying what the child can do in play enable the therapist to focus on the child's abilities rather than the disabilities.

Some of the disadvantages to play assessments have been summarized by Kielhofner and Barris (1984), Knox (1999), and Bundy (1993). Because play is an interaction between the child and the environment, the human and physical factors in the environment can substantially influence the child's play (Knox, 1999). Play assessments that are designed to take place in standardized settings with standardized toys significantly alter and may inhibit the child's play. Additionally, since play specifies its own purpose, observed behaviors may have different meanings and serve different purposes for different people. It is difficult for an observer to assess the meaning of play to the participant.

Another limitation is in the amount of time one observes the child. The therapist must determine if the sample of behavior is sufficient, typical, and representative of true play. Knox (1999) found that over a prolonged time, a child's play could be vastly different at different times. Also, children engaged in play episodes for prolonged times (up to one hour in some cases). In order to capture a variety of play behaviors, a therapist needs to observe a child multiple times and in a variety of settings.

Interpreting Play Assessments

Assessment of play should be a part of every occupational therapy evaluation in order to get a complete picture of an individual's competence in his or her occupational performance and to adequately plan intervention that focuses on helping that individual participate in meaningful and self-satisfying occupations. Such assessments provide the therapist with a picture of how the individual uses play in his or her daily life. In the child, an analysis of play also provides the therapist with a picture of the child's skills in motor, cognitive, and social areas (Figure 16-5). This is especially helpful when assessing a child who does not respond well to standardized developmental testing.

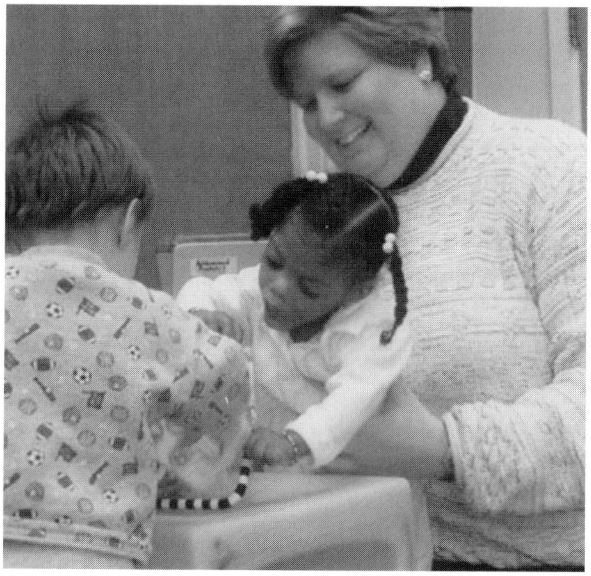

FIGURE 16-5 The occupational therapist assesses motor, cognitive, and social skills during a play activity. (Courtesy of Jayne Shepherd.)

Some of the newer assessments of affect, playfulness, or play style indicate how the individual approaches and gives meaning to the gamut of activities during the day. These instruments hold much promise in helping to determine how an individual balances his or her daily occupations in a meaningful way.

Evaluation in occupational therapy leads to intervention planning. Intervention should capitalize on abilities of the individual as well as remediate the deficits. Knowledge of the individual's skills, interests, and play style assists in this planning and guides treatment. Bundy (1993) offered a number of considerations when observing an individual's play that are useful in developing treatment goals. These include the following:

- In what activities does the child become totally absorbed?
- What does the child get from these activities?
- Does the child engage routinely in activities in which he or she feels free to vary the process, product, and outcome in whatever way he or she sees fit?
- Does the child have the capacity, permission, and support to do what he or she chooses to do?
- Is the child capable of giving and interpreting messages that "this is play; this is how you should interact with me now"?

CONSTRAINTS TO PLAY

As discussed earlier, play is always influenced by the environment. The effects of the environment on play can be seen in children who have experienced neglect or long hospitalizations. Extreme examples of constraints to play have been seen in some of the reports of children in Romanian orphanages (Cermak, 1996). These children showed severe sensory problems, extreme delay in developmental skills, and difficulties in interacting with others. Other characteristics of the play of deprived children included self-stimulation, limited repertoire of activities, decreased social play, and either increased or decreased fantasy play.

When children were hospitalized, they often experienced stress of separation, fear of illness, painful procedures, enforced confinement, and disruption of routines (Kaplan-Sanoff, Brewster, Stillwell, & Bergen, 1988). Some of the effects on play behavior included regression to earlier stages of development; decreased endurance and movement; decreased attention span, initiative, and curiosity; decreased resourcefulness and creativity; qualitatively less playful, decreased affect; and increased anxiety (Kielhofner, Barris, Bauer, Shoestock, & Walker, 1983).

Knox (1999), in her study of play styles of preschool children, discussed the importance of the environment on children's play. She found that when children's play styles matched the expectations of the environment, play flourished. When there was a mismatch between play style and the environment, play was stifled.

Effects of Disability on Play Behavior

The play of children with varying disabilities has been described often in the literature (Kaplan-Sanoff et al., 1988; Mogford, 1977). However, problems arise when generalizing across or within disabilities. Children are individuals and respond uniquely in different situations, even if they have a disability. Descriptions of the play of children with disabilities must be interpreted cautiously (Kaplan-Sanoff et al.). While it is helpful to examine some of the problems that certain conditions may impose on the child, in actual practice, each child must be considered individually. Bundy (1993) stated that although a child's play may not be typical, it was more important for "children to be good at what they want to do" (p. 218).

Some diseases and conditions limit physical interaction with the environment, with toys and other objects, and to some extent with people. The child with a physical impairment may display limited movement, strength, and pain when performing daily activities. Social contacts with family and peers may be disrupted by hospitalizations. The play characteristics of children with physical limitations may include fear of movement, decreased active play, and preferences for sedentary activities. The child may also have problems with manipulating toys and show decreased exploration (Figure 16-6). Opportunities for social play are often decreased due to

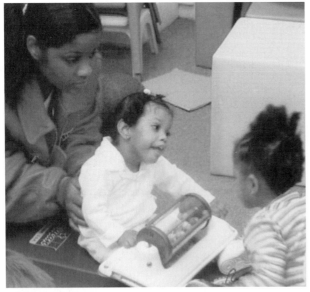

FIGURE 16-6 Impaired fine-motor skills limit exploratory play of this infant with cerebral palsy. Toys that activate to imprecise (full arm) movements are a good choice in play activities. (Courtesy of Jayne Shepherd.)

hospitalizations or routines that do not allow for social interaction (Johnson et al., 1999).

Children with cognitive impairment, such as those with mental retardation, often show delayed or uneven skills, difficulty in structuring their own behavior, or lack of sustained attention. These characteristics may be manifested in play in preferences for structured play materials, limited or inflexible play repertoires, decreased curiosity, destructive or inappropriate use of objects, decreased imagination, decreased symbolic play, decreased social interaction, decreased language, and increased observer play (Kaplan-Sanoff et al., 1988; Mogford, 1977). These children may need more structure and external cues in order to develop their play skills.

A number of studies have examined the effects of sensory impairment on play, particularly of children with visual or hearing impairments. Kaplan-Sanoff et al. (1988) and Mogford (1977) described how children with visual impairment have delays in developing an integrated perception of the world due to lack of vision and delayed motor exploration of surroundings and of objects. The play characteristics of these children are difficulty in constructive play, delays in developing complex play routines with others, and decreased imitative and role play.

The child with a hearing impairment is believed to have problems with decreased inner language, decreased social interactions, and decreased understanding of abstract concepts. These are manifested in play in that imagination becomes more restrictive with age and increased time is spent in noninteractive construction play. Children with hearing impairments demonstrate decreased symbolic play and increased solitary play (Kaplan-Sanoff et al., 1988; Mogford, 1977).

Children who have difficulty interpreting and integrating sensory input often have a limited or distorted perception of themselves and of their world, decreased ability to plan and execute motor and cognitive tasks, and poor organization of behavior. Play characteristics of these children include either excessive movement or avoidance of movement, decreased exploration, decreased gross motor or manipulative play, increased observation or solitary play, increased sedentary play, a restricted repertoire of play, resistance to change, distractibility, or destructiveness (Ayres, 1972, 1979; Bundy, 1991; Mogford, 1977).

Children with autism have severe sensory integrative problems as well as social and language deficits. Their play is characterized by lack of inner and expressive language, stereotyped movements or types of play, decreased imitation and imagination, lack of variety in play repertoires, motor planning problems, decreased play organization, decreased manipulation of toys, decreased construction and combining of objects, and decreased social play (Baranek, Reinhartsen, &

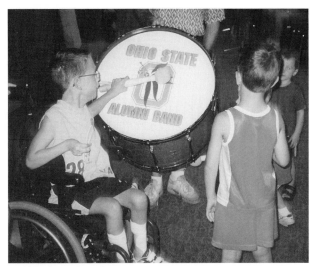

FIGURE 16-7   Michael, who has cerebral palsy, participates in the pregame rally by playing the drum. (Courtesy of Jill McQuaid.)

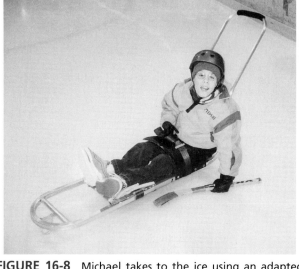

FIGURE 16-8   Michael takes to the ice using an adapted sled. (Courtesy of Jill McQuaid.)

Wannamaker, 2001). Children with autism appear to have a fundamental deficit in play greater than what would be expected when examining specific skills.

Children with cerebral palsy show difficulties in many areas (Figure 16-7). They may show limited and abnormal movement, sometimes have decreased cognitive abilities, may have sensory impairments, and often lack opportunities for social play (Finnie, 1975). In play, cognitive abilities are the most decisive factor in limiting play and children with good cognitive abilities can make adaptations to their physical limitations. Other problems include decreased physical interaction with environment and less interactive play time (Blanche, 1997).

Most of the studies of the play of children with disabilities stress the obstacles that the disabling conditions place on the children. Mogford (1977) summarized the problems that different disabling conditions have on children's play by stating that all children with disabilities have one thing in common—their ability to explore, interact with, and master the environment is impaired, depriving them of a normal childhood experience. The occupational therapy practitioner needs to explore supports for play. With adaptations, a child can overcome great obstacles in order to engage in a favorite activity.

PLAY IN INTERVENTION

What differentiates free play from therapeutic play? Free play is intrinsically motivated, fun, and is performed for its own sake rather than having a purpose. The child directs the play. However, in therapy, goals and objectives are established by the therapist and parents and they usually direct the play. When external constraints are placed on play, it is perceived as work and no longer contains playful elements. How then can play be used successfully in treatment? Rast (1986) stated:

> Play offers a practical vehicle to enlist a child's attention, to practice specific motor and functional skills, and to promote sensory processing, perceptual abilities, and cognitive development. It also serves to support social, emotional, and language development. In the therapeutic setting, play often becomes a tool used to work towards a goal, despite the fact that the goal-oriented, externally controlled aspects of the therapy situation conflict with the essence of play itself. (p. 30)

For play to be used successfully in intervention, the child should feel that he or she is choosing or directing the play episode. This is particularly important when the goal is to increase competence in play development. Play and leisure activities are important methods for promoting a child's performance and skills because they have meaning to the individual.

In a study by Couch (1996) investigating how pediatric occupational therapists use play in intervention, 91% of the therapists rated play as very important. For 95% of the respondents, play was primarily used to elicit motor, sensory, or psychosocial outcomes; only 2% used play as an outcome by itself. The therapists also primarily used adult-directed play versus child-directed play.

The way play is utilized in intervention is influenced by a number of factors: the therapist's frame of reference, the institution's emphasis on improving performance components and skills, and the family's values and concerns for the physical aspects of the child's disability.

Goals and objectives are established depending on how the child's disability affects his or her daily occupations and on analysis of occupational performance (AOTA, 2002). Play and leisure activities are used in occupational therapy in three ways: (1) as intervention modalities (to improve specific skills), (2) as an intervention goal (to improve play occupations), and (3) to facilitate playfulness.

Play as a Modality

Three frames of reference that use **play as a treatment modality** are the developmental, functional, and sensory integrative approaches. Play is most often used when a specific skill needs to be taught or when a specific goal needs to be met. Goals and objectives are established depending on how the disability affects the role performance of the child. Playful activities are used in a more structured or defined sense as a means to achieve the desired goal.

In the developmental frame of reference, play activities are used to develop physical, cognitive, emotional, or social abilities. The play materials are used to entice the child, such as when a toy is used to encourage a child to crawl or when a busy box is used to teach cause and effect concepts. Difficulty preserving the qualities of play may arise when therapy goals or techniques require a more structured "hands on" approach, such as when using a neurodevelopmental treatment technique. Use of play as a modality requires skill and imagination on the part of the therapist to combine approaches successfully and creatively. Anderson, Hinojosa, and Strauch (1987) and Blanche (1997) provided helpful suggestions for incorporating play into neurophysiological treatment approaches. Pierce (1997) described how objects can be used to develop children's negotiation in space, to address developmental goals, and to motivate children. Baranak et al. (2001) provided play engagement strategies for children with autism. These strategies included respecting the child's sensory processing capacities, scaffolding play, using imitation and modeling, and expanding play routines. They also offered suggestions for optimizing attention and organization and augmenting communication.

In the functional frame of reference, play is also used to meet a therapeutic end by adaptation of the activity, environment, or in therapeutic handling of the child while he or she is engaged in the activity. For example, a child's favorite toy might be positioned in such a way to improve the child's range of motion or adapted to increase the child's strength. In this sense, play is often used as a motivator for action.

In sensory integration, play is valued as the arena through which sensory integration develops (Ayres, 1972, 1979). To play successfully, children must have adequate sensory integration and be able to make adequate adaptive responses to environmental demands. In therapy, the therapist sets up and manipulates the environment (setting, objects, people) so that the child can choose among activities that potentially offer the "just right" challenge. During treatment, the therapist constantly adjusts the environment, child, or activity to bring about successful adaptation. Bundy (1991) provided an excellent description of the role of play within a sensory integrative framework. She concluded:

> Play is a powerful tool for treatment. For many individuals, the most important byproduct of occupational therapy may be the improved ability to play. If it is carefully planned and conducted, therapy using the principles of sensory integration may be very helpful in facilitating the development of play. Likewise, play as a part of a well orchestrated treatment plan, can result in improvements in sensory integration. (p. 67)

Mack, Lindquist, and Parham (1982) synthesized the commonalities of play from the occupational behavior and sensory integrative viewpoints. They stated:

> In practice, both approaches deem the therapist responsible for structuring adaptive behavior from the child. Thus, the potency of the environment's influence on development is confirmed by both. But from neither perspective does therapy rely solely on environmental manipulation. The child's initiative and active involvement are critical to the therapeutic process. From both perspectives, the intrinsic motivation or self direction of the child is primary in guiding therapy, for importance is placed on the child's inner drive toward mastery. Play, then, is the process through which therapeutic goals are achieved. (p. 367)

Play as an Intervention Goal

Burke (1993) stated, "An occupation-based view of play is built on basic notions concerning the importance of an occupation to an individual" (p. 201). The use of play as an intervention goal has been described within the occupational science and sensory integration frames of reference and most recently in the AOTA Practice Framework (AOTA, 2002). In occupational behavior and science, play is viewed as an occupation, determined by the individual and his or her interaction with the environment. The improvement of play skills and playfulness enables competent interaction with the world. Parham and Primeau (1997) stated that enhancement of play itself may be effective in promoting health and well-being.

In Primeau's (1995) study of play patterns in families, she suggested that parents modify the environment, incorporate play into the family's routine, and provide verbal suggestions to improve and increase the child's play. Knox (1999) emphasized the importance of considering children's play styles in choosing or setting up play environments.

Facilitating Playfulness

The third way play is used therapeutically is to facilitate playfulness in the child. As was stated in the section on assessment of play and leisure, often what individuals play with and how they play may not be as important as the affective quality of their play. Some children with significant or multiple disabilities manage to get great joy and benefit out of play. On the other hand, therapists often see children who are not playful and do not derive pleasure out of even the simplest play interaction. Facilitating playfulness in the child can be an important goal of therapy. Morrison and Metzger (2001) stated:

> The more playful child may generalize this flexible approach into environmental interaction beyond play and into other aspects of his or her life. For the child with a condition that impedes his or her ability to interact with the social or physical environment, a flexible (playful) approach may enable the child to succeed more frequently in these difficult situations. (p. 540).

Parham (1992) suggested strategies that a therapist can use to create a playful atmosphere. The therapist should express a playful attitude through speech, body language, and facial expressions (Figure 16-9). Also novelty and imaginary play should be used to facilitate playful participation on the part of the child. Bundy (1991) stated that the therapist must know how to play in order to be able to model play for the child. To develop playfulness, the child must develop intrinsic motivation, internal control, ability to suspend reality, and ability to give and read cues.

Facilitating playful interactions is important for any age child with or without disability. Holloway (1997) suggested strategies to encourage playfulness in parents and children within a neonatal intensive care unit. Helping parents learn to read their infant's cues and adapt to their infant's behavioral tempo helps to develop mutually positive experiences that form the basis for playful processes as the infant matures.

Whether the goals of therapy are to use play as media, to develop play skills, or to develop playfulness, planning intervention must always take into account the interaction among the therapist, the child, and the equipment and play objects in the environment. The therapist needs to create a playful atmosphere and attitude in order for the child to respond playfully. Six abilities important to facilitating play in a child appear to be that the adult can (1) apply theories of play, (2) analyze activities, (3) let go and let the child lead, (4) empathize, (5) demonstrate spontaneity, and (6) display creativity (Knox, Ecker, & Fitzsimmons, 2004). Their program focuses on helping therapists and parents follow the child's lead and develop

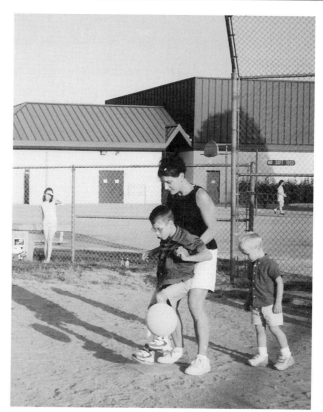

FIGURE 16-9 Mom adapts kickball so that Michael can play with his brother. (Courtesy of Jill McQuaid.)

the spontaneity and creativity necessary to weave play and therapy together.

Knowing what is motivating and pleasurable to the child is essential in order to accomplish goals through play episodes. Knox and Mailloux (1997) stated "When the therapist can make the match between an activity that is highly conducive to achieving a goal and is at the same time attractive to the child as a play experience, then the achievement of goals through play is most likely to occur" (p. 198).

Adaptations

Critical to creating a play atmosphere for children is considering the environment and the objects within it. Environmental spaces, toys, and equipment should have some flexibility in usage in order to foster play. In addition, toys and play equipment may need to be adapted in order for the child to access them optimally. Adaptation of toys and the environment is an important role of the occupational therapist, particularly for the severely involved child. Play spaces should offer a variety of experiences and allow for creativity, illusion, change, and chance. Children need to be able to control the space in terms of having objects, toys, and people to move and change, and also must have freedom to move (Chandler, 1997). The therapist must know the properties of toys as well as how to adapt them appropriately. Switches, adaptive keyboards, or provisions for sensory impairment may be necessary in order for the child to benefit from and be more independent in play. Play can be enhanced through a variety of augmentative devices ranging from very simple adaptations to complex electronic devices (Deitz & Swinth, 1997).

Parent Education and Training

Working with parents in relation to play is vitally important if there is to be carryover of the skills and abilities learned in therapy into the child's everyday life. Parents of children with disabilities often attempt to structure therapy into the child's routines. Children with physical disabilities may be involved in therapeutic regimens throughout the day and consequently are deprived of play opportunities. Four barriers to free play include (1) limitations imposed by caregivers, (2) physical and personal limitations of the child, (3) environmental barriers, and (4) social barriers (Missiuna & Pollock, 1991). Interventions that support the child's free play and include recommendations about playthings recognize the importance of play to overall development.

A goal of therapy is parent education—that is, helping parents to understand the importance of play for their child and helping them to interact with their child playfully. Often the parents need help in knowing how to create a balance between doing things for their child and allowing the child to form and carry out his or her own intentions. The therapist may need to model play behavior for the parent, encourage the parent to enter into and contribute to play sequences without directing or controlling them, and help the parent organize or adapt the play environment to meet the needs of the child. By actively involving the parents or caregivers, the therapist helps them appreciate their child's strengths, learn the fun of playing with their child, and develop play skills that will serve them well.

Hinojosa and Kramer (1997) stressed the importance of helping families to incorporate play into their lifestyles in order to strengthen interaction with their children and provide typical childhood experiences. They offered a framework for analyzing and understanding family play and provide suggestions to facilitate the inclusion of all members of the family in playful activities.

CASE STUDY

Ellen is a 1-year 3-month-old girl who was referred for home-based occupational therapy for developmental delay. She was born 1 month premature. She has a history of feeding problems with reflux following meals and when she gets upset. At the time she was referred, the reflux had partially resolved with small frequent feedings and positioning; however, her mother was reluctant to let her get upset, as she was afraid Ellen would vomit. Ellen is an only child and she lives with her parents in a single-family home.

Ellen's mother was interviewed using the Play History to provide information about her environment, daily schedule, and play experiences and interactions. She was also evaluated with the Knox Preschool Play Scale to provide information about developmental skills as observed in free and facilitated play. Ellen's mother's primary concerns were her reflux, her developmental skills, and that she did not know how to play with Ellen. Other mothers seemed to know what to do with their children, and she did not. Her preferred play with Ellen was to read her books.

The information gathered on the Play History is analyzed in terms of what is evidenced or not evidenced in the home environment and what is encouraged or discouraged by her parents. The child's play is compared to the appropriate "epoch" for her age. Ellen's play status worksheet is depicted in Box 16-1.

The information on the Knox Preschool Play Scale is described in terms of four dimensions: space management, material management, pretense/symbolic, and participation. Ellen's play age in each of the dimensions is described in Box 16-2.

Physical or neurological conditions were not interfering with her development, and it was felt that her delayed skills were due primarily to lack of experience or stimulation. Her feeding problems were resolving. Her home environment was conducive to play in terms of space, objects, and people. The parent-child relationships were warm and loving; however, her mother recognized that she had trouble stimulating Ellen and she was eager to learn.

Ellen's weaknesses included the following: Ellen was behind in all areas of development. She showed some mild hypersensitivities to tactile and auditory sensory stimuli. Ellen's mother lacked expertise and knowledge in facilitating development. She was apprehensive about Ellen's reflux and rarely allowed Ellen to challenge herself or get upset. Ellen's mother had few social and emotional supports.

The following goals were established for treatment: (1) improve developmental skills through play; (2) improve play and playfulness; (3) enable Ellen's mother to play with her, incorporate play into their daily routines, and scaffold play to encourage new skills and abilities; and (4) increase Ellen's mother's knowledge of developmentally appropriate play.

The intervention plan included weekly sessions with Ellen and her mother to teach them both play skills and playfulness. Her mother was also encouraged to seek out other resources in the community such as Mommy and Me classes and gym classes. She was also encouraged to

BOX 16-1 Play Status Worksheet

Expected Description
Epoch: Sensorimotor
Emphasis: Toys, objects for sensory experiences; cause and effect; container play; trial and error; gross motor—stand, sit, walk, pull, climb, pick up; fine motor—bang, carry, open/close, put in and take out, push, pull, relate two objects; people—parents, familiar adults; imitation—of simple actions; setting—home, yard

Evidence	Encouraged
Moderate variety of toys; blocks, nesting and stacking toys, books, stuffed toys, rattles, busy boxes, balls Freedom around the house for ambulation and exploration; generally plays in the bedroom, family room, and kitchen Generally likes to play in the same room as mother Outside grassy area available but not used much Long attention span for toys	Mother encourages looking at books while she reads to Ellen Watches *Sesame Street* Water play in tub with father; wading pool Rough-housing with father Container play, stacking, ball play Warm, loving relationship with both parents

No Evidence	Discouraged
Mother feels that she doesn't have the imagination or know-how to alter activities to meet Ellen's needs Little domestic play or imitative play Hypersensitive to grass and other textures, certain sounds, music Mother's major concerns have been with Ellen's physical growth, nourishment, and vomiting; as a result, she rarely lets Ellen cry or try things that might frustrate her	Little guiding of play or active participation in play on part of mother Little verbalizing during play by mother; doesn't encourage Ellen's verbalizations Concrete steps (3) leading out of house to patio; Ellen isn't allowed to creep up or down them yet

BOX 16-2 Knox Preschool Play Scale

SPACE MANAGEMENT: 6- TO 12-MONTH LEVEL
Ellen crawls, pulls to stance, and cruises. She sits with good balance and easily shifts weight in sitting. She plays in either sitting or supported stance against the coffee table. She is beginning to stand unsupported but flops down when balance is challenged. She walks with support from an adult.

MATERIAL MANAGEMENT: 12 TO 18 MONTHS
Ellen puts toys in and out of containers. She pulls and pushes, opens and shuts, bangs, stacks, and puts simple toys together. She puts together familiar single shape puzzles.

PRETENSE/SYMBOLIC: 12-MONTH LEVEL
Ellen imitates simple actions and novel movements. She is beginning to imitate schemas such as putting a spoon to the doll's face.

PARTICIPATION: 12 MONTHS
Ellen seeks attention from adults and seems to need the attention in order to prolong her play. She imitates, shows toys and shares toys. There is very little language.

set up play dates with other mothers. Ellen's father was included whenever he was available.

Both Ellen and her mother made striking gains with therapy. Ellen's development improved and she became very playful with both her mother and the therapist. Her mother became an active participant in the therapy sessions and became involved in community activities. Individual therapy was terminated when Ellen and her mother enrolled in an early intervention program. A few months later, the therapist visited Ellen and her mother and was pleased with her progress. Ellen was speaking a few words, and she showed the therapist some of the toys and games she played with her mother. Ellen's mother also seemed much happier and appeared to enjoy her daughter more. The experiences they described were typical, playful, and rewarding for both of them.

In this case, play was the primary goal as well as the therapeutic media used. It illustrates how effective an occupation-based approach can be.

STUDY QUESTIONS

1. Explain why the study of play is important to pediatric occupational therapists.
2. Describe play form, function, and meaning.
3. List the six characteristics of play.
4. Why is assessment of play important?
5. Describe three assessments of play developed by occupational therapists.
6. Describe the three ways play is used in treatment.
7. In Ellen's case, why was it so important to include her mother in the therapy?

REFERENCES

Alessandrini, N. (1949). Play—a child's world. *American Journal of Occupational Therapy, 3,* 9-12.

American Occupational Therapy Association. (2002). Occupational Therapy Practice Framework: Domain and process. *American Journal of Occupational Therapy, 56,* 609-639.

Anderson, J., Hinojosa, J., & Strauch, C. (1987). Integrating play in neurodevelopmental treatment. *American Journal of Occupational Therapy, 41* (7), 421-426.

Ayres, A.J. (1972). *Sensory integration and learning disorders.* Los Angeles: Western Psychological Services.

Ayres, A.J. (1979). *Sensory integration and the child.* Los Angeles: Western Psychological Services.

Baranek, G., Reinhartsen, D., & Wannamaker, S. (2001). Play: Engaging young children with autism. In R. Huebner (Ed.), *Autism: A sensorimotor approach to management* (pp. 313-351). Gaithersburg, MD: Aspen.

Barnett, L. (1990). Playfulness: Definition, design, and measurement. *Play and Culture,* 319-336.

Barnett, L. (1991). The playful child: Measurement of a disposition to play. *Play and Culture, 4,* 51-74.

Barnett, L., & Kleiber, D. (1982). Concomitants of playfulness in early childhood: Cognitive abilities and gender. *The Journal of Genetic Psychology, 141,* 115-127.

Barnett, L., & Kleiber, D. (1984). Playfulness and the early play environment. *The Journal of Genetic Psychology, 144,* 153-164.

Bateson, G. (1955). A theory of play and fantasy. *Psychiatric Research Reports, 2,* 39-51.

Behnke, C., & Fetokovich, M. (1984). Examining the reliability and validity of the play history. *American Journal of Occupational Therapy, 38,* 94-100.

Bergen, D. (1988). *Play as a medium for learning and development.* Portsmouth, NH: Heinemann.

Berlyne, D. (1966). Curiosity and exploration. *Science, 15,* 25-32.

Blanche, E. (1997). Doing with—not doing to: Play and the child with cerebral palsy. In L.D. Parham & L. Fazio (Eds.), *Play in occupational therapy for children* (pp. 202–218). St Louis: Mosby.

Bledsoe, N., & Shepherd, J. (1982). A study of reliability and validity of a preschool play scale. *American Journal of Occupational Therapy, 36* (12), 783-788.

Brown, C., & Gottfried, A. (Eds.) (1985). *Play interactions.* Skillman, New Jersey: Johnson & Johnson Baby Products.

Bruner, J. (1972). Nature and uses of immaturity. *American Psychologist, 27,* 687-708.

Bundy, A. (1991). Play theory and sensory integration. In A.G. Fisher, E.A. Murray, & A.C. Bundy (Eds.), *Sensory integration: Therapy and practice* (pp. 46-68). Philadelphia: F.A Davis.

Bundy, A. (1993). Assessment of play and leisure: Delineation of the problem. *American Journal of Occupational Therapy, 47,* 217-222.

Bundy, A. (1997). Play and playfulness: What to look for. In L.D. Parham & L. Fazio (Eds.), *Play in occupational therapy for children* (pp. 52-66). St. Louis: Mosby.

Burke, J. (1993). Play: the life role of the infant and young child. In J. Case-Smith (Ed.), *Pediatric occupational therapy and early intervention* (pp. 198-224). Boston: Andover Medical Publishers.

Caillois, R. (1958). *Man, play, and games.* New York: The Free Press of Glencoe.

Cermak, S. (1996). Ayres Memorial Lecture, presented at the Sensory International Annual Symposium, June 2, San Diego, CA.

Chandler, B. (1997). Where do you want to play? Play environments; an occupational therapy perspective. In B. Chandler (Ed.), *The essence of play* (pp. 159-174). Bethesda, MD: American Occupational Therapy Association.

Clark, F., Parham, D., Carlson, M., Frank, G., Jackson, J., Pierce, D., Wolfe, R., & Zemke, R. (1991). Occupational science: Academic innovation in the service of occupational therapy's future. *American Journal of Occupational Therapy, 45* (4), 300-310.

Clifford, J., & Bundy, A. (1989). Play preference and play performance in normal boys and boys with sensory integrative dysfunction. *Occupational Therapy Journal of Research, 9* (4), 202-217.

Cohen, D. (1987). *The development of play.* New York: New York.

Couch, K. (1996). *The role of play in pediatric occupational therapy.* Unpublished master's thesis, University of Washington, Seattle, WA.

Crowe, T. (1989). Pediatric assessments: A survey of their use by occupational therapists in northwestern school systems. *Occupational Therapy Journal of Research, 9,* 273-286.

Csikszentmihalyi, M., & Larson, R. (1984). *Being adolescent.* New York: Basic Books.

Deitz, J., & Swinth, Y. (1997). Accessing play through assistive technology. In L.D. Parham & L. Fazio (Eds.), *Play in occupational therapy for children* (pp. 219-232). St. Louis: Mosby.

Ellis, M.J. (1973). *Why people play.* Englewood Cliffs, NJ.

Erikson, E. (1963). *Childhood and society.* New York: Norton.

Finnie, N. (1975). *Handling the young cerebral palsied child at home* (2nd ed.). New York: E.P. Dutton & Company.

Florey, L. (1971). An approach to play and play development. *American Journal of Occupational Therapy, 25,* 275-280.

Franz, L. (1963). Introduction. In R. Hartley & R. Goldenson (Eds.), *The complete book of children's play* (pp. v-vi). New York: The Cornwall Press.

Garvey, C. (1977a). *Play.* London: Fontana/Open Books.

Garvey, C. (1977b). Play with language. In B. Tizard & D. Harvey (Eds.), *Biology of play.* Philadelphia: J.B. Lippincott.

Groos, K. (1976). The play of animals: play and instinct, and the play of man: Teasing and love play. In J. Bruner, A. Jolly, & K. Sylva (Eds.), *Play: Its role in development and evolution* (pp. 65-83). New York: Basic Books.

Harrison, H., & Kielhofner, G. (1986). Examining reliability and validity of the preschool play scale with handicapped children. *American Journal of Occupational Therapy, 40,* 167-173.

Hinojosa, J., & Kramer, P. (1997). Integrating children with disabilities into family play. In L.D. Parham & L. Fazio (Eds.), *Play in occupational therapy for children* (pp. 159-170). St. Louis: Mosby.

Holloway, E. (1997). Fostering parent-infant playfulness in the neonatal intensive care unit. In L.D. Parham & L. Fazio

(Eds.), *Play in occupational therapy for children* (pp. 171-183). St Louis: Mosby.

Howes, C., & Stewart, P. (1987). Child's play with adults, toys, and peers: An examination of family and child care influences, *Developmental Psychology, 23* (3), 423-430.

Huizinga, J. (1950). *Homo ludens*. Boston: The Beacon Press.

Hulme, I., & Lunzer, E.A. (1966). Play, language and reasoning in subnormal children. *Journal of Child Psychology and Psychiatry, 7,* 107.

Jacobs, E., & White, D. (1994). The relationship of child-care quality and play to social behavior in the kindergarten. In H. Goelman & E. Jacobs (Eds.), *Children's play in child care settings* (pp. 85-101). New York: State University of New York Press.

Johnson, J., Christie, J., & Yawkey, T. (1999). *Play and early childhood development.* New York: Longman.

Kaplan-Sanoff, M., Brewster, A., Stillwell, J., & Bergen, D. (1988). The relationship of play to physical/motor development and to children with special needs. In D. Bergen (Ed.), *Play as a medium for learning and development* (pp. 137-162). Portsmouth, NH: Heinemann.

Kielhofner, G., & Barris, R. (1984). Collecting data on play: A critique of available methods. *Occupational Therapy Journal of Research, 4* (3), 150-180.

Kielhofner, G., Barris, R., Bauer, D., Shoestock, B., & Walker, L. (1983). A comparison of play behavior in nonhospitalized and hospitalized children. *American Journal of Occupational Therapy, 37,* 305-312.

Knox, S. (1968). *Observation and assessment of the everyday play behavior of the mentally retarded child.* Unpublished master's thesis, University of Southern California, Los Angeles, CA.

Knox, S. (1974). A play scale. In M. Reilly (Ed.), *Play as exploratory learning* (pp. 247-266). Beverly Hills: Sage.

Knox, S. (1996). Play and playfulness in preschool children. In R. Zemke & F. Clark (Eds.), *Occupational science: The evolving discipline* (pp. 81-88). Philadelphia: F.A. Davis.

Knox, S. (1997). Development and current use of the Knox Preschool Play Scale. In L.D. Parham & L. Fazio (Eds.), *Play in occupational therapy for children* (pp. 35-51). St. Louis: Mosby.

Knox, S. (1999). *Play and playfulness of preschool children.* Unpublished doctoral dissertation, University of Southern California, Los Angeles, CA.

Knox, S., & Mailloux, Z. (1997). Play as treatment and treatment through play. In B. Chandler (Ed.), *The essence of play* (pp. 175-204). Bethesda, MD: American Occupational Therapy Association.

Knox, S., Ecker, C., & Fitzsimmons, L. (2004). *Play outside of the logical.* Paper presented at the Association for the Study of Play Conference, Atlanta, GA.

Lawlor, M., & Henderson, A. (1989). A descriptive study of the clinical practice patterns of occupational therapists working with infants and young children. *American Journal of Occupational Therapy, 43,* 755-764.

Levy, J. (1978). *Play behavior.* Malabar, FL: Robert E. Kruger.

Liebermann, J. (1977). *Playfulness: Its relationship to imagination and creativity.* New York: Academic Press.

Linder, T. (1993). *Transdisciplinary play-based assessment.* Baltimore: Paul H. Brookes.

Lindquist, J., Mack, W., & Parham, D. (1982). A synthesis of occupational behavior and sensory integrative concepts in theory and practice, part 2: Clinical applications. *American Journal of Occupational Therapy, 36,* 433-437.

Mack, W., Lindquist, J., & Parham, D. (1982). A synthesis of occupational behavior and sensory integrative concepts in theory and practice, part 1: Theoretical foundations. *American Journal of Occupational Therapy, 36,* 365-374.

McCree, S. (1993). *Leisure and play in therapy.* Tucson, AZ: Therapy Skill Builders.

Meyer, A. (1922). The philosophy of occupational therapy. *Archives of Occupational Therapy, 1,* 1-10.

Michelman, S. (1974). Play and the deficit child. In M. Reilly (Ed.), *Play as exploratory learning* (pp. 157-208). Beverly Hills, CA: Sage.

Miller, J. (1979). *Juvenile rheumatoid arthritis.* Littleton, MA: PSG.

Missiuna, C., & Pollock, N. (1991). Play deprivation in children with physical disabilities: The role of the occupational therapist in preventing secondary disability. *American Journal of Occupational Therapy, 45,* 882-888.

Mogford, K. (1977). The play of handicapped children. In B. Tizard & D. Harvey (Eds.), *Biology of play* (pp. 170-184). Philadelphia: J.B. Lippincott.

Morrison, C., & Metzger, P. (2001). Play. In J. Case-Smith (Ed.), *Occupational therapy for children* (4th ed., pp. 528-544). St Louis: Mosby.

Neulinger, J. (1981). *The psychology of leisure* (2nd ed.). Springfield, IL: Charles Thomas.

Neumann, E. (1971). *The elements of play.* New York: MSS Information.

Parham, D. (1992). Strategies for maintaining a playful atmosphere during therapy. *Sensory Integration Special Interest Section Newsletter, American Occupational Therapy Association, 15,* 2-3.

Parham, L.D., & Fazio, L.S. (1997). *Play in occupational therapy with children.* St. Louis: Mosby.

Parham, L.D., & Primeau, L. (1997). Play and occupational therapy. In L.D. Parham & L. Fazio (Eds.), *Play in occupational therapy with children.* St Louis: Mosby.

Parten, M. (1933). Social play among pre-school children. *Journal of Abnormal and Social Psychology, 28,* 136-147.

Piaget, J. (1952). *Play, dreams and imitation in childhood.* London: William Heinemann, Ltd.

Pierce, D. (1991). Early object rule acquisition. *American Journal of Occupational Therapy, 45,* 438-449.

Pierce, D. (1997). The power of object play. In L.D. Parham & L. Fazio (Eds.), *Play in occupational therapy for children* (pp. 86-111). St Louis: Mosby.

Primeau, L. (1995). *Orchestration of work and play within families.* Unpublished dissertation, University of Southern California, Los Angeles, CA.

Rast, M. (1986). *Play and therapy, play or therapy. Play: A skill for life.* Rockville, MD: American Occupational Therapy Association.

Reilly, M. (1974). *Play as exploratory learning.* Beverly Hills, CA: Sage.

Richmond (1960). Behavior, occupation and treatment of children. *American Journal of Occupational Therapy, 4,* 183-187.

Rosenblatt, D. (1977). Developmental trends in infant play. In B. Tizard & D. Harvey (Eds.), *Biology of play* (pp. 33-44). Philadelphia: J.B. Lippincott.

Rubin, K., Fein, G., & Vandenberg, B. (1983). Play. In P. Mussin (Ed.), *Handbook of child psychology,* Vol. IV (pp. 694-774). New York: John Wiley and Sons.

Rubin, K., Maioni, T.L., & Hornung, M. (1976). Free play behaviors in middle and lower-class preschoolers: Parten and Piaget revisited. *Child Development, 47,* 414-419.

Rubin, K.H. (1980). *Children's play.* San Francisco: Jossey-Bass.

Schiller, C. (1957). *Innate motor activity as a basis of learning, instinctive behavior.* New York: International Universities Press.

Schwartzman, H. (1978). *Socializing play: Functional analysis, transformations: The anthropology of children's play.* New York: Plenum Press.

Smilanski, S. (1968). *The effects of sociodramatic play on disadvantaged preschool children.* New York: John Wiley and Sons.

Takata, N. (1969). The play history. *American Journal of Occupational Therapy, 23* (4), 314-318.

Takata, N. (1971). The play milieu—a preliminary appraisal. *American Journal of Occupational Therapy, 25,* 281-284.

Takata, N. (1974). Play as a prescription. In M. Reilly (Ed.), *Play as exploratory learning* (pp. 209-246). Beverly Hills, CA: Sage.

Vygotsky, L. (1966). Play and its role in the mental development of the child. *Soviet Psychology, 12,* 62-76.

White, R. (1959). Motivation reconsidered: The concept of competence. *Psychological Review, 66,* 297-333.

Yerxa, E., Clark, F., Frank, G., Jackson, J., Parham, D., Pierce, D., Stein, C., & Zemke, R. (1989). An introduction to occupational science, a foundation for occupational therapy in the 21st century. *Occupational Therapy in Health Care, 6,* 1-17.

Prewriting and Handwriting Skills

Susan J. Amundson

Handwriting readiness
Functional written communication
Legibility
Domains of handwriting
Models of practice
Handwriting intervention outcomes

CHAPTER OBJECTIVES

1 Describe the role of the occupational therapist in the evaluation and intervention of children with handwriting difficulties.
2 Identify the factors contributing to handwriting readiness for young children.
3 Examine four aspects of functional written communication including the writing tasks in the classroom, legibility, speed, and ergonomic factors.
4 Discuss the student's performance skills, client factors, performance patterns, and context that influence his or her participation in the writing process.
5 Describe how handwriting fits into the educational writing process.
6 Develop remedial and compensatory strategies to improve a student's performance of written communication focusing on the actual occupation and the occupational context.
7 Examine the relationship of various pediatric occupational therapy models of practice and handwriting intervention programs.
8 Appreciate the need for gaining more evidence about the impact of occupational therapy intervention on children's handwriting.

INTRODUCTION

Occupational therapy practitioners view the occupations of children to be activities of daily living, education, work, play, and social participation. In the area of education, school-aged children's occupations encompass academic tasks, such as reading, writing, calculation, and problem-solving, as well as nonacademic or functional ones. Functional tasks might include navigating around classroom furniture and classmates, sharing school supplies with a peer, placing a notebook into a locker, constructing a papier-mâché globe, and writing words on paper—all of which support a student's academic performance in the classroom. These academic skills, functional abilities, and adaptive behaviors are expected to evolve and strengthen throughout a student's school years (Levine, 1994).

One common academic activity is writing, required when children and adolescents compose stories, complete written examinations, copy numbers for calculations, dictate telephone messages and numbers at home, and write messages to friends and family members. Although readily demanded of students, writing is a complex process requiring the synthesis and integration of memory retrieval, organization, problem solving, language and reading ability, ideation, and graphomotor function (Levine, 1994). The functional skill of handwriting supports the academic task of writing and allows students to convey written information legibly and efficiently while accomplishing written school assignments in a timely manner. Once developed, these skills continue to be used throughout adult life, as individuals write checks, schedule events on calendars, write directions to the dentist's office, scribble grocery lists, and jot down notes and messages to others.

Handwriting consumes much of a student's school day. McHale and Cermak (1992) examined the amount of time allocated to fine-motor activities and the type of fine-motor activities that school-aged children were expected to perform in the classroom. In their study of six classes consisting of two classes from grades 2, 4, and 6 in middle-income public schools, they found that 31 to 60% of the children's school day consisted of fine-motor activities. Of those fine-motor tasks, 85% of the time consisted of paper-and-pencil tasks, indicating that students may possibly spend up to one-quarter to one-half of their classroom time engaged in paper-and-pencil tasks.

When children are experiencing handwriting difficulty, problems with written assignments follow. Students with neurological impairments, learning problems, attention deficits, and developmental disabilities often expend enormous time and effort learning to write legibly (Amundson, 1992; Bergman & McLaughlin, 1988). School consequences of handwriting difficulties may include (1) teachers assigning lower marks for the writing quality of papers with poorer legibility but not poorer content (Chase, 1986; Sweedler-Brown, 1992), (2) students' slow handwriting speed limiting compositional fluency and quality (Graham, Berninger, Abbott, Abbott, & Whitaker, 1997), (3) students taking longer to finish assignments than do their peers (Graham, 1992), (4) students having problems with taking notes in class (Graham) and reading them later, (5) students failing to learn other higher-order writing processes such as planning and grammar, and (6) writing avoidance and, later, arrested writing development (Berninger, Mizokawa, & Bragg, 1991). Occupational therapists are frequently requested to evaluate handwriting when it interferes with a student's performance of written assignments. In fact, poor handwriting is one of the most common reasons for referring school-aged children to occupational therapy (Chandler, 1994; Oliver, 1990; Reisman, 1991). The role of the occupational therapist is to view the student's performance, in this case handwriting, by focusing on the interaction of the student, the school environment, and the demands of school occupations.

During the evaluation and intervention processes, the practitioner stays attuned to (1) the occupation of handwriting, determining which domains of handwriting (e.g., near-point copying or dictation) and which components (e.g., spacing or letter formation) are problematic for the student; (2) the school context (e.g., the curriculum or physical classroom arrangement related to the child's performance; (3) the student's personal context relating to cultural, temporal, spiritual, and physical features; and (4) the student's abilities, experiences, and performance skills that are interfering with handwriting production. Another role of the occupational therapist related to handwriting is the evaluation and intervention of children's prewriting and handwriting readiness skills (Oliver, 1990), particularly children of preschool and kindergarten age.

THE WRITING PROCESS

Writing Development of Children

Many children begin to draw and scribble on paper shortly after they are able to grasp a writing tool. As young children mature, they write intentionally meaningful messages, first with pictures and then proceed with scribbles, letter-like forms, and strings of letters (McGee & Richgels, 2000). The development of a child's writing process in the early elementary grades includes not only the mechanical and perceptual processes of graphics, but also the child's acquisition of language and the learning of spelling and phonology (Temple, Nathan, Temple, & Burris, 1993). Typically, children's writing and reading skills develop in a parallel process with one another (McGee & Richgels, 2000). Consequently, if a young child is unable to recognize letterforms and understand that these letterforms represent written language, occupational therapists and educators cannot expect the child to write.

As children develop, their scribbling and pictures evolve into the handwriting (i.e., language symbols) specific to their culture. Table 17-1 details the development of prewriting and handwriting in children in the United States. Age levels of handwriting progression listed are only approximations, as variation in skill development is to be expected among young children.

As for letter copying acquisition, very little information has been documented in the literature. One study by Tan-Lin (1981) examined the sequential stages of letter acquisition of 110 children between the ages of 3 and 5 years old. Children were observed copying numbers, letters, a few words, and a sentence three times over a period of four months. Her findings revealed the following sequential stages of prewriting and handwrit-

TABLE 17-1 Development of Prewriting and Handwriting in Young Children

Performance Task	Age Level
Scribbles on paper	10-12 months
Imitates horizontal, vertical, and circular marks on paper	2 years
Copies a vertical line, horizontal line, and circle	3 years
Copies a cross, right oblique line, square, left diagonal line, left oblique cross, some letters and numerals, and may be able to write own name	4-5 years
Copies a triangle, prints own name, copies most lowercase and uppercase letters	5-6 years

Modified from Bayley, N. (1993). *Bayley scales on infant development.* (Rev. ed.). San Antonio, TX: Psychological Corporation; Beery, K.E. (1982). *The Development Test of Visual-Motor Integration.* Cleveland: Modern Curriculum Press; Tan-Lin, A.S. (1981). An investigation into the developmental course of preschool/kindergarten aged children's handwriting behavior. *Dissertation Abstracts International, 42,* 4287A; Weil, M., & Amundson, S.J. (1994). Relationship between visual motor and handwriting skills of children in kindergarten. *American Journal of Occupational Therapy, 48,* 982-988.

ing: (1) controlled scribbles; (2) discrete lines, dots, or symbols; (3) straight-line or circular uppercase letters; (4) uppercase letters; and (5) lowercase letters, numerals, and words.

Handwriting Readiness

Some controversy exists as to when children are ready for formal handwriting instruction. Differing rates of maturity, environmental experiences, and interest levels are all factors that can influence children's early attempts and success in copying letters. Some children may exhibit handwriting readiness at 4 years of age while others may not be ready until they are 6 years old (Lamme, Laszlo & Bairstow, 1984). A number of authors (Alston & Taylor, 1987; Donoghue, 1975; Lamme; Wright & Allen, 1975) have stressed the importance of the mastery of handwriting readiness skills before handwriting instruction is initiated. These authors contend that children who are taught handwriting before they are ready may become discouraged and develop poor writing habits that may be difficult to correct later.

The readiness factors needed for handwriting require the integrity of a number of sensorimotor systems. Letter formation requires the integration of the visual, motor, sensory, and perceptual systems. Sufficient fine-motor coordination is also needed to form letters accurately (Alston & Taylor, 1987). Donaghue (1975) and Lamme (1979) identified six prerequisite skills of children necessary before handwriting instruction begins. These are (1) small muscle development; (2) eye-hand coordination; (3) the ability to hold utensils or writing tools; (4) the capacity to form basic strokes smoothly, such as circles and lines; (5) letter perception including the ability to recognize forms, notice likenesses and differences, infer the movements necessary for the production of form, and give accurate verbal descriptions of what was seen; and (6) orientation to printed language, which involves the visual analysis of letters and words along with right-left discrimination.

Other authors define readiness for handwriting on the basis of a child's ability to copy geometric forms. Beery (1992) and Benbow, Hanft, and Marsh (1992) suggested that instruction in handwriting be postponed until after the child is able to master the first nine figures in the Developmental Test of Visual-Motor Integration (VMI) (Beery, 1992, 1997). The nine figures are a vertical line, a horizontal line, a circle, a cross, a right oblique line, a square, a left oblique line, an oblique cross, and a triangle.

A study by Weil and Amundson (1994) examined 59 kindergarten children who were typically developing (aged 54 to 64 months) and their abilities to copy letterforms as well as the geometric designs on the VMI. The findings indicated that children who were able to copy the first nine forms of the VMI were able to copy significantly more letters than those who were not able to copy the first nine forms, thus providing support for the opinions of Beery (1992) and Benbow and others (1992).

Weil and Amundson (1994) also found that kindergarten children were, on average, able to correctly copy 78% of the letters presented, despite not having received formal handwriting instruction. Based on these results of the study, the authors concluded that most kindergarten children who are typically developing should be ready for actual handwriting instruction in the latter half of the kindergarten school year.

To develop children's handwriting readiness skills, the occupational therapy practitioner may incorporate activities into therapy sessions or the classroom. Selected activities should be aimed at improving fine-motor control and isolated finger movements, promoting prewriting skills, enhancing right-left discrimination, and improving orientation to printed language (Barchers, 1994; Benbow et al., 1992; Lamme, 1979; Myers, 1992; Wright & Allen, 1975).

Some children with significant cognitive or physical impairments may not acquire many of the prerequisite components needed for writing, and they are most successful in written communication using a computer with word processing and word prediction software programs. Other children, despite lacking the prerequisite components for handwriting, may be able to learn to write their name with drill and practice sessions. The occupational therapy practitioner must determine when it is appropriate for the child to work on prerequisite handwriting skills, the functional skill of handwriting, or both.

Activities are commonly used with young children to facilitate certain movements, experiences, and perception for handwriting development (Table 17-2). Movements and tasks to encourage handwriting development should be used in the context of what is meaningful and purposeful to the child.

Pencil Grip Progression

The development of pencil grip in young children follows a predictable course for typically developing children but may vary between cultures (Tseng, 1998). Children commonly begin by holding the pencil with a primitive grip. A primitive grip is characterized by holding the writing tool with one's whole hand or extended fingers, pronating the forearm, and using the shoulder to move the pencil. Later, a more transitional pencil grip is seen with the pencil being held with flexed fingers. Initially, the forearm is pronated (thumb side downward), but later the forearm is usually supinated. Finally, the mature pencil grip is marked with the pencil stabilized by the distal phalanges of the thumb, index,

TABLE 17-2 Activities to Promote Handwriting Readiness

Areas of Handwriting Readiness	Selected Readiness Activities
Improving fine-motor control and isolated finger movements	Roll one-quarter- to one-eighth-inch balls of clay or Silly Putty between the tips of the thumb and the index and middle fingers.
	Pick up small objects (e.g., Cheerios or raisins) with a tweezers.
	Pinch and seal a Ziplock bag using the thumb opposing each finger.
	Twist open a small tube of toothpaste with the thumb and index and middle fingers.
	Move a key from the palm to the fingertips of one hand.
Promoting graphic skills	Draw lines and copying shapes using shaving cream, sand trays, or finger paints.
	Draw lines and shapes to complete a picture story on blackboards.
	Form and color pictures of people, houses, trees, cars, or animals.
	Complete simple dot-to-dot pictures and mazes.
Enhancing right-left discrimination	Play "hokey-pokey."
	Maneuver through obstacles and focusing on the concept of turning right or left.
	Connect dots at the chalkboard with left-to-right strokes.
Improving orientation to printed language	Label children's drawings based on the child's description.
	Encourage book making with child's favorite topics (e.g., special places, favorite foods).
	Label common objects in the classroom.

middle, and possibly ring fingers, the wrist slightly extended yet dynamic, and the supinated forearm resting on the table (Erhardt, 1982; Rosenbloom & Horton, 1971; Schneck & Henderson, 1990; Tseng, 1998).

Traditionally, teachers and occupational therapy practitioners have stressed the importance of a dynamic tripod pencil grasp (Rosenbloom & Horton, 1971; Tseng & Cermak, 1993). The dynamic tripod grip appears with the writing utensil resting against the distal phalanx of the radial side of the middle finger while the pads of the thumb and index finger control it (Rosenbloom & Horton, 1971) (Figure 17-1). Recent studies (Bergmann, 1990; Dennis & Swinth, 2001; Koziatek & Powell, 2003; Schneck, 1991; Schneck & Henderson, 1990; Tseng, 1998; Ziviani & Elkins, 1984) have found that a variety of pencil grasp patterns exist among typical adults and children. Frequently observed mature pencil grips, besides the dynamic tripod grasp, include the lateral tripod, the dynamic quadripod, and the lateral quadrupod. Schneck and Henderson reported in their study of 320 children who were typically developing that by the age of 6.5 to 7 years old 95% of them had adopted a mature pencil grasp, either the dynamic tripod (72.5%) or the lateral tripod (22.5%). Outside of the United States, Tseng noted that the lateral tripod grip (42.9%) occurred almost as frequently as the dynamic tripod (44.1%) for typically developing Taiwanese children 5.5 to 6.4 years of age. In older elementary children, the dynamic quadrupod and lateral quadrupod grips have been identified as functional and mature pencil grasps (Dennis & Swinth; Koziatek & Powell). Thus, the lateral tripod, the dynamic quadrupod, and the lateral quadrupod grips may all be considered acceptable alternatives to the traditionally preferred dynamic tripod grip (see Figure 17-1).

HANDWRITING EVALUATION

When a child with poor handwriting has been referred to occupational therapy, the methods to gather evaluation information must be carefully selected and sequenced. An individual evaluation is needed as each child with handwriting dysfunction varies from every other child with handwriting problems. A comprehensive evaluation of a child's handwriting includes (1) examining written work samples; (2) discussing the child's performance with the teacher, parent, and other team members; (3) reviewing the child's educational and clinical records; (4) directly observing the child when he or she is writing in the natural setting (i.e., school, home); (5) evaluating the child's actual performance of handwriting; and (6) assessing any suspected performance skills interfering with handwriting.

Initially, the student's performance in the context of classroom standards should be the focus (before moving toward standardized testing). Assembling data and information from various sources gives the occupational therapist an integrated picture of the child's written communication. It also allows the therapist to examine the child's ability to perform other functional school tasks, such as handling school supplies and manipulatives, managing outdoor clothing and fasteners, and organizing school materials. Although poor handwriting is a common referring concern in the classroom, poor performance of other school tasks may have gone unnoticed and should also receive attention from the occupational therapist and educational team.

Work Samples

Oftentimes the referring person (e.g., the parent or educator) approaches the occupational therapist with the

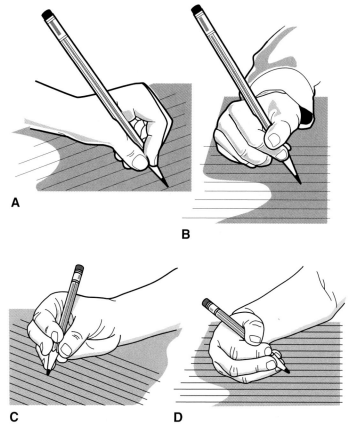

FIGURE 17-1 Elementary school children using mature pencil grips. **A,** Dynamic tripod; **B,** lateral tripod; **C,** dynamic quadrupod; and **D,** lateral quadrupod.

child's handwritten classwork or homework. Written work samples may include spelling lessons, mathematical problems, or a story. Ideally, these samples should represent a typical handwriting performance of the child. When reviewing the child's written product, a comparison of the writing samples of the child's peers is also warranted to understand the classroom standards and teacher expectations.

Interviews

Interviewing the child's parents, educator, and other team members serves as a mechanism for building rapport and gathering important data. Since teachers know a great deal about their students' performance in class, they can share information about the student's abilities and achievements, the classroom standards and curricula, and interactions with the student. A sampling of questions to facilitate discussion between the teacher and the occupational therapist is listed in Box 17-1. The educator can help provide a picture of the student's capabilities, behavior, and struggles at school.

Parents are also a valuable resource for occupational therapists; they provide a different perspective of the child and the child's handwriting abilities. Not only can parents relate the child's developmental, medical, and familial background to the educational team, they can

BOX 17-1   Questions to Facilitate Discussion among Educational Team Members

1   What are the student's educational strengths and concerns?
2   What is his or her handwriting performance in comparison with peers?
3   What handwriting method (D'Nealian, Zaner-Blöser, Palmer, italics) is being used and what is the student's history with this method?
4   What are the learning standards or curriculum of his or her grade?
5   What seems to be causing the poor handwriting?
6   When does he or she do his or her best written work?
7   When does the performance break down?
8   What strategies for improvement have been tried? Have they worked?
9   Is a student portfolio available on the student's writing development and progress?
10   Are there other daily tasks (e.g., using scissors, getting along with peers, keeping organized) that raise concern for the teacher?

share invaluable information about the child's interests, social competence, and attitudes toward learning and school.

Parents are considered educational team members, and they provide important perspectives that give the occupational therapist a comprehensive view of the child at home and at school. Questions asked of parents related to the child and his or her writing to facilitate discussion might include the following: (1) Do parents expect the child to complete school assignments or written work at home? (2) What is the child's response to written homework? (3) How does the child perform his or her written assignments at home, at school? and (4) What other writing tasks are expected of the child at home (e.g., corresponding with relatives, recording telephone messages)?

File Review

Relevant information regarding the child's past academic performance, special testing, or receipt of special services can be found in the referred child's educational cumulative file. Medical or clinical reports related to the child's education may also be located in the child's regular or special education files. The child's parents will be able to share academic records and reports with clinic- and hospital-based occupational therapists. This documentation may trigger further conversations among the child's parents and team members.

Direct Observation

Observing the student during a writing activity is an essential step in the evaluation process (Figure 17-2).

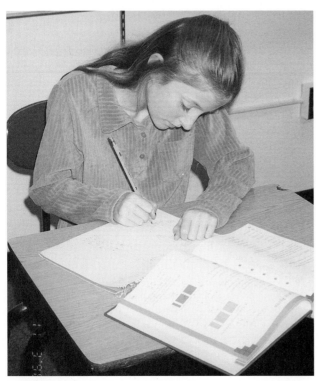

FIGURE 17-2 A girl completes a written assignment at her desk.

The referral of the child to occupational therapy is commonly made by the teacher or parent who observed the child struggling with handwriting. Thus, occupational therapists need to examine the child in this activity within the classroom. Skilled observation by the examiner usually occurs in the child's classroom and focuses on task performance, attention to task, problem solving, and behavior of the child (Hanft & Place, 1996). Practitioners also note the student's organizational abilities, movement through the classroom, interactions with the teacher and peers, transitions between activities, and overall performance of other school tasks. School contextual features (e.g., the classroom arrangement, lighting, noise level, and instructional media) as well as the actual instruction from school personnel should all be considered in relationship to the student's performance.

Besides a structured protocol for direct observation, questions for the occupational therapist might include the following:

1 Which writing tasks (for example, copying sentences from the chalkboard or composing a story) are most problematic for the child?
2 What behaviors are manifested when the child is required to write? For example, does the pupil chew on the eraser of the pencil or blow the pencil across the desktop to avoid writing?
3 Can the child engage in the task of writing independently, or does she or he need physical and verbal cues from the teacher or educational assistant?
4 Is the child easily distracted by visual and auditory stimuli during writing, such as the delivery truck driving by the school window?
5 Where does the child sit in the classroom?
6 What curriculum is being followed?
7 Where is the teacher located when he or she gives assignment directions?

MEASURING HANDWRITING PERFORMANCE

When evaluating the actual task of children's handwriting, the following areas need to be examined: (1) domains of handwriting, (2) legibility components, (3) writing speed, and (4) ergonomic factors. Whether the student writes in manuscript (print), cursive (joined script), or both, these four aspects will assist the educational team and parents to uncover problematic areas of handwriting and establish a baseline of handwriting function. With accurate and relevant handwriting assessment data, the occupational therapist, the child's parents, and the educational or clinical team will also be able to target specific goals and objectives for the development of written communication.

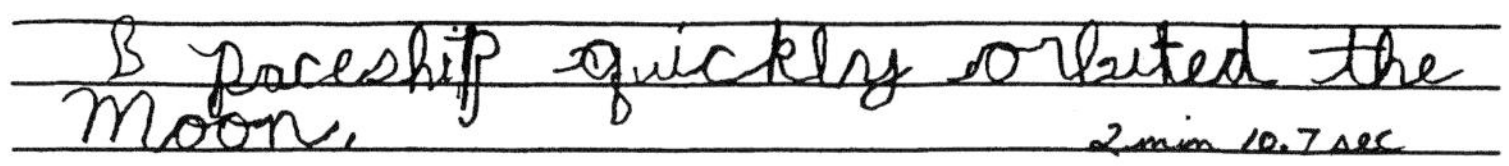

FIGURE 17-3 Cursive handwriting sample exemplifies improper letterforms and disproportionate letter size.

Domains of Handwriting

Evaluating the various domains of handwriting allows the occupational therapist to determine which tasks the child may be having difficulty with and address those tasks in the intervention plan. Handwriting tasks demanded of students, and helpful for intervention planning, include the following:

- Writing the alphabet in both uppercase and lowercase letters along with numbers requires the child to remember the motor engram, form each individual letter and numeral, sequence letters and numbers, and to use consistent letter cases.
- Copying is the capacity to reproduce numerals, letters, and words from a similar script model, either manuscript to manuscript or cursive to cursive.
- Near-point copying is producing letters or words from a nearby model, commonly on the same page or on the same horizontal writing surface as when an elementary pupil copies the meaning of a word from a nearby dictionary.
- Copying from a distant vertical model to the writing surface is termed far-point copying, demonstrated by early elementary students writing the words "Happy Valentine's Day" on construction paper cards from the teacher's modeled words on the class chalkboard.
- More advanced than copying, manuscript-to-cursive transition requires a mastery of letterforms in both manuscript and cursive as the child must transcribe manuscript letters and words to cursive letters and words. A higher-level handwriting task combining integration of auditory directions and a motoric response is dictation.
- Writing dictated words, names, addresses, and telephone numbers is a skill children will need at school and at home.
- Composition is the generation of a sentence or paragraph by the child demonstrated by writing a poem, a story, or a note to a friend. The composing process uses the cognitive functions of planning, sentence generation, and revision (Hayes & Flower, 1986); thus, this writing task involves complex integration of linguistic, cognitive, organizational, and sensorimotor skills.

Legibility

Legibility is often assessed in terms of its components (i.e., letter formation, alignment, spacing, size, and slant) (Alston, 1983; Amundson, 1995; Graham, Boyer-Shick,

Word legibility percentage =

$$\frac{\text{Total number of readable words}}{\text{Total number of written words}} = \frac{4}{8} = 50\%$$

FIGURE 17-4 Word legibility percentages are calculated using a simple mathematical formula.

& Tippets, 1989; Jackson, 1971; Ziviani & Elkins, 1984). However, the bottom line of legibility is readability. Of primary importance is whether what was written by the child can be read by the child, parent, or teacher. In a handwriting evaluation, both the components of legibility as well as readability need to be assessed.

The influence of legibility components on readability is significant (Graham et al., 1989; Jackson, 1971). In *letter formation*, Alston (1983) identified five features impacting legibility: (1) improper letterforms, (2) poor leading in and leading out of letters, (3) inadequate rounding of letters, (4) incomplete closures of letters, and (5) incorrect letter ascenders and descenders. *Alignment* or baseline orientation refers to the placement of text on and within the writing guidelines. *Spacing* includes the dispersion of letters within words and words within sentences (Larsen & Hammill, 1989) along with the text organization on the entire sheet of paper. Another component of legibility, *size* refers to the letter relative to the writing guidelines and to the other letters. Finally, the uniformity or consistency of the *slant* or the angle of the text should be observed. Figure 17-3 illustrates errors of letter formation and size in a child's cursive writing.

Although a child's writing sample may still be readable even though a legibility component (e.g., poor sizing) interferes with its appearance, some legibility components have a stronger impact on readability than others. Graham et al. (1989) found that the letter formation, spacing, and neatness of 61 grade 4 students with learning disabilities all significantly correlated with legibility. Typically, legibility is determined by counting the number of readable written letters or words and dividing it by the total number of written letters or words in a writing sample. For example, Figure 17-4 indicates the formula to determine word legibility percentage. As reflected in the figure, eight words were written in the child's writing sample; however, only four of them were legible, resulting in 50% word legibility.

Frequently, occupational therapy practitioners and educators want to determine what legibility percentage is appropriate for students at specific grade levels. Likewise, occupational therapists are interested in the "cut-off" legibility percentages for poor and good handwriting. The validity of readability and legibility percentages is reported in three studies with small samples.

Talbert-Johnson, Salva, Sweeney, and Cooper (1991) asked 15 upper-elementary, middle school, and high school students with special needs to copy a short passage in cursive writing. Through a sorting process, easy-to-read handwriting samples scored between 95 to 100% letter legibility with a mean of 99%. Conversely, difficult-to-read handwriting measured at 60 to 90% letter legibility with a mean of 78%. Reisman (1991) indicated that 51 second-grade students receiving handwriting intervention in occupational therapy averaged a 76% legibility rate on a pilot version of the Minnesota Handwriting Test. Recently, Graham, Berninger, Weintraub, and Shafer (1998), in their study of 900 children who were typically developing in grades 1 through 9, found that handwriting legibility showed little improvement in the first four elementary grades. Legibility gains were made in the upper-elementary grades and maintained through junior high school.

Most recently, Koziatek and Powell (2002) investigated four writing tasks from the Evaluation Tool of Children's Handwriting-Cursive (ETCH-C) with 101 grade 4 students. They found that the ETCH-C letter and word legibility scores were able to classify and predict children's handwriting grades on report cards. The 75% word legibility level of the ETCH-C could discriminate between satisfactory (A, B, C grades) and unsatisfactory cursive handwriting.

Although each of the above-mentioned studies examining legibility rates used different measures, implications for occupational therapy practice suggest that the range of 75 to 78% appears to discriminate between satisfactory and unsatisfactory handwriting legibility. This range of legibility percentages, however, is not the benchmark for which children warrant occupational therapy services. A student's handwriting legibility may be at the 75% legibility level and be unreadable. With recommended compensatory strategies from the occupational therapy practitioner, this same child might boost his or her handwriting into a readable text. Thus, no ongoing occupational therapy services may be needed. Determining appropriate educational and therapeutic services for children involves an entire team, including the child's parents, and, of course, should never be solely dependent on test scores. Thus, the occupational therapist must carefully and comprehensively assess the nature of the child's poor handwriting legibility and give recommendations based on this process.

Writing Speed

A child's rate of writing, or the number of letters written per minute, coupled with legibility are the two cornerstones of functional handwriting (Amundson, 1995). Students take longer to complete written assignments, have difficulty taking notes in class (Graham, 1992), lose their train of ideas for writing (McAvoy, 1996), and become frustrated when their handwriting speed is slower than their peers. Writing speed typically decreases when the amount of written work or complexity of the writing task increases (Rubin & Henderson, 1982; Weintraub & Graham, 1998). Upper-elementary and older students not only need an adequate writing speed but need to be able to adjust their speed from a hurried, rough draft to a neat, well-paced, final one (Weintraub & Graham).

Differences in methodologies, subjects, and data collection have resulted in a varied baseline of writing speeds for typically developing children (Tseng & Cermak, 1991; Ziviani & Elkins, 1984). Table 17-3 displays the

TABLE 17-3 Writing Speeds of Children (Letters Per Minute)

Grade	Graham et al. (1998) Girls	Graham et al. (1998) Boys	Hamstra-Bletz & Blöte (1990)	Phelps et al. (1984)	Ziviani & Elkins (1984)	Ziviani & Watson-Will (1998) Girls	Ziviani & Watson-Will (1998) Boys
1	21	17		32			
2	37	31	24	35		39	35
3	50	45	35	25	32	56	46
4	66	61	46	37	34	70	67
5	75	71	54	47	38	83	73
6	91	78	66	57	46	83	89
7	109	91		62	52	85	111
8	118	112		72			
9	121	114					

Graham, Berninger, Weintraub, & Shafer (1998): Copy a near-point paragraph for 1.5 minutes in preferred script of child. Hamstra-Bletz & Blöte (1990): Copy near-point paragraph for 5 minutes. Phelps, Stempel, & Speck (1984); Phelps & Stempel (1987): Copy 2 near-point sentences for 2 minutes. Ziviani & Elkins (1984): Copy phrase "cat and dog" repeatedly for 2 minutes in preferred script. Ziviani & Watson-Will (1998): Copy "cat and dog" repeatedly for 2 minutes in Australian modern script.

writing speeds of children in different studies of children's writing speeds, along with the methodologies used in each. All of the studies (Graham et al., 1998; Hamstra-Bletz & Blöte, 1990; Phelps & Stempel, 1987; Phelps, Stempel, & Speck, 1984; Ziviani & Elkins, 1984; Ziviani & Watson-Will, 1998) show that children's handwriting speeds develop gradually, becoming faster in each succeeding grade. However, the studies' findings also suggest that the increase in speed may not be linear but marked with various spurts and plateaus. Large ranges of handwriting speed per grade level are noted.

Due to the wide range of handwriting speeds, children's writing rates need to be considered individually within the context of their classroom. Teacher expectations and classroom standards may influence children's writing speeds. Thus, it's more appropriate to compare a student's writing speed performance with the rates of classroom peers. Generally, handwriting speed is problematic when a student is unable to complete written school assignments in a timely manner. When a student's written expression abilities (e.g., language, spelling) exceed handwriting rate, alternative forms (e.g., keyboarding, word prediction programs) should be considered.

Ergonomic Factors

Writing posture, upper-extremity stability and mobility, and pencil grip are all ergonomic factors that must be analyzed as the child writes. Sitting posture in the classroom should be observed. Does the child rest his or her head on the forearm or desktop when writing? Is the child falling and spilling out of his or her chair? Does the child stand beside the desk or kneel in the chair? Are the desktop and chair at suitable heights?

Stability and mobility of the upper extremities refer to the stabilization of the shoulder girdle, elbow, and wrist to allow the dexterous hand to manipulate the writing instrument. Does the child write with whole-arm movements? What are the positions of the trunk and writing arm? Does the nonpreferred hand stabilize the paper? Does the child apply excessive pressure to the writing tool?

An ergonomic focus for most occupational therapy practitioners is whether a child is holding his or her pencil properly or pencil grasp. Ziviani (1987) reported that different grasp variations are expected. Poor writers tend to demonstrate a greater variety of atypical grasp patterns than legible writers. Mature pencil grips of children now include the dynamic tripod, the lateral tripod, the dynamic quadripod, and the lateral quadrupod (Dennis & Swinth, 2001; Koziatek & Powell, 2003; Schneck & Henderson, 1990; Tseng, 1998). Unconventional pencil grips do not necessarily affect the speed or the legibility of a child's handwriting (Dennis & Swinth, 2001; Tseng & Cermak, 1993).

HANDWRITING INSTRUMENTS

Formal or standardized tests are important for assessing the performance of children, as they provide objective measures and quantitative scores, aid in monitoring a child's progress, assist professionals to communicate more clearly, and advance the field through research. Numerous standardized handwriting instruments are commercially available. Assessment tools commonly used by occupational therapists in the United States include the Children's Handwriting Evaluation Scale (Phelps et al., 1984), the Children's Handwriting Evaluation Scale-Manuscript (Phelps & Stempel, 1987), the Denver Handwriting Analysis (Anderson, 1983), the Minnesota Handwriting Test (Reisman, 1999), the Evaluation Tool of Children's Handwriting (Amundson, 1995), and the Test of Handwriting Skills (Gardner, 1998).

Each of these assessment tools possesses various features regarding domains of handwriting tested (e.g., far-point copying, dictation), age or grade of child (e.g., first and second grades), script examined (e.g., cursive), scoring procedures of the writing performance (e.g., legibility of manuscript), and scores obtained (e.g., percentiles). Typically, tests measure handwriting legibility and speed of handwriting. Scoring procedures for legibility use rating techniques ranging from global and subjective to detailed and specific (Tseng & Cermak, 1991). A description and publication information of handwriting instruments available to occupational therapists are presented in Appendix 17-A.

For tool selection, the occupational therapist should keep in mind the characteristics of each instrument as well as the strengths and limitations of the tests regarding normative data, reliability, validity, and other psychometric properties (see Chapter 8). Critiques and lengthier descriptions of handwriting instruments by several authors (Amundson, 1992; Daniels, 1988; Reisman, 1991; Tseng & Cermak, 1991) are worthy to consider when selecting the most appropriate test. A shortcoming of most handwriting instruments is the low reliability for measuring legibility due to the subjective nature of determining the readability of handwriting (Deikema, Deitz, & Amundson, 1998). The instrument chosen should match the areas of concern regarding the child's handwriting and should allow for effective intervention planning among the occupational therapist, the child's parents, and other team members.

Factors Restricting Handwriting Performance

To understand more fully which element might be interfering with a child's ability to produce text, the occupational therapist must consider a child's *performance skills, client factors, performance patterns,* and *contextual elements* (American Occupational Therapy Association,

2002). As occupational therapists build their clinical reasoning skills, they are able to observe a child struggling to write or view a child's distorted, unreadable handwriting and identify factors that might be interfering with the child's written communication. The following example indicates how various factors may restrict a child's handwriting performance. This example's complexity requires occupational therapists to be able to analyze the interactions of factors that influence children's occupations (e.g., handwriting).

Natasha, a 9-year-old girl with a traumatic brain injury, has an illegible script marked with overlapping letters, poor use of writing lines, and many dark erasures. When evaluating Natasha's writing performance in her classroom, the occupational therapist observes that her performance skills, particularly her fine-motor coordination, are limited. In-hand manipulation skills are poor as Natasha struggles to turn her pencil from the writing position to the erasing position, manages her worksheet, and uses her eraser for rubbing out errors. When she is engaging in classroom activities, the occupational therapist sees that Natasha has a short attention span and impulsiveness (client factors). Natasha has difficulty sustaining her attention to desktop work and the teacher's verbal instructions. Furthermore, when the occupational therapist examines a story that Natasha wrote earlier during the day, it's apparent that she has not incorporated the habit of writing her text on the lines of the paper. By not adopting this performance pattern, Natasha's text bumps above and below the writing baseline on her paper resulting in an unreadable story. Finally, the occupational therapist is told by a classroom paraprofessional that Natasha uses English as a second language due to her recent immigration to the United States. Consequently, the occupational therapy practitioner recognizes that her cultural context may be affecting her overall performance in the classroom.

As with Natasha, it's common for children with poor handwriting to have a web of factors restricting their handwriting performance. The occupational therapist must unravel each factor from the others to understand its influence as well as its interaction with other performance factors. For example, Natasha's client factors (i.e., short attention span, impulsiveness) and cultural context (i.e., English as a second language) are related and also interact with one another to restrict her handwriting performance. Natasha's short attention span not only diminishes her ability to learn handwriting but also her ability to learn new concepts including her second language, English. If she is unable to understand the language symbols, words, and syntax of the English language, she will have difficulty reading English. Furthermore, because reading and writing are parallel learning processes, Natasha's handwriting will be impeded. Natasha's handwriting is more likely to improve once effective compensatory and remedial techniques are in place to improve her attention span and her knowledge and use of the English language.

EDUCATOR'S PERSPECTIVE

Writing Process

When educators speak of the writing or composing process, they view it as a goal-directed activity using the cognitive functions of planning, sentence generation, and revision (Hayes & Flower, 1986). The actual text production occurs in sentence generation; thus, the child who needs to pay considerable attention to the mechanical requirements of writing may interrupt higher-order writing processes, such as planning or content generation. Hence, most educators view the mechanical requirements of handwriting as an integral subset of the writing process.

Handwriting Instruction Methods

During the past decade, an educational debate has focused on teaching handwriting systematically through commercially prepared or teacher-developed programs or learning it through a "whole-language" approach. The whole-language philosophy purports that both the substance (meaning) of writing and the form (mechanics) of writing are critical for learning to write (Graham, 1992). Thus, when using the whole-language method as children are learning and mastering handwriting, the teacher gives advice and assigns practice on an individual, as-needed basis. For example, if an educator sees a first-grader struggling to form the letter *m* while writing a story about monsters, he or she may instruct the child regarding the correct letter formation of *m* and encourage extra practice of the letter during the story composition period. Conversely, in a traditional handwriting instruction approach, students are introduced to letter formations and practice them outside of the context of writing. For children with learning disabilities and mild neurological impairments, regular practice in forming letters is essential in the early stages of handwriting development, yet handwriting should have a meaningful context. Thus, a combination of systematic handwriting instruction and whole-language methods may be most beneficial to this group of children (Graham).

In the United States, traditional handwriting instruction programs vary from school district to school district and occasionally from school to school and grade to grade. It's not uncommon for occupational therapy practitioners to receive a referral for a child with poor handwriting who has never had handwriting instruction! The most common instruction methods include Palmer, Zaner-Blöser, italics, and D'Nealian (Alston & Taylor, 1987; Duvall, 1985; Thurber, 1983). See Appendix 17-B for a list of handwriting curricula used in schools.

Unlike the United States, a few countries, such as the United Kingdom, New Zealand, and Australia (Alston, 1991; Alston & Taylor; Jarman, 1990; Ziviani & Watson-Will, 1998), have adopted national curricula for handwriting to improve the standards of handwriting assessment and instruction within their school systems.

Manuscript and Cursive Styles

A generally accepted sequence for handwriting instruction is manuscript writing for use in grades 1 and 2, with children transitioning to cursive writing at the end of grade 2 or the beginning of grade 3 (Barchers, 1994; Bergman & McLaughlin, 1988; Hagin, 1983). The need for manuscript writing may continue throughout life, when students label maps and posters, adolescents complete job or college applications, and adults compute federal income tax forms. By junior high age, many students have blended both manuscript and cursive to form their own style of handwriting. To date, no research has decisively indicated the superiority of one script style over the other.

Both manuscript and cursive possess complementary features, and these should be considered when the occupational therapist, child, child's parent, and educational team are collaboratively deciding which style might best serve the child.

Manuscript is endorsed for the following reasons:

1 Manuscript letterforms are simpler and hence are easier to learn.

2 It closely resembles the print of textbooks and school manuals.

3 It is needed throughout adult life for documents and applications.

4 Beginning manuscript writing is more readable than cursive.

5 Ball and stick strokes of manuscript letter formations are more developmentally appropriate than cursive letters for young children.

6 Manuscript letters are easier to discriminate visually than cursive ones (Barbe, Milone, & Wasylyk, 1983; Bergman & McLaughlin, 1988; Graham & Miller, 1980; Hagin, 1983).

Advocates of cursive writing pronounce the following:

1 Cursive movement patterns allow for faster and more automatic writing.

2 Reversal of individual letters and transpositions of words are more difficult than in manuscript.

3 One continuous, connected line enables child to form words as units.

4 Cursive is faster than manuscript.

5 Cursive allows the poor printer a new type of written format, which may be motivating at the child's present maturity level (Armitage & Ratzlaff, 1985; Bergman & McLauglin, 1988; Graham & Miller, 1980; Hagin, 1983).

HANDWRITING INTERVENTION

Planning

In school settings, if the referred child's educational team decides that functional written communication is a priority for the child's educational program, the occupational therapist may be instrumental in directing and guiding this aspect of the program. Typically, the team uses either a remedial or compensatory intervention approach or both to better the child's written communication. Compensatory strategies improve a student's participation in school with accommodations, adaptations, and modifications for certain tasks, routines, and settings (Amundson, 1998; Kemmis & Dunn, 1996; Swinth & Anson, 1998), whereas remedial ones are used to improve or establish a student's functional skills in a specific area.

When the team focuses on the occupation of written communication, generally both remedial and compensatory techniques are concurrently employed. For example, Hunter, a second-grader, has manuscript handwriting that is unreadable, about 60% of his written letters are not legible, and his writing speed is at the bottom of his class. While he participates in an intensive multisensory handwriting remediation program, he needs accommodations and strategies that assist him to be functional with his written communication in the classroom. Consequently, his teacher may need to adjust the time required to complete assignments, incorporate more oral reporting into his class assignments, or ask him to set a reasonable volume of work to be accomplished for each assignment that may differ from his peers. The teacher and occupational therapist might use other techniques to assist him with any legibility problems, such as spacing between words, sizing letters, and placing text on lines.

Initially, the child, the child's parents, and the educational team need to achieve consensus regarding the type of script (e.g., cursive) and the method of handwriting instruction (e.g., Zaner-Blöser) that seems most advantageous for the child to use. Specific intervention techniques should be generated and selected too. Subsequently, the type, frequency, and duration of service delivery along with the service providers (e.g., certified occupational therapy assistant) working with the child with handwriting problems may be determined within the planning meeting.

Occasionally when a child's handwriting is very illegible and slow, team members may decide to incorporate computer technology, such as a computer or portable word processor. Both the student and the team, particularly the occupational therapy practitioner, must work hard to find a technological system that allows the student proficiency of text generation (Swinth & Anson, 1998). As with paper and pencil, computer use requires adequate attention, motor control, sensory processing, visual functioning, and self-regulation from the student. Hence, the computer is not a magical tool but one that allows the child to acquire keyboarding and word processing skills through planning, routine instruction, and practice. Two studies of upper-elementary students with learning disabilities (Lewis, Graves, Ashton, & Kieley, 1998; MacArthur & Graham, 1987) indicated that handwriting was a quicker mode of generating text than was keyboarding, after several months of practice. Word processing with word prediction improved the legibility as well as the spelling of written assignments for two of three children with learning disabilities in a single-subject design study (Handley-More, Deitz, Billingsley, & Coggins, 2003). In this age of technology, it is important for all students to develop keyboarding skills as an additional academic basic for computer use in classrooms, workplaces, and homes. However, survival handwriting skills will continue to be needed throughout student and adult life.

Models of Practice to Guide the Occupational Therapist

Theories, strategies, and approaches of occupational therapists may seem unconventional to children, educators, parents, and other school personnel. Therefore, the occupational therapist must be able to (1) clearly articulate intervention techniques, activity modifications, and classroom accommodations being used; (2) collaborate with the teacher and others to provide service in the least restrictive environment; (3) implement therapeutic strategies for improving written communication; (4) train others to work with children with handwriting problems; and (5) closely monitor the progress of the child and change aspects of the program to continue improvement.

The overall focus of the educational program is the improvement of student performance in a particular area (e.g., written communication). Occupational therapy models of practice or frames of reference contributing to this occupational outcome include (1) neurodevelopmental, (2) acquisitional, (3) sensorimotor, (4) biomechanical, and (5) psychosocial. Surveys of occupational therapists in the United States (Woodward & Swinth, 2002) and Canada (Feder, Majnemer, & Synnes, 2000) indicate that the most applied theoretical approaches to children's handwriting intervention are multisensory (92%, United States) and sensorimotor (90%, Canada). However, using various theoretical approaches for handwriting intervention was found in Canada (Feder et al., 2000) and advocated in the pediatric occupational therapy literature (Amundson, 1992; Case-Smith, 2002; Peterson & Nelson, 2003).

When considering any intervention plan for handwriting, practitioners should consider the far-reaching parameters of each model of practice along with the overlap and the interplay between them. The occupational therapist must be skillful in the use of one or several models of practice concurrently and in teaching others to implement strategies originating from these models of practice. By remaining focused on the child's occupational outcome related to handwriting and applying various models of practice in the child's educational program, the occupational therapy practitioner can provide a conduit of opportunities for the child learning and mastering the skill of written communication.

Neurodevelopmental

The *neurodevelopmental theoretical approach* is based on neurological principles and normal development, focusing on an individual's ability to execute efficient postural responses and movement patterns (Howle, 2002). This model of practice provides an ideal orientation for addressing problems of children who have inadequate neurodevelopmental organization exhibited by poor postural control, automatic reactions, or limb control (Dutton, 1993a). Decreased, increased, or fluctuating muscle tone, inadequate righting and equilibrium responses, and poor proximal stability may interfere with successful performance in fine-motor activities (e.g., handwriting production at home and in school).

Postural and limb preparation activities are an important component of a comprehensive handwriting program for children with mild neuromuscular impairments and sensory processing problems. For these children, preparing their bodies and hands for handwriting becomes the preliminary ingredient of handwriting intervention before the instructional program begins. Selecting preparatory activities to address each child's specific deficits and carefully analyzing his or her response to these activities are both critical in the preparatory phase of the handwriting intervention program. The remaining paragraphs of this section include postural and upper-extremity activities for getting children's bodies ready to write. These activities can be used in the classroom or pullout therapy in the areas of (1) modulating muscle tone, (2) promoting proximal joint stability, and (3) improving hand function.

Postural preparation to modulate muscle tone may involve activities to increase, decrease, or balance muscle tone. Traditional activities to increase tone include jumping while sitting on a hippity-hop ball, spinning on a "sit-and-spin," and jumping on a mini-trampoline. In the classroom, activities to build tone and strength might include students placing their hands on the sides of their chairs and bouncing in place for a "popcorn ride." They may hold that position with arms extended for a chair pushup. They may perform simple calisthenics, such as pushing down on the top of their heads and shoulders with their hands while seated in a chair (Amundson,

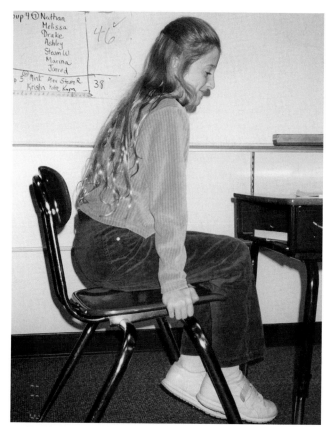

FIGURE 17-5 A girl demonstrates an arm pushup in her school chair.

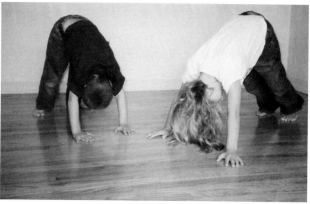

FIGURE 17-6 Two children participate in a yoga game to get ready for writing.

1998) or perform an arm pushup in a school chair (Figure 17-5).

For children whose muscle tone needs to be reduced, conventional slow rocking may be achieved by sitting astride a large bolster and moving from side to side to the rhythm of a child's poem recited aloud. In the classroom prior to writing, a child's postural tone may be decreased by rocking in a rocking chair to the beat of slow, rhythmic instrumental or vocal music from a headset, by snuggling into a bean bag chair, or by participating in a relaxing visual imagery exercise.

Children with poor handwriting frequently exhibit poor proximal stability and strength. To encourage co-contraction through the neck, shoulders, elbows, and wrists, young children may enjoy animal walks, such as the crab walk, the bear walk, the inchworm creep, and the mule kick. Older children may prefer calisthenics, such as pushups on the floor or against the wall, resistive exercises with elastic tubing or theraband, cooperatively pulling up a partner from a seated position on the floor, or yoga poses requiring weight bearing on the upper extremities. Figure 17-6 shows two children engaging in a yoga pose (London Bridge pose) to get ready for writing. Within the school setting, proximal stability also may be improved through everyday routines, such as cleaning blackboards and table tops, pushing heavy external doors open, or pushing and moving classroom furniture or physical education equipment.

Alternative positions during writing activities can enhance proximal stability during writing. The prone position requires weight bearing on the forearms for writing, which increases proximal joint stability and disassociation of the hand and digits from the forearm.

When preparing to write, some children may also benefit from developing more coordinated synergies of the intrinsic and extrinsic muscles of the hand to improve overall hand function. Typically, the hand needs to be stable and strong enough to provide support for fingers to manipulate tools. In-class hand strengthening activities include carrying heavy cases with thick handles, practicing knot-tying with thick rope, and participating in games, such as Felicity the Cat Scratch (Amundson, 1998). Prewriting, handwriting, and manipulative activities on vertical surfaces can assist children in developing more wrist extension stability to facilitate balanced use of the intrinsic musculature of the hand (Benbow, 1990b). Activities requiring in-hand manipulation or the adjustment of an object after placement within the hand (Exner, 1992) may be appropriate for children with deficits in handwriting (see Chapter 10). "Translation," moving the writing utensil from the palm to the fingers of the hand, "shifting" the shaft of the utensil within the hand for proper grasp, and "rotating" the pencil from the writing to the erasing position are all in-hand manipulation skills needed for writing tool management.

A study by Cornhill and Case-Smith (1996) of 48 first-graders found or demonstrated a moderate to high correlation between handwriting skills and in-hand manipulation, specifically translation and complex rotation. Boehme (1988) suggested that vertical excursion of the writing line is produced by the flexion and extension movements of the digits, whereas horizontal excursion originates primarily from lateral wrist movements. Hence, the balanced interaction of the intrinsic and extrinsic muscles of the hand is key to the dynamic, efficient, and fluid movements required for handwriting.

Acquisitional

Handwriting may be viewed as a complex motor skill that "can be improved through practice, repetition, feedback, and reinforcement" (Holm, 1986, p. 70). Instructional guidance of handwriting is recommended by Graham and Miller (1980) to be (1) taught directly; (2) implemented in brief, daily lessons; (3) individualized to the child; (4) planned and changed based on evaluation and performance data; and (5) overlearned and used in a meaningful manner by the child. When therapists and educators employ these conditions in a positive, interesting, and dynamic learning environment, children are more likely to become efficient, legible writers (Barchers, 1994; Graham & Miller; Milone & Wasylyk, 1981).

For occupational therapy practitioners, handwriting as a motor skill relates to theories of motor learning that impact the instructional process. Learning a new motor skill has been described as progressing through three phases: cognitive, associative, and autonomous (Fitts & Posner, 1967). First, in the *cognitive phase*, the child is attempting to understand the demands of the handwriting task and develop a cognitive strategy for performing the necessary motor movements. Visual control of fine-motor movements is thought to be important at this phase. A child learning handwriting in this phase may have developed some strategies for writing some of the easier manuscript letters, such as *o*, *l*, or *t*, but may have more difficulty writing complicated letters, such as *b*, *q*, or *g*.

In the *associative phase*, the child has learned the fundamentals of performing handwriting and continues to adjust and refine the skill. Proprioceptive feedback becomes increasingly important during this phase, whereas reliance on visual cues declines. For example, in the associative phase a child may have mastered the formations of letters but is engaged in improving the handwriting product by learning to space words correctly, to write letters within guidelines, or to maintain consistent letter slant. Children continue to need practice, instructional guidance, and self-monitoring strategies of handwriting performance.

In the final, *autonomous phase*, the child can perform handwriting automatically with minimal conscious attention. Variability of performance is slight from day to day and the child is able to detect and adjust for any small errors that may occur during the autonomous phase (Schmidt, 1982). Once the child has reached this level of handwriting, his or her attention can then be expended on other higher-order elements of writing (Graham, 1992) or it can be saved in order to alleviate fatigue (Schmidt).

Implications and strategies for handwriting instruction and remediation evolve from reviews of handwriting studies (Bergman & McLaughlin, 1988; Graham & Miller, 1980; Peck, Askov, & Fairchild, 1980) as well

as motor learning theory (Magill, 1985). Many handwriting intervention programs are commercially available (see Appendix 17-C for brief descriptions and ordering information of these programs; see Appendix 17-D for a list of Internet resources). Each should contain a scope and sequence of letter and numeral formations along with successive instructional techniques. To date, no empirical evidence reveals one commercial handwriting program to be more effective than another.

The scope and sequence of the handwriting intervention program should focus on a structured progression of introducing and teaching letter and numeral forms. Frequently, letters with common formational features are introduced as a family, such as the lowercase letters *e*, *i*, *t*, and *l*. After the child has mastered these letters, she or he can use them immediately to write the words, *eel*, *tile*, and *little*. Whether the chosen handwriting intervention method is a commercially available or a teacher- or therapist-prepared method, each child's program should be individualized to consist of the letters that he or she has not yet mastered. Thus, the focus of the child's program is to sequentially introduce new letters and use them with mastered letters, excluding letters the child is forming incorrectly or ones not known to the child, as this only reinforces unwelcome perceptual-motor patterns (Ziviani, 1987). Combining newly acquired letters with already mastered letters allows the child to write in a meaningful context (i.e., the formation of words and sentences). This immediate reinforcement of writing words is more powerful and purposeful for the child than writing strings of letters repeatedly.

Instructional approaches of handwriting intervention programs vary but tend to comprise a combination of sequential techniques including modeling, tracing, stimulus fading, copying, composing, and self-monitoring (Amundson, 1992; Bergman & McLaughlin, 1988; Milone & Wasylyk, 1987). When acquiring new letterforms, initially the child may need many visual and auditory cues. However, the service provider will want to fade the cues as soon as the child can successfully form the letter without them. Next, the child proceeds to copying letters and words from a model and then to writing letters and words from memory as they are dictated. Finally, the child will advance to generating words and sentences for practice. In each phase, the child should be expected to assume responsibility for correcting his or her own work, also known as self-monitoring (Bergman & McLaughlin). Older children might refer to a written checklist addressing spacing, size, alignment, letterforms, and slant during the self-assessment of their writing. However, younger children may need to verbally evaluate letter formation and overall appearance aloud to the service provider.

Acquiring handwriting skills and applying them in school life means the educational team not only focuses on teaching letter formation, it also focuses on the legibility and speed of the student's handwriting. Besides learning correct letterforms, other components of legibility include spacing, size, slant, and alignment. Spacing between letters and words, text placement on lines, and sizing letters often need direct attention. Size and placement of text on the writing lines relies on the width of writing guidelines.

An effective writing surface for assisting students with text placement and size is a color-coded, laminated sheet. This sheet provides immediate visual cues to the child learning letterforms, when accompanied by verbal cues from the service provider. Beneath the solid red writing baseline, the color brown represents the "soil" or "ground"; the space above the solid baseline and dashed black middle guideline is green for the "grass"; and above the dashed guideline to the top solid writing line is blue for the "sky." For example, the letter *h* would start at the top of the sky, head downward, and end in the grass. This same pictorial scheme can be applied to lined paper for classroom assignments, allowing students strong cues for learning letter placement and size (Amundson, 1998) (Figure 17-7). Various strategies for handwriting problems related to legibility components, classroom writing assignments, and speed are listed in Table 17-4.

Sensorimotor

The parameters for this model of practice, when applied by the occupational therapist with children with handwriting problems, include controlling sensory input through selected activities to enhance the integration of sensory systems at the subcortical level (Simon, 1993). By providing various sensory opportunities, the child's nervous system may integrate information more efficiently to produce a satisfactory motor output (e.g., legible letters in a timely manner). All sensory systems, including the proprioceptive, tactile, visual, auditory, olfactory, and gustatory senses, can be tapped within a handwriting intervention program, which is thought to enhance learning. Incorporating a sensory integrative approach into handwriting intervention equates to the use of a variety of sensory experiences, media, and instructional materials. Additionally, providing novel and interesting materials for children to practice letterforms may keep students motivated, excited, and challenged, thereby enhancing student success and learning. Children with handwriting difficulties who have experienced frustration with commonly used paper-and-pencil drills may be much more amenable to handwriting instruction utilizing this unique multisensory format.

Writing tools, writing surfaces, and positions for writing are all integral parts of a sensorimotor approach. Examples of writing tools to be used include felt-tip pens (regular, overwriter, changeable-color), crayons (scented, glittered, glow-in-the-dark), paintbrushes, grease pencils or china markers, weighted pens, mechanical pencils, wooden dowels, vibratory pens, and chalk. Lamme and Ayris (1983) examined the effects of five different types of writing tools on handwriting legibility. Results indicated that the type of writing tool did not influence legibility, but the educators involved in the study reported that children's attitudes toward writing were more positive when children were able to use a

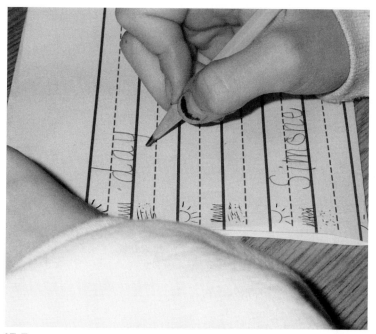

FIGURE 17-7 Line paper with diagrams helps with letter size and the placement of text.

TABLE 17-4   Strategies for Handwriting Problems

Handwriting Problems	Potential Solutions
Spacing between letters	Use finger spacing with index finger. Use fingerprint spacing by pressing on an ink pad before finger spacing. Teach the "no touching rule" of letters.
Spacing between words	Use adhesive strips (e.g., Post-it Notes) as spacers between words. Make spaces with a rubber stamp. Use a dot or a dash (Morse code) between words.
Spacing on paper	Use grid paper. Write on every other line of the paper. Draw colored lines to mark (e.g., green is left, red is right).
Placing text on lines	Use pictorial schemes on writing guidelines. Provide raised writing lines as tactile cues for letter placement. Remind students that unevenly placed letters are "popcorn letters."
Sizing letters and words	Use individualized boxes for each letter. Name letters with ascending stems, no stems, and descending stems, "birds," "skunks," and "snakes," respectively.
Near-point copying	Highlight the text on the worksheet to be copied. Teach the student to copy two or three letters at a time.
Far-point copying	Enlarge print for better viewing. Start with copying from nearby vertical models. Position the student to face the chalkboard.
Dictation	Attach an alphabet strip to a desktop for the student who cannot remember letter forms. Dictated spelling words would contain several but not all letters.
Composition	Be certain that students can form letters from memory. Provide magnetic words to write short poems or stories.
Speed	Allow students to begin projects early to finish with peers. Photocopy math problems from textbook to reduce copying. Preselect volume of work to be done that may be different from that of peers.

Modified from Amundson, S.J. (1998). *TRICS for written communication: Techniques for rebuilding and improving children's school skills.* Homer, AK: O.T. KIDS.

felt-tip pen rather than a No. 2 pencil. This suggests that children's feelings about writing might improve when allowed to use a wide variety of writing tools. Writing with chalk, grease pencils, or a resistive tool also provides additional proprioceptive input to children, as more pressure for writing is required than with the traditional media, paper and pencil. Unconventional writing tools can be easily incorporated into classroom assignments.

Writing surfaces may be in a vertical, a horizontal, or a vertically angled plane. Common vertical surfaces for writing include the chalkboard, painting easels, and poster board and laminated paper attached to the wall. These surfaces, along with desktop easels set at slanted inclines, facilitate a more mature grasp of the writing tool as a child's wrist extension may result in more arching of the hand and an open web space between the thumb and fingers (Benbow et al., 1992). Figure 17-8 shows a girl working on her homework assignment that is taped to a kitchen cupboard. An upright orientation may also decrease directional confusion of early writers when learning letter formations (Hagin, 1983). On the vertical plane, up means up and down means down, as opposed to working at a desktop where the direction up means away from the body and down means toward the body. Furthermore, standing in front of a chalkboard with the body in full extension and parallel to the writing surface may promote more internal stability of the trunk, increase the child's arousal, and provide more proprioceptive input throughout the arm and shoulder and allow the hand to move independently or dissociate from the arm (Amundson, 1992).

Handwriting practice on a horizontal surface at the table or on the floor might be performed using plastic freezer bags partially filled with colored hair styling gel, trays filled with sand, dry pudding mix, clay, or a light coat of hand lotion. Writing trays can be baking sheets or Styrofoam meat packaging trays, which provide children additional tactile and proprioceptive input when forming letters, numbers, and words with isolated fingers or wooden dowels. Other writing activities might occur on textured wall paper, nylon netting, finely meshed screen, or indoor-outdoor carpet squares to again provide proprioceptive input.

Biomechanical

In the truest sense, the biomechanical frame of reference addresses occupational performance in terms of range of motion, strength, and endurance (Dutton, 1993b).

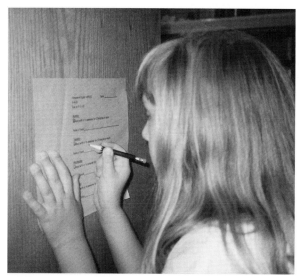

FIGURE 17-8 A girl works on a homework assignment that is taped to a vertical surface (i.e., kitchen cupboard).

This discussion, however, focuses on the ergonomic factors of sitting posture, paper position, pencil grasp, writing instruments, and type of paper. Compensatory strategies—including adaptive devices, procedural adaptations, and environmental modifications to improve the interaction and fit between a child's capabilities and the demands of the handwriting task—are presented. This model emphasizes modifications to the student's context rather than focusing on improving performance skills.

Sitting Posture. Although standing and lying prone may be encouraged as alternative writing positions, students continue to spend much of the school day seated at a desk. Therefore, the occupational therapist should immediately address the student's seated position in the classroom. While writing, the student should be seated with the feet firmly planted on the floor, providing support for weight shifting and postural adjustments (Benbow et al., 1992). The table surface should be 2 inches above the flexed elbows when the child is seated in the chair. In this position, the student can experience both symmetry and stability while performing written work. To ensure that students are appropriately seated, the occupational therapy practitioner may recommend adjusting heights of desks and chairs, providing needed foot rests for children, adding seat cushions and inserts, and repositioning a child's desk to face the chalkboard in the classroom.

Paper Position. Paper should be slanted on the desktop, so it is parallel to the forearm of the writing hand when the child's forearms are resting on the desk with hands clasped (Levine, 1991). This angle of the paper enables the student to see his or her written work and to avoid smearing his or her writing. Right-handed students may slant the top of their paper approximately 25 to 30° to the left with the paper just right of the

body's midline. Conversely, a slant of 30 to 35° to the right and paper placement to the left of midline are needed for students using a left-handed tripod grasp (Alston & Taylor, 1987). For the student with a left-handed "hooked" pencil grasp lacking lateral wrist movements, slanting the paper to the left as do right-handed students is appropriate (Benbow et al., 1992). The writing instrument should be held below the baseline, and the nonpreferred hand should hold the writing paper (Alston & Taylor).

Pencil Grip. Benbow (1990) defined the ideal grasp as a dynamic tripod with an open web space. With the web space open (forming a circle), the thumb, index, and middle fingers make the longest flexion, extension, and rotary excursions with a pencil (Benbow et al., 1992) during handwriting. Variations of grasps exist with some grips making handwriting more difficult and less functional (Tseng & Cermak, 1993). Educational team members may consider modifying a student's pencil grasp under the following conditions: (1) handwriting results in muscular tension and fatigue, also known as writer's cramp; (2) handwriting proficiency, such as letter formation or writing speed, is impeded; (3) the child's inability to use controlled and precise finger and thumb movements of the pencil stem from a tightly closed web space; and (4) the child holds the pencil with too much pressure or exerts too much pencil point pressure on the paper, resulting in breaking the pencil lead, making holes in the writing paper, and shaking out the writing hand repeatedly (Benbow).

When attempting to modify a grip pattern, characteristics of the child are an important consideration. The occupational therapy practitioner should encourage a mature grasp in young writers and recognize that the success in modifying a grasp pattern may be better with younger children (Ziviani, 1987). Once grip positions have been established, they are very difficult to change (Benbow, 1990). In fact, by the beginning of second grade, changing a child's grasp pattern may be stressful and near impossible (Benbow et al., 1992). Therefore, the educational team needs to highly regard a child's age, cooperation, and motivation along with the child's acceptance of the new grip pattern or prosthetic device before attempting to reposition the child's fingers permanently.

A variety of prosthetic devices and therapeutic strategies are available to assist the child in positioning his or her digits for better manipulation of the writing instrument (Amundson, 1998). The occupational therapist should be knowledgeable of hand functions to determine which adaptive devices and techniques are most appropriate for each individual child. Stetro grips, triangular pencils, moldable grips, and The Pencil Grip may facilitate tripod grasps. Writing muscle tension and fatigue may be reduced for some children by using a wider-barreled pencil. To gain more mobility of the radial digits, children may hold a small eraser against their palms with the ulnar digits, allowing for more dynamic movement of the pencil. For older children with hand hypotonicity, holding the pencil shaft between the web space of the index and middle fingers with thumb opposition may give them a viable pencil grasp (Benbow, 1990b). Other techniques to encourage the delicate stability-mobility balance of a functional pencil grasp include the use of external supports such as microfoam surgical tape supports, ring splints, and neoprene splints (Benbow, 1995) and should be used with a working knowledge of hand anatomy and kinesiology. A rubber band sling that encourages the student to use a slanted and relaxed pencil position for writing is shown in Figure 17-9.

Writing Tools. The type of writing instruments children use in the classroom also warrants consideration. In general, children should be allowed to choose among a variety of writing tools so parents and teachers may help the individual child determine which writing utensil is most efficient and comfortable. Traditionally, kindergarten and primary classrooms have promoted the use of a wide primary (or beginner's) pencil for beginning writers. Carlson and Cunningham (1990) examined tool usage among preschool children performing drawing, tracing, and writing tasks. They found that the readability of their written work was not enhanced by the use of a wider diameter pencil. This study suggests that the pervasive use of the primary pencil is probably not warranted for all kindergarten children as some children perform better with a No. 2 pencil whereas others do well with a primary pencil.

Paper. Various types of writing paper are available in the educational setting. Unlined paper and lined paper with a dashed middle guideline between the lower base-line and upper line are both commonly used in the early elementary grades. For the majority of children, most of the research confirms that lined paper improves the legibility of handwriting when compared to the use of unlined paper (Pasternicki, 1987). Children typically start out with wide-spaced (1-inch) guidelines. As handwriting proficiency improves, usually in grade 3 or 4, the child begins using paper with narrow-spaced ($\frac{3}{8}$-inch) lines (Barchers, 1994). The occupational therapist and educator can allow the student the opportunity to experiment with different-lined, sized, and textured paper to determine which offers the child the best medium for handwriting.

Psychosocial

Psychosocial approaches used for children's handwriting intervention typically focus on improving the student's self-control, coping skills, and social behaviors. In the area of handwriting, this means that a child may produce neatly written text when addressing an envelope to his or her residence, knowing that the occupational therapist will later use the envelope to send the child a small "surprise." Receiving a surprise, such as a bookmark, from the therapist is enjoyable and socially reinforcing for the child.

By sharing with children the importance of readable handwriting and the rationale for intervention, as well as providing positive, meaningful, everyday experiences using handwriting, children's behaviors to write more legibly may increase. Simple games at school and home, such as tic-tac-toe, can be played using the newly acquired letterforms rather than the traditional *X* and *O*. When a child presents a neatly drawn and written (relative to the child's ability) Thanksgiving Day card at home, the parents can provide social reinforcement. In addition, teachers might reward the child with typically poor handwriting with a special certificate for improved handwriting upon receipt of a readable spelling paper or written class assignment. By offering children choices, success, responsibility, and encouragement within an intervention program and the natural setting, handwriting may be viewed and practiced by children as a functional and socially valid skill.

Using a psychosocial approach, the occupational therapy practitioner may also enhance children's social competence within the framework of a handwriting intervention group. Currently, the use of small groups as a service delivery model for school-based handwriting intervention is limited. Woodward and Swinth (2002) found that school-based occupational therapists used small groups for handwriting intervention infrequently (12.4%) when compared to other types of service provision in school-based settings.

However, one successful group is a handwriting club of 4 to 6 students, who work on improving handwriting,

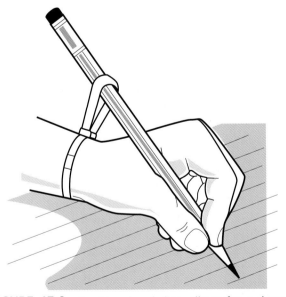

FIGURE 17-9 A rubber band sling allows for a slanted, relaxed pencil position.

developing social skills, and monitoring their own work and behavior (Amundson, 1998). Poor social performance is common among children with learning disabilities. Behaviors that interfere with social relations include poor eye contact, physical intrusiveness, lack of greeting others, and unawareness of verbal and nonverbal social cues, to name a few (Williamson, 1994). The service provider may aptly provide group experiences and teach children needed social skills, such as complimenting others, regulating the tone and volume of one's voice, accepting negative feedback, maintaining personal space, and giving and accepting apologies (Williamson) while involved with the handwriting group.

In a handwriting club, for example, when children are lying in prone position and practicing letterforms on a chalk mat, each of them can decide the amount of personal space they need to feel comfortable, as well as the amount of writing space required on the mat. The practitioner may introduce both of these space requirements, and he or she may assist the children in this problem-solving process. Another example related to building social skills in a handwriting intervention group might occur during an in-hand manipulation preparatory activity, such as in a competitive game as Kerplunk. While children remove plastic sticks supporting marbles from the game's cylinder, the occupational therapy practitioner can reinforce the social skills of taking turns, regulating one's behavioral state amid competition, and following the rules of a game.

Other strategies to enhance children's social performance within an intervention group may require a proactive role of the occupational therapist. Giving an overview of the intervention session at the beginning of the period and clearly delineating when activities are beginning and terminating may assist children who have difficulty with transitions between tasks and classes. Developing trust and a sense of cohesiveness among the children might be achieved by having the club or group members decide on a special name, logo, or handshake (Williamson, 1993). Finally, the interventionist should establish clear and reasonable rules and consequences, share them with the group members, and consistently and kindly manage the children's behavior. By overlaying the building of children's social skills within the framework of a handwriting intervention group, occupational therapy practitioners help children to be more socially competent with their peers and adults as well as to be more efficient and fluent in their handwriting.

Evidence of Occupational Therapy Intervention on Handwriting

Some children are good candidates for improving their actual manuscript or cursive handwriting through remediation. However, other children are not. The occupational therapist and the child's team need to con-

sider compensatory strategies that allow the child with poor handwriting the greatest opportunity for functional written communication. Alternatives to handwriting include keyboarding and word prediction, adapting and reducing the amount of written assignments, dictating assignments, and having study buddies to assist with written expression. In school settings, the educational team must determine which type of written communication is or will be most functional for the child and develop a short-term plan (e.g., learning essential manuscript words) and a long-term plan (e.g., learning word processing).

Although the field of occupational therapy assumes that occupational interventions improve children's handwriting, the professional literature continues to have a lack of controlled handwriting intervention studies. Two studies (Case-Smith, 2002; Peterson & Nelson, 2003), however, indicated that occupational therapy intervention positively affected elementary students' handwriting. Case-Smith investigated 29 children receiving occupational therapy services and 9 children who did not. Children ranged from grades 2 through 4. Occupational therapy intervention with the children focused on visual-motor skill improvement and handwriting practice. The occupational therapists reportedly used eclectic theoretical approaches during intervention sessions. Following 8.8 hours of direct occupational therapy, the intervention group made significant gains in handwriting legibility when compared to the control group. Although handwriting speed was not significantly affected for the intervention group, the students, on average, increased from 32 to 37 letters per minute. Pre- and posttesting was completed with the Evaluation Tool of Children's Handwriting (Amundson, 1995).

In the study by Peterson and Nelson (2003), 59 grade 1 students from low socioeconomic backgrounds participated. Thirty children randomly assigned to an occupational therapy group received 10 hours of handwriting intervention. The control group (n = 29) received regular academic instruction for handwriting. Children received handwriting intervention that was based on an integration of theoretical perspectives. Findings indicated that the children receiving handwriting intervention demonstrated a significant increase in scores on the Minnesota Handwriting Test (Reisman, 1999) than did those of the control group.

Both handwriting intervention studies (Case-Smith, 2002; Peterson & Nelson, 2003) give evidence that occupational therapy interventions significantly impact children's handwriting; however, both studies share limitations. One limitation in both studies is that the handwriting evaluators were not blind to the experimental conditions. Another limitation is that both of the handwriting instruments, the Evaluation Tool of Children's Handwriting (Amundson, 1995) and the Minnesota Handwriting Test (Reisman, 1999), have only fair to good test reliability. Finally, the small sample sizes and specific geographic regions limit the generalizability of either study.

Service Delivery

Providing occupational therapy services to children with handwriting dysfunction should be based primarily on the needs of the individual child as determined by the educational or clinical team. More and more educational teams in school-based practice are using a continuum of service delivery that allows for more flexibility, fluidity, and responsiveness to an individual child's needs (see Chapter 22).

For example, at the beginning of second grade, Tara, a girl with a learning disability, is assessed by the occupational therapist for poor handling of classroom manipulatives (e.g., glue stick, scissors, computer mouse) and handwriting. After a comprehensive occupational therapy evaluation, Tara's parents and the educational team decide to focus on assisting her to become a more proficient writer, with the occupational therapist and regular education teacher spearheading the intervention program.

The therapist and teacher met to develop classroom strategies to be implemented. These strategies included facing Tara's desk directly at the chalkboard, reducing the length of her written assignments, and providing her with an alphabet strip attached to her desktop and placed at the recommended angle of her writing paper (Figure 17-10).

The educator also requested that the occupational therapist help her with fun exercises to get the entire class "ready to write" before their daily creative writing period. The occupational therapist scheduled a time with the teacher and spent 10 to 15 minutes per week (for 4 weeks) teaching the entire class hand-dexterity games before a classroom writing activity. She also provided the teacher a written handout of games, so the teacher could ask questions and have a later reference.

Due to the extremely poor legibility of Tara's writing, the team chose to have her join an ongoing handwriting intervention group in the classroom. This group held 25-minute sessions, twice a week for 3 consecutive weeks. During this direct service time, the occupational therapist further assessed individual children. She trained the teacher's assistant to coordinate the handwriting group and address some of the individual problems. The occupational therapist returned to the handwriting intervention session once every 2 weeks to supervise the service provider, monitor the children's progress, and modify the programs when needed. A regular consultation time was established with the educator to evaluate Tara's progress in class, to strategize regarding new situations affecting her handwriting performance, and to write a progress note to her parent(s).

In Tara's case, during the first 4 weeks after the initial team meeting the occupational therapist implemented direct service, training of a teaching assistant, and consulting with the teacher. However, the provision of services was not locked into a set schedule (e.g., two 25-minute sessions per week of direct therapy). Consequently, by tapping into a continuum of service provision, the occupational therapist was able to respond to Tara's educational needs by initially working with the teacher, by orchestrating an ongoing intervention

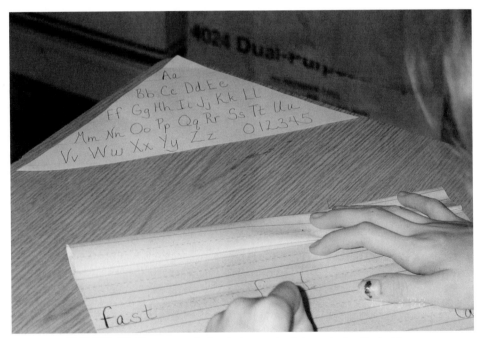

FIGURE 17-10   An angled strip is attached to a student's desktop.

program that another service provider could implement after training, and by continuing regular contact with Tara and the educational team members, including Tara's parents.

Most occupational therapists are comfortable with providing one-to-one or small-group therapy sessions; however, some are more challenged when consulting or training and supervising others to implement programs. Oftentimes, alternative service providers (e.g., educators, educational assistants, volunteers, high school students, and parents) are capable and willing to implement techniques and programs if the occupational therapist assumes responsibility for organizing and monitoring the methods and programs used. To do this, the occupational therapy practitioner must model the role of the service provider during the training, clearly articulate the rationale for the methods and approaches used in the program, and lay out the program in an organized fashion for easy use by the service provider.

By supplying (1) specific written and oral directions of the program; (2) a container, such as a basket, full of materials for the handwriting intervention program (e.g., Theraband, in-hand manipulation games, sequenced writing lessons, clay trays, and different writing tools; (3) data management sheets; and (4) a system to provide reinforcement and rewards, the program will be more user-friendly for the service provider. A user-friendly program may increase the likelihood that the directions provided by the occupational therapist are followed. If the occupational therapist regularly observes sessions implemented by the service provider, discusses the rationale for using specific methods, reviews the children's progress and the need for program changes, the training can be beneficial for the individual children receiving handwriting intervention. This training can also benefit other children in the classroom who may be struggling with handwriting.

SUMMARY

Handwriting is an important academic occupation for children. Children with mild neuromuscular impairments, learning disabilities, and developmental delays are often referred to occupational therapy for handwriting problems. The role of the occupational therapy practitioner includes evaluating a child's functional performance of prewriting and handwriting skills, along with the task demands and environmental features. The occupational therapist must also assist the educational or clinical team in determining and planning an integrated approach to promote a functional communication means for the child.

Handwriting intervention programs should be comprehensive, incorporating activities and therapeutic techniques from the neurodevelopmental, acquisitional, sensory integration, biomechanical, and psychosocial models of practice in the child's natural setting. Compensatory strategies may also be employed to provide the child a successful and efficient means for functional written communication.

STUDY QUESTIONS

1 If a 5-year-old girl cannot write her own name, is she ready for kindergarten, in which the class will be learning letters and letterforms throughout the academic year? Give your rationale for your decision.

2 Why is it inappropriate for an occupational therapist to evaluate a child's in-hand manipulation or visual perceptual skills as the first step of an occupational therapy evaluation focusing on handwriting performance?

3 Identify the models of practice utilized and the rationale for its selection when a child is involved in the following handwriting intervention activity:
  a Jade is building small clay figurines. He is pressing modeling clay flat on the tabletop, removing tiny pieces of clay with his fingers, and rolling them into small balls within one hand.
  b Ella is straddling a bolster while painting letters from the day's instructional lesson with an adapted-handled paintbrush during a tic-tac-toe letter game with Jesse.

4 Jamar is having difficulty with placing cursive letters on the writing line, spacing between words, and using margins properly. Which performance skill(s) seem to be interfering with his writing? What intervention modifications and techniques might be considered?

5 What would be the advantages of implementing a child's handwriting intervention program within the classroom in a small group setting rather than in a one-to-one "pullout" therapy session?

REFERENCES

Alston, J. (1983). A legibility index: Can handwriting be measured? *Educational Review, 35*, 237-242.

Alston, J. (1991). Handwriting in the new curriculum. *British Journal of Special Education, 18*, 13-15.

Alston, J., & Taylor, J. (1987). *Handwriting: Theory, research and practice.* London: Croom Helm.

American Occupational Therapy Association. (2002). Occupational therapy practice framework: Domain and process. *American Journal of Occupational Therapy, 56*, 609-639.

Amundson, S.J. (1992). Handwriting: Evaluation and intervention in school settings. In J. Case-Smith & C. Pehoski

(Eds.), *Development of hand skills in the child* (pp. 63-78). Rockville, MD: American Occupational Therapy Association.

Amundson, S.J. (1995). *Evaluation tool of children's handwriting*. Homer, AK: O.T. KIDS.

Amundson, S.J. (1998). *TRICS for written communication: Techniques for rebuilding and improving children's school skills.* Homer, AK: O.T. KIDS.

Anderson, P.L. (1983). *Denver handwriting analysis*. Novato, CA: Academic Therapy Publications.

Armitage, D., & Ratzlaff, H. (1985). The non-corrrelation of printing and writing skills. *Journal of Educational Research, 78,* 174-177.

Barbe, W.B., Milone, M.J., & Wasylyk, T. (1983). Manuscript is the write start. *Academic Therapy, 18,* 397-405.

Barchers, S.I. (1994). *Teaching language arts: An integrated approach.* Minneapolis, MN: West Publishing Company.

Beery, K.E. (1992). *The developmental test of visual-motor integration* (4th ed.). Austin, TX: Pro-Ed.

Beery, K.E. (1997). *The developmental test of visual-motor integration* (5th ed.). Austin, TX: Pro-Ed.

Benbow, M. (1990). Understanding the hand from the inside out. Handout distributed at a workshop, August 1990.

Benbow, M. (1995). Principles and practices of teaching handwriting. In A. Henderson & C. Pehoski (Eds.), *Hand function in the child: Foundations for remediation* (pp. 255-281). St. Louis: Mosby.

Benbow, M., Hanft, B., & Marsh, D. (1992). Handwriting in the classroom: Improving written communication. In C.B. Royeen (Ed.), *AOTA self-study series: Classroom applications for school-based practice* (pp. 1-60). Rockville, MD: American Occupational Therapy Association.

Bergman, K.E., & McLaughlin, T.F. (1988). Remediating handwriting difficulties with learning disabled students: A review. *Journal of Special Education, 12,* 101-120.

Bergmann, K.P. (1990). Incidence of atypical pencil grasps among nondysfunctional adults. *American Journal of Occupational Therapy, 44,* 736-740.

Berninger, V., Mizokawa, D., & Bragg, R. (1991). Theory-based diagnosis and remediation of writing disabilities. *Journal of School Psychology, 29,* 57-97.

Boehme, R. (1988.). *Improving upper body control.* Tucson, AZ: Therapy Skill Builders.

Carlson, K., & Cunningham, J. (1990). Effect of pencil diameter on the graphomotor skill of preschoolers. *Early Childhood Research Quarterly, 5,* 279-293.

Case-Smith, J. (2002). Effectiveness of school-based occupational therapy intervention on handwriting. *American Journal of Occupational Therapy, 56,* 17-25.

Chandler, B. (1994, December 15). The power of information: School based practice survey results, *OT Week, 18,* 24.

Chase, C. (1986). Essay test scoring: Interaction of relevant variables. *Journal of Educational Measurement, 23,* 33-41.

Cornhill, H., & Case-Smith, J. (1996). Factors that relate to good and poor handwriting. *American Journal of Occupational Therapy, 50,* 732-739,

Daniels, L.E. (1988). The diagnosis and remediation of handwriting problems: An analysis. *Physical and Occupational Therapy in Pediatrics, 8,* 61-67.

Dennis, J.L., & Swinth, Y. (2001). Pencil grasp and children's handwriting legibility during different-length writing tasks. *American Journal of Occupational Therapy, 55,* 175-183.

Diekema, S.M., Deitz, J., & Amundson, S.J. (1998). Test-retest reliability of the Evaluation of Children's Handwriting—Manuscript. *American Journal of Occupational Therapy, 52,* 248-254.

Donoghue, M. (1975). *The child and the English language arts* (2nd ed.). Dubuque, IA: William C. Brown.

Dutton, R. (1993a). Neurodevelopmental frame of reference. In H.L. Hopkins & H.D. Smith (Eds.), *Willard and Spackman's occupational therapy* (pp. 73-74). Philadelphia: Lippincott.

Dutton, R. (1993b). Biomechanical frame of reference. In H.L. Hopkins & H.D. Smith (Eds.), *Willard and Spackman's occupational therapy* (pp. 66-67). Philadelphia: Lippincott.

Duvall, B. (1985). *Evaluating the difficulty of cursive, manuscript, italic and D'Nealian handwriting* (No. CS 209 484). ERIC Document Reproduction Service No. ED 265 539.

Erhardt, R.P. (1982). *Developmental hand dysfunction: Theory, assessment, treatment.* Tucson, AZ: Therapy Skill Builders.

Exner, C.E. (1992). In-hand manipulation skills. In J. Case-Smith & C. Pehoski (Eds.), *Development of hand skills in the child* (pp. 35-45). Rockville, MD: American Occupational Therapy Association.

Feder, K., Majnemer, A., & Synnes, A. (2000). Handwriting: Current trends in occupational therapy practice. *Canadian Journal of Occupational Therapy, 67,* 197-204.

Fitts, P.M., & Posner, M.I. (1967). *Human performance.* Belmont, CA: Brooks/Cole.

Gardner, M.F. (1998). *Test of handwriting skills.* Hydesville, CA: Psychological and Educational Publications.

Graham, S. (1992). Issues in handwriting instruction. *Focus on Exceptional Children, 25,* 1-14.

Graham, S., Berninger, V., Abbott, R., Abbott, S., & Whitaker, D. (1997). The role of mechanics in composing of elementary school students: A new methodological approach. *Journal of Educational Psychology, 89,* 170-182.

Graham, S., Berninger, V., Weintraub, N., & Shafer, W. (1998). The development of handwriting fluency and legibility in grades 1 through 9. *Journal of Educational Research, 92,* 42-52.

Graham, S., Boyer-Shick, K., & Tippets, E. (1989). The validity of the Handwriting Scale from the Test of Written Language. *Journal of Educational Research, 82,* 166-171.

Graham, S., & Miller, L. (1980). Handwriting research and practice: A unified approach. *Focus on Exceptional Children, 13,* 1-16.

Hagin, R.A. (1983). Write right or left: A practical approach to handwriting. *Journal of Learning Disabilities, 15,* 266-271.

Hamstra-Bletz, L., & Blöte, A. (1990). Development of handwriting in primary school: A longitudinal study. *Perceptual and Motor Skills, 70,* 759-770.

Handley-More, D., Deitz, J., Billingsley, F.F., & Coggins, T.E. (2003). Facilitating written work using computer word processing and word prediction. *American Journal of Occupational Therapy, 57,* 139-151.

Hanft, B.E., & Place, P.A. (1996). *The consulting therapist: A guide for OTs and PTs in schools.* San Antonio, TX: The Psychological Corporation.

Hayes, J., & Flower, L. (1986). Writing research and the writer. *American Psychologist, 41,* 1106-1113.

Herrick, J.E., & Otto, W. (1961). Pressure on point and barrel of a writing instrument. *Journal of Experimental Education, 30,* 215-230.

Howle, J.M. (2002). *Neuro-developmental treatment approach: Theoretical foundations and principles of clinical practice.* Laguna Beach, CA: NDTA.

Jackson, A.D. (1971). A comparison of speed and legibility of manuscript and cursive handwriting of intermediate pupils. Unpublished doctoral dissertation. *Dissertation Abstracts, 31, 9.* 4383-A-4384-A.

Jarman, C. (1990). A national curriculum for handwriting? *British Journal of Special Education, 17,* 151-153.

Kemmis, B., & Dunn, W. (1996). Collaborative consultation: The efficacy of remedial and compensatory interventions in school contexts. *American Journal of Occupational Therapy, 50,* 709-717.

Koziatek, S.M., & Powell, N.J. (2002). A validity study of the Evaluation Tool of Children's Handwriting—Cursive. *American Journal of Occupational Therapy, 56,* 446-453.

Koziatek, S.M., & Powell, N.J. (2003). Pencil grips, legibility, and speed of fourth-graders' writing cursive. *American Journal of Occupational Therapy, 57,* 284-288.

Lamme, L.L. (1979). Handwriting in an early childhood curriculum. *Young Children, 35,* 20-27.

Lamme, L.L., & Ayris, B.M. (1983). Is the handwriting of beginning writers influenced by writing tools? *Journal of Research and Development in Education, 17,* 33-38.

Larsen, S.C., & Hammill, D.D. (1989). *Test of legible handwriting.* Austin, TX: Pro-Ed.

Laszlo, J.I., & Bairstow, P.J. (1984). Handwriting: Difficulties and possible solutions. *School Psychology International, 5,* 207-213.

Levine, K.J. (1991). *Fine motor dysfunction: Therapeutic strategies in the classroom.* Tucson, AZ: Therapy Skill Builders.

Levine, M. (1994). *Educational care: A system for understanding and helping children with learning problems at home and school.* Cambridge, MA: Educators Publishing Service.

Lewis, R.B., Graves, A.W., Ashton, T.M., & Kieley, C.L. (1998). Word processing tools for students with learning disabilities: A comparison of strategies to increase text entry speed. *Learning Disabilities Research and Practice, 13,* 95-108.

MacArthur, A., & Graham, S. (1987). Learning disabled students' composing under three methods of text production: Handwriting, word processing, and dictation. *Journal of Special Education, 21,* 22-42.

Magill, R.A. (1985). *Motor learning concepts and applications.* Dubuque, IA: William C. Brown.

McAvoy, C. (1996). Making writers. *Closing the Gap Newsletter, 15,* 1, 9.

McGee, L.M., & Richgels, D.J. (2000). *Literacy's beginnings: Supporting young readers and writers* (3rd ed.). Boston: Allyn & Bacon.

McHale, K., & Cermak, S. (1992). Fine motor activities in elementary school: Preliminary findings and provisional implications for children with fine motor problems. *American Journal of Occupational Therapy, 46,* 898-903.

Milone, M.N., Jr., & Wasylyk, T.M. (1981). Handwriting in special education. *Teaching Exceptional Children, 14,* 58-61.

Myers, C.A. (1992). Therapeutic fine-motor activities for preschoolers. In J. Case-Smith & C. Pehoski (Eds.), *Development of hand skills in the child* (pp. 47-62). Rockville, MD: American Occupational Therapy Association.

Oliver, C.E. (1990). A sensorimotor program for improving writing readiness skills in elementary-age children. *American Journal of Occupational Therapy, 44,* 111-124.

Pasternicki, J.G. (1987). Paper for writing: Research and recommendations. In J. Alston & J. Taylor (Eds.), *Handwriting: Theory, research and practice* (pp. 68-80). London: Croom Helm.

Peck, M., Askov, E.N., & Fairchild, S.H. (1980). Another decade of research in handwriting: Progress and prose in the 1970s. *Journal of Educational Research, 73,* 283-298.

Peterson, C.Q., & Nelson, D.L. (2003). Effect of an occupational intervention on children with economic disadvantages. *American Journal of Occupational Therapy, 57,* 152-160.

Phelps, J., & Stempel, L. (1987). *The children's handwriting evaluation scale for manuscript writing.* Dallas, TX: Texas Scottish Rite Hospital for Crippled Children.

Phelps, J., Stempel, L., & Speck, G. (1984). *The children's handwriting evaluation scale: A new diagnostic tool.* Dallas, TX: Texas Scottish Rite Hospital for Crippled Children.

Reisman, J. (1991). Poor handwriting: Who is referred? *American Journal of Occupational Therapy, 45,* 849-852.

Reisman, J. (1999). *Minnesota handwriting test.* San Antonio, TX: Psychological Corporation.

Rosenbloom, L., & Horton, M.E. (1971). The maturation of fine prehension in young children. *Developmental Medicine and Child Neurology, 13,* 3-8.

Rubin, N., & Henderson, S.E. (1982). Two sides of the same coin: Variations in teaching methods and failure to learn to write. *Special Education: Forward Trends, 9,* 17-24.

Schmidt, R.A. (1982). *Motor control and learning.* Champaign, IL: Human Kinetic.

Schneck, C.M. (1991). Comparison of pencil-grip patterns in first graders with good and poor writing skills. *American Journal of Occupational Therapy, 45,* 701-706.

Schneck, C.M., & Henderson, A. (1990). Descriptive analysis of the developmental progression of grip position for pencil and crayon control in nondysfunctional children. *American Journal of Occupational Therapy, 44,* 893-900.

Simon, C.J. (1993). Sensory integration frame of reference. In H.L. Hopkins & H.D. Smith (Eds.), *Willard and Spackman's occupational therapy* (pp. 74-75). Philadelphia: Lippincott.

Sweedler-Brown, C.O. (1992). The effects of training on the appearance bias of holistic essay graders. *Journal of Research and Development in Education, 26,* 24-88.

Swinth, Y., & Anson, D. (1998). Alternatives to handwriting: Keyboarding and text-generation techniques for schools. In J. Case-Smith (Ed.), *AOTA self-study series: Making a difference in school system practice.* Bethesda, MD: American Occupational Therapy Association.

Talbert-Johnson, C., Salva, E., Sweeney, W.J., & Cooper, J.O. (1991). Cursive handwriting: Measurement of function rather than topography. *Journal of Educational Research, 85,* 117-124.

Tan-Lin, A.S. (1981). An investigation into the developmental course of preschool/kindergarten aged children's handwriting behavior. *Dissertation Abstracts International, 42,* 4287A.

Temple, C., Nathan, R., Temple, F., & Burris, N.A. (1993). *The beginnings of writing.* Boston: Allyn & Bacon.

Thurber, D. (1983). *D'Nealian manuscript—An aide to reading development.* (Report No. CS 007 057). ERIC Document Reproduction Service No. ED 227 474.

Tseng, M.H. (1998). Development of pencil grip position in preschool children. *Occupational Therapy Journal of Research, 18,* 207-224.

Tseng, M.H., & Cermak, S.A. (1991, December). The evaluation of handwriting in children. *Sensory Integration Quarterly,* pp. 1-6.

Tseng, M.H., & Cermak, S.A. (1993). The influence of ergonomic factors and perceptual-motor abilities on handwriting performance. *American Journal of Occupational Therapy, 47,* 919-926.

Weil, M., & Amundson, S.J. (1994). Relationship between visual motor and handwriting skills of children in kindergarten. *American Journal of Occupational Therapy, 48,* 982-988.

Weintraub, N., & Graham, S. (1998). Writing legibly and quickly: A study of children's ability to adjust their handwriting to meet classroom demands. *Learning Disabilities Research and Practice, 13,* 146-152.

Williamson, G.G. (1993.). Enhancing the social competence of children with learning disabilities. *American Occupational Therapy Association Sensory Integration Special Interest Section Newsletter, 16* (1), 1-2.

Woodward, S., & Swinth, Y. (2002). Multisensory approach to handwriting remediation: Perceptions of school-based occupational therapists. *American Journal of Occupational Therapy, 56,* 305-312.

Wright, J.P., & Allen, E.G. (1975). Ready to write! *Elementary School Journal, 75,* 430-435.

Ziviani, J. (1987). Pencil grasp and manipulation. In J. Alston & J. Taylor (Eds.), *Handwriting: Theory, research and practice* (pp. 24-39). London: Croom Helm.

Ziviani, J., & Elkins, J. (1984). An evaluation of handwriting performance. *Educational Review, 36,* 251-261.

Ziviani, J., & Watson-Will, A. (1998). Writing speed and legibility of 7- to 14-year-old school students using modern cursive script. *Australian Occupational Therapy Journal, 45,* 59-64.

SUGGESTED READING

Campbell, S.K. (1989). Measurement in developmental therapy: Past, present, and future. *Physical and Occupational Therapy in Pediatrics, 9,* 1-14.

Johnson, D.J., & Carlisle, J.F. (1996). A study of handwriting in written stories of normal and learning disabled children. *Reading and Writing: An Interdisciplinary Journal, 8,* 45-59.

Lee-Corbin, H., & Evans, R. (1996). Factors influencing success or underachievement of the able child. *Early Child Development and Care, 117,* 133-134.

Taylor, J. (1985). The sequence and structure of handwriting competence: Where are the breakdown points in the mastery of handwriting? *British Journal of Occupational Therapy, 48,* 205-207.

Ziviani, J., & Elkins, J. (1986). Effect of pencil grip on handwriting speed and legibility. *Educational Review, 38,* 247-257.

Handwriting Instruments

CHILDREN'S HANDWRITING EVALUATION SCALE FOR MANUSCRIPT WRITING (CHES-M)

Description: Norm-referenced test that examines rate and quality of children's handwriting within a near-point copying task. Children's handwriting in grades 1 and 2 are examined qualitatively by letterforms, spacing, rhythm, and general appearance.
Authors: Joanne Phelps and Lynn Stempel (1987)
Publication: CHES
Information: 6031 St. Andrews
Dallas, TX 75205

CHILDREN'S HANDWRITING EVALUATION SCALE (CHES-C)

Description: Norm-referenced tool that assesses cursive writing of children in grades 3 through 8. Task consists of near-point copying of short paragraphs. Similar features of CHES-M.
Authors: Joanne Phelps, Lynn Stempel, and Gail Speck (1984)
Publication: CHES
Information: 6031 St. Andrews
Dallas, TX 75205

DENVER HANDWRITING ANALYSIS

Description: Criterion-referenced tool evaluating cursive handwriting of students in grades 3 through 8. Each of the following tasks has a time limit per grade: near-point copying, writing the alphabet from memory, far-point copying, manuscript-cursive transition, and dictation.
Author: Peggy L. Anderson (1983)
Publication: Academic Therapy Publications
Information: 20 Commercial Boulevard
Novato, CA 94947-6191

EVALUATION TOOL OF CHILDREN'S HANDWRITING (ETCH)

Description: Criterion-referenced test measuring a child's legibility and speed of children's handwriting in grades 1 through 6. Domains (manuscript or cursive) include alphabet writing of lowercase and uppercase letters, numeral writing, near-point copying, far-point copying, manuscript-to-cursive transition, dictation, and sentence composition.
Author: Susan J. Amundson, MS, OT (1995)
Publication: O.T. KIDS, Inc.
Information   P.O. Box 1118
Homer, AK 99603

MINNESOTA HANDWRITING TEST (MHT)

Description: Norm-referenced test that looks at quality and speed of manuscript handwriting of a near-point copying task. Models are in Zaner-Blöser or D'Nealian script for children in grades 1 and 2.
Author: Judith Reisman, PhD, OT (1999)
Publication: Therapy Skill Builders
Information: Psychological Corporation
195000 Bulverde Road
San Antonio, TX 79259
(800) 872-1726

TEST OF HANDWRITING SKILLS

Description: Norm-referenced test that examines both manuscript and cursive handwriting through dictation, near-point copying, and alphabet writing from memory. Normative data is provided for children 5 through 11 years old.
Author: Morrison F. Gardner (1998)
Publication: Psychological and Educational Publications, Inc.
Information: P.O. Box 520
Hydesville, CA 95547-0520

D'NEALIAN HANDWRITING PROGRAM

Target:	Manuscript, cursive
Author:	Scott Foresman Co.
Vendor:	Addison Wesley Longsman
	Division of Scott Foresman Addison Wesley
	1 Jacob Way
	Reading, MA 01867
	(800) 554-4411

ITALIC HANDWRITING SERIES

Target:	Manuscript, connected script
Authors:	B. Getty and I. Dubay
Vendor:	Portland State University
	Continuing Education Press
	P.O. Box 1394
	Portland, OR 97207-1394
	(800) 547-8887, ext. 4891

PALMER METHOD OF HANDWRITING

Target:	Manuscript, cursive
Author:	McGraw-Hill
Vendor:	McGraw-Hill
	220 E. Danieldale Road
	DeSoto, TX 75115
	(800) 442-9685

ZANER-BLÖSER HANDWRITING

Target:	Manuscript, cursive
Author:	Zaner-Blöser
Vendor:	Zaner-Blöser
	P.O. Box 16764
	Columbus, OH 43216-6764
	(800) 421-3018

HANDWRITING WITHOUT TEARS

This simple, developmentally-based handwriting curriculum was created by an occupational therapist. It is an award-winning, widely used curriculum for both special needs and regular education students. The program includes multi-sensory materials; workbooks for grades Pre-K through 4; teacher guides, and Spanish editions for grades K-4.

Author:	Janet Z. Olsen, OT
Vendor:	Handwriting Without Tears
	8001 Mac Arthur Boulevard
	Cabin John, MD 20818
Phone:	(301) 263-2700
Fax:	(301) 263-2707

Handwriting Intervention Programs

CALLIROBICS

Description: A program that sets paper and pencil exercises to children's songs as preparation for manuscript and cursive handwriting. Program cassette tapes accompany the student's workbook and can be implemented either individually or in groups.

Author: Liori Laufer
Vendor: Therapro, Inc.
          225 Arlington Street
          Framingham, MA 01702
          (800) 257-5376 or 508-872-9494

BIG STROKES FOR LITTLE FOLKS

Description: A developmental training program designed for children who already recognize most letters but have difficulty forming them. Its target group is children ages 5 through 9 for spontaneous, legible manuscript writing.

Author: B. Levine Rubell
Vendor: Therapy Skill Builders
          P.O. Box 839954
          San Antonio, TX 78283
          (800) 211-8378

HANDWRITING WITHOUT TEARS

Description: This Pre-K through Grade 4 program was developed by an occupational therapist. It is appropriate for all children, including those with special needs. The curriculum uses unique tactile and kinesthetic materials, music, and user-friendly student workbooks. The materials and teaching strategies are suitable for children who are struggling to write.

Author: Janet Z. Olsen, OT
Vendor: Handwriting Without Tears
          8001 Mac Arthur Boulevard
          Cabin John, MD 20818
Phone: (301) 263-2700
Fax: (301) 263-2707

LOOPS AND OTHER GROUPS: A KINESTHETIC WRITING SYSTEM

Description: This system was developed to enable second-grade children to learn the formations of all cursive lowercase letters in 6 weeks. Students learn four "families" of letters that share common movement patterns. Children visualize and verbalize the movement patterns while experiencing the "feel" of the letter.

Author: Mary Benbow, MS, OT
Vendor: Therapy Skill Builders
          P.O. Box 849954
          San Antonio, TX 78283
          (800) 211-8378

TRICS FOR WRITTEN COMMUNICATION: TECHNIQUES FOR REBUILDING AND IMPROVING CHILDREN'S SCHOOL SKILLS

Description: This resource manual provides more than 400 remedial and compensatory strategies for improving students' text production in the classroom. The focus is on students who experience mechanical and organizational difficulty during writing.

Author: Susan J. Amundson, MS, OT
Vendor: O.T. KIDS, Inc.
          P.O. Box 1118
          Homer, AK 99603
          (907) 235-0688

Internet Resources: Prewriting and Writing

www.hwtears.com (Handwriting Without Tears products and workshops)

www.alaska.net/~otkids (publications and information)

www.callirobics.com (Callirobics prewriting program)

www.firststrokeshandwriting.com (program, methods, and workshops)

www.handwritinghelpforkids.com (information and materials)

www.handwritinginterestgroup.org.uk (international group promoting children's handwriting)

www.ldoonline.org (section on handwriting for children with learning disabilities)

www.peterson-handwriting.com (practical strategies and methods)

Assistive Technology: Low Technology, Computers, Electronic Aids for Daily Living, and Augmentative Communication

Yvonne Swinth

Assistive technology (AT) has been an important tool since the origins of the occupational therapy profession. For years, therapists have used different types of low-tech devices, such as reachers, button hooks, pencil grips, and other pieces of adaptive equipment, to promote functional independence in their clients. However, within the past 10 to 15 years, with the technologic advances in society, occupational therapists have increasingly used a wide range of electronic devices, from simple switches to complex robotics, to promote functional independence. Additionally, Congress has enacted legislation supporting the procurement and use of AT for individuals with disabilities. This expansion in the use of AT opens new doors, creates opportunities, and enables individuals with disabilities to realize functional goals that were previously unattainable.

The Technology-Related Assistance for Individuals with Disabilities Act of 1988 (known as the Tech Act; Public Law 100-407) defines assistive technology as "any item, piece of equipment or product system whether acquired commercially off the shelf, modified, or customized that is used to increase or improve functional capabilities of individuals with disabilities." This is the same definition used in the Individuals with Disabilities Education Act (IDEA; Public Law 101-476), the federal legislation mandating services for students with disabilities in public schools. This definition includes low-tech adaptations, such as reachers and pencil grips, and high-tech devices, such as adaptive switches, adapted computers (computers set up for alternative access for individuals with disabilities), power wheelchairs, augmentative communication devices, and electronic aids for daily living (EADLs; formally known as environmental controls). Technology service delivery is categorized as assistive technologies, rehabilitative technologies, and learning technologies. Assistive technologies refer to technologies that are permanently used to compensate for limited skill. Rehabilitative technologies are used to remediate or restore function (e.g., cognitive retraining and crutches). Learning technologies are used to remediate or restore academic abilities (e.g., typing tutors and word banks). In this chapter, assistive technology is used as a broad term that includes all three concepts.

This chapter discusses general information regarding the use of AT with children, followed by specific examples on the use of computers and augmentative communication devices with children with disabilities. Other chapters in this text specifically address the other areas of AT (see Chapters 15 and 19). Many of the principles and decision-making strategies discussed in this chapter can be generalized to all areas of AT.

USE OF ASSISTIVE TECHNOLOGY WITH CHILDREN

Children as young as 6 months of age can learn to use simple AT devices (Swinth, Anson, & Deitz, 1993). For children with disabilities, introducing the appropriate types of technology systems as early as possible may enable the child to participate in important learning situations that otherwise, because of his or her disabilities, may not be possible. For more than 20 years, researchers and clinicians have documented and discussed the unique opportunities that all types of AT offer for teaching and for advancing the life choices of children with disabilities (Behrmann, 1984; Behrmann, Jones, & Wilds, 1989; Dickey & Shealey, 1987; Douglas, Reeson, & Ryan, 1988; Foulds, 1982; Judge, 2001; Lahm, 1989; Robinson, 1986; Sullivan & Lewis, 2000; Swinth, 1998). Many types of technology are available for children with disabilities, particularly those with limited motor control. The literature suggests that integration of AT in the lives of these children allows for increased productivity, independence and performance in the areas of occupation of activities of daily living (ADLs) and instrumental activities of daily living (IADLs), school and

work, play and leisure, and social participation (Bain & Leger, 1997; Judge, 2001; Parette & VanBiervliet, 1990; Smith, 1991; Swinth, 1998; Todis & Walker, 1993). Young children with disabilities may be able to learn basic contingencies, cause-effect, discrimination, turn taking, how to control the environment, and mobility and communication skills through the use of AT devices. All of these skills are foundational for higher-level conceptual learning. As these children grow, they can continue to use technology to develop independence in many ADLs/IADLs, complete written assignments in school, develop prevocational and vocational skills, increase opportunities for social participation, and play games or participate in leisure activities. The use of AT can create exciting opportunities for children with special needs to explore, interact, and function in their environments.

Because technology is constantly changing, this chapter presents problem-solving strategies, principles, and frameworks for decision making versus in-depth descriptions of specific devices or systems. Specific devices are used as examples; however, the reader is encouraged to focus on the principles versus the device itself. The frameworks and guides for decision making that are presented should not be viewed as limiting strategies. Rather, they are meant to be a starting point. Each practitioner needs to adjust the concepts given the individual needs of the client and family, teaming issues, availability of resources, and many other factors unique to each situation.

GUIDING THEORIES FOR DECISION MAKING

The occupational therapy practitioner must consider many factors when making decisions regarding the use of assistive technology. Throughout this process, the occupational therapy domain and process as described in the *Occupational Therapy Practice Framework: Domain and Process* (AOTA, 2002) serves as the foundation and guiding structure. During the decision-making process, procurement, use of the AT device, and follow-up, an occupational therapist considers the intrapersonal and interpersonal systems that influence the child's occupations. The client may be the child using the device, parents/caregivers, or other professionals working with the child and the systems in which the child participates (e.g., daycare, school). An alarming amount of literature documents the high rate of abandonment of AT devices, even viable devices (Batavia & Hammer, 1990; Bushrow & Turner, 1994; Garber & Gregorio, 1990; Scherer & McKee, 1989; Swinth, 1997). Approximately one third of the AT devices purchased or prescribed are abandoned by the user within 2 years. This may be because the individual no longer needs the device or because something better has become available. However, too often it appears that the high rate of abandonment is due to factors such as a mismatch between the user and the technology, complexity of the device, ineffectiveness of the device, lack of proper training on the use of the device, device failure, and amount of user input into the procurement of the device (Batavia & Hammer, 1990; Brooks & Hoyer, 1989; Bushrow & Turner, 1994; Phillips & Zhao, 1993; Scherer & McKee, 1989). By the time children with disabilities reach 21 years of age, they often have had experiences with many different types of AT devices. Given these factors, good AT decision making is crucial for the therapist to prevent device abandonment and to promote successful procurement and long-term use of AT devices by children with disabilities and their families.

The therapist begins effective decision making by viewing the child and his or her family as a system. Throughout the process, the occupational therapist considers the child, family, and environments in which the child participates, and the child's occupations (Dunn, Brown, & McGuigan, 1994; Law et al., 1996). These person-occupation-environment models emphasize the importance of contexts; client choice; and interactions among the child, context, tasks, performance, and therapeutic intervention.

Learned Helplessness and Self-Determination

Children with disabilities, physical or cognitive, can become passive and unmotivated because of a lack of learning opportunities or a lack of independent control over their environment. This can result in lack of interest or skills to interact with the environment (Douglas et al., 1988). When children learn that they have little control over outcomes within their environments, the phenomenon of learned helplessness can result. Learned helplessness is a secondary disability and is the belief that one cannot exert personal control over outcomes experienced when interacting with the environment (Abramson, Seligman, & Teasdale, 1978; Maier & Seligman, 1976). Children with learned helplessness exhibit low self-esteem, directly affecting how they interact and perform functional skills. They usually demonstrate a lack of initiation and an inability to cope with the events around them. Additionally, when opportunities for integrating basic cognitive and perceptual skills are missed in early childhood, these children do not develop a foundation for learning higher-level concepts. Strategies and adaptations that allow these children the maximum amount of independence possible as early as possible decrease the chance for them to learn that they have no control over their environment.

The opposite of learned helplessness is self-determination. Self-determination is defined as "acting as the primary causal agent in one's life and making choices and decisions regarding one's quality of life free from undue external influence or interference" (Wehmeyer, 1996, p. 24). Self-determination is an umbrella term that encompasses several common concepts used when describing children's personal, social, and skill development. These concepts include self-efficacy (outcome and efficacy expectations), self-esteem, and self-advocacy. Efficacy expectations are personal beliefs regarding one's capability to realize a desired behavior in a specific context (judgment of what one can do with the skills one has). Outcome expectations are personal beliefs about whether a particular behavior will lead to a particular consequence (being able to determine if one's goals are realistic). Self-esteem is the belief that one has in oneself or self-respect. Self-advocacy refers to an individual being able to speak for himself or herself, make decisions for himself or herself, and know what his or her rights are, particularly when those rights have been violated or diminished. The individual is able to take ownership of his or her needs rather than expect someone else to take responsibility for them because he or she has a disability (Swinth, 1997; Wehmeyer, 1996). Appreciating and being able to function with a sense of interdependence also is a crucial part of self-determination.

Self-determination is a set of skills that can be taught and learned. Key characteristics and components include autonomy, self-awareness, choice making (often children with disabilities are not given the opportunities to make effective choices), decision making, problem solving, goal setting and attainment, internal locus of control, positive attributions of efficacy and outcome expectations, and self-knowledge (Wehmeyer, 1996). With the increased emphasis on transition services and preparing children for life skills beyond school, occupational therapists should promote the development of self-determination for children of any age. This includes ensuring that services develop skills of interdependence and independence, addressing the participation and productivity of children, recognizing that self-determination can mean different things to different people, and recognizing that self-determination is a quality-of-life issue that can be addressed across settings, environments, and opportunities. AT devices, such as low-tech solutions, computers, EADLs, and augmentative communication devices (AAC), can help with the development, practice, and effective use of self-determining behaviors for children with disabilities.

Theories and Practice Models

The occupational therapist also uses theories and practice models to guide recommendations for procurement, implementation, and follow-up of AT intervention. Many different theories and practice models are discussed in Chapter 3. The ones most relevant to AT intervention include developmental theory and biomechanical, compensatory, acquisitional, and psychosocial frames of reference. Examples of AT interventions that apply these approaches are described in the following sections.

Developmental Theory

The therapist must maintain a developmental perspective when working with AT and children, especially young children, just as in any other area of pediatric practice. The child must acquire basic foundational skills before he or she can effectively use certain devices. Additionally, with some types of technology, a specific linear progression of learning and skill acquisition, both motorically and cognitively, must occur before the child can succeed with the device.

For technology to elicit an adaptive response, it must match the developmental skills of the child. For example, a child with spastic quadriparesis who requires complex adaptations to access a computer system may have the motor skills needed to access the system but may not have the cognitive skills needed to understand and independently use the system. Introducing the complex system before the development of appropriate skills can be frustrating for both the child and family, and it may discourage future use of AT devices.

Acquisitional Frame of Reference

When the team decides that the child is developmentally ready to learn AT, team members can apply the acquisitional frame of reference. The acquisitional frame of reference is commonly used during AT intervention. AT devices are provided when a child has significant motor or cognitive deficits that prevent him or her from performing a skill without the use of adaptations. Often the motor or cognitive delays prevent the child from reaching developmental milestones. Using the acquisitional frame of reference focuses on providing activities to help the child acquire specific skills both within and outside the typical developmental sequence. For example, a 14-year-old with cognitive delays may be taught how to enter numbers into a computer, using a predetermined format, from a piece of paper. Once the student has developed proficiency in this task, he or she begins to work in the school's front office entering attendance data into the computer. Eventually, he or she transitions into a community job entering data for a plumbing company.

Biomechanical Principles

Biomechanical principles address the musculoskeletal or neuromuscular needs of a child. If a child has musculoskeletal or neuromuscular dysfunction, then he or she may have difficulty maintaining postural alignment independently. Poor postural alignment affects the child's

ability to access and use most AT devices effectively and efficiently. Depending on the age of the child, the therapist may need to work on postural control before introducing a device. The therapist may need to provide external supports when the child's posture is unstable. For example, lateral supports, an H-strap, and shoulder protractors added to a wheelchair may help a child with spastic quadriparesis demonstrate improved arm control to independently access an expanded computer keyboard. When the child uses a voice recognition system, postural control is important for the child to maintain adequate voice quality. Using biomechanical principles, the therapist may also recommend or use different positions (e.g., standing versus sitting) to help enhance AT use.

Compensation/Adaptation Approach

The rehabilitation frame of reference capitalizes on a child's residual abilities as a means to compensate for a loss of skill/ability. Using this frame of reference, children adapt to their limitations by learning new methods for completing tasks. AT helps children compensate for the loss of skill. For example, a child who has had a head injury and has motor and organizational difficulties may use a computer with an adapted keyboard to complete written work at school. The computer also may be equipped with special software programs that will help the student organize his or her thoughts so that he or she can successfully write a paper.

Psychosocial Approaches

"The theoretical base for the psychosocial frame of reference is derived from the developmental theories related to temperament, attachment, peer interactive skills, play, ability to cope, and environmental interaction" (Olson, 1999, p. 323). When working with AT, the occupational therapist must consider the psychosocial implications of the choices being made. For example, school-age children may refuse to use certain computer access systems because the system makes them look "different." The psychosocial implications of AT use become increasingly important as children mature. What children will tolerate at younger ages often becomes taboo when they reach adolescence. AT can also enable the child to successfully master his or her environment in all the performance areas. Through application of AT, the child becomes more independent and competent, which positively affects his or her motivation, initiative, self-esteem, and self-identity. For some children and their families, even though an AT device may mean increased independence and freedom, they dismiss AT device use because of how it makes them feel or because of a comment of a peer (Swinth, 1997). The therapist must consider the effect that the AT device may have on the entire family system. A complex augmentative communication system can require hours of programming by a family member as the child's communication needs and skills change. This author has worked with several families in which handling the complex issues of a child's AT devices was among the reasons that one parent quit his or her job.

In most cases, therapists blend approaches and theories when designing AT intervention. For example, the therapist may use developmental and psychosocial theories when choosing an activity. The therapist uses the biomechanical frame of reference to position the child and equipment and uses the acquisitional frame of reference to develop strategies for teaching the child how to use the AT system. The therapist uses other practice models, experience, professional judgment, and the resources of other professionals to make recommendations regarding the use of AT devices.

BACKGROUND FOR UNDERSTANDING THE USE OF TECHNOLOGY WITH CHILDREN

Related Legislation

Since the 1970s, the United States Congress has passed several legislative acts that have directly affected the availability and use of AT for individuals with disabilities. The Rehabilitation Act, which was first introduced in 1973 and then rewritten in 1986 (Public Law 99-506), supports the use of AT for individuals with disabilities to (1) have greater control over their lives; (2) participate in home, school, and work environments; (3) interact with peers who do not have disabilities; and (4) otherwise do acts taken for granted by individuals without any known disability. The enactment of the Education for All Handicapped Children Act of 1975 (Public Law 94-142) provided support for designing, adapting, and using technology in the education of students with disabilities. This act encouraged private and public sectors to market new AT and provided incentives for the dissemination of information regarding AT.

In 1990, Congress amended the Education for All Handicapped Children Act and renamed it the Individuals with Disabilities Education Act (IDEA). These amendments call for the provision of AT devices and services as required to provide an appropriate public education for children with disabilities. The law defines an assistive technology device as any item, equipment, and system used "to increase, maintain, or improve functional capabilities of individuals with disabilities." AT services include any service that directly assists a child with a disability in the selection, procurement, and use of any AT device. Other AT services provided under the law are coordinating and using therapies, training, or technical assistance for individuals with disabilities.

The 1997 amendments to IDEA (Public Law 105-17) continue to emphasize the use of AT and AT services to enable the success of students with disabilities in their educational and school-to-career programs. Additionally, these amendments stated that teams must consider the need for AT for any child who is eligible for special education. This addition to the law has made it necessary for education teams (including occupational therapists who participate on these teams) to ensure that they have the expertise needed to make decisions regarding a student's need for assistive technology. These legislative acts have improved the access to and use of AT services by children with disabilities. They have also brought new options for therapeutic interventions when working with children with disabilities and their families.

Through the Tech Act of 1990 (Public Law 100-407), states have established resource centers and information systems for consumers of AT. These information systems offer consumers and their families technical assistance regarding obtaining and maintaining AT. In certain states, the Tech Act has supported training for consumers; other states have established central directories to facilitate access to AT. The goals of this legislation are to foster interagency cooperation, develop flexible and effective funding strategies, and promote access to AT for individuals with disabilities throughout their life spans.

The Assistive Technology Act (1998; P.L. 105-394) builds on the Tech Act. Its purpose is to increase access to, availability of, and funding for assistive technology through state efforts and national initiatives. The act affirms the federal role of promoting access to assistive technology devices and services for individuals with disabilities (Rehabilitation Society of North America [RESNA], 1999). Its three components are (1) state grant programs, (2) national activities, and (3) alternative financing mechanisms. Title I (State Grant Programs) supports public awareness program about assistive technology, promotes interagency coordination that improves access to assistive technology, provides technical assistance and training to promote access to assistive technology, and provides outreach support to statewide community-based organizations. The second component, Title II (National Activities), provides increased coordination of federal efforts and authorizes funding to support assistive technology grant. Title III (Alternative Financing Mechanisms) awards grant to states to help in establishing alternative funding mechanisms for assistive technology.

Teaming

As with many other specialty areas in pediatrics, the successful implementation of AT requires a cohesive and effective team that emphasizes shared vision and ownership. The team's input is critical in making decisions regarding AT because devices are used across the child's environments and address multiple performance goals that cross professional boundaries. Decisions based on teaming (i.e., the team and the family make decisions together) are most likely to meet the multifaceted needs of the child. In school-based practice, the law requires that a team of qualified professionals make decisions regarding the student's program. Thus, in this setting, by law, no single individual can make decisions about a student's assistive technology need(s).

The specific members of the team may be different in various situations depending on the type of device that they are introducing to the child, the expertise of the individuals involved, and the specific setting. For example, in a clinical setting, the team may include the child and family, occupational therapist, physical therapist, speech-language pathologist, doctor, nurse, rehabilitation engineer, and social worker. In a school setting, the team may include the child and family, occupational therapist, physical therapist, speech-language pathologist, educator, administrator, and psychologist. Table 18-1 illustrates the roles of some AT team members in different settings.

Often the introduction of an AT device, especially a complex device, can change the focus of a child's program. The therapist may need to spend time on training and practice within the child's educational program and at home as the family and professionals make efforts to integrate use of the device into the child's everyday activities. Thus, the development of skills needed to use the device often becomes the focus of intervention. Involvement by every member of the team encourages skill generalization in various settings and situations as the child becomes increasingly proficient using the new

AT device. The team's agenda may shift when the child learns a new AT system. Team input also is important to ensure that the AT device will not interfere with other priorities within the child's program. For example, if the use of an adaptive keyboard for writing limits a student's ability to complete a composition assignment, the teacher may select an alternate means for the student to complete the assignment.

The child (if appropriate) and the family are considered members of the team in all forms of service delivery. When the team working with a child begins to consider implementing AT, they must include the family in discussion and problem-solving sessions as early as possible. The family's financial resources, time, interests, and priorities can determine the success or failure of a particular AT device (Swinth, 1997). Depending on the family's resources, the procurement of an AT system can mean deciding between a family vacation or the possibility of the child communicating vocally. Additionally, for some families, AT can be confusing and overwhelming. The team can eliminate this obstacle by educating the family on the uses of AT and explaining the rationale for using it with the child. The parents' acknowledgment that their child must use AT devices can increase grief because it serves as a visual reminder that their child is not like other children. Explaining that AT facilitates the development of skills and compensates for the disability allows the family to view the use of AT positively.

Setting

The structure of an AT service delivery program is influenced by the services that team members provide, type of facility, funding sources, and sometimes particular

---

TABLE 18-1 Roles and Tasks of Some Common Assistive Technology (AT)*

Team Member	Setting	Example of Roles in Assistive Technology (AT)
Parent or older child	Clinic or school	Communicates and advocates for needs and preferences, provides follow-through at home
Occupational therapist	Clinic or school	Assesses functional needs in daily living, physical, and environmental needs; adapts and positions adaptive control systems; trains clients in use of equipment
Physical therapist	Clinic or school	Assesses mobility, seating, and positioning as it relates to the use of AT devices
Speech or language therapist	Clinic or school	Assesses receptive and expressive needs and abilities; determines appropriate symbol systems, techniques, and strategies; manages communication interventions
Funding specialist or social worker	Clinic	Secures funding for devices
Physician or nurse	Clinic	Manages medical needs
Rehabilitation engineer	Clinic	Designs, constructs, fits, and customizes devices and systems
Administrator	School	May become responsible to commit to district funding of systems
Special educator	School	Teaches academic and vocational skills; matches software programs with curriculum requirements
Psychologist	School	May serve as team leader; is responsible for eligibility criteria

*This is not meant to be an inclusive list of team members for any setting, nor is it meant as set criteria for any team member's role. Often these roles overlap depending on the child's need, the service delivery systems, and the individual professionals.
Modified from Beukelman, D.R., & Mirenda, P. (1992). *Augmentative and alternative communication: Management of severe communication disorders in children and adults.* Baltimore: Brookes; Church, G., & Glennen, S. (1992). Assistive technology programs. In G. Church & S. Glennen (Eds.), *The handbook of assistive technology* (pp. 1-26). San Diego: Singular Publishing Group.

disabilities specified in the agency's mission statement. Beukelman and Mirenda (1992) identified three categories of programs for children who need AT: medical centers, regional centers, and public schools. Occupational therapists are employed in all of these settings. The role of the occupational therapist in each of these settings is structured by our professional scope of practice, the expertise of other members of the team, and the agency/funding source.

Hospital or Medical Center

Some AT teams are based in hospitals that primarily serve children. A majority of these AT teams function in a predominantly evaluation role. The children may come in on an outpatient basis for a series of assessments by the AT team. The assessments may be completed in one or two visits, or they may require an inpatient stay of 2 to 3 weeks. Referrals and recommendations for specific equipment may be made to other agencies or third-party payers. After the initial assessment, team members often have limited access to the child for follow-up and training, and they have limited opportunities to consult with the teachers and parents (Beukelman & Mirenda, 1992). These activities are generally left to the agency (e.g., early intervention center, school district) where the child receives most of his or her services. Some AT teams in hospital settings also provide direct treatment to children with disabilities, especially for children under the age of 3 or children who have an acquired disability (e.g., a spinal cord injury).

Regional Center

As a result of the Tech Act and the Assistive Technology Act, many states have developed regional AT centers. In addition, some states have technology centers funded by the Department of Education or agencies for persons with developmental disabilities. Many of these regional centers have AT lending libraries. The child, the child's school, or the professionals working with the child in the community can borrow equipment on a short-term basis. The teams working at these centers have broad-based experience with various diagnoses, resources for obtaining equipment, types of AT, and adapted methods of AT use. Many of these centers are also involved in AT advocacy, consumer awareness, focus groups, and other activities related to efficient and effective use of AT by individuals with disabilities. Regional centers, like hospitals, often have limited follow-up care once the child has received the devices and may have minimal input into training the child, family, and educational team to use the device (Beukelman & Mirenda, 1992).

Public School

Most children who need AT service receive those services in school (IDEA, 1990, 1997). The demand for school occupational therapists to evaluate AT needs and help students learn to use AT has become a common feature of school-based practice. The large-scale growth of AT services in the school environment has evolved with new requirements through the IDEA amendments and the general increase in availability of AT in schools. In school, daily problem solving related to equipment use can occur and the child can receive support in using the device in the setting in which its use is most natural and important. Although the school-based team members have easy access to the child and the best understanding of the educational curriculum, they do not always have expertise or experience in AT. For this reason, collaboration among the school-based team and the regional or hospital AT teams is important. Currently, many school districts have instituted interdisciplinary assistive technology teams that provide comprehensive AT services throughout the district. Members of these teams provide support to other school personnel regarding AT decision making and the use of AT devices and AT services.

Funding

Occupational therapists working in the area of AT use with children are often involved in helping procure the appropriate devices, software programs, or adaptive peripherals. Funding can come from various sources, including Medicaid, grants, private insurance, nonprofit agencies such as United Cerebral Palsy, private foundations, schools, and individual payment. In some states, funds are available through the Department of Developmental Disabilities, Department of Health, or the Department of Social Services to help purchase AT devices. As students enter high school and begin the transition to work and career sites, the state's vocational rehabilitation agency also may consider assisting with the funding of devices. Occupational therapists must consider the complexity of the funding process. No matter what the funding source, the documentation must be complete and in proper order if a system is to be funded.

Additionally, there are some alternative sources of funding that the occupational therapist and client may want to consider (Carlson et al., 2003). These may include community service organizations, equipment loan programs, used and recycled equipment, and technical assistance projects. Often these alternative sources can take additional time and effort to research and contact. However, when a family or system has limited resources, pursuing creative funding options can result in the procurement of a device.

Funding of AT in school districts often raises unique issues. The school district is the payer of last resort, but it is ultimately responsible for AT devices that the child needs to learn in the school environment (Carlson et al., 2003; Swinth & Anson, 1998). Public or private insurance can be applied to the provision of a student's AT devices and services when they are determined to be medically necessary (Sibert, 1997; 34CFR §300.142(e), 34CFR §300.142(f), 34CFR §300.142(g)). The use of these funds must be voluntary on the part of the parents and with their written consent. School districts can also work with community service organizations or associations (e.g., the Muscular Dystrophy Association) to purchase AT devices or pay for services. Occupational therapists should learn about the different funding options available within their state and region to contribute to the team's effort to obtain funding for the AT device that is believed will best support the child's function. If the AT device is purchased with the parents' funds or insurance, then the device belongs to the child and the child's family. However, if the school district purchases the device through federal funds (e.g., IDEA), then the school district owns the device (Neighborhood Legal Services, 1999; Washington Assistive Technology Alliance [WATA], 1999).

Often the occupational therapist writes a letter of justification to support the funding of an AT device. Strong supporting documentation that clearly demonstrates the necessity of the device to strengthen the child's engagement in occupation is an important part of the process. This documentation is based on the evaluation data gathered by the occupational therapist and the team and takes into consideration the language and priorities of the funding agency (Carlson et al., 2003). If the letter is written to a health insurance agency, then the occupational therapist must address medical necessity; if it is directed to an education-related funding source, then it must address the child's ability to participate in educational programming. Requests to vocational agencies must address employment potential and skills (Carlson et al.; Schmeler, 1997; WATA, 1999). Other key elements in the letter may include information about the child, the device, the evaluation procedures, and the environment(s) in which it will be used; how the child will benefit from the device; alternative or potential outcomes of not being provided the device; supporting photos or measurements; and information about the cost of the device and other options considered.

Universal access has become an important concept that guides school and clinic purchase of new technology, particularly new computer systems. Most schools and clinics have established guidelines for ensuring universal access as they update and expand their computer systems. When all children, including those with disabilities, have equal access to technology, costly modifications for individuals can be avoided. Often the complexity of AT is not considered when general technology is purchased, which can result in computers that do not have enough memory to support some of the software programs or adaptive peripherals needed by children with disabilities. A team of professionals, consumers, technology developers, and standards organizations must plan together to assure that technology is accessible to all (Thompson, 2003).

One aspect of universal access that is gaining increased attention in the schools is "universal design for learning" (Rose & Meyer, 2002). School administrators have placed increased emphasis on the development and implementation of a universally designed curriculum that allows all children equal opportunity to learn and demonstrate what they have learned. AT and accessible software are important elements of a universally designed curriculum (Hitchcock & Stahl, 2003).

Sociocultural Factors

Sociocultural issues also may affect the procurement, implementation, and use of an AT system. Several authors have emphasized the various cultural influences on performance (Cook & Hussey, 2002; Krefting & Krefting, 1991). Box 18-1 summarizes some sociocultural factors that the therapist may need to consider when evaluating, designing, and selecting AT systems for children. Some cultures do not value the independence that AT provides individuals with disabilities, or an AT device may be abandoned if it replaces an important life function of another family member. For example, the grandmother who views communicating for a child with cerebral palsy as one of her roles may resist the child's use of an augmentative communication system.

OCCUPATIONAL THERAPY PROCESS AND ASSISTIVE TECHNOLOGY

When working with AT, the occupational therapist keeps in mind the theoretic frameworks of occupational

---

BOX 18-1 Examples of Sociocultural Factors That Can Affect Use of Assistive Technology

1 Financial resources of the family or cost of the device
2 Adaptability of the technology to enable higher levels of function as the child grows and matures
3 Use of time
4 Balance of work and play
5 Roles assumed in the family
6 Degree of importance attributed to independence
7 Sense of control over things that happen
8 Knowledge of disabilities and sources of information

Adapted from Cook, A., & Hussey, S. (2002). *Assistive technologies: Principles and practice* (2nd ed.). St. Louis: Mosby; Krefting, L.H., & Krefting, D.V. (1991). Cultural influences on performance. In C. Christiansen & C. Baum (Eds.), Occupational therapy: *Overcoming human performance deficits* (pp. 101-124). Thorofare, NJ: Slack Incorporated.

therapy and the aforementioned background information throughout the occupational therapy process. As in all areas of practice, the occupational therapy process follows what is outlined in the Occupational Therapy Practice Framework (2002) and involves evaluation (including gathering data for the occupational profile and the analysis of occupational performance), intervention (including planning, implementation and review) and outcomes. In AT service delivery, two additional steps are added to this process as distinct phases: (1) procurement of devices, which occurs before and as part of intervention, and (2) follow-up. Because of the complexity of many AT systems, especially computers, EADLs, and augmentative communication systems, the therapist needs a systematic procedure for follow-up and adjustments to help ensure the viability of the system over time. These steps of the process are dynamic rather than linear and sequential. For example, the therapist may begin intervention by addressing prerequisite skills for AT use before completing the AT evaluation and procuring a specific device. Once a system has been chosen and purchased, evaluation, monitoring, and decision-making processes continue throughout intervention.

Evaluation

The AT evaluation may be completed by the team who will also provide the intervention (e.g., fitting and training of the device) or a team that has been formed specifically for the purpose of completing AT evaluations. Many hospitals, clinics, and some community agencies and schools have a designated AT team because of the complexity of many AT systems. The occupational therapist who does not work with AT on a regular basis may have difficulty maintaining expertise on all the systems and devices available because of the number of devices and the rapid development of new systems. When a team that will not be providing the intervention evaluates a child, ideally the evaluation and intervention teams collaborate to make decisions and recommendations.

The occupational therapist has a key role on the AT evaluation team. The unique perspective on occupation and engagement in meaningful activities that the occupational therapist offers the team can often help with determining needs, problem-solving potential solutions, and evaluating outcomes. The assessment of client satisfaction/dissatisfaction has been one of the key factors in determining the effective implementation and usefulness of AT in the lives of individuals with disabilities (Demers, Weiss-Lambrou, & Ska, 2002; Demers, Wessels, Weiss-Lambrou, Ska, & De Witte, 1999; Scherer, 1993; Scherer & Lane, 1997; Swinth, 1997). Assessment tools and models to guide AT evaluation and service delivery have been developed (Bain & Leger, 1997; Bowser & Reed, 1998; Cook & Hussey, 2002; Scherer; Scherer &

Craddock, 2002; Smith, 1991; WATA, 1999; Zabala, 2002). Each of these models provides a framework for evaluating needs, making decisions, and implementing intervention. Using a model for service delivery helps ensure that the evaluation process is systematic and complete. Two of these models will be presented in this chapter (one in the following section and one later in the chapter when discussing issues specific to the school setting).

Human Activity Assistive Technology Model

In the Human Activity Assistive Technology (HAAT) model (Cook & Hussey, 2002), the assessment process is dynamic, and each step is interrelated. Figure 18-1 represents all the components of the model, each of which interacts with the other components and "plays a unique part in the total system" (Cook & Hussey, p. 38). In this model, the activity defines the goal of the AT system and "represents the functional result of human performance" (Cook & Hussey, p. 38). Activities are categorized within occupational performance areas. Each activity is carried out within a context, including social contexts, cultural context, physical settings, and the physical environment of a particular setting. Any of these contexts can influence how the technology is implemented. "The contexts in which the human carries out the activity are frequently forgotten when the assistive technology application is considered. However, the context is often the determining factor in the success or failure of the assistive technology system" (Cook & Hussey, p. 40). The human component represents the user of the technology system,

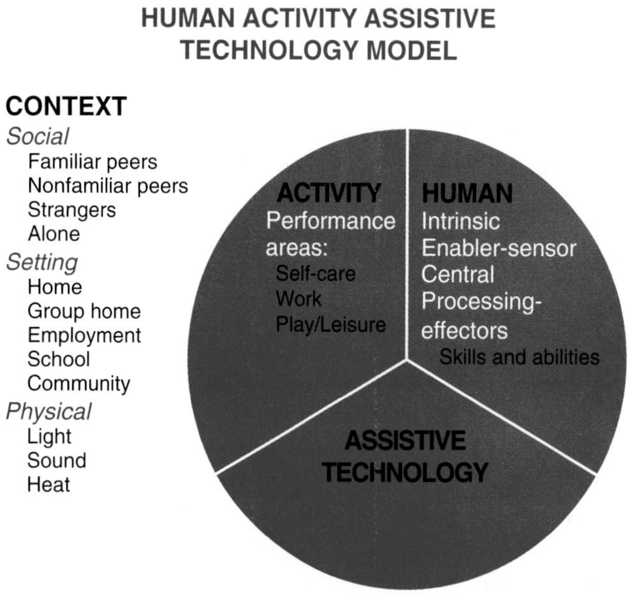

HUMAN ACTIVITY ASSISTIVE TECHNOLOGY MODEL

FIGURE 18-1 The Human Assistive Technology (HAAT) model. (From Cook, A., & Hussey, S. [2002]. *Assistive technologies: Principles and practice* [2nd ed.]. St. Louis: Mosby.)

or the child. The therapist must be able to determine the child's skills and abilities; "an ability is a basic trait of a person, what a person brings to a new task, while a skill is a level of proficiency" (Cook & Hussey, p. 39).

The HAAT model emphasizes the need to recommend AT devices that meet the specific needs of the child and the family by considering specific skills and activities that the child can or needs to perform and the contexts in which the child will perform the activities. In summary, an AT evaluation has the following steps (Swinth, 1998):

1 A team of multidisciplinary professionals is formed.
2 The team identifies family and child goals, priorities, and preferences.
3 The team identifies sociocultural considerations and concerns.
4 All team members evaluate the child. Elements of this evaluation include the following:
   a Performance skills and patterns of the child (developmental and functional, including motor [posture and positioning, fine motor, gross motor], sensory and perceptual, cognitive, communication, and psychosocial) (Box 18-2)
   b Activities (including activity demands) that the child needs or desires to perform
   c Contexts in which the technology will be used (see Box 18-2)
5 The team identifies and considers types of AT devices that can meet the child's needs.
6 The team provides trial opportunities for various appropriate AT devices.

Comprehensive and appropriate information gathered through the occupational profile and the analysis of occupational performance, coupled with trial periods with different types of AT, will result in a better match between the AT device or system and the child and family. The trial period may be one of the most important aspects of the AT evaluation. These trials can help prevent the costly procurement of an incorrect device. The cost of AT includes not only the purchase of the device, but also the ongoing costs for maintenance, upgrades to the system, and repairs. Questions that the therapist should address throughout assessment and intervention in relationship to cost include the following:

1 What financial resources are available to the family?
2 When the AT device is in need of repair, does the family have access to services?
3 Does the AT device significantly increase the child's level of independence and function?
4 Can the AT device be adapted to enable higher levels of function as the child grows and matures?
5 Can a less complex device meet the same needs just as well? (Swinth, 1998)

The team discusses these issues and others unique to each family in deciding whether the system is a

---

BOX 18-2 Guiding Questions When Evaluating a Child for Assistive Technology

MOTOR
- What body parts are capable of reliable, accurate, and controlled movement?
- Can the child be positioned adequately in and maintain an upright sitting posture?
- Does the child have sufficient range of motion, finger dexterity, strength, and endurance?
- What is the child's overall endurance and strength?
- What is the child's level of independence in daily living skills?

SENSORY AND PERCEPTUAL
- Can the child attend to visual feedback on the monitor?
- Can the child respond to auditory feedback?
- What are the child's strengths and limitations in visual perception and visual motor skills?
- Is the child easily distracted by visual stimuli?

COGNITIVE AND COMMUNICATION
- What is the child's cognitive level?
- What is the child's attention span?
- What are the child's receptive and expressive language skills? Potential?
- What are the child's face-to-face and written communication needs?
- Can the child sequence multiple-step directions?

PSYCHOSOCIAL
- Does the child seem motivated to use assistive technology (AT)?
- What activities does the child enjoy?
- Does the child see AT use as meaningful and rewarding?
- Will the child and family tolerate the influence of this AT device?

CONTEXT
- Where will the child use the AT device?
- How can the AT device or interface be positioned for optimal use?
- Do classroom or home environments allow for safe and easy access to educational materials and use of the AT devices?
- Does the child have any previous experience with AT?
- Are the individuals who work with the child (family and professionals) willing to use AT?
- What are the short- and long-term goals with the AT device?

---

reasonable and appropriate investment for the family that will result in increasing the child's functional independence. The team should present the child and family with objective and realistic information regarding investment in and use of AT. Given a complete description of the options and alternatives, the family and the team make the final decision as to what AT is implemented and how it is implemented into the child's program. Box 18-3 presents 11 criteria, developed by more than 700 AT consumers, that the team should use to evaluate different AT devices.

BOX 18-3 Criteria for Evaluating Assistive Technology Devices

1 *Effectiveness.* How much the device improves the user's living situation and enhances functional capability and independence

2 *Affordability.* The extent to which a person can purchase, maintain, and repair a device without financial hardship

3 *Reliability.* The degree to which a device is dependable, consistent, and predictable in its performance and levels of accuracy for a reasonable amount of time

4 *Portability.* The influence of the device's size and weight on the user's ability to move, carry, relocate, and operate it in varied locations

5 *Durability.* The extent to which a device delivers continued operation for an extended period of time

6 *Securability.* How well a consumer believes that a device affords physical control and is secure from theft or vandalism

7 *Safety.* How well a device protects the user, care provider, or family member from potential harm, bodily injury, or infection

8 *Learnability.* The perspective of the device's ease of assembly, initial learning requirements, and time and effort to master use

9 *Comfort and acceptance.* The extent to which a user feels physically comfortable with the device and does not experience pain or discomfort with use; how aesthetically appealing the user finds the device and the user's psychologic comfort when using it in private or public

10 *Maintenance and repairability.* The degree to which the device is easy to maintain and repair (either by the consumer, a local repair shop, or a supplier)

11 *Operability.* The extent to which the device is easy to use, is adaptable and flexible, and affords easy access to controls and displays

From Scherer, M.J., & Lane, J.P. (1997). Assessing consumer profiles of "ideal" assistive technologies in ten categories: An integration of quantitative and qualitative methods. *Disability and Rehabilitation, 19* (12), 528-535.

Decision Making

Occupational therapists use problem-solving and clinical reasoning skills throughout the process of procurement, implementation, and follow-up with AT. Problem solving should involve defining the situation or problem, determining the short- and long-term goals, and brainstorming potential processes to reach the determined goals. The therapist is often tempted to define the situation or problem and immediately jump to a possible technology for fixing the problem. However, if the therapist does not consider the short- and long-term goals before discussing potential solutions, the strategies implemented may not have a long-term benefit for the child. Many tools are available to support problem solving and decision making. For example, the Wisconsin Assistive Technology Initiative Project (2003) offers a variety of forms and checklists that can help therapists. Additionally, the Council on Exceptional Children (2004) offers a Consideration Wheel that can help teams

consider a wide range of options. Ablenet, a software company, has a CD-ROM available that provides information about low-tech and the use of simple communication aids for children with disabilities (www.ablenet.com). Finally, new information that supports effective decision making for children with disabilities is continually being added to the NCTI (National Center for Technology Innovation) website (www.nationaltechcenter.org). Due to the rapid changes with technology in our society, therapists working in this area of practice need to develop a strategy for keeping current with best practices related to effective decision making.

When working with children of any age, the occupational therapist should consider short- and long-term goals in terms of what the child's needs are at that time, 1 year later, 3 to 5 years later, and 7 to 10 years later. This can be difficult when working with young children, but the information can facilitate decision making, especially when addressing AT needs. When working with an adolescent, the focus becomes a successful transition plan, independence in the community, and participation in work roles. The procurement and use of the proper technology can be a critical part of a successful transition into future life roles for an adolescent (Burgstahler, 2003; Lamb, 2003; Stodden, Conway, & Chang, 2003). The team should revisit and rewrite goals systematically as the child grows and matures, as contexts change, as child and family needs and desires change, and if the child's medical condition changes.

Lahm and Sizemore (2002) interviewed AT teams to identify factors that influenced decision making when selecting assistive technology. The primary factors included client goals and environmental demands. Family/client demands and client diagnosis were also rated as important. Funding was considered but was lower in importance. The participants felt that it was important to understand environmental demands on the clients and recognized that evaluations completed in clinical settings did not provide sufficient information to make good decisions about AT (Lahm & Sizemore). Because distances, time, and funding often prohibit travel to the child, other strategies for gathering information about the environmental demands (e.g., phone interviews) were recommended in order to facilitate the best decision-making process.

Device Procurement

It can take months to procure an AT device. When funding issues stall the process, members of the team may be involved in writing letters of justification to insurance companies and other third party payers. Careful documentation during the trial periods with different devices can help with this process. Documentation can include videos or pictures of the child using the system that demonstrates how the system helps improve function.

Once the system has arrived, the therapist and team work to put the system together, test the system, and begin training. Some companies provide vendors that can help with the process, and others have videos that come with the system. However, it is not uncommon for a system to be delivered with minimal instructions. This can be daunting to the family if the system is delivered directly to their home and family members and other support providers are unsure how to use it. Comprehensive intervention and education are needed to help the child and family incorporate the device into their daily lives.

Intervention

Intervention involves the plan, the implementation, and the review. AT services, including device procurement, training, skill acquisition, monitoring, and other services, support and enable the child's participation in home, school, and community activities. The long-term goal of AT use should be social participation and productivity in the child's life roles and occupations of choice. Several authors have attempted to define specific prerequisite skills when introducing children to AT; however, empirical studies that define the skills needed to effectively use AT remain limited (Bowser, 1989; Symington, 1990). Behrmann et al. (1989) categorized the skills that children need to successfully use AT into four areas: motor skills, cognitive-language skills, visual perceptual skills, and social-emotional skills (Box 18-4). These skills are not prerequisites to using an AT device; the child can develop these skills while using the device.

Direct Service Delivery

Direct service delivery or therapeutic use of occupations and activities may or may not involve specialized training on the part of the occupational therapist. Therapists who specialize in AT may provide services to children for specified amounts of time that focus on helping the child develop proficiency with a system. Therapists who are not highly trained in AT should collaborate with specialists as needed. Frequently settings designate one therapist or a team of professionals to be the "AT experts." This designated expert can take a leadership role in learning how to operate the complex systems and in acquiring and reviewing updated information on AT for potential use by the team. Direct intervention may also include training the child and family how to use the device, customizing a system, and working on prerequisite skill acquisition so the child can successfully use the system. Whenever possible, training should occur in the environments in which the system will be used. This may require the therapist to travel or at times to function in

---

BOX 18-4 Categories of Skills Needed to Use Technology

MOTOR SKILLS
- Range of motion
- Strength and endurance
- Press and release
- Reliable and consistent motor movement

COGNITIVE-LANGUAGE SKILLS
- Cause-effect relationships
- Attention span (sustained or selected)
- Object permanence
- Means-ends causality
- Imitation
- One-on-one correspondence
- Intentional behavior (desire to communicate)
- Symbolic representation (recognize pictures)
- Reliable yes and no response
- Receptive understanding of commands
- Decision making

VISUAL PERCEPTUAL SKILLS
- Visual tracking and scanning
- Figure-ground
- Form discrimination

SOCIAL-EMOTIONAL SKILLS
- Initiating and terminating interactions
- Turn taking and waiting for turn
- Attending to an object or person
- Following one-step directions

From Behrmann, M.M., Jones, J.K., & Wilds, M.L. (1989). Technology intervention for very young children with disabilities. *Infants and Young Children, 1* (4), 66-77.

---

a consultative role when travel is not possible. Depending on the age, disability, program, and other child or family needs, the therapist provides direct intervention on regular or intermittent schedules for weeks, months, or, in some settings, years.

Consultation

Often after the occupational therapist has completed the evaluation process and set up the system, his or her services are primarily those of a consultant. For any child to be able to successfully use a system, the system must be implemented into his or her daily routine. Therefore, a major portion of the training to use technology should be implemented in the environment in which the child will use it. The therapist may work with the teachers to design a program that will allow the child to use the system in school. In addition, the therapist may design a home program so that the child can practice and develop increased proficiency with the system. The therapist then collaborates with the child, teacher, and family if any problems arise. Additionally, the therapist may systematically monitor the child's program at home and school and make changes, when needed, based on teacher, parent, or student input. If the therapist works in a preschool, he or she may help the teacher obtain a Touch Window and software program for the child to use to work on developing an understanding of cause-effect relationships and beginning computer skills. Once the therapist sets up the equipment and software programs, he or she consults with the preschool teacher as needed. As the child masters one skill, the teacher and therapist plan strategies, and sometimes new technology, to teach the next skill level.

In some settings, occupational therapy assistants and aides provide some of the AT service delivery. Assistants are particularly helpful in training a child to use a system once the therapist has set it up and established the program. Assistants and aides may also be involved in practicing use of the device with the child and helping others use the systems. Therapists working in AT service delivery must determine which activities are appropriate to delegate and which activities are specialized and require the training and skills of a therapist.

Education

Thorough training and education regarding AT systems are essential components in integrating AT into a child's daily life. Occupational therapists often function as educators for the child using the device and the family and other professionals involved in the child's program. The education that the therapist provides should be comprehensive and include use of the AT device, problem-solving potential difficulties, trouble-shooting when the device malfunctions, implementing the device in various settings, and, when needed, obtaining maintenance or repair services. Once the child has begun to successfully use an AT system, the therapist may continue to be a resource to address problems when they arise.

Advocacy

"Traditionally, occupational therapists have been advocates for consumers" (Trefler & Hobson, 1997, p. 501). Advocacy is part of the direct service, consultation, and educator roles of the occupational therapist. Occupational therapists work with other team members to increase the awareness of clients and families regarding their rights. Additionally, occupational therapists may use advocacy skills when working on funding issues and when helping other professionals understand the importance and function of AT in the lives of children with disabilities.

Outcomes

The intervention process includes intermittent evaluation of the child's performance with documentation of his or her progress toward the established goals. It is important that occupational therapists and the AT team select appropriate outcome measures to help them evaluate the appropriateness and effectiveness of the AT. Often, once the child and family have a basic understanding of the AT system and begin to use it independently, the occupational therapist may discharge the child from direct services. However, discharge from a regular routine of intervention should include a follow-up plan. The therapist can perform follow-up in several ways, from a telephone call to an extended clinic visit. The type of follow-up and when follow-up should occur depend on the complexity of the system and the skills of the child, family, and other professionals working with the child. "Follow-up provides valuable information. First, the effectiveness of the technology intervention can be monitored and/or measured. Second, if the intervention is not working smoothly, assistance can be provided before abandonment occurs, and finally, timing for changes in technology can be anticipated" (Trefler & Hobson, 1997, p. 499). A predetermined schedule for follow-up (sometimes at intervals of 6 months or less and sometimes 1 year or more) is a component of effective service delivery.

Evaluating the outcomes of AT takes a long-term commitment (DeRuyter, 1995) to ensure that it continues to support the child's engagement in purposeful activities. Often it is difficult to operationalize and define global outcomes specific to AT (Gelderblom & deWitte, 2002). Thus, it is important to determine how the effectiveness of a device or system will be evaluated for a specific client. Using the types of outcomes defined in the Framework (AOTA, 2002) can help occupational therapists and teams evaluate outcomes. Table 18-2 provides some examples.

Occupational Therapy Process and Assistive Technology in the Schools

Under the IDEA, assistive technology and AT services are provided if necessary for a child to receive a free appropriate public education (FAPE) in a least restrictive environment (LRE). All children who are eligible for special education must be considered for assistive technology. When AT is a necessary part of the student's program, then the school district is responsible to make sure that it is available to the child. It is not uncommon for the expertise of an occupational therapist or occupational therapy assistant to be requested as the team is considering AT for a student. Guides and models for considering AT for students in special education are available online. Appendix 18-A provides Internet resources to obtain this information.

A framework developed specifically for school settings is referred to as the SETT Framework: student, environment, task, and tools (Zabala, 2002; Zabala et al., 2000). This framework is designed to support good decision making that promotes collaboration,

TABLE 18-2 Examples of Types of Outcomes Specific to Assistive Technology

Types of Outcomes	Examples
Occupational performance	■ Improved ability to complete classroom assignments ■ Ability to participate in leisure activities with peers ■ Improved ability to communicate wants and needs ■ Ability to control environment (e.g., turn on lights and electronics)
Client satisfaction	■ Child is excited about new skill ■ Parents are pleased with child's progress ■ Child is motivated to use the device
Role competence	■ Able to meet the demands required of a preschooler ■ Able to participate as a fourth-grade student ■ Able to complete vocational activities
Adaptation	■ Change in the family's attitude about the use of assistive technology ■ Change in the adolescent's attitude about using software to compensate for a learning disability in reading and writing
Health and wellness Prevention	■ Student able to maintain psychosocial health in schools ■ Child develops needed typing skills to participate in third-grade assignments during second-grade ■ Child and family learn to use an alternate communication device in preschool so child can communicate with peers
Quality of life	■ Adolescent demonstrates self-determination skills across all environments and unfamiliar adults ■ Child is able to participate with peers across school environments ■ Child is able to go out in the community and order food from a server

Adapted from Swinth, Y.L., & Frolek-Clark, G. (2003). Overview of the occupational therapy practice framework and other considerations: Domain and process with school-based practice. In Y.L. Swinth (Ed), AOTA online course: Occupational Therapy in School-Based Practice: Contemporary Issues and Trends. Bethesda, MD: AOTA.

TABLE 18-3 SETT Framework Questions

The Student	The Environments	The Tasks	The Tools
■ What does the student need to do? ■ What are the student's special needs and current abilities?	■ What are the instructional and physical arrangements? Are there special concerns? ■ What materials and equipment are currently available in the environments? ■ What supports are available to the student and the people working with the student on a daily basis? ■ How are the attitudes and expectations of the people in the environment likely to affect the student's performance?	■ What activities occur in the student's natural environments that enable progress toward mastery of identified goals? ■ What is everyone else doing? ■ What are the critical elements of the activities? ■ How might the activities be modified to accommodate the student's special needs?	■ What no-tech, low-tech and high-tech options should be considered for inclusion in an assistive technology system for a student with these needs and abilities doing these tasks in these environments? ■ What strategies might be used to invite increased student performance? ■ How might the student try out the proposed system of tools in the customary environments in which they will be used?

communication, sharing of knowledge and perspectives, and flexibility. It supports a student's participation in curricular and extracurricular activities throughout the school day. SETT is a series of questions that are designed to guide discussion, evaluation, and intervention. Teams may choose to use a few or all of the questions, depending on the needs of the student. Table 18-3 outlines the SETT questions. Many of these questions are consistent with the type of information that an occupational therapist gathers as part of the occupational profile and analysis of occupational performance and may be applicable to other settings as well.

Outcomes in the school are generally based on the student's progress on IEP goals and objectives. Quality Indicators for Assistive Technology (QIAT) services in school settings have been developed (Zabala et al., 2000). The QIAT include administrative support, consideration of AT, AT assessment, documentation on the IEP, AT implementation, evaluation of the effectiveness of AT, transition, and professional development. Use of these indicators as guidelines can support good outcomes for the child, the family, the classroom and the system. These quality indicators can be used to help determine the effectiveness of services at a systems level as well as for individual students and finally for determining the level of expertise of the staff. They are designed specifically to address services that meet the requirements in the law, to improve effectiveness of services, to help consumers in evaluating AT services, and to assist in the development of policies related to AT.

APPLICATION OF ASSISTIVE TECHNOLOGY PRINCIPLES

This section describes how the previous principles of AT intervention can be applied to low-tech solutions, computers, EADLs, and augmentative communication. Occupational therapists are generally core members of a multidisciplinary team when a child requires the use of a low-tech solution to participate in occupations; a computer to play, learn, and work; an EADL to control the environment; or an augmentative communication device to communicate. Different types of systems are described, and examples are presented to illustrate principles in AT service delivery.

Low-Tech Solutions

Often occupational therapists and occupational therapy assistants work with very young children or children with significant disabilities. For these children, low technology, including the use of simple switches and cause-effect toys/appliances or software, may be the assistive technology system of choice. Therapists may use these devices to help a child learn cause-effect or to build foundational skills for future assistive technology systems. For some children with significant disabilities, simple devices that provide sensory input (e.g., fans, vibrators, music, lights) may be more motivating than some of the cause-effect toys or software (Figure 18-2). These devices can be hooked into an Ablenet Powerlink Control Unit and then a switch can be used to turn them on and off. This control unit can run electronically operated toys or appliances and has functions that allow the therapist to control how the switch is used (e.g., a timer can be used so the child has to hit the switch every 30 seconds) so that the system can be set up to help the child learn how to use a switch.

Often, low-tech solutions are controlled through a single switch. Typically, a touch switch that requires a press and release is used (Figure 18-3). However, for some children, this type of switch may not be motivating or the student may not have the physical skills needed to access the switch. Figure 18-4 shows an example of a switch that helps a student learn cause-effect relationships. Some children may not have the physical skills to press or to pull against resistance. These children may use a switch that is activated through a light touch (Figure 18-5, *A*). Switches can be mounted so that the position can be easily adjusted to improve access for a

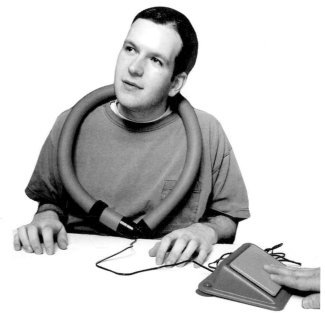

FIGURE 18-2   An example of a vibrating snake attached to a switch to provide independent control of sensory input. (Photo courtesy of Enabling Devices.)

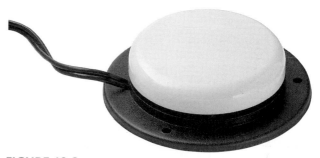

FIGURE 18-3   An example of a touch switch; the jelly bean switch. (Photo courtesy of Ablenet.)

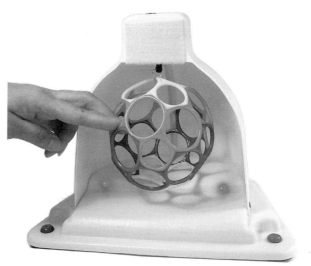

FIGURE 18-4   An example of a switch that is activated by pulling on the multicolored ball. (Photo courtesy of Enabling Devices.)

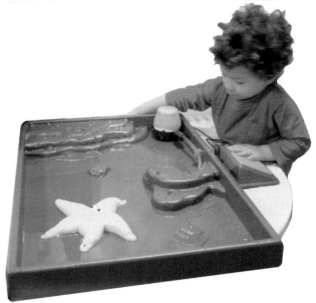

FIGURE 18-6 The child uses the switch to play with the water toy. (Photo courtesy of Enabling Devices.)

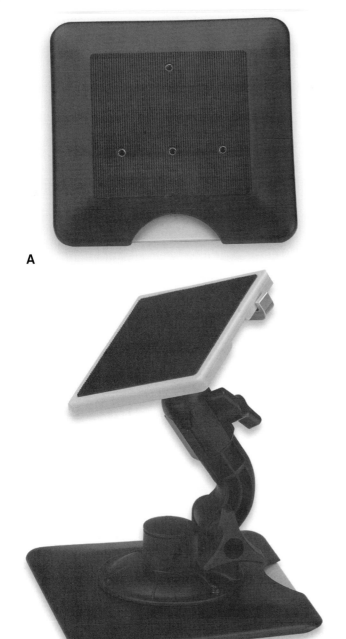

FIGURE 18-5 **A,** The Sensitrac flat pad switch by Ablenet. Switch is activated by a simple touch. **B,** The Sensitrac flat pad switch that can be easily positioned for a child to access. (Photos courtesy of Ablenet.)

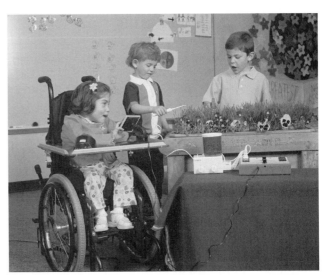

FIGURE 18-7 The child uses the switches to participate in a gardening activity with her peers. (Photo courtesy of Ablenet.)

student (Figure 18-5, *B*). Although this switch requires minimal controlled movement, its cognitive demand is greater than the switches pictured. The touch-free switch may be too abstract for students with low cognitive skills (Cole & Swinth, 2004).

Through the use of low-tech and simple cause-effect activities, children with disabilities can participate in a variety of learning activities in the classroom. Figure 18-6 shows an example of how a child with a disability can participate in a water play activity through a switch toy. Figure 18-7 shows how a child can participate in a gardening activity, and Figure 18-8 illustrates how a student with a disability can play the Bed Bugs game with his peers. Switches may allow partial participation, in which the student uses a switch to complete one step of the task. For example in Figure 18-8, the student pressed the switch to turn on the Water-Pik, then another student used the Water-Pik to water the flowers.

Children can participate in literacy activities using BookWorm (Figure 18-9 shows the BookWorm book). This device is set up to make almost any book a "talking book." After a book has been recorded into the Book-

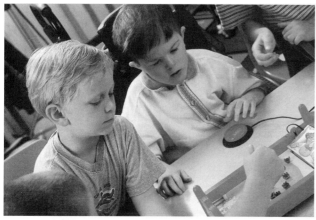

FIGURE 18-8   The child uses the switch to turn on the Bed Bugs game. (Photo courtesy of Ablenet.)

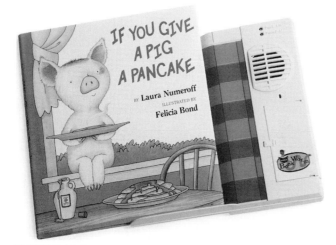

FIGURE 18-9   The BookWorm, by Ablenet. (Photo courtesy of Ablenet.)

Worm literacy tool, the child simply presses a keypad or an external switch to have the book read out loud. Another Ablenet program titled the Star Reporter uses low-tech devices such as switches, simple communication tools, and others to help children with disabilities collaborate with able-bodied peers to put out a school newspaper. The long-term goal of using low-technology devices with students with disabilities is full participation in typical classroom routines and activities.

Computers

Use of personal computers by individuals of all ages is becoming more prevalent in schools, homes, and work settings. Most children with and without disabilities have had some exposure to a computer system by the time they enter school. With the increase in personal computer use, children with disabilities have daily opportunities to use computers at home and school. Behrmann (1984) reported that children with the cognitive and

physical skills of a 3-month-old have the potential for electronic learning. In his study, 3-month-old infants activated a switch to hear their mothers' voices. Swinth and colleagues (1996) found that children as young as 6 months of age could access a switch to play a simple cause-effect game on the computer. Thus, it is realistic to consider beginning cause-effect activities when a child reaches a 7-month cognitive level. A computer can motivate children to learn and develop a large repertoire of skills. It provides simulations of experiences that children with motor disabilities cannot otherwise experience. For example, some adolescents with disabilities describe social networks and friendships that they have been able to develop using the computer, Internet access, and appropriate software programs (Swinth, 1997). The computer is also infinitely patient with drill and practice and can provide the repetition needed for some children to learn.

An almost endless variety of software programs, input devices, and output devices are available to customize computers to meet the individual needs of each child (Anson, 1997). If the therapist is working with a young child, he or she can introduce a progression of systems that follows the developmental and functional needs of the child. For a child who is born with a disability, success using simple systems precedes the use of more complex systems (e.g., use of a cause-effect program before a complex writing system). The successful use of a computer system requires that the user be able to provide input into the system, receive output (or information) from the computer, and process that information to use it in a functional, meaningful manner. Table 18-4 describes different computer options, hardware, and access systems.

Various types of computers are available in the home, school, clinical, and work settings (e.g., Macintosh or IBM-compatible computers). Macintosh computers tend to be the most commonly used systems in early intervention and grade-school settings, and families, facilities, and higher grades in schools more commonly use IBM-compatible machines. Before the therapist recommends the purchase of software programs or adapted access devices, he or she must evaluate the memory and technology of the system to determine its compatibility with the program. Now, many software programs are both PC and Mac compatible. For example, the IntelliKeys keyboard can be used on either machine without significant reconfiguration. However, because certain hardware and access devices remain specific to either the PC or the Mac, the therapist needs to attend to these specifications.

Input

When the therapist is looking at different input systems, he or she should use a least change principle. This means

Text continued on p. 637

TABLE 18-4 Problem Solving for Computer Access (Starting with a Standard Computer Workstation)

Name of System	Requirements and Considerations	Persons Who Benefit	Ordering Information
ALTERNATE KEYBOARDS			
IntelliKeys	■ Comes with some basic overlays, and customized overlays can be created using an IntelliTools program; numerous commercially produced overlays can also be used ■ Can be used in combination with IntelliTools to function as a talking word processor and communication tool or with IntelliPics to create accessible interactive computer programs ■ Can be used to run one-or two-switch programs ■ Works with Macintosh and IBM-compatible computers	■ Individuals with limited fine-motor control; access via mouth stick or head stick is possible ■ Individuals with decreased vision ■ Individuals who use a single switch to access single-switch software	IntelliTools, Inc., 55 Leveroni Court, Suite 9, Novato, CA 94949, Telephone: (800) 899-6687, E-mail: info@intellitools.com
Exanded keyboard: KeyLargo	■ Must have Ke:nx or some other type of software that allows the keyboard to communicate with the computer ■ Can be customized from single choice to 128 choices	■ Individuals with upper extremity control but limited fine-motor control; access via a mouth stick or head stick as well ■ Individuals with decreased vision	Infogrip, Inc., 1141 E. Main Street, Ventura, CA 93001, Telephone: (800) 397-0921, Web site: www.infogrip.com Madentec, 9935-29 A Avenue, Edmonton, Alberta, Canada T6N 1E5, Telephone (877) 623-3683, Web site: www.madentec.com
Expanded keyboard: Discover: Board	■ Talks so that it can be used for communication ■ Has basic overlays and software to create custom overlays ■ Can be used with educational programs ■ Can be used with Macintosh and IBM-compatible computers	■ Individuals with limited fine motor control ■ Individuals with limited speech or who are auditory learners	Don Johnston, Developmental Equipment, PO Box 639, 1000 N. Rand Road, Bldg. 115, Wauconda, IL 60084, Telephone: (800) 999-4660, Web site: www.donjohnston.com
Dvorak one-handed keyboard	■ Uses high-frequency keys under the fingers of the hand doing the typing (available in left-handed and right-handed versions) ■ Can be added to mainstream computers at little or no cost	■ Individuals who have one hand substantially more functional than the other; significantly diminishes finger travel as compared with QWERTY pattern for one-handed typists; may translate into faster typing or increased endurance for typing	Meeting the Challenge, 3630 Sinton Road, Suite 103, Colorado Springs, CO 80907, Telephone: (800) 864-4264 Microsoft Corporation, One Microsoft Way, Redmond, WA 98502, Telephone: (800) 876-4726 (ask for disk GA0650)
Chord keyboard	■ Uses a pattern of keys rather than a unique key for each letter ■ May be a replacement of the standard keyboard or an alternative driver for the standard keyboard	■ Individuals with limited upper-body strength but good hand coordination; allows the individual to type with little more than pressure changes on the keys rather than moving from key to key; requires the individual to learn the keyboard completely before typing because hunt-and-peck typing does not work	AccuCorp, Inc., P.O. Box 66, Christiansburg, VA 24073, Telephone: (703) 961-2001 Infogrip, Inc., 1141 E. Main Street, Ventura, CA 93001, Telephone: (800) 397-0921, Web site: www.infogrip.com
Mini keyboard	■ Requires Ke:nx or some other type of software that allows the	■ Individuals with limited upper-extremity control but	Tash International, Inc., Unit 1-91 Station Street,

TABLE 18-4   Problem Solving for Computer Access (Starting with a Standard Computer Workstation)—*cont'd*

Name of System	Requirements and Considerations	Persons Who Benefit	Ordering Information
	keyboard to communicate with the computer ■ Can be customized for the arrangement and size of choices	limited range of motion; depending on the size, requires fairly good fine-motor control; access via a mouth stick	Ajak, Ontario, Canada L1S3H2, Telephone: (800) 463-5685
Big Keys Plus	■ Is a simple keyboard with enlarged keys designed for young children or people who may require a large key-striking area ■ Has ABC or QWERTY layout ■ Has color-coded keys or black or white keys	■ Children with limited fine-motor control, particularly limited midrange arm movement	Greystone Digital, Inc., Telephone: (800) 249-5397, Web site: www.bigkeys.com
Little Fingers	■ Designed to fit children's smaller hands and fingers ■ Has trackball built into keyboard ■ Is only $12\frac{1}{2}$ inches wide including trackball ■ Is compatible with Macintosh or IBM-compatible computers	■ Children with small hands who need to use the keyboard as their primary method of written communication	Data Desk, Web site: www.datadesktech.com
MOUSE EMULATORS			
Headmaster Plus and Headmaster 2000	■ Works as a mouse emulator; a unit on top of the computer senses the position of a headset that the user is wearing ■ Requires an onscreen keyboard for typing ■ Is operated when user is attached to the computer through the headset; however, infrared wireless adaptations are available	■ Individuals with good-to-fair cognitive skills and no upper-extremity control; must have good head and breath control (lightly puffing into a tube connected to the headset is equivalent to mouseclick)	Prentke Romich, 1002 Heyl Road, Wooster, OH 44691, Telephone: (800) 262-1984
HeadMouse	■ Works as a wireless mouse emulator; a unit on top of the computer senses the position of a small sensor "dot" that the user is wearing ■ Requires an onscreen keyboard for typing ■ User can implement key press by dwelling over a key for a set time or by using an adaptive switch	■ Individuals with good-to-fair cognitive skills and no upper-extremity control; must have good head control and some motor movement to access a switch	Origin Instruments Corporation, 854 Greenview Drive, Grand Prairie, TX 75050, E-mail: Sales@orig.com
Tracker	■ Is a wireless mouse emulator; a unit on top of the computer works as an optical head tracking sensor via a tiny sensor attached to the user ■ Requires an onscreen keyboard for typing	■ Individuals with good-to-fair cognitive skills and no upper-extremity control	Medenta Communications, Inc., 9411A 20 Avenue, Edmonton, Alberta, Canada T6N 1ES, Telephone: (877) 623-3683, E-mail: madenta@ccinet.ab.ca
Hands-free mouse	■ Uses two foot pedals to control mouse direction, speed, and mouse clicks	■ Individuals who lack hand and arm movement but have adequate foot motion to activate pedals	Hunter Digital, 11999 San Vicente Boulevard, Suite 440, Los Angeles, CA 90049, Telephone: (800) 57-MOUSE
Touch Window	■ Provides easy, low-cost touch access ■ Requires dedicated software ■ Is compatible with Macintosh or IBM-compatible computers	■ Young children or those with limited cognitive skills	Riverdeep, 500 Redwood Boulevard, Novato, CA 94947, Telephone: (415) 763-4700, Web site: www.riverdeep.net

Continued

TABLE 18-4 **Problem Solving for Computer Access (Starting with a Standard Computer Workstation)**—*cont'd*

Name of System	Requirements and Considerations	Persons Who Benefit	Ordering Information
	▪ Allows user to interact directly with the computer screen; thought is not divided between the learning task and manipulating the computer		
OTHER INPUT SYSTEMS			
Dragon Naturally Speaking Dragon Dictate	▪ Is a voice recognition system available for MS-DOS and Windows-based computers ▪ Can create, edit, format, and move text by voice ▪ Can actuate a mouse by voice	▪ Individuals with limited motor control but good voice quality; does not work well in noisy environments	Dragon Systems, Inc., 320 Nevada Street, Newton, MA 02160, Telephone: (800) TALK-TYP, Web site: www.dragonsy.com
Eyegaze Computer System	▪ Is only available for MS-DOS computers	▪ User who has adequate vision to locate data on the computer screen and who is able to control one eye precisely; may not work well for someone with nystagmus	LC Technologies, 9455 King Court, Fairfax, VA 22031, Telephone: (800) 393-4293
KEYBOARDING SYSTEMS			
AlphaSmart 3000	▪ Is a small, lightweight, portable word processor for notetaking and simple compositions ▪ Allows user to see only four lines of text at a time ▪ Allows user to download to a Macintosh or IBM-compatible computer once he or she has entered data ▪ Allows user to print work via downloading to a computer or directing to most printers ▪ Can transfer data to a computer or printer using infrared	▪ Users with good motor control and visual perceptual skills ▪ Users who only require the computer or word processor for simple word processing (e.g., taking notes or completing papers) ▪ Users who need a system that they can easily transport	Intelligent Peripheral Devices, Inc., 20380 Town Center Lane, Suite 270, Cupertino, CA 95014, Telephone: (408) 252-9400, E-mail: alphasmart@cworld.com, Web site: www.alphasmart.com
Dana DreamWriter	▪ Is a portable word processor with functions that include editing, spell checking, grammar checking, text layout and formatting, and typing tutorials ▪ Allows user to see eight lines of text at a time ▪ Uses an icon and alphanumeric menu ▪ Allows students to store, recall, rename, copy, and delete files ▪ Comes with a calculator, calendar, electronic diary, address card system, and a world clock	▪ Users with good motor control and visual perceptual skills ▪ Users who only require the computer or word processor for simple word processing (e.g., taking notes or completing papers)	NTS Computer Systems, LTD, 20145 Stewart Crescent, #101, Maple Ridge, BC, Canada V2XOT6, Telephone: (800) 663-7163
Laser PC 4	▪ Is a portable word processor with functions that include editing, spell checking, grammar checking, text layout and formatting, and typing tutorials ▪ Allows user to see eight lines of text at a time ▪ Uses an alphanumeric menu ▪ Comes with a calculator, telephone directory, a program to write programs in BASIC, a database, and spreadsheets ▪ Is also available with a sticky key function	▪ Users with good motor control and visual perceptual skills ▪ Users of the computer or word processor for simple word processing (e.g., taking notes or completing papers), databases, spreadsheets, or desire to write programs in BASIC	Perfect Solutions, 12657 Coral Breeze Drive, West Palm Beach, FL 33414, Telephone: (561) 790-1070

TABLE 18-4 Problem Solving for Computer Access (Starting with a Standard Computer Workstation)—*cont'd*

Name of System	Requirements and Considerations	Persons Who Benefit	Ordering Information
SOFTWARE			
Word Prediction (Co:Writer, KeyWiz and EZ Keys, Aurora)	**Co:Writer** ■ Is available for Macintosh or IBM-compatible computers ■ Allows user to type into Co:Writer window; when a sentence is finished, it is exported to a word processor ■ Has grammar-sensitive prediction and is customizable **KeyWiz and EZ Keys** ■ Is available for MS-DOS and Windows ■ Works transparently into many word processors ■ Uses word frequency order of presentation **Aurora** ■ Is available for MS-DOS and Windows ■ Is a word prediction package that supports large vocabularies (greater than 100,000 words) ■ Offers special formatting to assist users with learning disabilities, including phonetic prediction and common misspelling prediction	■ Individuals with writing or spelling impairment	Co:Writer: Don Johnston, Developmental Equipment, PO Box 639, 1000 N. Rand Road, Bldg. 115, Wauconda, IL 60084, Telephone: (800) 999-4660, Web site: www.donjohnston.com KeyWiz and EZ Keys: Words + Inc., PO Box 1229, Lancaster, CA 95354, Telephone: (805) 949-8331 Aurora: Aurora Systems, 2647 Kingsway, Vancouver, BC, Canada V5R 5H4, Telephone: (604) 436-2694
Biggy	■ Is available for Macintosh and IBM-compatible computers	■ Individuals with visual deficits and visual perceptual challenges; enlarges the cursor so individuals can find it more easily on the screen	RJ Cooper & Associates, 24843 Del Prado, #283, Dana Point, CA 92629, Telephone: (800) RJCooper
Write:OutLoud	■ Is available for Macintosh and IBM-compatible computers ■ Is a word processing program with speech output ■ Contains a built-in Franklin spell checker and dictionary ■ Allows users to hear letters or words as they are typing or to have the computer read sentences to them when they are finished typing them ■ Highlights words as they are read ■ May enhance writing quality because user can hear if words are omitted or substituted ■ May help with comprehension	■ Individuals who can access a single switch; requires higher cognitive abilities	Don Johnston, Developmental Equipment, P.O. Box 639, 1000 N. Rand Road, Bldg. 115, Wauconda, IL 60084, Telephone: (800) 999-4660, Web site: www.donjohnston.com
Dana	■ Combines the affordability of a handheld device with the ergonomic benefits of a laptop ■ More cost-effective than a laptop ■ Runs with the Palm operating system ■ Compatible with Palm applications ■ Can write with a stylus on the screen or use the keyboard ■ Can adjust the font size on the screen ■ Downloads to PC and Macintosh computers	■ Users with good motor control and visual perceptual skills ■ Users who don't need all the functions of a laptop, but need to do more than just word processing ■ Users who need a system that is easily transportable	Intelligent Peripheral Devices, Inc., 20380 Town Center Lane, Suite 270, Cupertino, CA 95014, Telephone: (408) 252-9400, Web site: www.alphasmart.com

Continued

TABLE 18-4 Problem Solving for Computer Access (Starting with a Standard Computer Workstation)—*cont'd*

Name of System	Requirements and Considerations	Persons Who Benefit	Ordering Information
Balanced Literacy	■ Can access e-mail and the Web from the Dana ■ Multisensory literacy program ■ Provides opportunity for early reading and writing activities ■ Software is accessible via switch and expanded keyboard ■ Uses music/songs to reinforce learning ■ Does not go above the first-grade reading level ■ Comes with classroom activities/teacher's guide	■ Students who are pre-literate or beginning readers ■ Students with learning disabilities ■ Students who benefit from repetition and increased language opportunities to reinforce learning	Intellitools, Inc., 55 Leveroni Court, Suite 9, Novato, CA 94949, Telephone: (800) 899-6687, Web site: www.intellitools.com
Intellitalk 3	■ Available for Macintosh and PC ■ Word processing program with speech output ■ Highlights words as they are read ■ Can build customized activities for specific learning goals or classroom activities ■ May help with comprehension ■ May enhance writing quality because user can hear if words are omitted or substituted ■ Speaks words or sentences ■ Will give directions for a specific activity	■ Individuals with learning disabilities who benefit from auditory and visual input ■ Individuals with visual impairments	Intellitools, Inc., 55 Leveroni Court, Suite 9, Novato, CA 94949, Telephone: (800) 899-6687, Web site: www.intellitools.com
Kurzweil 3000	■ Scanning, reading, and writing software ■ Macintosh and PC compatible ■ Provides increased opportunities for independence during reading and writing in daily lives	■ Individuals with learning disabilities ■ Individuals who are visually impaired	Kurzweil Educational Systems, Inc., 14 Crosby Drive, Bedford, MA 01730-1402, Telephone: (800) 894-5374, Web site: www.kurzweiledu.com
WYNN	■ Scanning, reading, and writing software ■ PC compatible ■ Provides increased opportunities for independence during reading and writing in daily lives	■ Individuals with learning disabilities ■ Individuals who are visually impaired	Freedom Scientific Learning Group, 480 California Avenue, Suite 201, Palo Alto, CA 94035-0215, Telephone: 1-888-223-3344
SWITCH SYSTEMS			
Discover: Switch	■ Requires Ke:nx or other scanning software ■ Is slow and should be considered as a last resort ■ Allows computer to scan through various choices; user hits switch when computer reaches choice ■ Is available for Macintosh and IBM-compatible computers	■ Individuals who can access a single switch; requires higher cognitive abilities	Madentec, 9935-29 A Avenue, Edmonton, Alberta, Canada T6N 1E5, Telephone (877) 623-3683 Web site: www.madentec.com
TouchFree Switch	■ No touch switch system ■ Digital camera accepts any predetermined movement as a mouse click ■ Limited compatible software (mostly cause-effect) ■ Available for Macintosh and PC	■ Individuals with normal cognition and significantly poor motor skills ■ Individuals who fatigue easily	Riverdeep, 500 Redwood Boulevard, Novato, CA 94947, Telephone: (415) 763-4700, Web site: www.riverdeep.net

Modified from Swinth, Y.L., & Anson, D. (1998). Alternatives to handwriting: Keyboarding and text-generation techniques for schools. In J. Case-Smith (Ed.), *AOTA self-paced clinical course: Occupational therapy: Making a difference in school system practice.* Rockville, MD: AOTA; Contribution by J. Rogers (1999).

that if the child can use a standard keyboard and standard workstation with some modifications, this is preferred to purchasing an expanded keyboard or other type of input device (Table 18-5). For some children, using an ergonomic keyboard rather than a standard keyboard will increase their proficiency on the computer. For a child with slight tremors, defeating the autorepeat function or using a keyguard (plastic covers for the keyboard with a single hole) may enable independent use of the standard system (Figure 18-10). The therapist may need to consider a different type of mouse (e.g., trackball or touch pad) rather than the standard mouse. Software programs are available to redefine the keyboard versus using the standard QWERTY keyboard that comes with most computers. One commonly used keyboard is the Big Keys Plus, which offers as one of its keyboard layouts

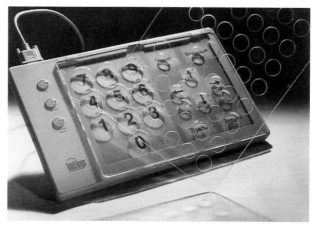

FIGURE 18-10 An example of a keyguard on an alternative keyboard. Keyguards also are available for standard keyboards. (Photo courtesy IntelliTools, Peta Luma, CA.)

TABLE 18-5 Problem Solving for Computer Access (Starting with a Standard Computer Workstation)

Problem	Potential Solutions
Difficulty pressing one or more keys	Change height of table or chair
	Change position of keyboard
	Change sensitivity of key or active delayed acceptance
	Use a keyguard
	Use an expanded keyboard with larger keys
	Use a stylus, mouthstick, or headstick
	Change size of letters on keyboard
Tendency to produce multiple characters rather than one	Change height of table or chair
	Change position of keyboard
	Change sensitivity of key or active delayed acceptance
	Deactivate autorepeat
Difficulty holding down more than one key simultaneously	Use Sticky Keys feature or utility
	Use a mechanical key latch
Ability to use only one hand	Teach student to use one-handed typing techniques for standard keyboard
	Use a chord keyboard
	Reconfigure the keyboard to use one-handed pattern
	Use onscreen keyboard and mouse for typing
Difficulty with the standard mouse	Use a trackball
	Use a trackpad
	Create a mouse track template
	Use MouseKeys feature of operating system
Slow or inefficient input	Increase keyboarding practice so that motor patterns are more automatic
	Set up templates for standard formats
	Use macros and abbreviation expansion for repeated words and phrases
	Use word prediction software programs
Drooling	Use a keyboard cover (Safe Skin)
	Use alternative keyboards that are not moisture sensitive
Difficulty seeing the screen or highlights	Ensure that the monitor is not facing a window or that the blinds are drawn
	Use an antiglare filter
	Reduce glare by turning down overhead lights
	Change size of font
	Change font (serif fonts are better for reading text; sans-serif fonts are better for letter recognition)
	Change attributes of font (bold)
	Change color of background or text for greater contrast
	Set screen to monochrome
	Use a large screen or lower screen resolution
	Use a screen magnifier (hardware or software)

Continued

TABLE 18-5   Problem Solving for Computer Access (Starting with a Standard Computer Workstation)—*cont'd*

Problem	Potential Solutions
Difficulty reading text	Ensure that the monitor is not facing a window or that the blinds are drawn
	Use an antiglare filter
	Reduce glare by turning down overhead lights
	Change size of font
	Change font (serif fonts are better for reading text; sans-serif fonts are better for letter recognition)
	Change attributes of font (bold)
	Change color of background or text for greater contrast
	Set screen to monochrome
	Use a large screen or lower screen resolution
	Use a screen magnifier (hardware or software)
	Use a voice output tool (screen reader)
Tendency to be distracted by sound	Turn off sound features of application
	Turn down volume from system control panel
	Use hearing protectors or noise-canceling ear protectors
Difficulty hearing feedback	Turn up volume (can use headphones)
	Use amplified speakers
Difficulty finding correct key on the keyboard	Use stickers or enlarged key letters to highlight correct keys
	Increase size or contrast of keyboard caps
	Use color coding for "landmark" keys
	Use Kids Keys Keyboard (for younger students)
	Mask inappropriate keys
Difficulty shifting between information on the screen, the keyboard, and the desktop	Use document clip to suspend printed page next to monitor
	Change position of keyboard
	Change position of monitor
	Use a Touch Window and on-screen keyboard
Difficulty remembering keyboard functions	Develop a "cheat sheet" of keyboard shortcuts to keep close by
	Develop keyboard mnemonics to aid memory of keyboard functions
Decreased motivation	Recheck student goals to ensure student involvement in goal-making process
	Try a different software program to address goal
	Change the purpose for which the computer is being used
	Change the access method
	Decrease the amount of time on the computer
	Scale the activity to the students' skills (up or down)

From Swinth, Y.L., & Anson, D. (1998). Alternatives to handwriting: Keyboarding and text-generation techniques for schools. In J. Case-Smith (Ed.), *AOTA self-paced clinical course: Occupational therapy: Making a difference in school system practice.* Rockville, MD: AOTA.

a color-coded alphabetic layout for younger children or children with cognitive delays who cannot find letters using the QWERTY layout. Additionally, the Dvorak Keyboard, in which the letters are arranged so that less motion is required for most common words, was developed to increase typing speed and reduce finger travel and strain for a two-handed typist. The Dvorak has a left- and right-hand version that can be used by children with hemiplegia. On a Chubon Keyboard, which is used for single-digit or mouth stick users, the letters with the highest frequency of use are placed in the center of the keyboard. Switches, adapted keyboards, and voice recognition systems offer alternative means for computer access to children with limited movement.

Alternate input systems come with their own software programs or a combination of unique hardware and software adaptations. Some alternate input systems allow for direct selection (the use selects letters, words, or phrases by touching or pointing to the desired key), and others allow indirect selection (an intermediate step is used when sending a command to the computer). Direct selection offers more choices to the child, requires less cognitive skill than indirect selection, and should be the first type of system that the therapist considers. An example of direct selection includes an expanded keyboard; indirect selection includes using letter scanning or Morse code and a switch.

Switches.   Switches allow access to the computer with a single movement. Many of the switches that can be used to access low-tech solutions (see Figures 18-3 to 18-5) can also be used to access the computer. Switches can be used for direct access (e.g., to make a choice in a cause-effect game) or indirect access (e.g., to move the cursor to a selection on the screen). Many of the more complex switch systems use indirect selection. When considering a switch-driven system, the therapist must consider the motoric and cognitive requirements of the system (Cole & Swinth, 2004). For example, a child who is able to accurately and reliably hit a switch at 9 months of age does not have the cognitive skills to understand the concept of scanning. In addition, research suggests that the placement of the switch (e.g., a head switch versus a switch that is struck with the hand) may have a cognitive component that affects a child's accuracy (Glickman, Deitz, Anson, & Stewart, 1996). A single (or dual) switch can be used to run systems such as Morse code and scanning. Morse code is faster than scanning but requires the user to learn a new language. However, once a user is proficient in Morse code he or she can typically type 20 words per minute or faster. Scanning is the slowest of the options available as an input method and should be considered as a last resort. Various scanning methods are available including row-column scanning, step scanning, and automatic scanning. The method that the therapist chooses depends on the skills of the child using the system. There are pros and cons to each of the methods. In row column scanning, the computer will scan down rows. Once the user selects the row in which the letter, number, or word resides, then the computer scans across the columns. This can be tedious but is more efficient than step scanning, which is when the user hits the switch for each step in the scan. Automatic scanning is when the computer scans through all the choices at a predetermined rate.

Alternate Keyboards. Alternate keyboards include programmable membrane keyboards, miniature keyboards, chord keyboards, and onscreen keyboards. Each type of alternate keyboard varies in size, layout, and complexity. The Discover:Board and IntelliKeys are membrane keyboards that allow the child with decreased fine-motor control or cognitive delays to successfully make choices on the computer. The Discover:Board allows for customization of overlays and provides voice output. The IntelliKeys (Figure 18-11) comes with inter-

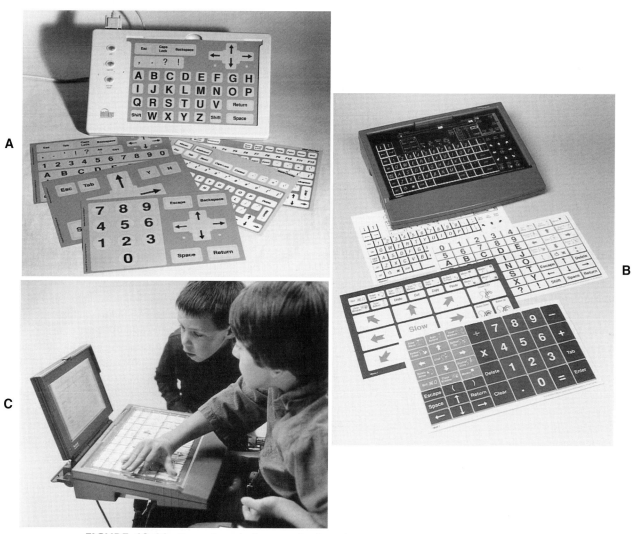

FIGURE 18-11 Examples of alternate keyboards. **A,** IntelliKeys with alphabet overlay. (Courtesy of IntelliTools, Peta Luma, CA.). **B,** KeyLargo and overlay examples. **C,** KeyLargo used with a powerbook. (Photo courtesy Don Johnston, Inc., Wauconda, IL.) Note: KeyLargo is now available from Infogrip.

changeable standard overlays and is compatible with Macintosh and PC computer systems. Each of these programmable keyboards allows the therapist to develop customized overlays and can be set up with "hotkeys" to allow the child to enter numbers, words, and phrases by hitting one key. Overlays are sheets of paper that have a graphic representation of a keyboard or functions of a software program (e.g., cursor keys). Changing the overlay, software program, and customization setup is relatively simple, making it easy to create new activities that align with the classroom curriculum or the current interests of the child. Miniature keyboards are smaller than the standard keyboard. An example is the Tash Mini Keyboard. Miniature keyboards are typically lightweight and designed to be used by children with limited range of motion or poor endurance. However, the user must have good fine-motor control because the keys are small and close together. Chord keyboards, like miniature keyboards, are designed to minimize finger travel. Use of these keyboards, similar to playing the piano, requires multiple simultaneous keystrokes to type letters and phrases. They require good hand coordination but allow for limited range of motion. They also require significant memory and cognitive skills to recall the chords assigned to a given letter. Onscreen keyboards (virtual keyboards) are software programs that provide the image of a standard or modified keyboard on the computer screen. The user can access these "keys" via different input systems such as a Tracker, Touch Window, trackball, joystick, and eye-gaze system.

Mouse Emulators. Mouse emulators are systems that the computer reads like a standard mouse. The most common type of mouse emulator is the different head-controlled pointing devices. The Touch Window also is a mouse emulator. Using this system, the child activates the computer by touching its transparent surface, which fits like a window over a computer monitor screen. Other mouse emulators include the Headmaster, HeadMouse, and Tracker (Figure 18-12). These systems work with a virtual keyboard often located at the bottom of the monitor screen. The child looks at the letter or word that he or she wishes to select or activate. A box on top of the monitor "reads" the child's head position and sends data to the computer. The cursor rests on the specific letter or picture on the screen. The child then hits a switch to make a choice or uses a dwell typing option (leaves the cursor on the letter for a specified amount of time so that the computer will select that letter as if it had been typed).

Voice Recognition. Voice (or speech) recognition systems, in which the computer recognizes and translates voice sounds into text or commands, are a good option for individuals with severe motoric limitations (e.g., high-level spinal cord injuries or spinal muscular atrophy). The user must have fair-to-good articulation

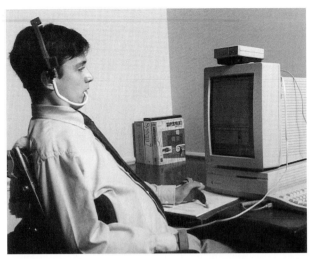

FIGURE 18-12 Young man using the Headmaster with a sip and puff switch. (Photo courtesy of Prentke Romich Co., Wooster, OH.)

to successfully operate a voice recognition system. The child speaks into a microphone to enter text, control the mouse, and execute computer commands. These systems are commonly available for IBM-compatible machines. Dragon Naturally Speaking is one example of a voice recognition system. These systems can be sensitive to environmental noise, especially in areas in which the noise level is high, such as a classroom. Voice recognition systems generally are not used with children under 12 years of age because of the complexity of the system.

Other Input Systems. Other types of input systems used with children include eye-gaze systems, Braille, Touch Free Switch, and a Tongue Touch Keypad. Eye-gaze systems are costly at this time. They require the child to visually focus on a desired position on the computer monitor. An optic light on the computer "reads" where the child gazes and makes the appropriate selection. When typing, eye-gaze systems use onscreen keyboards and other systems. Several programs allow a child who is blind or who has a significant visual impairment to input into the computer using Braille. The Touch Free Switch operates via a camera on top of the computer and is activated by a predetermined movement by the child. The Tongue Touch Keypad has nine tongue-activated keys that the child activates. Once the user activates the keys, a signal is sent to an interface box connected to the computer. The keypad fits into the mouth like an orthodontic retainer. Due to the cost and complexity of these systems, they are seldom used by children.

Output Systems and Information Processing

Computer output can also accommodate the needs of individuals with disabilities. Information (output) from the computer is visually displayed on the monitor or printed from the printer. Output can be auditory or auditory with visual. Monitors are the most common output devices, are available in various sizes, and can be mounted at various angles. For a child with a visual impairment, perceptual impairment, or cognitive impairment, the therapist may need to consider adaptations to the monitor. These may include the size of the monitor, whether it displays the data in color or black and white, the size of the text on the monitor, reduction of glare from the window or overhead lights, magnification of the screen, and change of contrast. The printer is the second most common way to receive information from the computer. Some printers provide Braille output, and several software programs provide voice output. Some of these programs read text, whereas others provide output regarding all the functions of the computer. Voice output systems can help support learning and computer use and exploration for students with learning disabilities, cognitive delays, autism, and visual impairments.

Output and successful processing of information are often closely related. Careful attention by the occupational therapist and team can mean the difference between success and failure with a device. If children with disabilities cannot successfully process and use the information received from the computer in a meaningful and functional manner, they will not use the system over time. With the increased screen resolution and the complexity of graphics now available in computers, some children with visual-perceptual difficulties are finding the visual information they receive distracting or overwhelming. For example, a child who has poor figure-ground skills may have difficulty with the Living Books Programs. This software program allows the computer to read popular stories to the child, but the graphics can be cluttered and complex. The therapist can also use this software program to help improve visual-perceptual skills, but he or she needs to be careful to provide the "just right challenge" so that the child does not become overwhelmed.

Software

With the burgeoning number of software programs available, from simple to highly complex, the therapist needs to make careful decisions to find programs that match children's interests and skills. Many children with disabilities can use common software programs that are available to everyone. Often software programs require that the child make specific, discrete responses to visual, auditory, or tactile stimuli. The child must be able to attend briefly and have the interest and motivation to activate a toy or a computer purposefully. Object permanence and understanding of cause-effect relationships are typically prerequisite skills for any computer program.

However, the therapist can also use computer activities and programs to teach some of these prerequisite skills, such as sustained attention and cause-effect relationships. Most computer programs also require skills in discrimination, matching, and directionality. Public domain software programs are available to work on cause-effect relationships and switch use.

Riverdeep, a software development company, has various learning programs appropriate for children of all ages. For example, the Early Learning House Series is a series of programs that work on early reading, math, science, and geography concepts through exploration and discovery. The educational version of these programs comes with a built-in single-switch scanning option. In addition to the concepts that the programs were designed to address, they also address skills such as visual perception, eye-hand coordination, visual motor skills, memory skills, sequencing skills, auditory processing, and listening skills. Another example of Riverdeep software is the Imagination Express Series, which teaches children story development and composition skills and allows children to create interactive stories using words and pictures. Sunburst, Davidson, Knowledge Adventure, and Laureate are other examples of software development companies that the therapist can consider when seeking different software programs appropriate for children with disabilities. Many companies such as Don Johnston and IntelliTools have developed software that can support early literacy (e.g., UkanDu series from Don Johnston), emerging literacy (e.g., Balance Literacy from IntelliTools), and more advanced literacy (e.g., Draft Builder from Don Johnston) development. Occupational therapists and occupational therapy assistants do not teach literacy, however, the therapist may be involved in helping to set up the system and customize it to meet the unique needs of the child. Two common software programs support advanced literacy skills and school participation for students with disabilities, particularly students with learning disabilities. These are Kurzweil 3000 and WYNN. Kurzweil is available for both the PC and Mac, and WYNN is only PC based. Both programs scan documents and books and will support reading and writing activities for students with disabilities. Computer software is also available that helps support the learning or computer use of children with disabilities. For example, therapists can use rate-enhancement software programs with standard or alternative input devices to increase the efficiency with which users complete written work or use alternative input devices. Examples of rate-enhancement software include abbreviation expansion and word prediction. Abbreviation expansion allows users to type in a short code that is later turned into a longer text. For example, a student with a spinal cord injury who uses a head-controlled pointing device may use abbreviation expansion to type his or her return address on college admissions applications. By typing "pra," the computer will expand this to include name, address, and phone number with correct spacing and spelling. Thus, by typing three letters, the user can make an entire entry of 50 or more characters. To use abbreviated expansion, the user will need to be able to remember the codes or refer to a list of codes when needed.

Word processing programs also use word prediction to increase efficiency with which a child types by decreasing the number of keystrokes needed to complete a word. They can also improve spelling because the child simply needs to recognize the word. Word prediction predicts words based on one to two letters the child types. As the child types the letters, a list of words appears on the computer screen (Figure 18-13). These words are typically a combination of commonly used words that fit the grammar of the sentence or the writing style of the child. For example, if the child types "s," the program lists "some," "someone," "speech," and "style." The lists generally include two to eight words and may be read to the user and presented visually. Once the program presents the list, the child either presses a number by the desired word or continues typing until the program presents the desired word. A child needs cognitive skills and a basic reading level to successfully use this system.

Computer Application and Intervention Techniques

With all the different input and output methods and software programs available, computers offer many ways to help children develop functional independence in life roles. The therapist should introduce children with disabilities who can benefit from the use of a computer as early as possible. They can have opportunities to use computers throughout their school careers and into their work settings. Children can also use computers as environmental control devices and for play and leisure exploration.

Early Intervention

As mentioned previously, therapists are using computers with 1- and 2-year-old children. In early intervention programs, therapists typically use the computer as an educational tool to help support and develop prerequisite skills for learning. Various early learning software programs and simple input systems are available. For many young children with and without disabilities, the standard keyboard may be too complex. Input systems such as the Touch Window, a switch, the Big Keys keyboard, or a mouse can simplify the cognitive and motor demands that the child faces when working on the computer. Young children can also learn simple computer functions such as putting in a disc, opening a program, and turning the computer on and off. Since many young children love to explore, there are software programs that limit the files and programs on a computer desktop that a child can access.

Case Study 1: Jeremy*

Jeremy is a 2-year-old with Down syndrome. His family wants to provide every opportunity for him to develop cognitive skills. They plan for him to attend regular education classrooms as he gets older. They were recently at a conference and heard about computers as tools for supporting learning and educational performance for some children with Down syndrome. They asked the early intervention team to recommend a computer system and software to use with Jeremy. What would you recommend?

School

Computers are used to help promote learning and productivity in the classroom. This includes activities such as writing, literacy, graphic designing, and searching the World Wide Web. Many high-quality programs support children with disabilities in science and math classes. Occupational therapists working in schools support team decision making regarding computer adaptations, software recommendations, and training and implementation. Children with learning disabilities, motoric

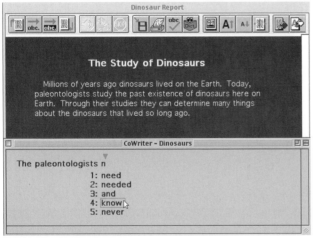

FIGURE 18-13 Co:Writer word prediction software. (Photo courtesy Don Johnston, Inc., Wauconda, IL.)

---

*There is no one correct response to any of the case studies in the following sections. Table 18-3 and Appendix 18-A provide resources that the therapist can use when problem solving potential solutions to each case study. Appendix 18-B provides solutions that one AT team recommended for each case study.

limitations, progressive illnesses, and cognitive limitations may have difficulties in written communication. It is often helpful for these children to transition from handwriting to text generation or word processing skills. Therapists combine hardware solutions (e.g., alternative keyboards) with software solutions (e.g., work prediction or talking word processors) to promote students' success in written communication.

In schools, it is common for various students to use one computer. This means that when changes are made to a base device, such as the addition of peripherals or software programs, the other students and teachers who use the system have to be willing to tolerate the changes. School-based occupational therapists are often involved in training other users of the systems how to work around the changes if the system is not dedicated to one student.

Case Study 2: Linnea

Linnea is a third-grade student with spinal muscular atrophy. She is fully included in her neighborhood school with support from related services as needed. Recently, she has been complaining to her parents and therapists that her hand gets tired when writing and that her handwriting looks "sloppy." Her teacher also has noticed that she seems irritable and lacks concentration during class. Linnea, her family, and her therapists have discussed using computers for written communication in the past, but Linnea and her family have always been reluctant to explore this at length because she does not want to "look different." Linnea has had experience with computers since kindergarten. Her class goes to the computer lab three times a week, and she began learning basic keyboarding skills in second grade. Her classroom has two computers that students use for drill, practice, and special projects. How would you address Linnea's handwriting problems?

Prevocational

When students use AT in school, there is often an emphasis on inclusion and "normalcy" versus production (Dudgeon, Massagli, & Ross, 1997). This becomes an issue as students transition from the classroom to a school-to-career program. Bersani, Fried-Oken, Anctil, Staehely and Bowser (1999) stated that for an adolescent to be successful at using AT in a work setting, the occupational therapist must carefully plan the transition with AT addressed at every step of the planning process. To support AT use, the therapist may work with the educational team in determining how to adapt the environment, task, or computer setup. When a student with cognitive disabilities expresses interest in a job that involves computer input and simple word processing, a therapist considers hardware and software adaptations,

environmental adaptations such as decreasing distractions, background color or font changes on the computer, and a consistent and predictable workspace. To ensure carryover with the student's caregivers and perspective employer, the therapist may develop step-by-step cheat sheets with words or pictures for directions, a drawing of a simple schematic, or color coding areas for attaching the peripherals. The student's success with AT can be critical to his or her success in employment and community living.

Case Study 3: Margy

Margy is 17 years old and has cognitive impairments and attention-deficit hyperactivity disorder (ADHD). During her last individualized transition plan (ITP), her family expressed the desire for Margy to get a job in the family carpet cleaning business. Margy enjoys greeting people, and others enjoy her bubbly and outgoing personality, so her dad and mom felt that it would be good if she could work with the receptionist in the front office of their business. Her dad felt that she should have more responsibility than simply greeting customers. He said that Margy has always enjoyed working on the computer and recommended that she learn data entry on the computer to make productive use of her down time when she was not talking with a customer. The team agreed that this could be a reasonable expectation for Margy and worked to develop a plan to reach this goal. Describe a plan that evidences multidisciplinary input.

Environmental Control

Some computer systems can double as environmental control units. Combining functions in the child's computer provides him or her with one system for several different functions and can be cost-effective since potentially fewer systems need to be purchased. Several different hardware and software systems support environmental control systems through the computer. These systems can be simple, such as operating a compact disc (CD) player or answering machine, or complex, such as operating several different environmental controls (e.g., unlocking and opening the front door; controlling lights and ceiling fans; and turning televisions, radios, and other small appliances on and off).

Case Study 4: Eric

Eric is 15 years old and has severe athetoid cerebral palsy. The only control that he has is dorsiflexion of his right foot. He attends general education classrooms and works independently on his computer. This year he received a new computer system. He completes all of his homework assignments via a row-column scanning system. He uses an IBM-compatible computer with Microsoft Office and word prediction software. He uses dorsiflexion of his right foot to execute the scanning. He is active on the Internet. He also writes plays for his high school football team. He would like to have some environmental control using his computer when he is in his room. What would you recommend?

Play and Leisure

Many individuals who have a personal home computer use them for play and leisure activities and for work. If a student has access to a computer at home or other frequently visited settings, the therapist and educational team may want to explore whether it would be a viable tool for leisure activities. Providing opportunities for play or leisure activities may help the student become more familiar with the system and its operation. Various software programs combine learning with leisure-type activities. The occupational therapist can work with children to determine which programs and leisure activities are most interesting and recommend adaptations for access (Swinth & Anson, 1998).

Case Study 5: Ryan

Ryan is 6 years old and has autism. His family is constantly looking for appropriate play activities that he can do independently for 5 to 6 minutes at a time. Many independent play activities are not appropriate because they would lead into his self-stimulation behaviors. Ryan is intrigued when his older siblings are doing their homework on the computer. He had erased several papers from the computer when a sibling turned his or her back and Ryan happened to hit the wrong button on the keyboard. Given Ryan's interests and behaviors, what would you recommend?

ELECTRONIC AIDS FOR DAILY LIVING (EADLs)

Originally, EADLs were known as ECUs (environmental control units). These are systems that allow a child to control appliances in the environment. EADLs allow the child to interact with and manipulate one or more electronic appliance, such as a television, radio, CD player, lights, telephone, and fan. This is accomplished using voice activation, switch access, a computer interface, or adaptations such as X-10 units. The EADL should meet the child's primary needs, and any long-range goals that might have been stated during the occupational profile. The system should also be fairly easy to assemble, learn to use, and maintain. As mentioned previously, EADLs can be integrated into a child's computer system. They also can be stand-alone systems. Some of these systems have discrete control interface (an electronic device is

either turned on or off), such as lights, fans, or a television set. Others are capable of continuous control interface, which results in successively greater or smaller degrees of control. For example, continuous control is lowering and raising of the volume on a television or dimming a light.

A common EADL used with children is the Powerlink by Ablenet (Figure 18-14). The Powerlink is a small box into which the desired electronic aid is plugged; it can control one or two devices. Many EADL options are available for a variety of settings.

ALTERNATIVE AND AUGMENTATIVE COMMUNICATION

Alternative and augmentative communication (AAC) is defined as communication that does not require speech and that can be individualized to the unique needs of the individual. An AAC system uses a combination of all the methods of communication available to a child. This can include "any residual speech, vocalizations, gestures, and communicative behaviors in addition to specific communication strategies and communication aids" (Doster & Politano, 1996, p. 7). The overall purpose of AAC is to enable an individual to transmit a message to another individual. As stated by the National Joint Committee for the Communications of Persons with Severe Disabilities (1992), "all persons, regardless of the extent or severity of their disabilities, have a basic right to affect, through communication, the conditions of their own existence." In addition to this basic right, the committee has outlined 12 specific communication rights that should be ensured during all daily communication acts with persons with disabilities (Box 18-5). According to Beukelman and Miranda (1992), even students with severe disabilities can benefit from AAC use.

AAC devices include low-tech systems, such as communication boards and picture exchange systems, and high-tech electronic devices. Often, both speech and language pathologists and occupational therapists work together to select and train children to use AAC. Both have unique perspectives and skills to offer in this specialized area. Occupational therapists should be familiar with terminology used in the area of AAC, such as single-switch scanning selection, encoding, directed scanning, and direct selection (Angelo & Smith, 1989). Additionally, occupational therapists working in the area of AAC should be able to use strategies that facilitate communication (Box 18-6). Continuing education courses and additional training can familiarize therapists with the terminology, communication strategies, and available hardware and software.

AAC can be viewed through several continuums, including aided or unaided communication methods and low-tech or high-tech devices. Depending on their age,

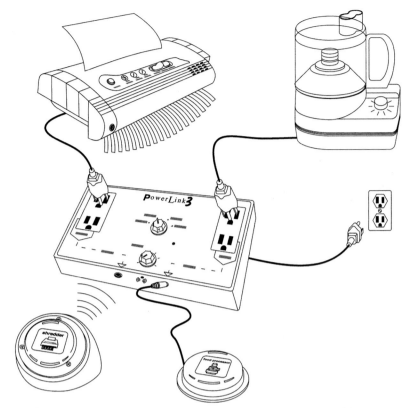

FIGURE 18-14   Schematic of an EADL set-up with the Powerlink. (Photo courtesy of Ablenet.)

contexts, and skills, children use a combination of aided and unaided communication and a combination of low- and high-tech devices. Unaided communication consists of vocalizations, gestures, facial expressions, sign language, and pantomime. All communicators use some sort of combination of unaided communication. Children with disabilities often use gestures, facial expressions, and body language as allowed by their functional skills.

Aided communication systems are also sometimes referred to as nonelectronic or electronic communication aids. Nonelectronic aids include communication boards and picture exchange communication systems (PECs), which use pictures, symbols, and words to communicate messages. PECs are being used increasingly with children in preschool, children with severe disabilities, and children with autism. To communicate his or her wants and needs, the child selects a picture of that item or activity, handing it to the adult. The adult acknowledges the child's communication attempt by naming of the picture and responding to the child's request. The child is encouraged to pair words with the picture cards with the goal of learning to use words with pictures and then using words alone.

Types of symbols include Blissymbolics, Rebus, and PicSyms (Figure 18-15). AAC users point to a picture or symbol to communicate messages and desires. As a child becomes more proficient in the use of pictures and symbols, complex communication boards can be developed to transmit messages (Figure 18-16). These systems can be mounted to a wheelchair tray, put in a notebook that the child carries, or mounted on a series of cards that the child gives to another individual when he or she wants to communicate ideas.

For children with severe disabilities or young children, several different types of simple AAC devices can be used. One example is a BigMac (Figure 18-17, *A*). This device has a recorded message that is activated each time the user presses the switch (Figure 18-17, *B*). Another simple AAC device that is good for individuals who are ambulatory is the TalkTrac (Figure 18-18, *A*), which is worn like a watch and can have several prerecorded messages. The messages are easy to change, and symbols can be used to help the user remember the messages (see Figure 18-18, *B*). Devices like a Supertalker (Figure 18-19) are good for children who may eventually use more high-tech AAC.

High-tech electronic communication aids generally are either computer-based systems or dedicated systems. Occupational therapists often consider computer-based systems for children who are using or will be using some sort of computer-assistive technology. Ideally,

BOX 18-5   Basic Communication Rights

1 The right to request desired objects, actions, events, and persons and to express personal preferences or feelings
2 The right to be offered choices and alternatives
3 The right to reject or refuse undesired objects, events, or actions, including the right to decline or reject all proffered choices
4 The right to request and be given attention from and interaction with another person
5 The right to request feedback or information about a state, object, person, or event of interest
6 The right to active treatment and intervention efforts to enable people with severe disabilities to communicated messages in whatever modes and as effectively and efficiently as their specific abilities will allow
7 The right to have communication acts acknowledged and responded to, even when the responder cannot fulfill the intent of these acts
8 The right to have access at all times to any needed augmentative and alternative communication devices and other assistive devices and to have those devices in good working order
9 The right to environmental contexts, interactions, and opportunities that expect and encourage persons with disabilities to participate as full communicative partners with other people, including peers
10 The right to be informed about the people, things, and events in one's immediate environment
11 The right to be communicated with in a manner that recognizes and acknowledges the inherent dignity of the person being addressed, including the right to be a part of communication exchanges about individuals that are conducted in his or her presence
12 The right to be communicated with in ways that are meaningful, understandable, and culturally and linguistically appropriate

From National Joint Committee for the Communication Needs of Persons with Severe Disabilities. (1992, March). Guidelines for meeting the communication needs of persons with severe disabilities. *ASHA, 34* (Supp. 7), 1-8.

BOX 18-6   Strategies to Facilitate Communicative Interaction

1 Structure the environment to foster interaction.
2 Attend to the child. Solicit a shared focus.
3 Provide meaningful opportunities for communication.
4 Have realistic expectations for the child.
5 Provide appropriate language input.
6 Avoid yes/no questions and "test" questions.
7 Pace the interaction. Give the student time to communicate. WAIT.
8 Follow the child's lead. Respond to his or her attempts to communicate.
9 Provide models for the child's expressive modes of communication. Coach the child as needed.
10 Prompt if necessary. Remember to fade prompts to natural cues. Enjoy communication.

Adapted from Special Education Technology Center, Ellensburg, WA.

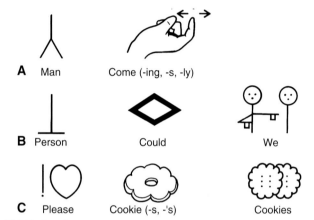

FIGURE 18-15   Examples of symbol systems. **A,** Bliss. **B,** Rebus. **C,** Picsyms.

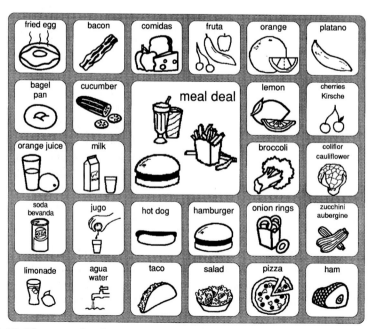

FIGURE 18-16   Example of a communication board that the child can use at meal time. (Photo courtesy of Mayer-Johnson Co.)

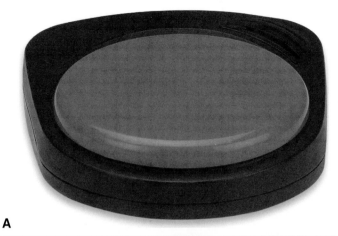

A

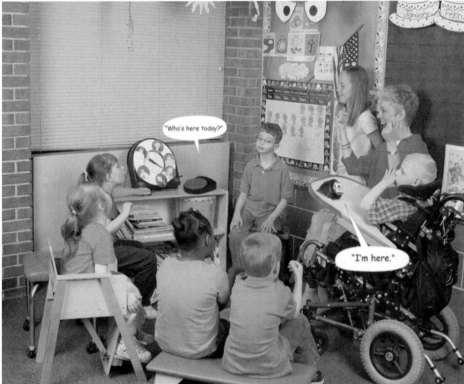

"Who's here today?"

"I'm here."

B

FIGURE 18-17 A, BigMac communication device. **B,** Using the BigMac to participate in circle time. (Photos courtesy of Ablenet.)

computer-based systems should be able to be mounted on wheelchairs or easily portable in some other manner. Dedicated systems operate primarily as electronic communication aids (Figure 18-20). These systems are available in various sizes and weights and provide auditory, visual, or printed output.

Examples of these high-tech electronic systems include devices such as the Intro Talker, the Voice Pal (Adapt Tech), the Delta Talker (formerly the Touch Talker), the Vanguard, the Pathfinder, and DynaVox. As with all other AT, communication systems are constantly being upgraded and changed. All electronic communication devices are programmed with individualized over-lays. The board's overlays can indicate as few as 2 and as many as 128 choices to the child. The Voice Pal is easy to program, durable, portable, and inexpensive. It works via pads attached to real objects. It is a simple and effective communication system that the occupational therapist can use to reinforce the learning of cause-effect relationships. The Delta Talker is activated by touch, whereas the Light Talker has numerous selection techniques, including direct selection using an optic light, row column scanning, direct scanning, and Morse code. Advanced systems include devices such as the Vanguard or DynaVox. The Pathfinder is an advanced communication system with the overlay options similar

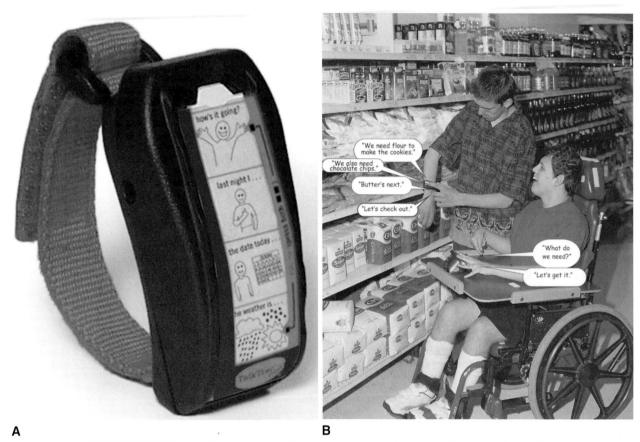

A

B

FIGURE 18-18 A, Talk Trac communication device. **B,** Using the Talk Trac and Step-by-Step communication devices to go shopping. (Photos courtesy of Ablenet.)

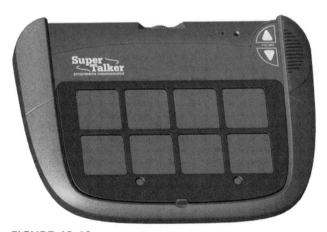

FIGURE 18-19 Supertalker. (Photo courtesy of Ablenet.)

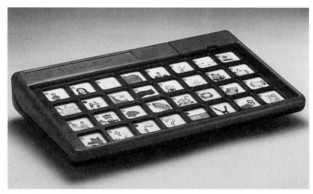

FIGURE 18-20 This dedicated augmentative and alternative communication device uses Minspeak on its keyboard. (Photo courtesy of Prentke Romich Co., Wooster, OH.)

to the Light Talker and Delta Talker. It is portable and flexible and can be activated either through touch or the optic light via direct selection or scanning. It is programmed similar to the Delta Talker and the Light Talker but has some additional computer-like functions, such as a notebook for taking notes. The Vanguard (Prentke Romich) and the DynaVox (Sentient Systems Technology, Inc.) have screens with dynamic liquid crystal displays. A dynamic display offers thousands of graphics (some that are electronically animated) and text options. The display on the DynaVox and the Vanguard changes (using the same message-formation process that produces natural speech) given the choices of the user. The user can input these devices via the touch screen; single, dual, and joystick switching; and visual and auditory scanning.

Computer-based and dedicated communication aids provide different types of voice outputs. Digitized speech is stored by recording the sound or message. The speech output of the system sounds like the voice of the person who dictates into the system. Synthesized speech sounds like a computerized voice but has the advantage of text-to-speech capabilities. The intelligibility of synthesized speech can vary depending on the type of system. As in computer-assistive technology, different rate enhancement options are available for high-tech, electronic communication systems. To allow a child to communicate faster than the rate of keying in text, encoding (or symbol) systems are used. A primary encoding system used in the Pathfinder and Vanguard is Minspeak. This language uses sequenced multiple-meaning icons to retrieve words, phrases, or sentences. Like word prediction, many communication systems come with message prediction. Some of the more advanced systems can learn the communication "style" of the user and begin to predict with greater accuracy.

Case Study 6: Lisa

Lisa is a 4-year-old preschool student with spastic tetraplegia cerebral palsy. She does not have cognitive delays. Her oral motor skills are poor, making vocalizations inconsistent and unintelligible. Lisa is able to communicate basic needs through gestures and facial expressions. She also has a communication board using PicSyms mounted on her wheelchair. She is efficient with these modes of communication within her home and preschool environment, but the team is concerned about her ability to communicate more complex messages as she moves on in her educational and community settings. What might the team consider for Lisa?

Case Study 7: Jim

Jim is a 16-year-old adolescent with a recent head injury from a motorcycle accident. He has poor expressive language, poor fine-motor skills, and poor oral motor control as a result of the brain damage. He is reluctant to use any type of electronic communication device. What would you recommend for Jim?

EVIDENCE-BASED PRACTICE AND ASSISTIVE TECHNOLOGY

Research has documented the benefits and limitations of devices (Edyburn, 2000; Edyburn, 2003; Scherer, 1996; Swanson, 1999). However, due to the ever-changing nature of this field, the complexity of the devices, and the need for individualized decisions, it is difficult to build a large evidence base in this area of practice that is consistent with the available technology (Edyburn). Some AT companies such as Kurzweil (www.kurzweiledu.com) and IntelliTools (www.IntelliTools.com) are adding research information regarding their products and AT outcomes to their web sites. Whenever possible, occupational therapists should use AT research to help with decision making and to gain further foundational knowledge about AT devices and services. When evidence is not available, occupational therapists working in this area must use good database decision making with each client to document whether the use of the device results in increased participation across environments.

SUMMARY

Because the technology available is rapidly changing, the therapist must make an ongoing effort to stay abreast of what is available and what technology has become obsolete. By reading the current literature and research on technology for children, the occupational therapist can effectively match the needs of clients with the available technology and can prepare children and families to use it to its greatest potential. Smith (1991) presented the following as competencies and responsibilities for occupational therapists who desire to work in the area of AT:

1 To become a technology problem solver by using AT to increase an individual's functional independence
2 To see oneself as the human technology and environmental expert
3 To gain a basic comfort level with low and high technology
4 To gain a basic literacy in technology-related areas
5 To understand one's limits in the area of AT
6 To understand the ethical issues surrounding the use of AT

Various resources on the World Wide Web can help occupational therapists stay current with all the changes in AT (see Appendix 18-A). Children who use AT at an early age have the advantage of developing with AT and using it to their benefit throughout their lives. Recent advances in AT allow many devices to grow and expand with the child during the developmental years and into adolescence and adulthood as they transition into higher education and community work experiences. With the current pace of progress and research, future AT will offer greater ease of use, wider application, assistance in additional areas of function, and more availability as a result of lower costs. Computer use, environmental control, and communication can enhance ADL skills, interaction with others, and learning capabilities of children with disabilities at all ages. Selecting and implementing an AT system for children with disabilities requires effective teaming, including the family in decision making and problem solving, and a solid match to the child's skills and limitations, the family's concerns and resources, the child's environments, and desired occupations.

STUDY QUESTIONS

1. The occupational therapist is asked to evaluate the computer lab of an elementary school for accessibility for all students. This school has a range of students with disabilities, including several with learning disabilities, mental retardation, and motor impairments. What aspects of the environment should the therapist evaluate? What recommendations should the therapist make regarding the computers, input devices, and output alternatives to improve accessibility for all students?

2. Give three alternative solutions so that children with ataxia and intentional tremor of their arms and hands can successfully use a computer keyboard and mouse.

3. List three types of scanning and methods of indirect selection. Describe the characteristics of a child who would benefit most from and be most successful with these methods.

4. The Touch Window is commonly available in preschool classrooms. Describe a child who would successfully use the Touch Window and would prefer this method of computer access over other methods.

5. List advantages of using a computer as an augmentative communication device. List disadvantages of using a computer rather than a dedicated augmentative communication device.

6. Explore the advantages and disadvantages of a speech therapist who has expertise in augmentative communication.

7. In the case study of Margy, a team of occupational, physical, and speech therapists worked with her so that she successfully entered employment. Describe potential roles of each therapist in her intervention program.

REFERENCES

Abramson, L.Y., Seligman, M.E.P., & Teasdale, J.D. (1978). Learned helplessness in humans: Critique and reformation. *Journal of Abnormal Psychology, 87* (1), 49-74.

American Occupational Therapy Association. (2002). Occupational therapy practice framework: Domain and process. *American Journal of Occupational Therapy, 56,* 609-639.

Angelo, J., & Smith, R.O. (1989). The critical role of occupational therapy in augmentative communication services. In *Technology review '89: Perspective on occupational therapy practice.* Rockville, MD: AOTA.

Anson, D.K. (1997). *Alternative computer access: A guide to selection.* Philadelphia: F.A. Davis.

Bain, B.K., & Leger, D. (1997). *Assistive technology: An interdisciplinary approach.* New York: Churchill Livingstone.

Batavia, A.I., & Hammer, G.S. (1990). Toward the development of consumer-based criteria for the evaluation of assistive devices. *Journal of Rehabilitation Research and Development, 27* (4), 425-436.

Behrmann, M.M. (1984). A brighter future for early learning through high tech. *The Pointer, 28* (2), 23-26.

Behrmann, M.M., Jones, J.K., & Wilds, M.L. (1989). Technology intervention for very young children with disabilities. *Infants and Young Children, 1* (4), 66-77.

Bersani, H., Fried-Oken, M., Anctil, T., Staehely, J., & Bowser, G. (1999). *Transitioning from high school with assistive technology: The good, the bad and the ugly.* Paper presented at the CEC conference on assistive technology. Portland: OR.

Beukelman, D.R., & Mirenda, P. (1992). *Augmentative and alternative communication: Management of severe communication disorders in children and adults.* Baltimore: Brookes.

Bowser, G. (1989). *Computers in the early intervention curriculum.* Oregon Technology Access Project, Oregon Department of Education.

Bowser, G., & Reed, P. (1998). *Education TECH points: A framework for assistive technology planning.* Winchester, OR: Coalition for Assistive Technology in Oregon.

Brooks, N.A., & Hoyer, E.A. (1989). Consumer evaluation of assistive devices. (Abstract). *Proceedings of the RESNA 12th Annual Conference* (pp. 358-359). New Orleans.

Burgstahler, S. (2003). The role of technology in preparing youth with disabilities for postsecondary education and employment. *Journal of Special Education Technology, 18* (4), 7-20.

Bushrow, K.M., & Turner, K.D. (1994). Overcoming barriers in the use of adaptive and assistive technology in special education. In D. Montgomery (Ed.), *Rural partnerships: Working together.* Proceedings of the Annual National Conference of the American Council on Rural Special Education (ACRES) (pp. 448-454).

Carlson, S.J., Clarke, C.D., Harden, B., Karr, S., Rosenberg, G.G., Swinth, Y.L., & Williams, E. (2003). *Assistive technology and IDEA: Effective practices for related services personnel.* American Speech-Language-Hearing Association. Rockville, MD: ASHA.

Cole, J., & Swinth, Y.L. (2004). Comparison of the touch-free switch to a physical switch, children's abilities and preferences: A pilot study. *Journal of Special Education Technology, 19* (2), 19-30.

Cook, A., & Hussey, S. (2002). *Assistive technologies: Principles and practice* (2nd ed.). St. Louis: Mosby.

Council on Exceptional Children (2004). *Assistive Technology Consideration Wheel.* Washington, DC: CEC.

Demers, L., Weiss-Lambrou, R., & Ska, B. (2002). The Quebec user evaluation of satisfaction with assistive technology (QUEST 2.0): An overview and recent progress. *Technology and Disability, 14,* 101-105.

Demers, L., Wessels, R.D., Weiss-Lambrou, R., Ska, B., & De Witte, L.P. (1999). An international content validation of the Quebec user evaluation of satisfaction with assistive technology (QUEST). *Occupational Therapy International, 6* (3), 159-175.

DeRuyter, F. (1995). Evaluating outcomes in assistive technology: Do we understand the commitment? *Assistive Technology, 7,* 3-16.

Dickey, R., & Shealey, S.H. (1987). Using technology to control the environment. *American Journal of Occupational Therapy, 41* (11), 717-721.

Doster, S., & Politano, P. (1996). Augmentative and alternative communication. In J. Hammel (Ed.), *AOTA self-paced clinical course: Technology and occupational therapy: A link to function.* Rockville, MD: AOTA.

Douglas, J., Reeson, B., & Ryan, M. (1988). Computer microtechnology for a severely disabled preschool child. *Child Care: Health and Development, 14,* 93-104.

Dudgeon, B.J., Massagli, T.L., & Ross, B.W. (1997). Educational participation of children with spinal cord injury. *American Journal of Occupational Therapy, 51,* 553-561.

Dunn, W., Brown, C., & McGuigan, A. (1994). The ecology of human performance: A framework for considering the effect of context. *American Journal of Occupational Therapy, 48,* 595-607.

Education for All Handicapped Children Act of 1975 (P.L. 94-142). 20 U.S.C. Secs. 1400-1485.

Edyburn, D.L. (2000) 1999 in review: A synthesis of the special education technology literature. *Journal of Special Education, 15* (1), 7-18.

Edyburn, D.L. (2003). Assistive Technology and evidence-based practice. *ConnSENSE Bulletin* at www.connsensebulletin.com.

Foulds, R.A. (1982). Applications of microcomputers in the education of the physically disabled child. *Exceptional Children, 49* (2), 143-162.

Garber, S.L., & Gregorio, T.E. (1990). Upper extremity assistive devices: Assessment of use by spinal cord-injured patients with quadriplegia. *The American Journal of Occupational Therapy, 44* (2), 126-131.

Gelderblom, G.J., & deWitte, L.P. (2002). The assessment of assistive technology outcomes, effects and costs. *Technology and Disability, 14,* 91-94.

Glickman, L., Deitz, J., Anson, D., & Stewart, K. (1996). Effect of switch control site on computer skills of infants and toddlers. *American Journal of Occupational Therapy, 50* (7), 545-553.

Hitchcock, C., & Stahl, S. (2003). Assistive technology, universal design, universal design for learning: Improved learning opportunities. *Journal of Special Education Technology, 18* (4), 45-52. IDEAPractices (2004). At www.ideapractices.org.

Individuals with Disabilities Education Act (P.L. 101-476). (1990). 20 U.S.C. Secs. 1400-1485.

Individuals with Disabilities Education Act Amendments of 1990 (P.L. 105-17). (1997). 62 Fed. Reg. 55068.

Judge, S.L. (2001). Computer applications in programs for young children with disabilities: Current status and future directions. *Journal of Special Education Technology, 16* (1), 29-40.

Kincaid, C. (1999, February). Alternative keyboards. *Exceptional Parent,* 34-35.

Krefting, L.H., & Krefting, D.V. (1991). Cultural influences on performance. In C. Christiansen & C. Baum (Eds.), *Occupational therapy: Overcoming human performance deficits* (pp. 101-124). Thorofare, NJ: Slack Incorporated.

Lahm, E.A. (Ed.). (1989). *Technology with low incidence populations: Promoting access and learning.* Reston, VA: The Council for Exceptional Children.

Lahm, E.A., & Sizemore, L. (2002). Factors that influence assistive technology decision-making. *Journal of Special Education Technology, 17* (1), 15-26.

Lamb, P. (2003). The role of the vocational rehabilitation counselor in procuring technology to facilitate success in postsecondary education for youth with disabilities. *Journal of Special Education Technology, 18* (4), 53-63.

Law, M., Cooper, B., Strong, S., Stewart, D., Rigby, P., & Letts, L. (1996). The person-environment-occupation model: A transactive approach to occupational performance. *Canadian Journal of Occupational Therapy, 63* (1), 9-23.

Maier, S.F., & Seligman, M.E. (1976). Learned helplessness: Theory and evidence. *Journal of Experimental Psychology: General, 105* (l), 3-46.

National Joint Committee for the Communication Needs of Persons with Severe Disabilities. (1992, March). Guidelines for meeting the communication needs of persons with severe disabilities. *ASHA, 34* (Supp. 7), 1-8.

Neighborhood Legal Services, Inc. (1999). *Funding of assistive technology: The public school's special education system as a funding source: The cutting edge.* Retrieved (11/7/03) from Neighborhood Legal Services, Inc., www.nls.org.

Olson, L.J. (1999). Psychosocial frame of reference. In P. Kramer & J. Hinojosa (Eds.), *Frames of reference for pediatric occupational therapy* (2nd ed., pp. 323-376). Baltimore: Lippincott Williams & Wilkins.

Parette, H.P., & VanBiervliet, A. (1990). A prospective inquiry into technology needs and practices of school-aged children with disabilities. *Journal of Special Education Technology, 10* (4), 198-206.

Phillips, B., & Zhao, H. (1993). Predictors of assistive technology abandonment. *Assistive Technology, 5* (1), 36-45.

Rehabilitation Society of North America (RESNA). (1992). *Assistive technology and the individualized education program.* Washington, DC: RESNA Press.

Rehabilitation Society of North America (RESNA). (1999). Assistive Technology Act of 1998, P.L. 105-394 (Summary). Technical Assistance Project: Library Laws, accessed on 1/27/2004 at www.resna.org/taproject/library/laws/ata98sum.html.

Robinson, L.M. (1986). Designing computer intervention for very young handicapped children. *Journal of the Division for Early Childhood, 103,* 209-213.

Rose, D.H., & Meyer, A. (2002). *Teaching every student in the digital age: Universal design for living.* Alexandria, VA: Association for Supervision and Curriculum Development.

Scherer, M.J. (1993). *Living in the state of stuck: How technology impacts the lives of people with disabilities.* Cambridge, MA: Brookline Books.

Scherer, M.J. (1996). Outcomes of assistive technology use on quality of life. *Disability and Rehabilitation, 18* (9), 439-448.

Scherer, M.J., & Craddock, G. (2002). Matching person & technology (MPT) assessment process. *Technology and Disability, 14,* 125-131.

Scherer, M.J., & Lane, J.P. (1997). Assessing consumer profiles of "ideal" assistive technologies in ten categories: An integration of quantitative and qualitative methods. *Disability and Rehabilitation, 19* (12), 528-535.

Scherer, M.J., & McKee, B.G. (1989). *But will the assistive technology device be used?* (Abstract). Proceedings of the

RESNA 12th Annual Conference. (pp. 356-357). New Orleans.

Schmeler, M.R. (1997, September). Strategies in documenting the need for assistive technology: An analysis of documentation procedures. *Technology Special Interest Section Quarterly, 7* (3), Bethesda, MD: American Occupational Therapy Association.

Sibert, R.I. (1997). Financing assistive technology: An overview of public funding sources. *Technology Special Interest Section Newsletter, 7* (2), 1-4.

Smith, R.O. (1991). Technological applications for enhancing human performance. In C. Christiansen & C. Baum (Eds.), *Human performance deficits.* Thorofare, NJ: Slack.

Stodden, R.A., Conway, M.A., & Chang, K.B.T. (2003). Findings from the study of transition, technology and postsecondary supports for youth with disabilities: Implications for secondary school educators. *Journal of Special Education Technology, 18* (4), 29-43.

Sullivan, M.W., & Lewis, M. (2000). Assistive technology for the very young: Creating responsive environments. *Infants and Young Children, 12* (4), 34-52.

Swanson, H.L. (1999). Instructional components that predict treatment outcomes for students with learning disabilities: Support for a combined strategy and direct instruction model. *Learning Disabilities Research and Practice, 14,* 129-140.

Swinth, Y.L. (1997). *The meaning of assistive technology in the lives of high school students and their families.* Unpublished doctoral dissertation, University of Washington, Seattle.

Swinth, Y.L. (1998). Assistive technology in early intervention: Theory and practice. In J. Case-Smith (Ed.), *Pediatric occupational therapy and early intervention* (2nd ed.). Woburn, MA: Butterworth-Heinemann.

Swinth, Y.L., & Anson, D. (1998). Alternatives to handwriting: Keyboarding and text-generation techniques for schools. In J. Case-Smith (Ed.), *AOTA self-paced clinical course: Occupational therapy: Making a difference in school system practice.* Rockville, MD: AOTA.

Swinth, Y.L., Anson, D. & Deitz, J., (1993). A descriptive study of young children using a single-switch system for computer access. *American Journal of Occupational Therapy, 47* (11), 1031-1038.

Symington, L. (1990, January/February). Pre-computer skills for young children. *Exceptional Children,* 36-38.

Technology-Related Assistance for Individuals with Disabilities Act of 1988 (P.L. 100-407). 34 C.F.R. Secs. 00.16.

Thompson, T. (2003). The interdependent roles of all players in making assistive technology accessible. *Journal of Special Education Technology, 18* (4), 21-27.

Todis, M., & Walker, H.M. (1993). User perspectives on assistive technology in educational settings. *Focus on Exceptional Children, 46* (3), 1-16.

Trefler, E., & Hobson, D. (1997). Assistive technology. In C. Christiansen & C. Baum (Eds.), *Occupational therapy: Enabling function and well-being* (2nd ed., pp. 482-506). Thorofare, NJ: Slack.

Washington Assistive Technology Alliance [WATA] (1999). *Paying for the assistive technology you need: A consumer guide to funding sources in Washington State.* Retrieved (11/5/2003) from Washington Assistive Technology Alliance: www.wata.org.

Wehmeyer, M.L. (1996). Self-determination as an educational outcome: Why is it important to children, youth, and adults with disabilities? In D.J. Sands & M.L. Wehmeyer (Eds.), *Self-determination across the life span: Independence and choice for people with disabilities* (pp. 17-36). Baltimore: Paul H. Brookes.

Wisconsin Assistive Technology Initiative Project (2003). available at www.wati.org

Zabala, J.S. (2002). *2002 update of the SETT Framework.* Retrieved (9/5/03) from University of Kentucky, sweb.uky.edu/~jszabala/JoySETT.html.

Zabala, J., Bunt, M., Carl, D., Davis, S., Deterding, C., Foss, T., Hamman, T., Bowser, G., Hartsell, K., Korsten, J., Marfilius, S., McCloskey-Dale, S., Nettleton, S., & Reed, P. (2000). Quality indicators for assistive technology services in school settings. *Journal of Special Education Technology, 15* (4), 25-36.

Additional Resources Available on the World Wide Web

The primary goal of this chapter is to present general principles for decision making and problem solving for occupational therapy practitioners when providing assistive technology (AT) services. The author has endeavored to offer guidelines and thoughts for providing services in this area rather than a cookbook of specific strategies. Each child an occupational therapist encounters is special and unique. Thus, each AT solution is as unique as the child who uses the system. New systems and software continually become available. However, because of funding issues and the appropriateness of some of the older systems, many of these systems will continue to be used by children with disabilities for years to come. Thus, service delivery in this specialty area often is a blending of the old and the new.

To be an effective service provider, occupational therapists must develop and use strategies to stay current with a rapidly changing field. One way to do this is to use the vast amount of information available on the World Wide Web. The following are some web sites to consider. Many of these sites have links to other sites and will support both the novice and the expert in this service area to provide quality services to the children and families with whom they work.

GENERAL

Apple Computer's Worldwide Disability Solutions Group
www.apple.com/disability

IBM's Special Needs Solutions
www.austin.ibm.com/pspinfo/snshome.html

Assistive Technology OnLine (provides extensive information on AT, including research)
www.asel.udel.edu/

Information regarding online AT classes and other resources
snow.utoronto.ca/coursereg.html

Resource pages with links to other popular AT sites and examples of student projects
otpt.ups.edu/AT/home.html

Information regarding AT and links to additional resources
www.abledata.com

Family Center on Technology and Disability
http://fctd.ucp.org/

Parents Helping Parents–iTECH Center
www.php.com

The PACER Center, Inc.
www.pacer.org

Center on Information Technology Accommodation
www.gsa.gov/coca

Trace Center
www.trace.wisc.edu

Assistive technology funding and systems through United Cerebral Palsy
www.ucp.org

Alliance for technology access
www.ataccess.org

Closing the Gap
www.closingthegap.com

Council on Exceptional Children
www.cec.sped.org

George Adams Consulting
www.coexceptional.com

National Assistive Technology Advocacy Project: A project of neighborhood Legal Services
www.nls.org

Rehabilitation and Engineering and Assistive Technology Society of North America
www.resna.org

Center for Assistive Technology
http://cat.buffalo.edu/

Resources for Schools
(includes information and forms regarding legislation, AT consideration and evaluation, service delivery, funding and IEPs specific to AT services)
National Technology Center
www.nationaltechcenter.org

Education Tech Points
www.edtechpoints.org

Georgia Project
www.gpat.org

Iowa Project
Lserver.aea14.k12.ia.us/atteam/at/iowa

SETT Framework
www2.edc.org/NCIP/workshops/sett3/SETT.html
sweb.uky.edu/~jszabala0/SETT2.html

Quality Indicators for Assistive Technology Services
www.qiat.org

Wisconsin Project
www.wati.org

Potential Solutions for Case Studies

CASE STUDY 1: JEREMY

The occupational therapist began her evaluation by asking the parents if they just wanted Jeremy to use the computer at the early intervention program or if they would be using it at home. The family stated that money was not an object and that they would purchase whatever Jeremy needed. Jeremy's father said that he has a Macintosh with a color monitor and CD-ROM drive at home. The therapist and team then evaluated Jeremy's skills on the computer. They found that he could touch individual keys on the standard keyboard but that he would become distracted and play with the keyboard versus watching the computer screen. They also tried several different mice but found them to be too complex for Jeremy. However, when they tried the Touch Window with Jeremy, he demonstrated sustained interaction with a cause-effect program for 4 minutes. The speech therapist commented that this was one of the longest times that she had seen Jeremy maintain on-task behavior.

The team decided to start with a Touch Window input device and use software that provided both visual and auditory output for Jeremy. In addition to his Macintosh at home, the team had a Macintosh computer with a Touch Window that Jeremy could use when at the early intervention center. The family and therapists decided to use various types of early learning and interactive software with Jeremy.

The parents wanted to make sure that Jeremy would have the opportunity to learn the standard keyboard and mouse as computer input systems. The occupational therapist stated that it was too early to determine if these would be viable options for Jeremy, but the team agreed to meet again in 6 months to discuss his progress and goals for computer access and use.

CASE STUDY 2: LINNEA

With the changes in Linnea's performance in the classroom, she and her family began discussing other options for written communication in addition to the traditional paper and pencil. Linnea and her family felt that her irritability and lack of concentration in the classroom may be due to fatigue, and her therapists agreed. The team decided to work with a local AT center and provide Linnea and her family with opportunities to explore different options.

Linnea's father is a computer specialist and wanted to be actively involved with the process. Because Linnea is in general education classrooms and has a full schedule when at school, the team decided to set up the trial systems to be used at home. The school occupational therapist, physical therapist, and speech therapist received permission from their administrator to provide Linnea's individualized education program (IEP) services at home to support the family's decision-making process. Linnea's teacher agreed to allow Linnea to dictate her work as needed to help prevent fatigue until a viable system is determined (some input systems require 2 to 3 weeks to achieve a level of comfort and a month to reach proficiency).

Linnea and her team explored many devices, including voice activation and several ergonomic keyboards with surfaces to rest her hands and smaller keys (e.g., Tash Mini Keyboard) to reduce the need to move her hands over the keys. All of the systems included word prediction and abbreviated expansion to help increase efficiency and prevent fatigue. Throughout the decision-making process, the team discussed the potential progression of her disease and future academic environments. Linnea and her family liked the voice-activated system, but they were concerned about her voice quality over time. Reducing keystrokes (using word prediction) and abbreviated expansion seemed to improve her endurance, enabling her to type several pages. The Tash Mini Keyboard supported two of Linnea's long-term goals: word processing and Internet access.

CASE STUDY 3: MARGY

The occupational therapist, physical therapist, speech therapist, and teacher worked with Margy and her family to set up a program to help her learn simple receptionist and computer data entry skills. Margy did not have motor limitations, so she could use a standard keyboard and mouse. However, she did require external organization to complete the computer tasks. After much trial and error experimentation, the team found that a standard environmental setup that was free from extra papers and clutter and used a large font and a strong contrast on the computer monitor supported Margy's success when entering data on the computer. Margy's parents purchased a special paper holder that allowed her to keep her place on the paper when copying data so that she could quickly find her place again when she looked up to talk with customers.

Once the team found a successful system in the computer, she was registered as an office assistant as one of her classes in school. This allowed the team to be close to help problem-solve any unforeseen difficulties and for Margy to practice her new skills in a familiar environment. As her skills continued to improve, she began to generalize the skills to the family business. The entire team continued to be available to problem-solve any difficulties and help rearrange the reception area so that Margy could be successful. The team worked closely with Margy and her family during the transition to the family business and with the receptionist to ensure that the environmental modifications would work for Margy and the receptionist with whom Margy would work.

CASE STUDY 4: ERIC

His computer system has a CD-ROM and speakers. A family member or his assistant loads his compact discs (CDs) into his computer at his request. Once the CDs are loaded, he can use his scanning system to turn the CDs on and off, select the songs he wishes to hear, and control the volume. In addition, he has an answering machine hooked into his computer so that he can receive phone calls from his friends.

The occupational therapy assistant working with Eric collaborated closely with Eric, his family, and other community therapists to help come up with this system. She collaborated with the occupational therapist in drafting letters for funding and researching different options for Eric.

CASE STUDY 5: RYAN

Because of Ryan's interest in the computer and the fact that all the other family members used the computer, the team decided to explore computer options for play activities for Ryan. Through experimentation, the team discovered that Ryan enjoyed having the computer read different Living Books to him. He also enjoyed the exploration and cause-effect experiences when he was able to interact with pages of the book. Because Ryan seemed to enjoy being in the room when other family members worked on the computer, the family used some of their respite funds from the Department of Developmental Disabilities to purchase a second computer for Ryan's use. This computer was set up in the same room as the original family computer. When siblings were working on their homework, Ryan would "work" on his computer for up to 10 minutes at a time. Ryan used earphones so that his program would not interrupt his sibling's work, but he generally resisted using them. The family referred to this as "social time" because it gave Ryan an opportunity for activity-focused interaction with the other family members.

CASE STUDY 6: LISA

Given Lisa's poor oral motor skills and her cognitive potential, the team has decided to begin to train her to use a Pathfinder. This dynamic communication system will be able to grow with her as she matures so that she can continue to communicate at increasingly more advanced levels over time. It also will support her in her academic environments and can be used as a computer interface system when she begins to work more on the computer to produce written assignments. At this time she will use direct selection with her dominant hand to access the system.

CASE STUDY 7: JIM

Jim and his therapists work together to make a communication wallet. This wallet consists of various laminated pictures and phrases that are bound together. The occupational therapist worked with Jim and the speech pathologist to design the size and shape of the wallet and the thickness of the pages so that Jim's poor fine-motor skills do not hinder his ability to communicate. In addition, the occupational therapist has worked with Jim in the clinic, community, and home settings as he has developed proficiency with the system.

Mobility

Christine Wright-Ott

Developmental theory of mobility
Augmentative mobility
Mobility evaluation models
Alternative powered mobility devices
Seating and positioning
Manual wheelchairs
Power wheelchairs

CHAPTER OBJECTIVES

1 Understand the importance of mobility to development.
2 Apply a mobility assessment model to children with different levels of motor function.
3 Identify alternative methods of mobility appropriate to meet the child's developmental and functional needs.
4 Describe wheelchair features and designs that meet the needs of children with various levels of motor control.
5 Explain the biomechanical principles important to positioning and seating.
6 Identify power mobility devices currently available for children.
7 Describe power mobility assessment and intervention.
8 Describe new technology in assessing seating and positioning and new equipment available to children with unique seating and positioning needs.

The information in this chapter is intended to clarify the importance of mobility for growth and development and the implications of impaired mobility. Responsibilities of the occupational therapist for evaluating and recommending appropriate mobility devices are emphasized. Guidelines and criteria for selecting mobility equipment are defined, and descriptions of mobility devices are provided. This chapter also describes the importance of positioning and other factors that influence successful use of assistive devices.

Mobility is fundamental to an individual's overall development and functioning in the occupations of self-care, work, and leisure and is essential to quality of life. The definition of *functional mobility* includes moving from one position or place to another (e.g., bed mobility, wheelchair mobility, and transfers [wheelchair, bed, car, tub or shower, toilet, or chair]), performing functional ambulation, and transporting objects. *Community mobility* is defined as moving oneself in the community and using public or private transportation (e.g., driving or accessing buses, taxi cabs, or other public transportation systems). This chapter primarily addresses mobility as a means of locomotion, with an emphasis on evaluation and intervention principles.

DEVELOPMENTAL THEORY OF MOBILITY

The newborn has little independent control of any part of the body. Gradually, symmetry and midline orientation begin, followed by controlled purposeful movements and the beginning of alternating coordinated movements. The first form of mobility that the infant experiences is rolling, first from side to supine, then prone to supine, and finally in either direction. The 6-month-old infant achieves mobility by pivoting in the prone position. The infant continually becomes more active against gravity (Figure 19-1). Most 8-month-old infants creep and move from sitting to quadruped and back. By the ninth to tenth month the infant experiences a strong desire to move upward. First infants pull to stand and cruise along furniture, such as a coffee table; then they hold onto someone or something as they take their first steps. The average age of independent walking is 11.2 months, and most children achieve independent upright ambulation between 9 and 15 months of age (Bly, 1994; Cech & Martin, 1995).

With the developmental theory of mobility, developmental theorists accept that physical and psychologic development are interrelated and that early experiences influence subsequent behavior. "Through their motor interactions infants and toddlers learn about things and people in their world and also discover they can cause things to happen" (Butler, 1988b, p. 18). During the first months of life, children seek physical control of their environment and continue to do so by building and enhancing their motor skills day by day.

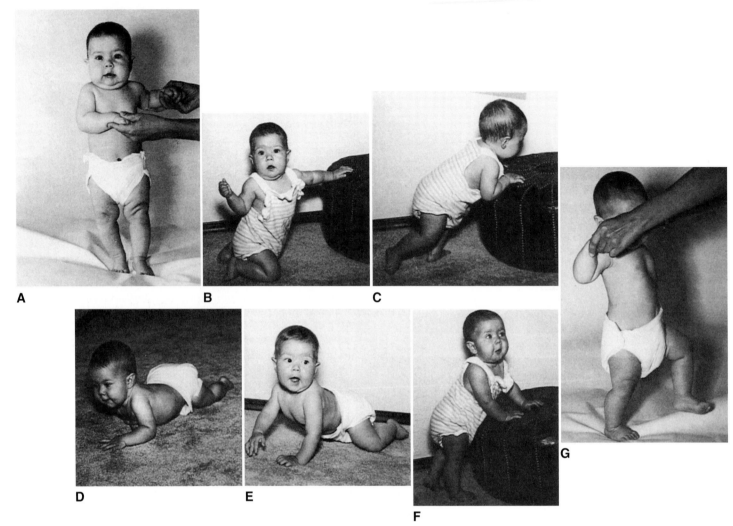

FIGURE 19-1 Development of locomotion. **A,** Infant bears full weight on feet by 7 months of age. **B,** Infant can maneuver from sitting to kneeling position. **C,** Infant can pull himself or herself to standing position. **D,** Infant crawls with abdomen on floor and pulls himself or herself forward. **E,** Infant creeps on hands and knees at 9 months of age. **F,** Infant can stand holding onto furniture at 9 months of age. **G,** While standing, infant takes deliberate steps at 10 months of age. (From Wong, D.L. [1995]. *Whaley and Wong's essentials of pediatric nursing* [4th ed., p. 274]. St. Louis: Mosby.)

During the first 4 years of life, the child gains independence through mastery of important life tasks such as locomotion, ability to manipulate, bowel and bladder control, language development, and social interactions. The most fundamental of these, with the widest influence in all spheres of development, are learning to move about the environment and to use language as a communicative and information processing system.

Children gain various learning experiences as they move about. Locomotion and other motor skills, which develop rapidly during the first 3 years of life, become the primary vehicles for learning and socialization and for the healthy growth of a sense of independence and competence. Piaget (1954) viewed self-produced movement as a crucial building block of knowledge. He theorized that the intercoordination of vision and audition with movements, including locomotion, laid the basis for the child's understanding of space, objects, causality, and the self. The ability of children to influence their environment and to affect or alter it through their own actions is intrinsically motivating. Early experiences are believed to foster curiosity, exploration, mastery, and persistence and therefore are important for later intellectual functioning.

IMPAIRED MOBILITY

Children with physical disabilities, who have difficulty achieving independent motor control, are often deprived of opportunities for self-initiated or self-produced mobility. When these children do experience mobility, it is of a passive nature, as when being held or pushed in a stroller. Because they lack the necessary movements to explore and act on their environment, important learning opportunities are hindered. Mobility impaired toddlers who cannot move across a room to reach out and touch an object or interact with a person are at a great disadvantage. They cannot experience the sensory motor and developmental activities of their peers who have achieved upright mobility such as pushing and pulling toys, opening and closing drawers, or moving around and under objects. Psychologists who have studied normal development have observed improvements in social-emotional, cognitive, perceptual, and motor functioning in infants when they first gain mobility (Woods, 1998). Researchers who have studied the impact of early exploration on a child's development have also suggested that self-produced locomotion and active choice are important for the development of perception and cognition (Campos & Bertenthal, 1987; Foreman, Foreman, Cummings, & Owens, 1990; Kermoian, 1997; Telzrow, Campos, Shepherd, Bertenthal & Atwater, 1987). Young children who seek stimulation in their environment at a young age demonstrate increased cognitive, scholastic, and neuropsychologic test performance at 11 years (Raine, Reynolds, Venables, & Mednick, 2002).

"When development along any line is restricted, delayed, or distorted, other lines of development are adversely affected as well" (Butler, 1988a, p. 66). Restricted experiences and mobility during early childhood can have a diffuse and lasting influence. Long-term physical restriction during infancy or early childhood can significantly alter and disrupt the entire subsequent course of emotional or psychologic development in the involved child (Becker, 1975; Hundert & Hopkins, 1992). Such deprivation of physical and social contingencies can lead to secondary developmental problems, which are motivational. Infants born with motor impairments quickly "begin to lose interest in a world which they do not expect to control" (Brinker & Lewis, 1982, p. 113). This motivational effect is termed *learned helplessness,* a condition in which the child gives up trying to control his or her own world because of motor disability and diminished expectations of caregivers (Everand, 1997; Seligman, 1975). Butler (1988a) found that children whose mobility is limited during early childhood develop a pattern of apathetic behavior, specifically a lack of curiosity and initiative. These character traits are believed to have a critical influence on intellectual performance and social interaction. The detrimental effects of limited early exploration were identified in a study comparing shortcut choices in a simulated maze of able-bodied teenagers with those of physically disabled teenagers who had varying histories of mobility impairment. Despite equivalent levels of mobility, disabled participants whose mobility was more limited early in development were poorer in the task than those whose mobility had deteriorated with age. The results suggest that early independent exploration is important in the development of spatial knowledge and that the detrimental effects of limited early exploratory experience may persist into the teenage years (Stanton, Wilson, & Foreman, 2002).

In children with severe physical disabilities, newly gained independent mobility can have a positive effect on emotional, social, and intellectual states (Douglas & Ryan, 1987; Furumasu, Tefft, & Guerette, 1998). Paulsson and Christoffersen (1984) found that children with disabilities using mobility devices became less dependent on controlling their environment through verbal commands, more interested in all mobility skills, and more active in peer activities. Butler (1986) found that children who had some means of ambulation could and would make choices, but those who did not ambulate were much less likely to exercise available options. The lack of ambulation appeared to severely restrict the child's opportunities to practice decision making, thus giving him or her no reason to express an opinion or desire.

Intervention for young children with physical disabilities often includes the provision of adapted equipment: supported chairs, standers, bath seats and adapted strollers. This equipment provides a means for properly and safely positioning a child, but it does not provide a means for accessing the environment or experiencing the stages of development that occur with self-initiated mobility. Children who have a means for self-initiated mobility decide where, when, and how to move. It is the responsibility of the occupational and physical therapist to determine how young children with disabilities can access their environment, explore their surroundings, and experience developmentally appropriate activities. Mobility devices, which provide a physically disabled child with a means to access and explore the environment, not only provide a means for mobility, but also facilitate psychosocial, language, and cognitive development. Such devices include prone scooters, hand-held walkers, support walkers, manual and powered wheelchairs, and alternative powered mobility devices. However, professionals lack agreement whether mobility devices for very young children, particularly support walkers and powered devices, are appropriate. A support walker provides moderate to maximum support at the pelvis, trunk, and sometimes the head. If the walker does not fit or function properly, the child may use undesirable movements to propel it. Continued use of undesirable postures and movements are viewed as contradicting the child's therapy goals and delaying or impairing the quality of motor development. However, most support walkers are now designed with various adjustments and features that provide more desirable positioning than has been available in the past (Figure 19-2) (Paleg, 1997). Professionals may believe that use of a support walker for a child with cerebral palsy will increase the child's spasticity due to the resistive exercise children may

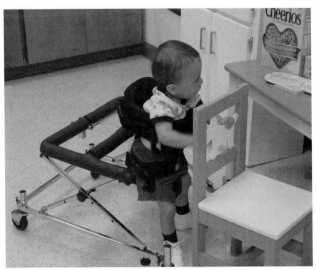

FIGURE 19-2 The Pommel Walker allows an 18-month-old child with a developmental delay to explore his environment. (Available from the Rehabilitation Center for Children in Winnipeg, Manitoba, Canada.)

experience when trying to move the walker. Several studies contradict the premise that resistive exercise can increase spasticity in individuals with cerebral palsy (Blundell, Shepherd, Dean, Adams & Cahill, 2003; Fowler, Ho, Nwigwe, & Dorey, 2001). In fact one study concluded that a progressive strength-training program can improve muscle strength and walking ability without increasing spasticity in persons with cerebral palsy (Andersson, Grooten, Hellsten, Kaping & Mattsson, 2003).

Professionals and third-party payers may resist providing a young physically disabled child with a powered mobility device, particularly under the age of 5 years. Indeed, most children born with congenital mobility impairments are not given their first wheelchair until at least 3 years of age and most of these do not receive a chair they can propel independently until age 5 (Furumasu et al., 1998). Children with a physical disability under the age of 5 years are often denied the opportunity for using a powered mobility device because they are too young to have the cognitive skills to understand how to use it. However, "Clinical experience and research projects have established that powered mobility devices offer children at least as young as 17 months of age a safe and efficient method of independent locomotion" (Butler, 1988b, p. 18). Research continues to substantiate the fact that children as young as 18 months can achieve independent skills in powered mobility (Furumasu et al., 1996; Jones, McEwen, & Hansen 2003).

Caregivers often believe that use of a power wheelchair will reduce the likelihood of their child achieving independent mobility through ambulation. Research has not demonstrated that use of a powered mobility device

prevents or delays the child's acquisition of motor skills. On the contrary, researchers have found positive changes in children's development after the introduction of a powered mobility device (Nilsson & Nyberg, 2003; Paulsson & Christoffersen, 1984; Wright-Ott, 1997). During mobility training, children with severe motor disabilities have demonstrated improved head control and trunk stability, increased motivation, and more self-confidence in movement (Butler, 1986). Deitz, Swinth, and White (2002) concluded that for some young children with severe motor impairments and developmental delay, use of a powered mobility device might increase self-initiated movement occurrences during free play. Nilsson and Nyberg (2003) analyzed case studies of preschool children with profound cognitive disabilities participating in powered wheelchair training experiences. They concluded that the training experiences increased wakefulness and alertness, stimulated a limited use of arms and hands, and promoted the understanding of very simple cause-and-effect relationships.

In another study, children 15 months to 5 years of age with physical disabilities who participated in a 2-week mobility exploration day camp demonstrated a variety of positive behavioral changes (Wright-Ott, 1997). The children experienced mobility by using the GoBot (formerly known as the Transitional Powered Mobility Aide [TPMA]), a standing powered mobility device, to explore the environment. They participated in daily $1\frac{1}{2}$-hour sessions for 2 weeks. Behavioral changes that caregivers and occupational therapists observed in some children included increased eye contact, increased verbalization and communication, improved sleeping patterns, increased active arm use, and a more positive disposition.

The current trend is for mobility devices to be recommended at young ages, when typical children are first ambulating. Many professionals believe that if self-initiated mobility does not occur in the first year, the use of devices for mobility should be considered. Mobility appears to be a priority issue for children with disabilities and others in their environment. When researchers surveyed the occupational performance needs of school-age children with physical disabilities in the school system and community, most teachers, parents, and children identified mobility as their greatest area of concern (Pollock & Stewart, 1998). However, it can be a challenging task for a therapist to suggest to a family of a young mobility impaired child, consideration of a mobility device, particularly a power wheelchair. Many caregivers consider the suggestion as a symbol of giving up hope for independent ambulation. For this reason, use of a walker, support walker, or alternative powered mobility device may be more accepted by the families of very young children. The therapist must convey to the family the concept that all children need a means of mobility to access the environment for exploration to encourage development in the visual perceptual, language, social, and cognitive domains. The mobility device is intended to assist the child in achieving independence in exploration until and if another method is acquired.

AUGMENTATIVE MOBILITY

Butler (1988b) introduced the term augmentative mobility, which refers to all types of mobility that supplement or augment ambulation. "Given augmentative mobility, disabled children can experience more success in directly controlling their environment, thereby reducing or avoiding secondary social, emotional and intellectual handicaps" (p. 18).

The concept of augmentative mobility for functional mobility can be expanded to include transitional mobility. Transitional mobility allows the child to use a mobility device to experience self-initiated movement without the expectation that it must be functional. The child may not consistently move the mobility device in a desired direction but uses it as a means for exploring the effects of movement and learning how to move. The therapist can best provide transitional mobility by allowing the child to move the device in a large room with open space where the child is free to explore. These experiences can then help the child make the transition to a more functional level of purposeful mobility. Not all children are able to achieve functional mobility; in these instances, transitional mobility remains an important means for the child to explore the environment.

The team must consider several factors before selecting the type of mobility device that is appropriate for a child. These factors include the purpose or goals for using the device, environments for intended use, and the child's physical and psychosocial abilities and limitations. When selecting a mobility device, the team considers the advantages and disadvantages of the device, the modifications that may be needed for comfort and control, the congruence to intervention goals, and the cost/benefit ratio. Ideally a mobility-impaired child should have more than one type of mobility device for use in indoor and outdoor environments. Any methods that are chosen for mobility require close cooperation among all professionals working with the child and family.

ASSESSMENT AND INTERVENTION

Classification of Mobility Skills

Children's mastery of functional mobility skills has been classified and categorized in several ways. Hays (1987) examined current existing diagnostic conditions of children without locomotion and divided them into four functional subgroups:

1 *Children who will never ambulate.* This includes children with cerebral palsy with severe involvement and spinal muscular atrophy types I and II. Generally,

these children have no opportunity for independent mobility unless a power wheelchair is prescribed.

2 *Children with inefficient mobility who ambulate but are unable to do so at a reasonable rate of speed or with acceptable endurance.* This includes children with cerebral palsy with less involvement and myelomeningocele with upper-extremity involvement. For these children, the power wheelchair may provide an efficient means of mobility above that which they are capable of producing themselves. Warren (1990) uses the term *marginal ambulators* for this group.

3 *Children who have lost their independent mobility.* This includes victims of trauma and children with progressive neuromuscular disorders. The developmental implications may be less critical than in the first two groups, and the issue is acceptance of assisted mobility as an adaptation to the acquired disability.

4 *Children who temporarily require assisted mobility and often progress to independent mobility with age.* This includes many children with osteogenesis imperfecta and arthrogryposis. Functional considerations in this group are both developmental and practical.

There are significant differences among these groups that may have implications for mobility and its integration into the child's overall concept of disability, as well as for evaluation and intervention.

Evaluation

Evaluation of children has traditionally focused on the achievement of developmental milestones. Occupational therapists have discussed the limitation of such evaluations because underlying impairments (e.g., motor control deficits) cannot fully explain the extent and form of functional difficulties seen in children with disabilities (Coster, 1998). Furthermore, the tasks that are most relevant for daily independence in mobility function have not been well defined in traditional developmental milestone tests. Recently therapists have advocated the use of a top-down evaluation process that focuses on what the child needs or wants to do, the context in which he or she typically engages occupations, and the limitations that he or she may experience (Coster, 1998; Fisher, 1998). Therapists assess underlying performance abilities only to the extent that is needed to help clarify the possible sources of limitations in occupational performance. In mobility evaluation, occupational therapists should focus on the child's overall pattern of locomotion and transfer skills in relation to a particular performance context.

Two instruments focus on the evaluation of functional abilities, including mobility, in children. The Pediatric Evaluation of Disabilities Inventory (PEDI) (Haley, Coster, Ludlow, Haltiwanger & Andrellos, 1992) rates two dimensions of performance: capability to perform functional skills and the level of caregiver assistance needed. The functional mobility subscale measures basic transfer skills (e.g., getting in and out of a car) and body transportation activities (e.g., walking up and down stairs). The Functional Independence Measure for Children (WeeFIM; Uniform Data System for Medical Rehabilitation, 1999) is based on the Functional Independence Measure (FIM) and is for children from 6 months to 7 years of age. It includes six subscales, three of which address mobility: transfers, locomotion, and stairs. The WeeFIM provides useful information in progress assessment, program planning, and communication with caregivers.

The Canadian Occupational Performance Measure (COPM) (Law et al., 1994) is a semistructured interview that focuses on the identification of problems in self-care, productivity, and leisure. It provides a framework to help clients articulate the difficulties that they are encountering in their daily lives and appears to be responsive to change after occupational therapy intervention (Law et al.). In the case of mobility, the COPM can address the concerns of children and caregivers, help them identify what is important to them, and help them prioritize goals. The COPM also provides a baseline assessment for measuring outcomes on reassessment.

Tefft and colleagues (1992, 1993, 1995, 1997, 1999), a research team at the Rehabilitation Engineering Research Center on Technology for Children with Orthopedic Disabilities at Rancho Los Amigos Medical Center, developed a cognitive assessment battery and a wheelchair mobility training and assessment program to help clinicians determine a young child's readiness to drive a power wheelchair. The Pediatric Powered Wheelchair Screening Test (PPWST) and the Powered Mobility Program (PMP) were developed and validated for children ages 20 to 36 months with orthopedic disabilities who used a joystick to control their wheelchair (Guerette, Tefft, Furumasu, & Moy, 1999). Through this research, the cognitive domains of spatial relations and problem solving were found to be significant predictors of powered wheelchair mobility performance (Tefft et al., 1999). The research team continues to study the validity of the assessment battery for children with neurologic conditions such as cerebral palsy who use a joystick or switches to drive power wheelchairs.

Occupational therapists need to evaluate several components of performance that may influence mobility control, such as motor, perceptual, and cognitive factors. This may include neuromotor status, orthopedic conditions, and psychosocial considerations. The therapist must also address the performance context of chronologic and developmental age and environment. The therapist must make the mobility devices and positioning system available during the evaluation process so that the child and caregivers have an opportunity to gain experience using potential mobility devices. These trials provide the caregivers and child with information and experience that will assist them in becoming informed consumers and full participants in deciding which mobility device best meets their needs.

Mobility Evaluation Models

Selection of the most appropriate positioning and mobility device requires the skills of a therapy team working in close collaboration with the school team, prescribing physician, child, parent or caregiver, and assistive technology supplier (ATS). The ATS is a specialist who is trained and experienced in providing durable medical rehabilitation equipment and is credentialed through the Rehabilitation Engineering and Assistive Technology Society of North America (RESNA). This organization also provides the assistive technology practitioner (ATP) credential for professionals. The ATS is responsible for maintaining updated knowledge of available equipment and assisting in identifying choices of mobility devices according to the features that the child requires to use it optimally.

The physical or occupational therapist, together with the child and family, identifies the needs of the child and establishes goals to identify the features and options in a mobility device or devices that will meet the desired outcomes and assist the family in setting appropriate goals and expectations for using the mobility device. The therapist is responsible for assisting the family in becoming informed consumers who can make decisions regarding a mobility device. Once the mobility device is selected and provided to the family, the therapist is responsible for periodically reevaluating the fit and function of the device to determine if it meets the stated goals and objectives.

Most funding agencies do not approve replacement of a mobility device, such as a wheelchair, within 3 to 5 years of the purchase date. If the equipment is not appropriate, the child and family may not have another option for several years. The limitations in reimbursement become critical when a misunderstanding during the evaluation or ordering process results in a device that does not meet the predetermined outcomes. It is imperative that the therapists, ATS, and family immediately decide on how to best resolve these issues.

The occupational therapist selects among a variety of mobility evaluation models to evaluate a child for a mobility device. The most common is for the therapists to request a local supplier of durable medical equipment or ATS to bring the device under consideration to the therapy session. The ATS offers input as to what features and options are available on the device and how to properly adjust it. The difficulty encountered with this model is that one supplier typically has a limited selection of devices available for demonstration, so only one device can be evaluated at each session. Therefore, the therapist does not have the opportunity to compare the child's performance in various types of mobility devices. Without direct comparison of the mobility devices, decisions about which devices are optimal for the child are difficult for the therapist to make. The decision is less risky when side-by-side comparisons of each device are available during the evaluation. This method enables comparison of performance of each mobility device under consistent child and environmental conditions.

Several assistive technology (AT) centers and rehabilitation engineering centers throughout the country use a multidisciplinary team approach and side-by-side evaluation methods to assess seating and mobility needs, particularly with individuals who have severe disabilities. The teams consist of occupational therapists, physical therapists, rehabilitation engineers, speech pathologists, and ATSs working with the child's therapy team, school team, physician, and family. These centers offer the advantage of being able to consider all the needs of the child and offering a concentrated level of expertise.

MOBILITY DEVICES

Selection of a specific type of a mobility device depends on several factors. The team must first decide on the purpose for using the mobility device or devices. Does the child need a means for exploring and accessing the environment (self-propelled manual, power wheelchair, or support walker) or do the caregivers need a convenient way to transport the child (stroller or manual wheelchair)? The next most critical aspect of evaluating a mobility device is to consider the environments where it is to be used by the child and caregivers. If the child's home has high pile carpet, propelling a manual wheelchair or using a walker will be quite difficult. The force needed to traverse a wheelchair over various surfaces has been measured. Using concrete as the baseline, the increase in force needed to cross each surface is +3% for linoleum, +20% for low-pile carpet, and +62% for high-pile carpet (ADA/IT, Americans with Disabilities Act & Accessible Information Technology Center, 2003). The effort required by the individual to use the device will affect functional performance. If the mobility device is too complicated or the child must exert too much effort, it will not be used.

The occupational therapist must consider the individual's positioning needs when selecting features as well as adaptations for optimal use in functional activities such as eating, transfers, augmentative communication, personal hygiene, and school activities. The team also considers the needs and concerns of the caregivers and school personnel who will be transferring the child into and out of the device, transporting it and maintaining the equipment, and costs versus benefits.

The occupational therapist must use the skills of an investigator during the mobility assessment process.

Thoughtful planning and careful analysis of person-device-environment fit is necessary for the therapist to ensure that the child and family receive the optimal device. A wheelchair that will not fit into the family van with the user in it, tips over when the augmentative communication device is mounted on it, or cannot be self-propelled outside because the family lives in a hilly area are examples of problems incurred when a device is ordered without a comprehensive mobility evaluation. The following is an example of a child whose mobility device, a support walker, is not evaluated properly:

Brian is 5 years old and has severe spastic cerebral palsy. He is dependent on others for mobility in his manual wheelchair. He is fully included in a kindergarten classroom. His mother believes Brian will have more peer interaction if he can use a support walker in the classroom, which places him at his peer's height. She also believes he had better digestive function when he previously used a walker at a younger age. Brian was evaluated at his medical therapy session to determine what type of walker would provide him with mobility in the classroom. His parents expressed interest in a particular walker, and the therapist borrowed one from an ATS for Brian to use during the evaluation at the medical therapy unit. The family was excited when they observed Brian slowly propelling the walker forward. The therapist recommended the walker for purchase with custom modifications, which included a higher backrest, a headrest, and a custom thigh length seat to reduce adduction. The family ordered the walker and Brian began to use it in his classroom.

After 5 months of trying to use the support walker in the classroom, he had not yet successfully used it. The therapist determined that he did not have the ability to maneuver the walker in the classroom because of the high degree of resistance from the carpeted surfaces. The therapist initially evaluated Brian in a room with linoleum, without consideration of the classroom environment. The therapist reevaluated Brian in another walker that had a higher quality, 5-inch caster, which made it easier for him to maneuver over carpet. At this time additional funding to purchase another walker is not available. He would have benefited from a side-by-side evaluation of several types of walkers with consideration of the characteristics of the environments in which he would use the walker.

Initial Mobility Devices for Young Children
Tricycles

Tricycles (Figure 19-3) are a means for mobility, although third-party funding is typically not available because tricycles are not considered a medical necessity. However, they can provide mobility outdoors and in hallways and corridors, such as for moving from class to class or from class to therapy. Many types of tricycles are available with adaptations, such as trunk supports, and hand-propelled models are available for children who do not have the ability to pedal with their legs (e.g., children with spina bifida).

Prone Scooters

Prone scooters (Figure 19-4) require use of the arms and the ability to lift the head while moving. The advantages of using a prone scooter include access for participating in play activities on the floor, the ability to get on and off independently, and the ability to change direction more easily than with other types of manual mobility devices. Disadvantages include fatigue from maintaining neck and back extension, vulnerability of the head to hitting objects, possibility of the hands getting caught in the casters or rubbed on rough surfaces, and difficulty viewing the environment above the ground level. Children with spina bifida may find the prone scooter functional because they have the upper-extremity function to propel it and it can support their legs. A battery-powered prone scooter from Enabling Devices allows a child to move either in a circular motion with one switch input or in all directions using several switches (Figure 19-5).

Caster Carts

Caster carts offer another means of mobility to children with upper-extremity function (e.g., those with spina bifida) (Figure 19-6). Children can use caster carts

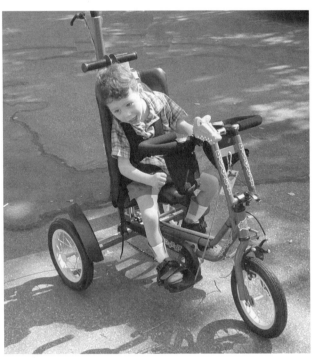

FIGURE 19-3   The Discovery Trike can fit a child as young as 12 months. An adult can assist the child by steering the front wheel with the push handle. (Manufactured by Freedom Concepts, Canada.)

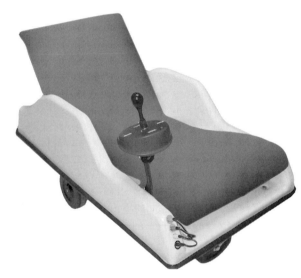

FIGURE 19-5   Motorized prone scooter. (Courtesy of Enabling Devices, Hastings-on-Hudson, New York.)

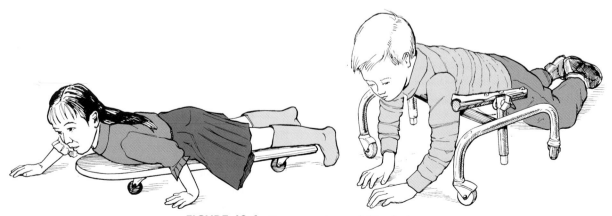

FIGURE 19-4   Prone scooter mobility devices.

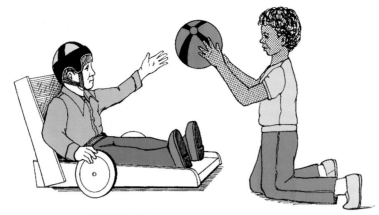

FIGURE 19-6 Caster cart mobility device.

indoors or on flat outdoor surfaces, such as playgrounds. Some children may be able to transfer on and off independently because of the close proximity to the floor. The device requires a considerable amount of energy expenditure for propelling long distances because of the small diameter of the wheels. Children with lower-extremity muscle contractures or tightness, such as in the hamstring muscles, may find it difficult to sit comfortably and securely because they are often unable to tolerate long leg sitting. These children may feel more comfortable with a triangular-shaped wedge placed under the knees to support their legs in knee flexion.

Aeroplane Mobility Device

The *aeroplane mobility device* was designed for children with cerebral palsy who can move their legs but need support of the upper body (Figure 19-7). The device provides developmentally appropriate positioning, particularly for children with spasticity, because the child is positioned with hip abduction and extension with knee flexion and the upper extremities are in a weight-bearing position. This position often assists in reducing undesirable posturing in children who have spastic cerebral palsy, especially for children who exhibit extensor posturing in standing. Other advantages include ease in viewing the environment, the handmade nature of the device, and acceptance by parents, because it looks like a toy rather than an assistive device. The aeroplane mobility device is not commercially available but can be fabricated from wood. Disadvantages include lack of adjustability for growth, difficulty turning and moving backward, and heaviness.

Mobile Stander

If a child has upper-extremity function to push and maneuver wheels, a *mobile stander* may provide another means for mobility. These devices allow the child to experience lower extremity weight bearing in a standing

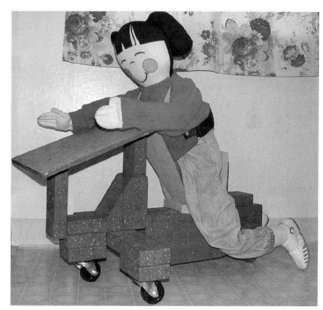

FIGURE 19-7 The aeroplane mobility device can be hand-made and is designed for children younger than 3 years of age.

position. The child achieves mobility using large hand-held wheels for self-propulsion (Figure 19-8).

Walkers

Children who have the ability to pull to a standing position and maintain a grip may be able to use a *hand-held walker*. These walkers are designed for use either in front of (*anterior walker*) or behind the child (*posterior walker*) (Figure 19-9). Children with mild to moderate cerebral palsy or lower levels of spina bifida with leg bracing most commonly use hand-held walkers. Walkers can have three or four wheels and are available in various wheel sizes. The smaller the caster, the more difficult it is for use outdoors and over uneven surfaces. Posterior walkers are available with a feature in which the casters lock when the walker is pushed backward, such as when

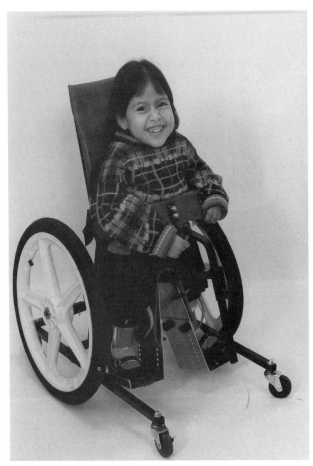

FIGURE 19-8 The ABLER, a mobile stander. (Courtesy of Jennie Company, Bakersfield, California.)

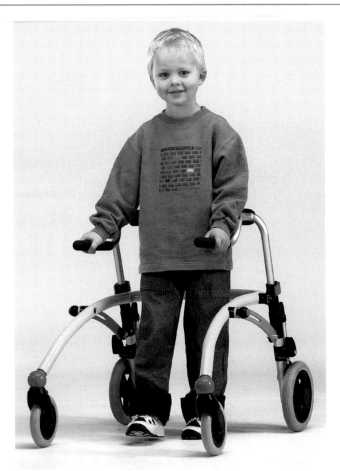

FIGURE 19-9 The Crocodile posterior walker is designed for children from 2 to 14 years of age. It incorporates a design that encourages active postural control while promoting more natural movement during ambulation. (Manufactured by Snug Seat.)

a child leans into it. This feature enables the child to stand and lean against the walker for rest periods; however, it makes maneuvering the walker backward more difficult. Casters can be fixed rather than swiveled, which allows movement only in the forward direction so the user must lift the walker to turn it. Swivel casters allow the child to turn the walker without lifting it, but this feature requires more postural control from the child to direct the walker. The advantages of hand-held walkers are the low cost and convenient transportability. The disadvantages for some users include poor body alignment when pushing a walker and hands are not free for performing tasks.

Support walkers are designed for children who have some ability to move their legs reciprocally but need support at the pelvis, chest, and possibly the upper extremities and head (see Figure 19-2). Selection of appropriate features and adjustments that provide optimal positioning for the child are critical to functional use of these types of walkers. Support walkers that provide a seat with an abduction pad between the legs at the thighs tend to reduce adduction or scissoring of the legs in children with spasticity, making it more efficient for the child to propel the walker. Another

desirable feature in support walkers is adjustable pitch, which allows the child's upper body to be placed in a slight forward lean position. This position places the feet behind the pelvis and trunk, which may make it easier for the child to initiate forward movement. If the feet are positioned in front of the pelvis, the child often moves only backward. Walkers designed with a frame that extends below the seat and between the ankles may be more appropriate for children who widely abduct their legs than children who adduct, because the feet might get caught in the hardware during movements.

Other features include adjustability for growth and wheel locks to brake the wheels for stability during transfers. Walkers with optional trays may be appropriate for children who need upper body support, such as those with muscle weakness or low muscle tone (Figure 19-10). If a tray is needed, it is best to use a clear tray so the child can view the floor and feet while moving. Walkers without trays or hardware in front of the child have the advantage of providing the child with greater access to the environment because it allows the child

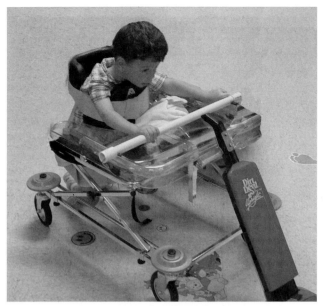

FIGURE 19-10 A 2-year-old boy with spastic cerebral palsy uses the Pommel Walker with a tray and hand grip to provide support while pushing a toy vacuum. (Manufactured by the Rehab Centre for Children, Winnipeg, Manitoba, Canada.)

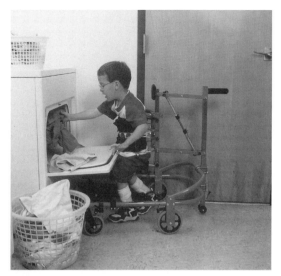

FIGURE 19-11 Walkabout is a weight-relieving walker. (Manufactured by Mulholland Positioning Systems, Inc.)

to be within arm's reach of an object for exploration (Figure 19-11).

Support walkers can provide children with the opportunity to explore their environment in an upright, hands-free, weight bearing position while providing active range of motion. However, many support walkers have limitations in maneuverability and are difficult to turn in a limited space due to a large turning radius. The Transitional Ortho-Therapeutic Walker (TOTWalker) is a new type of indoor mobility device designed at the Rehabilitation Engineering Center, Lucile Packard Children's Hospital at Stanford, Palo Alto, California.* It is designed with minimal hardware in front of the child so the child can be within arms reach to access and explore the environment. The TOTWalker allows for a high degree of maneuverability due to a small turning radius, because placement of the wheel is located near the axis of the child's body (Figure 19-12).

Alternative Powered Mobility Devices

A variety of alternative powered mobility devices are available. Motorized toy vehicles are available for children to provide early mobility experiences using either a joystick or adapted models with special electronics for using up to four switches. Joystick-driven go carts are available for use outdoors (Figure 19-13). From the

* The TOTWalker was funded through a research grant from the U.S. Department of Education, OSERS, NIDRR,. PR Award # H133G99010301.

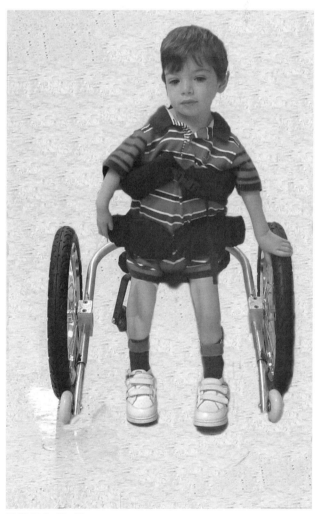

FIGURE 19-12 An 18-month-old boy with arthrogryposis supported in the TOTWalker.

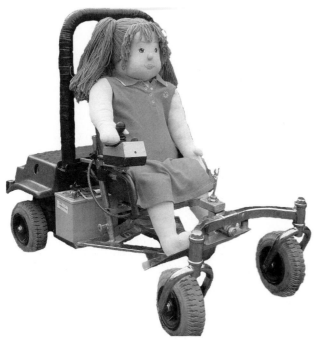

FIGURE 19-13 GOCART Photo: Custom designed gocart with joystick control. (Courtesy of RJE designs).

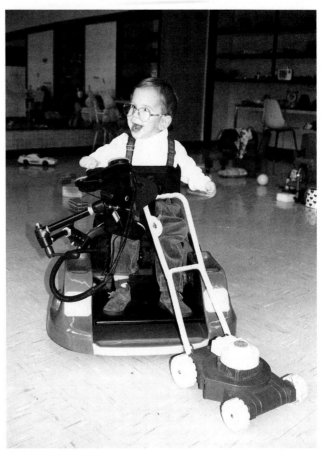

FIGURE 19-14 A 20-month-old boy with cerebral palsy pushes a toy during exploratory play while using the Transitional Powered Mobility Aide. He operates it using switches under his right hand. (Manufactured by Innovative Products, Inc.)

caregiver's perspective, the greatest advantage for use of these toy vehicles is that they look like a toy that any other child would use rather than an assistive device. They are also an option for providing a child with the opportunity to learn how to drive a motorized device in preparation for using a power wheelchair. Disadvantages include difficulty using these vehicles indoors because of limited maneuverability; large size, which prevents the child from getting close to objects in the environment for reaching, exploring, and interacting with others; and sometimes noisy operation.

The Transitional Powered Mobility Aide (TPMA) was developed at the Rehabilitation Technology and Therapy Center, Lucile Packard Children's Health Services at Stanford (Figure 19-14) (Wright-Ott, 1998, 1999). The TPMA is a powered mobility device designed to enable physically challenged preschool children from 12 months to about 6 years of age to move in an upright position and explore the environment by getting close enough to objects and peers to reach and touch. It is intended for transitional mobility indoors or for use outdoors on flat surfaces. The child can be positioned in either a standing, semistanding, or seated position. A joystick or multiple switches can be positioned at any location at which the child can reach the controls for driving the device. The TPMA is not a power wheelchair; it is a therapeutic and educational tool intended to provide developmental opportunities equivalent to those experienced by able-bodied peers, such as pushing or pulling toys, kicking balls, moving fast, moving slowly, and problem solving. The TPMA is intended to increase the child's

opportunities for hands-free exploration and provide new sensory experiences (particularly vestibular, visual motor, and spatial relations). The TPMA is now commercially available from Innovative Products as the GoBot and Mini-Bot and is intended for children who would otherwise spend their early developmental years passively sitting in a stroller or manual wheelchair (Figure 19-15).

WHEELCHAIRS

Wheelchairs are either manual or powered. Manual wheelchairs depend on the user or an assistant for propulsion, whereas powered devices depend on a motorized unit that the individual accesses using a joystick or alternative control methods such as pneumatic sip-and-puff, ultrasonic head controls, proximity switches, or multiple switches. Wheelchairs are available in standard or custom sizes as measured by the seat width and depth, height of the seat from the floor, and backrest height. The therapist must carefully consider features and options on wheelchairs and select the wheelchair to

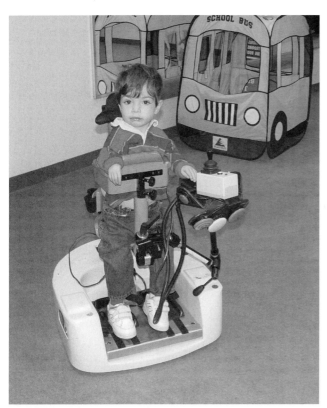

FIGURE 19-15 The Mini-Bot provides early, exploratory, self-initiated mobility experiences. A 2-year-old child with arthrogryposis stands and moves in the Mini-Bot using a joystick or switches. (Manufactured by Innovative Products, Inc.)

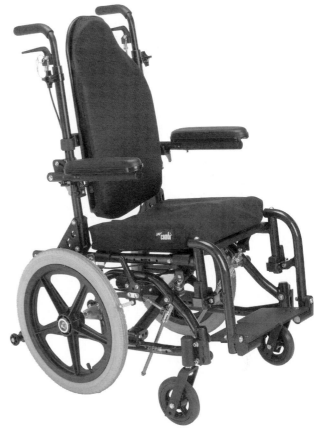

FIGURE 19-16 The Zippie TS is available in both a rigid and folding frame to accommodate the widest possible variety of seating, and features a simple system for tilting in space up to 45° for proper positioning and comfort. (Courtesy of Sunrise Medical, Inc.)

accommodate the child's growth and physical and functional needs as well as the needs of the caregivers. The therapist should begin selection of a wheelchair by evaluating and documenting the child's current physical and functional abilities with consideration of physical changes that may occur and the positioning and mobility goals for the child. Wheelchair selection depends on the type of seating and positioning system the individual requires. He or she must also consider the environments in which the child will use the wheelchair, how the caregivers will transport it, and the sources of funding. The therapist is responsible for providing a medical justification for the seating and mobility system.

Once the therapist has identified the child's needs, he or she matches them to the specific features available in a wheelchair. For example, if a child cannot shift weight independently and is at risk for developing pressure-related problems, then a wheelchair with a pressure relief cushion and either a manual or powered tilt-in-space feature may be necessary to shift weight from under the buttocks to the back (Figure 19-16). The manual tilt-in-space feature allows the caregiver to press levers, which tilts the frame of the wheelchair backward while the seating positioning system maintains the same seat-to-back angle. This differs from a reclining wheelchair, which opens the seat-to-back angle so that the person is

lying supine with hip extension. Powered tilt-in-space is an option available on either manual or power wheelchairs so that the user has independent control of tilting the frame. A tilt-in-space feature can also provide an anterior tilt to position the child slightly forward, which may affect changes in posture.

The therapist must consider the following wheelchair features during an evaluation:

- Style of frame: Folding manual wheelchair (has lots of flex; folds side to side or forward onto the seat); non-folding or rigid manual wheelchair (lightest weight, has "tightest" responsive ride, back folds down and wheels are removable); modular folding (frames come apart, separating the seating system from the base, which folds for manual and power wheelchairs); modular nonfolding (can be disassembled into several parts for manual and power wheelchairs).
- Tilt-in-space: Tilt adjusts the seat backward as an entire unit while maintaining the same seat-to-back angle. It can be manual or powered for independent operation by the user. Tilt ranges are 45 to 65°. Tilt can accommodate users with insufficient head and trunk control, those who need dynamic seating

varying from the upright "'ready" position to a more relaxed position, individuals who require pressure relief under the pelvis or who have back or hip pain. The greater the degree of tilt, the greater the weight is distributed from the pelvis to the back.

- Recline: Recline positions the user in a reclined position in which the seat-to-back angle opens from the seated angle to about 170°. It can be manually operated by a caregiver or operated with power by the user.
- Footrest style: Footrests support the user's feet and may act as a step for some users to transfer in and out. Features include single plate or double plate, fixed, pull up, swing away, and elevating leg rests. The angle of footrests can be standard at 90° or adjustable to various angles to accommodate fixed positions of the feet.
- Armrest style: Armrest styles can be full length, which makes it difficult to get under a desk or desk arm style, which is designed with a notched area in the frame of the armrest for getting under surfaces. Armrests can be height adjustable, either fixed or removable, with pull-out or swing-away option. Some users may benefit from wider, contoured armrest pads for more arm support when using an input method for driving a power wheelchair.
- Backrest height: A high backrest may be needed to support the seating and positioning needs of a client with a severe disability or for tilt and recline. A low backrest may be more functional for a client with good upper body function.
- Height of push handles for the adult pushing the wheelchair.
- Floor-to-seat height: Seat height is important for transfers and getting under surfaces like tables. A lower seat height is typically preferred for younger children, particularly if a seating system will be integrated into the chair, which may raise the user higher.
- Style and location of wheel locks or brakes.
- Type, size, and placement of tires and casters on a manual wheelchair for maximum efficiency during propulsion and to accommodate weight distribution: An adjustable axle plate can provide individualized wheel placement for the child to reach the tire. This may also assist children who are positioned forward of the push wheel due to a short seat depth, which places too much weight over the forward casters thereby increasing resistance during propulsion. Tires can be pneumatic (air filled for a cushioned ride); semipneumatic (gel insert for flat-free maintenance), or solid (no maintenance but provides the stiffest ride and may add extra weight).
- Additional features include sit-to-stand in a manual wheelchair (Figure 19-17) or a power wheelchair (Figure 19-18).

Specialized strollers are similar to infant strollers but are available with seating components for postural

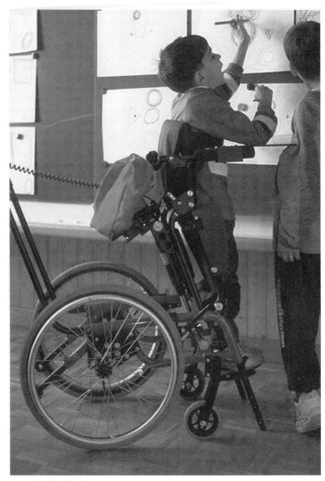

FIGURE 19-17 The LEVO KID wheelchair provides a sit-to-stand feature in a manual wheelchair with the touch of a button. (Available through LEVO USA, Inc.)

support. They are considered dependent mobility devices because the child is dependent on others for mobility. Specialized strollers are available with small casters or larger 8-inch wheels for maneuvering over rugged terrain. The greatest disadvantage of strollers for young children is that opportunities for independent mobility are not readily available. If the child cannot reach the wheel in an attempt to propel it, the child may never get the opportunity to do so as motor performance improves. Strollers that have the option of adding a larger wheel in the future for the opportunity to self-propel may be more beneficial for the child. Parents often prefer the ease of use of a stroller and feel the appearance is more acceptable than that of a wheelchair (Cook & Hussey, 2002).

POSITIONING CONSIDERATIONS

Positioning is critical to the successful use of any mobility device because posture and task performance are interrelated (Cooper, 1998). How an individual is

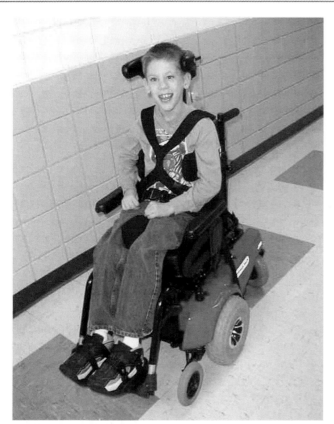

FIGURE 19-18 Power Wheelchair. Luke, age 10, uses the proximity array from Adaptive Switch Labs, Inc., as the input method to drive his Quantum Dynamo Power wheelchair. (Courtesy of Quantum Rehab, a division of Pride Mobility Products, Exeter, Penn.)

positioned in a mobility device, whether it be standing or sitting, can have an effect on several physiologic factors, including visual and motor performance, postural control (Myhr & Wendt, 1991), ranges of movement, muscle tone (Nwaobi, 1986), endurance, comfort, respiration, and digestion. These factors can affect functional performance activities such as hand function (Nwaobi, 1987), levels of independence in mobility, self-care, activities of daily living (ADLs) such as transfers, and social interaction with others (Hulme, Poor, Schulein, & Pezzino, 1983).

Understanding the Biomechanics of Seating

To identify the positioning needs of a child, the occupational therapist must first have a thorough understanding of the biomechanical forces and neurophysiologic factors that can influence posture and movement. Biomechanical considerations are critical to obtaining proper alignment of the pelvis, spine, and head when postures are flexible or when accommodating individuals who no longer have active or passive ranges of movement due to contractures. The position and stability of the pelvis is

---

BOX 19-1 Exercises to Understand the Biomechanics of Seating

SITTING IN POSTERIOR PELVIC TILT
While in a sitting position, place your hands on the anterior crest of your pelvis (the two hip bones). Bend forward by rounding your back. You will feel your pelvis rolling backward into a posteriorly tilted position. Hold your pelvis in this position and try to sit upright by extending your back. You may be able to move your head upright, but moving your trunk into a vertical position is dependent on placing your pelvis in a neutral or anteriorly tilted position. To view your environment with your pelvis in the posteriorly tilted position, you would either need to hyperextend your neck (an undesirable position) or slide your pelvis forward in the seat until your head achieves an upright position. Try maintaining a rounded or kyphotic back position and slide your pelvis forward in the seat. Feel the excessive pressure at the cervical and upper thoracic levels and the coccyx. Imagine being positioned like this for hours at a time and experiencing the discomfort, fatigue, and limited range of your upper extremities if you were in a wheelchair without a proper positioning system to improve or accommodate your posture.

ASYMMETRIC PELVIC POSITION
Place your buttocks at the edge of your seat, lean only onto one side of your pelvis, and lift your feet so they are unsupported. Hold your pencil at its top edge and try to write. It is difficult to have accurate and efficient movements of your arm and hands because you do not have a stable base for the movements to occur. Imagine trying to accurately and safely operate the joystick of a power wheelchair in this position.

---

critical to movements that occur above and below the pelvis. Box 19-1 presents exercises that stress the importance of good alignment in sitting. Neurophysiologic factors include the child's reaction to tactile input, body reactions to orientation in space, and movement.

Seating Guidelines

The goal of seating is to provide a stable place for the child's pelvis and spine from which a range of controlled movements for achieving functional tasks can occur. Seating is not static. Rather, it is a series of active movements an individual utilizes to accomplish a series of tasks, such as maintaining the pelvis, trunk, and head upright against gravity for using the eyes, arms, and hands to manipulate the joystick of a power wheelchair and then adjusting the position to rest by moving the pelvis and trunk onto a supported surface, such as the backrest or headrest. For this reason, a series of postures must be made available to the child, not by restraining the child with straps and harnesses, but rather by supporting the child with an appropriate seating system in combination with independently adjustable wheelchair options such as tilt-in-space. A seating evaluation should consider biomechanical forces of an individual's postures and accommodate stiff postures that are no longer flexible. While accommodating these postural problems, the positions should provide maximum weight distribution for stability, comfort, and skin integrity.

The therapist can achieve stability at the pelvis by providing support at three contact points. The therapist first evaluates the type of support needed underneath the pelvis. The therapist determines whether the child can sit on a flat surface or is more stable using a contoured seat (a recessed seat that provides a recessed pocket for the pelvis and blocks forward movement of the ischial tuberosities). Some individuals require support at the sides of the pelvis to maintain a symmetric position and reduce pelvic shift to one side. Support at the sides of the pelvis can be contoured into the seat or added as lateral hip guides. Stability can be provided above the pelvis to reduce sliding in an upward and forward direction. The therapist typically accomplishes this by placing a positioning belt at a 45° angle to the seat or placing it closer to the thighs. A new device for dynamically positioning the pelvis while allowing for functional pelvic movements is the HipGrip Pelvic Stabilization Device from Body Point. Made of a contoured padded harness, the HipGrip attaches to the lower part of the wheelchair backrest and around the sacral area of the pelvis. A positioning belt is secured in front of the pelvis. A rotational mechanism at the sides of the HipGrip allows the user to move the pelvis anteriorly and posteriorly as when reaching or propelling the wheelchair, while maintaining postural stability. The therapist can also improve stability of the pelvis and trunk by ensuring that the femur is properly supported along its entire length, from the back of the pelvis to approximately 1 inch from the popliteal area under the knee. One exception to this is to utilize a much shorter seat depth for a client who can propel a wheelchair using the legs and feet. In this situation, a shorter seat with a slight anterior tilt would be preferred. Other components, such as footplates, lap trays, arm rests or troughs, a contoured backrest, and headrests, provide additional support.

The areas for the therapist to consider when evaluating the type of seating system that an individual needs in a wheelchair include (1) the angle between the seat and the back surfaces, (2) the tilt of the system in space (orientation), and (3) the type of surface on which the child will be seated (Bergen, Presperin, & Tallman, 1990).

The three types of seating surfaces are planar, contoured, and custom molded. *Planar seating* consists of flat surfaces with no contours. This type of seating may be more appropriate for individuals with mildly affected development who require only minimal body contact with the support surfaces of the seat. *Contoured seating* systems allow the body to have more contact with the support surface because its shape conforms to the curves of the spine, buttocks, and thighs. The therapist can accomplish a contoured seat by layering various densities of foam, which respond to the height and weight of the person, thereby contouring around the bony pro-

minences and other body curves. The therapist can recommend a standard size contoured back and seat cushion from a manufacturer that can be adjusted to fit individual needs (Figure 19-19). *Custom-molded* seat cushions are designed specifically for an individual by taking an impression of the body and making a mold, which is sent to the manufacturer for fabrication of the cushions. Another method uses a computer-generated graphic picture taken from the impression, which is sent to the manufacturer, who then uses a computer-assisted milling machine to fabricate the cushions. Cushions can also be custom molded using foam-in-bag technology in which liquid foam is poured into an upholstered bag that is positioned around the person's body, providing a molded and finished cushion. This technique is more difficult to use because the individual's position must be held in place while the foam is being formed. If the child moves, the quality of the foam is negatively affected.

The use of orthotics, or bracing of the extremities or body, may also assist in achieving optimal positioning in the seated and standing positions. Ankle-foot orthoses are most commonly recommended to align the foot and ankle and assist in either reducing muscle tone or supporting a weak limb. A thoracic lumbar sacral orthosis (TLSO), or body jacket, may be another alternative for individuals with scoliosis to use for support in the seated position. Young children who exhibit an increase in extensor movements and asymmetry when being evaluated for a seating system may benefit from using a "barrier" vest as proposed by Kangas (2001). The vest is made from plastazote, which is not strong enough to

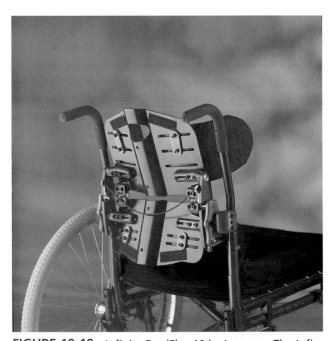

FIGURE 19-19 Infinity DualFlex 10 by Invacare. The Infinity DualFlex 10 is a modular seating system that accommodates a wide range of position needs. (Courtesy of Invacare, Elyria, Ohio.)

totally support the child, but does allow the child to experience some movement. It is worn to decrease the child's sensitivity to individual points of contact from hands touching the body during handling or from pads on a seating system, which can set off the extensor body reaction. The child wears the vest for up to 6 months while learning to become more posturally secure.

METHODS FOR EVALUATING SEATING AND POSTURING

The therapist should begin the initial assessment by observing the child using any existing seating and mobility systems to note posture, movements, comfort, satisfaction with the equipment, and other factors that may affect function. The therapist should then position the child on a low mat table so that he or she can complete a postural assessment to determine whether any limitations in ranges of movement exist that may interfere with the upright and seated position. The therapist obtains further information by positioning the child in a sitting position while using his or her hands to support the child to identify key points of control and positions that provide a desirable change in posture, muscle tone, and movements. These key points become the necessary components of the seating system. The positions, such as the angle of hip flexion and the orientation in space of the child, become the pitches and angles of the components necessary in the seating system (Cooper, 1998).

Once the therapist gathers information from the postural assessment, other methods are also available that use evaluation equipment for assessment of a child's position to determine what components, angles, and sizes are needed in a seating system. Simulators are self-contained, adjustable fitting chairs that the therapist can adjust to fit a child or adult to determine what type of seating components and angles are appropriate (Trefler, 1999). The simulator allows the therapist to "evaluate the client in the system, alter angles of the seat to the back, try varying positions in space, and determine component sizes and accessories that are required before making recommendations for a particular system" (Trefler, Hobson, Taylor, Monahan & Shaw, 1993, p. 73).

The therapist can use simulators to evaluate planar, contoured, and molded seating. The therapist first completes a postural evaluation of the individual to determine which seating components are necessary and then adjusts the simulator to the individual's size. The therapist selects angles, which include seat-to-back and tilt. He or she can make further adjustments to determine how position influences movement and function. The advantages of using a seating simulator include (1) use as a single evaluation tool for various ages, sizes, and diagnoses; (2) source of information about the various types of seating systems, such as planar versus molded; and (3) options to motorize simulators to evaluate powered mobility access and the effect of positioning on motor control. The problem that the assessment team often encounters when using simulators is difficulty in transferring the information from the simulator into an actual seating system and knowing how that system will integrate into a mobility base. Another disadvantage occurs when the seating system is used in a manual wheelchair; the biomechanics of propelling the wheels while positioned in the simulator cannot be assessed. Children may respond negatively to the simulator because its mechanical appearance and large size intimidate them.

Another method for evaluating seating and positioning is use of a modular mockup or adjustable evaluation seat system that can be placed in a mobility base. These are typically available in planar or contoured seating devices rather than in custom-molded devices. The advantages of using this method include the ability for the child to use the mobility device while seated in the mockup seat. This is particularly important because positioning can influence body movements and therefore functional outcomes. The disadvantages are that more equipment must be available to fit a range of individuals, and pitches and angles cannot always be accurately assessed.

Children with hypotonia, such as those with muscle diseases or cerebral palsy, have specific needs. A useful positioning system includes a back design that supports the sacrum in a neutral position but angles about 15° away from the back at the posterior superior iliac spine. This provides a resting position of the trunk behind the pelvis and accommodates the forces of gravity in the upright position. Consideration of a tilt-in-space feature in the mobility base may also provide the hypotonic or weak child with greater tolerance for sitting upright.

Children with increased muscle tone and spasticity who tend to adduct their legs and extend their hips and spine are often more difficult to position. The therapist must identify key points of control for positioning these children. For example, the therapist determines the desired degree of hip and knee flexion, hip abduction, and reduction of asymmetric positioning that positively influences muscle tone and control of extremity movement. The critical factor for reducing the degree and frequency of extensor posturing is to determine what factors contribute to these undesirable movements. Kangas (2001) believes extensor posturing and leg adduction indicate postural insecurity in the child and the inability to modulate the sensory and tactile systems. Some children become more asymmetrical as hypertonus increases, which may occur when they feel pressure behind their head or neck from a headrest, which seems to stimulate the response. These children may also have better postural control in the upright position rather than reclined or tilted (Nwaobi, 1986).

The therapist must frequently reevaluate a child's position, particularly in a seated mobility device, to accommodate postural, developmental, and physiologic changes. Once a child receives a seating mobility system, the therapist should reevaluate its fit and function every 6 months. Positioning and mobility literature and support materials are available (Cook & Hussey, 2002; Engstrom, 1993; Trefler et al., 1993; Trefler, 1999), and more specific information and techniques on positioning are available through additional reading and workshops.

Manual Wheelchairs

A manual wheelchair is appropriate for a child who has the ability to functionally and efficiently propel it. It is also used as a means of transportation by caregivers or as a backup wheelchair when the child's power wheelchair is not working. Great strides in manual wheelchair design have resulted in lightweight and ultra-lightweight wheelchairs that provide higher performance during propulsion (Figure 19-20).

Wheelchairs with large rear tires are most common, but models with large front tires and small back casters are available (Figure 19-21). Propelling a wheelchair with large front tires may be more efficient for the child because more surface area of the tire is exposed for gripping the wheel and pushing. However, the large front

tires can limit access to the environment, such as when transferring and sitting at tables. The wheelchair with large front tires is also more difficult to push over curbs and uneven surfaces due to interference from the rear casters.

If a child will be independently propelling the wheelchair, it is critical that the wheelchair and seating are designed to allow the child to use proper biomechanics for efficient propulsion. The therapist achieves this by

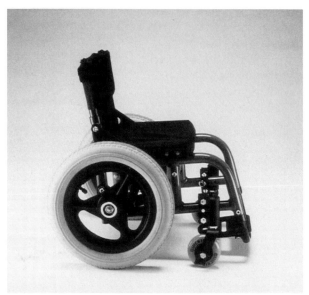

A

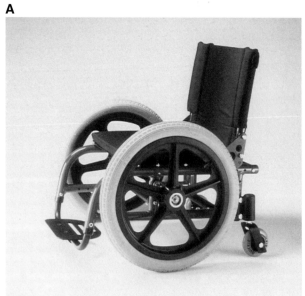

B

FIGURE 19-21 Quickie Kidz manual wheelchair features wider rear wheels for maximum pushing surface (**A**) and standard or reverse wheel configurations (**B**) so that the chair can be propelled with either a push or pull motion. (Courtesy of Sunrise Medical, Carlsbad, Calif.)

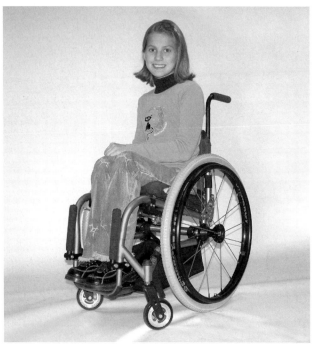

FIGURE 19-20 Chelsea, age 9 years with paraplegia at the L1 level, selects a TiLite TR for its lightweight feature, durability, and a smooth ride. (Courtesy of TiLite.)

selecting the proper size of wheelchair frame and an appropriate seating system. Most wheelchair manufacturers include wheelchair growth kits, which accommodate the need to widen or lengthen the frame without entirely replacing the wheelchair. The therapist must select a wheelchair that fits the child's present needs rather than a wheelchair that is too large with the goal the child will grow into it. A wheelchair that is too wide is more difficult for the child to propel. If the seat is too long, the child's pelvis cannot achieve a neutral position; it will be pulled into a posterior tilt position, causing the child to sit on the sacrum with a rounded back.

The therapist simultaneously considers what type of seating or positioning system is needed and how it will interface with the mobility base for optimal function and performance. For example, one mistake is use of a seat cushion without consideration of the frame size of the manual wheelchair. When the cushion is placed on top of the wheelchair frame, it may position the child too far from the wheels for reaching and propelling them efficiently. If the therapist had considered the height of the wheelchair seat when ordering the cushion, alternatives could have been used to prevent this situation (e.g., a narrower cushion that can be recessed into the wheelchair frame).

Another common situation that reinforces the need to assess seating and mobility simultaneously is acquiring a backrest cushion for a child after selecting the manual wheelchair. The cushion may position the child too far forward of the axle's wheel. If the child's center of gravity is forward of the rear wheels instead of directly over the rear wheel axle, propulsion is more difficult and inefficient. Many wheelchairs have a standard axle plate where the hub of the wheel is mounted to the frame and the wheels cannot be relocated within the child's reach. However, if the therapist orders an adjustable axle plate for the wheelchair in combination with the appropriate front caster size, the wheels can be relocated and mounted in the best location for the child to reach the wheels for propulsion.

Manual wheelchairs for playing court sports such as tennis and basketball or racing are designed specifically for the sport (Cooper, 1998). These wheelchairs have a rigid frame, a high degree of camber in the rear wheels, and use small rollerblade type casters in front.

Wheelchairs can be retrofitted with a one-arm drive mechanism that is intended for users who have a single functional arm for propulsion. A variation of a one-arm drive wheelchair is the Mono-drive wheelchair by Snug Seat. The wheelchair is propelled by pushing and pulling a hand lever for driving and steered by turning the handle.

Alternative manual wheelchairs include the EZ Chair by Premier Designs, a foot propelled, lightweight, transportable wheelchair the user steers with handles attached

to the front casters. Another innovation in wheelchair mobility is a power assist unit designed into the hub of a special wheel attached to a manual wheelchair. The power assist unit provides the convenience of a manual wheelchair without the extra effort involved with propulsion (Figure 19-22). The LEVO Kid wheelchair includes a powered sit-to-stand feature, which can provide peer height interaction and the benefits of conveniently standing throughout the day (see Figure 19-17).

Power Wheelchairs

If a child cannot propel a wheelchair long distances at the same speed and efficiency as the average person walks, then the therapist should consider recommending a power wheelchair to increase the child's independence and function. The advantages of a power wheelchair over a manual are increased speed capability, ease of maneuvering, and less energy expenditure required for moving, particularly for long distances. Some children who use a power wheelchair also have a manual wheelchair for use in environments that are not accessible to a power wheelchair or when the power wheelchair is being repaired.

Power wheelchairs are available in several styles with various options and are differentiated by the placement

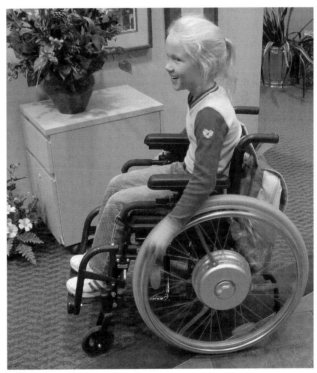

FIGURE 19-22 Quickie Xtender provides power assist to a manual wheelchair by designing a motor unit into the hub of the quick release wheel. (Courtesy of Sunrise Medical, Carlsbad, Calif.)

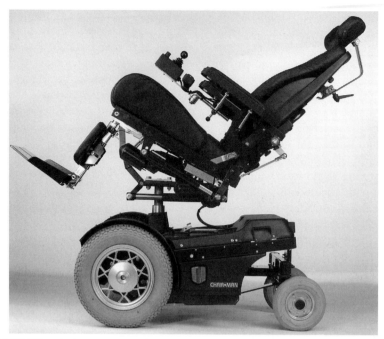

FIGURE 19-23 Chairman Corpus by Permobile is a front-wheel drive power wheelchair with tilt-in-space, recline with shear reduction, and an 8-inch seat elevator. (Courtesy of Permobil, Lebanon, Tenn.)

of the drive wheel, which may be front-wheel (Figure 19-23), mid-wheel (Figure 19-24), or rear-wheel drive. Attributes that are affected by the drive wheel position include maneuverability, stability, traction, and performance (speed, efficiency, obstacle climbing, and crossing a side slope). Maneuverability depends on the turning radius. Mid-wheel drive wheelchairs tend to have greater maneuverability because of the smaller turning radius. However, mid-wheel drive wheelchairs require a third set of stabilizing wheels that may pitch the user forward when going downhill or over curbs, affecting stability of the user. The recent trend in power wheelchair design is to provide a full suspension system in the front and rear casters or tires. This allows the user to move over a variety of terrains up to 2 inches in height, even at slow speeds.

The most common approach to selecting a power wheelchair begins by describing the environments in which the child will use it and determining which make and model offers the type of features needed to access those environments. The next consideration is to determine how the child will access or drive the power wheelchair and which models provide the access methods that the child needs now and will need in the future. Most wheelchair manufacturers provide a choice of several types of wheelchair models that are intended for joystick operation and models that include sophisticated microcomputer electronics for alternative input methods for driving and for remotely operating environmental devices. Different models offer various features to

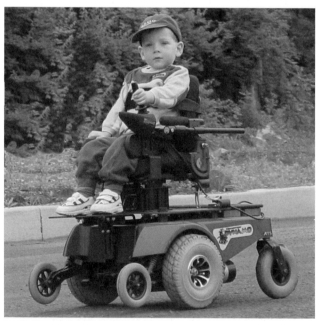

FIGURE 19-24 Alex, age 2, independently rides in his Quantum Dynamo ATS, which utilizes a midwheel drive system. (Courtesy of Quantum Rehab, a division of Pride Mobility Products, Exeter, Penn.)

accommodate the needs of each user. Such features include adjustments for torque, tremor dampening for children experiencing difficulty directing the joystick, a short-throw joystick option for users with muscle weakness who do not have the strength to push the joystick to its end range, speed adjustments, and acceleration settings so that the wheelchair can be set to increase speed rapidly or gradually. Speeds can be as high as 15 mph, but typically range from 3 to 10 mph. Distance traveled on one battery charge can be as far as 25 miles.

A joystick is the standard and preferred method for the individual who can efficiently and accurately maneuver it. The user can operate a joystick using a hand, foot, forearm, chin, head pointer, or even the back of the head by using an adaptation that connects the joystick to a bracket that is attached to a moveable headrest. Some children may find it difficult to accurately use a joystick placed in its traditional location at the front end of the armrest. These children may have better motor control if the joystick is placed inside the armrest, in midline, or rotated toward their body several degrees. A remote or attendant joystick, which is smaller in size than a standard joystick, may be necessary for these types of situations and are available for most power wheelchairs. The remote joystick is easier to position in midline or under the chin. Another feature that can assist in improving control or efficiency during joystick use is a support (such as a wide armrest or trough) under the elbow, forearm, or wrist. During the evaluation for joystick operation, the therapist must consider the positioning needs of the child, placement of the joystick, type of joystick, type of joystick knob, and desired location of the on/off switch for independent access by the user. An attendant joystick is another option for a power wheelchair. It is a second joystick, which is mounted to the back of the wheelchair and is accessed by the caregivers who need to drive the power wheelchair when accuracy is required, such as moving up a narrow ramp.

A proportional joystick allows the driver to increase acceleration and speed of the wheelchair in relationship to the distance that he or she moves the joystick. The further the user pushes the proportional joystick, the more rapidly the wheelchair moves. A nonproportional joystick (digital or microswitch) does not affect the wheelchair's speed; any amount of force used to push the joystick results in the same speed.

Joystick knobs are available in various styles, shapes, and sizes to accommodate various hand and wrist positions. The most common shapes are round, T-shaped, and I-shaped joysticks. A child with weakness of the upper extremities may find it more efficient to use a U-shaped joystick so that the hand is supported in the palm and at the sides. Joysticks can be so sensitive that they require only slight movement of one finger, which may be useful for a child with muscle disease. Selection of the most appropriate style of joystick and its placement directly affects the ability to accurately and efficiently drive a power wheelchair.

Children with severe physical disabilities may be able to operate a power wheelchair but often are not given the opportunity because they are physically unable to operate a joystick. Alternative input or access methods are available for these individuals. An input method frequently used by individuals with spinal cord injuries is pneumatic sip-and-puff, which the user activates by gently inhaling or exhaling into a strawlike device held in the mouth. Another alternative method is the head-switch sensing array, which consists of proximity switches embedded into a headrest that detect head movements for driving the wheelchair (see Figure 19-18). The Tongue Touch Keypad by New Abilities is a custom-made retainer in which small switches are imbedded. The user activates each switch by touching it with the tongue. Multiple switch access is available in which push switches are placed around the body part that is able to reach the switches. The wheelchair is driven in one of four directions, depending on which switch is activated. It is even possible for the individual to drive a power wheelchair with one switch, which operates a scanning light on a display. The following is an example of a child who uses an alternative input device.

Matthew is 14 years old and has severe spastic cerebral palsy (Figure 19-25). He uses a custom seating system composed of a contoured seat cushion, a biangular back cushion with lateral hip and trunk pads, and an occipital neckrest with anterior chest support. This position has increased his ability to activate a push switch placed on the right side of his head. He operates his power wheelchair by using special electronic controls in the wheelchair that are connected to the switch and a small scanning light box mounted in front of him. When he presses the switch, the light begins to scan in one of four directions. Another press of the switch stops the light on the arrow indicating the direction of the desired movement. A third press of the switch stops the wheelchair. He uses the same switch to operate a scanning light on his augmentative communication device, mounted in front of him on his wheelchair.

Switches can be placed around any part of the body, such as the hand, head, elbows, or feet, where the child has the most reliable, accurate, and efficient movements. However, the quality of motor control and accuracy is directly dependent on the child's position and the extent to which the position influences stability, mobility, muscle tone, and energy expenditure. Therefore an evaluation of power wheelchair mobility control must simultaneously include a seating evaluation to determine how the child's motor control is influenced by body position.

Several features can be made available on power wheelchairs to increase a child's function and level of independence. Technology-dependent children who require oxygen support can become mobile by using portable ventilator carts attached to the wheelchair (Backer & Howell, 1997). Another recently developed feature enables the child to independently move from a sitting to a standing position and drive around while

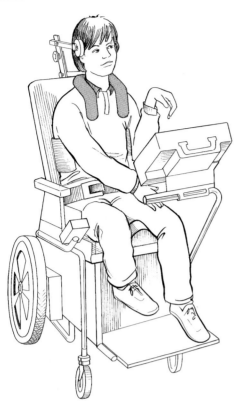

FIGURE 19-25 Young man with severe spastic cerebral palsy drives a power wheelchair using a switch mounted at each side of his head to operate the scanning display.

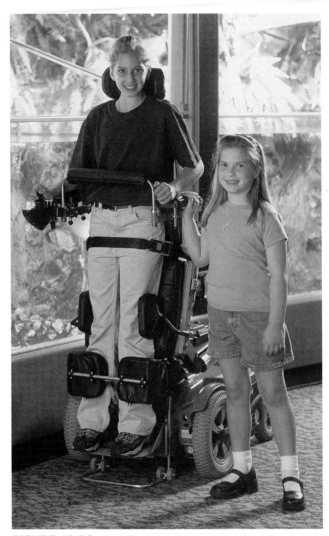

FIGURE 19-26 The Chairman 2K Stander. Standing can be achieved from a sitting position or gradually from supine. (Courtesy of Permobil, Lebanon, Tenn.)

standing (Figure 19-26). A powered elevating seat, which raises the child to various heights for greater accessibility in the environment, is also available (Figure 19-27). Additional features include power tilt-in-space, which tilts the seat backward to about 45° while maintaining the same seat-to-back angle (Figure 19-28), and power recline, which places the child in the supine position by reclining the back of the chair. These two features are useful for individuals who need independent and frequent relief of pressure under their buttocks, such as those with spinal cord injury and muscle weakness or for those with back and neck pain. Most wheelchair manufacturers offer securement points on the frame of the wheelchair to secure the wheelchair to the floor of a vehicle for safely transporting the user while seated in the wheelchair.

A manual wheelchair can be converted to a power wheelchair by purchasing an add-on unit that includes two motors that are placed on the tires to rotate them, batteries, an electronic control unit, and a joystick. The electronic controls for the add-on units are not as sophisticated or adjustable as those found on standard power wheelchairs. This makes it more difficult for some children with impaired motor responses to accurately

operate an add-on unit. They are also not highly recommended for individuals who use their wheelchairs outdoors and over rough terrain because they are not designed to withstand the forces that a power wheelchair must endure.

Power wheelchairs do not typically fold for transporting in a vehicle. Accessible vans that have been modified with a lift are required for transporting the user and power wheelchair in a vehicle. However, there is a pediatric power wheelchair, the Starlight from Global Power Systems, Inc., which folds quite readily so that it can be transported in a vehicle without the need for a van. Another lightweight, transportable power wheelchair is the EZ Power by Premier Designs (Figure 19-29). If the child can be transferred to a car seat, there are covered trailers that can be hitched to the back of a vehicle for transporting a power wheelchair.

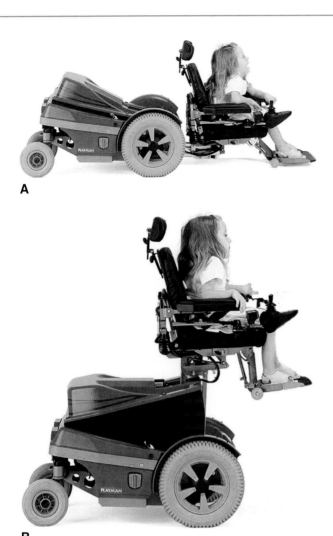

A

B

FIGURE 19-27 Playman Robo's seat will lower to the ground and elevate, covering a total of 25 inches height difference for vertical mobility. (Courtesy of Permobil, Lebanon, Tenn.)

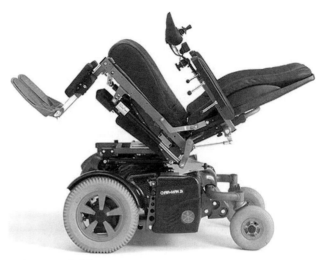

FIGURE 19-28 Chairman 2K front wheel drive power wheelchair with the Corpus seating system and 45° of tilt in space. (Courtesy of Permobil, Lebanon, Tenn.)

Three-wheeled scooters are another option for power mobility. The individual who uses a scooter typically has good sitting balance, requires minimal positioning adaptation, and can understand and physically operate the tiller handle bar controls.

POWER MOBILITY EVALUATION AND INTERVENTION

The therapist, teacher, child, and caregivers must first define the goals for using a powered mobility device. Are the goals to provide functional and independent mobility or are the goals to provide transitional mobility experiences so that the child can have new opportunities to learn how to move, explore, and interact within the environment? Maneuverability features of the powered

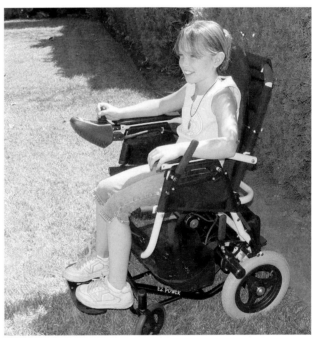

FIGURE 19-29 The EZ Power Chair is pedal powered and steered with a handle connected to the casters. (Courtesy of Premier Designs.)

device are important when considering the various environments in which the device will be used (e.g., indoors, outdoors, school, home, or playground). If it is necessary for the child to reach various heights in the wheelchair then a power lift seat may be justified. Will the child need the ability to tilt-in-space or recline? How will the mobility device be transported? Will it need to fold to fit inside the trunk of a vehicle? If the wheelchair is to be transported in a van, is head clearance sufficient for the child when entering the vehicle? Will the environments need to be made accessible with ramps into doorways or lifts into vehicles?

The most common method for evaluating a person's ability to use a power mobility device is to have the device available for trial use during the evaluation. A facility typically cannot afford to purchase power wheelchairs for evaluation purposes. Fortunately, ATSs often lend power wheelchairs to a clinical therapy unit for short-term evaluation purposes. The positioning and mobility equipment with the specific features that the child will need to use the device should be available during the evaluation. Equipment used during an evaluation should be in optimal working condition. The therapist should begin the evaluation by test-driving the equipment to learn the forces and movements required to drive it, select the best speed for the client, and set any other adjustments, such as sensitivity of the controls.

The therapist begins an evaluation of the child's ability to drive a power wheelchair by evaluating the child's position to determine how to optimize motor function for efficient and accurate access of the controls. Several strategies are available to improve the ability of a child to use a joystick. If the child has difficulty moving the joystick in the desired direction, the therapist can place a template with a cross shape cut out inside the control box to limit deviation of the joystick to the desired directions. The therapist can also position the joystick with proper hardware to another location where control might be enhanced. The following is an example of a child whose position is evaluated for more accurate use of a powered mobility device.

Erin, a 4-year-old child who is unable to communicate, was experiencing difficulty driving the power wheelchair using a joystick placed at the end of her right armrest. The teacher questioned Erin's ability to drive safely and accurately, believing that bumping into objects was purposeful. The occupational therapist observed Erin's arm and hand movements and noted that she seemed to have difficulty pushing the joystick forward and to the right side. She tended to internally rotate her arm and pull it toward her body. The joystick was then mounted on an adjustable bracket that positioned it in midline, close to her chest. It also enabled the joystick box to be rotated about 30° toward her body. After several more attempts at driving, her accuracy immediately improved. Once the most reliable placement was located, she became a functional driver.

If a child does not have the physical ability to control a joystick with the hand, foot, or head, the therapist can consider alternative means of switch operation, particu-

larly for individuals with cerebral palsy. Before the therapist selects the type of switch, he or she should determine the movements that the child can use to access a switch. If the child can nod his or her head "yes" and "no," then he or she may have the ability to use switches around the back of the head.

The therapist may need to evaluate switch placement by allowing the child to first use switches to operate modified battery-operated toys (Wright & Nomura, 1991). The therapist first identifies the most reliable and efficient movements that the child can voluntarily use to access the switches. Switches are either momentary or latched. Momentary switches require the user to maintain contact on the switch to activate it. The child needs to be able to maintain contact on the switch long enough to move the wheelchair in a desired direction. A latching mode allows the individual to press the switch one time to activate it rather than holding it in the on position. A second activation turns the switch off. If the child needs to use switches to drive a power wheelchair, at least three switch sites are preferred: for driving forward, turning both directions, and moving in reverse. If the child can operate only one or two switches, the therapist may need to consider a scanning method; however, the scanning method requires a higher degree of cognitive function and concentration because of the complexity of the task.

Switch placement should begin at the hands and proceed to the head, elbows, feet, and any other location determined appropriate. An adjustable mounting bracket, such as that available through AbleNet Incorporated, is extremely helpful for positioning a switch in multiple locations. Once the therapist has determined an accurate and reliable motor response, he or she can assess the switch on a powered mobility device. Several factors can interfere with a person's ability to drive a powered mobility device. If a child has difficulty, the therapist first evaluates whether the type or placement of the controls is appropriate. The therapist then evaluates the child's position to determine if changes in the child's posture influence motor control. Other considerations include undetected visual and perceptual difficulties, impairment in response time, seizures, motivation, and behavior.

Many children may not initially be successful using a power wheelchair because of the overwhelming amount and degree of sensory input that is required. Imagine being a child with a severe disability who has difficulty with motor planning, coordination, visual perception, and communication and is experiencing movement in a powered device for the first time. It would be overwhelming to experience the excitement and vestibular sensation of moving while trying to view the surroundings, which are quickly passing by, and simultaneously listen to an adult telling you how and where to move.

The therapist should assess a young child for powered mobility, whenever feasible, by providing a method that promotes exploration, problem solving, and self-learning for the child. Such a method requires an open space with activities and toys strategically placed around the room to facilitate experiences in movement and exploration. The therapist should "limit physical and verbal commands as much as possible to avoid sensory overload on the part of the child" (Taylor & Monahan, 1989, p. 85). If a child is trying to move toward an object, the therapist should state the desired outcome, such as "come closer," rather than specific commands, such as "push the joystick left" or "push the red switch and come over here." Feedback should also be positive, such as "you found the wall" rather than "oops, you crashed again" (Wright-Ott, 1997). If further assistance is needed to help the child understand the operation of the control, the therapist can facilitate the proper response by physically guiding the child's movements for the desired response. The therapist must understand that children respond to visual, auditory, and sensory demands at different rates. A child with spastic cerebral palsy, quadriplegia, may require much longer to make a visual motor response than a child with a spinal cord injury.

It may also be beneficial to lend or rent a power wheelchair to children and their families for an extended evaluation. This allows more time for the child to learn how to use the controls and for the family to become familiar with the features of a power wheelchair to assist them in becoming more informed consumers. It also provides an opportunity for the family to experience the responsibilities of maintaining and transporting a power wheelchair.

Computer programs are also available for powered mobility assessment and training (Taplin, 1989). R.J. Cooper and Associates have developed a joystick and mouse training program and a wheelchair simulation program. The programs display a power wheelchair on the screen that the user must navigate through a maze or room. Hasdai, Jessel, and Weiss (1998) studied whether a driving simulator would help a child master skills that are comparable with those required to drive a powered wheelchair. Their results indicated benefits from using such a program to prepare children for powered mobility.

Researchers have explored the use of virtual reality for assessing and training powered mobility skills (Trimble, Morris, & Crandall, 1992). The user wears a helmet that has a screen display of a three-dimensional room through which the person must navigate by using a joystick. More research is needed to determine if virtual reality is an effective means for assessing and training powered mobility and to determine if children will integrate the skills of wheelchair driving if they have not participated in the actual task.

FACTORS THAT INFLUENCE THE SUCCESSFUL USE OF MOBILITY DEVICES

Successful use of mobility devices depends on the fit of the child to the device, the features of the device, and the physical and social environments. Studies have shown a significant relationship between certain standardized tests of cognition and perception and use of powered mobility. Specific functional performance tasks correlate to ability to use a power wheelchair. Preliminary findings indicate a relationship between specific cognitive scales and readiness for powered mobility, particularly in the areas of spatial relations and problem solving (Tefft et al., 1999; Verburg, Field, & Jarvis, 1987).

Another factor that influences a child's ability to use a powered device is the ability of the professional or caregiver to determine the most accurate and efficient means for the child to access the device. If a child is having significant difficulty successfully maneuvering a powered mobility device, the therapist must first evaluate the position of the child and the access method to determine if it is the most effective means. The longer it takes a child to successfully demonstrate use of a control, the more likely it is that either the access method is inappropriate or the child's seating needs have not been met. The following example best describes this type of situation.

Stephanie is a 15-month-old girl with cerebral palsy who successfully used a switch-operated Go Bot to maneuver and explore her surroundings. It took her about 5 hours to become proficient at using a set of four press switches with her hand and to understand the relationship to directionality. However, when she entered another therapy program, the therapist did not consider information on her ability to use switches for driving. Instead, the therapist placed her in a wheelchair training program using the only equipment available, a joystick-operated power wheelchair. After 6 months of training for 3 hours each week, Stephanie demonstrated no improvement in her ability to drive the power wheelchair. Upon reevaluation of her access method, the therapist provided her with four switches at her hand and evaluated a switch array behind her head. She was able to use both access methods but when questioned, preferred using switches behind her head. The head switch array provided her with immediate success in driving the power wheelchair. Had the therapist provided her with the appropriate control method (switch access instead of a joystick, which she could not operate because of her impaired motor function), she may have demonstrated the ability to use the power wheelchair in significantly less time.

The therapist must consider changes that the child will be experiencing in the future, both unexpected and expected, when recommending equipment. For example, the therapist must determine whether the system can be readily changed as the child gains new skills, grows, or experiences other physical changes. This is particularly important for the therapist to consider when ordering a power wheelchair. For example, a child with a progressive disability may be able to operate a joystick at the time the chair is ordered. However, the therapist needs to determine whether the power wheelchair can be economically reconfigured to operate using another method, if the child's strength diminishes. Several options may need to be included in the wheelchair, such as the ability to readily change the input method if the child's functional status changes, the ability to connect interfaces to remotely control appliances in the environment, or the ability to add features such as tilt-in-space or recline. It is more economical in most cases to initially order options on equipment rather than retrofit the equipment at a later date.

Another issue for the therapist to consider when recommending mobility and positioning equipment is where and how augmentative communication equipment is mounted to the child's wheelchair. Selection of the appropriate mounting bracket depends on the tube size of the wheelchair frame and locations on the wheelchair where it can be attached. A problem that therapists often encounter with manual wheelchairs is positioning the child or rear wheels too far forward of the center of gravity in the wheelchair, which often causes the wheelchair to tip forward when the communication device is mounted. The most frequent problem encountered with power wheelchairs is the communication device's interference with the field of vision required for driving. There are now motorized mounting systems for augmentative communication devices, which the user can independently reposition for communicating and for driving.

The therapy team and ATS have a responsibility to assist the family and child in selecting the most appropriate device by presenting several alternatives. The family makes the final decision on the specific type of mobility device after considering the options that the therapy team presents. The most important and significant contribution that the therapist can make is to evaluate access methods and help caregivers develop and implement strategies to meet identified goals. The therapist must reevaluate the outcome as the child progresses. This includes periodic evaluation of fit and function of the equipment.

SUMMARY

The literature indicates that independent mobility plays a facilitative role in cognitive, language, and social development (Jones et al., 2003). Therefore when mobility is severely delayed or restricted, emotional and psychosocial development are affected. Augmentative

mobility devices can provide either functional or transitional mobility. These devices can provide children with physical disabilities with greater opportunities to develop and become initiators and active participants in daily occupations and experiences. Occupational therapists emphasize methods of adapting the child's environments to maximize his or her functional mobility. The occupational therapist is responsible for ensuring that children with physical disabilities receive opportunities for mobility at the earliest age possible to promote participation and development more equal to their able-bodied peers.

Case Studies

These case studies include comprehensive information about the children's equipment and adapted environments. These descriptions demonstrate how mobility equipment is integrated with other assistive technology (AT) and environmental adaptations to best meet the children's functional needs.

Case Study 1: David and Eric

David is 11 years of age, and he was diagnosed with Duchenne's muscular dystrophy at 4 years of age. Shortly afterward, his little brother, Eric, was diagnosed with the same condition at 5 months of age. The two brothers and an older sister live with their parents in a small town.

Duchenne's muscular dystrophy is an inherited X-linked disease that affects the voluntary skeletal musculature with progressive weakness and degeneration of the muscles that control movement. The muscle weakness begins in the proximal and axial musculature and slowly progresses distally. Frequently children with Duchenne's muscular dystrophy require a wheelchair by 12 years of age. Breathing becomes affected during the later stages of the disease, leading to severe respiratory problems. Respiratory infections commonly claim the client's life during the early twenties.

When receiving David's diagnosis, the family was introduced to a team of professionals that specialize in different aspects of musculoskeletal weaknesses. The family received support to help them deal with the initial shock and necessary information about the disease. Twice a year the family continued to meet with the team for medical and orthopedic evaluations. Social and psychologic concerns were also addressed.

Last year David had an Achilles tendon lengthening to release a tight heel cord. Today he walks with a long leg orthosis. It is important to lengthen the walking phase in boys with Duchenne's muscular dystrophy to delay hip and knee flexion deformities and equinovarus deformity of the foot and ankle. For 2 years, David used a standard lightweight manual wheelchair for traveling long distances or when he was fatigued. Currently, the therapy team and David's family are considering a power wheelchair for David to allow him to conserve energy for social and educational activities. The team plans spinal stabilization when David's scoliosis exceeds 25° and normal forced vital capacity (FVC) pulmonary function drops below 50%.

Eric is now 7 years of age. The progression of his disease is following the same course as David's, although somewhat slower. The early signs of Duchenne's muscular dystrophy are becoming prominent, such as the waddling gait, tendency to fall, and difficulty rising from a sitting or lying position.

At the time of Eric's diagnosis, the family lived in an apartment but soon decided to build a house. The occupational therapist provided recommendations for designing the house for wheelchair accessibility to maximize function and independence.

The family has been living in the house for 2 years, and they are pleased with the features that enable the boys to be independent. The outdoor surfaces (sidewalks and ramps) are firm, stable, and slip resistant. The floor plan is spacious, doorways are wide, and there are no thresholds. A few sliding doors have been installed to allow maximum door width and to eliminate floor swing space requirements. Controls, levers, and switches are placed low to be within reach from a wheelchair. The window's lower edge is only 20 inches above the floor for the same reason. The bathrooms are spacious, and there is a bathtub and a shower. The boys love taking baths because they stay warmer and move more freely in the water. The sink is freestanding so the boys can get close to the sink. An automatic faucet has been installed, which is turned on when the hands are placed under the faucet. A full-length mirror is on the wall.

The family continues to need a lot of support and assistance to adjust to new challenges. In addition to direct service to the family, the occupational therapist continues to work closely with the schools to ensure that accessibility is available.

Case Study 2: Jason

Jason is a 7-year-old boy with cerebral palsy, which has affected his ability to speak, move his body with control, and eat. Although he demonstrates severe delays in his motor skills, he appears alert and attentive and understands what is said to him. From his early days, his family was motivated to ensure that Jason has a childhood as normal as possible. They were creative in designing simple devices and tools to accomplish these goals. His grandfather designed the first mobility device for him. It was a push cart used to hold golf clubs, but he mounted a car seat to the frame and placed foam pieces in the seat to help align Jason's body and prevent him from leaning over. His mother would use it to push him around the neighborhood during her daily jogging routine. He also used a standard stroller but required a positioning system to assist him in sitting upright by providing support at the pelvis, trunk, and head. The first seating system was made of triwall, a three-layer thickness cardboard that can be used to fabricate temporary seat inserts for children. Another seat insert was fabricated from triwall, but this one could be placed on the dining room chair so that he could eat at the family table instead of a high chair.

By the time he was 12 months of age, Jason's family built him an aeroplane mobility device (see Figure 19-7) to use at home. When he outgrew this by 2 years of age, his therapist evaluated him for a support walker and he could effectively use the Walkabout by Mobility Plus. He continued to use this for indoor mobility and for playing in Little League for special needs children when he was 5 years of age. He and his teammates used an automatic device to hit the ball, and Jason ran around the field using his walker.

When Jason was $2\frac{1}{2}$ years of age, his family decided that the walker alone was not adequately meeting his mobility needs. His therapist evaluated him for a power wheelchair, and he could operate the joystick once he was positioned with maximal support at his feet, pelvis, trunk, and head. His therapist and family determined the features that he needed so that he could use a power wheelchair. They determined that he needed a molded seating system for support and alignment. To increase independence, the system needed to include the ability to elevate the seat from the floor to various heights. The therapist identified a power wheelchair with these features and recommended a custom-molded seating system.

The family made the home environment accessible to Jason in many ways. When he was 2 years of age they decided that it was important for him to roll out of bed in the morning and try to roll on the floor. They placed a low-height mattress on the floor in the corner of his bedroom and made it his bed. They lined the sides of it with his stuffed toys to protect him from unintentionally hitting his arms against the walls. This arrangement allowed him to get out of bed on his own. They also extended the light switch in his room so that he could reach it from his walker or wheelchair.

Positioning in the bathtub when he was a toddler was a challenge, but his mother made a bath seat for him from a milk crate. She placed foam around the edges and the seat for comfort. When he outgrew this, his family acquired a bath seat designed for children with disabilities. His occupational therapist recommended an adapted toilet seat with a high backrest. It provided Jason with the ability to begin toilet training at 2 years of age. His family also installed a flip-down bar in front of the toilet so Jason could stand at the toilet "like his dad."

During these early years, Jason's therapist introduced him to augmentative communication symbols and aids. By the time he was 12 months of age, he could point to symbols in his communication book and soon progressed to using an augmentative communication device with voice output by accessing it with a light pointer on his head. The communication device was mounted on his power wheelchair. Today Jason is fully included in a second grade class. He uses AT to do his schoolwork and has an attendant with him throughout the day. Both simple and sophisticated AT devices have enabled him to function within a regular education classroom and to participate in most of the activities of his peers.

STUDY QUESTIONS

1 What questions should be answered before selecting a mobility device?
2 A child with cerebral palsy (spastic diplegia) uses a push walker but needs a manual wheelchair for mobility in the community and at school. He is expected to learn how to transfer in and out of it in the future. What features will be needed on his manual wheelchair for optimal independence?
3 What type of wheelchair control would an individual with a spinal cord injury at the C_3 level be most likely to use?
4 If a child has less than 90° of passive range of movement in knee extension because of tight hamstring muscles, explain how this would affect his ability to sit upright in a wheelchair using standard footrest hangers (60° angle).
5 Why is it important for the therapist to simultaneously consider a child's positioning needs when assessing a mobility device?

REFERENCES

ADA/IT, Americans with Disabilities Act & Accessible Information Technology Center, 2003. Bulletin #4, www.adaproject.org.

Andersson, C., Grooten, W., Hellsten, M., Kaping K., & Mattsson E. (2003). Adults with cerebral palsy: Walking ability after progressive strength training. *Developmental Medicine and Child Neurology, 45* (4), 220-228.

Backer, G., & Howell, B. (1997). Physical therapy goals and intervention for the ventilator-assisted child or adolescent. In L. Driver, V. Nelson, & S. Warschausky (Eds.), *The ventilator assisted child.* San Antonio, TX: Communication Skill Builders.

Becker, R.D. (1975). Recent developments in child psychiatry: The restrictive emotional and cognitive environment reconsidered: A redefinition of the concept of the therapeutic

restraint. *Israel Annals of Psychiatry and Related Disciplines, 13,* 239-258.

Bergen, A., Presperin, J., & Tallman, T. (1990). *Positioning for function: Wheelchairs and other assistive technologies.* New York: Valhalla Rehabilitation Publications.

Blundell S., Shepherd, R., Dean C., Adams R., & Cahill B. (2003). Functional strength training in cerebral palsy: a pilot study of a group circuit training class for children aged 4-8 years. *Clinical Rehabilitation, 17* (1), 48-57.

Bly, L. (1994). *Motor skills acquisition in the first year.* Tucson, AZ: Therapy Skill Builders.

Brinker, R.P., & Lewis, M. (1982). Making the world work with microcomputers: A learning prosthesis for handicapped infants. *Exceptional Children, 49,* 163-170.

Butler, C. (1986). Effects of powered mobility on self-initiated behaviors of very young children with locomotor disability. *Developmental Medicine and Child Neurology, 28,* 325-332.

Butler, C. (1988a). High tech tots: Technology for mobility, manipulation, communication, and learning in early childhood. *Infants and Young Children, 2,* 66-73.

Butler, C. (1988b). Powered tots: Augmentative mobility for locomotor disabled youngsters. *American Physical Therapy Association Pediatric Publication, 14,* 21.

Campos, J.J., & Bertenthal, B.I. (1987). Locomotion and psychological development in infancy. In K.M. Jaffe (Ed.), Childhood powered mobility: Developmental, technical, and clinical perspectives. In *Proceedings of the RESNA First Northwest Regional Conference* (pp. 11-42). Washington, DC: RESNA Press.

Cech, D., & Martin, A. (1995). *Functional movement development across the life span.* Philadelphia: W.B. Saunders.

Cook, A.M., & Hussey, S.M. (2002). Seating and positioning systems as extrinsic enablers for assistive technologies. In A.M. Cook & S.M. Hussey (Eds.), *Assistive technologies: Principles and practice* (2nd ed.). St. Louis: Mosby.

Cooper, R. (1998). Biomechanics and ergonomics of wheelchairs. In R. Cooper (Ed.), *Wheelchair selection and configuration.* New York: Demos.

Coster, W. (1998). Occupation-centered assessment of children. *American Journal of Occupational Therapy, 52,* 337-344.

Deitz, J., Swinth, Y, & White, O. (2002). Powered mobility and preschoolers with complex developmental delays. *American Journal of Occupational Therapy, 56,* 86-96.

Douglas, J., & Ryan, M. (1987). A preschool severely disabled boy and his powered wheelchair: A case study. *Child Care, Health and Development, 13,* 303-309.

Engstrom, B. (1993). *Ergonomics, wheelchairs and positioning.* Hasselby, Sweden: Posturalis Books.

Everand, L. (1997). Early mobility means easier integration. *Canadian Review of Sociology and Anthropology, 34,* 224-234.

Fisher, A.G. (1998). Uniting practice and theory in an occupational framework. *The American Journal of Occupational Therapy, 52,* 509-521.

Foreman N., Foreman D., Cummings A., & Owens, S. (1990). *Journal of General Psychology, 117* (2), 215-233.

Fowler, E.G., Ho T.W., Nwigwe A.I., & Dorey F.J. (2001). The effect of quadriceps femoris muscle strengthening exercises on spasticity in children with cerebral palsy. *Physical Therapy, 81* (6), 1215-1223.

Furumasu, J., Tefft, D., & Guerette, P. (1998). Pediatric powered mobility: Readiness to learn. *Technology and Disability, 5,* 41-48.

Guerette P., Tefft, D., Furumasu, J., & Moy F. (1999). Development of a cognitive assessment battery for young children with physical impairments. *Infant-Toddler Intervention: The Transdisciplinary Journal, 9,* 169-184.

Haley, S.M., Coster, W.J., Ludlow, L.H., Haltiwanger, J., & Andrellos, P. (1992). *Pediatric Evaluation of Disability Inventory (PEDI).* San Antonio, TX: Psychological Corp.

Hasdai, A., Jessel, A.S., & Weiss, P.L. (1998). Use of computer simulator for training children with disabilities in the operation of a powered wheelchair. *American Journal of Occupational Therapy, 52,* 215-220.

Hays, R. (1987). Childhood motor impairments: Clinical overview and scope of the problem. In K.M. Jaffe (Ed.), Childhood powered mobility: Developmental, technical, and clinical perspectives. *Proceedings of the RESNA First Northwest Regional Conference.* Washington, DC: RESNA Press.

Hulme, J., Poor, R., Schulein, M., & Pezzino, J. (1983). Perceived behavioral changes observed with adaptive seating devices for multi-handicapped developmentally disabled individuals. *Physical Therapy, 62* (4), 204-208.

Hundert, J., & Hopkins, B. (1992). Training supervisors in a collaborative team approach to promote peer interactions of children with disabilities in integrated preschools. *Journal of Applied Behavioral Analysis, 25,* 385-400.

Jones, M., McEwen I., & Hansen, L. (2003). *Physical Therapy, 83,* 253-262.

Kangas, K. (2001). *Chest supports: Why they are not working.* Seventeenth International Seating Symposium, February 22-24, 41-44.

Kermoian, R. (1997). Locomotion experience and psychological development in infancy. In J. Furumasu (Ed.), *Pediatric powered mobility: Developmental perspectives, technical issues, clinical approaches* (pp. 7-22). Arlington, VA: RESNA Press.

Law, M., Baptiste, S., Carswell, A., McColl, M.A., Polatajko, H., & Pollock, N. (1994). *The Canadian Occupational Performance Measure* (2nd ed.). Toronto, ON: CAOT Publications.

Myhr, U., & Wendt, L. (1991). Improvement of functional sitting position for children with cerebral palsy. *Developmental Medicine and Child Neurology, 33,* 246-256.

Nilsson, L., & Nyberg, P. (2003). Driving to learn: a new concept for training children with profound cognitive disabilities in a powered wheelchair. *American Journal of Occupational Therapy, 57* (2), 229-233.

Nwaobi, O. (1986). Effects of body orientation in space on tonic muscle activity of patients with cerebral palsy. *Developmental Medicine and Child Neurology, 28,* 41-44.

Nwaobi, O. (1987). Effect of unilateral arm restraint on upper extremity function in cerebral palsy. In *Proceedings of the Annual RESNA Conference* (pp. 311-313). Washington, DC: RESNA Press.

Paleg, G. (July, 1997). Made for walking: A comparison of gait trainers. *Team Rehab Report,* 41-45.

Paulsson, K., & Christoffersen, M. (1984). Psychological aspects of technical aids: How does independent mobility affect the psychological and intellectual development of children with physical disabilities. In *Proceedings of the Second Annual Conference on Rehabilitation Engineering* (pp. 282-286). Washington, DC: RESNA Press.

Piaget, J. (1954). *The construction of reality in the child.* New York: Basic Books.

Pollock, N., & Stewart, D. (1998). Occupational performance needs of school-aged children with physical disability in the community. *Physical and Occupational Therapy in Pediatrics, 18* (1), 55-68.

Raine A., Reynolds, C., Venables, P.H., & Mednick, S.A. (2002). Stimulation seeking and intelligence: A retrospective longitudinal study. *Journal Personality and Social Psychology, 82,* 663-674.

Seligman, M. (1975). *Helplessness: On depression, development, and death.* San Francisco: W.H. Freeman.

Stanton, D., Wilson, P.N., & Foreman, N. (2002). Effects of early mobility on shortcut performance in a simulated maze. *Behavioral Brain Research, 136* (1), 61-66.

Taplin, C.S. (1989). Powered wheelchair control, assessment, and training. In *RESNA '89: Proceedings of the 12th annual conference* (pp. 45-46.) Washington, DC: RESNA Press.

Taylor, S., & Monahan, L. (1989). Considerations in assessing for powered mobility. In C. Brubaker (Ed.), *Wheelchair IV: Report of a conference on the state of the art of powered wheelchair mobility, December 7-9, 1988.* Washington, DC: RESNA Press.

Tefft, D., Furumasu, J., & Guerette, P. (1992). *Cognitive readiness for powered mobility in the very young child* (Unpublished manuscript). Downey, CA: Rancho Los Amigos.

Tefft, D., Furumasu, J., & Guerette, P. (1993). Cognitive readiness for powered wheelchair mobility in the young child. In *Proceedings of the RESNA 1993 Annual Conference* (pp. 338-340). Las Vegas, NV: RESNA Press.

Tefft, D., Furumasu, J., & Guerette, P., (1995). Development of a cognitive assessment battery for evaluating readiness for powered mobility. *In Proceedings of the RESNA 1995 Annual Conference* (pp. 320-322). Vancouver, Canada: RESNA Press.

Tefft, D., Furumasu, J., & Guerette, P. (1997). Pediatric powered mobility: Influential cognitive skills. In J. Furumasu (Ed.), *Pediatric powered mobility: Developmental perspectives, technical issues, clinical approaches* (pp. 70-91). Washington, DC: RESNA Press.

Tefft, D., Guerette, P., & Furumasu, J. (1999). Cognitive predictors of young children's readiness for powered mobility. *Developmental Medicine and Child Neurology, 41* (10), 665-670.

Telzrow, R., Campos, J., Shepherd, A., Bertenthal, B., & Atwater, S. (1987). Spatial understanding in infants with motor handicaps. In K. M. Jaffe (Ed.), *Childhood powered mobility: Developmental, technical and clinical perspectives.* Proceedings of the RESNA First Northwest Regional Conference (pp. 62-69). Seattle, WA: RESNA Association for the Advancement of Rehabilitation Technology.

Trefler, E. (1999). Then & now: Saving time with simulators. *Team Rehab,* February, 32-36.

Trefler, E., Hobson, D., Taylor, S., Monahan, L, & Shaw, C. (1993). *Seating and mobility.* Tucson, AZ: Therapy Skill Builders.

Trimble, J., Morris, T., & Crandall, R. (1992). Virtual reality: Designing accessible environments. *Team Rehab Report, 3,* 8-12.

Uniform Data System for Medical Rehabilitation. (1999). *Functional Independence Measure for Children (WeeFIM)* (Outpatient version 5.0.). Buffalo, NY: State University of New York at Buffalo.

Verburg, G., Field, D., & Jarvis, S. (1987). Motor, perceptual, and cognitive factors that affect mobility control. In *Proceedings of the 10th Annual Conference on Rehabilitation Technology*, Washington, DC: RESNA Press.

Warren, C.G. (1990). Powered mobility and its implications, *Journal of Rehabilitation Research and Development. Clinical Supplement, 27*(2), 74-85.

Woods, H. (1998, Fall). Moving right along: Young disabled children can now experience the developmental benefits of moving and exploring on their own. *Stanford Medicine,* 15-19.

Wright, C., & Nomura, M. (1991). *From toys to computers, access for the physically disabled child.* San Jose, CA: Author.

Wright-Ott, C. (1997). The transitional powered mobility aid: A new concept and tool for early mobility. In J. Furumasu (Ed.), *Pediatric powered mobility* (pp. 58-69). Washington, DC: RESNA Press.

Wright-Ott, C. (1998). Designing a transitional powered mobility aid for young children with physical disabilities. In D. Gray, L. Quatrano, & M. Lieverman (Eds.), *Designing and using assistive technology: The human perspective* (pp. 285-295). Baltimore: Brooks.

Wright-Ott, C. (1999) A transitional powered mobility aid for young children with physical disabilities. In *ICORR 99 Sixth International Conference on Rehabilitation Robotics,* July 1999, Stanford, CA.

SUGGESTED READING

Bertenthal, B.I., Campos, J.J., & Barrett, K.C. (1984). Self-produced locomotion: An organizer of emotional, cognitive, and social development in infancy. In R.N. Emde & R.J. Harmon (Eds.), *Continuities and discontinuities in development.* New York, Plenum Press.

Furumasu, J., Guerette, P., & Tefft., D. (1996). The development of a powered wheelchair mobility program for young children. *Technology and Disability, 5* (1), 41-48.

Tefft, D., Furumasu, J., & Guerette, P. (1996*). Ready, set, go: Powered mobility with young children.* Downey, CA: Los Amigos Research and Education Institute, Rancho Los Amigos Medical Center.

WEB SITES

www.abledata.com/ resources for assistive technology products

www.assistivetech.net/

www.resna.org: The Rehabilitation Engineering and Assistive Technology Society of North America

www.irsc.org: Internet resources for special children

www.medgroup.com/rehab Adrienne Bergen, RPT provides an informative newsletter on new seating/mobility products shown annually at the MedTrade Exhibits.

www.enablingdevices.com: adapted toys and switches.

www.freedomconcepts.com: adapted trikes

www.iphope.com: market the MiniBot, Gobot and modified powered toys

www.blvd.com:

www.mobilityfordiscovery.com articles and resources on early mobility

www.rjedesigns.com: custom modifications and joystick go carts.

www.abilitiesexpo.com: Regional exhibits of adaptive technology devices

www.medtrade.com: National annual conference and exhibit where new seating and mobility products are demonstrated.

www.pediatricpowernetwork.com: sponsor a national annual conference

www.wheelchairnet.org: lists resources of the RERC on wheeled mobility

Areas of Pediatric Occupational Therapy Services

20 Neonatal Intensive Care Unit

Jan G. Hunter

CHAPTER OBJECTIVES

1 Understand the scope of knowledge required for competent practice in the neonatal intensive care unit (NICU).
2 Compare the traditional occupational therapy approach of rehabilitation and developmental stimulation with current concepts of individualized developmentally supportive care in the NICU.
3 Define and compute postconceptional, chronologic, and corrected age.
4 Explain why preterm infants are so susceptible to heat loss and how heat loss can occur.
5 Define common medical conditions in the preterm and high-risk infant.
6 Identify potential negative effects of light, sound, and caregiving practices in the NICU.
7 Describe interventions to modify light, sound, and caregiving practices in the NICU so that preterm infants are protected from excessive and inappropriate stimulation.
8 Discuss the factors that complicate parenting in the NICU.

9 Describe the roles and potential interventions of the NICU therapist in providing family support through family-centered neonatal care.
10 Discuss factors that should be considered in the evaluation of an infant in the NICU and identify published neonatal assessments.
11 Explain the synactive theory of development proposed by Heidi Als.
12 Describe neurobehavioral and neuromotor development in preterm infants.
13 Identify and describe the six neurobehavioral states.
14 Describe common positional deformities of preterm infants, their potential influence on future development, and how they can be prevented.
15 Explain the advantages and disadvantages of different positioning options.
16 Explain the indications for and applications of neuromotor interventions that involve range of motion and splinting.
17 Explain why nonnutritive sucking is beneficial to preterm infants.
18 Describe organized and disorganized nutritive sucking patterns observed during infant feeding.
19 Summarize key factors that can facilitate successful breast feeding in the NICU.
20 Apply methods of modifying the sensory environment to a case study of an extremely preterm infant with multiple medical problems and neurobehavioral difficulties.

Kimberly underwent an emergency cesarean delivery at 26 weeks' gestation when intrauterine circulation problems developed between two of her three triplets. Savannah was born prematurely to a 15-year-old student who concealed her pregnancy from her parents. Tonya, with a history of three previous miscarriages, had a cerclage (a surgical procedure to keep the cervix closed during pregnancy), and was able to carry Darren until 32 weeks' gestation. Brittney was born at 28 weeks to a mother addicted to crack cocaine who received no prenatal care. Dylan, born at term to a febrile mother, became critically ill with pneumonia and developed respiratory failure during his first day of life. Myesha was delivered by an emergency cesarean section after a motor vehicle accident in which the placenta was partially torn from the wall of her mother's uterus. Maria's prenatal ultrasound revealed an infant with multiple congenital anomalies.

In all these cases, the infants were admitted to a neonatal intensive care unit (NICU) after delivery; all but one baby survived. These real life examples represent the urgency and wide range of skilled medical care needed to optimize both survival and functional outcome in preterm and high-risk infants.

EVOLUTION OF NEONATAL INTENSIVE CARE

The NICU is a complex, highly specialized hospital unit designed to care for infants born prematurely or those who are critically ill (Figure 20-1). Today's state-of-the-art NICU bears little resemblance to the "Special Department for Weaklings," the first special care unit for preterm newborns established by Dr. Pierre Budin in 1893, when medical care consisted of providing warmth, small feedings, and protection from infection (Hodgman, 1985). Technologic advances have prompted the observation that being a newborn *preterm infant* in a modern NICU is like being abducted from a warm, comfortable home by "aliens" or "terrorists" and subjected to an overwhelming barrage of continuous bright lights and jarring noises while fruitless attempts

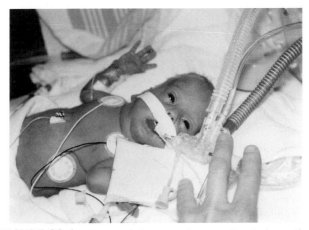

FIGURE 20-1 Preterm infant receives mechanical ventilation in a neonatal intensive care unit (NICU). Three cardiorespiratory leads and a temperature probe are visible; a percutaneous catheter for intravenous infusions is in the infant's right arm. (Courtesy Infant Special Care Unit, University of Texas Medical Branch, Galveston, Texas; photograph by Candy Cochran.)

at sleep are repeatedly interrupted by frequent invasive and painful procedures performed by "huge creatures" (White & Newbold, 1995). An increased awareness of the influence of environmental and caregiving factors on the vulnerable newborn has enlarged the scope of NICU care to encompass infant developmental support and family issues in addition to primary medical concerns (Als & Gilkerson, 1997; Altimier, 2002; Glass, 1999; Gottfried & Gaiter, 1985; McGrath & Conliffe-Torres, 1996). This chapter discusses the knowledge and skills an occupational therapist needs to work within this expanded focus of high-tech neonatal care.

Nursery Classification and Regionalization of Care

Advances in medical technology and specialized care for preterm and high-risk infants have skyrocketed since the early 1960s. However, the spiraling expense and complexity of medical care also gave rise to a growing discrepancy between neonatal mortality rates at major medical centers and those at smaller hospitals. In the early 1970s, the concept of regionalization of perinatal care emerged; this allowed the provision of advanced health care to any mother or infant in a particular perinatal region while avoiding unnecessary duplication of services (American Medical Association, 1971). Patient care generally was provided at the nearest hospital, with transfer to a higher level facility as needed for more complex problems.

Area hospitals traditionally have been designated by the level of care they provide (Pettett, Sewell, & Merenstein, 2002). A level I nursery (e.g., in a small community hospital) manages uncomplicated pregnancies with expected normal deliveries and well infants. Level II nurseries are designed to care for newborn infants who require some additional medical management, such as phototherapy for jaundice, intravenously administered (IV) antibiotics, or tube feedings. A neonatologist is usually on staff, but these units typically lack the equipment and additional expertise, such as a pediatric surgeon or cardiologist, to care for all medical emergencies and severe neonatal problems. Level III nurseries have the necessary equipment and trained personnel in the NICU and other hospital departments to care for all potential neonatal conditions and emergencies. "Level IV" is an unofficial classification used to designate NICUs that offer "rescue" technology (e.g., extracorporeal membrane oxygenation [ECMO] for infants in respiratory failure that is unresponsive to conventional medical management), although some technologies used initially for rescue (e.g., nitric oxide [NO] administration) become more widely available as a routine standard of care with continued proven success.

Since the 1980s, the economic forces of an increasingly competitive health care market have compromised the traditional concepts of regionalization of care (Pettett et al., 2002). The growth of managed health care, advocacy efforts to increase the number of children with health insurance (including Medicaid), and the availability of neonatal technology and specialists have encouraged many hospitals to expand their perinatal services, resulting in fragmentation of services and a wide disparity in the level of care provided. Renewed analysis and modification of regionalization policies to achieve better outcomes at a lower cost (e.g., routine provision of mechanical ventilation in level II units) have been suggested (Meadow et al., 1996).

Long-term responsibility for an individual infant's medical care may also be determined by economics. Some managed care programs may reimburse only an infant's transfer to a higher level nursery, precluding a "back transfer" to a hospital closer to the parents when the infant's condition is more stable and the baby is convalescing. Some neonatal units may refuse to accept transfer of a stable but chronically medically fragile infant because of expected long-term costs that will exceed reimbursement. Achieving a balance between cost control and universal quality patient access is the current dilemma and necessity facing organizers and providers of perinatal health care (Pettett et al., 2002).

NICU Outcome Indicators: Mortality and Morbidity

Infant survival initially was the primary indicator of NICU success. As innovations in medical science, technology, and caregiving skills increased the survival rate of younger, smaller, and sicker infants, concerns emerged about the effects of the NICU on preterm infants and about the long-term developmental outcome of NICU survivors. These concerns facilitated the entry of occupational therapists and other neonatal developmental specialists into the critical care arena of the NICU. Researchers continue to explore preterm infant development, the effects of acute and chronic illness, animate and inanimate NICU environmental factors, family dynamics when newborns are hospitalized because of prematurity or illness, the ultimate outcome of NICU survivors, and NICU cost containment with improved use of resources (Blackburn, 2003; Hendricks-Munoz, Predergast, Caprio, & Wasserman, 2002: Peabody & Martin, 1996; Yu, 2000).

Sensory Deprivation Versus Stimulation

Changing theories about sensory stimulation in the NICU have also promoted occupational therapists' entry into the intensive care nursery. Understanding the evolution of thought regarding stimulation in the NICU, as outlined below, can help the new neonatal therapist progress more efficiently to a state-of-the-art practice approach:

1 *Minimal stimulation.* Special care nurseries in the 1940s and 1950s were strictly minimal stimulation units with low lights, quiet environments, and restricted access by families and even physicians.

2 *Sensory deprivation theory.* The paucity of stimuli in these early nurseries precipitated the sensory deprivation theory espoused in the 1960s and 1970s. Infants in the NICU were thought to be at increased developmental risk from deprivation of normal sensory stimulation that occurs naturally in the womb or at home after birth.

3 *Sensory stimulation programs.* Sensory deficit proponents advocated compensation for perceived deprivation of beneficial sensory stimuli with selected regimens of patterned stimuli in a "one size fits all" approach. These supplemental stimulation programs generally consisted of massage, stroking, passive range of motion, vestibular input, and/or auditory input. Concerns have been raised that extra stimulation may have benefited larger, stable infants but possibly stressed more fragile babies; behavioral responses of individual infants were not reported in the studies of this era.

4 *Sensory overload theory.* The sensory deficit model failed to recognize that the explosion of knowledge and technology in the 1960s and 1970s actually created an abundance of disorganized, noncontingent stimuli that were disturbing to infants in the NICU. Intensive care nurseries had become large, brightly lit rooms filled with noisy monitors and equipment. Additional technology required more staff members, who engaged in more frequent handling of infants for procedures and who greatly increased the general noise and activity level in the unit. The sensory overload theory, which began to emerge in the 1970s, hypothesized that NICU infants were actually overwhelmed by a constant bombardment of inappropriate stimuli.

5 *Environmental neonatology.* Increasing concerns about the significant number and variety of random stimuli prompted the rise in the 1980s and 1990s of environmental neonatology, in which the short-term and long-term influences of animate and inanimate environmental factors on NICU infants are explored.

6 *Individualized, relationship-based, family-centered developmental care.* This approach strives continually to structure the NICU environment and caregiving practices according to the ongoing neurobehavioral cues of each infant and to promote the involvement of family members as primary caregivers and integrated team members for their infant.

CHANGING FOCUS OF NEONATAL OCCUPATIONAL THERAPY

Traditional Occupational Therapy: Rehabilitation and Stimulation

In the 1980s, traditional neonatal occupational therapy consisted solely of rehabilitation and developmental stimulation, an approach still used in some NICUs. Infants were identified as appropriate for occupational therapy by specific risk factors (e.g., very low birth weight, prenatal drug exposure), diagnosis of pathology (e.g., congenital anomalies, severe asphyxia), or performance indicators (e.g., abnormal tone, poor feeding, chronic illness with developmental delay). Therapy goals and intervention activities targeted specific problems, such as limited range of motion, high or low muscle tone, extreme irritability, poor feeding, or developmental delay (Rapport, 1992).

Rehabilitation continues to be an appropriate component of therapy for a select group of medically stable NICU infants with definitive diagnoses, such as arthrogryposis multiplex congenita (see Case Study 1) or myelomeningocele with hydrocephalus. Older chronically ill infants who need developmental therapy may remain in some NICUs, but they increasingly are being transferred to step-down units or discharged with home health services at much earlier ages and with greater acuity than was done previously.

State-of-the-Art Occupational Therapy: Developmental Support

With advances in developmental knowledge pertinent to the NICU, the parameters of neonatal occupational therapy have expanded beyond traditional rehabilitation services to encompass *individualized developmentally supportive care*. This approach is based on the recognition that any infant young enough or sick enough to require intensive care has inherent developmental risks and vulnerabilities, that parenting an infant in the NICU is stressful and difficult, and that both infant and family must receive individualized support throughout the NICU hospitalization for optimal outcome (Aita & Snide, 2003; Ashpaugh & Leick-Rude, 1999; Gressens, Rogido, Paindaveine, & Sola, 2003; Heermann & Wilson, 2000).

Developmental support includes a protective and preventive component of care that is not inherent in the traditional rehabilitation model. In contrast to the traditional approach, which emphasized direct, "hands-on" contact, protecting the fragile newborn from excessive or inappropriate sensory input often is a more urgent priority than direct intervention or interaction with the infant (American Occupational Therapy Association [AOTA], 2000).

Therapist Trust and Acceptance in the NICU

As the neonatal therapist expands beyond conventional stimulation and rehabilitation techniques to include the practice of individualized developmental care, closer working relationships are cultivated with nursery medical staff. NICU caregivers are rightfully very protective of their tiny, vulnerable patients. Professional credentials and a patient referral may allow an unfamiliar therapist access to the unit, but medical staff can still hinder access to the infant. Trust, acceptance, and respect from the NICU team develop gradually as the neonatal therapist consistently demonstrates competency in knowledge, skills, and interpersonal professional relationships. An understanding of the transitional stages in the development of collaborative partnerships between therapists and neonatal nurses can be helpful to the therapist who is in the process of moving from "guest" to "family" in the NICU (Sweeney, 1993). The following are the four stages leading to collaborative partnership:

- *Stage 1:* Professional guest (involves independent consultation with minimal interaction)
- *Stage 2:* Competitive or protective posturing (occurs during the period the co-worker's competence is evaluated)
- *Stage 3:* Integrated NICU team member (involves building trust and mutuality in joint caregiving and problem solving)
- *Stage 4:* Committed partnership (provides opportunities for peak creative experiences)

Competencies for the Neonatal Therapist

Practice standards to promote relevant competencies for NICU developmental specialists have been documented (AOTA, 2000; Browne, VandenBerg, Ross, & Elmore, 1999; VandenBerg, 1993; Vergara & Bigsby, 2003). Occupational therapy in the NICU is considered a specialized area of practice that requires advanced knowledge and skills. Specialized knowledge requirements include a familiarity with relevant neonatal medical conditions, procedures, and equipment; an understanding of the unique developmental abilities and vulnerabilities of term, preterm, and ill infants; a familiarity with theories and clinical applications of neonatal neuromotor and neurobehavioral development, family systems, and NICU ecology; and an appreciation of the manner in which these factors interact to influence infant and family behavior and development. The occupational therapist develops the necessary knowledge and skills through continuing education and supervised clinical experience in assessment and intervention specific to the NICU (Dewire, White, Kanny, & Glass, 1996; Hunter, 1996).

The remainder of this chapter is divided into four distinct but interrelated sections. The first section emphasizes the development of a NICU medical foundation. The remaining three sections cover the NICU environment, NICU family, and NICU infant; each of these sections discusses foundation information, evaluation, and intervention strategies pertinent to the focus topic. Evaluation of and intervention for the infant are discussed last to symbolize the ethical neonatal therapist who conscientiously prepares before touching the NICU infant.

DEVELOPING A MEDICAL FOUNDATION

Abbreviations and Terminology

It is essential that the neonatal occupational therapist learn the language of the NICU. Documentation typically contains many abbreviations, as illustrated by this medical summary:

> Cody is a 39 wk pca wm born at 25 WBD, 27 WBE by SVD to a 18-yo now $G_2P_1Ab_1$, A+,VDRL– mom with hx of IVDA, smokes 1 PPD, PIH and PTL tx'd with $MgSO_4$, PPROM 72° PTD. Pt. had TCAN X 1 (reduced PTD), was SGA at 505 g, Apgars $1^1,3^5,6^{10}$. Significant medical complications have included RDS, BPD, PIE, PDA (ligated), hyperbilirubinemia, anemia, MRSE sepsis, NEC, AOP, BIH, R gr. 3 and L gr. 4 IVH with PVL, ROP stage III OD (regressing) and stage III + OS (s/p laser OS). Pt. was on SIMV for 41 days, NCPAP for 32 days, and remains on FiO_2 1.0 at 0.5 L by NC.

Understanding abbreviations and the terms they represent is a prerequisite for neonatal practice. Appendix 20-A lists some common NICU abbreviations.

Classification by Age

Gestational age (GA) refers to the total number of weeks the infant was in utero before birth. The determination of gestational age may be based on dating the last menstrual period (LMP), on ultrasound results (USG), or on a physical examination of the infant. The range for a full-term pregnancy is 38 to 42 weeks at some hospitals and 37 to 42 weeks at others. An infant born before 37 to 38 weeks is considered preterm; an infant born after 42 weeks is postterm. Once the infant is born, the GA remains the same.

Calculation of the GA by ultrasound or physical assessment generally is considered accurate within a plus or minus 2-week range. Gestational age assessment is useful for determining problems that may have occurred in utero (e.g., an unusually small term infant may have experienced placental insufficiency or a prenatal infection) and for anticipating potential problems after birth

(e.g., the risk of respiratory distress or intraventricular hemorrhage is higher for extremely preterm infants born at less than 28 weeks' gestation and low for babies born at term).

Postconceptional age (PCA) refers to the infant's age in relation to conception and thus continually changes over time. The PCA is obtained by adding the weeks since birth to the infant's gestational age. When the infant born at 27 weeks reaches his or her expected due date, the PCA is 40 weeks (27 weeks' gestation plus 13 weeks since birth). PCA is commonly used until 40 to 44 weeks, equivalent to term or 1 month corrected age, respectively.

Chronologic age refers to the infant's actual age since birth. Chronologically, the infant born at 27 weeks' gestation is 3 months old on the expected due date and 12 months old on the first birthday. The chronologic age of preterm infants is usually "corrected for prematurity" to better correlate with developmental expectations and performance (e.g., the infant born at 27 weeks' gestation will not developmentally look the same at 3 months' chronologic age as the infant born at term).

Corrected age refers to how old the infant would be if born at term rather than prematurely. The number of weeks of prematurity is first determined (gestational age in weeks is subtracted from the term equivalent of 40 weeks), and that figure is then subtracted from the chronologic age. The infant born at 27 weeks' gestation was born 13 weeks prematurely (40 weeks – 27 weeks = 13 weeks early). The corrected age of this infant on the first birthday is 9 months, because the actual birth was 3 months earlier than the expected due date. Corrected age typically is used until 2 years of age when assessing developmental status.

Classification by Birth Weight

Infants born weighing more than 2500 g (5.5 pounds) are considered average in size. A birth weight of 1,500 to 2,500 g is a *low birth weight (LBW)*. A *very low birth weight (VLBW)* is 1,000 to 1,500 g; *extremely low birth weight (ELBW)* is less than 1,000 g, and *ultra-low birth weight (ULBW)* is less than 750 g.

A birth weight that falls between the 10th and the 90th percentiles on a standardized growth chart is *appropriate for gestational age (AGA)*. A birth weight below the tenth percentile is *small for gestational age (SGA)*, and a birth weight above the 90th percentile is *large for gestational age (LGA)*. These categories apply equally to preterm, term, and postterm infants. Any infant growing normally in utero will be AGA. If a mother has severe pregnancy-induced hypertension (PIH) and the infant experiences intrauterine growth retardation (IUGR), he or she may be born SGA. The infant of a mother with diabetes is often LGA.

Thermoregulation

Preterm infants are predisposed to excessive heat loss and are vulnerable to cold stress from several causes. Extended postures, thin skin, and, in very premature infants, a reduced amount of insulating subcutaneous fat allow heat to transfer from the body to the air. A specialized *brown fat* used by newborns to metabolize heat is not produced until the last trimester of gestation. Pulmonary dysfunction, central nervous system (CNS) immaturity, and frequent caregiving interventions may also contribute to heat loss. The infant may lose heat by *convection* (heat loss to surrounding air), *conduction* (body contact with a cooler solid surface), *radiation* (heat loss to a cooler solid object not in direct contact with the infant, such as incubator walls), and *evaporation* (heat that is lost as liquid from the respiratory tract and permeable skin and is converted into a vapor).

Radiant warmers, incubators, positioning aids that provide containment, clothes, and swaddling in blankets help conserve heat in NICU infants (Seguin & Vieth, 1996). The neonatal therapist must diligently protect NICU infants from heat loss during all evaluations and interventions. Cold stress can burn calories needed for growth and healing, cause behavioral and physiologic complications, and, in severe cases, result in death.

Medical Conditions and Equipment

Learning NICU medical terminology is a continuing process that progresses from a general familiarity with terms and definitions to an understanding of the pathophysiology of diseases and the biomechanics of equipment. Medical complications and technology both have profound effects on preterm and high-risk infants, with subsequent implications and precautions for neonatal therapists (Hunter, Mullen, & Dallas, 1994; Vergara & Bigsby, 2003). For the occupational therapist, developing a basic medical foundation is essential to the ability to address an infant's developmental needs safely. Appendix 20-B presents selected neonatal medical complications that are frequently encountered in the NICU. Therapists should also develop a working knowledge of maternal conditions associated with premature delivery and perinatal problems.

Table 20-1 lists medical equipment commonly used in the NICU. In addition to the life support equipment listed in the table, other devices help monitor the physiologic status of the ill newborn. For example, pulse oximetry is a noninvasive method of continually assessing blood oxygen saturation via a sensor wrapped around an infant's hand or foot. The cardiorespiratory monitor provides ongoing visual tracings and numeric correlates of heart and breathing rates, an auditory and/or visual alarm if these rates are not within a preset range, and the capability to analyze trends over time; additional functions, such as pulse oximetry and blood pressure measurement, are often included with cardiorespiratory monitors. Neonatal physiologic monitoring capabilities are continually increasing and improving with advances in medical knowledge and technology (Figure 20-2).

NICU ENVIRONMENT

"Mismatch" of Immature Infant and High-Tech Environment

The sensory components of the extrauterine environment in the NICU are different from those in the womb (Table 20-2). Barring complications, before birth the fetus is in a warm, snug, dark environment in which basic needs are automatically met and a normal sequence of development is supported. After birth, demands are suddenly made on the preterm newborn to breathe, regulate body temperature, move against the effects of gravity, adjust to bright light and unmuffled noise, and cope with invasive or painful procedures and frequent sleep deprivation. The preterm infant's immature central nervous system is generally competent for protected intrauterine life, but it is not sufficiently developed to adjust to and organize the overwhelming stimuli and demands of the NICU. This creates a "mismatch" between the neonate and the high-tech world in which he or she now needs to survive (Als, 1986).

Continual overwhelming stimuli created by the NICU environment and caregiving practices may stress the highly sensitive preterm infant's already vulnerable and disorganized central nervous system. Excessive sensory stimulation can cause insults to the developing brain (e.g., from repeated hypoxic episodes related to stress) and can create maladaptive behaviors that later contribute to a poor developmental outcome (Als et al., 1986; Black, 1998; DiPietro, 2000; Gressens, Rogido, Paindaveine, & Sola, 2002).

Because the sick preterm infant experiences significant stress (e.g., agitation, autonomic instability, excessive use of calories) when incoming stimuli exceed the ability of the immature CNS to respond and adapt, it becomes a priority to reduce avoidable stressors and to help the infant remain calm and organized (Blackburn, 2003). The neonatal therapist facilitates this goal by promoting NICU light and sound modifications, a reduction in handling, and alteration of caregiver techniques so that the infant is protected from stressful stimuli and allowed to remain quiet and inactive. These modifications facilitate recovery and an improved long-term neurodevelopmental outcome in very preterm infants (Als et al., 1994; Als, Buehler, Duffy, McAnulty, & Liederman, 1995; Byers, 2003; Fieisher et al., 1995; VandenBerg, 1995).

TABLE 20-1 Medical Equipment Commonly Found in the Neonatal Intensive Care Unit

Item	Description	Purpose
THERMOREGULATION EQUIPMENT		
Radiant warmer	Open bed with overhead heat source.	Typically used during medical workup of new admission or for critically ill infants requiring easy access for frequent or complicated medical care.
Incubator (Isolette)	Clear plastic, heated box that encloses the mattress and infant.	Used to provide warmth so that calories can be used for growth and healing; preferred location for infant if attempts are being made to reduce environmental stimuli, discourage unnecessary handling, and protect sleep. Infant may or may not be dressed, depending on specific NICU's protocol. Depending on design, access is though portholes or a door on the front, or the entire top of the Isolette flips open.
Open crib	Bassinet-style bed; no external heat source is provided; infant is dressed in clothes and swaddled in blankets.	Used for larger and more stable infants; caregivers (including occupational therapist) must be careful to avoid cold stress during baths, assessments, and procedures.
OXYGEN THERAPY WITH ASSISTED VENTILATION		
Bag and mask ventilation	Bag attached to face mask is rhythmically squeezed to deliver positive pressure and oxygen.	Used for resuscitation of an infant at delivery, during acute deterioration, or to increase oxygenation if necessary after apneic spell.
CPAP	Steady stream of pressurized air given through an endotracheal tube, nasopharyngeal tube, nasal prongs, or small nasal mask; supplemental oxygen may or may not be used.	Positive pressure is used to keep the alveoli and airways from collapsing (i.e., to keep them open) in an infant who is breathing spontaneously but has a disorder such as respiratory distress syndrome, pulmonary edema, or apnea.
Mechanical ventilation	Machine controls or assists breathing by mechanically inflating the lungs, increasing alveolar ventilation, and improving gas exchange.	Used for infants with depressed respiratory drive, pulmonary disease with increased work of breathing and suboptimal oxygenation and ventilation (i.e., MAS, RDS), and frequent apnea despite CPAP; infant is usually orally or nasally intubated but may have a tracheostomy if ventilator dependence will be prolonged.
ECMO	Sophisticated life support system that uses modified heart-lung bypass to provide nearly total lung rest and minimize barotrauma (lung damage that can occur with prolonged high ventilator settings).	Used as "rescue" technology for qualifying infants in critical respiratory failure who are unresponsive to conventional medical management, or at times for preoperative support during cardiac surgery. These infants meet medical criteria for a >80% mortality risk; survival rate with ECMO averages about 80%. Most (~75%) do well developmentally, although school-age sequelae may occur. Use of ECMO has decreased with advent of therapies such as high-frequency ventilation and nitric oxide (NO) inhalation (NO is a pulmonary vasodilator drug).
OXYGEN THERAPY WITHOUT ASSISTED VENTILATION		
Vapotherm	Respiratory therapy device attached to a nasal cannula that allows very high nasal flows of warmed and moist air or air/oxygen blends.	Used to improve gas exchange or reduce work of breathing. High flow rates may reduce the need for intubation and mechanical ventilation or may replace less well-tolerated nasal CPAP. Very high humidity (saturated without condensation) allows higher flow rates (compared to nasal cannula) without drying nasal mucosa.
Oxygen hood (oxyhood)	Plastic hood that provides a flow of warm, humidified oxygen; it is placed over infant's head.	Used for infants who are breathing independently but need a higher concentration of oxygen than 21% room air; higher humidification allows delivery of oxygen that is less drying to nasal mucosa than with a nasal cannula.
Nasal cannula (NC)	Humidified oxygen delivered by flexible NC with small prongs that fit into the nares.	Used for infants requiring supplemental oxygen without positive pressure support, generally for prolonged periods. NC offers easier handling and better portability than an oxyhood.

CPAP, Continuous positive airway pressure; *ECMO,* extracorporeal membrane oxygenation; *NICU,* neonatal intensive care unit; *MAS,* meconium aspiration syndrome; *RDS,* respiratory distress syndrome.

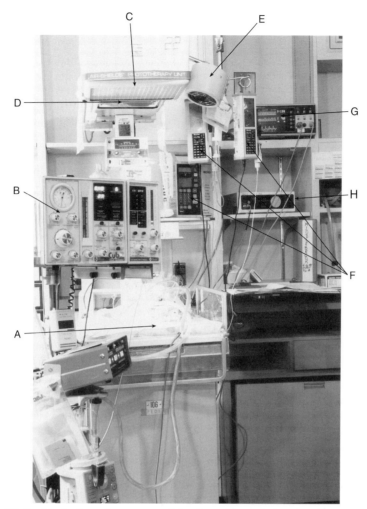

FIGURE 20-2 Medical equipment used in the NICU includes a radiant warmer (bed) **(A)**, mechanical ventilator **(B)**, phototherapy lights (may also be freestanding) **(C)**, radiant heat source **(D)**, procedure light **(E)**, infusion pumps for fluids and medications **(F)**, cardio-respiratory monitor **(G)**, and pulse oximeter **(H)**. (Courtesy Infant Special Care Unit, University of Texas Medical Branch, Galveston, Texas; photograph by John Glow.)

TABLE 20-2 Comparison of Intrauterine and Extrauterine Sensory Environments

System	Intrauterine	Extrauterine
Tactile	Constant proprioceptive input; smooth, wet, usually safe and comfortable; circumferential boundaries	Often painful and invasive; dry, cool air; predominance of medical touching with relative paucity of social touching
Vestibular	Maternal movements, diurnal cycles; amniotic fluid creates gently oscillating environment; flexed posture with boundaries to movements	Horizontal, flat postures; rapid position changes; influence of gravity, restraints, and equipment
Auditory	Maternal biologic sounds, muffled environmental sounds	Loud, noncontingent, mechanical, frequent (sometimes constant), harsh intermittent impulse noise
Visual	Dark; may occasionally have very dim red spectrum light	Bright lights, eyes unprotected; often no diurnal rhythm
Thermal	Constant warmth, consistent temperature	Environmental temperature variations, high risk of neonatal heat loss

Light in the NICU
Light and Vision

Determination of the appropriate lighting for an infant in the NICU is a complex issue that involves the physiologic impact of illumination, the ongoing development of the visual system in preterm infants, and the effects of lighting on the biologic circadian clock. NICU caregivers also have specific lighting needs for providing care and for personal biorhythms that may conflict with the lighting needs of fragile, underdeveloped infants.

Some have expressed concern about the exposure of inadequately shielded immature infants to frequent or continuous bright light from ceiling and procedure lights, phototherapy, heat lamps, and sunlight (Gardner & Goldson, 2002; Graven et al., 1992) (Figure 20-3). In contrast to the dark womb and compared with the standard adult office lighting level of 40 to 50 footcandles (fc), ambient lighting in the NICU has been measured at 30 to 150 fc, with peaks exceeding 1,500 fc if sunlight is present (Glass, 1993).

Continuous, intense, white fluorescent ambient light has been linked to chromosomal damage, disruption of diurnal biologic rhythms, changes in endocrine gland and gonadal function, and alteration of vitamin D synthesis in humans and other mammals (Wurtman, 1975). Increased light intensity has been shown to increase the heart and respiratory rates and decrease oxygen saturation for preterm infants in the NICU (Peng, Mao, Chen, & Chang, 2001). Overstimulation of the immature CNS, with resultant physiologic instability and subsequent potential effects on developmental outcome, has also been suggested (Gorski, Davidson, & Brazelton, 1979; VandenBerg, 1995).

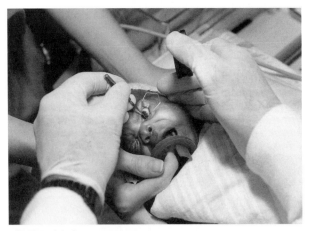

FIGURE 20-3 Ophthalmologist examines the eyes of an infant in the NICU for the development of retinopathy of prematurity. Swaddling and sucking on a pacifier dipped in 24% sucrose solution provide some relief for procedural discomfort. (Courtesy Infant Special Care Unit, University of Texas Medical Branch, Galveston, Texas; photograph by John Glow.)

Structural and functional immaturity suggests that the preterm infant is extremely vulnerable to light in the NICU. The growth of the eye in utero is genetically coded and needs no light; the infant's visual system continues to develop during the last trimester of gestation, with significant maturation and differentiation occurring in the retina and visual cortex (Gonzalez & Dweck, 1994; Graven, 2002). The eyelids remain fused until 24 to 26 weeks' gestation, with little spontaneous eye opening occurring until after 29 weeks, further indicating that the eyes of the preterm infant are not yet ready to process visual input at this stage of development. Preterm infants are unable to protect themselves from room light because they are unable to close their eyelids tightly until after 30 weeks, their thin eyelids do not filter light adequately, and the iris does not significantly constrict until 30 to 34 weeks (Fielder & Moseley, 2000).

Early light exposure has not been shown to increase the incidence of retinopathy of prematurity (ROP) (Reynolds et al., 1998). However, ambient NICU illumination may be implicated in subtle visual pathway sequelae and visual processing problems that cannot be attributed to other major complications of preterm birth such as ROP, strabismus, or myopia (Fielder & Moseley, 2000; Graven, 2002; Lickliter, 2000).

Light and Circadian Rhythm

Circadian rhythm regulates cyclic daily functions such as sleep, alertness, mood, temperature, and hormone levels. A fetus in utero is continuously receiving time-of-day signals from maternal cues such as hormone secretion, activity patterns, and feeding cycles. By at least the third trimester of pregnancy, the fetus has a functioning biologic clock (suprachiasmatic nuclei in the hypothalamus) capable of generating circadian rhythms in response to maternal day-night cues; these maternal circadian entrainment signals are disrupted when birth occurs prematurely (Mirmiran & Ariagno, 2000).

Light affects the infant's circadian system through a different neuronal pathway from that used for vision, and it becomes important in the regulation of circadian biorhythms after preterm birth. It has been suggested the circadian system of a preterm infant is responsive to light very early (perhaps by 25 to 28 weeks' gestation) and that low-intensity light can entrain the developing circadian clock (Graven, 2002; Rivkees & Hao, 2000). Cycled lighting, as opposed to near darkness, has been shown to improve weight gain in young preterm infants (Brandon, Holditch-Davis, & Belyea, 2002; Robison, 2003). Although the effects and specific timing of cycled lighting remain under investigation, support is increasing for controlled environments and cycled lighting in the NICU (Lynam, 2003; Mirmiran & Ariagno, 2000).

Environmental Modifications of Light in the NICU

Guidelines for appropriate lighting levels in the NICU continue to be updated; the current trends are for lower levels of general illumination and for the introduction of cycled lighting (White et al., 2003). NICU lighting levels should be very dim for at least part of the day for some babies, whereas moderate lighting might be better for staff caregiving and to facilitate the development of a diurnal cycle (Mirmiran & Ariagno, 2000; White et al.). Significant flexibility in lighting levels is required to accommodate both caregiver needs and the variable needs of babies at differing stages of development and at various times throughout the day; ambient lighting in the NICU should be adjustable through a range of at least 1 to 60 fc (White et al.).

Light in the NICU can be controlled by a general lowering of ambient room light and by shading external windows and shielding an infant's bed space. In older NICUs, rheostats, track lighting, or removing one light tube from each bank of fluorescent lights can help control room brightness without compromising visibility (Figure 20-4). Individual bedside lighting, indirect and deflected lighting, and the use of natural light from windows or skylights are options in NICUs being built or remodeled.

The eyes of a preterm infant should always be protected from bright and direct light. Shielding from ambient room light and direct procedure lights can be achieved at each infant's bedside by draping the infant's eyes with a cloth or phototherapy eye mask (Figure 20-5) and by using a light-blocking Isolette cover (Figure 20-6). Shielding does not mean occluding the eyes; no evidence supports the use of patching beyond what is necessary for phototherapy (Glass, 2002).

Because infants sleep at least 80% of the time, it has been recommended that lighting at the immediate bedside be controlled to 10 fc or lower at night and 25 to 30 fc during the day to promote sleep (White, 1999). Infants 32 weeks or older need some light for retinal stimulation, but not light so bright it wakes them up; light in the 30 to 40 fc range for intermittent periods has been suggested for these infants (White, 1999). The ability to attend visually emerges at 32 to 34 weeks PCA and is enhanced in low lighting. Providing opportunities for spontaneous eye opening in dim or dark conditions may be advantageous after this age (Glass, 1993, 1999). Infants at term gestation and beyond need light and visual stimulation for appropriate visual development and state regulation.

Lighting of 25 fc that is free of glare and shadows is adequate for staff charting. Caregiver assessment of the infant requires light between 50 and 100 fc. Lighting of 100 to 200 fc may be necessary for tasks that require visual acuity, such as insertion of an IV line. A procedure light can be focused narrowly on the task area rather than allowed to encompass the infant. The infant's eyes should be shielded during the procedure, and bright lights should be turned off after the task has been

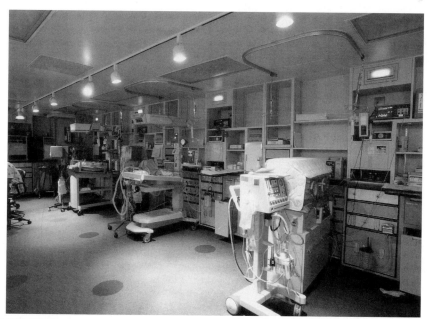

FIGURE 20-4 Overview of an older NICU shows an incubator and a mechanical ventilator in the foreground and radiant warmers in the background. Track lighting allows the option of turning off overhead ceiling lights to reduce room light levels. (Courtesy Infant Special Care Unit, University of Texas Medical Branch, Galveston, TX; photograph by John Glow.)

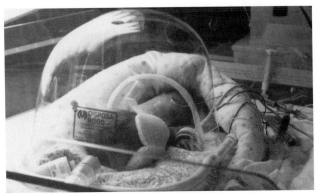

FIGURE 20-5 Preterm infant wears protective eye shields during phototherapy for the treatment of jaundice. Oxygen hood is large enough to encompass the upper body and allow hand-to-face (or hand-to-mouth) movement for self-calming. Snuggle-Up provides boundaries for foot bracing but is left open to allow maximum skin exposure to bili lights. (Courtesy Infant Special Care Unit, University of Texas Medical Branch, Galveston, Texas; photograph by Al Romeo.)

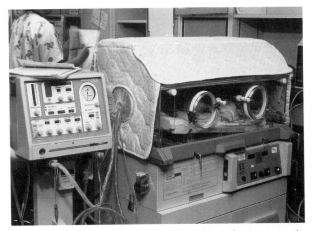

FIGURE 20-6 Isolette cover provides infant protection from room light without eliminating visibility of the infant by neonatal intensive care unit staff. Some NICUs totally cover the Isolette for maximum protection from light. (Courtesy Infant Special Care Unit, University of Texas Medical Branch, Galveston, Texas; photograph by John Glow.)

completed. Periodic "light showers" (e.g., two or three 15-minute breaks in a brightly lit room of 200 to 500 fc) can reset body clocks, restore alertness, and allow efficient functioning for staff members who become drowsy in a dim NICU (Bullough & Rea, 1996).

Sound in the NICU

Noise is undesirable sound (American Academy of Pediatrics, [AAP] 1997); environmental noise can stress NICU infants and cause significant changes in their behavioral and physiologic states. The hearing threshold

has been reported to be 40 decibels (dB) at 28 to 34 weeks' gestation, 30 dB at 35 to 38 weeks' gestation, and less than 20 dB at term; these thresholds are greatly exceeded in the NICU (AAP), 1997; Lary, Briassoulis, de Vries, Dubowitz, & Dubowitz, 1985). NICU baseline sound levels of 50 to 90 dB (comparable with street traffic and light machinery, respectively), with peaks of 90 to 120 dB (comparable with heavy machinery), have been documented (AAP; Robertson, Cooper-Peel, & Vos, 1998). Sound levels of 50 to 55 dB are considered moderately annoying by adults (Vergara & Bigsby, 2003), and the federal Occupational Safety and Health Administration (OSHA) has imposed an industrial standard limit of 90 dB for 8 hours as the highest safe level for adult workers (AAP).

In a typical NICU, environmental noise is constant throughout the day and night, mechanical versus social, and noncontingent to individual infants. Sound inside the Isolette is characterized by continuous white noise and nonspeech sounds; harsh, mechanical noises penetrate clearly and reverberate, whereas speech sounds are indistinct (Berens & Weigle, 1997). Newer incubators attenuate sound better than older models (Robertson, Cooper-Peel, & Vos, 1999).

Noise can be highly arousing for preterm and ill infants in the NICU. The resultant agitation and crying can decrease oxygenation and increase vasoconstriction, blood pressure, intracranial pressure, and the heart and respiratory rates; apnea and bradycardia may also occur (Gardner & Goldson, 2002; Morris, Philbin, & Bose, 2000). Noise may disrupt sleep and may adversely affect the newborn's recovery and growth (DePaul & Chambers, 1995; Philbin, 2000). Loud or prolonged sounds may contribute to hearing loss, affecting the frequency range that corresponds to the frequency of the damaging sound; preterm infants are at risk for hearing loss in both low-frequency (speech) and high-frequency ranges (Thomas, 1989).

Critical development of the human auditory system occurs in the third trimester; sensory interference may occur when immature sensory systems are stimulated out of order or bombarded with inappropriate stimuli. Animal studies support a connection between atypical patterns of early sensory experience (e.g., chaotic environmental noise, or excessive light exposure prior to term gestation when auditory system development should be occurring without competition) and disruption of early perceptual and behavioral development (Lickliter, 2000).

Long-term difficulties in auditory processing can occur with normal intelligence and hearing sensitivity; behaviors associated with disturbed auditory processing have been noted in NICU graduates (Graven, 2000). Auditory processing problems may be manifested by poor listening skills ("Huh?" "What?"), difficulty following multistep directions, poor discrimination of specific auditory signals amid other background or impulse noise, distractibility, short attention span, or poor reading and spelling skills (Chermak, Somers, & Seikel, 1998; Jerger & Musiek, 2000).

Environmental Modifications of Sound in the NICU

Although definitive safety standards for sound exposure have not been established for infants, recommendations have been made for maintenance of a general sound level in the NICU of 45 to 50 dB, with 55 dB allowed 10% of the time and transient peaks not to exceed 70 dB (AAP, 1997; Philbin, Robertson, & Hall, 1999; White et al., 2003). Measuring sound levels in the NICU with a sound dosimeter can be helpful for identifying noise sources and problems, especially when the measurements are taken at different times throughout 24-hour days, with varying caregivers, and during different levels of activity and patient acuity (Gray & Philbin, 2000; Robertson, Cooper-Peel, & Vos, 1998).

Theoretically, sound in the NICU should be easy to reduce. However, because most peak noise is related to human activity (Chang, Lin, & Lin, 2001), change can be surprisingly difficult. Staff education, unit policies, peer pressure, and patience may be helpful; sometimes just dimming the lights has a calming effect and reduces noise.

Because efforts at changing behavior have not been fully successful in reducing NICU noise, inclusion of physical noise-abatement alterations has been recommended (Philbin, 2000; Philbin & Gray, 2002). Bacteriostatic carpeting, acoustic ceiling tiles, soundproof or sound-absorbing building materials, central vacuum systems, and "pods" that divide space for use by individual or a small number of infants can be considered in remodeling and new unit design. Radios are often against NICU policy, although enforcement varies. Pagers should be switched to "vibrate" upon entry into the NICU. Parents and staff members can view instructional videos away from patient areas. Telephones that flash instead of ring, personal message pagers or cordless phones that allow nurses to communicate without having to call across or between rooms, visual alarms, and quieter equipment (e.g., ventilators, incubators) are emerging as additional options for modifying noise.

Bed spaces for extremely ill or sensitive infants should be located away from sinks, ice machines, telephones, high-traffic areas, and vocal infants. Staff members can reduce the volume of auditory alarms and can silence all alarms quickly to reduce infant exposure to piercing impulse noise; remote control devices to silence some alarms are available. Respiratory tubing and water traps can be positioned to promote drainage; accumulated water can be emptied frequently to prevent bubbling (60 to 70 dB).

Isolette covers can significantly reduce the noise level in an incubator (Saunders, 1995). Staff members should avoid tapping on the Isolette (80 dB), abruptly closing incubator doors or portholes (90 to 100 dB), or using the incubator top as a work surface or storage area (AAP, 1997; VandenBerg, 1995). Conversations, including medical rounds, should be held away from the bedside. Plastic trash cans are quietest, and trash can lids can be padded if necessary. Musical toys and tape recordings can reverberate inside the Isolette; extreme caution and very low volume are recommended (DePaul & Chambers, 1995).

Some have suggested implementation of a quiet hour and the use of earmuffs to reduce noise in the NICU (Strauch, Brandt, & Edwards-Beckett, 1993; Zahr & de Traversay, 1995). However, if staff members believe that such modifications are sufficient, less active effort may be made to reduce personal and environmental noise; a better option would be to keep noise in the NICU to a minimum at all times.

Caregiving in the NICU

NICU caregiving patterns differ significantly from the fetal intrauterine environment and the normal home setting (Gressens, Rogido, Paindaveine, & Sola, 2002). The sense of touch is highly developed in utero, and gentle human touch normally provides consistent, positive tactile input after term birth; touch in the NICU, however, usually is related to medical care rather than social nurturing (Lynam, 2003). NICU interventions often are intrusive or painful and typically occur constantly throughout a 24-hour span.

Examples of medical touch include physical examinations, drawing of blood, application or removal of tape, measurements (temperature, blood pressure, weight, and circumference of head or abdomen), repositioning, IV insertion, gavage feedings, transfusions, injections, bag and mask ventilation, intubation, tube adjustments, chest percussion, and suctioning. Caregiving procedures have been related to increased heart rate, fluctuations in blood pressure, alterations in cerebral blood flow, and hypoxemia (Lindh, Wiklund, Snadman, & Hakansson, 1997; Long, Alistar, Phillip, & Lucey, 1980; Porter, Wolf, & Miller, 1998).

Preterm infants are extremely vulnerable to pain. Diminished ability to attenuate pain may allow even relatively benign procedures to be perceived as painful, especially if they occur just after handling or another painful experience (Porter, Wolf, & Miller, 1998). Immediate consequences of severe or repetitive painful experiences in the NICU may include physiologic instability, medical complications, sleep disturbances, feeding problems, and poor self-regulation; long-term changes, such as a decreased pain threshold and hypersensitivity to pain, may also occur (Grunau, 2002; Mitchell & Boss,

2002). Repetitive or prolonged pain has been implicated in increased neuronal cell death in the immature brain, which creates concerns for future neurodevelopmental outcome (Bhutta & Anand, 2002).

Caregiving based primarily on external criteria, such as fixed schedules for measurement of vital signs and for feeding, often ignores or delays the caregiver's response to the infant's cues that he or she needs care; caregiving thus becomes noncontingent to the infant's efforts to communicate. Eventually this may discourage the infant's efforts to communicate needs, may lead to emotional detachment from the sensation of needs, and possibly may contribute to the development of distrust (Gardner & Goldson, 2002).

Sleep deprivation of NICU infants has also been recognized. Studies in the 1970s revealed that NICU infants were disturbed 80 to 132 times per day (Gottfried, 1985; Korones, 1976); more recent evidence suggests that few modifications have been made in NICU handling patterns, frequency, and trends (Peters, 1999). Because secretion of human growth hormone is associated with regular recurrence of sleep-wake cycles and peaks during active sleep (rapid eye movement [REM] sleep), sleep deprivation in the NICU may interfere with optimal infant growth and development (Gardner & Goldson, 2002).

Modifications of Caregiving in the NICU

Developmentally supportive caregiving in the NICU strives to minimize avoidable stressors, facilitate infant medical and neurobehavioral stability, protect sleep, promote self-regulation, foster normal developmental sequences, and encourage family participation. Although the general trend is toward developmental care in the NICU (Byers, 2003), implementation remains inconsistent while evidence-based caregiving strategies continue to emerge.

The individual infant (rather than the nursery routines) should determine the timing and sequencing of caregiving. For example, does the infant tolerate and benefit from caregiving procedures that are clustered together (allowing longer undisturbed periods for rest and sleep), or should caregiving procedures be interspersed because of low stress tolerance and prolonged recovery times? Two caregivers may be needed for some procedures, with one adult performing the task while the other adult (staff member or parent) supports the infant (Figure 20-7).

Procedures and interventions for each infant should be based on necessity rather than habits, and unnecessary handling and movement should be avoided. For example, must weights and baths be done daily? Can some vital signs be taken from monitors? Can suctioning be performed on an as-needed basis? Does the infant really need an occupational therapy evaluation requiring

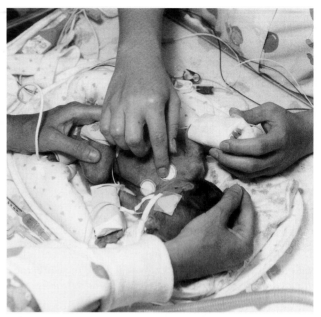

FIGURE 20-7 Having a second person provide containment helps minimize stress in this preterm infant during a caregiving procedure. (Courtesy Infant Special Care Unit, University of Texas Medical Branch, Galveston, Texas; photograph by John Glow.)

handling now? Those who handle the infant should prepare him or her for touch or movement by speaking softly first and containing the infant's extremities during movement and lifting. Table 20-3 summarizes considerations for caregiving related to the infant's state of arousal.

Bath time frequently is stressful and exhausting to NICU infants (Peters, 1996, 1998). Bathing by immersion in warm water usually is more soothing than sponge bathing if the infant's body is well supported with the extremities contained; "swaddled" bathing has proved successful even with irritable and disorganized infants. The swaddled infant is immersed to the shoulders in a tub of warm water, and the face is washed first with clean water. Next, one body section is unwrapped for bathing and rinsing and then is rewrapped in the wet cloth before another section of the body is washed (e.g., right upper body, then left upper body, then legs and buttocks) (Fern, Graves, & L'Huillier, 2002). The warmth and proprioceptive weight of a wet blanket seem calming, and infants usually are quiet and alert throughout this bath, making swaddled bathing a successful and enjoyable caregiving experience for parents (Figure 20-8).

Even social touch and noninvasive caregiving procedures can disturb and stress vulnerable infants, requiring caregiver efforts to console and facilitate infant recovery. Examples of supportive measures include comfortable bedding, containment (e.g., using a Snuggle-Up, blanket swaddling, or the hands of the parent or second caregiver) (Figure 20-9), parental skin-to-skin holding

TABLE 20-3 Newborn States and Considerations for Caregiving

Newborn State	Comments
SLEEP STATES	
Deep sleep (non–rapid eye movement [NREM])	Infant is very difficult if not impossible to arouse. Infant will not breast-feed or bottle-feed in this state even after vigorous stimulation. Infant is unable to respond to environment; frustrating for caregivers.
Slow state changes	Term infants may exhibit a "slow" heart rate (80 to 90 beats per minute), which may
Regular breathing	trigger heart rate alarms and result in unnecessary stimulation by NICU staff.
Eyes closed; no eye movements	
No spontaneous activity except startles and jerky movements	At birth, preterm infants have altered states of consciousness. Early dominant states are light sleep, quiet, and active alert. *Protective apathy* enables the preterm to remain
Startles with some delay and suppresses rapidly	inactive, unresponsive, and in a sleep state to conserve energy, grow, and maintain physiologic homeostasis.
Lowest oxygen consumption	
Light sleep (rapid eye movement [REM] sleep)	Full-term infants begin and end sleep in active sleep; preterm infants are more responsive (than term infants) to stimuli in active sleep.
Low activity level	Infants may cry or fuss briefly in this state and be awakened to feed before they are
Random movements and startles	truly awake and ready to eat.
Respirations irregular and abdominal	
Intermittent sucking movements	
Eyes closed; rapid eye movement	
Higher oxygen consumption	Oxygenation states are lower and more variable.
AWAKE STATES	
Drowsy or semidozing	Infant may awaken further or return to sleep if left alone.
Eyelids fluttering	Quietly talking and looking at the infant or offering a pacifier or an inanimate object
Eyes open or closed (dazed)	to see and listen to may arouse the infant to the quiet alert state.
Mild startles (intermittent)	Less mature infants (30 weeks) demonstrate a more drowsy than quiet alert state than
Delayed response to sensory stimuli	older infants (36 weeks).
Smooth state change after stimulation	
Fussing may or may not be present	
Respirations more rapid and shallow	
Quiet alert, with bright look	Immediately after birth, term newborns exhibit a period of quiet alertness, their first
Focuses attention on source of stimulation	opportunity to "take in" their parents and the extrauterine environment. Dimmed lights, quiet talking, and stroking optimize this time for parents.
Impinging stimuli may break through; may have some delay in response	This is the best state for learning to occur, because infant focuses all of attention on visual, auditory, tactile, and sucking stimuli; best state for interaction with parents,
Minimal motor activity	because baby is maximally able to attend and reciprocally respond to parents.
Active alert—eyes open	Infant has decreased threshold (increased sensitivity) to internal (hunger, fatigue) and
Considerable motor activity—thrusting movements of extremities; spontaneous startles	external (wet, noise, handling) stimuli. Infant may quiet self, may escalate to crying, or, with consolation from caretaker, may become quiet, alert, or go to sleep.
Reactions to external stimuli with increase in movements and startles (discrete reactions are difficult to differentiate because of generally higher activity level)	Infant is unable to maximally attend to caretakers or environment because of increased motor activity and increased sensitivity to stimuli.
Respirations irregular	
May or may not be fussy	
Crying—intense and difficult to disrupt with external stimuli	Crying is infant's response to unpleasant internal and/or external stimulation (i.e., infant's tolerance limits have been reached and exceeded). Infant may be able to
Respirations rapid, shallow, and irregular	quiet self with hand-to-mouth behaviors; talking may quiet a crying infant; holding, rocking, or putting infant upright on caretaker's shoulder may quiet infant.

From Gardner, S.L., & Goldson, E. (2002). The neonate and the environment: Impact on development. In G.B. Merenstein & S.L. Garner (Eds.), *Handbook of neonatal intensive care* (5th ed., p. 225). St. Louis: Mosby.

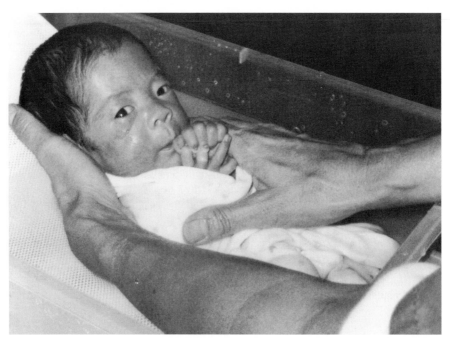

FIGURE 20-8 Swaddled preterm infant is immersed in a tub of warm water for a developmentally supportive bath. (Courtesy NICU, Medical Center of Plano, Plano, Texas; photograph by Dana Fern.)

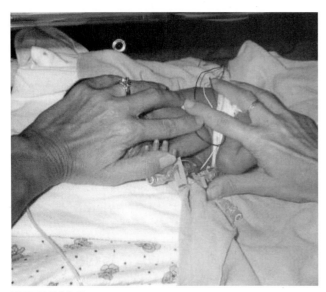

FIGURE 20-9 Facilitative tuck (gentle but firm hand swaddling) is calming to a stressed or disorganized preterm infant. This type of touch is well tolerated, in contrast to highly stimulating stroking. (Courtesy NICU, Medical Center of Plano, Plano, Texas; photograph by Vicky Leland.)

(kangaroo care), and reduction of environmental light and sound. Nonnutritive sucking often is successful for soothing and self-regulation; a pacifier dipped in a 24% sucrose solution can be used to help manage "minor" procedural pain (Benis, 2002; Gibbins et al., 2002).

FAMILIES IN THE NICU

Families in Crisis

Admission of an infant to the NICU frequently puts the family in crisis, facing an intense onslaught of confusing emotions (Siegel, Gardner, & Merenstein, 2002; Spear, Leef, Epps, & Locke, 2002). The delivery often was unexpected, and the family unit now is separated. The appearance of the infant can be frightening and the NICU environment overwhelming. Unknown staff members and unfamiliar terminology can hinder effective communication. Some mothers have continued physical complications or illness from the pregnancy or delivery. Financial considerations, transportation or travel issues, and conflicting needs of siblings can be worrisome. Parental shock, denial, and grief over loss of the ideal birth and perfect infant are compounded by concerns for the recovery of a critically ill infant; maternal depression increases stress and hinders coping (Hummel, 2002; Spear et al., 2002).

NICU vision statements, staff hiring and appraisal practices, caregiving guidelines, and new unit design increasingly reflect the growing emphasis on family-centered care (Moore, Coker, DuBuisson, Swett, & Edwards, 2003; Van Riper, 2001; White, 2003). Progression from the philosophic mental image of full family support and inclusion to actual consistent implementation is a challenging process that requires a change to unit culture, including staff beliefs and practices. Unit-based developmental specialists can promote this change from traditional provider-centered, task-directed care to holistic, individualized, relationship-based, family-centered care (Ballweg, 2001).

The many facets of understanding and working with families who have an ill or special needs child are discussed in depth in Chapter 5. Parental responsibilities (occupations) have been described as those of provider, protector, caregiver, educator, and facilitator of the child's development (Vergara & Bigsby, 2003). Many areas of normal parental control, however, are relinquished to medical staff members because the new mother and father are unprepared for and uncertain about parenting an infant in the NICU. Policies that prohibit access to the infant (e.g., restricted visiting hours or denial of entry during medical rounds or shift change) or that limit the presence of supportive family members or friends can further limit and isolate parents (Siegel et al., 2002). Conversely, family coping, satisfaction, confidence and competence can be facilitated through positive relationships with NICU staff members who openly communicate and consistently include parents in decision making and caregiving throughout the infant's hospitalization (VandenBerg, 2000; Van Riper, 2001).

Communication and Collaboration

Medical care and concerns, the complexity of high-tech NICU environments, and the neurobehavioral immaturity of preterm infants undermine the role of families in the NICU (Gale & Franck, 1998; Shields-Poe & Pinelli, 1997). Parents can be encouraged to ask questions about what they understand and want to know; staff responses need to be honest, consistent, and understandable. Parents are often frustrated when information appears to be contradictory; much of their anxiety stems from incomplete information or a perceived lack of truth. Printed resources (Albritton et al., 1998; Fern & Graves, 1996; Madden, 2000; Smith, 1999; Zaichkin, 2002) can be made available for parents in a waiting room, in a parents' library, or for individual checkout. Some NICUs have computers available with parent education and support resources or Internet access. Parent groups can also be helpful in providing information, comfort, and support.

When parents make requests that are unusual or that differ from the preferences of the NICU staff, the NICU caregiver needs to remember that parents have emotional and legal rights to make decisions on behalf of their infant. Baker (1995) suggested a four-question approach to handling conflicts that allows both parents and staff members to feel respected:

1 What is the staff's goal?
2 What is the parent's goal?
3 Will the parent's request harm the infant?
4 What options are available to meet both goals?

In most cases the parent's choice will achieve the same outcome, and staff members can maintain their standards for safe, effective, quality care. Family cultural, religious, and other beliefs often can be respected and accommodated with this approach.

Family Inclusion in Developmental Support

Nonjudgmental support adapted to parental coping mechanisms, learning styles, personalities, and cultural background is challenging but essential. For neonatal occupational therapists, the shift in the NICU is away from "therapist as expert, child as client, parents as students" to family-centered mutual collaboration. Developmental support services with families in the NICU are based on relationship; the therapist talks *with* rather than *to* the parents and facilitates the family's active role with their infant and on the NICU team. The father, as well as the mother, should be encouraged to participate in discussions and caregiving.

Therapists can support collaboration with families by creating frequent opportunities for two-way dialog, such as seeking and valuing parents' opinions and insights in addition to sharing their own, being sensitive to possible hidden messages in parent-professional communications, addressing parent concerns, planning joint infant observations and interventions, avoiding judgments, and acknowledging that the parent has the infant's best interests at heart (Holloway, 1994). Recognizing parental skills, celebrating successes, and facilitating parents' expertise can be invaluable, as illustrated by one parent's comment, "Seeing others follow through on our suggestions . . . bolstered our confidence in our parenting skills, knowledge of our baby, and ability to develop a closeness with him" (Holloway, 1994).

Some family-friendly changes in NICU routines and practices automatically facilitate parenting. Placing twins next to each other (or co-bedding them, with both twins in the same Isolette or crib) rather than in separate parts of the nursery helps create a family space. Staff efforts to make the infant as comfortable and as "normal" looking as possible (e.g., positional nesting, using baby clothes, adding a hair bow, providing a cute name tag) help parents look beyond the diagnosis and technology. Diligence in using the infant's name and correct gender demonstrate to families that NICU staff members acknowledge their baby as a real person, not just a sick premie (Maroney, 1994). Feeding schedules and other types of caregiving can be arranged to accommodate parents' schedules as much as possible. The inclusion of siblings, extended family members, and other support persons should be encouraged during the infant's NICU stay.

A behavioral and developmental assessment of an infant by the neonatal therapist can be educational for the parents (Figure 20-10). The therapist also assesses and nurtures parents' understanding and skill in recognizing and responding appropriately to their infant's cues of stress or stability, providing therapeutic positioning and developmentally supportive handling (e.g.,

containing extremities in flexion, cupping the infant's head and lower body in the parent's palms in a "hand swaddle" or "facilitative tuck," letting the infant hold onto the parent's finger), regulating sensory input to avoid overstimulation, facilitating functional oral feeding, and meeting the infant's long-term developmental needs.

If parents cannot come frequently to the NICU, the therapist can make or encourage regular phone calls, send photographs (printed or digital) or notes sharing significant events or behaviors, or keep a bedside journal in which staff members can record observations or note progress for parents to read when they arrive (Costello, Bracht, Van Camp, & Carman, 1996). Working a non-traditional schedule that includes some evenings, weekends, and holidays greatly increases a therapist's availability and benefit to families. Promoting parent-infant attachment and helping the family grow in their ability to know, love, and respond to their infant as a unique person yield greater benefits than any other intervention by the NICU therapist.

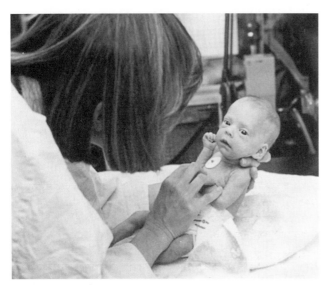

FIGURE 20-10 Assessment of this stable preterm infant includes evaluation of neuromotor and neurobehavioral functioning. Assessment can be a valuable teaching tool when performed jointly with the infant's parents. (Courtesy Neonatal Intensive Care Unit, John N. Dempsey Hospital, University of Connecticut Health Center, Farmington, Connecticut; photograph by Gregory Kriss.)

Skin-to-Skin Holding (Kangaroo Care)

Kangaroo care refers to the practice of parents holding their diaper-clad, premature infant beneath their clothing, chest-to-chest and skin-to-skin (Figure 20-11). Kangaroo care originated in Bogota, Colombia, as a response to overcrowded nurseries and insufficient medical equipment; the practice spread throughout Western Europe

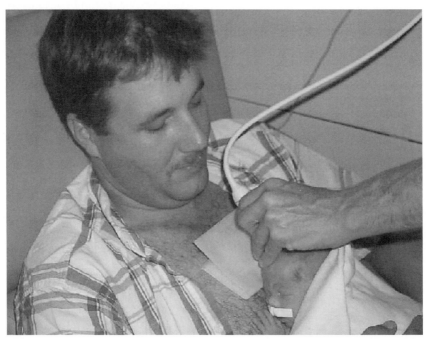

FIGURE 20-11 Father using skin-to-skin holding technique (kangaroo care) while preterm infant undergoes a head ultrasound examination to rule out intraventricular hemorrhage. (Courtesy Infant Special Care Unit, University of Texas Medical Branch, Galveston, Texas; photograph by Jan Hunter.)

and has gained increased acceptance in the United States. The initiation, frequency, and duration of kangaroo care varies among individual NICUs according to the age, weight, and acuity of the NICU infant; skin-to-skin holding is more widely accepted for stable infants not on ventilators but is also implemented with younger and sicker infants (Byers, 2003; Engler et al., 2002; Franck, Bernal, & Gale, 2002).

Although continued caution is urged because of the poor methodology of some studies and conflicting findings of others (Bohnhorst, Heyne, Peter, & Poets, 2001; Conde-Agudelo, Diaz-Rossello, & Belizan, 2003; Smith, 2001), multiple benefits to both infant and parents from kangaroo care have been reported.* Reported infant benefits of skin-to-skin holding include more stable heart and breathing rates, reduced apnea, stable body temperature, decreased agitation and random motor activity, less distress from environmental disturbances and medical interventions, improved state control, maturation of the circadian system, improved growth, decreased or less severe infections, easier transition to breast feeding, earlier hospital discharge, and a positive effect on neurodevelopmental outcome. Benefits to the parents include facilitation of maternal milk production and longer duration of breast feeding, increased awareness of their infant's cues of well-being or distress, increased parental attachment and feelings of closeness to their infant, more positive touch of the infant, less focus on technical care, more confidence in their own caregiving ability, and decreased maternal stress.

Discharge Planning

Discharge planning begins on the day of admission. Facilitation of the infant's behavioral stability, sleep-wake cycle organization, and self-regulation capacities by consistent environmental modifications and sensitive caregiving eases the transition to home for the infant and family. Inclusion and support of parents in active caregiving roles throughout the infant's hospitalization are essential. The American Academy of Pediatrics (1998) has proposed detailed guidelines for hospital discharge of high-risk newborns (e.g., preterm infant, infant requiring technologic support, infant at risk primarily from family issues, infant whose irreversible condition will result in an early death).

After downsizing closed some patient care areas, one innovative hospital allowed NICU parents to stay in unoccupied rooms and thus be readily available to help care for their infant; nighttime breast feeding was a common occurrence in their NICU. Many hospitals provide accommodations for parents to stay with their infant overnight in a NICU parent room before discharge.

Parents should be familiar with their infant's specific developmental strengths and needs (VandenBerg, 1999). The therapist can provide information about community resources and parent support groups. If indicated, the infant should be referred to a local early childhood intervention program, but this is not routinely necessary for every NICU graduate. Arranging for parents to meet community resource personnel before their infant is discharged from the hospital, as well as a follow-up telephone call from an NICU staff member after discharge, can help reduce parental "separation anxiety" from the NICU.

It is highly recommended that neonatal therapists actively participate in NICU follow-up clinics. Besides allowing reinforcement and continuation of developmental teaching, preventing some infants from "falling through the cracks," and continuing relationships with NICU families, the therapist gains valuable knowledge from countless opportunities to observe infant outcomes from various diagnoses and clinical courses. Many infants do surprisingly well after a long NICU stay, whereas others develop unanticipated problems. This information helps the therapist appreciate the unpredictable nature of NICU infant development and understand the variables that contribute to developmental outcomes.

INFANTS IN THE NICU

Evaluation of the NICU Infant

The golden rule of occupational therapy evaluation and intervention with the NICU infant is, "Above all, do no harm!" Safety for the infant takes priority over convenience for the therapist in all aspects of care. The following suggestions can help ensure infant protection:

1 Before administering any hands-on items, learn a new evaluation tool thoroughly (e.g., read and reread the manual, observe an experienced colleague evaluate appropriate infants of varying ages and medical status, practice on a doll and then on healthy term infants). Many therapists use a structured assessment that is supplemented with data gathering and clinical observations relevant to occupational therapy. Administration of some structured neonatal assessments requires the therapist to have specialized training; others may be used after independent study of the manual (Table 20-4 and Box 20-1).

2 Gather baseline information before performing the evaluation. This can include demographics, relevant family history (e.g., socioeconomic and cultural factors, support systems), maternal prenatal history, birth history, subsequent medical history and current

---

* Aucott, Donohue, Atkins, & Atten, 2002; Charpak, Ruiz-Pelaez, de Figueroa, & Charpak, 2001; Feldman & Eidelman, 2003; Feldman, Eidelman, Sirota, & Weller, 2002; Gardner & Goldson, 2002; Luddington-Hoe, Thompson, Swinth, Hadeed, & Anderson et al., 1994; Ohgi, Fukuda, & Moriuchi, et al., 2002.

TABLE 20-4   Neonatal Assessments Requiring Certification for Administration*

Assessment	Contact
NATURALISTIC OBSERVATIONS OF NEWBORN BEHAVIOR (NONB) (NIDCAP LEVEL I)	Heidelise Als, PhD
Based on Als' Synactive Theory of Development.	Children's Hospital
For preterm and term infants too fragile for handling.	300 Longwood Ave.
Structured observations of specific behaviors are repeated at 2-minute intervals before, during, and after routine caregiving.	Boston, MA 02115
Assessment of the maturation and interplay of infant neurobehavioral subsystems (autonomic, motor, state, attention and interaction, and self-regulation), as evidenced by behavioral cues to environmental and caregiving events over time. Signs of stress and stability can be cataloged as avoidance or approach behaviors, and attempts at self-organization (including failure, success, and cost of the effort) are noted. The degree of caregiver facilitation required to promote infant neurobehavioral organization may be observed if developmentally supportive care is being provided.	
ASSESSMENT OF PRETERM INFANT BEHAVIOR (APIB) (NIDCAP LEVEL II)	Heidelise Als, PhD
Based on Als' Synactive Theory of Development.	Children's Hospital
For stable preterm (>30 to 32 weeks) and term infants.	300 Longwood Ave
Complex assessment that provides an integrated subsystem profile of the infant, identifying current level of functioning with varying environmental demands. The therapist handles the infant in a structured progression of test items to assess neurobehavioral organization and methods of attaining self-regulation, as well as the type and amount of caregiver support needed for the infant to achieve and maintain organized behavior.	Boston, MA 02115
Used more as a research tool than for everyday clinical purposes.	
NEONATAL BEHAVIORAL ASSESSMENT SCALE (NBAS)	The Brazelton Institute
For term healthy infants (used in 36- to 44-week range).	1295 Boylston St., Suite 320
Evaluates infant neurobehavioral capabilities in the context of a dynamic relationship with the caregiver. Supplemental items can be used with high-risk infants.	Boston, MA 02215
Four stages to certification include self-study phase, skill test phase, practice phase, and certification session.	
Certification is valid for 3 years.	
Provided the model for the Assessment of Preterm Infant Behavior.	
Used more as a research tool than for everyday clinical purposes.	
NICU NETWORK NEUROBEHAVIORAL SCALE (NNNS)	Infant Development Center
Assesses neurologic integrity and behavioral function of healthy term, stable preterm, or at-risk infants (e.g., prenatal drug exposure).	Women & Infants' Hospital of Rhode Island
Provides a separate scale for signs of stress and withdrawal in the at-risk drug-exposed infant.	101 Dudley St.
Used primarily for infants in the 34- to 45-week range.	Providence, RI 02905
	www.infantdevelopment.org
INFANT BEHAVIORAL ASSESSMENT (IBA)	Rodd Hedlund, MEd
Used from birth to 6 months of age; can be used for follow-up.	Washington Research Institute
Evaluates infants within the synactive theory framework to sensitize parents or caregivers to the infant's behavioral states and organizational abilities, so that caregiver interactions can be modified accordingly	150 Nickerson St., Suite 305
	Seattle, WA 98104

*Each certification process requires formal training and assessment of rater reliability.
NIDCAP, Neonatal Individualized Developmental Care and Assessment Program.

status of the infant (including medical equipment in use, feeding method and schedule, current medications, and level of physiologic homeostasis).

3 Appreciate the nurse's role in protecting the infant and obtain clearance for evaluation if the infant will be handled.

4 Use astute clinical observations of the infant and surrounding environment before any touching. Very fragile infants can be assessed entirely by skilled observations (Als, 1986).

5 Weigh the value of any hands-on evaluation procedures against potential stressful effects on the infant: what is truly necessary and important? Avoid evaluation items done simply to fill in the blanks on an evaluation form. Co-assessments with other disciplines may reduce unnecessary duplication of items that require handling.

6 Time evaluations according to the infant's sleep cycle, feeding schedule, caregiving routine, and medical status. Respect the infant's signs of stress during

BOX 20-1   Structured Neonatal Assessments That Do Not Require Certification for Administration

NEUROLOGIC ASSESSMENT OF THE PRETERM AND FULL-TERM NEWBORN INFANT (NAPFI)
Description
- For preterm and term infants who can tolerate handling.
- Administered per instruction manual; can give partial or total assessment based on infant's specific situation.
- Designed to record the functional status of an infant's nervous system by assessing habituation, posture, muscle tone, head control, spontaneous movements, abnormal movements, selected reflexes, state transition, level of arousal and alertness, auditory and visual orientation, irritability, consolability, and cry.
- Provides a baseline at initial assessment for comparison of continued developmental maturation and progression during sequential assessments.

Reference
Dubowitz, L., Dubowitz, V., & Mercuri, E. (2001). *The neurological assessment of the preterm and fullterm newborn infant* (2nd ed.). New York: Cambridge University Press.

NEONATAL NEUROBEHAVIORAL EVALUATION (NNE)
Description
- For preterm and term infants who can tolerate handling.
- Closely resembles the NAPFI but can establish quantifiable indicators of the infant's neurobehavioral maturation over time in the areas of tone and motor patterns, reflexes, and behavioral responses. Standardization was done on term infants at 2 days of age and on preterm infants around term equivalency.

Reference
Morgan, A.M., Koch, V., Lee, V., & Aldag, J. (1988). Neonatal neurobehavioral examination: A new instrument for quantitative analysis of neonatal neurological status. *Physical Therapy, 68,* 1352.

NEUROBEHAVIORAL ASSESSMENT FOR PRETERM INFANTS (NAPI)
Description
- For medically stable preterm infants functioning in the range of 32 to 42 weeks postconceptional age. Test items were selected from existing evaluations by Amiel-Tison, Brazelton, Dubowitz, and Prechtl.
- Purpose is to assess neurobehavioral maturity of infant over time and to detect neurologically suspect performance.
- Neurobehavioral areas evaluated include motor development and vigor, scarf sign, popliteal angle, alertness and orientation, irritability, vigor of crying, and percentage of time spent sleeping.
- Training video and manual are available; contact web site: NAPI@med.stanford.edu

Reference
Korner, A.F., Constantinou, J., Dimiceli, S., & Brown, B.W., Jr. (1991). Establishing the reliability and developmental validity of a neurobehavioral assessment for preterm infants: A methodological process. *Child Development, 62,* 1200.

NEONATAL NEUROLOGICAL EXAMINATION (NEONEURO)
Description
- For normal and abnormal term infants during the first week of life only; cannot be used with infants born at less than 37 weeks' gestation.
- Examines posture, tone, reflexes, and auditory/visual orientation to assess infant's neurologic integrity.

Reference
Sheridan Pereira, M., Ellison, P.H., & Helgeson, V. (1991). The construction of a scored neonatal neurological examination for assessment of neurologic integrity in full-term neonates. *Journal of Developmental and Behavioral Pediatrics, 12,* 25.

---

handling; switch to an observational assessment if the infant does not readily return to a calm, organized state even with caregiver assistance.

Performing an evaluation is easier than accurately analyzing the results; overinterpretation and mistaking immaturity for pathology are frequent errors of new neonatal therapists. The following sections on preterm infant development and interventions can help the neonatal therapist more accurately interpret evaluation findings. Routine, continual reassessment in the NICU and in a follow-up clinic as infants mature and recover is essential to the development of sound clinical judgment about the meaning of early clinical findings.

Neurobehavioral Organization of the Preterm Infant
Synactive Theory of Development

Preterm infants are continually affected by and responsive to environmental influences. Als has proposed a model for understanding these emerging capabilities of preterm infants to organize and control their behavior (Als, 1986). The synactive theory of development identifies five separate but interdependent subsystems in the infant (autonomic, motor, state, attention-interaction, and self-regulation) that constantly interact with one another and with the environment. Figure 20-12 illustrates the unfolding of these subsystems as the infant continues to mature before and after birth. Through recognizable approach and avoidance behaviors that occur in these subsystems, infants continually communicate their level of stress and stability in relation to what is happening to and around them (Table 20-5 and Figure 20-13). Maturation and improved (or declining) health are reflected in sequential observation of subsystem development (Table 20-6).

Synaction refers to the process by which stable functioning or decompensation in one subsystem can affect the organization and integrity of other subsystems (Als, 1982). For example, Marissa, who is now physiologically and motorically stable and able to maintain quiet alertness for about 10 minutes, can reasonably be expected to attend to and interact with specific social stimuli. However, if the caregiver simultaneously smiles and nods while talking to and stroking her, Marissa becomes

TABLE 20-5 Synactive Theory of Development: Neurobehavioral Subsystems, Signs of Stress and Stability

Subsystem	Signs of Stress	Signs of Stability
AUTONOMIC	**Physiologic instability**	**Physiologic stability**
Respiratory	Pauses, tachypnea, gasping	Smooth, regular respiratory rate
Color	Changes to mottled, flushed, pale, dusky, cyanotic, gray, or ashen	Pink, stable
Visceral	Hiccups, gagging, spitting up, grunting, straining (as if producing bowel movement)	Stable viscera with no hiccups, gags, emesis, or grunting
Motor	Tremors, startles, twitches, coughs, sneezes, yawns, sighs, seizures	No sign of tremors, startles, twitches, coughs, sneezes, yawns, sighs, or seizures
MOTOR	**Fluctuating tone, uncontrolled activity**	**Consistent tone, controlled activity**
Flaccidity	Gape face, low tone in trunk, limp lower and upper extremities	Muscle tone consistent in trunk and extremities and appropriate for postconceptional age
Hypertonicity	Leg extensions and sitting on air; upper extremity salutes, finger splays, and fisting; trunk arching; tongue extensions	Smooth, controlled posture Smooth movements of extremities and head
Hyperflexions	Trunk, lower and/or upper extremities Frantic, diffuse activity in extremities	Motor control can be used for self-regulation (hand and foot clasp, leg and foot bracing, hand to mouth, grasping, tucking, sucking)
STATE	**Diffused or disorganized quality of states, including range and transition between states**	**Clear states; good, calming, focused alertness**
During sleep	Twitches, sounds, whimpers, jerky movements, irregular respiratory rate, fussy, grimaces	Clear, well-defined sleep states Good self-quieting and consolability Robust crying
When awake	Abrupt state changes Eye floating, glassy eyed, staring, gaze aversion, worried or dull look, hyperalert panicked expression, weak cry, irritability	Smooth transition between states Focused clear alertness with animated expressions (e.g., frowning, cheek softening, "ooh" face, cooing, smiling)
ATTENTION-INTERACTION	**Effort to attend to and interact with specific stimulus elicits stress signals of other subsystems**	**Responsive to auditory, visual, and social stimuli**
Autonomic	Irregular respiratory rate, color changes, visceral responses, coughs, yawns, sneezes, sighs, straining tremors, twitches	Clear and prolonged responsivity to auditory, visual, and social stimuli
Motor	Fluctuating tone; frantic, diffuse activity	Actively seeks out auditory stimulus; able to shift attention smoothly from one stimulus to another
State	Eye floating, glassy eyed, staring; worried or dull look; hyperalert, panicked expression; gaze aversion; weak cry; irritability Becomes stressed if two or more types of stimuli are given simultaneously Abrupt state changes	Face demonstrates bright-eyed, purposeful interest, varying between arousal and relaxation

SELF-REGULATION

Defined as infant's efforts to achieve, maintain, or regain balance and self-organization in each subsystem as needed. Examples include motor strategies (e.g., foot clasp, leg and foot bracing, finger folding, hand clasping, hand to mouth, grasping, tucking, sucking, postural changes); state strategies (e.g., lowers state of arousal or releases energy with rhythmic, robust crying); and attention and orientation strategies (e.g., visual locking). The success of various strategies may vary among infants.

Modified from Als, H. (1982). Toward a synactive theory of development: Promise for the assessment and support of infant individuality. *Infant Mental Health Journal, 3,* 229-243; and Als, H. (1986). A synactive model of neonatal behavior organization: Framework for the assessment of neurobehavioral development in the premature infant and for support of infants and parents in the neonatal intensive care environment. *Physical and Occupational Therapy in Pediatrics, 6,* 3-55.

TABLE 20-6 Neurobehavioral Development of Preterm Infants by Gestational Age

Neurobehavioral System	Developmental Behaviors

≤30 WEEKS' GESTATION

Autonomic	May exhibit periodic breathing, apnea, and bradycardia.
	Color changes common with stimulation.
	Eyelids are thin; infant has minimal ability to achieve or maintain protective tightening of eyelid against bright light.
	Eyes flutter open, often with rapid, uncoordinated eye movements or diffuse, unfocused gaze.
Motor	Reflex smiling and startle response are present.
	Muscle tone is low; limp extension of extremities and flat resting postures are predominant.
	Uncontrolled spontaneous movements (e.g., extremity twitches, tremors) are common.
	Active movements of extremities are jerky.
	Infant is unable to coordinate sucking, swallowing, and breathing.
State	Light sleep states predominate, with rapid eye movement (REM) and frequent tonguing/mouthing apparent.
	States are not yet well defined; drowsy or awake "alert" periods are brief.
	Visual acuity is poor, with little accommodation.
	Apnea may result when visual stimuli are intense.
Attention/interaction	Hearing is well developed; may show preference for mother's voice.
	Usually easily stressed by environmental and caregiving stimuli.
Self-regulation	Self-regulation efforts are immature and ineffective.

INFANTS AT 30-33 WEEKS' GESTATION

Autonomic	May exhibit periodic breathing, apnea and bradycardia.
	Reflexive ability to constrict iris emerges.
	Able to keep eyelids shut, but eyelids still thin.
Motor	Muscle tone improving and more flexion is apparent, better in lower extremities than in upper extremities motor tone.
	Motor activity becoming smoother, but startles and tremors still common.
	Improved head control is evident.
State	Active sleep predominant, but quiet sleep increasing.
	Increase in alert awake time.
	States more distinct as sleep-wake organization emerges.
	Arousal with feeding readiness cues may be observed.
	Emerging coordination of sucking, swallowing, and breathing.
Attention/interaction	Brightens to sound; preference for human voice.
	May be able to briefly visually focus (with much effort) on specific stimulus.
	Limited capacity for social contact.
	Still often stressed by environmental and caregiving stimuli.
Self-regulation	Self-regulation efforts (i.e. grasping, foot bracing, hand-to-mouth) increasing with variable effectiveness.

34 TO 36 WEEKS' GESTATION

Autonomic	Generally more stable heart rate, respiratory rate, and oxygen saturation.
Motor	Muscle tone, activity level, and motor control continue to improve.
	Able to right head forward and backward.
	Tremors decreased.
	Usually able to breast- or bottle-feed.
State	Increase in quiet sleep, with more regular respiration and decreased random activity.
	Smoother transition between sleep and awake states.
	Usually awakens to stimulation, although duration and quality of alertness may vary.
	Arousal and crying more frequent in response to discomfort, pain, or hunger.
Attention/interaction	More consistent behavioral responsiveness to auditory stimuli.
	Visual orientation (focus, brief tracking) is present, but infant may become overstimulated or fatigued with the effort.
Self-regulation	Increased capacity for social attentiveness and responsiveness.
	May tolerate just one type of sensory or social stimulation at a time.
	Efforts and success at self-consoling and self-regulation are improving.

37 TO 40 WEEKS' GESTATION

Motor	Extremity flexor tone present; movements are increasingly smooth and controlled.
	Wide variety of movements are observed.
	Takes feedings by breast or bottle.

Continued

TABLE 20-6 Neurobehavioral Development of Preterm Infants by Gestational Age—*cont'd*

Neurobehavioral System	Developmental Behaviors
State	Well-defined range of states with smooth transitions.
	Quiet sleep increases, with equal periods of active sleep.
	Sleep-wake cycles are shorter, with less mature sleep-wake organization than infant born at term.
	Crying more closely approximates that of term infant.
Attention/interaction	Increasingly consistent behavioral responsiveness to auditory stimuli; prefers human voice.
	Active "looking" behaviors increase during quiet alert periods.
	Infant displays preferences for visual stimuli (usually human face) and tracks objects; best visual focus is at 8 to 10 inches.
Self-regulation	More reciprocal social interaction.
	Self-regulation efforts are more organized and successful.

Modified from Hadley, M.A., West, D., Turner, A., & Santangelo, S. (1999). *Developmental and behavioral characteristics of preterm infants.* Petaluma, CA: NICU; and Yecco, G.J. (1993). Neurobehavioral development and developmental support of premature infants. *Journal of Perinatal and Neonatal Nursing, 7,* 56-65.

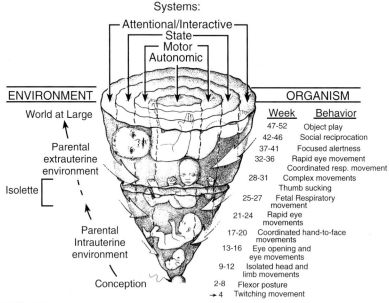

FIGURE 20-12 Emerging and expanding capabilities of the developing infant, beginning at conception, are illustrated in this model of synactive organization of behavioral development. (From Als, H. [1982]. *Infant Mental Health Journal, 3,* 229-243.)

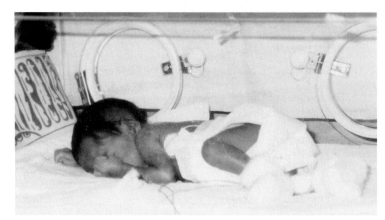

FIGURE 20-13 Preterm infant using motor strategies of hand-to-face, extremity tucking, and foot bracing on mattress surface to maintain calm, organized state. Although competent enough to demonstrate these behaviors, this infant is expending extra energy in self-regulation because no boundaries or protection from light were provided. (Courtesy Infant Special Care Unit, University of Texas Medical Branch, Galveston, Texas.)

overwhelmed by the effort required to integrate all these incoming stimuli and responds with avoidance and stress behaviors such as gaze aversion, motor flaccidity, and possibly apnea (Figure 20-14).

Synactive theory forms the basis for individualized developmentally supportive and family-centered care. Caregivers are trained to be sensitive to each infant's fragility and stress (versus robustness and stability) behaviors. The caregiver then uses these observations to promote modification of the immediate environment and caregiving practices to facilitate the infant's organization and well-being. The caregiver also notes and facilitates the infant's attempts to maintain or return to a calm, organized state. The infant and family are seen as an integral unit, and the parents are supported in assuming an active role with their infant in the NICU.

Medical, developmental, and financial gains have been attributed to provision of developmentally supportive care (Als, 1998; Buehler, Als, Duffy, McAnulty, & Lieberman, 1995; Fleisher et al., 1995; VandenBerg, 1995; Westrup, Kleberg, von Eichwald, Stjernqvist, & Lagercrantz, 2000). Reported benefits include decreased severity of chronic lung disease, fewer days on assisted ventilation and supplemental oxygen, reduced incidence of intraventricular hemorrhage (IVH), reduced need for sedation, earlier transition to oral feedings, improved weight gain, shorter hospital stays with significant cost savings, improved cognitive and motor development compared with control infants, and increased family involvement and confidence.

Preterm Neurobehavioral Organization: In-Turning, Coming-Out, and Reciprocity

Another description of preterm infant behavioral organization (Gorski, Davidson, & Brazelton, 1979) facilitates rule-of-thumb guidelines for the occupational therapist seeking to determine appropriate interventions for specific infants. Infants in the *in-turning stage* generally are immature or critically ill; these infants need minimal handling with maximal environmental and caregiving protection. Infants in the *coming-out stage* remain fragile and vulnerable but have brief periods of availability to attend to their environment; graded, unimodal stimulation may be appropriate in small doses based on observed infant tolerance. The more mature and stable infant in the *reciprocity stage* is able to attend and interact when in an appropriate quiet alert state, but the caregiver must still respect approach and avoidance signals. Advancing postconceptional age and medical status (acuity and chronicity) affect an individual infant's progression through these stages. Table 20-7 summarizes and compares the stages and characteristics of preterm behavioral organization presented in this theory and those of Als' synactive theory of development.

States of Arousal

The term *state* refers to the infant's degree of consciousness or arousal, and the quality and consistency of state differentiation in preterm infants generally improve with age and maturation (Blackburn, 2003). State significantly affects other areas, such as muscle tone, feeding performance, and reaction to stimuli. State is most frequently classified into six categories (Als, 1982):

- *State 1:* Deep sleep (i.e., eyes are closed with no REM; breathing is regular; movement is absent except for isolated startles)
- *State 2:* Light sleep (i.e., eyes are closed, REM may be observed under eyelids; breathing may be irregular; movements are more frequent; responsivity to external stimuli is increased)
- *State 3:* Transitional state of dozing or drowsiness (i.e., eyes open and close, appearing heavy lidded; activity level is variable; infant either returns to deeper sleep or becomes increasingly alert)
- *State 4:* Quiet and alert (i.e., eyes are open; movement is minimal). The quality of the quiet alert state is important. An infant with bright-eyed, "robust" alertness is in an optimal state to attend and interact with specific environmental stimuli (Figure 20-15). Conversely, an infant may be in state 4 but unavailable for interaction if the alertness is of poor quality.

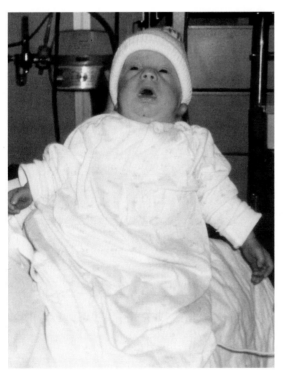

FIGURE 20-14 Flaccid muscle tone, gape face, and low-level diffuse alertness are signs of stress in this preterm infant. (Courtesy Infant Special Care Unit, University of Texas Medical Branch, Galveston, Texas.)

TABLE 20-7 Stages and Characteristics of Behavioral Organization in Preterm Infant

Als	Gorski, Davidson, & Brazelton
Physiologic homeostasis: Stabilization and integration of temperature control, cardiorespiratory function, digestion, and elimination. *Characteristics:* Becomes pale, dusky, cyanotic; heart and respiratory rates change—all symptoms of disorganization of autonomic nervous system.	**In turning:** Physiologic stage of mere survival. *Characteristics:* Autonomic nervous system responses to stimuli (rapid color changes caused by swings in heart and respiratory rates); no or limited direct response; inability to arouse self spontaneously; jerky movements; asleep (and protecting the central nervous system from sensory overload) 97% of the time. Preterms (<32 weeks) are easily physiologically overwhelmed by stimuli.
Motor development may infringe on physiologic homeostasis, resulting in defensive strategies (vomiting, color change, apnea, and bradycardia). State development becomes less diffuse and encompasses full range: sleep, awake, crying. States and state changes may affect physiologic and motor stability.	**Coming out:** First active response to environment may be seen as early as 34 to 35 weeks (provided some physiologic stability has been achieved). *Characteristics:* Remains pink with stimuli; has directed response for short periods; arouses spontaneously and maintains arousal after stimuli ceases; if interaction begins in alert state, maintains quiet alert for 5 to 10 minutes, tracks animate and inanimate stimuli; spends 10% to 15% of time in alert state with predictable interaction patterns.
Alert state is well differentiated from other states; state changes may interfere with physiologic and motor stability.	**Reciprocity:** Active interaction and reciprocity with environment develop at 36 to 40 weeks. *Characteristics:* Directs response; arouses and consoles self; maintains alertness and interacts with both animate and inanimate objects; copes with external stress.

Modified from Als, H. (1986). A synactive model of neonatal behavior organization: Framework for the assessment of neurobehavioral development in the premature infant and for support of infants and parents in the neonatal intensive care environment. *Physical and Occupational Therapy in Pediatrics, 6,* 3-55; and Gorski, P.A., Davidson, M.F., & Brazelton, T.B. (1979). Stages of behavioral organization in the high-risk neonate: Theoretical clinical considerations. *Seminars in Perinatology, 3,* 61-72.

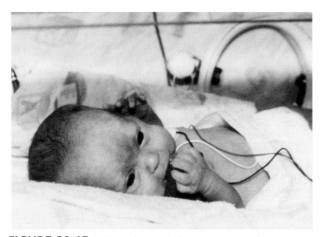

FIGURE 20-15 This calm and alert preterm infant is in an appropriate state of arousal for the therapist to assess her ability to attend and interact with specific environmental stimuli. (Courtesy Infant Special Care Unit, University of Texas Medical Branch, Galveston, Texas; photograph by Dottie Jones.)

This is generally noted as a diffuse, low-level alertness with a dull, glassy-eyed gaze (see Figure 20-14) or hyperalertness with a wide-eyed stare that makes the infant appear somewhat panicked.

- *State 5:* Active alert (i.e., eyes are open; motor activity is increased; infant may be fussy without really crying and often is unable to focus and interact with specific stimuli)

- *State 6:* Crying (i.e., eyes may be open or closed; motor activity is increased; infant is obviously distressed; cry may be lusty with a stable or larger infant, weak in a preterm infant, or inaudible in an intubated infant; autonomic and motor stress signals are common [see Table 20-5])

Whether the infant transitions smoothly or with abrupt fluctuation between states, both spontaneously and during handling, provides information on neural organization and control (Blackburn, 2003). The infant who cannot be aroused, who is excessively irritable, or who has wide swings between sleep and cry states with no interim alert periods may be demonstrating either immaturity or pathology. A gradual awakening with smooth transition from sleep to alertness and eventually back to sleep is one of the signs of maturation and neurologic integrity.

State modulation (i.e., the infant's ability to make smooth transitions between states, arouse when appropriate, and sustain sleep states) requires appropriate regulation and response to a variety of sensory input (Blackburn, 2003). The infant's ability to modulate state is affected by intrinsic factors (e.g., pain, stress, immaturity, illness, intrauterine drug exposure) and extrinsic factors (e.g, light, noise, caregiving activities). Individual temperament may also be a variable in the infant's state of arousal; some infants are more active and demanding, whereas others are more relaxed (Gardner & Goldson, 2002). Sleep is essential for body and brain growth and development; supporting and protecting undisturbed sleep should be a caregiving priority.

Sensory System Development and Sensory Stimulation
Sensory System Development

Development of fetal sensory systems occurs in a chronologic but overlapping order. The infant's sensory systems of touch, movement, taste, smell, and hearing are structurally complete but functionally immature at the age of viability. Table 20-8 summarizes highlights of fetal brain and sensory system development at advancing gestational ages, with corresponding implications for environmental and caregiving modifications.

Supplemental Sensory Stimulation

Much of the early research on supplemental stimulation with preterm infants was based on the sensory deprivation theory and the subsequent desire to provide additional stimuli. This research has been criticized because of the use of small samples, exclusive application to healthy preterm infants, the wide age span of infants treated as a homogeneous group, failure to take into account individual differences of infants, and methodologic discrepancies that preclude comparisons among studies.

With sensory stimulation in the NICU, protecting the fragile newborn from excessive or inappropriate sensory input is a more compelling priority than direct interven-

---

TABLE 20-8 Fetal Sensory System Development: Implications for Environmental and Caregiving Modifications

BASIC BRAIN DEVELOPMENT

- *First trimester:* Formation of neural tube and prosencephalon. Disruption of normal development during this period can result in major malformations, such as neural tube defects and agenesis of corpus callosum.
- *2 to 4 months' gestation:* Proliferation of neuronal and glial cells, which are stored in the germinal matrix.
- *3 to 8 months' gestation:* Migration of cells from germinal matrix to cerebral cortex.
- *5 months' gestation through childhood:* Organization (alignment, orientation, layering) of cortical neurons; arborization (differentiation and branching of axons and dendrites to increase cell connection possibilities); increased complexity in brain surface convolutions (sulci) as different areas develop for specific functions.
- *8 months' gestation (peak time):* Myelinization.

Most fetal sensory systems (tactile, vestibular, taste, smell) are functioning at the age of viability	NICU Implications
Tactile: Even youngest NICU infant has sophisticated perioral sensation and perceives pressure, pain, and temperature. Back and legs are very sensitive to touch, especially prior to 32 weeks, when modulation improves.	Coordinate care among disciplines to reduce handling, minimize sleep disturbances, accommodate feedings. Help support infant during examinations and procedures: ■ Contain extremities (use hands, blanket, Snuggle-Up) ■ Encourage sucking on pacifier or on own hand ■ Brace feet against boundaries or palm of your hand ■ Have baby grasp tubing, strap, adult finger ■ Observe for signs of overstimulation; can you pause and help infant reorganize before proceeding?
Vestibular: System is structurally complete but still functionally immature. Movement and position changes can be overstimulating and stressful.	Contain infant's extremities flexed against his or her body during smooth, slow position changes. Use soft, fluid boundaries; amount of support needed will vary but is greater for younger, sicker infants. Firm, steady touch (i.e., containment) is better tolerated than light, moving touch (stroking). Young infants may tolerate holding better skin-to-skin (versus swaddled) and without vestibular stimulation (rocking).
Taste: Infant withdraws from bitter taste at 26 to 28 weeks and calms to sweet taste at 35 weeks.	Protective gloves may have unpleasant taste; wash and rinse first if inserting finger into infant's mouth.
Taste can be affected by sense of smell.	Consider giving oral medications by gavage or mixing with feedings.
Smell: Infant responds to odors with approach or avoidance.	
Noxious odor can prompt physiologic instability and behavioral stress.	Protect infant from noxious smells (e.g., disinfectant).
Infant can recognize mother via smell.	Placing mother's breast pad, or Snoedle, near infant may be calming and may facilitate feeding.

Continued

TABLE 20-8 Fetal Sensory System Development: Implications for Environmental and Caregiving Modifications—*cont'd*

Auditory/Visual Sensory System Fetal Development (Age of Viability)

System Development During Gestation	NICU Implications
AUDITORY SYSTEM 24 weeks: Ear (outer, middle, inner) and cortical auditory center essentially formed and functional. 26 weeks: Can elicit brain stem evoked potentials. *Note:* Preterm infants have an increased incidence of sensorineural hearing loss. Auditory processing problems also occur; some animal studies implicate "sensory interference" (inappropriate timing and intensity of exposure to sensory stimuli related to critical periods of development).	Preterm infants are sensitive to NICU noise. Auditory overstimulation can cause physiologic stress. "People" noise is the hardest to reduce and control. Isolettes can be protective (*Note:* Mechanical noises penetrate incubators more easily than speech sounds.). Efforts to reduce noise can occur at many levels: ■ Environmental modifications (e.g., use sound-absorbing ceiling tiles and carpet; pad bottoms and lids of trash cans; use padded Isolette covers; remove radios) ■ Activity relocation (e.g., move clerk, main phone, medical rounds away from bedside areas) ■ Caregiving practices (e.g., silence alarms quickly, speak softly, close Isolette doors quietly) ■ Technologic devices (e.g., use visual alarms, vibrating beepers) Neonates demonstrate preference for mother's voice. Relaxing music may be effective with older infants.
VISUAL SYSTEM 22 weeks: All retinal layers present. 25 weeks: Can distinguish rods and cones; light elicits blink reflex. 25-26 weeks: All neurons of visual cortex present. 26-28 weeks: Eyelids open (no longer fused). 27 weeks: May have brief spontaneous wakefulness; unable to focus visually. 28-30 weeks: Eyes may remain open occasionally; eye movements typically rapid and jerky. 30-32 weeks: Closes eyes to bright light; brief quiet alert state; visual attention still often stressful; vision is monocular. 32-35 weeks: Demonstrates visual preference; visually tracks horizontally past midline; efforts at visual attention may cause fatigue. 36-40 weeks: Retinal vascularization and optic nerve development complete; visually tracks in horizontal, vertical, and circular directions; head and eye movements not well coordinated; preference for curved lines and shapes (versus angular or straight); can see colors.	Visual system is the least mature of all sensory systems at preterm birth; infant must be consistently protected while visual maturation continues. Eyelids are thin and do not block out all room light; decrease NICU room light, cover bed space, and/or shield infant's eyes from direct or bright lighting (including during procedures). Avoid abrupt increases in lighting levels. Lower light levels to help reduce staff noise, activity, and stress. Studies suggest benefits in altering NICU light levels to provide day-night cycles. Supplemental visual stimulation does not seem to accelerate visual system maturation; can fatigue young premies and can create significant neurobehavioral stress, including apnea and bradycardia. Allow infant to indicate readiness for visual stimulation (in quiet alert state, already attending to environment). Lower light levels to facilitate eye opening for attention. Black and white designs are overstimulating for immature infants; the human face is the best model for visual stimulation when baby is mature and stable. Black and white may be therapeutic for infants with significant visual impairment.

tion or interaction with the infant. Stimulation is not therapeutic if it does not promote state regulation and neurobehavioral organization (Dieter & Emory, 1997). In general, a preterm infant is not ready for "extra" stimulation until autonomic stability is present; motoric and state subsystem stability should be emerging intrinsically (e.g., under the infant's control) but may be facilitated by the caregiver during the transitional coming-out stage (see Table 20-7). For example, providing postural security (e.g., swaddling for limb containment and trunk support) and looking quietly at the infant without facial animation may help maintain infant alertness and minimize stress related to sensory input at this stage (Figure 20-16).

Therapists must continually modify sensory stimulation in the NICU according to each infant's postconceptional age, medical status, current state of readiness and responsiveness, and ongoing cues of stress or stability. In other words, the therapist provides graded sensory input when the infant is ready and seeking, not because "it's time for OT." A 32- to 35-week-old infant may respond to visual, auditory, and social stimuli, but at a physiologic cost. Early stimulation for these younger preterm infants may be safest if it replicates normal

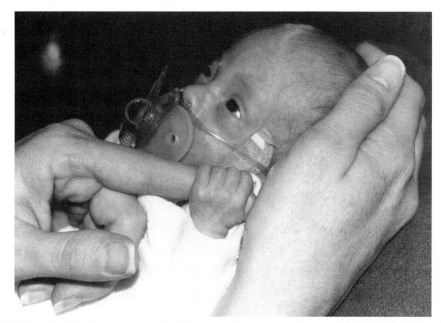

FIGURE 20-16 Support provided by containment, sucking, and grasping help this preterm infant establish eye contact with her mother for a period of quality interaction. (Courtesy NICU, Medical Center of Plano, Plano, Texas; photograph by Vickly Leland.)

parenting activities such as being held, listening to the caregiver's soft voice, or looking at the caregiver's face. Young infants tolerate stimulation best if it is unimodal (one sensory input at a time). Ideally, family members provide this contact.

Infant Massage.   It seems logical for sensory stimulation to begin with the more mature sensory systems, such as the sense of touch (Dieter & Emory, 1997). Massage, which provides tactile stimulation and reduces stress in other populations, increasingly has been recommended as an intervention to promote the growth and development of preterm and low birth weight infants in the NICU. Major considerations include the following:

- Massage is an art and a science, best performed by a caregiver appropriately trained in infant massage techniques, precautions, and warning signs. The caregiver can (and should) train the parents.

- Massage is an active engagement between the infant and the caregiver; it is done "with" (rather than "to") the baby. As with any type of stimulation, the therapist should closely monitor the infant's physiologic and neurobehavioral responses and modify handling accordingly.

- Massage in the NICU consists of gentle but firm human touch (not light stroking) that is given (or discontinued) according to the infant's responses.

- Traditional massage can be physiologically stressful and behaviorally disorganizing to preterm infants younger than about 32 weeks PCA or who are not yet medically stable (Browne, 2000; Burns, Cunningham, White-Traut, Silvestri, & Nelson, 1994; Scafidi, Field, & Schanberg, 1993). These younger or medically

fragile infants may benefit more from the gentle human touch of a static hand swaddle *(facilitative tuck)* (Figure 20-17; see also Figure 20-9) (Harrison, Olivet, Cunningham, Bodin, & Hicks, 1996).

- Preterm infants with the prerequisite degree of medical stability for infant massage are often approaching hospital discharge. Therapists can teach parents infant massage techniques to use with their infant at home, because massage can be calming for older infants (Field, 1995).

- Reported benefits of massage include increased weight gain, decreased stress levels, improved alertness and activity levels, enhanced Brazelton developmental scores, better quality sleep, earlier hospital discharge, and increased parent-infant attachment.*

- Authors of a *Cochrane Review* (a nonprofit collaborative organization that explores the evidence for and against the effectiveness and appropriateness of treatments) found that deficiencies in the methodology of infant massage studies weakened the credibility of study findings. The reviewers' concluded that evidence of developmental benefits from massage for preterm infants is weak and does not currently warrant wider use of preterm infant massage (Vickers, Ohlsson, Lacy, & Horsley, 2002).

- Despite the lack of endorsement from the Cochrane Library, clinically there seems to be interest in and

---

* Griffin, 2000; Ferber et al., 2002; Hernandez-Reif, Field, Diego, & Beutter, 2001; Mainous, 2002; Beachy, 2003; Modrcin-Talbott, Harrison, Groer, & Younger, 2003.

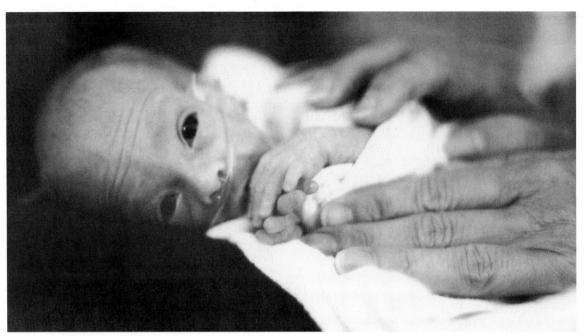

FIGURE 20-17 This preterm infant, who would be highly stressed by infant massage at this age, relaxes with the gentle pressure of hand swaddling. (Courtesy NICU, Medical Center of Plano, Plano, Texas; photograph by Vickly Leland.)

cautious use of limited infant massage in an increasing number of NICUs.

Auditory Stimulation. Use of supplemental auditory stimulation in the NICU is another topic that currently lacks sufficient evidence from well-designed clinical studies specific to the preterm population (Graven, 2000; Philbin & Klaas, 2000). Baseline noise levels in the NICU tend to exceed decibel recommendations even before other sources of sound are added; in-turning preterm infants who are less than 34 weeks PCA probably receive enough auditory input just from being in the NICU and may be overstimulated with more auditory stimulation (Gardner & Goldson, 2002). In addition, recordings require the use of a nonresponsive machine and may reduce exposure to a caring, contingent human voice (Graven, 2000; Philbin, Lickliter, & Graven, 2000).

The maternal heartbeat is widely assumed to be a calming, familiar sound because of the infant's intrauterine exposure, but the maternal heartbeat actually may not be distinct to a fetus floating in amniotic fluid. Earlier researchers who performed animal studies identifying maternal heartbeat as a fetal auditory stimulus had drained the amniotic fluid before placing an intrauterine sensor; this allowed the sensor to rest on the uterine wall, detecting sounds that are not as obvious when the sensor is floating in fluid (Gerhardt & Abrams, 1996).

Soothing music has been recommended in the NICU (Jones & Kassity, 2001), although most studies have focused on older stable preterm infants. The potential benefits of music stimulation have been reported to be decreased stress behaviors, improved weight gain, increased feeding intake, increased parent participation, and shorter hospitalization (Burke, Oehler, Walsh, & Gingras, 1995; Caine, 1991; Kaminski & Hall, 1996; Whipple, 2000). Music facilitated physiologic and behavioral recovery after heel stick in preterm infants over 31 weeks PCA (Butt & Kiselevsky, 2000).

The human voice is a preferred infant sound that is known to be important for early attachment; speech sounds are diminished and indistinct in an incubator. Exposure to human speech is important but can be arousing to the preterm infant (Standley & Moore, 1995); a soothing, high-pitched voice using typical speech patterns (not baby talk) is preferred (Gardner & Goldson, 2002).

Current guidelines for auditory stimulation in the NICU can be summarized as follows (Gardner & Goldson, 2002; Graven, 2000):

1 Although little evidence supports the use of recorded music or speech in the NICU, ample opportunities should be provided for the infant to hear live and interactive parent voices at the bedside.
2 Earphones and other devices that would be attached to the infant's ears for sound transmission should never be used.
3 Any auditory stimulus should be played only for brief periods, should be less than 55 dB, and should be placed at a reasonable distance from the infant's ear. Audio recordings should not be used routinely or left unattended in the environment of the high-risk infant.

4 Supplemental auditory stimulation can be used if the infant remains soothed and stable with adequate protected sleep, but it should be discontinued if the infant becomes distressed (i.e., stressed, restless, or agitated).

Visual Stimulation. Glass (1993, 1999, 2002) raises several issues regarding visual stimulation for preterm infants, emphasizing that even the best-intended interventions may have unexpected consequences beyond the immediate goal of enhancing visual attention. Vision is the least mature sensory system at preterm birth, but it nevertheless often receives excessive and uncontrolled input in the NICU.

Numerous neural connections that normally are transient in the fetal and newborn brain may persist if sensory input is sufficiently altered by atypical environmental stimulation (Glass, 2002; Lickliter, 2000). Visual stimulation too early in life interferes with the development of normal auditory dominance and processing (Gottlieb, Tomlinson, & Radell, 1989; Lickliter, 2000) and may have the unexpected consequence of decreased attention to normal auditory input (speech) (Glass, 2002).

An infant's ability to respond to a stimulus does not necessarily mean that stimulation is beneficial. An immature infant may stare at a stimulus because of an inability to break away; obligatory visual attention is not a preferred behavior. Increased attention to high-contrast stimuli (black and white; brightly colored mobiles with flashing lights and moving parts) does not mean that infants cannot see still forms and pastel colors; the stronger response is considered obligatory rather than preferential. Use of black and white patterns or toys should be limited to infants past term age equivalency who are visually impaired and are unable to attend to a face or toy and who have already received other forms of sensory intervention. As soon as the therapist can elicit a visual response with the high-contrast pattern, the transition should be made to typical infant toys.

The human face is the most appropriate visual stimulus in early infancy and bears no resemblance to black and white patterns. A face is three-dimensional; has some contrast at the hairline or at facial features; provides slow, contingent movement around the eyes and mouth; is situated at variable distances from the infant; changes to arouse or quiet the infant; and is not always present (Glass, 1993). It may be beneficial to incorporate some of these same features into any nonhuman visual stimuli presented to preterm infants (Figure 20-18).

Dim light enhances spontaneous eye opening. Softer, simpler forms and three-dimensional objects are preferred to high-contrast designs; placement of a visual stimulus that the infant cannot escape should be avoided. The incubator has edges and contrasts that provide visual input. The interior of the Isolette cover should be plain, or a plain blanket can be placed under a brightly colored quilt brought from home to cover the incuba-

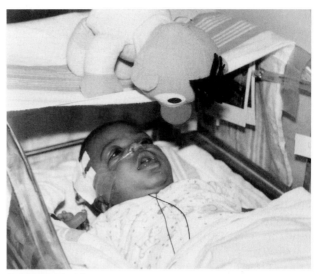

FIGURE 20-18 Softer, three-dimensional objects may be a more appropriate visual stimulus for preterm infants than high-contrast designs. Even though this competent infant could look at or away from "Ernie" at will, the doll was removed after 2 to 3 minutes. Placement of visual stimuli that the infant cannot escape is avoided. (Courtesy Infant Special Care Unit, University of Texas Medical Branch, Galveston, Texas; photograph by Candy Cochran.)

tor. Opportunities for hand regard occur in a supported side-lying position.

Because the visual system is the least mature at birth, Glass (2002) suggests an approach to stimulation that is based on the hierarchical organization of sensory systems, with direct visual stimulation the least emphasized modality. Early tactile stimulation (i.e., massage) can enhance later visual information processing. Soft, rhythmic talking elicits a quiet alert state in the infant, which in turn invites a response (voice, touch) by the caregiver. The interplay between the baby's early efforts at attention and a contingent response by the adult facilitates reciprocal interaction and a normal developmental progression.

Traditional Developmental Stimulation. Traditional developmental stimulation generally is not appropriate until the infant is both nearing (or past) term equivalency and sufficiently medically stable to seek attention and interaction (Figure 20-19). Infants vary significantly, therefore the therapist must be sensitive to each infant's cues.

Stable infants approaching or exceeding term PCA may demand more attention with varying success; it is worrisome if prolonged crying is ignored. For auditory stimulation of these infants, the occupational therapist may provide mobiles, mirrors, or toys for visual stimulation and musical toys or tape recorders with lullabies or tapes of family members singing or reading stories. Baby swings or bouncy infant seats can provide vestibular input and a different view of the world. Even the

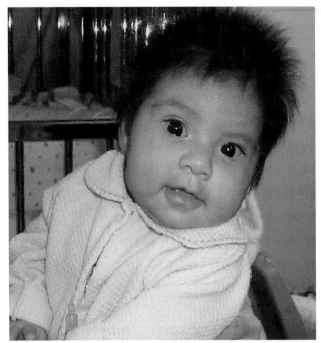

FIGURE 20-19 This term infant remains in the NICU because of an intestinal anomaly but demands to be treated like a "real" baby! Traditional development stimulation is necessary and appropriate. (Courtesy Infant Special Care Unit, University of Texas Medical Branch, Galveston, Texas; photograph by Jan Hunter.)

variation of being placed in a standard infant seat may calm some infants. Portable infant carriers may be options for stable infants who can be temporarily separated from (or have portable) medical equipment. Supporting families to be available, involved, and knowledgeable is the best way the therapist can meet the infant's developmental and emotional needs, both in the NICU and after discharge.

Neuromotor Development and Interventions
Reflex Development

Neonatal reflex development is well documented in medical and therapy literature (Amiel-Tison & Grenier, 1986; Dargassies, 1977; Vergara & Bigsby, 2003). Although reflex testing is a popular method of assessing an infant's maturation and CNS integrity, complete reflex testing is extremely stressful for young or acutely ill NICU infants and is unnecessary as an early routine evaluation. Self-regulatory reflexes, such as suck and grasp, often are sufficient indicators of primitive reflex integrity in young and ill infants. Testing of selected additional reflexes may be appropriate for older stable infants before discharge (Amiel-Tison, 2002) or for an infant who has or is suspected of having neuromuscular

pathology (e.g., spina bifida, congenital neuropathy). The therapist can observe many reflexes (e.g., grasping, sucking, head righting) in the context of normal handling, which often provides functional information with less stress than generalized formal reflex testing.

Muscle Tone

Hypotonia is normal for extremely preterm infants. Muscle tone in preterm infants gradually increases with age and proceeds in a caudocephalic (feet to head) and a distal to proximal (extremities to trunk) direction (Amiel-Tison & Grenier, 1986; Blackburn, 2003). Active muscle tone, observed during spontaneous movement or elicited by righting reactions when the infant is handled, develops before passive flexor tone is seen at rest (Blackburn, 2003); an extremely preterm infant at term equivalency typically demonstrates greater extension and less physiologic flexion than a newborn full-term infant. Twitches, tremors, and startles are common in preterm infants (Grunau, Holsti, Whitfield, & Ling, 2000), but movements typically become smoother and tremors less prevalent as term equivalency nears.

In addition to postconceptional age, state of arousal and medical status are significant variables in the assessment of muscle tone. A preterm infant may be active and feisty when awake but may appear hypotonic if assessed while drowsy or asleep. Muscle tone in an acutely ill infant cannot be accurately evaluated except for that point in time; the underlying muscle tone usually changes as the infant recovers. The therapist should also check whether an infant's medications have neuromotor side effects. For example, phenobarbital given for seizures initially may make the infant lethargic; theophylline or caffeine given for apnea may make the infant jittery; and Versed (midazolam) given for sedation may cause tremors.

The influence of evolving muscle tone on resting posture and the degree or quality of movement has implications for positioning and caregiving needs. The therapist should note and monitor atypical findings or asymmetric responses; often unusual movement patterns resolve with maturation and physical recovery.

Importance of Therapeutic Positioning

Developmental support in the form of environmental and caregiving modifications is provided in the NICU because preterm and sick infants lack the maturity, health, or competence necessary to cope easily with life in the NICU. Therapeutic positioning, for example, attempts to promote the normal neuromotor control and structural alignment necessary for optimal development of motor and exploratory skills. Conversely, lack of caregiver attention to an infant's developing movement patterns and postures can, by default, create short-term and long-term functional problems even in the absence of overt brain pathology.

A fetus in the womb typically is flexed and contained, with midline orientation of the head and extremities. Healthy term newborns maintain this general posture because of (1) physiologic flexion (i.e., posture is biased toward flexion, with temporary "contractures" of the knees/hips/elbows, because of the limited intrauterine space) and (2) the formation and reinforcement of important neural connections during the last trimester of pregnancy that emphasize flexion and midline as the "normal" baseline resting posture.

Preterm infants in the NICU tend to assume flattened postures (trunk, pelvis, and extremities flat on the bed surface) because of the effects of gravity, prematurity, illness, weakness, low tone, primitive reflexes, and immature neuromotor control (Fay, 1988; Sweeney & Gutierrez, 2002) (Figure 20-20). In addition, *active extension*, a strong prenatal motor pattern that develops as the fetus kicks and stretches in the womb, is no longer counterbalanced by the consistent uterine boundaries that compelled the fetus to return to a flexed midline position. Arching often evolves in the NICU from these dominant extensor movements and from postural asymmetry as gravity and primitive reflexes pull the head out of midline and to one side. Preterm infants left in unsupported extended positions frequently exhibit increased stress and agitation and decreased physiologic stability; persistent and extreme extensor posturing may interfere with caregiving and with the infant's ability to attend and interact appropriately in his or her environment.

Therapeutic positioning in the NICU tends to simulate the flexed/contained/midline intrauterine posture for the immature infant (Figure 20-21); external controls are provided as a temporary substitute for the infant's diminished internal motor control. Therapeutic positioning is important for the following reasons:

- Activity-dependent development (Heijst, van Touwen, & Vos, 1999): Much CNS development occurs during the last trimester of pregnancy as cortical neurons layer, organize, specialize, and form vital connections and pathways; the womb allows a much more controlled and predictable progression of this neuronal development than does the NICU. Formation of synaptic connections is particularly vulnerable to circumstances and environment; the principle of activity-dependent development basically states that "neurons that fire together, wire together; neurons that don't, won't" (Penn & Schatz, 1999).

Flexion and symmetry are the neuronal pathways that are reinforced in utero; active fetal extension is always followed by a return to flexion because of uterine constraints. The resting posture of a NICU infant *without* therapeutic positioning, however, is flat, extended, asymmetric with the head to one side (usually to the right), and with the extremities abducted and externally rotated. Active extension of the trunk and extremities still occurs, but without

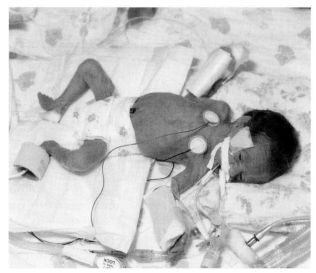

FIGURE 20-20 Hypotonic posture of premature infant. Without therapeutic positioning, the W configuration of the arms, frogged posture of the legs, and asymmetric head position may lead to positional deformities. Tiny premie diaper (Wee-pee) prevents forced hip abduction from diaper bulk. (Courtesy Infant Special Care Unit, University of Texas Medical Branch, Galveston, Texas; photograph by John Glow.)

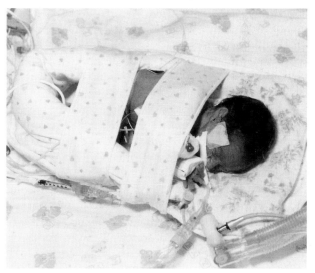

FIGURE 20-21 Small preterm infant (same baby as Figure 20-20) supported in side-lying position with midline orientation and flexion of extremities. Snuggle-Up bunting maintains the contained posture; Squishon I gel pillow under the head facilitates comfort and minimizes head flattening. (Courtesy Infant Special Care Unit, University of Texas Medical Branch, Galveston, Texas; photograph by John Glow.)

boundaries, spontaneous return to a flexed midline posture is absent. Over time, those neuronal connections are reinforced; that is, a flat, externally rotated, asymmetric resting posture becomes the baseline for the infant; active extension and arching become unopposed dominant motor patterns.

- Neurobehavioral organization: Therapeutic positioning promotes improved rest and neurobehavioral organization; the baby is calmer and easier to care for.
- Musculoskeletal factors: Abnormal body alignment over time promotes musculoskeletal changes and acquired positional deformities (detailed in the following section) that can affect the NICU graduate's future motor development, play skills, attractiveness, and social attachment.

Iatrogenic Positional Deformities of Preterm Infants in the NICU

Common positional deformities have been identified and related to inappropriate nursery positioning (Semmler, 1989; Sweeney & Gutierrez, 2002).

Head Position. Preterm and full-term infants demonstrate preferential head turning to the right, both spontaneously and in response to stimulation; infants with this preference keep their head to the right 70% to 80% of the time when supine (Hopkins et al., 1990; Konishi, Mikawa, & Suzuki, 1986). Preferential head turning has been linked to asymmetric skull deformation (a flattened occiput on the preferred side with or without corresponding bulging of the forehead), torticollis, lateral trunk curvature that does not disappear on ventral suspension, early right hand preference (because that hand is constantly in the visual field), and asymmetric gait patterns with increased external rotation of the left lower extremity (Boere-Boonekamp, vander Linden-Kuiper, & van Es, 1997; Dias, Klein, & Blackstrom, 1996; Geerdink, Hopkins, & Hoeksma, 1994). These findings are more prevalent and prolonged in preterm than in full-term infants (Konishi et al.) and have been accentuated by recommendations concerning sudden infant death syndrome (SIDS); that is, that infants be placed supine for sleeping (Chadduck, Kast, & Donahue, 1997). Some infants with this preferential head turning and early right hand preference have been mistakenly referred and treated in early intervention programs for a left hemiparesis, a misuse of scarce resources that causes the parents considerable anxiety in the process.

Deformational Plagiocephaly. *Deformational plagiocephaly* refers to the development of an abnormal head shape in infants resulting from externally applied molding forces, which may occur either prenatally or postnatally. The skull of a preterm infant is thinner, softer, and more vulnerable to postural deformation than the skull of a full-term infant (Huang, Cheng, Lin, Liou, & Chen, 1995). Plural birth infants have an increased

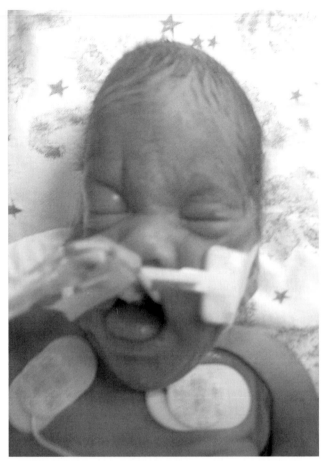

FIGURE 20-22   Critically ill micropremie who can tolerate only the prone position; severe lateral head flattening (dolichocephaly) is evident. (Photograph by Teri Tullous, Galveston, Texas.)

risk of deformational plagiocephaly because of in utero constraints, prematurity, supine sleeping position, and torticollis (Littlefield et al., 1998).

Dolichocephaly (also called *scaphocephaly**) refers to progressive lateral skull flattening that can result in a narrow and elongated "premie-shaped" head (Rutter, Hinchcliffe, & Cartlidge, 1993) (Figure 20-22). Lateral head flattening has implications for infant attractiveness, which may affect social attachment and consequently may increase the risk of abuse (Budreau, 1989). Mechanical factors associated with this narrow head shape have been linked to a persistent lateralized position of the head in supine with prolonged motor asymmetries (Geerdink, Hopkins, & Hoeksma, 1994; Konishi et al., 1986). No effect on brain development has been reported (Elliman, Bryan, Elliman, & Starte, 1986).

---

* *Note:* The term *scaphocephaly* may be used to denote actual craniosynostosis with early fusion of the sagittal suture, as opposed to positional skull molding from external forces; the clinical implications and medical management differ.

There is speculation regarding potential vision or temporomandibular joint (TMJ) problems related to head shape, but current scientific literature on this topic is limited to individuals with actual craniosynostosis, especially if the condition is left untreated or is related to syndromes.

The supine sleeping position recommended in the SIDS "Back to Sleep" initiative has resulted in an increase in brachycephaly, or lambdoid positional molding (Argenta, David, Wilson, & Bell, 1996; Dewey, Fleming, & Golding, 1998; Huang, Mouradian, Cohen, & Gruss, 1998). Clinical features include unilateral occipital flattening with alopecia (bald spot) and forward displacement of the ear, forehead, and maxilla on the same side. Head tilt with tightness of the ipsilateral sternocleidomastoid muscle (torticollis) is common and usually right sided; male infants tend to be affected more often than females (Chadduck et al., 1997). Potential interventions have included surgery, head-shaping helmets, and physical therapy (Kelly et al., 1999; Persing, 1997; Taylor & Norton, 1997); prevention is easier and cheaper. In addition to supine sleeping, overutilization of infant carriers (including car seats, bouncy seats, and swings), plus neonatal medical problems resulting in relative immobility, may contribute to posterior positional molding. Although many infants with this deformation have associated developmental delays and mobility problems (Davis, Moon, Sachs, & Ottoline, 1998; Jantz, Blosser, & Fruechting, 1997; Ratliff-Schaub et al., 2001), there is no evidence of compressive brain pathology (Chadduck et al., 1997).

Extensor Tone and Asymmetry. Neck hyperextension, often inadvertently reinforced in NICU infants with endotracheal tubes and oversized cloth neck rolls, overstretches and weakens anterior neck flexor muscles; this can contribute to later problems with balanced (centered) head control and with the chin tucking necessary for downward visual gaze (Sweeney & Gutierrez, 2002). Increased active extension of the trunk and neck with subsequent motor asymmetries well past term age equivalency is more common in preterm infants with a low risk for neurologic impairment than in term babies; this is especially true of infants who were SGA and/or less than 32 weeks' gestation (de Groot et al., 1997). Of the infants with asymmetry at 4 months' corrected age in this study, about one half displayed asymmetric oculomotor responses at 52 weeks, and a third remained asymmetric in voluntary hand and gross motor performance (de Groot, Hopkins, & Touwen, 1997). It has been suggested that sensory feedback from early movement patterns is incorporated into developing neural networks (principle of activity-dependent development) (Heijst, Touwen, & Vos, 1999) and that repetitive use of specific developing neural pathways strengthens those connections while lesser used pathways weaken (principle of activity-dependent development)

(Hadders-Algra, Brogren, & Forssberg, 1997; Penn & Schatz, 1999); thus early abnormal movement patterns become even more significant in the preterm population.

Upper Extremities. Shoulder external rotation and retraction with scapular adduction are common upper extremity external rotation deformities (see Figure 20-20) (Georgieff & Bernbaum, 1986; Monfort & Case-Smith, 1997; Sweeney & Gutierrez, 2002). A persistent W arm position can do the following:

- Affect hand-to-mouth activity used for self-calming.
- Reinforce a tendency for arching by facilitating increased tone in the neck and trunk; the increased tone in turn may contribute to persistent motor asymmetry (de Groot et al., 1997).
- Interfere with forearm propping in the prone position and with subsequent gross motor skills (sitting, hands-and-knees crawling, transitional movements from floor to upright).
- Delay the development of shoulder co-contraction (necessary for distal fine motor control, reaching against gravity, and midline hand play in the supine and sitting positions). By default these delays in fine and gross motor skills also interfere with the spontaneous play and exploration needed for optimal cognitive development during the first year (or more) of life.

Lower Extremities. Lower extremity hip abduction, external rotation, knee flexion, and ankle eversion are common when legs rest on the surface in a frog-leg or M shape (see Figure 20-20); external tibial torsion (rotation of the tibia) has also been reported. (Davis, Robinson, Harris, & Cartlidge, 1993; Downs, Edwards, McCormick, Roth, & Stewart, 1991; Lacey, Henderson-Smart, & Edwards, 1990; Sweeney & Gutierrez, 2002). These positional deformities have been implicated in a variety of sequelae, including the following:

- Disadvantages for the weight-bearing forefoot, leading to delays in motor skills such as crawling and walking during the first year (Fay, 1988; Monterosso, Coenen, Percival, & Evans, 1995) and possible association with toe walking up to 18 months of age (Bottos & Stefani, 1982).
- Persistence of out-toeing, which does not resolve by 3 to $4\frac{1}{2}$ years of age (Davis, Robinson, Harris, & Cartlidge, 1993)
- Excessive external tibial torsion until 6 years of age (Katz, Krikler, Wielunsky, & Merlob, 1991)
- Impaired development of children with neurologic abnormalities and possibly delayed walking in neurologically normal children due to difficulty achieving good balance (Davis et al., 1993).

Lower extremity positional deformities frequently prompt referrals to early intervention programs, physical therapists, and orthopedic surgeons. Parental concerns and anxiety are prolonged, because the extent of residual sequelae often cannot be determined definitively until long after the first birthday, when the child is walking well independently.

Grooved Palate. The relationship between grooved palates and prolonged oral intubation continues to be investigated, with sometimes conflicting conclusions (Ash & Moss, 1987; Monteli & Bumstead, 1986; Procter, Lether, Oliver, & Cartlidge, 1998; Seow, 1997; VonGonten, Meyer, & Kim, 1995; Watterberg & Munsick-Bruno, 1986). A persistently grooved palate may cause future problems with feeding, some speech sounds, and dental development, requiring orthodontic intervention.

Therapeutic Positioning

General Positioning Goals

Position changes and therapeutic positioning techniques in the NICU have been widely suggested as possible means of reducing acquired positional deformities and the resultant postural and functional sequelae. The primary purpose of therapeutic positioning with young preterm infants is to provide comfortable, secure containment with the extremities flexed and toward the midline. A flexed midline posture facilitates hand-to-mouth/hand-to-face activity, helps the infant remain more calm and organized, promotes the development of flexor tone, and minimizes positional deformities. Clinical experience suggests that the appropriate degree of containment is whatever is needed for each infant to remain calm and sleep peacefully; "too much" positional support often is better than "too little" temporarily for very young, ill, and/or irritable infants until they gain more maturity and motor control. Increased freedom of movement and more upright postures become options with older, more stable infants.

General Positioning Guidelines

1 Efforts at nesting babies in flexed, contained postures historically have involved blanket and/or sheepskin rolls, with variable success. Concave "nests" made from a blanket or from sheepskin over blanket rolls frequently are too wide and shallow to provide adequate containment, flexion, and/or midline orientation. To be effective, any nest needs to have high, steep boundaries that closely surround the baby, with the ends securely tucked to help prevent the infant from pushing the boundary aside. Boundaries work only if they have enough contact with the infant to promote flexion and containment.

2 A soft surface, secure nesting with deep boundaries (e.g., Snuggle-Up, high blanket rolls), and swaddling somewhat simulate the intrauterine environment and may help the infant settle in to rest more peacefully. A gel mattress may be useful for a baby with enforced prolonged immobility in one position; some pressure relief can be achieved by gently pressing on the mattress surrounding the baby to displace the gel and alter pressure points.

3 Commercial positioning devices (e.g., Snuggle-Up) can significantly reduce variability among caregivers while improving the ease and consistency of providing therapeutic positioning, but even the best equipment can be used inappropriately (Figure 20-23).

4 Motor disorganization generally is most pronounced in the supine and unsupported side-lying positions, especially if the limbs are not contained. Motor organization may be improved by the following measures:

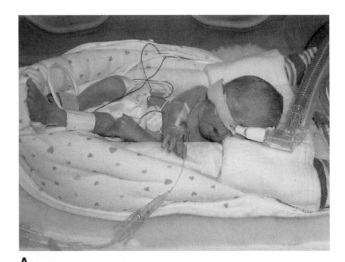

A

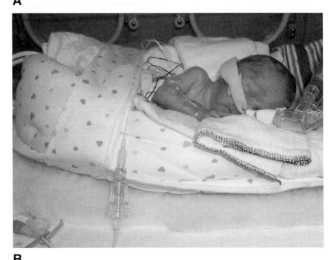

B

FIGURE 20-23 Commercial positioning devices, such as Snuggle-Up, make positioning easier, but the caregiver must still be aware of positioning guidelines and use positioning aids correctly to ensure secure and therapeutic positioning. Note the more relaxed posture and facial expression of this infant after suboptimal positioning was corrected. (Courtesy Infant Special Care Unit, University of Texas Medical Branch, Galveston, Texas; photograph by Jan Hunter.)

(a) Prone positioning. This position increases physiologic stability through improved oxygenation and ventilation and provides better postural security from facilitation of trunk and extremity flexion via the tonic labyrinthine reflex.

(b) Side-lying positioning. This position is easiest to support with the baby swaddled and/or tucked securely into a Snuggle-Up, especially with a Bendy Bumper or blanket roll positioned firmly along the entire length of the baby's back. A single blanket roll behind the back with no other support is inadequate. The hands should be together in the midline, preferably up by the face.

(c) Use of boundaries around the entire body, including the head (as in utero).

(d) Swaddling. This provides the easiest and most secure containment, especially when used with other positioning aids. Swaddling provides neutral warmth that helps relax the infant, reduces extraneous movement, promotes the development of flexor tone by containing the extremities in flexion, can improve the neuromuscular development of preterm infants, and may be useful in managing infant pain (Mouradian & Als, 1994; Short, Brooks-Brunn, Reeves, Yeager, & Thorpe, 1996). Swaddling with lightweight cotton (e.g., a bandana) can provide containment without excessive heat for infants who get too warm if blanket swaddled in an incubator.

5 Most infants undergoing phototherapy can and should have some postural support, at minimum a surface against which to brace the feet, and side supports to prevent the arms and legs from resting completely flat on the mattress.

6 Infants should be repositioned at least every 2 to 4 hours or when behavioral cues suggest discomfort that may be relieved by a position change.

7 Infant individuality and emerging capabilities must be respected (e.g., the occasional baby who seems to fight all efforts at containment and rests better when an extremity or two is allowed to sprawl, or the maturing infant who can maintain a flexed posture without firm swaddling). *Note:* Remember that a fetus forcefully extends in utero and is passively brought back into flexion by the uterine wall. After preterm birth, active extension occurs frequently and is not yet balanced by purposeful flexion of the extremities. This imbalanced motor control should not be confused with infant preference (e.g., "He doesn't like to be contained; he always pushes out of his Snuggle-Up."). Often this infant needs more boundaries, ones that are more secure and/or circumferential (surrounding the whole body, including up around the head).

8 Oversized diapers on a small preterm infant passively maintain the hips in an exaggerated externally rotated and abducted frog-leg position. Excessive diaper bulk between the legs can prevent more normal hip alignment even when side supports (boundaries) are provided around the infant. Conversely, consistent use of appropriately sized diapers combined with therapeutic positioning to maintain normal hip alignment can help reduce or prevent this typical premie positional deformity of the lower extremities.

9 Before hospital discharge, the baby should be transitioned to positioning that will be used in the home.

10 The infant should always be handled gently, with the extremities contained during and after slow position changes.

Flexion, midline, containment, comfort; implementing these four keywords in all positions ensures the most consistent and supportive therapeutic positioning.

Specific Positioning Suggestions
Supine Position

- Some NICUs implement micropremie protocols that mandate that the infant be kept supine with the head in the midline for the first several days of life. However, keeping the head in the midline *whenever* the baby is supine, regardless of gestational or postconceptional age, is the only regular opportunity to relieve weight-bearing pressure on the sides of the skull and help minimize lateral skull flattening (scaphocephaly/dolichocephaly). Foam donuts or blanket rolls can maintain midline head positioning with small, lethargic, or sedated infants; Freddie the Frog (a beanbag positioning device available from Children's Medical Ventures, Norwell, Mass.) is effective with most infants. Orotracheal ventilator tubing should be secured at the level of the mid-oral cavity to minimize contact between the endotracheal tube and the baby's palate; nasotracheal ventilator tubing should be secured so as to avoid soft tissue pressure that distorts the nares. All ventilator tubing should be positioned to avoid pulling the infant's head to one side (Figure 20-24).

- Unless the infant is on a waterbed (Fowler, Kum-Hji, Wells, & Mangrem, 1997), the head should be cushioned with a gel pillow to minimize head flattening; to prevent conductive heat loss, the pillow should be warmed before it is placed underneath the infant. When a gel pillow is used with a supine infant, excessive neck flexion that can cause airway occlusion should be avoided by extending the pillow at least to nipple level. A gel pillow may be used as a mattress under the head and body of a micropremie to maintain proper body alignment and eliminate excessive neck flexion. Gel can be displaced from the sides to the middle of a pillow while it is underneath an infant

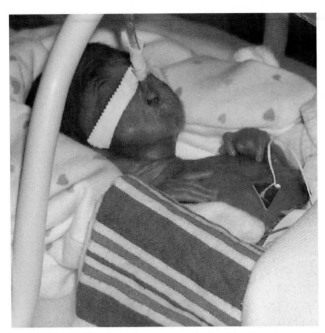

FIGURE 20-24 The importance of attention to small details is illustrated by this extremely premature infant who is securely positioned in the supine position with a flexed midline orientation. Tension on the endotracheal tube places deforming pressure on his gum ridge and palate. The curved bar over his body is the inner rod of a Bendy Bumper, which has been bent into a freestanding frame; a blanket is draped over this frame to shield infants on radiant warmers from light. (Courtesy Infant Special Care Unit, University of Texas Medical Branch, Galveston, Texas; photograph by Jan Hunter.)

by exerting downward pressure simultaneously on the two ends of the pillow.

- The upper extremities should be tucked in by the body, with the shoulders gently rounded (not flat on the surface) and the elbows in flexion; surrounding boundaries can be used to support this position (see Figure 20-24). Elbow flexion past 90 degrees may cause occlusion of some percutaneous catheters.
- The hips should be partly flexed and adducted toward the midline (*not* medial to neutral alignment, because adduction with internal rotation places the neonate's hips in an unstable, dislocatable position). "Nipples and knees in alignment" is an easily remembered general guideline.
- The knees should be partly flexed with the feet *inside* surrounding boundaries, rather than having the boundary under the baby's thighs with the lower part of the legs dangling over, which may compromise circulation and does not provide a support for the infant to use foot bracing as a self-regulatory strategy.
- Theoretically, neck rolls help maintain airway patency by preventing hyperflexion of the neck. In practice, neck rolls tend to be overused and oversized. Intubated infants rarely benefit from the addition of a neck roll. If an occasional nonintubated baby (usually

one who is extremely hypotonic or sedated and/or has lateral head flattening with a prominent occiput) seems to need the extra support of a neck roll in the supine position, the roll should be small enough to provide neutral alignment of the head and trunk without neck hyperextension. Proper use of a gel pillow to reduce the development of scaphocephaly and to maintain neutral alignment of the head, neck, and upper trunk is preferred.

Prone Position

- The infant's head should be supported on a gel pillow or prone roll and alternately rotated to the right and left during position changes by the caregiver.
- A gel pillow should not be placed such that it creates excessive neck extension and shoulder retraction; putting the bottom edge of the pillow at the infant's nipple level helps keep the neck properly aligned. The arms can be tucked around the sides of the pillow to facilitate shoulder protraction (rounding). Using the gel pillow lengthwise as a mattress under a micropremie or folded in half lengthwise as a prone roll may be a solution if the softer surface does not compromise respiratory function.
- The only way to get some flexion of the extremities in the prone position without excessive pressure on the fragile skin of the knees and elbows is to raise up the baby's body a bit (from the umbilicus to the top of the head) from the surface. Use of a prone roll the width of the infant's torso (i.e., the gel of a pillow is pushed to one side lengthwise, and excess urethane is folded over and taped in place) under the infant's head and extending to the umbilicus allows the infant's arms and legs to flex forward gently toward the midline over the edges of the roll. Stopping the prone roll at the hips prevents abduction, which would occur if the baby's legs straddled the roll. Stable external boundaries (e.g., swaddling, bunting, Bendy-Bumper) are needed to help the infant maintain a secure, balanced, and flexed position on the prone roll (Figure 20-25); this is especially crucial if the infant is intubated to prevent inadvertent extubation.
- Secure lower boundaries must be provided for the baby to use in foot bracing.
- In the past, hip flexion has been promoted by the placement of a small roll under the lower pelvis; however, many infants do not appear to tolerate this well, and midline orientation is not facilitated by a hip roll.

Side-Lying Position

- Some neonatologists do not advocate prolonged side-lying positioning for micropremies (except in the treatment of specific air leaks, such as pulmonary interstitial emphysema [PIE]) because of concern that excessive time in this position may promote atelectasis of the dependent (lower) lung. Staff members must check with the attending physician.

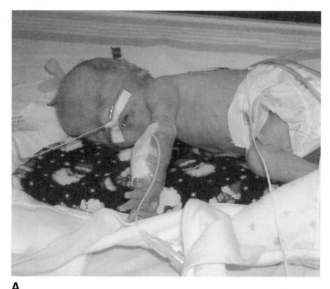

A

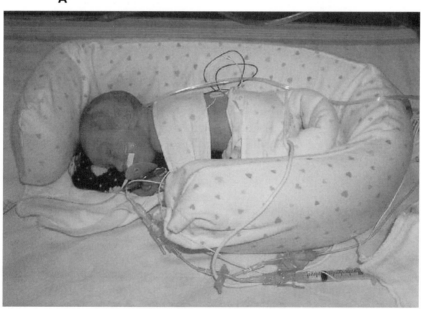

B

FIGURE 20-25 **A,** Preterm infant without secure positional support shows stress cues of arm extension, finger splay, gape face, tongue protrusion, and facial grimace. **B,** Preterm infant on a gel prone roll to facilitate flexed posture, with appropriate-size Snuggle-Up and Bendy Bumper, which make this position secure. (Courtesy Infant Special Care Unit, University of Texas Medical Branch, Galveston, Texas; photographs by Jan Hunter.)

- When used appropriately, the side-lying position decreases the extensor effects of gravity, facilitates midline orientation of the head and extremities, and encourages hand-to-hand, hand-to-mouth, or hand-to-face activity (see Figure 20-23).
- To maintain the side-lying position (and to avoid extremity extension and retraction, as well as increased infant stress from positional instability), the infant's top hip and shoulder should be positioned slightly forward of the weight-bearing hip and shoulder. Small rolls along the chest for the baby to "hug" (e.g., a

diaper roll or Beanie Baby) can encourage forward flexion. *Note:* Beanie Babies may not be allowed in some NICUs that may want to avoid a potential mixed message regarding the SIDS prevention guideline of no stuffed toys in the bed. A folded diaper placed lengthwise slightly under the back and hip of the weight-bearing side might also help keep the baby's center of gravity forward.
- A single blanket roll behind the infant's back is inadequate. Side-lying position is most secure with swaddling and/or a Snuggle-Up. A Bendy Bumper

can be used alone or as additional support with a Snuggle-Up; the Bendy Bumper can be custom bent (not just loosely curved) if used for side-lying support. Care must be taken not to trap the bottom arm in an uncomfortable position beneath the baby's body, and bundling should not be so tight that chest expansion is compromised by forceful upper extremity midline orientation.

Medical and Developmental Considerations in Positioning. To summarize, a well-positioned infant has gently flexed extremities with a midline orientation within secure but flexible surrounding boundaries. Positioning may need to be modified temporarily to accommodate medical equipment or conditions. For example, conventional phototherapy requires more exposed body surface; the multiple lines and needs for caregiver access to a supine infant may restrict positioning options during ECMO, generalized edema may limit flexion of the extremities, or severe extremity contractures associated with arthrogryposis multiplex congenita can make any therapeutic positioning a challenge.

Supine is usually the position of choice for the following:

- First several days of micropremie protocol in some NICUs
- Infant with unrepaired or newly repaired abdominal defect (e.g., gastroschisis, omphalocele, bladder exstrophy)
- Acute abdominal distention; known or suspected necrotizing enterocolitis (NEC)
- Severe sepsis, septic shock

Prone is often the position of choice for the following:

- Infant with respiratory distress
- Infant with agitation and motor disorganization (Grenier, Bigsby, Vergara, & Lester, 2003)
- Infant with Pierre Robin sequence
- Newborn with spina bifida (before and after surgery)
- Infant with contractures (gravity and body weight are used for gentle, sustained stretch)

Side-lying position is useful for the following:

- Agitated, arching infant (positioning must be done correctly and securely)
- To promote midline orientation of the extremities
- To facilitate hand-to-hand, hand-to-mouth, and hand-to-face activity

No position is totally benign in its effects on the NICU infant. Although medical stability is the top priority, developmental issues also merit consideration. A summary of the medical and developmental advantages and disadvantages of various positioning options is presented in Appendix 20-C.

SIDS and Positioning Transition from the NICU to Home. Familiarity with current guidelines on the prevention of SIDS can help the neonatal therapist successfully transition the infant from the NICU to home while reinforcing optimal development after hospital discharge (Hunter & Malloy, 2002; Lockridge, Taquino, & Knight, 1999). According to the American Academy of Pediatrics (AAP, 2000), SIDS is second only to prematurity and congenital anomalies as a cause of infant death, and it is the leading cause of infant death from age 1 month to 1 year. The number of cases of SIDS in the United States has decreased more than 40% since 1992; prone positioning has decreased from 70% to about 20%. Mothers from low socioeconomic status or minority groups or who are single or adolescents are less aware of SIDS recommendations and/or are less compliant; additional effort in teaching these populations may be warranted. The supine position currently is recommended for nearly all infants for sleeping; most previous exceptions (e.g., gastroesophageal reflux) have been eliminated. The side-lying position is preferred over prone for sleeping, but it is not considered as safe as the supine position.

There is neither a "one size fits all" answer nor a current common standard among NICUs on how to transition infants from commercial positioning aids into supine sleeping in preparation for discharge to home. The general sequence is to move from very secure boundaries to looser positioning of aid support, to swaddling without positioning aids, to just covering the clothed infant with a blanket. The timing varies, and the last step may occur after the infant is home.

Although it has been suggested that gross motor development norms be "adjusted" (i.e., lowered) to reflect "normal variation" (i.e., delays) from supine sleeping (Jones & McMurray, 2003), prevention of developmental gaps and delays and positional deformities is both possible and easier than remediation. Saying, "Your baby needs some belly time for play when awake" is not as effective as teaching parents the developmental consequences of inadequate belly play time during infancy; the therapist shouldn't just say, "Do it"; he or she should teach the parent *why* it should be done. Parents are less likely to neglect tummy time if discharge teaching includes basic information on normal development and parents come to truly understand the consequences of neglecting tummy time when the baby is awake and supervised. Infant tolerance of prone positioning is not a problem when tummy play time is routinely encouraged from birth. The therapist should consider using pictures, handouts, and/or videos to reinforce the verbal message of "supine to sleep, prone to play."

Parents should be instructed to alternate placing the infant's head to the right and left sides for supine sleeping. If a tendency toward a preferential side is noted (usually the head turned to the right), visual attention to the opposite side should be encouraged when the infant is awake (e.g., mobiles or toys can be attached on the left side of the crib; the infant can be placed in the crib so that a blank wall is to the right and the center of the room is to the left; the parent can approach the infant from the left side) (Hunter & Malloy, 2002).

Range of Motion

Passive range of motion (PROM) is primarily indicated for infants who would benefit from a rehabilitation approach because of structural or neuromuscular limitation of movement (see Case Study 1) or for infants who are demonstrating abnormal tone. PROM incorporated into therapeutic handling is preferable to conventional ranging techniques for most infants. Examples of diagnoses appropriate for PROM include congenital malformations and deformations (Figure 20-26); trauma, such as a brachial plexus injury during delivery (Hunter, 1990); or hypertonicity associated with severe asphyxia. Infants usually do not need PROM after treatment for osteomyelitis because they begin to move the affected extremity spontaneously once the pain and swelling have subsided (Hunter).

PROM occasionally may be appropriate for an infant who is sedated or chemically paralyzed for prolonged periods. However, experience suggests that prevention of positional deformities with therapeutic positioning may be sufficient intervention for infants whose movement is temporarily restricted (see Case Study 2). Therapists should *never* consider PROM a routine NICU intervention, because it is unnecessary and often stressful to the general preterm population.

Splinting

Splinting also is rarely needed with NICU infants. Significant contractures are uncommon, and infants are

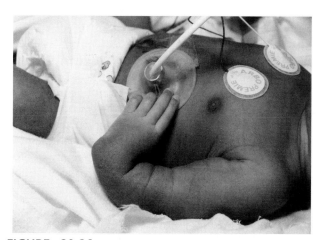

FIGURE 20-26 Term infant with multiple congenital anomalies that require rehabilitation approach, including passive range of motion and splinting. Gastrostomy feeding tube is visible. (Courtesy Infant Special Care Unit, University of Texas Medical Branch, Galveston, Texas; photograph by John Glow.)

notably pliable over time. Therapists usually achieve significant rapid improvement with gentle ranging, therapeutic positioning, the effects of gravity, and spontaneous movement of the infant. Conversely, spontaneous movement is inhibited while the infant is wearing a splint.

If the therapist makes the decision to splint an NICU infant, protecting skin integrity is a top priority. Thermoplastic splints may create pressure points unless well padded, including the edges. It can also be difficult to maintain correct joint alignment on a rigid splint because extremity movement of $\frac{1}{4}$-inch can significantly alter placement of a tiny hand on a splint. A safer and still effective option is to make neonatal splints entirely from creative combinations of various foams, occasionally incorporating (enclosing) a rigid reinforcing bar if needed for some types of splints. Pliable molding compounds, such as those used in dentistry or even in children's crafts (e.g., Crayola Model Magic) may offer additional alternatives for form-fitting splints that do not create pressure points.

The therapist should begin initial trials with the splint for short intervals to ensure tolerance, and he or she should gradually increase wearing time to correspond with other routine caregiving. Because multiple caregivers greatly increase the probability of error, a photograph of proper splint application should be attached to bedside instructions. The posted written directions, wearing schedule, and precautions should be large enough to read easily and easy to understand. Staff and family education is essential but does not replace careful monitoring by the therapist.

Feeding

Parents often ask when their baby can go home; the standard response for an "uncomplicated" discharge historically has been "When your baby can (1) breathe independently, (2) feed well by bottle and/or breast, and (3) maintain body temperature while still gaining weight without the added heat from an incubator." All these abilities generally improve with maturation; babies used to stay in the NICU as long as necessary for these skills to develop.

Two major differences are evident in the NICU population between "then" and "now." First, much younger and sicker babies are surviving, thus increasing the medical and neurodevelopmental complexity of the current population of NICU infants. Second, health care reforms and cost containment measures have encouraged hospital discharge at younger ages and lower weights. For infants who go home on apnea medications, monitors, and oxygen rather than outgrowing their breathing problems in the NICU, oral feeding often is the last remaining obstacle to hospital discharge (Eichenwald et al., 2001). Consequently, oral feeding routinely is being initiated at earlier ages (Lemons, 2001; Simpson, Schanler, & Lau, 2002). The daily challenge for current NICU caregivers is to facilitate safe, successful oral feeding by carefully balancing the infant's readiness factors with environmental modifications and sensitive feeding techniques.

Because NICU caregiving has a cumulative effect on each infant, preparation for successful oral feeding begins at birth. Consistent developmentally supportive care strives to optimize the infant's medical, neuromotor, and neurobehavioral outcome. The infant with less severe lung disease, normal neurologic status, and better neurobehavioral organization obviously has an advantage when mastering the complex task of feeding. Therapeutic positioning to prevent shoulder retraction and neck hyperextension facilitates the neuromuscular control and postural alignment needed for coordinated suck, swallow, and breathing. Attention to minimizing aversive oral stimulation, providing pleasurable sucking experiences, and facilitating a normal sucking pattern during the early weeks or months expedites the later transition to oral feeding. Parents who already know their baby's cues and are comfortable in providing care have an advantage when learning to feed their infant.

The neonatal therapist who understands the components and complex interactions inherent in infant feeding will become more proficient at assessing and facilitating safe oral feeding with preterm and high-risk infants.

Nonnutritive Sucking

Nonnutritive sucking (NNS) or "dry" sucking, such as on a fist or pacifier, is present but disorganized in infants younger than 30 weeks; sucking rhythm generally improves by 30 to 32 weeks' postconception. The ability to suck nonnutritively is considered a sign of CNS integrity (Medoff-Cooper, Verklan, & Carlson, 1993), and individual infants demonstrate a fairly predictable sucking pattern; that is, a personal "sucking signature."

Because nonnutritive sucking does not interrupt breathing, it usually (but not always) is established before an infant has the neurologic maturation to coordinate sucking with swallowing and breathing. Clinically, however, the presence of a strong, rhythmic nonnutritive suck does not guarantee that an infant will orally feed well, and some infants with a poor nonnutritive suck may actually feed without difficulty. Table 20-9 compares the characteristics of nonnutritive and nutritive sucking.

Benefits of Nonnutritive Sucking

- NNS has been described as a self-soothing activity that improves state control, reduces stress, promotes weight gain by reducing fussing and restless activity, promotes faster return to the sleep state, improves oxygenation, and increases arousal (DiPietro, Cusson, Caughy, & Fox, 1994; Pickler, Frankel, Walsh, & Thompson, 1996; Shiao, Brooker, & DiFiore, 1996).

- Evidence suggests that NNS lessens the behavioral distress seen in response to iatrogenic stressors (DiPietro, et al., 1994). NNS on a pacifier dipped in a 24% sucrose solution is advocated for the relief of procedural pain (Benis, 2002; Gibbins et al., 2002).

- NNS during gavage feedings of preterm infants has been recommended to increase the maturation of the sucking reflex, decrease intestinal transit time, cause more rapid weight gain, and facilitate the transition from gavage to oral feeding, thereby contributing to a shorter hospital stay (Bernbaum, Pereira, Watkins, & Peckman, 1983).

- NNS can facilitate the initiation and duration of the first nutritive sucking burst (Pickler et al., 1996).

A *Cochrane Review* from evidence-based medicine databases summarized the benefits of NNS as increased oxygenation, faster transition to nipple feeding, better bottle-feeding performance, less time in fussy and awake states, quicker settling after feedings, less defensive behaviors during tube feeding, and a significantly decreased hospital stay. No short-term negative effects were identified (Pinelli & Symington, 2002).

Nutritive Sucking

The obvious difference between nutritive and nonnutritive sucking is the presence of fluid that must be swallowed, creating the need to coordinate suck and swallow with breathing. The most common feeding difficulties in preterm and ill infants are immaturity, respiratory compromise, and inadequate endurance. Nutritive sucking, which occurs when liquid is available to swallow, often is disorganized because of the immature infant's inability to rhythmically coordinate breathing with sustained sucking and swallowing (Lau, Smith, & Schanler, 2003; Palmer, 1993; Palmer & VandenBerg, 1998; Wolf & Glass, 1992). This disorganization often persists in the infant with chronic lung disease because the need to breathe supersedes the infant's efforts to suck.

Nutritive Sucking Patterns. The two organized nutritive sucking patterns, mature and immature, differ in timing and rhythmicity but imply coordination of sucks and swallows with breathing. Disorganized sucking patterns, characterized by difficulty coordinating sucks and swallows with breathing, are common in preterm or ill NICU infants transitioning to oral feeding. Although a fourth pattern is labeled dysfunctional because of abnormal movements of the jaw and tongue, oral feeding may still be possible (Palmer, 1993; Palmer & VandenBerg, 1998). Determination of an infant's nutritive sucking pattern has implications both for feeding safety and for the selection of appropriate interventions. The four sucking patterns are as follows:

- *Mature (Organized) Pattern:* Typical of healthy term infants, the mature sucking pattern demonstrates

TABLE 20-9   Comparison of Nonnutritive and Nutritive Sucking

Trait	Nonnutritive sucking (NNS)	Nutritive sucking (NS)
Development (progression)[1,2,4,7,8]	27-28 weeks: Weak single sucks with long variable pause (random, disorganized). 30-33 weeks: Short but stable sucking bursts (1-$1\frac{1}{2}$ sucks/sec), with long irregular pauses. Respiratory rate may increase. ≥34 weeks: Longer sucking bursts and more regular pauses. Stability of sucking rate and pattern same as term infants by 37 weeks. Intermittent swallowing after ≤6-8 sucks.	Sucking and swallowing occur in utero after the first trimester, but breathing is not yet a factor. Suck-swallow-breathe (s-s-b) coordination has been demonstrated as early as 32 weeks, but smoothness and consistency of $1:1:1$ s-s-b ratio improve with increasing maturity. Mature pattern usually is present by 37 weeks. Suck-swallow-breathe coordination may be adequate for breast feeding earlier than for bottle feeding.
Rate[1,8]	2 sucks/sec	1 suck/sec
Pattern[1,7,8]	Alternating sucking bursts (4-13 sucks) and rest periods (3-10 sec)	If mature, initially continuous stream of sucks (10-30), then variable bursts and rest periods toward end of feeding
Stimulus[1,8]	Occurs in sleep as spontaneous mouthing movements or in response to "dry" stimulus (e.g., pacifier, finger)	Liquid obtainable from nipple
Arousal[1,5,8]	Able to elicit in all states except deep sleep and crying	Occurs most efficiently in arousal episodes
Feeding[2-4,6,7]	Nonnutritive sucking in a preterm infant may help facilitate initiation of a nutritive sucking burst, but the presence of a rhythmic NNS does not guarantee an effective nutritive suck.	Suck elicits swallow. Maturation is more important than age, weight, or practice in achieving suck-swallow-breathe coordination.
Suck-swallow-breathe ratio[2,4,7,8]	At least 6-8 nonnutritive sucks prior to a swallow	$1:1:1$ ratio. May be higher (more sucks) if suck is inefficient, at end of feeding, or with preterm infant. Infant (preterm more than term) may take multiple swallows without breathing.
Respiration[2,4]	Improved oxygenation in preterm infants up to 35 weeks and in noncrying term infants. Breathing frequency, tidal volume, and minute ventilation remain unchanged in term infants.	Breathing frequency, tidal volume, and minute ventilation become depressed in both term and preterm infants during oral feeding; apnea and cyanosis are relatively common.
Indicator of neurologic impairment[8]	Because of its predictive and measurable qualities, NNS has been suggested as a potential early indicator of neurologic impairment in an infant with perinatal distress but a normal traditional neurologic evaluation.	Because NS is sensitive to factors such as arousal and environmental distractions, it is not interchangeable with NNS as an early measurable index of neurologic function. (Persistent poor feeding often is a positive indicator.)

1 Bosma, J.F. (1986). Development of feeding. *Clinical Nutrition, 5,* 210-218.
2 Bu'Lock, F., Woolridge, M.W., & Baum, J.D. (1990). Development of coordination of sucking, swallowing and breathing: Ultrasound study of term and preterm infants. *Developmental Medicine and Child Neurology, 32,* 669-678.
3 Comrie, J.D., & Helm, J.M. (1997). Common feeding problems in the intensive care nursery: Maturation, organization, evaluation and management strategies. *Seminars in Speech & Language, 18,* 239-261.
4 Hanlon, M.B., Tripp, J.H., Ellis, R.E., Flack, F.C., Selley, W.G., & Shoesmith, H.J. (1997). Deglutition apnea as indicator of maturation of suckle feeding in bottle-fed infants. *Developmental Medicine and Child Neurology, 39,* 534-542.
5 McCain, G. (1997). Behavioral state activity during nipple feedings for preterm infants. *Neonatal Network, 16,* 43-47.
6 Medoff-Cooper, B., Verklan, T., & Carlson, S. (1993). The development of sucking patterns and physiologic correlates in very-low-birth-weight infants. *Nursing Research, 42,* 100-105.
7 Wolf, L.S., & Glass, R.P. (1992). *Feeding and swallowing disorders in infancy: Assessment and management.* Tucson: Therapy Skill Builders.
8 Wolff, P.H. (1968). The serial organization of sucking in the young infant. *Pediatrics, 1,* 943-955.

continuous sucking bursts of 10 to 30 sucks, a smooth $1:1:1$ suck-swallow-breathe rhythm in which respiration appears continuous and uninterrupted, and brief respiratory pauses between sucking bursts (Bu'Lock, Woolridge, & Baum, 1990; Medoff-Cooper, Verklan, & Carlson, 1993). Sucking bursts are usually longest at the beginning of a feeding (continuous sucking), followed by intermittent sucking with more opportunities for breathing as the feeding continues (Mathew, 1991).

- *Immature (Organized) Pattern:* Observed in healthy preterm infants as young as $32\frac{1}{2}$ weeks, the immature nutritive sucking pattern consists of short sucking bursts (3 to 5 sucks) with respirations and swallows occurring before and after the sucking burst (Meier & Anderson, 1987). The respiratory pause is equal in length to the short sucking burst, with suck-swallow alternating with breathing in a coordinated manner (Brake & Fifer, 1988). Instead of having the $1:1:1$ suck-swallow-breathe coordination seen in term babies, these infants cluster sucks together and breaths together; this breath-holding during sucking is believed to be related to the infant's instinct to protect the airway from penetration by the liquid bolus (Mathew, 1991; Shiao, 1997).

■ *Transitional (Disorganized) Pattern:* Some preterm infants and older, medically fragile infants (up to 45 weeks PCA) may display a disorganized pattern characterized by variable sucking bursts (generally 6 to 10 sucks per burst), with bursts and pauses of equal duration and apneic periods after longer sucking bursts (Palmer, 1993). This pattern occurs when the infant tries to use the continuous sucking burst of a mature pattern but does not yet have a smooth rhythm of suck-swallow with breathing (Palmer, 1993; Palmer & VandenBerg, 1998). Infants who demonstrate more than one sucking pattern (e.g., frequent and significant variability in the length of sucking bursts during the same feeding) are also considered transitional. Disorganized transitional sucking is the most common feeding pattern observed in NICU infants and is the one with the most potential for caregiver intervention.

■ *Dysfunctional Pattern:* Dysfunctional sucking is characterized by abnormal movements of the tongue and jaw and has been linked to future speech and language delays (Palmer, Crawley, & Blanco, 1993).

Nutritive Sucking Pressures. Liquid is removed (stripped) from the nipple by a combination of suction (negative pressure) and compression (positive pressure) (Glass & Wolf, 1998; Wolf & Glass, 1992). *Suction* refers to negative intraoral pressure generated as the infant (1) enlarges the oral cavity by lowering the jaw and (2) prevents air entry by sealing the lips around the nipple and elevating the soft palate to close off the nasopharynx. *Compression* occurs when the nipple is squeezed against the premaxilla (gums) and palate by the tongue and lower jaw and is exerted by repetitive peristaltic motions of the tongue that strip fluid from the nipple.

Nutritive Sucking and Respiration. Oxygenation and ventilation are compromised during nutritive sucking because the airway briefly closes during every reflexive swallow (Hanlon et al., 1997; Mathew, 1988; Shivpuri, Martin, Carlo, & Fanaroff, 1983). This compromise is more significant during continuous sucking than during intermittent sucking (Mathew, 1991; Shiao, 1997) and worse with an indwelling nasogastric tube than without the tube (Shiao, Brooker, & DiFiore, 1996; Shiao, 1997). Continuous sucking may result in blood chemistry changes that trigger the baby to shift to an intermittent sucking pattern (Shivpuri et al., 1983).

Improvement in feeding-induced apnea (deglutition apnea), often associated with multiple swallows without breathing, appears to correlate more with advancing age (maturation) than with practice (Hanlon et al., 1997). Traditionally this has been interpreted to mean that additional time to mature is more beneficial than more

frequent opportunities to "practice" oral feeding for younger preterm infants. Deglutition apnea may be seen in term infants, but it occurs more frequently and is more prolonged in preterm infants reaching term equivalency than in infants born at term (Hanlon et al., 1997). Preterm infants with chronic lung disease typically have more difficulty coordinating suck and swallow with breathing (Craig, Lee, Freer, & Laing, 1999) and take longer to transition to full oral feeding (Pridham et al., 1998).

Nutritive Sucking and Aspiration. In addition to the suck-swallow reflex, a term neonate has anatomic and physiologic "safety features" that offer some natural protection against aspiration (Bosma, 1986; Wolf & Glass, 1992). These include proportionately large soft tissue structures (i.e., tongue, epiglottis, and vocal folds), relatively small openings, shorter passageways of smaller diameter, and a higher resting position of the larynx under the base of the tongue, providing an "umbrella" or "watershed" protective effect. A preterm infant with less mature development and function of these structures may not have the same degree of protection from aspiration during feeding (Comrie & Helm, 1997).

Clinical experience suggests that trace aspiration may occur frequently in NICU infants, and frank aspiration often is silent (e.g., no clinical signs of choke, cough, color change) in this population (Comrie & Helm, 1997). The clinical significance of trace or frank aspiration that occurs during oral feeding (as opposed to aspiration from reflux) is not well documented, and medical and feeding management of infants with known intermittent aspiration varies considerably among hospitals, units, and physicians. In addition to potential aspiration pneumonia, preterm infants are at higher risk for reactive airway disease, which raises the question of whether airway irritation caused by frequent mild aspiration during oral feeding could be a contributing factor.

Some researchers (Pickler & Reyna, 2003; Simpson, Schanler, & Lau, 2002) and NICU medical caregivers suggest facilitating earlier transition to oral feeding by beginning bottle feeding at 30 to 33 weeks' PCA. Although this additional practice may enhance earlier development of oral-motor skills, the possibility of silent aspiration during bottle feeding at 30 to 32 weeks' PCA has not yet been addressed or studied, therefore the ultimate safety of these early feedings currently is not known.

Feeding Readiness and Cue-Based Feeding

Historically, most NICUs have not had specific policies for initiation of oral feedings (Siddell & Froman, 1994). Traditional NICU criteria for starting oral feedings usually require the relatively stable preterm infant to reach a certain age and/or weight, although this target age and weight may vary considerably among physicians and hospitals. Feedings typically have been based on a set number of calories and fluid volume per kilogram of body weight and have been given on a set schedule around the clock.

In contrast, an individualized approach to feeding readiness considers such factors as each infant's medical status, general neurobehavioral organization (i.e., vigor, sleep/wake cycle, ability to achieve some stable alert periods, autonomic/motor/state stability), and feeding readiness cues (e.g., awakening and/or fussing prior to feedings, spontaneous rooting and sucking behaviors, gagging with gavage tube insertion) (Hubler et al., 1997; Kinneer & Beachy, 1994; Mentro, Steward, & Garvin, 2002; Ross & Browne, 2002; Shaker, 1999). One study reported that preterm infants of 32 to 33 weeks' gestation showed feeding readiness cues during 92% of recorded trials but that these cues did not coincide with a scheduled feeding 70% of the time (Cagan, 1995). Since then, results from an increasing number of studies support a cue-based or semidemand approach to feeding in the NICU.

Cue-based feedings of stable preterm infants beginning at 32 to 33 weeks resulted in transition to full oral feedings at earlier ages, better weight gain on a lower volume intake, and earlier hospital discharge (Hubler et al., 1997; McCain, 2003; Waber, Hubler, & Padden, 1998). The improved weight gain might be related to calorie conservation from avoidance of prolonged agitation when the baby appears ready to eat at a time when a feeding is not scheduled and to fewer interruptions of sleep, during which growth hormone is secreted. (*Note:* Physical activity accounts for up to 17% of a neonate's total caloric energy expenditure, and a crying preterm infant uses about 30 times more energy for physical activity than does a quietly sleeping preterm baby [Thureen, Phillips, Baron, DeMarie, & Hay, 1998]).

In another study of ad lib feedings in response to infant cues of hunger and satiation, fully nipple-fed preterm infants who were fed ad lib initially lost weight but appeared to gain skill in regulating intake with experience and approached the caloric intake of infants with prescribed feeding volumes within the 5 days of the study (Pridham et al., 1999; Pridham et al., 2001). Two additional groups of preterm infants 32 to 34 weeks' PCA (81 and 89 infants, respectively) demonstrated that a semidemand feeding method contingent on infant behavior shortened the time for infants to achieve oral feeding by 5 days (compared to the standard practice of gradually increasing scheduled oral feedings), with no differences in weight gain between the study groups (McCain, Gartside, Greenberg, & Lott, 2001; Stade & Bishop, 2002).

Possible guidelines for semidemand, cue-based feedings might include the following:

1 Approval by a bedside nurse or occupational therapist determines an infant's readiness to attempt cue-based feeding.

2 Physician's order for cue-based feeding is written in the infant's medical record.

3 A small indwelling nasogastric tube (NGT) (5 or 6.5 French) should be placed and secured along the infant's cheek, avoiding tape near the upper lip. If the infant shows feeding readiness cues, offer feeding by bottle (or mother may breastfeed) until cues suggest stress or fatigue.

4 The infant does *not* need to feed for a preset maximum time or volume. Give remainder of feed by NGT (via pump if 5 French NGT).

This approach allows opportunities for the infant to feed orally without pressure or compromised nutrition; the frequency, duration, and volume of feedings will vary according to the infant's tolerance. For example, an infant who does not arouse with caregiving or initiate sucking on the nipple will receive a NGT feeding; an infant who does well initially before becoming disorganized and tachypneic can feed orally for a few minutes, with the remaining volume given by NGT. Staff members can offer oral feedings more often but can avoid prolonged sessions of trying to force-feed preset volumes.

Clinical Assessment of Oral Feeding

Oral feeding assessments of NICU infants require close attention and continual observations. The Clinical Feeding Evaluation of Infants (CFEI) has seven categories: behavior and state, motor control, tactile responses, oral-motor function, suck-swallow-breathe, physiologic stability, and general observations (Glass & Wolf, 1994; Wolf & Glass; 1992). The Neonatal Oral-Motor Assessment Scale (NOMAS), which requires training for certification, classifies characteristics of jaw and tongue movement into categories of normal, disorganized, and dysfunctional (Palmer et al., 1993). Disorganization reflects difficulty coordinating breathing with suck-swallow, is associated with age, and generally improves with maturation; dysfunction has not correlated with gestational or postconceptional age (Palmer et al., 1993). The NOMAS can help distinguish disorganization from dysfunction during early feeding and can measure the effectiveness of interventions for poor feeders in the NICU.

General Factors in a Neonatal Feeding Assessment. General factors the therapist should consider during a neonatal feeding assessment include the following:

1 *Nursery environment:* General level of and infant proximity to light, sound, activity, and traffic in the room

2 *Seating:* Comfortable for caregiver; conducive to caregiver providing adequate support for baby; nonrocker for ill or preterm infant just learning to feed orally

3 *Anatomic factors:* Facial anomalies (e.g., micrognathia, asymmetry, cranial nerve involvement, cleft lip

and/or palate); history of other anomalies or complications that can influence feeding, including gastrointestinal motility (e.g., repaired tracheoesophageal fistula, diaphragmatic hernia, duodenal or jejunal atresia or stenosis, necrotizing enterocolitis [NEC], gastrointestinal reflux)

4 *Physiologic factors:* Pertinent infant medical complications (e.g., cardiopulmonary, neurologic, genetic); baseline color, respiratory rate, heart rate, and oxygen saturation; changes from baseline during feeding

5 *Behavioral factors:* Identifiable sleep-wake cycle?; timing, duration, and quality of arousal/alertness (spontaneous, in response to caregiving, and whether infant awakens with apparent hunger cues); sensitivity to environmental stimuli (e.g., distractibility, disorganization, shut-down); response and tolerance to caregiver touch and handling; acceptance or avoidance of pacifier or bottle nipple

6 *Neuromuscular factors:* Muscle tone and posture at rest (especially head, neck, shoulders, and trunk); differences in tone, posture, and movement with handling or change of position; general activity level (frequency, intensity, and quality of movements normal for age?); muscle tone and spontaneous movements of oral musculature (cheeks, lips, tongue, and jaw)

Oral-Motor Factors.   Clinical observations of oral-motor function during a feeding may be guided by the following questions.

■ Does the infant latch on to nipple (i.e., tongue grasps nipple and forms central groove to cup nipple, lips close, jaw elevates)? Is latching on immediate or delayed? Do the lips remain around nipple? (*Note:* The labial seal typically is loose in young infants.) Does sucking occur spontaneously, without caregiver facilitation? Is initiation of a sucking burst immediate or delayed? Are sucking bursts rhythmic and sustained or irregular and disorganized? Do sucking bursts alternate with rest pauses? Are rest pauses too long?

■ Can the infant coordinate suck-swallow with breathing or is external pacing by the caregiver necessary to avoid feeding-induced apnea, bradycardia, and desaturations? What changes occur in the respiratory rate and saturations at the beginning of and throughout the feeding? How much recovery time is needed for the infant to return to the baseline respiratory rate and oxygen saturation level? Does increasing oxygen during the feeding (if applicable) improve the baby's respiratory rate, saturation, and endurance?

■ Does the infant hold the tongue retracted or hold the tongue tip elevated against the hard palate? Does the tongue show midline grooving and rhythmic peristalsis during sucking? Is there excessive tongue protrusion during sucking? (*Note:* Some preterm infants who push the tongue forward against an endotracheal tube during prolonged oral intubation also tend to use this pattern of exaggerated tongue protrusion to inadvertently push the nipple from the mouth during early oral feedings.) Are tongue movements rhythmic or disorganized?

■ Are jaw movements rhythmic? Is there excessive jaw excursion (i.e., excursion is visible, or a smacking sound may be heard as the lip seal is broken during excessive jaw excursion)? Is the baby able to strip milk efficiently (i.e., bubbles appear in the bottle; liquid is consumed at a reasonable rate)? Are swallows occurring (i.e., observed, palpated, audible, heard by cervical auscultation)? Is excessive liquid lost? Is this loss by passive leakage (drooling), by forceful pushing of liquid from mouth in small spurts, by wet burps, or by actual emesis during or after the feeding? Is the infant's endurance sufficient (i.e., adequate volume is consumed within a reasonable time without undue physiologic compromise)? Does the infant start well but finish poorly or start out slowly but "warm up" and improve as the feed progresses?

Facilitating Feeding Success in the NICU

Some preterm infants do well with oral feeding from the beginning, and many have only transient feeding difficulties that improve spontaneously with maturation. Long-term feeding problems are encountered most often, although not exclusively, in infants with persistent cardiorespiratory, gastrointestinal, and/or neurologic compromise. Box 20-2 presents multiple considerations and suggestions the therapist can use to facilitate successful feeding of the preterm or high-risk infant in the NICU, but these suggestions should not be used as a "cookbook." An infant who demonstrates physiologic stability and adequate intake during oral feeding with basic environmental modifications and postural support may not need additional physical caregiver interventions, such as chin or cheek support. Caregiver manipulations during feeding should always be individualized based on demonstrated need and never done routinely with the rationale that "this is the way we feed premies."

Breast Feeding the Preterm Infant

This section presents a basic summary of breast feeding. Selected comprehensive texts, such as *The Breastfeeding Answer Book* (Mohrbacher & Stock, 2002) and others (Riordan & Auerbach, 1999) present additional information.

Benefits of Breast Feeding in the NICU.   Numerous studies report significantly improved health and developmental outcomes for preterm infants fed their own mother's milk, with and without human milk fortifiers (Mohrbacher & Stock, 2002). Benefits to the infant include less physiologic stress during breast feeding (as opposed to bottle feeding) (Meier & Anderson, 1987;

BOX 20-2 Considerations and Suggestions for Facilitating Feeding in the NICU

- Facilitation of potential for successful oral feeding begins upon admission. Provide consistent developmentally supportive care for all infants from birth.
- Encourage pacifier sucking throughout hospitalization. The Wee Thumbie works well with small infants (Engebretson, 1997). Transition to a pacifier shaped like a bottle nipple for nonnutritive sucking during later gavage feeds.
- Be patient. Feeding difficulties with most preterm infants are transient; they improve with maturation (most important) and practice as the infant learns to sustain sucking and to coordinate suck-swallow with breathing.
- If excessive caregiver facilitation is consistently required to elicit nutritive sucking, it may be prudent to defer oral feeding temporarily; maturation takes time. Pushing an infant to do too much, too fast may deplete the infant's energy reserves, resulting in a setback that actually delays the onset of successful oral feeding.
- Check the environment. A calm, quiet atmosphere with dimmed (not dark) lighting is best; subtle physiologic color changes *can* be detected without bright overhead lights.
- Some preterm infants seem to feed reflexively regardless of their state of arousal (Medoff-Cooper, McGrath, & Bilker, 2000), whereas other preterm infants do better with oral feeding when awake (Figure 20-27). Gently arouse the infant prior to feeding, such as by stroking (Gaebler & Hanzlik, 1996), changing the diaper, talking in a soft voice, or changing the infant's position. The more upright position and the tactile stimulation (rubbing, patting) used to facilitate burping may improve or restore arousal during a feeding.
- Feeding of the preterm infant should be nurturing but *not* overtly social. Unnecessary auditory and visual stimulation may overwhelm and disorganize the preterm infant who is just learning to nipple feed. Caretakers therefore must avoid direct social interaction when feeding a young infant *and* resist the urge to using feeding time with an immature or compromised infant as an opportunity to socialize with peers.
- Provide good postural stability; swallowing is mechanically difficult if the neck is extended, shoulders retracted, and arms dangling. Efficient swallowing is easier when the baby is swaddled with the arms and legs tucked in toward the midline or with the hands by the face, the neck in neutral alignment or slight flexion (neutral may be better if the infant still has respiratory compromise), and *firm* thoracic support that straightens/supports the trunk (Comrie & Helm, 1997). Some infants demonstrate significantly improved sucking organization when given the opportunity to "hold on" (e.g., to the caregiver's finger or the edge of a blanket) during feeding.
- Support the infant either in a semiupright position (45 to 60 degrees) (Shaker, 1990) or in an even more upright position (Lewallen-Matthews, 1994). The semiupright side-lying position (i.e., approximating the angle at which a breast-fed baby is held) has been helpful for facilitating coordination of suck-swallow-breathing with many preterm infants (Comrie & Helm, 1997).
- The use of milk odor to stimulate smell, sucking, and the release of digestive hormones has been suggested (Bingham, Abassi, & Sivieri, 2003). Use a cotton-tip swab to dab a "milk mustache" on the upper lip or applied directly to the nose.

- Consider a 2- to 3-minute prefeeding warm-up using perioral/intraoral stimulation (e.g., stroking or tapping around mouth, stroking a pacifier on tongue, and especially pacifier sucking) with selected babies *if* necessary (Case-Smith, 1988; Gaebler & Hanzlik, 1996). Dripping a drop of milk onto the tongue once or twice before the nipple is inserted into the mouth may also help some infants prepare for oral feeding.
- Firm, steady jaw support under the base of the tongue (*not* up-and-down pumping action of the jaw) and firm but gentle cheek support (inward and slightly forward) may help provide stability to the infant who has difficulty latching, a weak lip seal, liquid loss, and/or excessive/poorly graded jaw excursion during the transitional stage of learning to feed (Einarsson-Backes, Deitz, Price, Glass, & Hays, 1994; Hill, Kurkowski, & Garcia, 2000). Not all infants need this assistance, and the extra touch and stimulation may be disorganizing to a few sensitive babies.
- Frequent twirling or twisting of the nipple in the baby's mouth creates a moving target and can prevent the infant from achieving and/or maintaining a firm latch on the nipple.
- Warm or cold temperature may increase sensory awareness of the presence of milk in the mouth. Reported effects of formula temperature vary. One study of healthy premies weighing 1,500 to 2,000 g found that gastric emptying time was not affected by cold or warm feeding temperature (Blumenthal, Lealman, & Shoesmith, 1989). Another study of preterm infants showed significantly smaller gastric residuals after feedings with milk warmed to body temperature, but no significant difference in residuals when cold and room temperature milk was used (Gonzales, Duryes, Vasquez, & Geraghty, 1995). Refrigerator-chilled liquid has been suggested to improve the speed of the swallowing reflex in infants, and most young infants will take chilled formula without protest (Wolf & Glass, 1992). No significant differences in body temperature were found after using milk that was chilled, room temperature, or warm (Gonzales et al., 1995).
- Flow rate is often the key to failure or success. A slow-flow nipple frequently is best to avoid overwhelming the baby's ability to manage a liquid bolus. Avoiding soft, fast-flow premie nipples may help reduce feeding-induced apnea. However, a premie nipple may be helpful toward the end of a feeding for a baby who fatigues or with a weak, low-energy infant who has an intact suck-swallow but poor stripping of milk from the nipple.
- Carefully observe the infant's rhythm of sucking and breathing, watching for respiratory pauses and monitoring for increased heart rate/respiratory rate with a decline in oxygen saturation. Continuous sucking is more likely at the beginning of a feeding and thus may require special caregiver vigilance of infant stability (Shiao, 1997).
- If sucking is vigorous and prolonged without a respiratory pause, the caregiver may need to externally pace the baby to provide breathing breaks and avoid feeding-induced apnea with subsequent desaturation and bradycardia. Caregiver pacing can be done by removing the nipple from the baby's mouth (VandenBerg, 1990) or, if nipple removal distresses or disorganizes the infant, by tilting the bottle downward to drain milk from the nipple (Comrie & Helm, 1997) (Figure 20-28). Continuation of rhythmic external

Continued

BOX 20-2 Considerations and Suggestions for Facilitating Feeding in the NICU—*cont'd*

---

pacing that mimics an immature sucking pattern (alternating sucking bursts of 3 to 4 sucks with enforced rest pauses of 3 to 4 seconds) has been suggested to limit bolus size and facilitate regular breathing in infants with a transitional sucking pattern (Palmer, 1993).

(*Note:* There is some debate over whether external pacing by tipping the bottle or removing it is better for the infant. An air-hungry baby will respond with a gasping inhalation when the nipple is pulled from the mouth, creating the risk of laryngeal penetration and/or aspiration of residual milk that has not yet been swallowed. Conversely, there are concerns that tilting the bottle causes the infant to swallow excessive air or that air in the pharynx may be disorganizing [Shaker, 1999]).

Babies seem to have two distinct responses to bottle tilting. Some clear the milk remaining in the mouth with a swallow or two and then stop sucking for a rest pause. Others keep sucking but revert to a nonnutritive sucking pattern in the absence of fluid (i.e., "dry" sucking) (Comrie & Helm, 1997). Remember that nonnutritive sucking improves oxygenation (the infant can still breathe and recover), and at least 6 to 8 sucks (or more) occur before a swallow is elicited (see Table 20-9), which suggests that additional air intake is minimal with bottle tipping.

- Some infants may compensate for respiratory compromise with very short sucking bursts during nipple feeding. Try regulating the flow rate by using a slow-flow nipple (premie and NUK nipples have a faster flow rate than term nipples, making it harder for the baby to stop and breathe), by putting the infant in a side-lying positioning, and by using external pacing to allow breathing breaks.

- Subtle, gentle outward traction on the nipple by the caregiver during the suction component of sucking may stimulate a longer, stronger suck with infants who tend to bite or to suck in a rapid, inefficient pattern (Comrie & Helm, 1997).

- The Haberman feeder, designed for infants with cleft lip and/or cleft palate, can be used with some NICU babies who don't have clefts, but they definitely are not appropriate for all NICU "difficult feeders." The purpose of the Haberman feeder is to get milk into the mouth of a baby who has an intact suck-swallow but who cannot get milk adequately from the nipple (poor stripping). Babies with clefts obviously have difficulty because both the negative and the positive intraoral pressure (suction and compression) used in stripping milk from the nipple are compromised. Other babies who may benefit from a Haberman feeder are those with very low energy, strength, and endurance, such as babies who are lethargic from chronic lung disease or cardiac defects. A Haberman feeder can be used until the infant's stripping or endurance improve sufficiently to allow functional use of a regular nipple, i.e. intake of an adequate amount of milk in a reasonable time without undue fatigue. A Haberman is not a good choice for a "typical" immature baby who is learning to coordinate suck-swallow with breathing or for a neurologically compromised infant known to have or suspected of having oropharyngeal discoordination. It should never be used by any caregiver to "just get the milk into" a baby who is a passive or inactive feeder.

- Plan for success (Daley & Kennedy, 2000). If possible, orally feed when the infant is showing readiness cues (e.g., awakening, fussing, hand to mouth, rooting, sucking). Avoid trial oral feedings after stressful procedures such as eye examinations. Reduce environmental distractions as much as possible. Avoid too many simultaneous physical and/or physiologic demands on the infant (e.g., significantly increasing feeding volume or frequency and weaning from Isolette at the same time).

- Feedings generally should be completed within 15 to 20 minutes for most preterm babies by discharge; longer may be acceptable for certain infants with anomalies or chronic illness.

- For truly physiologically compromised infants, consider decreasing the work of feeding by giving or increasing supplemental oxygen during oral feedings, if needed, by giving stable submandibular and/or cheek support; by nipple choice (including Haberman feeder); by increasing the volume of gavage feeds so that oral feedings can be smaller; or by using modular additives (e.g., Polycose, microlipids, corn oil) or concentrating the formula to increase caloric density and thus decrease the required volume.

- Slightly thickened feedings may be considered for some infants who have difficulty with thin liquids. *Note:* Enfamil AR (added rice) thickens in the acidity of the stomach but is *not* as viscous in the bottle as standard formula with dry rice cereal added.

- For thickened feedings, 1 tablespoon of baby rice cereal flakes can be added to 1 to 2 ounces of formula or breast milk, with the cereal pulverized in a blender before mixing to avoid lumps (Wolf & Glass, 1992; Comrie & Helm, 1997). The nipple hole may be enlarged slightly with a sterilized darning needle (Comrie & Helm, 1997) or No. 11 surgical blade (Wolf & Glass, 1992). If cleaning and reuse are allowed, store-bought nipples with larger holes may eliminate inconsistencies in the size of nipple holes enlarged by different caregivers. The lower viscosity of prepared Enfamil AR allows the use of a standard nipple. Commercial thickeners are emerging but have not yet been designed specifically for NICU infants.

- Thickened feedings as part of a gastrointestinal reflux protocol vary among hospitals and physicians. Some caregivers believe this is helpful for some infants; others believe that thickened feedings delay gastric emptying and thus increase the risk of reflux.

- Consistency from primary nursing (or daily parental involvement) is often helpful with difficult feeders, especially if frequent disorganization or aversive behaviors are problematic. With some older chronic infants, the relationship with the caregiver can become just as important in oral feeding performance as specific feeding techniques.

- Documentation of infant oral feedings on the nursing flowsheet must include qualitative data and clear terminology, not just the volume consumed and the duration of feeding (Ancona, Shaker, Puhek, & Garland, 1998; Panniers, 2002).

- Despite caregivers' earliest and best efforts, some NICU graduates have long-term feeding problems that require prolonged, multidisciplinary management to facilitate physical growth, optimal development, and healthy parent-child interactions (Burklow, McGrath, & Kaul, 2002; Jones, Morgan, & Shelton, 2002; Mathisen, Worral, O'Callaghan, Wall, & Shepherd, 2000). Neonates with prolonged respiratory support, delayed enteral and oral feeding, and disorganized or dysfunctional feeding patterns near term age equivalency have the highest rate of persistent feeding dysfunction (Hawdon, Beauregard, Slattery, & Kennedy, 2000). Thankfully, these infants are the exception rather than the rule.

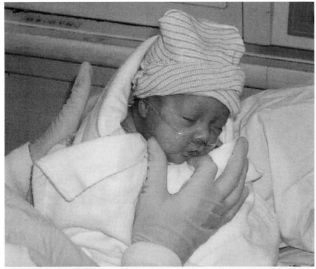

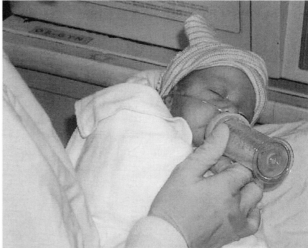

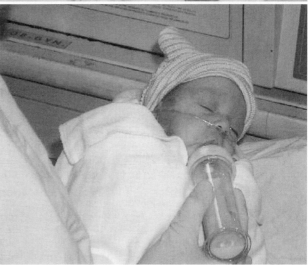

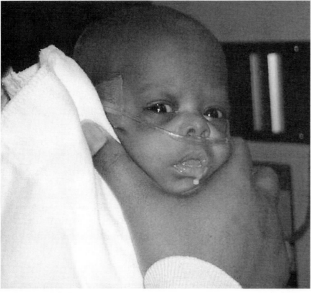

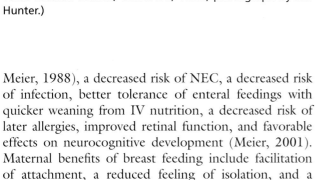

FIGURE 20-27 Oral feeding often is more successful once the preterm infant can achieve and maintain an awake state of arousal. (Courtesy Infant Special Care Unit, University of Texas Medical Branch, Galveston, Texas; photograph by Jan Hunter.)

FIGURE 20-28 *Top,* Preterm infant with transitional sucking pattern is fed in modified side-lying (breast-feeding) position. *Bottom,* Infant is externally paced as the caregiver tips the bottle to force a breathing break. (Courtesy Infant Special Care Unit, University of Texas Medical Branch, Galveston, Texas; photograph by Jan Hunter.)

Meier, 1988), a decreased risk of NEC, a decreased risk of infection, better tolerance of enteral feedings with quicker weaning from IV nutrition, a decreased risk of later allergies, improved retinal function, and favorable effects on neurocognitive development (Meier, 2001). Maternal benefits of breast feeding include facilitation of attachment, a reduced feeling of isolation, and a decreased sense of helplessness.

Challenges to Breast Feeding Success in the NICU. Breast feeding provides unique benefits to both mother and infant and is obviously a desirable family and infant–focused activity in the high-tech NICU. However, most mothers who want to breast-feed their preterm infants give up before the infant is discharged from the NICU or quit soon after going home.

Some common obstacles to successful breast feeding in the NICU include continued medical complications of the mother and/or infant, separation of parents and infant, and maternal stress or fear. Many mothers of preterm or ill infants lack adequate breast-feeding education on access to pumps, milk expression techniques, safe collection and storage of expressed breast milk, transportation of milk to the hospital, and maintenance of an adequate milk supply after preterm delivery. Inadequate milk production is the reason most often cited for halting breast-feeding efforts; appropriate staff interventions and support can minimize this problem.

The NICU environment, policies, and staff attitudes may also not be conducive to breast feeding. Conflicting advice, lack of breast-feeding knowledge, and a perceived lack of support by NICU staff members have been cited (Hill, Hanson, & Mefford, 1994). Professional responsibility is no longer limited to implementing a mother's decision on whether to breast-feed her infant in the NICU; it should facilitate well-informed parental decisions by providing research-based evidence on the health benefits of breast feeding and alternatives to exclusive long-term breast feeding (Meier, Brown, & Hurst, 1999).

It has been suggested that breast feeding at hospital discharge is not necessarily the best or only marker for breast-feeding success in the NICU; rather, an NICU infant's receiving his or her own mother's milk for the first 30 days is probably the most important criterion for measuring success (Meier, 2002). This concept can be comforting for mothers who have been diligent but are unable to maintain an adequate milk supply or transition the baby to full breast feeding.

Facilitating Breast Feeding in the NICU
Early Education and Pumping

Options and details of breast feeding are optimally discussed with the parents before delivery or as soon as possible afterward (Meier, 2001). One hospital reports a 99% pumping rate in their NICU, partly because physicians give at-risk mothers the following explanation before delivery: "Have you considered providing milk for your baby? If your baby is born now (early), I'm going to need two things: a ventilator to manage the baby's breathing, and your milk to manage feeding. Your early milk, called colostrum, is like medicine for your baby. How long you pump and whether you actually breast-feed is up to you, but it will really help me do the best for your baby if your milk is available for at least the first several days and hopefully the first month." Having the physician say, "I need your milk" has had the most impact on changing the minds of mothers who had not intended to pump or breast-feed (Meier, 2002).

Preterm mothers who are indecisive should begin pumping in the interim because lactation is easiest to stimulate in the early postpartum period (compared to several days later) and because early milk and colostrum are highest in antiinfective properties (Meier et al., 1999). The mother can stop pumping at any time, but she will have had the opportunity, and her infant will benefit. Some mothers may wish to pump and feed breast milk by bottle to provide the benefits of breast milk without actually putting the infant to the breast; this can be done indefinitely or on a short-term basis.

Parent education needs to include a reasonable pumping schedule and arrangements for a postdischarge pump. The goal is to obtain maximum milk volume with minimal expenditure of energy without incurring breast or nipple pain or trauma. Hospital-grade electric pumps with a double collection kit should be standard for NICU mothers with infants weighing less than 1,500 g, those whose infants will not feed directly at the breast for at least 2 weeks, and those with multiple births (Auerbach & Walker, 1994). Increasing the frequency of pumping is more effective than increasing the duration of each episode. With double pumping, the greatest milk volume is obtained in about 10 to 12 minutes; double pumping facilitates more milk production than pumping each breast separately (Auerbach & Walker, 1994). Each breast needs to be completely emptied to stimulate milk production and because the last portion of milk (hindmilk) contains the highest lipid and calorie content (Mohrbacher & Stock, 2002). Maximal milk production generally requires eight to 10 pumping sessions per day; five or six pumpings a day may be adequate for mothers who plan to supplement breast feeding with formula or who intend to breast-feed for only a limited time (Meier et al., 1999). Techniques that encourage rest and relaxation, reduce stress and tension, and promote pleasurable thoughts of the infant can facilitate more successful pumping (Feher, Berger, Johnson, & Wilde, 1989); privacy to allow pumping at the infant's bedside is also helpful.

Nonnutritive Nuzzling at the Breast. The easiest transition to breast feeding begins with initiation of skin-to-skin holding (kangaroo care) as soon as possible under nursery guidelines (Hurst, Valentine, Renfro, Burns, & Ferlic, 1997). Nonnutritive suckling (nuzzling, licking, and mouthing) at the breast during skin-to-skin holding can be encouraged by having the mother pump her breasts just before providing kangaroo care for stable infants who are not yet orally feeding; kangaroo care with nonnutritive nuzzling is helpful in maintaining the mother's interest in breast feeding and facilitating milk production. Nonnutritive nuzzling can be a "get acquainted" period for the mother and infant to become familiar and comfortable with each other without the pressure of trying to get the infant to latch on and feed. Many clinicians are more comfortable with young preterm infants nuzzling only at pumped breasts, although others promote self-regulatory access to breast feeding at very early ages; root and latch at the breast by 28 weeks postconception and nutritive sucking of 10 sucks or more per burst by 32 weeks have been reported (Nyqvist, Sjödén, & Ewald, 1999).

Breast Feeding Readiness. Research suggests that suck-swallow-breathe coordination may occur earlier with breast feeding than with bottle feeding and that early breast feeding is physiologically less stressful (e.g., less hypoxemia, apnea, bradycardia, cyanosis) than bottle feeding for preterm infants (Meier & Anderson, 1987; Meier, 2001). A Swedish study of early breast feeding with 71 preterm infants concluded that initiation of breast feeding should be based on cardiorespiratory stability, irrespective of current maturity, age, or weight; nutritive sucking at the breast was reported as early as 30.6 weeks (Nyquist et al., 1999).

NICU caregivers can reduce concerns regarding actual intake by weighing the infant on a sensitive scale before and after breast feeding (Meier, Sjödén, & Ewald, 1999; Meier, 2001). Prefeeding and postfeeding weighing is not routine for healthy term infants, but it can help the caregiver determine what a preterm infant received so that other fluids and nutrients can be adjusted.

Methods for Introducing and Sustaining Breast Feeding. The primary goals in initial breast feedings are for the preterm infant to achieve proper positioning at the breast and to remain physiologically stable during the feeding; significant volume intake is not as important during this stage. A comfortable chair, pillows that raise the infant to chest height and support the mother's arm, and a privacy screen or separate breast-feeding room should be provided. The mother should be educated on how to support her breast, position the infant, and facilitate latch-on to the nipple. Monitoring and documentation of the infant's responses and stability during breast feeding are important; a charting system specifically for breast feeding can be useful (Jensen, Wallace, & Kelsay, 1994).

Optimally, some measurable nutritive intake (as determined by test weights) occurs within a week after the start of early breast feeding. Measurable intake greater than 5 ml suggests that the mother's milk has "let down" in response to the infant sucking at the breast. Once measurable intake occurs and the infant remains physiologically stable during early breast feeding, the goal changes to developing interventions that allow the infant to consume adequate volumes of breast milk in anticipation of hospital discharge. Interventions in this phase of breast feeding may include test weights, transition to cue-based feeding schedules, and specific techniques for intake-related problems (Meier et al., 1999).

Although intake volume increases progressively from earlier to later breast feeding, the amount of milk consumed at each breast-feeding session varies for both term and preterm infants. However, a trend of inadequate volume intake at each breast feeding over several days requires determination of the cause (e.g., low maternal milk supply, improper positioning, difficulty with milk ejection, problem with the strength and endurance of the infant's sucking effort) and initiation of appropriate interventions (Meier, 2001). For example, if the infant has a mature sucking pattern but sucks only for a few minutes, having the mother use a breast pump at one breast while the infant feeds at the other breast will maintain the milk flow, which may encourage the infant to continue feeding. The mother can also use a supplemental feeder (bottle with breast milk hung from the mother's neck with small flexible tubing taped to extend slightly beyond the nipple) to increase milk intake during

the actual sucking time. Pumping the breasts for a few minutes immediately before breast feeding allows the infant with limited sucking time to receive calorie-rich hindmilk rather than less dense foremilk (Valentine, Hurst, & Schanler, 1994). Specific suggestions have been developed for each identified root cause of consistently inadequate milk intake (Mohrbacher & Stock, 2002; Riordan & Auerbach, 1999).

Transition to Cue-Based Feeding Schedules. Although term breast-fed infants frequently are fed on demand, the necessary self-regulation of sleep and feeding behaviors is still developing in preterm infants. If a premie's need for sleep overrides the ability to feed, poor weight gain or dehydration may result; the NICU staff needs to individualize and carefully monitor any transition from a regular (i.e., 3-hour) feeding schedule to cue-based feedings while the infant is still in the hospital rather waiting until discharge (Meier et al., 1999; Meier, 2001).

Breast Feeding Hot Topics

Nipple Confusion

The term *nipple confusion* refers to the belief held by many breast-feeding advocates that use of artificial nipples (both bottle nipples and pacifiers) interferes with successful initiation of breast feeding (Neifert, 1998). Nipple confusion remains a hypothesis that has not yet been scientifically validated, but it often is a passionately debated topic (Fisher & Inch, 1996; Menahem, 1997; Neifert, Lawence & Seacat, 1995). It is important to remember that what might be advocated for healthy term neonates does not necessarily apply to sick or preterm NICU infants.

Pacifiers. Although pacifiers are not given to term breast-feeding infants in a "baby friendly" hospital (Saadeh & Akre, 1996), it generally is felt that preterm infants in the NICU should not be denied the comfort and self-regulation offered by sucking on pacifiers (Drosten, 1997; Meier, 2001). A double-blinded, randomized control study in Montreal did not support the common belief that pacifier use interfered with breast feeding or led to early weaning (Kramer et al., 2001).

NUK Nipples. Because NUK nipples have been advertised as being more like a mother's own nipple, nurses frequently choose them for intermittent or supplemental bottle feeding of breast-feeding preterm infants. It has been radiographically demonstrated, however, that the NUK nipple has a higher flow rate than other standard nipples, has different mechanical characteristics than other artificial nipples and the human breast, and facilitates an up-and-down chewing motion to express milk from the nipple (Nowak, Smith, & Erenberg, 1994).

Nipple Shields. The use of ultrathin silicone nipple shields increases milk transfer during breast feeding with preterm infants, facilitates the wide-open mouth latch needed for breast feeding, and generally increases the duration of breast feeding (Clum & Primomo, 1996; Meier et al., 1999; Meier, 2001). Most infants tend to wean from the nipple shield at around term age equivalency, therefore weaning from the shield often is not a priority before hospital discharge.

Supplementation by Tube versus a Bottle.
Compared with infants receiving bottle supplements, preterm infants receiving NGT supplements were more likely to be breast feeding at discharge and at 3 days, 3 months, and 6 months of age (Kliethermes, Cross, Lanese, Johnson, & Simon, 1999).

Alternative Feeding Methods and Cup Feeding.
Alternative feeding methods (e.g., cup feeding, syringe with tubing, feeding tube taped to caregiver's finger, eye dropper, spoon) have been suggested to avoid bottles and prevent nipple confusion (Kuehl, 1997; Lang, Lawrence, & Orme, 1994; Neifert, 1998). Although some researchers report physiologic stability on measured parameters (i.e., respiratory rate, heart rate, oxygen saturation) of preterm infants during cup feeding (Marinelli, Burke, & Dodd, 2001), others have stated that cup feeding is an inefficient means of supplementing the milk intake of preterm infants and that more clinical trials are needed to ensure safety and efficacy before cup feeding is used routinely in the special care nursery (Freer, 1999; Meier, 2001; Meier et al., 1999; Shaker, 1998). The possibility of silent aspiration with alternative feeding methods of preterm infants has not been addressed. Clinical experience suggests that the current emphasis on skin-to-skin holding, early nonnutritive nuzzling at the breast, and breast feeding initiated for the first oral feedings reduce both the opportunity and the need to consider alternative feeding methods for preterm infants in the NICU.

Although mothers of term infants often want to breast-feed exclusively, many mothers of preterm infants do not object to some bottle feedings while the infant is hospitalized; they report that the transition from gavage to all-oral feeding (breast or bottle) is a major milestone and an important step toward discharge. Many of these mothers plan for the infant to have one or more bottles daily at home so that the father can participate, to ensure adequate intake, or to allow the mother additional time.

Discharge Planning

Most NICU mothers report at least one major breast-feeding problem in the first month after discharge, and many stop breast feeding during this time (Kavanaugh, Mead, Meier, & Mangurten, 1995). In-hospital support should include preparation of the mother for breast feeding after discharge and especially should address common maternal concerns about milk supply, whether the infant is getting enough milk during breast feeding,

and conflicting demands on her time (e.g., infant's medical needs, family, cooking, laundry, cleaning, job).

A common breast-feeding error after discharge is immediately returning the electric pump. Because the trend is toward earlier discharge of younger and smaller infants who do not yet empty the breast as efficiently as a pump, the mother's milk supply often decreases, the infant has to work harder, and the milk ejection response may be less effective. Generally speaking, the mother should continue using the pump after each breast feeding until the infant is emptying the breasts well and gaining weight on breast feeding alone, often around term age equivalency.

Feeding Scenarios

Darian

Darian was born at 36 weeks' gestation with initial respiratory depression from maternal medications and a right cleft lip that extended through the alveolar (gum) ridge but not into the palate. He was admitted to a level II nursery and was kept under an oxygen hood for 48 hours and in an incubator for 8 days. Oral feedings were begun on the third day of life, with good results; all feedings were taken by mouth with a regular nipple that was placed to occlude the cleft in his lip.

The occupational therapist was contacted on the tenth day of life because of an acute decline in oral feeding. Darian had taken less than 30 ml in the last several oral feedings, and gavage feedings had been started. He was lethargic and difficult to arouse, which nurses reported as a change. Darian showed no signs of illness other than lethargy and poor feeding, but a complete blood count had been done that morning, with normal results, and a sepsis workup was being considered.

A trial feeding by the occupational therapist showed normal suck-swallow-breathing coordination but extremely low arousal with no active feeding effort after the first 2 minutes. Darian's nurse said that he had been awake and active for about 20 minutes $1\frac{1}{2}$ hours before this scheduled feeding. Review of medical records showed two caregiving changes just before the decline in feeding performance; Darian's feeding schedule had been changed from every 3 hours to every 4 hours, and he had been weaned from his Isolette to an open crib.

Collaboration with the nurse and physician produced a consensus that even though Darian was "old enough and big enough," he possibly was not ready for all the changes and "demands"; he was placed back in the Isolette and allowed to rest. Oral feedings were offered whenever Darian was awake and appeared ready to eat (cue-based feeding), with gavage feeding supplements as needed for 24 to 48 hours. Oral feedings were then advanced according to his performance. Darian was back on all-oral feedings within 4 days and weaned from the incubator 2 days later. In the interim, his mother had made care arrangements for her other children and was able to stay at the nearby Ronald McDonald house. She expressed a desire to breast-feed Darian, and this transition was successfully made before his discharge on the seventeenth day of life. Darian's feeding problem was real but was related to autonomic and state factors rather than feeding mechanics; oral stimulation and specialized feeding techniques would not have been the most helpful approach.

Emile

Emile was born at 29 weeks' gestation with a birth weight of 1,030 g (2 pounds, 4 ounces). Medical complications included a patent ductus arteriosus, respiratory distress syndrome (RDS) that progressed to oxygen-dependent bronchopulmonary dysplasia (BPD), severe apnea, a bilateral grade I IVH, suspected sepsis, retinopathy of prematurity (ROP), and significant feeding intolerance. She remained medically fragile and was still in the NICU as she approached term age equivalency; developmental concerns at that time included Emile's fluctuating muscle tone, persistent tremors, irritability, and low responsiveness to auditory and visual stimuli even when held and calm.

At 39 weeks' PCA, oral feedings were attempted once a day. Emile demonstrated intermittent and inefficient sucking effort; maximal caregiver support and facilitation were required to complete the feedings. A deep midline ridge in her palate was diagnosed as a submucous cleft but was not believed to be the cause of her feeding difficulty. As the frequency and volume of oral feedings were slowly advanced, Emile began to desaturate during feedings.

A modified barium swallow was requested. Emile's disorganized suck expressed only small amounts of liquid from a regular nipple, therefore a Haberman feeder was used to complete the study. Emile demonstrated the following:

1 Oral disorganization, as observed clinically
2 Incomplete elevation of the soft palate with occasional regurgitation of barium into the nasopharynx, possibly related to the submucous cleft
3 A prompt swallow reflex with complete clearance of barium from the pharynx, even when "challenged" with large or continuous boluses squeezed from the Haberman feeder
4 One or two incidences of threatened airway penetration (a trace amount of barium entered the opening of the larynx but cleared immediately during a subsequent swallow)
5 A significant fatigue factor with increasing need for longer rest periods to allow for extra breathing and recovery of energy
6 No significant gastroesophageal reflux

Feeding recommendations included the following:

1 Continuation of oral feedings with gavage supplements as needed
2 Decreasing work of feeding by use of the Haberman feeder
3 Allowing feedings to continue 20 to 30 minutes if rest periods were needed
4 Increased supplemental oxygen during feedings
5 Consideration of formula additives to increase calories with less volume (deferred initially because of feeding intolerance).

Emile's improvement was slow, but feeding became functional, and she gained weight. Her teenage, married mother visited frequently and was loving toward her daughter, but she had difficulty with caregiving. She appeared mentally slow to the staff members, required repetitive explanations and demonstrations of all aspects of care, and needed structure and encouragement to care for Emile. At 1 month corrected age, Emile was transferred to an extended care unit, where her mother could be eased into full responsibility for the infant's care under supervision.

Because concerns still existed at discharge, plans were made for the husband to drop Emile and her mother off at the grandmother's house on his way to work each morning for continued assistance and support. A check 1 week after hospital discharge showed excellent weight gain. Feeding and developmental progress were monitored at follow-up clinics, and the submucous cleft was managed by the cleft palate team.

Destiny

Destiny was triplet C born SGA (420 g) at 25 weeks' gestation. Her most significant medical complications included patent ductus arteriosus, pulmonary insufficiency, RDS, severe BPD, hypertension, bilateral IVH (right = grade 2, left = grade 3), posthemorrhagic hydrocephalus with a ventriculoperitoneal shunt, moderate ROP, and a humeral fracture secondary to bone demineralization from her body's inability to use nutrients efficiently.

Destiny remained oxygen dependent and consistently demonstrated poor growth. Her muscle tone was mildly increased but appeared related to frequent irritability. Oral feeding was delayed because of Destiny's medical status until she was nearly 5 months of age (5 weeks' corrected age). Noted problems during oral feeding included difficulty latching on to the nipple, weak stripping, a humped tongue with poor intraoral bolus control, difficulty propelling a bolus posteriorly to swallow, excessive leakage that totaled 20% to 25% of the feeding, and intermittent crying. Oxygen was increased during oral feedings because of desaturations during sucking bursts and rest periods.

Several factors contributed to the therapist's growing concerns about Destiny's feeding safety. Her reduced oral control of a liquid bolus increased her risk of aspiration before a reflexive swallow. Her neurologic history (pulmonary insufficiency with resultant hypoxic episodes, IVH, and hydrocephalus) put Destiny at increased risk for neuromotor dysfunction. Mild desaturations during sucking bursts are common occurrences in the NICU, but her desaturations during rest pauses were worrisome. Destiny did not adjust easily to new caregivers, responding with increased irritability when fed by an unfamiliar person. A major concern was potential aspiration during forceful inhalation from intermittent crying during oral feedings.

A modified barium swallow was requested, during which Destiny demonstrated oral incoordination, a delayed swallow reflex, and gross silent aspiration (e.g., no changes in respirations, oxygen saturations, color; no choking or coughing). A feeding gastrostomy was subsequently placed, and Destiny went home to join her sisters as a nonoral feeder. Follow-up modified swallow studies 6 and 12 months later continued to show silent aspiration. Last seen at $2\frac{1}{2}$ years of age, Destiny was orally aversive and totally gastrostomy fed. She exhibited continued failure to thrive, global developmental delays, immature play and motor patterns, and a short attention span.

FUTURE OF OCCUPATIONAL THERAPY IN THE NICU

Developmental specialists and developmentally supportive care are currently accepted standards in the NICU. Although some physicians and nurses remain reluctant or resistant to this approach, often reflecting an erroneous view of developmental intervention as "stimulation" that is not wise or proven with fragile infants (Shannon & Gorski, 1994), most NICUs are providing at least some components of developmental care. Newer NICUs are designed and engineered to facilitate family-centered developmentally supportive care (Figure

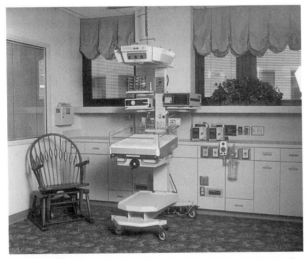

FIGURE 20-29 Individual infant rooms protect the infant from the many environmental stressors of crowded NICUs and facilitate the development of the parent-infant relationship. (Courtesy Neonatal Intensive Care Unit, Baptist Medical Center of Oklahoma, Oklahoma City, Oklahoma.)

20-29). At Children's Hospital in Dayton, Ohio, the NICU entrance and patient bed spaces were constructed to resemble a Victorian house in an effort to help families feel more comfortable in this "home away from home."

Ongoing changes in health care that emphasize a bottom line of cost containment and savings may be an obstacle in some NICUs. Neonatal therapists are firmly convinced that developmental care is both beneficial and cost-effective and that savings appreciated from a therapist's services are many times greater than the salary expended. Data collection and research studies that document positive outcomes are important to the long-term future of occupational therapy in the NICU.

Occupational therapists are ideal for the varied roles appropriate in the NICU because of their unique blend of psychosocial and neurophysiologic training, but occupational therapy is not the only profession that currently fulfills the role of NICU developmental specialist. As a profession of clinicians, educators, and administrators, occupational therapists must develop a more efficient system to provide training to aspiring neonatal therapists that will ensure both baseline and advanced competencies.

Case Study 1: Kevin
Medical History

Kevin was a TSGA (2,340 g) male born to a 40-year-old married mother by cesarean section because of an omphalocele diagnosed on prenatal ultrasound; Apgar scores were $5^{1}/7^{5}$. He quickly developed respiratory distress from airway obstruction due to severe micrognathia (small jaw) and neck rigidity in forward flexion; he was unable to be intubated, and a tracheostomy was performed soon after birth.

The following multiple congenital anomalies were noted:

1 Omphalocele: Surgically repaired on his day of birth.
2 Arthrogryposis: Kevin had significant contractures and extreme paucity of spontaneous movement. PROM measurements were taken while Kevin was still chemically paralyzed after his tracheostomy surgery to determine maximal range without active resistance to movement. Both shoulders and elbows had moderate limitations. The wrists and hands were immobile, and the wrists were flexed and in ulnar deviation. The fingers were rigid in metacarpophalangeal (MP) flexion and interphalangeal (IP) extension; they were also swollen and fusiform (muscle atrophy makes joints appear enlarged). Both thumbs were "digitalized" (high placement without true web space, giving the appearance of additional digits). The legs were severely deformed, in a modified tailor position but very adducted with the left leg overlapping the right; washing or inserting a diaper between his legs was difficult. Bilateral greater trochanter prominence

suggested teratologic hip dislocation (occurs early in fetal development and requires surgical correction rather than treatment with a Pavlik harness). The knees were fusiform; clubfeet were rigid.

3 Cervical vertebral anomalies: These limited neck extension, requiring the tracheostomy.

4 Craniofacial anomalies: Webbed neck, severe micrognathia, bilateral complete cleft palate, and significant ankyloglossia ("tongue tied") involving muscular connection in addition to a tight lingual frenulum were noted. The ankyloglossia probably proved beneficial to Kevin after birth by preventing his tongue, already posteriorly placed because of micrognathia, from falling into his pharynx and totally obstructing his airway before the tracheotomy tube was placed.

Occupational Therapy Intervention

Multiple areas of intervention were appropriate for Kevin from birth.

Tracheostomy Ties.   Velfoam ties were made in tan for the tracheostomy tube and in blue for the tracheostomy collar (small oxygen face mask held in place over the tracheostomy tube to provide humidified supplemental oxygen) to avoid confusion and increase safety. The two sets of ties were different lengths; securing the tracheostomy tube with a tie that was too long (i.e., if both sets had been the same color) could allow the tracheostomy tube to pop out.

Splinting.   Bilateral hand splints from three layers of different-density foams were designed for stability without pressure points. These splints encompassed the wrists and MPs, leaving the fingers free. Each splint took only a few seconds to put on or remove; the wearing schedule was 3 hours on, 3 hours off, with good tolerance and no compromise of skin integrity. The splinting goal in the NICU was to provide sustained stretch toward more normal alignment; wrist extension/radial deviation and MP extension increased to almost neutral. A mild increase in IP flexion was obtained with PROM, but spontaneous finger movement was minimal. At the time of transfer to a step-down unit, Kevin's splints maintained wrist and MP correction but no longer provided additional stretch; his therapists in the new unit would continue efforts toward further correction.

Therapeutic Positioning and Passive Range of Motion.   Therapeutic positioning and PROM were important because vigorous early therapy often can improve functional range with arthrogryposis (Hunter, 1990). A thick "bolster" of rolled blankets was wedged between Kevin's legs in the supine and side-lying positions to facilitate hip abduction with hip/knee extension and to prevent skin breakdown where his legs had been folded upon each other. Lateral positioning boundaries attempted to increase leg extension in the supine position; prone positioning on a gel mattress (initially with the hips dangling over the edge of the mattress because

of hip flexion contractures) was initiated a few weeks after birth for variety and to use the combined force of body weight and gravity to further stretch out Kevin's legs.

PROM with sustained stretch was performed by the therapist two or three times a day, initially coordinated with scheduled sedation and then graded according to Kevin's tolerance. Soft relaxation music, rest breaks, NNS with sucrose, and social contact (e.g., touch, talking, eye contact) were used to soothe Kevin during PROM as needed. Nurses did some stretching at each diaper change; the therapist taught Kevin's family PROM techniques, but they were reluctant to assume this part of his care in the NICU. The combined effects of gravity, caregiving, some spontaneous movement, therapeutic positioning, and PROM resulted in significant increases in hip range (extension and abduction) and knee extension (Figure 20-30).

Development.   Monitoring of Kevin's neurobehavioral status with appropriate environmental and caregiving modifications and developmental stimulation were ongoing priorities. Although Kevin was born at term, the NICU still is an overwhelming environment, and he initially required protection from avoidable stressors of light, noise, and caregiving practices. He was easily stressed by caregiving but calmed to his pacifier, containment, holding, and eventually to both gavage and oral feeding.

Kevin's facial expression lacked variety and typically appeared "worried." He was able to visually focus, but visual tracking was poor because of his limited neck mobility and perhaps because of decreased ocular mobility, noted by an ophthalmologist. Kevin calmed to gentle voices and soothing music. He enjoyed being held and recognized his family and familiar caregivers.

Feeding.   After thorough tracheotomy suctioning by his nurse (because of excessive secretions with respiratory distress and agitation), the potential for oral feeding was first assessed at 2 weeks of age. A drop of blue food dye was added to the formula; blue froth bubbling from the tracheostomy tube or blue-tinged secretions suctioned from his tracheostomy tube after nippling would be a clear indication of aspiration below the level of his vocal cords.

Kevin demonstrated normal rooting, latched on to the nipple, and had weak but rhythmic sucking bursts of 6 to 8 sucks with intermittent rest pauses. Feeding considerations included the following:

- Medical status: Kevin had good days and bad days regarding physiologic stability, which invariably affected feeding.
- Positioning: Kevin could orally feed only when held in an upright sitting position; he became agitated and disorganized if anyone tried to feed him semireclined.
- Weak stripping of formula from the nipple: This resulted from compromised suction and compression

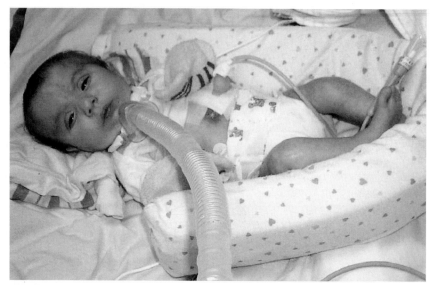

FIGURE 20-30 Term small for gestational age (SGA) infant, who was born with multiple anomalies and required a combined approach of rehabilitation and developmental support, now is ready to go home. (Courtesy Infant Special Care Unit, University of Texas Medical Branch, Galveston, Texas.)

from the cleft palate; a Haberman feeder was used to compensate.

- Ankyloglossia: Tongue mobility (elevation, protrusion, retraction) was significantly limited, resulting in poor oral bolus control and excessive leakage during oral feeding. A plastic surgeon and the cleft palate team did not consider surgical release necessary at this time.
- Endurance: Kevin consistently tired quickly even with increased oxygen during oral feeding.

After suctioning, Kevin calmed to oral feeding if fed by a familiar caregiver. Kevin was fed to tolerance because of his limited and variable endurance, typically taking 30 to 35 ml in 10 minutes for the therapist and 10 ml in 10 minutes for his mother. Because Kevin was unable to consume sufficient volume for nutritional needs, a feeding gastrostomy was placed, with the recommendation that it be used exclusively for night feedings (to allow the family maximal rest) and that daytime feedings include oral intake to tolerance with the remainder given by gastrostomy. Once Kevin recovered from surgery for the gastrostomy, he was transferred from the NICU to a step-down unit to allow active family participation in preparation for discharge.

Parent Support and Education. Family education and support were ongoing and challenging. Travel time was 2 hours each way, Kevin's father worked 6 days a week, and his teenage siblings were in school; the family usually was able to come to the hospital only during evenings and weekends until school was out for the summer.

The family was accepting and involved but overwhelmed by Kevin's functional problems and medical needs. They were more comfortable observing care than participating; involvement of the family in Kevin's routine daily care was slow and took precedence over their involvement in therapy needs. Kevin's mother was emotionally fragile and easily overwhelmed; she required much patient reinforcement over several weeks. Kevin's sister was very attentive, willing to help care for "her baby," and definitely the most successful in eliciting social responsiveness in Kevin.

Because Kevin's care was complex and the family was hesitant to assume full responsibility, he was transferred to a step-down unit for 5 weeks before eventual hospital discharge. Full-time home nursing care was arranged for the first week at home to further ease the transition and to provide medical support and backup to the family.

Referral to Early Intervention. Kevin was referred to early intervention at hospital discharge and was scheduled for ongoing follow-up in a hospital chronic care clinic that coordinates medical and developmental services for medically complex children. A future muscle biopsy was planned to assess muscle composition and assist with formulation of a realistic functional prognosis.

Case Study 2: Elizabeth
Medical History

Elizabeth was a PTSGA/IUGR female born at 27 weeks' gestation to a 27-year-old married mother with PIH and oligohydramnios. Her birth weight was 500 g; Apgar scores were $8^1/9^5$.

Elizabeth's hospital course was complicated. Her extreme prematurity and fetal compression from maternal oligohydramnios resulted in pulmonary hypoplasia;

she developed respiratory distress syndrome (RDS), which progressed to severe bronchopulmonary dysplasia (BPD) with atelectasis. She required a double-volume exchange blood transfusion for hyperbilirubinemia and several transfusions for anemia. A right atrial mass, thought to be a thrombus, was discovered several weeks after birth but resolved spontaneously. Multiple episodes of suspected sepsis required antibiotics. She developed stage 3, zone I ROP and underwent successful laser surgery of both eyes to prevent retinal detachment.

Chronic abdominal distention and feeding intolerance required long-term total parenteral nutrition (TPN), which contributed to progressive cholestatic jaundice with subsequent ascites and hepatosplenomegaly. A barium enema at 5 months suggested partial obstruction caused by scarring or global dysfunction compatible with prematurity. Advancement of enteral feedings by continuous drip progressed at a conservative rate; bone demineralization from Elizabeth's compromised nutritional status and prolonged illness was a concern.

Elizabeth remained ventilator dependent because of severe BPD and bilateral atelectasis, caused in part by internal compression from continued abdominal distention. Weaning from the ventilator was finally successful $6\frac{1}{2}$ months after birth, with rapid subsequent medical progress and discharge to home 7 weeks later with an apnea monitor and oxygen by nasal cannula (NC). Elizabeth's chronologic age was 8 months (corrected age, 5 months) at the time of discharge.

Occupational Therapy Intervention

First $6\frac{1}{2}$ Months: Orally Intubated and Ventilator Dependent

Elizabeth's extreme prematurity and immature CNS severely compromised her ability to cope within the NICU, a situation complicated by prolonged critical illness requiring intensive nursing care and aggressive respiratory treatments. The balance between medical priorities and attempts to reduce stimuli and protect sleep was often elusive.

Neonatal Individualized Developmental Care and Assessment Program (NIDCAP) observations documented frequent physiologic and motoric stress signals in response to direct caregiving and environmental impulse noise (e.g., monitor alarms, telephones). Elizabeth's early care plan emphasized protection, with environmental (light, noise) and caregiving modifications.

She eventually was moved to a small, glass-enclosed room that allowed greater flexibility in protecting her from excessive traffic and environmental stresses; she remained in "Elizabeth's room" for several months.

Therapeutic positioning was provided to reduce stress from postural insecurity, minimize positional deformities, facilitate development of extremity flexor tone, and encourage midline orientation. Because Elizabeth

developed an increasing tendency to self-extubate in the prone position as her energy and activity level improved, prone opportunities were limited after the first few months; side-lying, supine, and reclining in a bouncy infant seat were the primary positioning options. She was typically swaddled in blankets in a Snuggle-Up to conserve heat, facilitate growth, prevent extubation, facilitate flexion, and provide calming. Spontaneous movement was restricted, therefore Elizabeth was unwrapped for supervised "exercise" periods of free movement several times a day. At 3 months' corrected age, fine motor activities were incorporated into free play time to encourage reach, grasp, hand-to-hand, and supervised hand-to-mouth activities.

As state regulation improved, Elizabeth appeared to recognize favorite caregivers and calmed to a human voice or soft music. Toys were changed frequently to provide novelty of visual and auditory stimuli. Propping in a Boppy pillow or reclining in the bouncy infant seat gave Elizabeth different perspectives on her world.

Elizabeth demonstrated low tolerance and significant stress to any tactile input, including social touch, possibly because of months of necessary medical procedures and constant swaddling that provided proprioceptive input but minimal tactile variety. This problem was approached slowly, first by giving gentle pressure or patting through the swaddling, doing swaddled baths, and having Elizabeth hold on to an adult's finger. Her extremities initially were contained to prevent a startle response when she was unswaddled for "exercise time," and some gentle but firm massage techniques gradually were incorporated. The therapist, nurses, and Elizabeth's parents held her when possible.

Elizabeth became more tolerant of touch but exhibited tongue thrusting with no sustained or rhythmic NNS on a pacifier. Prefeeding oral stimulation was complicated by prolonged oral intubation, an indwelling orogastric feeding tube for drip feedings, and the tape securing these tubes. It was anticipated that eventual transition to oral feedings would be slow.

Transportation difficulties limited hospital visits by Elizabeth's family. Phone calls between parents and staff members were frequent, and pictures of Elizabeth were taken regularly.

From $6\frac{1}{2}$ Months to Hospital Discharge: Off the Ventilator.
Elizabeth finally weaned from the ventilator to an oxyhood to a nasal cannula. She was on continuous drip feedings of Pregestamil with additives to increase the caloric density of the formula.

Elizabeth's developmental progress and paucity of anticipated problems during this stage were impressive. She tolerated handling without difficulty. She was given loose boundaries but seemed to enjoy the new freedom to move. The "imposed" flexion from prolonged swaddling had minimized positional deformities and now seemed to facilitate motor skill development. Elizabeth had normal tone with good midline orientation. In the supine position she demonstrated upper extremity antigravity flexion in the midline, hand-to-hand play, mouthing of the hands, and visual observation of hand movements. Leg lifting into the air developed within a month; she also had no head lag in pull-to-sit at this time. Initially Elizabeth would tolerate the prone position only while sleeping, but by the time of discharge, 7 weeks after extubation, she was propping on the forearms, lifting her head consistently to 45 degrees (90 degrees with visual stimuli), and rolling purposely from prone to supine with appropriate quality and components of movement.

Surprisingly, Elizabeth had minimal aversive behaviors to oral stimulation. She mouthed her hands frequently, mouthed toys when assisted, and accepted oral stimulation used to decrease excessive tongue protrusion and increase tongue shaping (midline grooving). Strong tongue protrusion is common in infants with prolonged oral intubation because they lick and push against the endotracheal tube; this is different from the neurologic tongue thrust seen in cerebral palsy. Elizabeth's pacifier sucking remained poor because of tongue protrusion.

Oral feeding, begun less than 2 weeks after extubation, initially was difficult because of her thick, protruding tongue. Within a week of the start of oral feedings, the therapist was able intermittently to inhibit tongue protrusion and elicit sucking bursts of 10 to 12 sucks, with good rhythm and efficient stripping. Because these sucking bursts were not consecutive, the feeding time was long (40 ml in 20 minutes). Within 2 to 3 weeks, Elizabeth began oral feedings eagerly but would abruptly stop and fight nipple insertion. The neonatologist agreed to a trial switch from Pregestamil to stock formula (initially diluted until tolerance was established); that feeding was completed in 5 minutes. Elizabeth's feeding resistance vanished, which suggests that taste was the problem. She continued to feed with good coordination, taking 90 ml in 20 minutes when discharged.

Although many infants with BPD tend to be irritable, Elizabeth had a delightful personality (Figure 20-31). She was social, loved to be held, and would generally fuss only if left to entertain herself for longer than 20 to 30 minutes. She took "field trips" with her therapist to visit staff members in other sections of the NICU and even went outside to see a Christmas tree (no snow; 75° F).

Initially rare smiles became spontaneous and frequent; vocalizations remained soft and infrequent. Elizabeth progressed so rapidly that she was not transferred to a step-down unit before hospital discharge. Her family came to the hospital more often as discharge approached and readily assumed Elizabeth's care; she went home at 8 months of age (5 months' corrected age) with a pictorial "biographic poster" assembled by the staff.

Because of Elizabeth's increased risk for developmental delay secondary to prematurity and severity of illness,

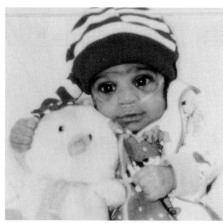

FIGURE 20-31 Elizabeth, who weighed 500 g (1 pound, $1\frac{1}{2}$ ounces) at birth, is finally ready to go home after 8 months in the NICU. Her development was nearly appropriate for her corrected age at the time of discharge. (Courtesy Infant Special Care Unit, University of Texas Medical Branch, Galveston, Texas; photograph by Jackie Lohner.)

she was referred to a local early intervention program. She developed into a charming and social child; she wears glasses for nearsightedness, demonstrates a speech delay and mild learning disabilities, and occasionally is somewhat clumsy.

Case Study 3: Connor
Hospital Course

Connor was born at 22 weeks' gestation by spontaneous vaginal delivery to a teenage mother with a history of polysubstance abuse, preterm labor, and suspected chorioamnionitis. His birth weight was 540 g, and his Apgars were 1^1 at 1 and 5 minutes. He was limp and blue and had a very low heart rate and two agonal respirations in 5 minutes. As per parental agreement for no heroics at this stage of extreme prematurity, Connor was dried, wrapped, held by his parents, then taken to the NICU for observation and comfort care. Over the next hour, he defied all odds as his heart rate spontaneously increased to 110 beats per minute and his respiratory rate to 37; life support measures were then initiated, with much staff concern.

Connor initially was extremely fragile, responding to even gentle caregiving with tachypnea, desaturations, and a variable heart rate; spontaneous movement was minimal. By 28 weeks PCA, Connor had been weaned to nasal continuous positive airway pressure (CPAP); he remained on mild sedation but was motorically more active, with frequent squirming and jerky extremity movements. Mild dolichocephaly and external rotation of the upper and lower extremities were emerging despite positioning efforts. He was now awake for brief periods, with unfocused alertness; some weak vocalization and mouthing movements were noted.

By 32 weeks PCA, Connor was on a nasal cannula and was assessed by an occupational therapist, who used the Dubowitz Neonatal Neurological Examination. Muscle tone was variable, depending on the state of arousal, but it generally was good for his age. Flexor tone was greater in the lower than the upper extremities, demonstrating the expected caudocephalic progression of tone development. He had minimal head lag in pull-to-sit (advanced for age), with head righting forward and backward. Movements were primarily generalized stretching or large excursion and jerky. Connor stirred and occasionally fussed with caregiving; he calmed to containment and a pacifier, although his NNS was weak and irregular, with increased tongue protrusion.

At $33\frac{1}{2}$ weeks, movements continued to be large excursion, jerky, and tremulous; head control remained increased for his age. Smoother transitions were noted between sleep and awake states, and definitive "brightening" was noted to a rattle. Although NNS remained poor, Connor was stable enough for a trial of oral feeding. Feeding was better than expected; Connor demonstrated fairly sustained rhythmic sucking bursts of 8 to 20 sucks and good autonomic stability. Stripping of milk from the nipple was decreased because of lingual mechanics (decreased central groove, increased protrusion) and "chomping"; leakage was excessive at 8 ml of a 34 ml volume.

Connor did surprisingly well with several oral feedings over the next 3 days, progressing to 34 ml in 10 minutes with only mild leakage. At this point, major desaturations, with very slow recovery, after eye dilation and an eye examination at 34 weeks PCA caused oral feedings to be deferred for several days; Connor generally was asleep, with decreased energy and motor activity, during this time. When bottle feedings resumed the following week, Connor took 43 ml in 9 minutes. He started with an immature sucking pattern and required external pacing because of eagerness, then progressed to a mature sucking pattern with self-pacing; leakage was minimal with chin support.

Connor was on an apnea countdown (apnea free for 7 days) for an intended hospital discharge at 36 weeks' PCA when he began having significant desaturations associated with feedings; upper gastrointestinal and modified barium swallow studies were ordered to rule out gastroesophageal reflux and aspiration. He demonstrated frequent laryngeal penetration (formula penetrating the laryngeal vestibule, or voice box, without moving below the vocal cords); occasional flash aspiration to the lower level of the vocal cords, which cleared spontaneously; and significant reflux to the oropharynx. No physiologic instability was noted until desaturation occurred with reflux. Connor was placed on formula with added rice, desaturations decreased, and he was discharged from the hospital 4 days later at $36\frac{1}{2}$ weeks PCA.

Connor's medical diagnoses included extreme prematurity, ULBW, hypotension, metabolic acidosis, pulmonary insufficiency, RDS, BPD, PIE, PDA, PPS, AOP, adrenal suppression, glucose intolerance, hyperbilirubinemia, anemia, thrombocytopenia, clinical sepsis, GER, stage 1-2 ROP, and colpocephaly by head ultrasound ×3 (prominent ventricles). He passed his BSER.

Developmental Outcome

The initial emphasis of occupational therapy was solely protective developmental support (i.e., therapeutic positioning, environmental modifications to reduce light and noise, infant support during procedures, parent education and support). Connor's evolving medical status, neuromotor activity, emerging arousal/attention, and generally disorganized (but gradually improving) behaviors guided advancement of occupational therapy interventions and goals (i.e., tolerance to handling, therapeutic positioning and neuromotor control, attention/interaction, self-regulation, oral feeding). His mother worked but came to the hospital regularly and was comfortable and confident caring for Connor. Developmental concerns at discharge included mild hypertonicity, tremors, irritability, poor self-regulation, and questionable visual attention. He was referred to an early childhood intervention (ECI) program; his mother reported that phone contact was made, but no assessment was ever completed.

Connor returned for developmental follow-up at premie clinic at 34 weeks' chronologic age with a corrected age of 16 weeks; skills in all areas were within the 16- to 20-week range (Figure 20-32). Muscle tone was globally increased (i.e., some fisting, strong shoulder retraction, intermittent scissoring in standing) with decreased ease of movement, increased active effort, and occasional tremors), but tone had not yet interfered with achievement of developmental skills appropriate for corrected age.

Connor is a happy, social infant who easily smiles, laughs, squeals, and grunts. He visibly excites to a novel toy, reaches against gravity with both hands, tries to hold his bottle, looks at a toy held in his hand, takes the toy to his mouth when supine, and looks for a dropped toy. He lifts his head to 90 degrees with partly extended arms in the prone position, lifts his legs against gravity in the supine position, has no head lag in pull-to-sit, holds his head steady in supported sitting, and can maintain propped sitting briefly once placed.

Because he is developmentally appropriate for his corrected age, he does not currently qualify for a re-referral to ECI. A home program was established with his very involved mother, and Connor will be reassessed at the clinic in 2 months. Concerns still exist, but Connor has once more amazed the adults in his life with his incredible progress against very stiff odds. His outcome is not

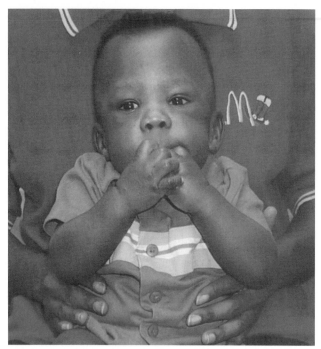

FIGURE 20-32 Infant born at 22 weeks' gestation is brought to premie clinic for developmental follow-up at corrected age of 16 weeks (chronologic age of 34 weeks). (Photograph courtesy Teri Tullous, Galveston, Texas.)

typical, but not impossible, for the extremely small and premature infant.

STUDY QUESTIONS

1 Using the description of Cody (see p. 692 and Appendices 20-A and 20-B), provide the medical terms for each of the abbreviations. Explain the implications of each medical condition that represents a potential threat to Cody's development.
2 Explain how environmental light and sound levels pose a threat to the vulnerable newborn. Describe several intervention strategies that modify light and auditory input for an individual infant.
3 What issues complicate parenting in the NICU?
4 Describe published assessments and informal methods for evaluating the following aspects of infant function and behavior:
   a Neurobehavioral organization
   b Neuromotor development
5 For each general positioning goal listed below, describe how to meet the goal using a prone, supine, or side-lying position.
   a To provide proprioceptive input to increase the infant's sense of containment

b To reduce premie positional deformities, increase postural flexion, and facilitate midline orientation
   c To promote calming and behavioral organization
   d To assist in the development of hand-to-mouth movements
6 What are common feeding problems for preterm infants in the NICU? Describe appropriate interventions to help resolve these problems.

REFERENCES

Aita, M., & Snide, L. (2003). The art of developmental care in the NICU: A concept analysis. *Journal of Advanced Nursing, 41,* 223-232.

Albritton, S., Acosta, D., Bellinger, D., Farmer, D., Goodwin, L., Heinrich, R., Hollingsworth, C., Kakimoto, J., Lotter, S., Raval, D.S. (Ed.), Campbell, S. (Ed.), Ratzan, P. (Ed.), McGinnis, J. (Ed.), Urrutia, I. (1998). *You are not alone: The NICU experience.* Norwell, MA: Children's Medical Ventures.

Als, H. (1982). Toward a synactive theory of development: Promise for the assessment and support of infant individuality. *Infant Mental Health Journal, 3,* 229-243.

Als, H. (1986). A synactive model of neonatal behavior organization: Framework for the assessment of neurobehavioral development in the premature infant and for support of infants and parents in the neonatal intensive care environment. *Physical and Occupational Therapy in Pediatrics, 6,* 3-55.

Als, H. (1998). Developmental care in the newborn intensive care unit. *Current Opinion in Pediatrics, 10,* 138-142.

Als, H., & Gilkerson, L. (1997). The role of relationship-based developmentally supportive newborn intensive care in strengthening outcome of preterm infants. *Seminars in Perinatology, 21,* 178-189.

Als, H., Lawhon, G., Brown, E., Gibes, R., Duffy, F., McAnulty, G., & Blickman, J. (1986). Individualized behavioral and environmental care for the very low birth weight preterm infant at high risk for bronchopulmonary dysplasia: Neonatal intensive care unit and developmental outcome. *Pediatrics, 78,* 1123-1132.

Als, H., Lawhon, G., Duffy, F.H., McAnulty, G.B., Gibes-Grossman, R., & Blickman, J.G. (1994). Individualized developmental care for the very low-birth-weight preterm infant. *Journal of the American Medical Association, 272,* 853-858.

Altimier, L. (2002). Management of the NICU environment. In C. Kenner & J.W. Lott (Eds.), *Comprehensive neonatal nursing care* (pp. 229-235). St. Louis: Mosby.

American Academy of Pediatrics. (1998). Policy statement: Hospital discharge of the high-risk neonate—proposed guidelines (RE9812). *Pediatrics, 102,* 411-417.

American Academy of Pediatrics, Committee on Environmental Health. (1997). Policy statement: Noise, a hazard for the fetus and newborn (RE9728). *Pediatrics, 100,* 724-727.

American Academy of Pediatrics, Task Force on Infant Sleep Position and SIDS. (2000). Changing concepts of sudden infant death syndrome: Implications for infant sleeping environment and sleep position. *Pediatrics, 105,* 650-656.

American Medical Association (AMA). (1971). *Centralized community or regionalized perinatal intensive care* (Report J). Adopted by the AMA House of Delegates, June, 1971.

American Occupational Therapy Association. (2000). *Knowledge and skills for occupational therapy practice in the neonatal intensive care unit* (Rev.). Bethesda, MD: AOTA.

Amiel-Tison, C. (2002). Update of the Amiel-Tison neurologic assessment for the term neonate or at 40 weeks' corrected age. *Pediatric Neurology, 27,* 196-212.

Amiel-Tison, C., & Grenier, A. (1986). *Neurological assessment during the first year of life.* New York: Oxford University Press.

Ancona, J., Shaker, C.S., Puhek, J., & Garland, J.S. (1998). PI3: Performance improvement, ideas and innovations. Improving outcomes through a developmental approach to nipple feeding. *Journal of Nursing Care Quality, 12,* 1-4.

Argenta, L., David, L., Wilson, J., & Bell, W. (1996). An increase in infant cranial deformity with supine sleeping position. *Journal of Craniofacial Surgery, 7,* 5-11.

Ash, S.P., & Moss, J.P. (1987). An investigation of the features of the preterm infant palate and the effect of prolonged oral intubation with and without protective appliances. *British Journal of Orthodontics, 14,* 253-261.

Ashpaugh, A., & Leick-Rude, M.K. (1999). Developmental care teams in the neonatal intensive care unit: Survey on current status. *Journal of Perinatology, 19,* 48-52.

Aucott, S., Donohue, P.K., Atkins, E., & Allen, M.C. (2002). Neurodevelopmental care in the NICU. *Mental Retardation and Developmental Disabilities Research Reviews, 8,* 298-308.

Auerbach, K.G., & Walker, M. (1994). When the mother of a premature infant uses a breast pump: What every NICU nurse needs to know. *Neonatal Network, 13,* 23-29.

Baker, J.G. (1995). Commentary: Parents as partners in the NICU. *Neonatal Network, 14,* 9-10.

Ballweg, D.D. (2001). Implementing developmentally supportive family-centered care in the newborn intensive care unit as a quality improvement initiative. *Journal of Perinatal and Neonatal Nursing, 15,* 58-73.

Beachy, J.M. (2003). Premature infant massage in the NICU. *Neonatal Network, 22,* 39-45.

Benis, M.M. (2002). Efficacy of sucrose as analgesia for procedural pain in neonates. *Advances in Neonatal Care, 2,* 93-100.

Berens, R.J., & Weigle, C.G.M. (1997). Noise analysis of three newborn infant Isolettes. *Journal of Perinatology, 17,* 351-354.

Bernbaum, J.C., Pereira, G.R., Watkins, J.B., & Peckman, G.J. (1983). Non-nutritive sucking during gavage feeding enhances growth and maturation in premature infants. *Pediatrics, 71,* 41-45.

Bhutta, A.T., & Anand, K.J. (2002). Vulnerability of the developing brain: Neuronal mechanisms. *Clinics in Perinatology, 29* (3), 357-372.

Bingham, P.M., Abassi, S., & Sivieri, E. (2003). A pilot study of milk odor effect on nonnutritive sucking by premature newborns. *Archives of Pediatrics and Adolescent Medicine, 157,* 72-75.

Black, J.E. (1998). How a child builds its brain: Some lessons from animal studies of neural plasticity. *Preventive Medicine, 27,* 168-171.

Blackburn, S.T. (2003). Neuromuscular and sensory systems. In *Maternal, fetal, and neonatal physiology: A clinical perspective* (2nd ed., pp. 546-598). Philadelphia: WB Saunders.

Blumenthal, I., Lealman, G., & Shoesmith, D. (1989). Effect of feeding temperature and phototherapy on gastric emptying. *Archives of Disease in Childhood, 55,* 562-574.

Boere-Boonekamp, M.M., vander Linden-Kuiper, A.T., & van Es, P. (1997). Preferential posture in infants: Serious demands on health care. *Nederlands Tijdschr voor Geneeskd, 141,* 769-772.

Bohnhorst, B., Heyne, T., Peter, C.S., & Poets, C.F. (2001). Skin-to-skin (kangaroo) care, respiratory control, and thermoregulation. *Journal of Pediatrics, 138,* 193-197.

Bosma, J.F. (1986). Development of feeding. *Clinical Nutrition, 5,* 210-218.

Bottos, M., & Stefani, D. (1982). Postural motor care of the premature baby. *Developmental Medicine and Child Neurology, 5,* 706-707.

Brake, S.C., & Fifer, W.P. (1988). The first nutritive sucking responses of premature newborns. *Infant Behavior and Development, 11,* 1-19.

Brandon, D.H., Holditch-Davis, D., & Belyea, M. (2002). Preterm infants born at less than 31 weeks' gestation have improved growth in cycled light compared with continuous near darkness. *Journal of Pediatrics, 140,* 192-199.

Browne, J.V. (2000). Developmental care: Considerations for touch and massage in the neonatal intensive care unit. *Neonatal Network, 19,* 61-64.

Browne, J.V., VandenBerg, K., Ross, E.S., & Elmore, A.M. (1999). The newborn developmental specialist: Definition, qualifications and preparation for an emerging role in the neonatal intensive care unit. *Infants and Young Children, 11,* 53-64.

Bu'Lock, F., Woolridge, M.W., & Baum, J.D. (1990). Development of coordination of sucking, swallowing and breathing: Ultrasound study of term and preterm infants. *Developmental Medicine and Child Neurology, 32,* 669-678.

Budreau, G.K. (1989). The perceived attractiveness of preterm infants with cranial molding. *Journal of Obstetric, Gynecologic, and Neonatal Nursing, 18,* 38-44.

Buehler, D., Als, H., Duffy, F., McAnulty, G., & Liederman, J. (1995). Effectiveness of individualized developmental care for low-risk preterm infants: Behavioral and electrophysiologic evidence. *Pediatrics, 96,* 923-932.

Bullough, J., & Rea, M. (1996). Lighting for neonatal intensive care units: Some critical information for design. *Lighting Research Technology, 28,* 189-198.

Burke, M., Oehler, J., Walsh, J., & Gingras, J. (1995). Music therapy following suctioning: Four case studies. *Neonatal Network, 14,* 41-49.

Burklow, K.A., McGrath, A.M., & Kaul, A. (2002). Management and prevention of feeding problems in young children with prematurity and very low birth weight. *Infants and Young Children, 14,* 19-30.

Burns, K., Cunningham, N., White-Traut, R., Silvestri, J., & Nelson, M.N. (1994). Infant stimulation: Modification of an intervention based on physiologic and behavioral cues.

Journal of Obstetric, Gynecologic, and Neonatal Nursing, 23, 581-589.

Butt, M.L., & Kisilevsky, B.S. (2000). Music modulates behaviour of premature infants following heel lance. *Canadian Journal of Nursing Research, 31,* 17-39.

Byers, J.F. (2003). Components of developmental care and the evidence for their use in the NICU. *American Journal of Maternal and Child Nursing, 28,* 174-180.

Cagan, J. (1995). Feeding readiness behavior in preterm infants (abstract). *Neonatal Network, 14,* 82.

Caine, J. (1991). The effects of music on the selected stress behaviors, weight, caloric and formula intake, and length of hospital stay of premature and low birth weight neonates in a newborn intensive care unit. *Journal of Music Therapy, 28,* 180-192.

Case-Smith, J. (1988). An efficacy study of occupational therapy with high-risk neonates. *American Journal of Occupational Therapy, 42,* 499-506.

Chadduck, W.M., Kast, J., & Donahue, D.J. (1997). The enigma of lambdoid positional molding. *Pediatric Neurosurgery, 26,* 304-311.

Chang, Y.J., Lin, C.H., & Lin, L.H. (2001). Noise and related events in a neonatal intensive care unit. *Acta Paediatrica, 42,* 212-217.

Charpak, N., Ruiz-Pelaez, J.G., de Figueroa, C.Z., & Charpak, Y. (2001). A randomized, controlled trial of kangaroo mother care: Results of follow-up at 1 year of corrected age. *Pediatrics, 108,* 1072-1079.

Chermak, G., Somers, E., & Seikel, J. (1998). Behavioral signs of central auditory processing disorder and attention deficit hyperactivity disorder. *Journal of the American Academy of Audiology 9,* 78-84.

Clum, D., & Primomo, J. (1996). Use of a silicone nipple shield with premature infants. *Journal of Human Lactation, 12,* 287-290.

Comrie, J.D., & Helm, J.M. (1997). Common feeding problems in the intensive care nursery: Maturation, organization, evaluation and management strategies. *Seminars in Speech & Language, 18,* 239-261.

Conde-Agudelo, A., Diaz-Rossello, J.L., & Belizan, J.M. (2003). Kangaroo mother care to reduce morbidity and mortality in low birthweight infants (Cochrane Review). In *The Cochrane Library,* Issue 1. Oxford: Update Software.

Costello, A., Bracht, M., Van Camp, K., & Carman, L. (1996). Parent information binder: Individualizing education for parents of preterm infants. *Neonatal Network, 15,* 43-46.

Craig, C.M., Lee, D.N., Freer, Y.N., & Laing, I.A. (1999). Modulations in breathing patterns during intermittent feeding in term infants and preterm infants with bronchopulmonary dysplasia. *Developmental Medicine and Child Neurology, 41,* 616-624.

Daley, H.K., & Kennedy, C.M. (2000). Meta analysis: Effects of interventions on premature infants feeding. *Journal of Perinatal and Neonatal Nursing, 14,* 62-77.

Dargassies, S.S. (1977). *Neurological development in the full-term and premature neonate.* New York: Excerpta Medica.

Davis, B.E., Moon, R.Y., Sachs, H.C., & Ottoline, M.C. (1998). Effects of sleep position on infant motor development. *Pediatrics, 102,* 1135-1140.

Davis, P.M., Robinson, R., Harris, L., & Cartlidge, P.H.T. (1993). Persistent mild hip deformation in preterm infants. *Archives of Disease in Childhood, 69,* 597-598.

de Groot, L., Hopkins, B., & Touwen, B. (1997). Motor asymmetries in preterm infants at 18 weeks' corrected age and outcomes at 1 year. *Early Human Development, 48,* 35-46.

DePaul, D., & Chambers, S.E. (1995). Environmental noise in the neonatal intensive care unit: Implications for nursing practice. *Journal of Perinatal and Neonatal Nursing, 8,* 71-76.

Dewey, C., Fleming, P., & Golding, J. (1998). Does the supine sleeping position have any adverse effects on the child? Development in the first 18 months. *Pediatrics Electronic Pages, 101,* E5.

Dewire, A., White, D., Kanny, E., & Glass, R. (1996). Education and training of occupational therapists for neonatal intensive care units. *American Journal of Occupational Therapy, 50,* 486-494.

Dias, M.S., Klein, D.M., & Backstrom, J.W. (1996). Occipital plagiocephaly: Deformation or lambdoid synostosis. I and II. *Pediatric Neurosurgery, 24,* 61-68.

Dieter, J.N.I., & Emory, E.K. (1997). Supplemental stimulation of preterm infants: A treatment model. *Journal of Pediatric Psychology, 22,* 281-295.

DiPietro, J.A. (2000). Baby and the brain: Advances in child development. *Annual Review of Public Health, 21,* 455-471.

DiPietro, J.A., Cusson, R.M., Caughy, M.O., & Fox, N.A. (1994). Behavioral and physiologic effects of nonnutritive sucking during gavage feeding in preterm infants. *Pediatric Research, 36,* 207-214.

Downs, J.A., Edwards, A.D., McCormick, D.C., Roth, S.C., & Stewart, A.L. (1991). Effect of intervention on development of hip posture in very preterm babies. *Archives of Disease in Childhood, 66,* 797-801.

Drosten, F. (1997). Pacifiers in the NICU: A lactation consultant's point of view. *Neonatal Network, 16,* 47, 50.

Eichenwald, E.C., Blackwell, M., Lloyd, J.S., Tran, T., Wilker, R.E., & Richardson, D.K. (2001). Inter-neonatal intensive care unit variation in discharge timing: Influence of apnea and feeding management. *Pediatrics, 108,* 928-933.

Einarsson-Backes, L.M., Deitz, J., Price, R., Glass, R., & Hays, R. (1994). The effect of oral support on sucking efficiency in preterm infants. *American Journal of Occupational Therapy, 48,* 490-498.

Elliman, A.M., Bryan, E.M., Elliman, A.D., & Starte, D. (1986). Narrow heads of preterm infants: Do they matter? *Developmental Medicine and Child Neurology, 28,* 745-748.

Engebretson, J. (1997). Development of a pacifier for low-birth-weight infants' nonnutritive sucking. *Journal of Obstetric, Gynecologic, and Neonatal Nursing, 26,* 660-664.

Engler, A.J., Ludington-Hoe, S.M., Cusson, R.M., Adams, R., Bahnsen, M., Brambaugh, E., Coates, P., Grieb, J., McHargue, L., Ryan, D.L., Settle, M., & Williams, D. (2002). Kangaroo care: National survey of practice, knowledge, barriers, and perceptions. *MCN, American Journal of Maternal Child Nursing, 27,* 146-153.

Fay, M.J. (1988). The positive effects of positioning. *Neonatal Network, 8,* 23-29.

Feher, S.D.K., Berger, L.R., Johnson, J.D., & Wilde, J.B. (1989). Increasing breast milk production for premature infants with a relaxation/imagery audiotape. *Pediatrics, 83,* 57-61.

Feldman, R., & Eidelman, A.I. (2003). Skin-to-skin contact (kangaroo care) accelerates autonomic and neurobehavioural maturation in preterm infants. *Developmental Medicine and Child Neurology, 45,* 274-281.

Feldman, R., Eidelman, A.I., Sirota, L., & Weller, A. (2002). Comparison of skin-to-skin (kangaroo) and traditional care: Parenting outcomes and preterm infant development. *Pediatrics, 110(1 Pt 1),* 16-26.

Ferber, S.G., Kuint, J., Weller, A., Feldman, R., Dollberg, S., Arbel, E., & Kohelet, D. (2002). Massage therapy by mothers and trained professionals enhances weight gain in preterm infants. *Early Human Development, 67,* 37-45.

Fern, D., & Graves, C. (1996). *Infants in the NICU.* Norwell, MA: Children's Medical Ventures.

Fern, D., Graves, C., & L'Huillier, M. (2002). Swaddled bathing in the newborn intensive care unit. *Newborn and Infant Nursing Reviews, 2,* 3-4.

Field, T. (1995). Massage therapy for infants and children. *Developmental and Behavioral Pediatrics, 16,* 105-111.

Fielder, A.R., & Moseley, M.J. (2000). Environmental light and the preterm infant. *Seminars in Perinatology, 24,* 291-298.

Fisher, C., & Inch, S. (1996). Nipple confusion: Who is confused? (letter). *Journal of Pediatrics, 129,* 174-175.

Fleisher, B., VandenBerg, K., Constantinou, J., Heller, C., Benitz, W., Johnson, A., Rosenthal, A., & Stevenson, D. (1995). Individualized developmental care for very-low-birth-weight premature infants. *Clinical Pediatrics, October,* 523-529.

Fowler, K., Kum-Nji, P., Wells, P.J., & Mangrem, C.L. (1997). Water beds may be useful in preventing scaphocephaly in preterm very low birth weight neonates. *Journal of Perinatology, 17,* 397.

Franck, L.S., Bernal, H., & Gale, G. (2002). Infant holding policies and practices in neonatal units. *Neonatal Network, 21,* 13-20.

Freer, Y. (1999). A comparison of breast and cup feeding in preterm infants: Effect on physiological parameters. *Journal of Neonatal Nursing, 5,* 16-21.

Gaebler, C.P., & Hanzlik, J.R. (1996). The effects of a prefeeding stimulation program on preterm infants. *American Journal of Occupational Therapy, 50,* 184-192.

Gale, G., & Franck, L.S. (1998). Toward a standard of care for parents of infants in the neonatal intensive care unit. *Critical Care Nurse, 18,* 62-74.

Gardner, S.L., & Goldson, E. (2002). The neonate and the environment: Impact on development. In S.L. Merenstein & G.B. Gardner (Eds.), *Handbook of neonatal intensive care* (5th ed., pp. 219-282). St. Louis: Mosby.

Geerdink, J.J., Hopkins, B., & Hoeksma, J.B. (1994). The development of head position in preterm infants beyond term age. *Developmental Psychobiology, 27,* 153-168.

Georgieff, M., & Bernbaum, J. (1986). Abnormal shoulder girdle muscle tone in premature infants during their first 18 months of life. *Pediatrics, 77,* 664-669.

Gerhardt, K.J., & Abrams, R.M. (1996). Fetal hearing: Characterization of the stimulus and response. *Seminars in Perinatology, 20,* 11-20.

Gibbins, S., Stevens, B., Hodnett, E., Pinelli, J., Ohlsson, A., & Darlington, G. (2002). Efficacy and safety of sucrose for procedural pain relief in preterm and term neonates. *Nursing Research, 51,* 375-382.

Glass, P. (1993). Development of visual function in preterm infants: Implications for early intervention. *Infants and Young Children, 6,* 11-20.

Glass, P. (1999). The vulnerable neonate and the neonatal intensive care environment. In G.B. Avery, M.A. Fletcher, & M.G. MacDonald (Eds.), *Neonatology: Pathophysiology and management of the newborn* (5th ed.). Philadelphia: JB Lippincott.

Glass, P. (2002). Development of the visual system and implications for early intervention. *Infants and Young Children, 15,* 1-10.

Glass, R.P., & Wolf, L.S. (1994). A global perspective on feeding assessment in the neonatal intensive care unit. *American Journal of Occupational Therapy, 48,* 514-526.

Glass, R.P., & Wolf, L.S. (1998). Feeding and oral-motor skills. In J. Case-Smith (Ed.), *Pediatric occupational therapy and early intervention* (2nd ed., pp. 127-166). Boston: Butterworth-Heinemann.

Gonzales, I., Duryes, E.J., Vasquez, E., & Geraghty, N. (1995). Effect of enteral feeding temperature on feeding tolerance in preterm infants. *Neonatal Network, 14,* 39-43.

Gonzalez, L., & Dweck, H.S. (1994). Eye of the newborn: A neonatologist's perspective. In S.J. Isenberg (Ed.), *The eye in infancy* (pp. 1-8). St. Louis: Mosby.

Gorski, P.A., Davidson, M.F., & Brazelton, T.B. (1979). Stages of behavioral organization in the high-risk neonate: Theoretical clinical considerations. *Seminars in Perinatology, 3,* 61-72.

Gottfried, A.W. (1985). Environment of newborn infants in special care units. In A.W. Gottfried & J.L. Gaiter (Eds.), *Infant stress under intensive care* (pp. 23-54). Baltimore: University Park Press.

Gottfried, A.W., & Gaiter, J.L. (1985). *Infant stress under intensive care.* Baltimore: University Park Press.

Gottlieb, G., Tomlinson, W.R., & Radell, P.L. (1989). Developmental intersensory interference: Premature visual experience suppresses auditory learning in ducklings. *Infant Behavior and Development, 12,* 1.

Graven, S.N. (2000). Sound and the developing infant in the NICU: Conclusions and recommendations for care. *Journal of Perinatology, 20,* S88-S93.

Graven, S.N. (2002). Early visual development in preterm and term infants. Paper presented at conference on the Physical and Developmental Environment of the High-Risk Infant, Clearwater Beach, FL, January 27-30.

Graven, S.N., Bowen, F., Brooten, D., Eaten, A., Graven, M., Hack, M., Hall, L., Hansen, N., Hurt, H., Kavavhuna, R., Little, G., Mahan, C., Morrow, G., Oehler, J., Poland, R., Ram, B., Sauve, R., Taylor, P., Ward, S., & Sommers, J. (1992). The high-risk environment: I. The role of the neonatal intensive care unit in the outcome of high-risk infants. *Journal of Perinatology, 12,* 164-172.

Gray, L., & Philbin, M.K. (2000). Measuring sound in hospital nurseries. *Journal of Perinatology, 29,* S100-S104.

Grenier, I.R., Bigsby, R., Vergara, E.R., & Lester, B.M. (2003). Comparison of motor self-regulatory and stress behaviors of preterm infants across body positions. *American Journal of Occupational Therapy, 57,* 289-297.

Gressens, P., Rogido, M., Paindaveine, B., & Sola, A. (2002). The impact of neonatal intensive care practices on the developing brain. *Journal of Pediatrics, 14,* 646-653.

Griffin, T.M. (2000). Introduction of a positive touch programme: The value of infant massage. *Journal of Neonatal Nursing, 6,* 112, 114-116.

Grunau, R. (2002). Early pain in preterm infants: A model of long-term effects. *Clinics in Perinatology, 29,* 373-394.

Grunau, R., Holsti, L., Whitfield, M.F., & Ling, E. (2000). Are twitches, startles, and body movements pain indicators in extremely low birth weight infants? *Clinical Journal of Pain, 16,* 37-45.

Hadders-Algra, M., Brogren, E., & Forsberg, H. (1997). Nature and nurture in the development of postural control in human infants. *Acta Paediatrica Supplement, 422,* 48-53.

Hanlon, M.B., Tripp, J.H., Ellis, R.E., Flack, F.C., Selley, W.G., & Shoesmith, H.J. (1997). Deglutition apnea as indicator of maturation of suckle feeding in bottle-fed infants. *Developmental Medicine and Child Neurology, 39,* 534-542.

Harrison, L., Olivet, L., Cunningham, K., Bodin, M.B., & Hicks, C. (1996). Effects of gentle human touch on preterm infants: Pilot study results. *Neonatal Network, 15,* 35-42.

Hawdon, J.M., Beauregard, N., Slattery, J., & Kennedy, G. (2000). Identification of neonates at risk of developing feeding problems in infancy. *Developmental Medicine and Child Neurology, 42,* 235-239.

Heermann, J.A., & Wilson, M.E. (2000). Nurses' experiences working with families in a NICU during implementation of family-focused developmental care. *Neonatal Network, 19,* 23-29.

Heijst, J.J., van Touwen, B.C.L., & Vos, J.E. (1999). Implications of a neural network model of sensorimotor development for the field of developmental neurology. *Early Human Development, 55,* 77-95.

Hendricks-Munoz, K.D., Predergast, C.C., Caprio, M.C., & Wasserman, R.S. (2002). Developmental care: The impact of Wee Care developmental care training on short-term infant outcome and hospital costs. *Newborn and Infant Nursing Reviews, 2,* 39-45.

Hernandez-Reif, M., Field, T., Diego, M., & Beutler, J. (2001). Evidence-based medicine and massage. *Pediatrics, 108,* 1053.

Hill, A.S., Kurkowski, T.B., & Garcia, J. (2000). Oral support measures used in feeding the preterm infant. *Nursing Research, 49,* 2-10.

Hill, P.D., Hanson, K.S., & Mefford, A.L. (1994). Mothers of low birthweight infants: Breastfeeding patterns and problems. *Journal of Human Lactation, 10,* 169-176.

Hodgman, J.E. (1985). Introduction. In A.W. Gottfried & J.L. Gaiter (Eds.), *Infant stress under intensive care* (pp. 1-6). Baltimore: University Park Press.

Holloway, E. (1994). Parent and occupational therapist collaboration in the neonatal intensive care unit. *American Journal of Occupational Therapy, 48,* 535-538.

Hopkins, B., Lems, Y.L., Van Wulften Palthe, T., Hoeksma, J., Kardaun, O., & Butterworth, G. (1990). Development of head position preference during early infancy: A longitudinal study in the daily life situation. *Developmental Psychobiology, 23,* 39-53.

Huang, C-S., Cheng, H-S., Lin, W-Y., Liou, J-W., & Chen, Y-R. (1995). Skull morphology affected by different sleep positions in infancy. *Cleft Palate–Craniofacial Journal, 32,* 413-419.

Huang, M.H., Mouradian, W.E., Cohen, S.R., & Gruss, J.S. (1998). The differential diagnosis of abnormal head shapes: Separating craniosynostosis from positional deformities and normal variants. *Cleft Palate–Craniofacial Journal, 35,* 204-211.

Hubler, E., Demare, D., Cabral, L., Stahl, G., Waber, B., & Imaizumi, S. (1997). Infant regulation of nipple feeding progression. *Pediatrics, 100,* 508S-509S.

Hummel, P. (2002). Parenting the high-risk infant. *Newborn and Infant Nursing Reviews, 3,* 88-92.

Hunter, J.G. (1990). Orthopedic conditions. In C.J. Semmler & J.G. Hunter (Eds.), *Early occupational therapy intervention: Neonates to three years* (pp. 72-123). Gaithersburg: Aspen.

Hunter, J.G. (1996). Clinical interpretation of "education and training of occupational therapists for neonatal intensive care units." *American Journal of Occupational Therapy, 50,* 495-503.

Hunter, J.G., & Malloy, M.H. (2002). Effect of sleep and play positions on infant development: Reconciling developmental concerns with SIDS prevention. *Newborn and Infant Nursing Reviews, 2,* 9-16.

Hunter, J., Mullen, J., & Dallas, D.V. (1994). Medical considerations and practice guidelines for the neonatal occupational therapist. *American Journal of Occupational Therapy, 48,* 546-560.

Hurst, N.M., Valentine, C.J., Renfro, L., Burns, P., & Ferlic, L. (1997). Skin-to-skin holding in the neonatal intensive care unit influences maternal milk volume. *Journal of Perinatology, 17,* 213-217.

Jantz, J.W., Blosser, C.D., & Fruechting, L.A. (1997). A motor milestone change noted with change in sleep position. *Archives Pediatric and Adolescent Medicine, 151,* 565-568.

Jensen, D., Wallace, S., & Kelsay, P. (1994). LATCH: A breastfeeding charting system and documentation tool. *Journal of Obstetric, Gynecologic, and Neonatal Nursing, 23,* 27-32.

Jerger, J., & Musiek, F. (2000). Report of the consensus conference on the diagnosis of auditory processing disorders in school-aged children. *Journal of the American Academy of Audiology, 11,* 467-474.

Jones, J.E., & Kassity, N. (2001). Varieties of alternative experience: Complementary care in the neonatal intensive care unit. *Clinical Obstetrics and Gynecology, 44,* 750-768.

Jones, M.W., & McMurray, J.L. (2003). The other side of "Back to Sleep." *Neonatal Network, 22,* 49-53.

Jones, M.W., Morgan, E., & Shelton, J.E. (2002). Follow-up of the high-risk infant: Dysphagia and oral feeding problems in the premature infant. *Neonatal Network, 21,* 51-57.

Kaminski, J., & Hall, W. (1996). The effect of soothing music on neonatal behavioral states in the hospital newborn nursery. *Neonatal Network, 15,* 45-54.

Katz, K., Krikler, R., Wielunsky, E., & Merlob, P. (1991). Effect of neonatal posture on later lower limb rotation and gait in premature infants. *Journal of Pediatric Orthopedics, 11,* 520-522.

Kavanaugh, K., Mead, L., Meier, P., & Mangurten, H.H. (1995). Getting enough: Mothers' concerns about breastfeeding a preterm infant after discharge. *Journal of Obstetric, Gynecologic, and Neonatal Nursing, 24,* 23-33.

Kelly, K.M., Littlefield, T.R., Pomatto, J.K., Ripley, C.E., Beals, S.P., & Joganic, E.F. (1999). Importance of early recognition and treatment of deformational plagiocephaly with orthotic cranioplasty. *Cleft Palate–Craniofacial Journal, 36,* 127-130.

Kinneer, M.D., & Beachy, P. (1994). Nipple feeding premature infants in the neonatal intensive care unit: Factors and decisions. *Journal of Obstetric, Gynecologic, and Neonatal Nursing, 23,* 105-112.

Kliethermes, P.A., Cross, M.L., Lanese, M.G., Johnson, K.M., & Simon, S.D. (1999). Transitioning preterm infants with nasogastric tube supplementation: Increased likelihood of breastfeeding. *Journal of Obstetric, Gynecologic, and Neonatal Nursing, 23,* 264-273.

Konishi, Y., Mikawa, H., & Suzuki, J. (1986). Asymmetrical head-turning of preterm infants: Some effects on later postural and functional lateralities. *Developmental Medicine and Child Neurology, 28,* 450-457.

Korones, S.B. (1976). Disturbance and infants' rest. In T.D. Moore (Ed.), *Sixty-Ninth Ross Conference on Pediatric Research: Iatrogenic Problems in Neonatal Intensive Care.* Columbus, OH: Ross Laboratories.

Kramer, M.S., Barr, R.G., Dagenais, S., Yang, H., Jones, P., Ciofani, L., & Jane, F. (2001). Pacifier use, early weaning, and cry/fuss behavior: A randomized controlled trial. *Journal of the American Medical Association, 286,* 322-326.

Kuehl, J. (1997). Cup feeding the newborn: What you should know. *Journal of Perinatal and Neonatal Nursing, 11,* 56-60.

Lacey, J.L., Henderson-Smart, D.J., & Edwards, D.A. (1990). A longitudinal study of early leg postures of preterm infants. *Developmental Medicine and Child Neurology, 32,* 151-163.

Lang, S., Lawrence, C.J., & Orme, R.L. (1994). Cup feeding: An alternative method of infant feeding, *Archives of Disease in Childhood, 71,* 365-369.

Lary, S., Briassoulis, G., de Vries, L., Dubowitz, L., & Dubowitz, V. (1985). Hearing threshold in preterm and term infants by auditory brainstem response. *Journal of Pediatrics, 107,* 593-599.

Lau, C., Smith, E.O., & Schanler, R.J. (2003). Coordination of suck-swallow and swallow-respiration in preterm infants. *Acta Paediatrica, 92,* 721-727.

Lemons, P.K. (2001). From gavage to oral feeding: Just a matter of time. *Neonatal Network, 20,* 7-14.

Lewallen-Matthews, C. (1994). Supporting suck-swallow-breathe coordination during nipple feeding. *American Journal of Occupational Therapy, 48,* 561-562.

Lickliter, R. (2000). The role of sensory stimulation in perinatal development: Insights from comparative research for care of the high-risk infant. *Journal of Developmental & Behavioral Pediatrics, 21,* 437-447.

Lindh, V., Wiklund, U., Snadman, P.O., & Hakansson, S. (1997). Assessment of acute pain in preterm infants by evaluation of facial expression and frequency domain analysis of heart rate variability. *Early Human Development, 48,* 131-142.

Littlefield, T.R., Beals, S.P., Manwaring, K.H., Pomattor, J.K., Joganic, E.F., Golden, K.A., & Ripley, C.E. (1998). Treatment of craniofacial asymmetry with dynamic orthotic cranioplasty. *Journal of Craniofacial Surgery, 9,* 11-17.

Lockridge, T., Taquino, L.T., & Knight, A. (1999). Back to sleep: Is there room in that crib for both AAP recommendations and developmentally supportive care? *Neonatal Network, 18,* 29-33.

Long, J.G., Alistar, G.S., Phillip, A.G.S., & Lucey, J.F. (1980). Excessive handling as a cause of hypoxemia. *Pediatrics, 65,* 203-207.

Luddington-Hoe, S.M., Thompson, C., Swinth, J., Hadeed, A.J., & Anderson, G.C. (1994). Kangaroo care: Research results and practice implications and guidelines. *Neonatal Network, 13,* 19-27.

Lynam, L. (2003). The impact of the microenvironment on newborn care: A facility report—Christiana Care Health System. *Neonatal Intensive Care, 16,* 13-20.

Madden, S.L. (2000). *The preemie parents' companion: The essential guide to caring for your premature baby in the hospital, at home, and through the first years.* Boston: Harvard Common Press.

Mainous, R.O. (2002). Infant massage as a component of developmental care: Past, present, and future. *Holistic Nursing Practice, 16,* 1-7.

Marinelli, K.A., Burke, G.S., & Dodd, V.L. (2001). A comparison of the safety of cup feedings and bottle feedings in premature infants whose mothers intend to breastfeed. *Journal of Perinatology, 21,* 350-355.

Maroney, D. (1994). Helping parents survive the emotional "roller coaster ride" in the newborn intensive care unit. *Journal of Perinatology, 14,* 131-133.

Mathew, O.P. (1988). Regulation of breathing pattern during feeding: Role of suck, swallow, and nutrients. In O.P. Mathew & G. Sant'Ambrogio (Eds.), *Respiratory function of the upper airway* (pp. 535-560). New York: Marcel Dekker.

Mathew, O.P. (1991). Breathing patterns of preterm infants during bottle feeding: Role of milk flow. *Journal of Pediatrics, 119,* 960-965.

Mathisen, B., Worral, L., O'Callaghan, M., Wall, C., & Shepherd, R.W. (2000). Feeding problems and dysphagia in 6-month-old extremely low birth weight infants. *Advances in Speech Language Pathology, 2,* 9-17.

McCain, G.C. (2003). An evidence-based guideline for introducing oral feeding to healthy preterm infants. *Neonatal Network, 22,* 45-50.

McCain, G.C., Gartside, P.S., Greenberg, J.M., & Lott, J.W. (2001). A feeding protocol for healthy preterm infants that shortens time to oral feeding. *Journal of Pediatrics, 139,* 374-379.

McGrath, J.M., & Conliffe-Torres, S. (1996). Integrating family-centered developmental assessment and intervention into routine care in the neonatal intensive care unit. *Nursing Clinics of North America, 31,* 367-386.

Meadow, W., Mendez, D., Makela, J., Malin, A., Gray, C., & Lantos, J.D. (1996). Can and should level II nurseries care for newborns who require mechanical ventilation? *Clinics in Perinatology, 23,* 551-561.

Medoff-Cooper, B., McGrath, J.M., & Bilker, W. (2000). Nutritive sucking and neurobehavioral development in preterm infants from 34 weeks PCA to term. *American Journal of Maternal Child Nursing, 25,* 64-70.

Medoff-Cooper, B., Verklan, T., & Carlson, S. (1993). The development of sucking patterns and physiologic correlates in very-low-birth-weight infants. *Nursing Research, 42,* 100-105.

Meier, P. (1988). Bottle and breast feeding: Effects on transcutaneous oxygen pressure and temperature in preterm infants. *Nursing Research, 37,* 36-41.

Meier, P.P. (2001). Breastfeeding in the special care nursery: Prematures and infants with medical problems. *Pediatric Clinics of North America, 48,* 425-442.

Meier, P.P. (2002). Rush Mother's Milk Club. Paper presented at conference on the Physical and Developmental Environment of the High-Risk Infant, Clearwater Beach, FL, January 27-30.

Meier, P., & Anderson, G.C. (1987). Responses of small preterm infants to bottle and breast feeding. *American Journal of Maternal Child Nursing, 12,* 97-105.

Meier, P., Brown, L.P., & Hurst, N.M. (1999). Breastfeeding the preterm infant. In J. Riordan & K.G. Auerbach (Eds.), *Breastfeeding and human lactation* (2nd ed., pp. 440-481). Boston: Jones & Bartlett.

Menahem, S. (1997). Confusion re: Nipple confusion (letter). *Journal of Pediatrics, 130,* 1012.

Mentro, A.M., Steward, D.K., & Garvin, B.J. (2002). Infant feeding responsiveness: A conceptual analysis. *Journal of Advanced Nursing, 37,* 208-216.

Mirmiran, M., & Ariagno, R.L. (2000). Influence of light in the NICU on the development of circadian rhythms in preterm infants. *Seminars in Perinatology, 24,* 247-257.

Mitchell, A., & Boss, B.J. (2002). Adverse effects of pain on the nervous systems of newborns and young children: A review of the literature. *Journal of Neuroscience Nursing, 34,* 228-236.

Modrcin-Talbott, M.A., Harrison, L.L., Groer, M.W., & Younger, M.S. (2003). The biobehavioral effects of gentle human touch on preterm infants. *Nursing Science Quarterly, 16,* 60-67.

Mohrbacher, N., & Stock, J. (2002). *The breastfeeding answer book* (3rd ed.). Schaumburg, IL: La Leche League International.

Monfort, K.P., & Case-Smith, J. (1997). The effects of a neonatal positioner on scapular rotation. *American Journal of Occupational Therapy, 51,* 378-384.

Monteli, R.A., & Bumstead, D.H. (1986). Development and severity of palatal grooves in orally intubated newborns. *American Journal of Diseases in Children, 140,* 357-359.

Monterosso, L., Coenen, A., Percival, P., & Evans, S. (1995). Effect of a postural support nappy on "flattened posture" of the lower extremities in very preterm infants. *Journal of Paediatric and Child Health, 31,* 350-354.

Moore, K.A., Coker, K., DuBuisson, A.B., Swett., B., & Edwards, W.H. (2003). Implementing potentially better practices for improving family-centered care in neonatal intensive care units: Successes and challenges. *Pediatrics, 112,* e450-e460.

Morris, B.H., Philbin, M.K., & Bose, C. (2000). Physiological effects of sound on the newborn. *Journal of Perinatology, 2,* S55-S60.

Mouradian, L.E., & Als, H. (1994). The influence of neonatal intensive care unit caregiving practices on motor functioning of preterm infants. *American Journal of Occupational Therapy, 48,* 527-533.

Neifert, M.R. (1998). The optimization of breast-feeding in the perinatal period. *Clinics in Perinatology, 25,* 303-326.

Neifert, M.R., Lawrence, R., & Seacat, J. (1995). Nipple confusion: Toward a formal definition. *Journal of Pediatrics, 126,* S125-S129.

Nowak, A.J., Smith, W.L., & Erenberg, A. (1994). Imaging evaluation of artificial nipples during bottle feeding. *Archives of Pediatric and Adolescent Medicine, 148,* 40-42.

Nyquist, K.H., Sjöden, P.O., & Ewald, U. (1999). The development of preterm infants' breastfeeding behavior. *Early Human Development, 55,* 247-264.

Ohgi, S., Fukuda, M., Moriuchi, H., Kusumoto, T., Akiyama, T., Nugent, J.K., Brazelton, T.B., Arisawa, K., Takahashi, T., & Saitoh, H. (2002). Comparison of kangaroo care and standard care: Behavioral organization, development, and temperament in healthy, low-birth-weight infants through 1 year. *Journal of Perinatology, 22,* 374-379.

Palmer, M.M. (1993). Identification and management of the transitional suck pattern in premature infants. *Journal of Perinatal and Neonatal Nursing, 7,* 66-75.

Palmer, M.M., & VandenBerg, K.A. (1998). A closer look at neonatal sucking. *Neonatal Network, 17,* 77-79.

Palmer, M.M., Crawley, K., & Blanco, I.A. (1993). Neonatal oral-motor assessment scale: A reliability study. *Journal of Perinatology, 13,* 28-35.

Panniers, T.L. (2002). Practice applications of research: Refining clinical terminology for expert system development—An application in the neonatal intensive care unit. *Pediatric Nursing, 28,* 519-523, 529.

Peabody, J.L., & Martin, G.I. (1996). From how small is too small to how much is too much: Ethical issues at the limits of neonatal viability. *Clinics in Perinatology, 23,* 473-489.

Peng, N., Mao, H., Chen, Y., & Chang, Y. (2001). Effects of light intensity on the physiological parameters of the premature infant. *Journal of Nursing Research, 9,* 333-343.

Penn, A.A., & Schatz, C.J. (1999). Brain waves and brain wiring: The role of endogenous and sensory-driven neural activity in development. *Pediatric Research, 45,* 447-458.

Persing, J. (1997). Controversies regarding the management of skull abnormalities. *Journal of Craniofacial Surgery, 8,* 4-5.

Peters, K. (1999). Infant handling in the NICU: Does developmental care make a difference? A review of the literature. *Journal of Perinatal and Neonatal Nursing, 13,* 1-12.

Peters, K.L. (1996). Dinosaurs in the bath. *Neonatal Network, 15,* 71-73.

Peters, K.L. (1998). Bathing premature infants: Physiological and behavioral consequences. *American Journal of Critical Care, 7,* 90-100.

Pettett, G., Sewell, S., & Merenstein, G.B. (2002). Regionalization and transport in perinatal care. In G.B. Merenstein & S.L. Gardner (Eds.), *Handbook of neonatal intensive care* (5th ed., pp. 31-45). St. Louis: Mosby.

Philbin, M.K. (2000). The influence of auditory experience on the behavior of preterm newborns. *Journal of Perinatology, 20,* S77-S87.

Philbin, M.K., & Gray, L. (2002). Changing levels of quiet in an intensive care nursery. *Journal of Perinatology, 22,* 455-460.

Philbin, M.K., & Klaas, P. (2000). Evaluating studies of the behavioral effects of sound on newborns. *Journal of Perinatology, 20,* S61-S67.

Philbin, M., Lickliter, R., & Graven, S. (2000). Sensory experience and the developing organism: a history of ideas and view to the future. *Journal of Perinatology, 20,* S2-S5.

Philbin, M., Robertson, A., & Hall, J. (1999). Recommended permissible noise criteria for occupied, newly constructed, or renovated hospital nurseries. *Journal of Perinatology, 19,* 559-563.

Pickler, R.H., & Reyna, B.A. (2003). A descriptive study of bottle-feeding opportunities in preterm infants. *Advances in Neonatal Care, 3,* 139-146.

Pickler, R.H., Frankel, H.B., Walsh, K.M., & Thompson, N.M. (1996). Effects of nonnutritive sucking on behavioral organization and feeding performance in preterm infants. *Nursing Research, 45,* 132-135.

Pinelli, J., & Symington, A. (2002). Non-nutritive sucking for promoting physiologic stability and nutrition in preterm infants (Cochrane Review). In *The Cochrane Library,* Issue 3. Oxford: Update Software.

Porter, F.L., Wolf, C.M., & Miller, J.P. (1998). The effect of handling and immobilization on the response to acute pain in newborn infants. *Pediatrics, 102,* 1383-1389.

Pridham, K., Brown, R., Sondel, S., Green, C., Wedel, N.Y., & Lai, H-C. (1998). Transition time to full nipple feeding for premature infants with a history of lung disease. *Journal of Obstetric, Gynecologic, and Neonatal Nursing, 27,* 533-545.

Pridham, K., Kosorok, M.R., Greer, F., Carey, P., Kayata, S., & Sondel, S. (1999). The effects of prescribed versus ad libitum feedings and formula caloric density on premature infant dietary intake and weight gain. *Nursing Research, 48,* 86-93.

Pridham, K.F., Kosorok, M.R., Greer, F., Kayata, S., Bhattacharya, A., & Grunwald, P. (2001). Comparison of caloric intake and weight outcomes of an ad lib feeding regimen for preterm infants in two nurseries. *Journal of Advanced Nursing, 35,* 751-759.

Procter, A.M., Lether, D., Oliver, R.G., & Cartlidge, P.H.T. (1998). Deformation of the palate in preterm infants. *Archives of Disease in Childhood: Fetal and Neonatal Edition, 78,* F29-F32.

Rapport, M.J.K. (1992). A descriptive analysis of the role of physical and occupational therapists in the neonatal intensive care unit. *Pediatric Physical Therapy, 4,* 172-178.

Ratliff-Schaub, K., Hunt, C.E., Crowell, D., Golub, H., Smok-Pearsall, S., Palmer, P., Schafer, S., Bak, S., Cantey-Kiser, J., & O'Bell, R. (CHIME Study Group). (2001). Relationship between infant sleep position and motor development in preterm infants. *Journal of Developmental & Behavioral Pediatrics, 22,* 293-299.

Reynolds, J.D., Hardy, R.J., Kennedy, K.A, Spencer, R., van Heuven, W.A.J., & Fielder, A.R. (for the LIGHT–ROP Cooperative Group). (1998). Lack of efficacy of light reduction in preventing retinopathy of prematurity. *New England Journal of Medicine, 338,* 1572-1576.

Riordan, J., & Auerbach, K.G. (1999). Breastfeeding and human lactation (2nd ed.). Boston: Jones & Bartlett.

Rivkees, S.A., & Hao, H. (2000). The development of circadian rhythmicity. *Seminars in Perinatology, 24,* 232-242.

Robertson, A., Cooper-Peel, C., & Vos, P. (1998). Peak noise distribution in the neonatal intensive care nursery. *Journal of Perinatology, 18,* 361-364.

Robertson, A., Cooper-Peel, C., & Vos, P. (1999). Sound transmission into incubators in the neonatal intensive care unit. *Journal of Perinatology, 19,* 494-497.

Robison, L. (2003). Cycled light and growth of preterms. *Journal of Pediatrics, 142,* 451-452.

Ross, E.S., & Browne, J.V. (2002). Developmental progression of feeding skills: An approach to supporting feeding in preterm infants. *Seminars in Neonatology, 7,* 469-475.

Rutter, N., Hinchcliffe, W., & Cartlidge, P.H.T. (1993). Do preterm infants always have flattened heads? *Archives of Disease in Children, 68,* 606-607.

Saadeh, R., & Akre, J. (1996). Ten steps to successful breast-feeding: A summary of the rationale and scientific evidence. *Birth, 23,* 154-160.

Saunders, A.N. (1995). Incubator noise: A method to decrease decibels. *Pediatric Nursing, 21,* 265-268.

Scafidi, F.A., Field, T., & Schanberg, S.M. (1993). Factors that predict which preterm infants benefit most from massage therapy. *Developmental and Behavioral Pediatrics, 14,* 176-180.

Seguin, J.H., & Vieth, R. (1996). Thermal stability of premature infants during routine care under radiant warmers. *Archives of Disease in Childhood: Fetal and Neonatal Edition, 74,* F137-F138.

Semmler, C. (1989). Positioning and deformities. In C. Semmler (Ed.), *A guide to care and management of very low birth weight infants: A team approach.* Tucson, AZ: Therapy Skill Builders.

Seow, W.K. (1997). Effects of preterm birth on oral growth and development. *Australian Dental Journal, 42,* 85-91.

Shaker, C.S. (1990). Nipple feeding premature infants: A different perspective. *Neonatal Network, 8,* 345-350.

Shaker, C.S. (1998). Letter to the editors re: Cup feeding the newborn: What you should know (JPNN 11, 56-60, September 1997). *Journal of Perinatal and Neonatal Nursing, 12,* vi.

Shaker, C.S. (1999). Nipple feeding preterm infants: An individualized, developmentally supportive approach. *Neonatal Network, 18,* 15-22.

Shannon, J.D., & Gorski, P.A. (1994). Health-care professionals' attitudes toward the current level and need for developmental services in neonatal intensive care units. *Journal of Perinatology, 14,* 467-472.

Shiao, S-YPK. (1997). Comparison of continuous versus intermittent sucking in very-low-birth-weight infants. *Journal of Obstetric, Gynecologic, and Neonatal Nursing, 26,* 313-319.

Shiao, S-YPK., Brooker, J., & DiFiore, T. (1996). Desaturation events during oral feedings with and without a nasogastric tube in very low birth weight infants. *Heart & Lung, 25,* 236-245.

Shields-Poe, D., & Pinelli, J. (1997). Variables associated with parental stress in neonatal intensive care units. *Neonatal Network, 16,* 29-37.

Shivpuri, C.R., Martin, R.J., Carlo, W.A., & Fanaroff, A.A. (1983). Decreased ventilation in preterm infants during oral feeding. *Journal of Pediatrics, 103,* 285-289.

Short, M.A., Brooks-Brunn, J.A., Reeves, D.S., Yeager, J., & Thorpe, J.A. (1996). The effects of swaddling versus standard positioning on neuromuscular development of very low birth weight infants. *Neonatal Network, 15,* 25-31.

Siddell, E.P., & Froman, R.D. (1994). A national survey of neonatal intensive care units: Criteria used to determine readiness for oral feedings. *Journal of Obstetric, Gynecologic, and Neonatal Nursing, 23,* 783-789.

Siegel, R., Gardner, S.L., & Merenstein, G.B. (2002). Families in crisis: theoretical and practical considerations. In S.L.

Merenstein & G.B. Gardner (Eds.), *Handbook of neonatal intensive care* (5th ed., pp. 725-753). St. Louis: Mosby.

Simpson, C., Schanler, R.J., & Lau, C. (2002). Early introduction of oral feeding in preterm infants. *Pediatrics, 110,* 517-522.

Smith, S.L. (2001). Physiologic stability of intubated VLBW infants during skin-to-skin care and incubator care. *Advances in Neonatal Care, 1,* 28-40.

Smith, T. (1999). *Miracle birth stories of very premature babies: Little thumbs up!* Westport, CT: Bergin & Garvey.

Spear, M.L., Leef, K., Epps, S., & Locke, R. (2002). Family reactions during infants' hospitalization in the neonatal intensive care unit. *American Journal of Perinatology, 19,* 205-213.

Stade, B., & Bishop, C. (2002). A semidemand feeding protocol reduced time to full oral feeding in healthy preterm infants. *Evidence-Based Nursing, 5,* 74.

Standley, J.M., & Moore, R.S. (1995). Therapeutic effects of music and mother's voice on premature infants. *Pediatric Nursing, 21,* 509-512, 574.

Strauch, C., Brandt, S., & Edwards-Beckett, J. (1993). Implementation of a quiet hour: Effect on noise levels and infant sleep states. *Neonatal Network, 12,* 31-35.

Sweeney, J.K. (1993). Assessment of the special care nursery environment: Effects on the high-risk infant. In I.J. Wilhelm (Ed.), *Physical therapy assessment in early infancy* (pp. 13-34). New York: Churchill Livingstone.

Sweeney, J.K., & Gutierrez, T. (2002). Musculoskeletal implications of preterm infant positioning in the NICU. *Journal of Perinatal and Neonatal Nursing, 16,* 58-70.

Taylor, J.L., & Norton, E.S. (1997). Developmental muscular torticollis: Outcomes in young children treated by physical therapy. *Pediatric Physical Therapy, 9,* 173-178.

Thomas, K.A. (1989). How the NICU environment sounds to a preterm infant. *American Journal of Maternal Child Nursing, 14,* 249-251.

Thureen, P.J., Phillips, R.E., Baron, K.A., DeMarie, M.P., & Hay, W.W. (1998). Direct measurement of the energy expenditure of physical activity in preterm infants. *Journal of Applied Physiology, 85,* 223-230.

Valentine, C.J., Hurst, N.M., & Schanler, R.J. (1994). Hindmilk improves weight gain in low-birth-weight infants fed human milk. *Journal of Gastroenterology and Nutrition, 18,* 474-477.

Van Riper, M. (2001). Family-provider relationships and well-being in families with preterm infants in the NICU. *Heart & Lung: Journal of Acute & Critical Care, 30,* 74-84.

VandenBerg, K.A. (1990). Nippling management of the sick neonate in the NICU: The disorganized feeder. *Neonatal Network, 9,* 9-16.

VandenBerg, K.A. (1993). Basic competencies to begin developmental care in the intensive care nursery. *Infants and Young Children, 6,* 52-59.

VandenBerg, K.A. (1995). Behaviorally supportive care for the extremely premature infant. In L.P. Gunderson & C. Kenner (Eds.), *Care of the 24-25 week gestational age infant (small baby protocol)* (pp. 145-170). Petaluma, CA: Neonatal Network.

VandenBerg, K.A. (1999). Developmental care: What to tell parents about the developmental needs of their baby at discharge. *Neonatal Network, 18,* 57-59.

VandenBerg, K.A. (2000). Supporting parents in the NICU: Guidelines for promoting parent confidence and competence. *Neonatal Network, 19,* 63-64.

Vergara, E.R., & Bigsby, R. (2003). *Developmental and therapeutic interventions in the NICU.* Baltimore: Brookes.

Vickers, A., Ohlsson, A., Lacy, J.B., & Horsley, A. (2002). Massage for promoting growth and development of preterm and/or low birth-weight infants. In *The Cochrane Library,* Issue 3. Oxford: Update Software.

VonGonten, A.S., Meyer, J.B. Jr., & Kim, A.K. (1995). Dental management of neonates requiring prolonged oral intubation. *Journal of Prosthodontics, 4,* 221-225.

Waber, B., Hubler, E.G., & Padden, M.L. (1998). Clinical observations: A comparison of outcomes in demand versus schedule formula-fed premature infants. *Nutrition in Clinical Practice, 13,* 132-135.

Watterberg, K., & Munsick-Bruno, G. (1986). Incidence and persistence of acquired palatal groove in preterm neonates following prolonged oral intubation. *Clinical Research, 34,* 113A.

Westrup, B., Kleberg, A., von Eichwald, K., Stjernqvist, K., & Lagercrantz, H.A. (2000). A randomized, controlled trial to evaluate the effects of the newborn individualized developmental care and assessment program in a Swedish setting. *Pediatrics, 105(1 Pt) (1),* 66-72.

Whipple, J. (2000). The effect of parent training in music and multimodal stimulation on parent-neonate interactions in the neonatal intensive care unit. *Journal of Music Therapy, 37,* 250-268.

White, R., & Newbold, P.A. (1995). Reinventing the newborn ICU. *Healthcare Forum Journal, 38,* 30-33.

White, R.D. (1999). Light: Use and control in the NICU. Paper presented at conference on the Physical and Developmental Environment of the High-Risk Infant, Clearwater Beach, FL, January 27-30.

White, R.D. (2003). Individual rooms in the NICU: An evolving concept. *Journal of Perinatology (Supplement), 23,* S22-S24.

White, R.D., Browne, J., Cicco, R., Erickson, D.S., Graven, S.N., Greer, M., Gregory, S., Hall, J., Harell, J.W., Jaeger, C.B., Kenner, C., Kolberg, K.J.S., Little, G.A., Marshall-Baker, A., Martin, G.L., McGlone, C.A., Philbin, M.K., & Smith, J.A. (2003). Recommended standards for newborn ICU design. Report of the Fifth Consensus Conference on Newborn ICU Design. *Journal of Perinatology, 23,* S3-S21. Available at http://www.nd.edu/~kkolberg/DesignStandards.htm

Wolf, L.S., & Glass, R.P. (1992). *Feeding and swallowing disorders in infancy: Assessment and management.* Tucson, AZ: Therapy Skill Builders.

Wurtman, R.J. (1975). The effects of light on the human body. *Scientific American, 233,* 68-77.

Yu, V.Y.H. (2000). Developmental outcome of extremely preterm infants. *American Journal of Perinatology, 17,* 57-61.

Zahr, L.K., & de Traversay, J. (1995). Premature infant responses to noise reduction by earmuffs: Effects on behavioral and physiologic measures. *Journal of Perinatology, 15,* 448-455.

Zaichkin, J. (2002). *Newborn intensive care: What every parent needs to know* (2nd ed.). Petaluma, CA: NICU, Inc.

Medical Abbreviations Commonly Used in the Neonatal Intensive Care Unit

A

A: apnea
Ab: abortions (includes spontaneous)
ABG: arterial blood gas
ABR: auditory brain stem response
AD: right ear
AEP: auditory evoked potential
AGA: appropriate for gestational age
A-line: arterial line
AOP: apnea of prematurity
APIP: Assessment of Preterm Infant Behavior (Als)
AROM: assisted rupture of membranes
AS: left ear
As & Bs: apnea and bradycardia
ASD: atrial septal defect
AU: both ears

B

B: bilateral, or bradycardia
BAEP: brain stem auditory evoked potential
BAER: brain stem auditory evoked response
BIH: bilateral inguinal hernia
BPD: bronchopulmonary dysplasia
BPM: beats per minute (pulse)
BSER: brain stem evoked response (same as ABR, AEP, BAER, or BAEP)
BW: birth weight

C

CAN: cord around neck (nuchal cord)
CBC: complete blood count
CDH: congenitally dislocated hip
CHD: congenital heart disease
CHF: congestive heart failure
CLD: chronic lung disease
CMV: cytomegalovirus
CNGF: continuous nasogastric feeding
CNS: central nervous system
COGF: continuous orogastric feeding
CPAP: continuous positive airway pressure
CPT: chest physical therapy
C/S: cesarean section

CSF: cerebrospinal fluid
CTF: continuous tube feeding
CXR: chest x-ray

D

D_5W: 5% glucose solution
$D_{10}W$: 10% glucose solution
DIC: disseminated intravascular coagulation
DTGV: transposition of the great vessels

E

ECMO: extracorporeal membrane oxygenation
ELBW: extremely low birth weight (<1,000 g)

F

FEN: fluids, electrolytes, nutrition
FHR: fetal heart rate
FiO_2: fraction of inspired oxygen (percentage of oxygen concentration)
FT: full term

G

G: gravida (pregnancies)
GA: gestational age
GBS: group B streptococcus
GER: gastroesophageal reflux
GERD: gastroesophageal reflux disease

H

HAL: hyperalimentation (same as TPN)
HC: head circumference
HFV: high-frequency ventilation
HFJV: high-frequency jet ventilation
HFOV: high-frequency oscillating ventilation
HIE: hypoxic-ischemic encephalopathy
HMD: hyaline membrane disease
HR: heart rate
HSV: herpes simplex virus
HTN: hypertension
HUSG: head ultrasound

I

ICH: intracranial hemorrhage
ICN: intensive care nursery
IDM (or IODM): infant of a diabetic mother
IDV: intermittent demand ventilation
IH: inguinal hernia
IMV: intermittent mandatory ventilation
I/O: intake/output
IPPB: intermittent positive pressure breathing
IRV: inspiratory reserve volume
IUGR: intrauterine growth retardation
IV: intravenous
IVDA: intravenous drug abuse
IVF: in vitro fertilization; intravenous feeding
IVH: intraventricular hemorrhage

K

Kcal: kilocalories

L

L (or LC): living children
LA: left atrium
LBW: low birth weight (<2,500 g)
LGA: large for gestational age
LMP: last menstrual period
L/S ratio: lecithin/sphingomyelin ratio
LTGV: physiologically corrected transposition of the great vessels
LV: left ventricle

M

MAP: mean airway pressure
MAS: meconium aspiration syndrome
MCA: multiple congenital anomalies
MDU: maternal drug use
MRSA: methicillin-resistant *Staphylococcus aureus*
MRSE: methicillin-resistant *Staphylococcus epidermidis*

N

NB: newborn
NBAS: Newborn Behavioral Assessment Scale (Brazelton)
NC: nasal cannula
NCPAP: nasal continuous positive airway pressure
ND: nasoduodenal
NEC: necrotizing enterocolitis
NG: nasogastric
NGT: nasogastric tube
NICU: neonatal intensive care unit
NIDCAP: Neonatal Individualized Developmental Care and Assessment Program (Als)
NNS: Neonatal Network Neurobehavioral Scale

NNS: nonnutritive sucking
NO: nitric oxide
NP: nasopharyngeal
NPCPAP: nasopharyngeal continuous positive airway pressure
NPO: nothing by mouth
NS: nutritive sucking
NTE: neutral thermal environment

O

O_2 sats: oxygen saturation
OD: oral-duodenal; right eye
OG: oral gastric
OGT: oral gastric tube
OS: left eye
OU: both eyes

P

P: pulse; para (births)
P_1: primipara (first birth)
$PaCO_2$: arterial partial pressure of CO_2 (concentration of CO_2 in peripheral arteries)
PaO_2: arterial partial pressure of O_2 (concentration of O_2 in peripheral arteries)
PCA: postconceptional age
PDA: patent ductus arteriosus
PEEP: positive end expiratory pressure
PFC: persistent fetal circulation (more correctly called persistent pulmonary hypertension of the newborn [PPHN])
PICC: percutaneously inserted central catheter (previously called PerQ cath, or percutaneous catheter)
PIE: pulmonary interstitial emphysema
PIH: pregnancy-induced hypertension (preeclampsia, eclampsia)
PIP: pulmonary insufficiency of the preterm; peak inspiratory pressure
PO: by mouth
PPD: packs per day (refers to smoking)
PPHN: persistent pulmonary hypertension of the newborn (previously called persistent fetal circulation [PFC])
PROM: premature rupture of membranes
PPROM: prolonged premature rupture of membranes
PS: pulmonic stenosis
PPS: peripheral pulmonic stenosis
PT: preterm
PTL: preterm labor
PVL: periventricular leukomalacia

Q

q: every
qh: every hour

qid: 4 times a day

R

RA: right atrium
RBC: red blood cell
RDS: respiratory distress syndrome
ROM: rupture of membranes
ROP: retinopathy of prematurity (formerly called retrolental fibroplasia [RLF])
RPR: rapid plasma reagin (can be used to test for syphilis)
RRR: rate, rhythm, respiration
RV: right ventricle

S

SA: substance abuse
sats: oxygen saturation levels
SCN: special care nursery
SGA: small for gestational age
SIMV: synchronized intermittent mandatory ventilation
s/p: status post
SROM: spontaneous rupture of membranes
SVD: spontaneous vaginal delivery

T

TA: truncus arteriosus
TAPVR: total anomalous pulmonary venous return
TCAN: tight cord around neck
TCM: transcutaneous monitor
TcPO$_2$: transcutaneous oxygen pressure

TLC

TLC: total lung capacity
TOF: tetralogy of Fallot
TORCH: congenital viral infections (toxoplasmosis, rubella, cytomegalovirus, and herpes)
TPF: toxoplasmosis fetalis
TPN: total parenteral nutrition
TPR: temperature, pulse, respiration
TRDN: transient respiratory distress of the newborn
TTN: transient tachypnea of the newborn

U

UAC: umbilical artery catheter
UAL: umbilical artery line
ULBW: ultra low birth weight (<750 g)
URI: upper respiratory infection
USG: ultrasound
UTI: urinary tract infection
UVC: umbilical venous catheter

V

VDRL: Venereal Disease Research Laboratory
VEP (VER): vision evoked potential (response)
VLBW: very low birth weight (<1,500 g)
VSD: ventricular septal defect

W

WBC: white blood cell
WBD: weeks by dates (for gestational age)
WBE: weeks by examination (for gestational age)

Medical Complications of Preterm and High-Risk Infants

BOX 20B-1 Congenital Cardiac Defects

Review of Normal Heart Anatomy and Physiology

The normal heart consists of two upper chambers (right and left atria) and two lower chambers (right and left ventricles) divided by septums into the right and left sides, along with outflow arteries and inflow veins for both pulmonary and systemic (body) circulation. Blood flow progression is as follows:

1 From the body, the blood returns through the inferior and superior vena cava to empty into the right atrium
2 It passes through the tricuspid valve into the right ventricle
3 It leaves the right ventricle through the pulmonary semilunar valve to the main pulmonary artery
4 The blood is oxygenated in the lungs and returns to the left atrium of the heart through four major pulmonary veins
5 It passes from the left atrium through the mitral valve into the left ventricle
6 It leaves the left ventricle through the aortic semilunar valve to the ascending aorta
7 It travels through the systemic vasculature network

Congenital Heart Disease

Congenital cardiovascular malformations occur in 8 per 1,000 live births. Most of these defects are simple left-to-right shunts that are acyanotic and pose relatively low risk to the infant, such as a patent ductus arteriosus or ventricular septal defect. Approximately 25% of congenital heart disease is serious enough to require cardiac catheterization and other medical diagnostic procedures during the first year. Early surgical intervention typically is more common (and sometimes imperative) with cyanotic congenital heart disease.

Acyanotic Congenital Heart Defects
Aortic Stenosis
The aortic valve (or the areas immediately above or below the actual valve) is stenosed, with resultant obstruction to outflow from the left ventricle to the aorta. The degree of stenosis is progressive (from fibrin deposits, fibrosis, and calcification), and stenosis tends to recur even after surgical correction.
Atrial Septal Defect (ASD)
ASD is a defect in the septum separating the right and left ventricles. The size and site of the lesion may vary. Spontaneous closure is rare unless the defect is small; surgical sutures or a patch is typical.
Atrioventricular (AV) Canal: Endocardial Cushion Defect
AV refers to a spectrum of malformations that includes defects in the lower part of the interatrial septum, the upper part of the interventricular septum, and the portions of the AV (tricuspid and mitral) valves closest to the atrial and ventricular septa. AV valve regurgitation differentiates this anomaly from a simple ventricular septal defect or an ASD. Large defects require surgery.

Coarctation of the Aorta
Narrowing or constriction of a portion of the aorta that causes elevated blood pressure proximal to the stricture and decreased blood flow or blood pressure distal to the obstruction. Surgical repair is indicated but may not be urgent.
Partial Anomalous Pulmonary Venous Return
One, but not all, of the pulmonary veins does not empty into the left atrium. The pulmonary veins on the right may connect directly to the superior vena cava, or the pulmonary veins on the left may communicate with the innominate vein. This defect may occur in isolation or in conjunction with an ASD. It usually requires surgical correction if at least two veins are involved.
Patent Ductus Arteriosus (PDA)
A PDA is a short fetal blood vessel that connects the main pulmonary artery to the descending aorta. It is a normal component of fetal circulation, but failure of the PDA to close soon after birth allows direct shunting of blood between the main pulmonary artery and the aorta. This shunt is right to left if the infant is in respiratory distress and left to right with potential congestive heart failure if no significant respiratory illness exists. PDAs may close spontaneously or may require medication or surgical ligation.
Physiologically Corrected Transposition of the Great Vessels (LTGV)
The origins of the great vessels are reversed (aorta from the right ventricle, pulmonary artery from the left ventricle), but discordant atrioventricular and ventriculoarterial connections result in misalignment such that the right atrium drains into the left ventricle and the left ventricle drains into the right pulmonary artery. Thus systemic blood still returns to the lungs for oxygenation. Oxygenated blood proceeds to the left atrium through the right ventricle, out the aorta, and back into systemic circulation. LTGV frequently occurs with more complex lesions. The need for surgical intervention varies.
Pulmonic Stenosis
Constriction of the pulmonary artery or pulmonic semilunar valve can result in obstructed outflow from the right ventricle through the pulmonary arteries to the lungs. Stenosis is not progressive. Severe cases may require surgical intervention.
Ventricular Septal Defect (VSD)
VSD is a defect in the septum separating the right and left ventricles. A VSD may be an isolated defect or it may occur as part of complex heart disease; the size and exact location of the lesion can vary. Most VSDs close spontaneously; some require surgery.

Cyanotic Congenital Heart Defects
Double Inlet Ventricle (Single Ventricle)
With a double inlet ventricle, either the right or left ventricle is incompletely formed, and the remaining ventricle is dominant; the connection is described as double inlet when one, and at least 50% of the other, atrioventricular valve feeds into

BOX 20B-1 Congenital Cardiac Defects—Cont'd

the dominant ventricle. Although rare, a single primitive ventricle with no dividing septum may occur.

Double Outlet Right Ventricle

With a double outlet right ventricle, both the aorta and the main pulmonary artery originate from the right ventricle; a VSD and varying degrees of cyanosis are always present. Surgical repair is necessary.

Ebstein's Anomaly

Ebstein's anomaly involves a malformation of the tricuspid valve in which the leaflets of the valve are displaced downward and adhere to the inflow portion of the right ventricle. This incorporates a portion of the right ventricle into the right atrium; the remaining ventricular cavity may be small. Tricuspid insufficiency is present in varying degrees, and the condition eventually may require surgery.

Hypoplastic Left Heart

With a hypoplastic left heart, the left ventricle and ascending aorta are underdeveloped, and the mitral and aortic valves are atretic or stenotic. Multistage surgery may be attempted (the survival rate is 10%), but this defect usually is fatal without a heart transplant.

Interrupted Aortic Arch

In this condition, the aortic arch is interrupted at some point between the innominate artery and the left subclavian artery; a VSD typically is present. Severe congestive heart failure, cyanosis, and respiratory distress appear early. Classic clinical findings are a strong pulse in the right upper extremity but weak or absent pulses from the lower extremities and left upper extremity. The lower body becomes hypoxemic and acidotic; subsequent organ damage and death result if surgical repair is delayed.

Pulmonary Atresia with Intact Ventricular Septum

In pulmonary atresia with an intact ventricular septum, forward flow through the usually hypoplastic right ventricle is not possible because of agenesis of the pulmonary valve. Blood returning from the body is shunted from the right atrium to the left atrium and mixed with whatever blood is returning from the lungs. Blood then passes into the left ventricle and back into systemic circulation. Surgical intervention is required.

Tetrology of Fallot (TOF)

Tetrology of Fallot (TOF) comprises a constellation of defects that include a large VSD, right ventricular outflow obstruction (pulmonary stenosis), an aorta that overrides the VSD, and right ventricular hypertrophy. The degree of pulmonary stenosis typically dictates the severity and course of TOF. The term *Tet spells* refers to hypoxic episodes of suddenly increasing cyanosis and agitation that usually are associated with arising, eating, activity, or crying. Surgical intervention is usually required, although the timing can vary significantly.

Total Anomalous Pulmonary Venous Return (TAPVR)

In TAPVR none of the four pulmonary veins empties into the left atrium; drainage occurs indirectly through various routes into the right atrium. An ASD must always be present to permit function of the left side of the heart. Early surgical correction is usually required.

Transposition of the Great Vessels (DTGV)

With transposition of the great vessels, the origins of the aorta and main pulmonary artery are reversed from a normal presentation; the aorta arises from the right ventricle, and the pulmonary artery arises from the left ventricle. DTGV may occur in an isolated form or with complex heart disease. Early surgery is required.

Tricuspid Atresia

In this condition, the tricuspid valve between the right atrium and right ventricle is either absent or not patent, resulting in obstruction of blood flow into the right ventricle. The right ventricle may be fully formed if a VSD is present, or it may be hypoplastic. Surgical repair is required.

Truncus Arteriosus (Types I-IV)

When normal separation of the aorta and main pulmonary artery do not occur during fetal development, both the right and left ventricles empty into a single large vessel. Types I and IV truncus arteriosus are common; types II and III are not. The pulmonary arteries are connected to the aorta in types I, II, and III. In type IV the pulmonary arteries have no connection to the common trunk (single large vessel), and pulmonary perfusion occurs from collateral circulation. A VSD is always present. Surgical repair is required.

American Heart Association. (2001). *If your child has a congenital heart disease: A guide for parents.* Dallas: American Heart Association; Artman, M., Mahony, L., & Teitel, D.F. (2002). *Neonatal cardiology.* Columbus, OH: McGraw-Hill; Brook, M.M., Heymann, M.A., & Teitel, D.F. (2001). The heart. In M.H. Klaus & A.A. Fanaroff (Eds.), *Care of the high-risk neonate* (5th ed., pp. 393-424). Philadelphia: W.B. Saunders; Montoya, K.D., & Washington, R.L. (2002). Cardiovascular diseases and surgical interventions. In G.B. Gardner & S.L. Merenstein (Eds.), *Handbook of neonatal intensive care* (5th ed., pp. 576-608). St. Louis: Mosby.

TABLE 20B-1 Common Respiratory Complications

Diagnosis	Description	Implications for Occupational Therapists
Transient respiratory distress of the newborn (TRDN)	Also called transient tachypnea of the newborn (TTN), TRDN refers to delayed resorption of fetal lung fluid. It usually occurs with a term or near-term infant who has undergone a rapid delivery or cesarean section or who has neonatal depression. The baby breathes rapidly to clear excess fluid and may initially require supplemental oxygen.	The infant typically is receiving oxygen ≥40% from an oxyhood. TRDN generally resolves within 24 to 48 hours and is not usually associated with lasting complications.
Respiratory distress syndrome (RDS); also called hyaline membrane disease (HMD)	RDS is an acute lung disease of primarily preterm infants in which the lungs cannot inflate or function correctly because of a lack of surfactant. Chronic intrauterine stress may facilitate lung maturation and decrease RDS severity; female and black infants may also be less affected. Surfactant replacement therapy is common. Atelectasis (incomplete expansion of the lungs at birth) and collapse of the lungs after expiration are primary problems. Typical symptoms of respiratory distress (tachypnea, nasal flaring, grunting, chest retractions, apnea, and cyanosis), poor air entry, and right-to-left shunting often worsen for 36 to 48 hours. RDS may plateau and then improve, or it may progress to bronchopulmonary dysplasia.	Supplemental oxygen can be given with or without assisted ventilation. Physiologic instability is apparent; protection from avoidable stress is indicated to facilitate recovery (Latini, De Felice, & Presta, Rosati, & Vacca, 2003).
Pulmonary insufficiency of the preterm (PIP)	PIP is lung immaturity that results from extreme prematurity. The lungs are underdeveloped and need assistance to provide adequate oxygenation and ventilation for the infant.	This condition usually affects extremely premature infants (i.e., <1,000 g). The infant may be ventilated mechanically or placed under an oxyhood. These infants must be protected from avoidable stress.
Meconium aspiration syndrome (MAS)	Meconium, the fecal matter passed by neonates in early bowel movements, may be released into the amniotic fluid before delivery under certain conditions of stress (e.g., postterm or IUGR infant, complicated delivery, fetal hypoxia, and acidosis). A baby may be "meconium stained" without aspirating the tarlike substance into the tracheobronchial tree. Not all infants who aspirate meconium are symptomatic. MAS most accurately refers to infants with meconium found below the vocal cords and typical changes on x-rays. MAS complications may include pulmonary hypertension, the need for mechanical ventilation, secondary bacterial infection, and pulmonary or cerebral hemorrhages.	Symptomatic MAS infants can be critically ill. Mechanical ventilation is required for symptomatic infants; large infants who "fight the vent" may be sedated or chemically paralyzed. Mortality increases if persistent pulmonary hypertension (PPHN) occurs; less severe cases may improve within a week. Progression to chronic lung disease may occur. Acutely ill MAS infants need to be protected from avoidable stress.
Persistent pulmonary hypertension (PPHN); also called persistent fetal circulation (PFC)	When respiratory distress (from any cause) and the resultant hypoxia or acidosis leads to constriction of pulmonary vasculature, the increased resistance to pulmonary blood flow allows the ductus arteriosus to remain functionally open or to reopen. As blood is shunted away from the lungs, right-to-left shunting through the foramen ovale and ductus arteriosus continues, and the fetal pattern of circulation persists.	Infant ventilation and oxygenation are severely compromised. This is a potentially life-threatening complication, and these critically ill infants typically are on minimal stimulation protocols. Extracorporeal membrane oxygenation (ECMO) is possible if the infant does not respond to medical management.
Bronchopulmonary dysplasia (BPD) and chronic lung disease (CLD)	The original "classic" definition of BPD from the late 1960s described progressive lung changes (inflammation, fibrosis, and smooth muscle hypertrophy in the airways) evident on x-rays in larger, more mature preterm infants with severe HMD. Classic BPD was strongly related to mechanical injury from positive pressure ventilation and prolonged high oxygen concentrations. Antenatal steroids, surfactant administration, less aggressive parameters of mechanical ventilation (e.g., lower pressures and oxygen concentrations, earlier	Chronic pulmonary compromise is common, often requiring prolonged mechanical ventilation or NCPAP. Oxygen supplementation by nasal cannula may be required for several weeks or months. These infants have an increased susceptibility to recurrent respiratory infections and asthma. Some CLD infants tend to be irritable and demonstrate increased muscle tone (aggravated by frequent agitation); other

TABLE 20B-1 Common Respiratory Complications—*cont'd*

Diagnosis	Description	Implications for Occupational Therapists
	weaning to nasal continuous positive airway pressure [NCPAP]), and survival of extremely premature infants have altered the severity and characteristics of BPD; it now occurs primarily in infants under 1,200 g and <30 weeks' gestation. Immaturity, perinatal infection, and persistent ductus arteriosus are contributing factors to the "new BPD." Lung fibrosis and inflammation are reduced in new BPD, but lung anatomic development is altered, with hypoplasia of the alveoli (fewer in number, larger in size) and of the pulmonary microvasculature. New BPD may be less severe than classic BPD, but pulmonary hypertension can still develop. One distinction has emerged that refers to infants requiring oxygen at 28 days as having BPD, and to infants requiring oxygen at 36 weeks as having chronic lung disease. *CLD* is a less specific term that includes BPD but also recognizes that chronic lung problems can occur from other causes (e.g., heart defects, diaphragmatic hernia, and MAS).	CLD infants tend to be low energy, lethargic, and difficult to arouse. Difficulty with oral feedings may occur, especially if the infant remains tachypneic, has excessive secretions, is lethargic and difficult to arouse, or has developed oral hypersensitivity. The infant usually needs extra calories for growth. There is an increased risk of long-term neurodevelopmental sequelae.
Apnea	With apnea, cessation of breathing occurs for longer than 20 seconds. The etiology may be: ■ Central (i.e., related to nervous system immaturity in a preterm infant or to CNS pathology, such as seizures or encephalopathy) ■ Obstructive (e.g., tracheomalacia, tracheal stenosis from repeated or prolonged intubation, micrognathia, and posterior tongue placement in Pierre Robin sequence) ■ Associated with illness (e.g., RDS, infection, anemia, cold stress, and reflux) ■ Related to stress (e.g., after eye dilation and examination ■ Caused by medications (e.g., maternal magnesium sulfate for preterm labor; oversedation) ■ Incoordination of suck, swallow, and breathing during oral feeding ■ Vagal response to gastroesophageal reflux ■ Idiopathic (cause unknown)	The infant may require prolonged mechanical ventilation or NCPAP. Apnea medication is common. Severe apnea increases the risk both of central nervous system (CNS) damage from hypoxia and of necrotizing enterocolitis (NEC) from disturbed perfusion of the intestine. Apnea is more common during periods of active sleep than when awake. Feeding-induced apnea decreases with maturation; external pacing and a slow-flow nipple may be required when the infant is learning to feed orally. The infant may go home on an apnea monitor.
Pneumonia	The causes of pneumonia include infectious exposure to various organisms across the placenta or during delivery; and nosocomial infection (hospital-acquired infection, [e.g., transmission from inadequate hand washing]); or the disease may occur in association with sepsis or meningitis. The clinical presentation may include signs of respiratory distress (grunting, flaring, retractions, tachypnea, or cyanosis), shock, and signs of sepsis (temperature instability, apnea, hypoglycemia, lethargy, poor feeding, or seizures).	A seriously or critically ill infant requires mechanical ventilation and intravenous (IV) antibiotics. Enteral feedings may be temporarily discontinued. The infant must be protected from avoidable stress.

Agrawal, V., David, R.J., & Harris, V.J. (2003). Classification of acute respiratory disorders of all newborns in a tertiary care center. *Journal of the National Medical Association, 95*, 585-595; Bhatt-Mehta, V., & Schumacher, R.E. (2003). Treatment of apnea of prematurity. *Paediatric Drugs, 5*, 195-210; Clark, R.H., Gerstmann, D.R., Jobe, A.H., Moffitt, S.T., Slutsky, A.S., & Yoder, B.A. (2001). Lung injury in neonates: causes, strategies for prevention, and long-term consequences. *Journal of Pediatrics, 139*, 478-486; Eber, E., & Zach, M.S. (2001). Long-term sequelae of bronchopulmonary dysplasia (chronic lung disease of infancy). *Thorax, 56*, 317-323; Enzman-Hagedorn, M.I., Gardner, S.L., & Abman, S.H. (2002). Respiratory diseases. In G.B. Gardner & S.L. Merenstein (Eds.), *Handbook of neonatal intensive care* (5th ed., pp. 485-575). St. Louis: Mosby; Jobe, A.H., & Ikegami, M. (2001). Prevention of bronchopulmonary dysplasia. *Current Opinion in Pediatrics, 13*, 124-129; Latini, G., De Felice, C., Presta, G., Rosati, E., & Vacca, P. (2003). Minimal handling and bronchopulmonary dysplasia in extremely low-birth-weight infants. *European Journal of Pediatrics, 162*, 227-229; Martin, R.J., Sosenko, I.R.S., & Bancalari, E. (2001). Respiratory problems. In M.H. Klaus & A.A. Fanaroff (Eds.), *Care of the high-risk neonate* (5th ed., pp. 243-276). Philadelphia: W.B. Saunders.

TABLE 20B-2 Common Neurologic Complications

Diagnosis	Description	Implications for Occupational Therapists
Brachial plexus injuries	Transient or permanent upper extremity paralysis may result from damage to the brachial plexus during a difficult birth. The nerve roots and trunks of the plexus may be bruised, stretched, or torn.	Treatment in the acute stage is primarily aimed at preventing further damage to traumatized structures and preventing contractures of involved joints.
Erb's palsy	Erb's palsy is caused by damage to the upper trunk of the brachial plexus at the junction of nerve roots C-5 and C-6. It is the most common brachial plexus injury and has the best prognosis.	Caregivers are taught positioning and handling techniques that protect the extremity, as well as passive range of motion that emphasizes absent movements.
Erb-Duchenne-Klumpke's palsy	The injury occurs at nerve roots C-5 to T-1. This is the next most common injury to brachial plexus injuries, and the prognosis generally is good.	As for Erb's palsy
Klumpke's palsy	This condition arises from an injury to nerve roots C-8 to T-1. It is the least common type of nerve injury, and often less recovery is seen.	As for Erb's palsy
Periventricular hemorrhage (PVH) and intraventricular hemorrhage (IVH)	Infants weighing <1,500 g and <30 weeks' gestation are at highest risk for these conditions; most bleeding episodes occur within the first few days of life. Causes may have intravascular factors (i.e., fluctuating or increased cerebral blood flow, increased venous pressure or blood flow, platelet and coagulation disturbances); vascular factors (fragile capillaries and immature vascular network are vulnerable to rupture); and extravascular factors (poor structural support of capillary bed; fibrinolytic activity that extends bleeding). There are four grades of IVH: Grade I: Subependymal germinal matrix bleeding occurs. Grade II: Bleeding extends into the ventricles. Grade III: Ventricles are so full of blood they become dilated Grade IV: Bleeding extends beyond the cavity of the ventricle into the surrounding parenchyma; hydrocephalus is typical	Symptoms may include apnea, temperature instability, poor sucking or feeding, vomiting, lethargy, irritability, pallor or mottling, hypotension or shock, bulging and tense fontanel, and seizures. Stress and improper handling may contribute to an IVH in a vulnerable infant (e.g., abrupt position changes or elevation of the hips during a diaper change can cause intracranial pressure fluctuations in a micropremie). Infants with grade I or grade II IVH usually do well developmentally; infants with grade III or grade IV IVH are more likely to have developmental problems, especially if there is associated periventricular white matter destruction (periventricular leukomalacia [PVL]) or posthemorrhagic hydrocephalus.
Periventricular leukomalacia (PVL)	PVL is a widely recognized ischemic brain lesion frequently associated with developmental sequelae. Infants with asphyxia or who are born to mothers with chorioamnionitis or prolonged rupture of the membranes have an increased risk of PVL, which literally means the loss of white matter around the ventricles. PVL is characterized by necrosis and residual scarring of the white matter and may be responsible for extension of an IVH into a grade IV condition.	Areas of increased echodensity on head ultrasound examinations that resolve over time do not represent true PVL. Repeat ultrasound studies of PVL typically show cystic formation from white matter destruction. Developmental sequelae are seen in most (but not all) infants with PVL; the extent and specific location of the PVL determine subsequent clinical findings.
Hydrocephalus, posthemorrhagic hydrocephalus	Inflammation from blood in the ventricles may impede the normal circulation and resorption of cerebrospinal fluid (CSF); fibrin or other debris may occlude the pathways for CSF drainage, leading to hydrocephalus.	The infant may need a ventriculoperitoneal shunt to allow drainage of CSF. If the infant is too small or if the blood protein level is too high for immediate surgery, the baby may have frequent lumbar or ventricular taps to relieve accumulating pressure.
Congenital obstructive hydrocephalus	Aqueductal stenosis: Obstruction of the aqueduct of Sylvius before the fourth ventricle occludes CSF flow, causing the lateral and third ventricles to dilate. Arnold-Chiari malformation (ACM): Displacement of the medulla inferiorly through the foramen magnum into the cervical spinal canal (type I), at times with the fourth ventricle (type II, the classic form of ACM associated with spina bifida) or the cerebellum (type III). Obstructive hydrocephalus results.	The infant may be irritable or lethargic. Brain stem dysfunction may occur with ACM, especially after repair of myelomeningocele and possibly several months after birth. The infant may have silent aspiration with feedings; surgical decompression may relieve pressure on brain stem. Developmental sequelae are common.
Hypoxic-ischemic encephalopathy (HIE)	Numerous maternal, placental, obstetric, fetal, and neonatal factors can reduce oxygen transfer to the baby. HIE is the neurologic syndrome resulting from perinatal asphyxia.	The infant initially may be on a minimal stimulation protocol. Monitoring of the early presentation and subsequent changes

TABLE 20B-2 Common Neurologic Complications—*cont'd*

Diagnosis	Description	Implications for Occupational Therapists
	The clinical manifestations and prognosis depend primarily on the severity and duration of asphyxia. The Sarnat classification is a common prognostic indicator, with higher staging and longer duration associated with poor outcome.	is recommended. Irritability, hyperactive tendon reflexes, and absence of seizures indicate mild asphyxia. Infants with moderate asphyxia show hypotonia, increased tendon reflexes, weak suck, and seizures with an abnormal electroencephalogram (EEG). Severely asphyxiated infants are unconscious, with absent reflexes and unreactive pupils; the prognosis is poor. The infant may show signs of more than one stage and may progress to another stage, indicating recovery or deterioration.
Neonatal seizures	Seizures are the most common sign of neurologic problems in the neonate. Abnormal electrical discharges in the brain may occur with various medical complications, such as hypoxemia, ischemia, metabolic disturbances, and CNS infection. Manifestations of seizure activity depend on brain maturation and may be subtle in preterm infants. Repetitive eye movements, prolonged staring, lip smacking, posturing, cyclic extremity movements, and apnea are common indicators of neonatal seizure activity.	Seizures greatly increase neuronal energy consumption and may contribute to subsequent CNS hypoxia and hypoglycemia. Neonatal seizures, especially if prolonged or repetitive, increase the risk of developmental sequelae.

Blackburn, S.T. (2003). Neuromuscular and sensory systems. In *Maternal, fetal, and neonatal physiology: A clinical perspective* (2nd ed., pp. 546-598). St. Louis: W.B. Saunders; Medlock, M.D., & Hanigan, W.C. (1997). Neurologic birth trauma, *Perinatology, 24,* 845-857; Paige, P.L., & Carney, P.R. (2002). Neurologic disorders. In G.B. Gardner & S.L. Merenstein (Eds.), *Handbook of neonatal intensive care* (5th ed., pp. 644-678). St. Louis: Mosby; Sarnat, H.B., & Sarnat, M.S. (1976). Neonatal encephalopathy following fetal distress: A clinical and electroencephalographic study. *Archives of Neurology, 33,* 696-705; Volpe, J.J. (2001). *Neurology of the newborn* (4th ed.). Philadelphia: W.B. Saunders.

TABLE 20B-3 Hemolytic and Infectious Complications

Diagnosis	Description	Implications for Occupational Therapists
Anemia	Anemia is a low hemoglobin content of the blood. In the NICU, anemia most commonly results from blood loss (i.e., frequent intermittent blood sampling; perinatal or postnatal hemorrhage) or from hemolysis (breakdown of red blood cells [RBCs]). Immune hemolytic disorders (e.g., ABO incompatibility or Rh incompatibility) and hereditary RBC disorders are some of the other causes.	Mild anemia is common; severe anemia can be life-threatening. Jaundice may occur with hemolytic anemia (i.e., bruising from delivery causes hemolysis with subsequent hyperbilirubinemia). Pallor and increased lethargy are common; cardiorespiratory distress is possible. The infant should not be disturbed during blood transfusions because of the presence of a large-bore catheter in small, fragile veins.
Disseminated intravascular coagulation (DIC)	DIC is an acquired pathologic process that occurs when various underlying disorders or disease processes trigger intravascular clot formation. This clot formation consumes platelets and plasma clotting factors; additional biochemical mechanisms contribute to platelet and RBC destruction. DIC usually results in generalized bleeding from puncture sites, the gastrointestinal tract, CNS, and skin. Anticoagulant measures to prevent major vessel thrombus or skin necrosis from thrombi can complicate medical management.	An infant with DIC is seriously or critically ill. Bruising or petechiae (tiny hemorrhages within the skin or subcutaneous layers that appear as small, flat, red or purple spots) are warning signs; oozing from puncture sites or hemorrhage is a definite red flag. The infant is typically on a minimal stimulation protocol to protect him or her from avoidable stress.
Hyperbilirubinemia	Hyperbilirubinemia is physiologic jaundice resulting from an excess of the bile pigment bilirubin in the blood. Immaturity of the liver and destruction of fetal RBCs are common causes. Jaundice may resolve spontaneously if it is mild, may require phototherapy if it is moderate, or may require phototherapy and exchange blood transfusions if it is severe. Phototherapy converts bilirubin into a form that can be excreted; in severe cases exchange blood transfusions may be indicated to reduce blood levels of bilirubin or to correct severe anemia. In some infants, bilirubin levels may rebound after phototherapy is discontinued and the infant is put back under the bili lights. Untreated severe neonatal hyperbilirubinemia may lead to a condition called kernicterus, which can produce mental retardation as well as sensory and motor disturbances.	Hyperbilirubinemia requiring phototherapy is common in the NICU. An infant under bili lights may appear lethargic or irritable. Positioning is often looser to allow maximal skin exposure to the bili lights. Fiberoptic bili blankets currently provide too firm a surface but allow more secure boundaries. The infant's eyes are patched for protection (neighboring infants also need to be protected from this light source). An oral feeder generally can be removed from the lights during feedings but must remain under phototherapy the rest of the time.
Sepsis	Bacterial sepsis in neonates is characterized by systemic signs of infection associated with bacteria in the blood (bacteremia); multiple organisms can be responsible. NICU infants are susceptible to infection because of prematurity, immature immune systems, stress, medical complications, and surgical procedures. Blood-borne bacteria can localize to produce focal disease such as osteomyelitis (bone infection); pneumonia or meningitis also may result from neonatal sepsis.	Inadequate hand washing is the primary cause of nosocomial infection (infection acquired during hospitalization). Symptoms vary according to the severity of the disease but may include sudden deterioration, metabolic acidosis, temperature instability, apnea, and seizures. The infant must be protected from avoidable stress.

Frank, C.G., Cooper, S.C., & Merenstein, G.B. (2002). *Jaundice.* In G.B. Gardner & S.L. Merenstein (Eds.), *Handbook of neonatal intensive care* (5th ed., pp. 443-461). St. Louis: Mosby; Isaacs, D., & Moxon, E.R. (2000). *Handbook of neonatal infections: A practical guide.* Philadelphia: W.B. Saunders; Manco-Johnson, M., Rodden, D.J., & Collins, S. (2002). Neonatal hematology. In G.B. Gardner & S.L. Merenstein (Eds.), *Handbook of neonatal intensive care* (5th ed., pp. 419-442). St. Louis: Mosby; Merenstein, G.B., Adams, K., & Weisman, L.E. (2002). Infection in the neonate. In G.B. Gardner & S.L. Merenstein (Eds.), *Handbook of neonatal intensive care* (5th ed., pp. 462-484). St. Louis: Mosby.

TABLE 20B-4 Vision and Hearing Complications in Preterm/High-Risk Infants

Diagnosis	Description	Implications for Occupational Therapists
Retinopathy of prematurity (ROP)	ROP designates a pathologic condition that occurs primarily (not exclusively) in preterm infants when injury to the still-developing blood vessels of the retina causes subsequent abnormal vascular formation. ROP description is based on the following factors. *Location:* Zone 1: Innermost circle with the optic disc at its center Zone 2: Donut-shaped circle surrounding zone 1 Zone 3: Crescent-shaped outer zone *Extent:* The retina is divided into clock hours to help describe the extent of the disease. *Stage:* The stage indicates the severity of vascular abnormality, from least severe (stage 1) to partial or total retinal detachment (stages 4 and 5). *PLUS* disease refers to increasingly dilated, tortuous peripheral retinal vessels. Prematurity with low birth weight, oxygen toxicity, vitamin E deficiency, high light intensity, blood transfusions, and infant medical complications that affect oxygen perfusion or vascular constriction and dilation all have been mentioned as potential factors in ROP.	At least 80% of infants with ROP have spontaneous regression, minimal scarring, and little or no visual loss. A high incidence of subsequent refractive errors (astigmatism, myopia, or asymmetric refractive errors), amblyopia, and strabismus (i.e., esotropia and exotropia) does occur. Of the 10% that progress to fibrous scar tissue formation, about one fourth will be blind and the rest will have some degree of significant vision impairment. In general, the prognosis for vision worsens the more posterior the location (i.e., zone 1), the more clock hours involved (extent), and the higher the stage.
Hearing loss; auditory processing disorders	The incidence of confirmed hearing loss in NICU graduates has been reported as 2% to 10%. Medical risk factors include birth weight less than 1,500 g, congenital infection (e.g., cytomegalovirus, rubella, herpes, toxoplasmosis, and herpes), severe sepsis, bacterial meningitis, severe asphyxia, persistent pulmonary hypertension of the newborn, anatomic malformations of the head and neck, severe hyperbilirubinemia, and prolonged hospitalization. Certain medications can damage inner ear structures, causing permanent sensorineural hearing loss. A family history of childhood hearing impairment or parent consanguinity are additional risk factors for some infants. Long-term difficulties in auditory processing can occur in the presence of normal intelligence and hearing sensitivity; behaviors associated with disturbed auditory processing have been noted in NICU graduates (Graven, 2000).	Hearing screening is mandatory and is usually done by a noninvasive technique that measures the brain stem auditory pathway response to sound. Decreased infant responsiveness to auditory parental stimulation may interfere with an optimal parent-infant relationship. Even an intermittent hearing loss (i.e., from fluid accumulation in the middle ear) or a mild hearing loss can adversely affect later speech and language development. Sensory processing problems can occur without hearing loss.

American Academy of Pediatrics, Committee on Environmental Health. (1997). Policy statement: Noise, a hazard for the fetus and newborn. *Pediatrics, 100,* 724-727; Enzman-Hagedorn, M.I., Gardner, S.L., & Abman, S.H. (2002). Respiratory diseases. In G.B. Gardner & S.L. Merenstein (Eds.), *Handbook of neonatal intensive care* (5th ed., pp. 485-575). St. Louis: Mosby; Gardner, S.L., & Goldson, E. (2002). The neonate and the environment: Impact on development. In S.L. Merenstein & G.B. Gardner (Eds.), *Handbook of neonatal intensive care* (5th ed., pp. 219-282). St. Louis: Mosby; Graven, S.N. (2000). Sound and the developing infant in the NICU: Conclusions and recommendations for care. *Journal of Perinatology, 20,* S88-S93; Repka, M.X. (2002). Ophthalmological problems of the premature infant. *Mental Retardation and Developmental Disabilities Research Reviews, 8,* 249-257; Volpe, J.J. (2001). *Neurology of the newborn* (4th ed.). Philadelphia: W.B. Saunders.

TABLE 20B-5 Nutritional and Gastrointestinal Complications

Diagnosis	Description	Implications for Occupational Therapists
Rickets of prematurity (osteopenia)	Preterm infants (especially very low birth weight infants) miss the period of most rapid intrauterine accumulation of calcium and phosphorus, which cannot be duplicated in parenteral nutrition because of insolubility. Some medications also increase urinary calcium losses. For these reasons, preterm infants are at risk for metabolic rickets of prematurity secondary to poor bone mineralization.	Osteopenia increases the risk of fractures. Caregivers must handle the infant gently and be alert for signs of possible fractures (e.g., bruising, swelling, and tenderness).
Necrotizing enterocolitis (NEC)	NEC occurs primarily in preterm infants (90%) and is a major cause of mortality in the NICU. The exact cause and pathogenesis of NEC are unknown; infection, enteral feedings, and local vascular compromise of the gastrointestinal tract (e.g., ischemia from cold stress or persistent apnea) have all been implicated in the resultant mucosal injury. Bacterial invasion and the formation of gas bubbles in the intestinal linings are common. Some cases respond to medical management, although sequelae may still occur. Surgery is indicated if the intestine ruptures or if portions of the intestine become gangrenous.	"NEC watch": Enteral feedings are stopped; antibiotics and total parenteral nutrition (TPN) are started. The infant is positioned for comfort if abdominal distention is present. Comfort measures with gentle handling are appropriate. An infant with actual NEC will no longer receive enteral feeding, will have continuous gastric suction, will be on TPN and antibiotics, and may be on a ventilator. Functional or structural obstruction may occur with or without surgery. Short bowel syndrome with failure to thrive may result, depending on the location and amount of bowel surgically removed.
Gastroschisis	Gastroschisis results from a defect in the abdominal wall of the embryo, usually on the right side near (but not involving) the umbilicus. The intestines and possibly other abdominal organs (stomach, liver, and spleen) develop outside the body and are exposed at birth, with no membranous covering. Gastroschisis often has an associated intestinal malrotation and occasionally atretic portions of the externalized bowel are seen, but malformations of other organ systems are not typical. The exposure of internal organs increases the risk of infection.	Surgery usually is done on day of birth but may be done in stages if not all the organs can fit inside the abdominal cavity immediately (the remainder is sterilely wrapped and suspended above the supine infant in a "silo"); gravity and manual manipulation gradually reduce the contents, and final surgical repair usually is performed at about 1 to 2 weeks of age. Residual problems with gastrointestinal motility or absorption may affect feeding.

Bensard, D.D., Calkins, C.M., Partrick, D., & Price, F.N. (2002). Neonatal surgery. In G.B. Gardner & S.L. Merenstein (Eds.), *Handbook of neonatal intensive care* (4th ed., pp. 702-724). St. Louis: Mosby; Fanaroff, A.A. (2001). Selected disorders of the gastrointestinal tract. In M.H. Klaus & A.A. Fanaroff, (Eds.), *Care of the high-risk neonate* (5th ed., pp. 178-186). Philadelphia: W.B. Saunders; Wilson-Costello, D., Kliegman, R.M., & Fanaroff, A.A. (2001). Necrotizing enterocolitis. In M.H. Klaus & A.A. Fanaroff, (Eds.), *Care of the high-risk neonate* (5th ed., pp. 186-189). Philadelphia: W.B. Saunders.

Medical and Developmental Considerations in Neonatal Positioning

Primary medical staff and developmental specialists who are aware of both the medical and developmental considerations regarding neonatal positioning options can reinforce common goals of maximizing physiologic stability, increasing the infant's comfort, minimizing premie positional deformities, and facilitating normal muscle tone and movement patterns.

TABLE 20C-1 Advantages and Disadvantages of Positioning Options in the NICU

Prone Position	
Medical Advantages	**Developmental Advantages**
Improved oxygenation and ventilation (despite increased work of breathing) with and without ventilatory support.[4,8,18,19,34]	Facilitates development of flexor tone.
Better gastric emptying than in supine position or on left side (unless feedings pool regardless).[46]	Facilitates hand-to-mouth activity for self-calming.
Reduced reflux, especially if head of bed is elevated 30 degrees.[9,39]	Facilitates active neck extension and head raising, forearm propping, and subsequent floor-based gross motor skills.[27]
Decreased episodes of bradycardia and hypoxemia with head of bed elevated 15 degrees versus prone horizontal.[28]	Improved coping with extrauterine environment (i.e., infants sleep more, cry less).
Recommended sleep position for infants with complicated reflux unresponsive to medical and dietary measures.[1,17]	With early placement of head to alternating sides, may decrease persistent head turning to right that results in skull asymmetry.
Decreased risk of aspiration.[23]	Can be used to gently reduce occasional abnormal hip flexion contractures (e.g., potentially with arthrogryposis or fetal compression syndrome) without extra handling for passive range of motion by combined effect of body weight and gravity when legs are extended in neutral alignment.
Term and preterm infants sleep more and cry less in prone than in supine position.[37]	
Less energy expenditure in prone than in supine position.[33]	
Less sleep apnea in prone than in supine position in term and preterm infants.[22,30]	
Increased heart rate during sleep.[41]	
Allows exposure of diaper rash to air or heat lamp.	
Medical Disadvantages	**Developmental Disadvantages**
Access for some acute medical procedures is more difficult.	Flattened, frog-leg posture if no intervention is done.[16,19,35]
Agitated or active infant may self-extubate.	Contributes to dolichocephaly, lateralized head position, and potential prolonged motor asymmetries.[21]
Prone sleep position is associated with increased risk of SIDS.[1,2,17,31,40]	Visual exploration is more difficult for baby.
	Face-to-face social contact between baby and caregiver is more difficult.

Continued

TABLE 20C-1 Advantages and Disadvantages of Positioning Options in the NICU—*cont'd*

Supine Position

Medical Advantages	Developmental Advantages
Easier access to infant for medical care. Supine position in hammock (versus "flat" supine position) increases sleep time for preterm infants.[9] Recommended position for reducing risk of sudden infant death syndrome (SIDS) (when infant is near and after discharge).[1,2,17,31,40] Decreased arterial oxygen tension, lung compliance and tidal volume compared to prone position. More reflux than in prone position at any time or than in upright sitting if infant is awake.[39] Greater risk of aspiration than in prone or right side-lying position.[23] Term and preterm infants sleep less and cry more in supine than in prone position.[37] Supine position (in hammock) may decrease respiration if infant has decreased lung compliance (i.e., respiratory distress syndrome).[9] Greater energy expenditure in supine than in prone position.[33]	Easier visual exploration by infant. Facilitates face-to-face social contact between baby and caregiver. Supine position (in hammock) may facilitate midline position.[9] Head can be positioned in the midline to reduce lateral head flattening. Encourages extension rather than flexion (i.e., increased muscle tone with hyperextension of head, neck, and shoulders). Encourages external rotation positional deformities of arms and legs (with subsequent delay in hands-to-midline and reaching activities, plus out-toeing gait). Supine sleep position (per SIDS recommendations) has been correlated with posterior plagiocephaly[3,14,15,22-24,26,27,29,36,38] and later developmental delays in motor skills.[27]

Side-Lying Position

Medical Advantages	Developmental Advantages
Right side: Better gastric emptying than in supine or left side-lying position (about same as in prone position).[45] Better oxygenation for infant with unilateral lung disease with good lung positioned uppermost.[11] Can be used to treat pulmonary interstitial emphysema by placing affected lung in dependent (bottom) position.[42]	Encourages midline orientation of head and extremities. Counteracts external rotation of limbs; promotes extremity flexion and adduction. Facilitates hand-to-mouth pattern for self-calming. Facilitates hand-to-hand activity.

Medical Disadvantages	Developmental Disadvantages
Left side: Decreased gastric emptying compared to prone or right side-lying position.[44] May contribute to atelectasis of dependent (bottom) lung in micropremie. Side sleeping is linked to increased risk of SIDS compared with supine position.[2,31,40]	May be difficult to maintain flexed side-lying position with active, irritable, and/or hypertonic extended infant.

Semireclined/Sitting Position

Medical Advantages	Developmental Advantages
Alternative position (e.g., for variety, skin integrity). Increased lung compliance and decreased pulmonary resistance (possibly due to increased pulmonary functional residual capacity) in semisitting versus supine position.[13]	An alerting posture. Encourages infant visual exploration. Encourages social interaction. May allow use of swing for older NICU infants. May help temporarily inhibit (relax) high tone (i.e., with hips flexed ≥90 degrees).

Medical Disadvantages	Developmental Disadvantages
Infant seat or car seat elevated 60 degrees increases frequency and duration of reflux.[39] More upright position (95 degrees) increases heart rate and mean arterial pressure in preterm infants compared to more reclined car seat positions of 110 degrees and 140 degrees.[43] Decreased oxygen saturation, apnea, and bradycardia may occur in smaller premature infants and some healthy term infants in semireclined/car seat positioning.[5,6,12]	May be difficult to maintain proper head, neck, and trunk alignment because baby is more upright.[13] Neck flexion (if it occurs) increases airway resistance and predisposes infant to obstructive apnea.[12,13] Overuse of infant carriers may contribute to development of posterior plagiocephaly.[14] Unless infant's head is supported in the midline, asymmetric head position will predominate.

Continued

TABLE 20C-1 Advantages and Disadvantages of Positioning Options in the NICU—*cont'd*

Head Position/Head in Midline

Medical Advantages	Developmental Advantages
Keeping head in midline seems to decrease intracranial pressure and intraventricular hemorrhage.[20]	Head in midline may reduce lateral head flattening and asymmetric plagiocephaly.
Elevation of head of bed 30 degrees may reduce intracranial pressure.[20]	Midline positioning reduces postural asymmetry and encourages development of antigravity flexion.
	Water beds (and water pillows) may reduce head flattening (dolichocephaly, scaphocephaly).[19,32]
Pressure sore may develop on occiput if head remains in midline too long on firm surface without pressure relief.	Head midline positioning is not possible in prone position.

References

1 American Academy of Pediatrics. (1992). Policy Statement: Positioning and SIDS (RE9254). *Pediatrics, 89,* 1120-1126.

2 American Academy of Pediatrics. (1996). Policy Statement: Positioning and Sudden Infant Death Syndrome (SIDS) Update (RE9254). *Pediatrics, 98,* 1216-1218.

3 Argenta, L., David, L., Wilson, J., & Bell, W. (1996). An increase in infant cranial deformity with supine sleeping position. *Journal of Craniofacial Surgery, 7,* 5-11.

4 Baird, T.M., Paton, J.B., & Fisher, D.E. (1992). Improved oxygenation with prone positioning in neonates: Stability of increased transcutaneous PO_2. *Neonatal Intensive Care, 5,* 43-44, 46.

5 Bass, J.L., Mehta, K.A., & Camara, J. (1993). Monitoring premature infants in car seats: Implementing the American Academy of Pediatrics policy in a community hospital. *Pediatrics, 91,* 1137-1141.

6 Bass, J.L., & Mehta, K.A. (1995). Oxygen saturation of selected term infants in car seats. *Pediatrics, 96,* 288-290.

7 Beckmann, C.A. (1997). Use of neonatal boundaries to improve outcomes. *Journal of Holistic Nursing, 15,* 54-67. (*Note:* The Snuggle-Up was not used correctly in this study, i.e. "... The *head* is supported by a rounded rim of material filled with batting," p. 60).

8 Bjornson, K., Deitz, J., Blackburn, S., Billingsly, F., Garcia, J., & Hays, R. (1992). The effect of body position on the oxygen saturation of ventilated preterm infants. *Pediatric Physical Therapy,* 109-115.

9 Bottos, M., Pettenazzo, A., Giancola, G., Stefani, D., Pettena, G., & Viscolani, B., et al. (1985). The effect of a containing position in a hammock versus the supine position on the cutaneous oxygen level in premature and term babies. *Early Human Development, 11,* 265-273.

10 Bozynski, M., Naglie, R., Nicks, J., Burpee, B., & Johnson, R.V. (1988). Lateral positioning of the stable ventilated very low birthweight infant. *American Journal of Diseases in Children, 142,* 200-202.

11 Callahan, C.W., & Sisler, C. (1997). Use of seating devices in infants too young to sit. *Archives of Pediatric and Adolescent Medicine, 151,* 233-235.

12 Carlo, W.A., Beoglos, A., Siner, B.S., & Martin, R.J. (1989). Neck and body position effects on pulmonary mechanics in infants. *Pediatrics, 84,* 670-674.

13 Chaduck, W.M., Kast, J., & Donahue, D.J. (1997). The enigma of lambdoid positional molding. *Pediatric Neurosurgery, 26,* 304-311.

14 Chan, J.S.L., Kelley, M.L., & Khan, J. (1995). Predictors of postnatal head molding in very low birth weight infants. *Neonatal Network, 14,* 47-52.

15 Downs, J.A., Edwards, A.D., McCormick, D.C., Roth, S.C., & Stewart, A.L. (1991). Effect of intervention on the development of hip posture in very preterm babies. *Archives of Disease in Childhood, 66,* 197-201.

16 Faure, C., Leluyer, B., Aujard, Y., deBethmann, O., Bedu, A., & Briand, E., et al. (1996). Sleeping position, prevention of sudden infant death syndrome and gastroesophageal reflux. *Archives de Pediatrica, 3,* 598-601.

17 Fox, M., & Molesky, M. (1990). The effects of prone and supine positioning on arterial oxygen pressure. *Neonatal Network, 8,* 25-29.

18 Fox, R., Viscardi, R., Tackiak, V., Niknafs, H., & Cinoman, M.I. (1993). Effect of position on pulmonary mechanics in healthy preterm newborn infants. *Journal of Perinatology, 13,* 205-211.

19 Fowler, K., Kum-Nji, P., Wells, P.J., & Mangrem, C.L. (1997). Water beds may be useful in preventing scaphocephaly in preterm very low birth weight neonates. *Journal of Perinatology, 17,* 397.

20 Geerdink, J.J, Hopkins, B., & Hoeksma, J.B. (1994). The development of head position in preterm infants beyond term age. *Developmental Psychobiology, 27,* 153-168.

21 Goldberg, R.N., Joshi, A., Moscoso, P., & Castillo, T. (1983). The effect of head position on intracranial pressure in the neonate. *Critical Care Medicine, 11,* 428-430.

22 Heimler, R., Langlois, J., Hodel, D., Nelin, L., & Sasidharan, P. (1992). Effect of positioning on the breathing pattern in premature infants. *Archives of Disease in Childhood, 67,* 312-314.

23 Hewitt, V. (1976). Effect of posture on the presence of fat in tracheal aspirate in neonates. *Australian Pediatric Journal, 12,* 267.

24 Huang, C-S, Cheng, H-S, Lin, W-Y, Liou, J-W, & Chen, Y-R. (1995). Skull morphology affected by different sleep positions in infancy. *Cleft Palate–Craniofacial Journal, 32,* 413-419.

25 Huang, M.H., Mouradian, W.E., Cohen S.R., & Gruss, J.S. (1998). The differential diagnosis of abnormal head shapes: Separating craniosynostosis from positional deformities and normal variants. *Cleft Palate–Craniofacial Journal, 35,* 204-211.

26 Hunt, C.E., & Puczynski, M.S. (1996). Does supine sleeping cause asymmetric heads? *Pediatrics, 98,* 127-129.

27 Jantz, J.W., Blosser, C.D., & Fruechting, L.A. (1997). A motor milestone change noted with a change in sleep position. *Archives of Pediatric and Adolescent Medicine, 151,* 565-568.

28 Jenni, O.G., von Siebenthal, K., Wolf, M., Keel, M., Duc, G., & Bucher, H.U. (1997). Effect of nursing in the head elevated tilt position (15°) on the incidence of bradycardic and hypoxemic episodes in preterm infants. *Pediatrics, 100,* 622-625.

29 Kane, A.A., Mitchell, L.E., Craven, K.P., & Marsh, J.L. (1996). Observations on a recent increase in plagiocephaly without synostosis. *Pediatrics, 97,* 877-885.

30 Kurlak, L.O., Ruggins, N.R., & Stephenson, T.J. (1994). Effect of nursing position on incidence, type, and duration of clinically significant apnea in preterm infants. *Archives of Disease in Childhood, 71,* F16-F19.

31 Lockridge, T. (1997). Now I lay me down to sleep: SIDS and infant sleep positions. *Neonatal Network, 16,* 25-31.

Notes to Table 20C-1 (Cont'd)

32 Marsden, D.J. (1980). Reduction of head flattening in preterm infants. *Developmental Medicine and Child Neurology, 22,* 507-509.
33 Masterson, J., Zucker, C., & Schulze, K. (1987). Prone and supine effects on energy expenditure and behavior of low birth weight neonates. *Pediatrics, 80,* 689-692.
34 Mizuno, K., Itabashi, K., & Okuyama, K. (1995). Effect of body position on the blood gases and ventilation volume of infants with chronic lung disease before and after feeding. *American Journal of Perinatology, 12,* 275-277.
35 Monfort, K.P., & Case-Smith, J. (1997). The effects of a neonatal positioner on scapular rotation. *American Journal of Occupational Therapy, 51,* 378-384.
36 Mulliken, J.B., VanderWoude, D.L., Hansen, M., LaBrie, R.A., & Scott, R.M. (1999). Analysis of posterior plagiocephaly: Deformational versus synostotic. *Plastic & Reconstructive Surgery, 103,* 371-380.
37 Myers, M.M., Fifer, W.P., Schaeffer, L., Sahni, R., Ohira-Kist, K., & Stark, R.I., et al. (1998). Effects of sleeping position and time after feeding on the organization of sleep/wake states in prematurely born infants. *Sleep, 21,* 343-349.
38 Najarian, S.P. (1999). Infant cranial molding deformation and sleep position: Implications for primary care. *Journal of Pediatric Health Care, 13,* 173-177.
39 Orenstein, S., Whitington, P., & Orenstein, D. (1983). The infant seat as treatment for gastroesophageal reflux. *New England Journal of Medicine, 309,* 760-763.
40 Oyen, N., Markestad, T., Skaerven, R., Irgens, L.M., Helweg-Larsen, K., & Alm, B., et al. (1997). Combined effects of sleeping position and prenatal risk factors in sudden infant death syndrome: The Nordic epidemiological SIDS study. *Pediatrics, 100,* 613-621.
41 Sahni, R., Schulze, K.F., Kashyap, S., Ohira-Kist, K., Myers, M.M., & Fifer, W.P. (1999). Body position, sleep states, and cardiorespiratory activity in developing low birth weight infants. *Early Human Development, 54,* 197-206.
42 Schwartz, A., & Graham, B. (1986). Neonatal tension pulmonary interstitial emphysema in bronchopulmonary dysplasia: Treatment with lateral decubitus positioning. *Radiology, 161,* 351-354.
43 Smith, P., & Turner, B. (1990). The physiologic effects of positioning premature infants in car seats. *Neonatal Network, 9,* 11-15.
44 Tobin, J.M., McCloud, P., & Cameron, D.J. (1997). Posture and gastro-esophageal reflux: A case for left lateral positioning. *Archives of Disease in Childhood, 76,* 254-258.
45 Victor, Y.H. (1975). Effect of body position on gastric emptying in the neonate. *Archives of Disease in Childhood, 50,* 500-504.
46 Willett, L., Leuschen, M.P., Nelson, L.S., & Nelson, R.M. (1986). Risk of hypoventilation in premature infants in car seats. *Journal of Pediatrics, 109,* 245-248.

Early Intervention

Linda C. Stephens ■ Susan K. Tauber

CHAPTER OBJECTIVES

1 Describe the early intervention legislation and
   program regulations.
2 Explain family-centered early intervention philosophy and principles.
3 Define the components of an individualized
   family service plan (IFSP).
4 Explain models of evaluation, and describe specific assessments.
5 Describe developmentally appropriate and family-
   centered intervention approaches.
6 Define areas of emphasis in occupational therapy.
7 Explain strategies and activities used by occupational therapists in working with infants and
   children.

WHAT IS EARLY INTERVENTION?

The term early intervention connotes different meanings to different professionals. In this chapter, *early* refers
to the most critical period of a child's development
between birth and 3 years of age. *Intervention* refers
to program implementation designed to maintain or
enhance the child's development in natural environments
and as a member of a family. The authors also use early
intervention to describe services for children from birth
to 3 years of age who have an established risk, have a
developmental delay, or are considered to be environmentally or biologically at risk. The goal of early
intervention is "to prevent or minimize the physical, cognitive, emotional, and resource limitations of young children disadvantaged by biological or environmental risk
factors" (Blackman, 2002, p. 11).

LEGISLATION RELATED TO EARLY INTERVENTION

The 1980s brought widespread acceptance and support
for family-centered care for children with special needs
(Shonkoff & Meisels, 1990). Family-centered care is
based on the principle that an infant is dependent on his
or her mother and other family members for daily care
and meeting his or her physical and emotional needs. At
the same time, the birth of an infant with special health
care needs affects the entire family emotionally, socially,
and economically. In 1986, amendments to the Education of the Handicapped Act (EHA) established incentives for states to develop systems of coordinated care for
infants with disabilities and their families. These incentives were strengthened in 1990, when the EHA was
further amended and retitled the Individuals with
Disabilities Education Act (IDEA, 1990; P.L. 101-476).
Through Part C of IDEA, all children from birth
through 2 years of age who experience developmental
delays are entitled to services. The revisions to IDEA in
1990 and again in 1997 expand and clarify the roles
of parents, promote well-planned and well-coordinated
transitions of children from early intervention programs to preschool, emphasize assistive technology, and
strengthen obligations of other agencies to provide
services to students in school.

Part C of IDEA: Infants and Toddlers with Disabilities

**Part C of the Individuals with Disabilities Education
Act** delineates the policies and regulations that participating states must follow in establishing early intervention services and systems. Table 21-1 summarizes the
differences between Part C, which defines early intervention services for children between birth and 3 years
of age, and Part B, which defines school programs for
eligible students between 3 and 21 years of age (see
Chapter 22). Part C is an entitlement program, and
Part B defines mandated services. An entitlement simply
acknowledges one's rights to something; a mandate
establishes programs and services that are obligatory
by law.

TABLE 21-1 Comparison of Educational Programs by Age Group

	0 to 2 Years	**3 to 5 Years**	**6 to 21 Years**
Legislation	IDEA, Part C	IDEA, Part B	IDEA, Part B
Program	Early intervention	Special education	Special education
Type	Entitlement	Mandate	Mandate
Eligibility	Noncategorical	Categorical	Categorical
Services Provided	16 Primary services, including occupational therapy, physical therapy, speech therapy, and special instruction	Related services only as support to special education	Related services only as support to special education
	Interdisciplinary and transdisciplinary assessment	Discipline-specific assessment	Discipline-specific assessment as related to education
	Individualized Family Service Plan	Individualized Education Program	Individualized Education Program
	Family-centered	Family-focused in theory, child-focused in practice	Child-focused with emphasis on curricular standards
	Service coordination	Service coordination recommended but not mandated	Service coordination recommended but not mandated
Location	Natural settings	Home, center, or school-based	School-based

IDEA, Individuals with Disabilities Education Act.

The purpose of Part C of IDEA is to give each state support in maintaining and implementing comprehensive, coordinated, multidisciplinary, interagency systems of early intervention services for infants and toddlers with disabilities and their families. Each state is required to establish a system that meets the following requirements:

1 Officially defines *developmental delay*
2 Establishes a state policy that ensures that appropriate early intervention services are available to all infants and children with disabilities and their families
3 Provides timely, comprehensive, multidisciplinary evaluations of the functioning of each infant and toddler with a disability
4 Allows the families of children who are recipients of early intervention services to identify their family priorities
5 Establishes a process for implementing individualized family service plans (IFSPs) that include service coordination
6 Develops a comprehensive child find system
7 Implements a public awareness program
8 Creates a central directory with information on early intervention services, resources, and experts and makes it available to families and others
9 Designs and implements a comprehensive system of personnel development; establishes policies and procedures for personnel standards
10 Puts procedure safeguards into place
11 Designates and establishes a single line of authority in a lead agency; establishes a policy for contracting or coordinating with local service providers
12 Establishes procedures for timely reimbursement of funds

13 Designs and implements a system for compiling data regarding early intervention programs
14 Defines policies and procedures to ensure that (a) to the maximum extent appropriate, early intervention services are provided in a natural environment and (b) provision of early intervention services occurs in a setting other than the infant's natural environment only when early intervention cannot be achieved satisfactorily for the infant or child in a natural environment
15 Establishes a state interagency coordinating council composed of parents, government officials, agency representatives, and service providers (this body advises and assists the lead agency in administering and coordinating the state early intervention system)

Eligibility

Infants or toddlers are eligible for early intervention services if they fall into the following categories:

- *Established risk.* Infants and toddlers are eligible for early intervention services if they have a diagnosis associated with developmental delay, such as Down syndrome or cerebral palsy.
- *Developmental delay.* Results of an "appropriate" diagnostic instrument or procedure or informed clinical opinion indicate delay in one or more of the following developmental areas: cognitive, motor (includes vision and hearing), communication, social-emotional, and adaptive. States differ in the criteria chosen to determine "appropriate" instruments or procedures.
- *At risk.* This category is included at state discretion and refers to a child who is considered to be at risk

for the occurrence of a substantial developmental delay unless early intervention services are provided. Causation may be a result of environmental or biologic risk factors (e.g., infants born to teen mothers or drug- or alcohol-addicted mothers and infants with very low birth weight [VLBW] or failure to thrive [FTT]). Intervention strategies and programs are intended to prevent or ameliorate developmental delays and deformities, maximize each child's potential, and assist the family in adjusting to the challenges of daily living in the home and community.

Required Services

Families with infants with disabilities are eligible for 16 early intervention services provided by qualified personnel under public supervision and in conformity with the IFSP. Services should be family-centered, inclusive, and culturally sensitive. The services are as follows:

1 Assistive technology devices and services
2 Audiology
3 Family training, counseling, and home visits
4 Health services
5 Medical services for diagnostics and evaluation only
6 Nursing
7 Nutrition
8 Occupational therapy
9 Physical therapy
10 Psychological services
11 Service coordination
12 Social work
13 Special instruction
14 Speech and language therapy
15 Transportation
16 Vision services

Identification

The first step in the early intervention process is public awareness and a state system of Child Find that effectively identifies children at risk for developmental delay who would benefit from early intervention. This system must include standard referral procedures to be used by all primary referral sources and assignment of a service coordinator for the child and family as soon as possible after receiving the referral.

Evaluation Requirements

As stated in IDEA (1997):

(1) Evaluation means the procedures used by appropriate qualified personnel to determine a child's initial and continuing eligibility under this part, consistent with the definition of "infants and toddlers with disabilities" in Sec. 303.16.

(2) Assessment means the ongoing procedures used by appropriate qualified personnel throughout the period of a child's eligibility under this part to identify—
    (i) The child's unique strengths and needs and the services appropriate to meet those needs, and
    (ii) The resources, priorities, and concerns of the family and the supports and services necessary to enhance the family's capacity to meet the developmental needs of their infant or toddler with a disability.

In this chapter the term *evaluation* refers to both evaluation and assessment procedure. The multidisciplinary team who evaluates the child includes the professionals listed previously whose services seem warranted or are desired by the family. The team must obtain parental permission before the evaluation. The team must complete the evaluation process within 45 days of identification.

The service coordinator is responsible for ensuring that the evaluation process (1) is conducted by trained personnel; (2) is based on the state's adopted criteria of standard deviations or informed clinical opinion; (3) includes the child's medical and health history; (4) includes levels of functioning, unique needs, and recommended services related to the five developmental areas (cognition, physical, communication, social and emotional, and adaptive); and (5) takes place in natural environments.

The therapist documents the family resources, priorities, and concerns as they relate to the child's development. Collection of this information is family-directed and voluntary. The evaluation procedures must be nondiscriminatory as to race, ethnicity, and socioeconomic background and in the family's native language or mode of communication to the best extent possible.

Individualized Family Service Plan

The IFSP follows completion of the evaluation. It is a written plan that delineates the family's desired outcomes for the child and the services that will be provided to reach those outcomes. The IFSP must be written during a meeting of the parents or caregivers and the team members within 45 days after the referral. The IFSP is a map of the family's services and informs anyone who will be working with the child and family, which services will be provided, where they will be provided, and who will provide them. IDEA specifies that services must be provided in the infant's natural settings. The IFSP defines the environments in which the child is to be served and provides a statement of justification if services are not provided in natural environments. The IFSP also identifies the service coordinator who will be responsible for working with the family.

The role of a service coordinator in the IFSP process is a unique Part C provision. The service coordinator assists the family in accessing information and resources and coordinates implementation of the IFSP. Box 21-1 lists the required components as they are stated in IDEA.

If the child requires preschool special education or other services, the therapist must write the services into the IFSP's transition procedures. This step requires contact with the local education agency (LEA) and requires parental consent to provide records to the LEA for continuity of services and evaluation, as well as for assessment information. The IFSP is reviewed every 6 months, with an annual reevaluation.

The IFSP is not a treatment plan; it is both a planning process and a document that identifies child and family outcomes. Specific services are listed as they relate to the hoped-for outcomes. For example, occupational therapy services may be listed on the IFSP as they relate to desired developmental goals that the parents identified. The therapist often writes specific occupational therapy intervention objectives and procedures that will support the family and infant or child outcomes on a separate document. This additional document can give specific guidance to the therapist by maintaining a record of the child's performance. The therapist may also submit the document to third-party reimbursement agencies.

BOX 21-1   Required Components of the Individualized Family Service Plan

The IFSP shall be in writing and shall contain the following (IDEA, sec. 636):

1. A statement of the infant's or child's present level of motor, cognitive, communication, social-emotional, and adaptive development, based on objective criteria
2. A statement of the family's resources, priorities, and concerns related to enhancing the development of their infant or child
3. A statement of the major outcomes expected to be achieved for the infant or child and the family, and the criteria, procedures, and timelines used to determine the degree to which progress toward achieving the outcomes is being made and whether modifications or revisions of the outcomes or service are necessary
4. A statement of specific early intervention services necessary to meet the unique needs of the infant or child and the family, including the frequency, intensity, and method of delivering services
5. A statement of the natural environments in which early intervention services shall appropriately be provided, including a justification of the extent, if any, to which the services will not be provided in a natural environment
6. The projected dates for initiation of service and the anticipated duration of the services
7. The identification of the service coordination from the profession most immediately relevant to the infant's or family's needs who will be responsible for the implementation of the plan and coordination with other agencies and persons
8. The steps to be taken to support the transition of the child with a disability to preschool or other appropriate services

---

Procedural Safeguards

The parents must be informed of their rights that underlie the early intervention process. All states that use federal funds for early intervention services have specified procedural safeguards that protect the rights of parents and infants. The procedural safeguards required in a statewide system under section 635(1)(13) of IDEA include the following:

1. Timely administrative resolution of complaints by parents
2. Right to confidentiality of personally identifiable information, including the right of parents to written notice of and written consent to the exchange of information among agencies
3. Right of parents to determine whether they, their infant or toddler, or other family members will accept or decline any early intervention service
4. Opportunity for parents to examine records relating to assessment, screening, eligibility determinations, and the development and implementation of the IFSP
5. Written prior notice to the parents of the infant or toddler with a disability whenever a service provider proposes to initiate or change the identification, evaluation, or placement of the infant
6. Notice of any change fully informing the parent in the parents' native language

During a period in which proceedings or action involving a complaint by the parents is pending, the infant or toddler continues to receive the appropriate early intervention services.

Transition into Preschool Services

A transition plan should be identified and documented in the IFSP as soon as possible and as soon as relevant. A referral to the LEA should be made 6 months before the child's third birthday or at 30 months of age. This helps the school system analyze all existing evaluation and assessment information and determine if further testing or information is necessary. It also enables the LEA to determine eligibility under Part B (which in some cases may differ from Part C eligibility) and, if eligible, plan for appropriate placement. In the case of a child who may not be eligible for preschool services, with the approval of the family, the early intervention service providers should convene to discuss the appropriate services that the child may receive.

Funding and State Administration

Through the Part C program, states receive federal funds based on their census of infants and toddlers compared with the total number of infants and toddlers nationally. Part C funds are used as the "payer of last resort" for services for eligible children only after other available funds through another federal, state, local, or private sources have been used. The lead agency is responsible for identifying and coordinating all funding resources and must enter into formal interagency agreements with other state agencies that provide services to young children and their families. Families are entitled to the following services at no cost: Child Find, evaluation and assessment, service coordination, and administration and coordination of IFSP activities. As in Part B of IDEA, families are entitled to all procedural safeguards.

An Interagency Coordinating Council (ICC) is to advise and assist the lead agency in the implementation of a statewide early intervention system. The system is to be a "comprehensive, coordinated, collaborative, multidisciplinary, program for infants and toddlers with disabilities and their families." The ICC assists the lead agency and the state education agency (SEA) in coordinating Part C and Part B of IDEA. Members of the state ICC, who are appointed by the governor, include parents, public and private providers, a member of the legislature, a representative from personnel preparation, and members from the state agencies involved in administering early intervention services, paying for services, administering preschool programs and head start, and administering the state governance of insurance (e.g., Medicaid).

In addition to the state ICC, each district or county has a local ICC (LICC), which includes parents and public and private providers. Each LICC is responsible for identifying and coordinating services within its geographic area. The LICC or local collaborative groups often help families identify and access infant evaluation and intervention services that are available within the county or region.

IMPLICATIONS OF LEGISLATION FOR THE OCCUPATIONAL THERAPIST

Part C of IDEA considers occupational therapy to be a "primary service" for eligible infants and toddlers from birth through 2 years of age who qualify for early intervention services. As a primary service, occupational therapy can be provided as the only service a child receives or in addition to other early intervention services. By its legal definition, occupational therapy includes services to address the functional needs of the child related to adaptive development; adaptive behavior and play; and sensory, motor, and postural development. It includes adaptation of the environment and selection, design, and fabrication of assistive and orthotic devices to facilitate development and promote the acquisition of functional skills. The therapist designs these services to prevent or minimize the influence of initial or future impairment, delay in development, or loss of functional ability.

The practice of occupational therapy in early intervention has been influenced by public legislation in the following ways:

- *Team coordination and interagency communication.* The occupational therapist practices as part of an interdisciplinary team and contributes occupational therapy findings and recommendations to the IFSP. With parental permission and observation of confidentiality, the therapist shares therapy reports with other agencies that are delivering services to the family (Garland & Linder, 1994; Harbin, McWilliam, & Gallagher, 1998).
- *Family service plan versus child-centered treatment plan.* The occupational therapist provides services according to family priorities. The family determines the intervention goals, which may focus on the child or the family as a whole (Miller & Hanft, 1998; McWilliam & Strain, 1993; Odom & McLean, 1993).
- *Indirect versus direct treatment.* The occupational therapist may consider various service delivery models, including those that may be transdisciplinary or consultative in nature. The model of direct, individual, child-centered services often is not the most appropriate one in early intervention (McWilliam, 1996).
- *Concern with generalization of skills.* The occupational therapist is concerned with the functional use of skills in the child's natural environment rather than the development of skills in isolation (Hanft & Pilkington, 2000).
- *Ability to practice role release.* Professionals in early intervention often find it advantageous to use role release in the provision of services. In role release, one professional may be trained to take over functions that traditionally have been performed by another professional (Bruder & Bologna, 1993; McGonigel & Garland, 1988).
- *Variety of settings.* Natural environments include the home and community settings in which children without disabilities participate. Occupational therapists are more likely to provide services in community settings, such as the home or a childcare center, than in medical settings (Hanft & Pilkington, 2000; Trivette, Dunst, & Deal, 1997).
- *Wide range of disabilities.* As state lead agencies and Child Find services identify children who qualify for services, the occupational therapist is expected to work with children with various special needs. These may include biologically or environmentally at-risk populations that traditionally may not have received intervention (Garbarino & Ganzel, 2000).
- *Work in small groups.* Traditional methods of individual or one-on-one treatment are often replaced by the delivery of services to small groups of children or small parent-infant groups (Figure 21-1).

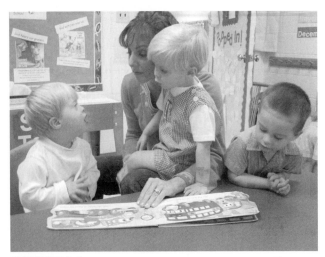

FIGURE 21-1   The occupational therapist uses small groups that include children with an IFSP and peer models.

- *Knowledge about the educational and community service delivery models.* Occupational therapists must be competent in working outside the traditional medical model and need to understand educational and family-centered models of practice (McWilliam, 1996; Turnbull, Turbiville, & Turnbull, 2000).
- *Addressing family concerns and priorities.* The occupational therapist must be sensitive to family needs and have respect for the parents' priorities. For example, the parent who is homeless or jobless may not be concerned about occupational therapy for the child. Another parent may believe that certain skills or goals are more important than those identified by the therapist. The occupational therapist should also be cognizant of the effect of factors, such as criteria imposed by third-party payers that limit a family's access to services.

FAMILY-CENTERED PROGRAMS

The early intervention system recognizes that families can be and often are knowledgeable consumers and effective change agents for the child. It also acknowledges that families have specific needs related to a child with disabilities and that families may be the recipients of services (Mahoney & Filer, 1996; Turnbull et al., 2000). The family's early intervention team helps each family identify its unique resources, priorities, and concerns. The team then identifies outcomes and goals that enable the family to function more effectively and help the child as a member of the family unit. Acknowledging that families are both participants and consumers of early intervention services, Simeonsson and Bailey (1990) identified four different ways in which interven-

tion could be provided for infants with special needs and their families:

1 Therapy administered to the infant, with the parent as a passive observer
2 Parents involved as members of the intervention team, participating in the planning process and involved in the child's program
3 Parents trained to carry out therapeutic activities as co-therapists or as the primary intervention agents
4 Families viewed as important recipients of services in their own right

The nature and extent of family involvement may vary and depends on family needs, values, lifestyles, and variables within the structure of the early intervention program itself. The degree of family involvement may fluctuate and change in response to external or internal factors that affect family functioning and coping. Some examples are degree of acceptance of the child's disability, job status of one or both parents, a new infant in the family, or changes in the family's support networks, such as grandparents, friends, or church groups.

The occupational therapist who works within a family-centered model develops goals collaboratively with parents or primary caregivers. Using a family systems perspective, the therapist recognizes the influence and interrelationships of the family within various systems, such as extended family, neighborhood, and early intervention programs. By thinking broadly about families and their subsystems, the therapist can help parents communicate their concerns and identify their priorities for the child. Effective listening and interviewing skills are essential, as is the ability to communicate with sensitivity the therapist's own concerns about the child's development. Families who have children with special needs highly value services in which professionals provide clear, understandable, complete information; demonstrate respect for the child and family; provide emotional support; and provide expert, skillful intervention (Featherstone, 1980; Rosenbaum, King, Law, King, & Evans, 1998). Box 21-2 lists principles of family-centered intervention.

EARLY INTERVENTION TEAM

The success of an early intervention program depends largely on the integration of the child's individual program components into a comprehensive system carried out by a cooperative team of professionals. Teamwork is critical because of the interrelated nature of the problems of the developing child and the need for skills and resources from many professionals to meet the needs of the child and family. The emphasis of intervention should be the child within the family unit rather than the child alone and should be carried out through collaboration among all professionals involved. (Models of teamwork are described in Chapter 2.) The two team

BOX 21-2   Principles of Family-Centered Intervention

The following principles have been generally accepted in the implementation of family-centered care (McGonigel, 1991, p. 9):

1 Infants and children are uniquely dependent on their families for their survival and nurturance. This dependence necessitates a family-centered approach to early intervention.

2 Programs should define *family* in a way that reflects the diversity of family patterns and structures.

3 Each family has its own structure, roles, values, beliefs, and coping styles. Respect for and acceptance of this diversity is a cornerstone of family-centered early intervention.

4 Early intervention systems and strategies must honor the racial, ethnic, cultural, and socioeconomic diversity of families.

5 Respect for family autonomy, independence, and decision making means that families must be able to choose the level and nature of early intervention's involvement in their lives.

6 Family and professional collaboration and partnerships are the keys to family-centered early intervention and to successful implementation of the IFSP process.

7 An enabling approach to working with families requires that professionals reexamine their traditional roles and practices and develop new practices when necessary (practices that promote mutual respect and partnerships).

8 Early intervention services should be flexible, accessible, and responsive to family-identified needs.

9 Professionals should provide early intervention services according to the normalization principle (i.e., families should have access to services provided in as normal a fashion and environment as possible and that promote the integration of the child and family within the community).

10 No one agency or discipline can meet the diverse and complex needs of infants and children with special needs and their families. Therefore a team approach to planning and implementing the IFSP is necessary.

---

models of interaction most appropriate in early intervention are interdisciplinary and transdisciplinary.

Team Models of Interaction
Interdisciplinary

In the interdisciplinary model of interaction, a team of professionals from several disciplines involved with the child collaborates with the family to develop and implement an intervention program. These professionals have continuing direct involvement with the child and collaborate with one another in carrying out the child's program. The team members perform evaluations independently or together and set goals in collaboration with professionals and parents. With this approach the child and family can receive coordinated services and are able to benefit from the expertise of professionals from several disciplines who are directly involved (Case-Smith & Wavrek, 1998).

Each member of an interdisciplinary team is accountable to the team as a whole, although the degree and amount of involvement may vary and change depending on the child and family needs. The family's service coordinator is usually the person responsible for the coordination of team members to avoid fragmentation or duplication of services. To ensure the success of this approach, the team members must respect one another's roles, develop effective formal and informal communication patterns, and be flexible in response to family preferences. This requires a willingness to share expertise and knowledge and to assume accountability for intervention procedures (Bailey, 1991; see Chapter 2).

Transdisciplinary

In the transdisciplinary model of interaction, various disciplines interact as a team, but one member is usually designated to provide direct intervention with other team members who act as consultants. This approach is based on the belief that the family benefits from having intervention primarily from one professional rather than multiple interventions from several professionals. All team members contribute to assessment and program planning, and then the designated person implements the plan with consultation and training from other members of the team. Therefore, the transdisciplinary model enables each professional to perform functions that are normally outside the scope of practice of his or her discipline. Implementation of this model requires role release, or the relinquishing of some or all of one professional's functions to another professional (Figure 21-2). Role release has been defined as a process of sharing and the exchange of certain roles and responsibilities among team members (McGonigel, Woodruff, & Roszmann-Millican, 1994).

Giangreco (1986) described the transdisciplinary approach as "indirect, integrated, and decentralized; it limits the number of people carrying out a program but makes use of the expertise of a variety of professionals" (p. 9). However, this approach was not intended to promote a team in which each professional developed the same skills across discipline lines, but rather to promote frequent and regular sharing of knowledge and skills. For example, a transdisciplinary team evaluated a 2-year-old child with spina bifida. The team determined that the home was the preferred location for intervention and that the physical therapist would act as the direct service provider. The occupational therapist, speech pathologist,

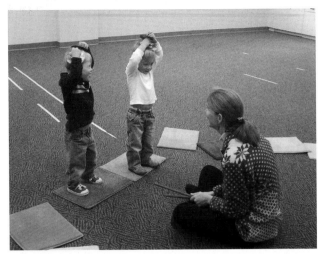

FIGURE 21-2 A music therapist helps children enhance their body awareness, a goal that is a primary responsibility of the occupational therapist.

and early childhood specialist taught the physical therapist techniques to use for feeding, language stimulation, and cognitive development. As a result, the physical therapist was able to provide various intervention strategies on her weekly visits, with periodic monitoring and consultation from the other professionals on the team. Successful functioning as a transdisciplinary team takes commitment and willingness to cross traditional discipline boundaries and effective communication and consultative skills. To implement this approach, the therapist must be highly skilled in analyzing the child's developmental function and synthesizing the family and home situation given a limited amount of information (Case-Smith & Wavrek, 1998).

Although the transdisciplinary model may seem to be the most appropriate in early intervention, several barriers or obstacles have been identified in this approach (Bruder, 1993; McGonigel et al., 1994; Orelove & Sobsey, 1991; Ottenbacher, 1983). These obstacles include philosophic and professional differences, legal liabilities and licensure limitations, variable background education of designated service providers, and inconsistent mastery of skills practiced through role release (Buysse & Wesley, 1993; Klein & Gilkerson, 2000). In addition, reimbursement from third-party payers may dictate intervention based on a medical model with direct provision of services by each professional. Regardless of which approach the team uses, effective teamwork does not come easily. It requires a flexible administration based on a sound philosophic framework and honest, hard work on the part of each team member.

EVALUATION OF INFANTS AND TODDLERS

Teti and Gibbs (1990) traced the interest in infancy and infant assessment back to the 1800s and the Child Study Movement and the efforts of Stanley Hall, founder of normative study of child development. Normative study of development is the basis for norm-referenced assessment, which assesses a particular behavior or attribute of children of a particular age group, establishing a mean age of development and an accompanying developmental curve with which other children can be compared.

An assumption of the developmental theory is that there is continuity of function from the infancy stages of sensorimotor development through the early childhood stages of verbalization and representational functioning. However, environmental and physiologic factors influence this development. The knowledge that environmental factors influence the infant's development and the belief that neurodevelopment of the infant is plastic and malleable supports the concept of early intervention (Teti & Gibbs, 1990).

The developmental approach to infant assessment involves a multidimensional, holistic method in which each developmental domain is individually examined and then the influence that the domains have on one another and on the child as a whole is assessed. For example, infants with motor impairments are restricted in their ability to explore their environment, a critical component to sensorimotor development, which in turn can affect other developmental areas of cognition, language, and socialization.

The functional approach focuses on the child's functional abilities in interaction with environmental activities, contexts, and conditions. To implement a functional approach, the therapist gathers information about the types of activities in which the child is to participate, methods of the child's participation, and expected goals for each activity. Using this information, the therapist analyzes competencies and barriers to the child's independent participation in relevant activities.

The functional approach relies on an ecologic framework that emphasizes skills and behaviors. The developmental approach documents the child's isolated skills (e.g., motor or cognitive) by referencing developmental milestones or domains, whereas the functional approach documents the child's behaviors by referencing skill clusters that describe functions (e.g., feeding or playing).

Early intervention evaluation consists of a series of steps and is an ongoing, collaborative process of collecting, analyzing, and gathering information about the infant and the family to identify specific needs and develop goals in the IFSP (Case-Smith, 1998a; Greenspan & Meisels, 1994). The evaluation, combined with a treatment program and ongoing reassessment, is a problem-solving process that continues throughout the period that the infant or toddler is eligible for Part C services.

Therapists can use developmental evaluations for screening, diagnosing or evaluating, and program planning. These processes are defined in Chapters 7 and 8 of this book. Family involvement with the evaluation is encouraged and varies from observation to full participation.

Evaluation

The process of evaluation is the gathering and interpreting of information on the child's health status and medical background, current developmental levels of functioning, and family resources to maximize the child's development. There are two major goals in the evaluation of infants and toddlers: (1) determination of eligibility for early intervention programs and (2) development of outcomes and goals to guide the early intervention program.

Eligibility Determination

Infants and toddlers who have *established risk* because of their diagnosis are automatically eligible for Part C services. This category includes diagnoses associated with developmental delay, such as cerebral palsy, Down syndrome, or spina bifida. Infants and toddlers without a specific diagnosis who are suspected of having developmental delay are entitled to an evaluation, which must be timely and comprehensive and must include input by a multidisciplinary team. The occupational therapist may be a member of the evaluation team. The team should be responsive to the family's needs and desires when determining the time and location of the evaluation and which individuals should be present. The family's involvement is central to the evaluation process and the information that they share about the child influences how assessments are implemented and results are interpreted. The focus of the evaluation should be on the process itself (i.e., engaging the child and eliciting representative performance). In addition to test scores, the evaluation should result in a list of strengths and weaknesses (Miller, 1994).

The developmental areas that the team evaluates to determine eligibility are cognition, communication, motor, social-emotional, and adaptive. Play is another area of importance for the team to assess but is not part of most assessment instruments. However, play assessments demonstrate how well the child integrates separate skill areas and how he or she playfully interacts with social and physical environments. Some of the most frequently used instruments for the team assessment approach are the *Bayley Scales of Infant Development*, 2nd edition (BSID-II) (Bayley, 1993) and the Battelle Developmental Inventory (BDI)(Newborg, Stock,

Wnek, Guidubaldi, & Svinicki, 1988). Several more recently developed scales are listed in Appendix 7-A. The Hawaii Early Learning Profile (HELP) (Furuno et al., 1994; Parks, 1992) is a well-used developmental curriculum-based assessment.

Standardized assessments should never be the sole source for determining eligibility for early intervention services (McLean & McCormick, 1993). Furthermore, few reliable, comprehensive standardized assessments are available for children between birth and 2 years of age. A standardized test provides merely a sampling of a child's abilities and behaviors observed at a particular time and situation, from a particular perspective, and with a particular instrument (Greenspan & Meisels, 1994). Assessment results that do not reflect the child's typical functioning or behavioral characteristics are neither meaningful nor accurate. Therefore professional judgment is a critical element of assessment. The test instruments chosen and the use of professional judgment may vary from state to state and may be specified by policies of the state lead agency.

Evaluation and Goal Development

Once the interdisciplinary team has defined a child's eligibility for early intervention services, further assessment is important for the therapist to determine what intervention strategies and services are of greatest value to the child and family. At this point, evaluation becomes a comprehensive decision-making process to identify social-emotional, cognitive, motor, and communication problems; develop goals; and define an early intervention program plan. Miller (1994) made the following recommendations for evaluation of infants and young children:

- The therapist should base the assessment on an integrated developmental model. Parents and professionals must observe the child's range of functions in different contexts to identify how the child can best be helped, rather than just coming up with a test score.
- Assessment involves multiple sources and multiple components of information. Parents and professionals contribute to forming the total picture of the child.
- An understanding of typical child development is essential to the interpretation of developmental differences among infants and young children.
- The assessment should emphasize the child's functional capacities, such as attending, engaging, reciprocating, interacting intentionally, organizing patterns of behavior, understanding his or her environment symbolically, and having problem-solving abilities (Greenspan, 1992).
- The assessment process should identify the child's current abilities, strengths, and areas of need to attain desired developmental outcomes (Figure 21-3).

- The therapist should not challenge young children during the assessment by separating them from their parents or caregivers. The parents' presence supports the child and begins the parent-professional collaborative process.
- An unfamiliar examiner should not assess young children. The therapist should give the child a "warmup" period. Assessment by a stranger when the parent is restricted to the role of a passive observer represents an additional challenge.
- Assessments that are limited to easily measurable areas, such as certain motor or cognitive skills, should not be considered complete.
- The therapist should not consider formal or standardized tests the determining factor of the assessment for the infant or young child. Most formal tests were developed and standardized on typically developing children and not on those with special needs. Furthermore, many young children have difficulty attending to or complying with the basic expectations of formal tests. Formal test procedures are not the best context in which to observe functional capacities of young children. Assessments that are intended for intervention planning should use structured tests only as part of an integrated approach (Figure 21-4).

OCCUPATIONAL THERAPY INTERVENTION

Occupational therapists are important members of the early intervention team and can provide services in various settings using one of several models of intervention. Occupational therapists promote a child's independence, mastery, and sense of self-worth and self-confidence in their physical, emotional, and psychosocial development. These services are designed to help families and other caregivers improve children's functioning within their environments. Therapists use a developmental framework in assessing the following domains: play, adaptive skills, sensorimotor, posture, fine-motor manipulation, and oral motor feeding. Purposeful activity is then used to expand the child's functional abilities in these areas (Brown & Rule, 1993; Kramer & Hinojosa, 1999).

Case-Smith (1998b) has identified general goals of occupational therapy intervention with infants and children:

- Facilitate change in the child's developmental function (Figure 21-5).
- Interpret and redefine behavioral responses.
- Compensate for and adapt to the effects of a disability (Figure 21-6).
- Provide support to family members

Occupational therapy is provided in collaboration with other members of the team and is specified as part of the IFSP.

Settings

Part C of IDEA specifies that early intervention services are provided in the child's natural environment. Natural environments are defined as settings that are natural or normal for children without disabilities and include the home and community settings. To enable the child to remain an integral part of the family and for the family to be integral parts of the neighborhood and community, services should be community based and in locations convenient to the family (Dunst, 1991; IDEA, 1997; Turnbull et al., 2000). Ideally, the therapist should offer the family a range of options so that they can choose those that best fit their priorities, lifestyle, and values. These options should include those that provide the least restrictive settings in situations that would be

FIGURE 21-3 The therapist can assess perceptual motor skills through observation of puzzle completion.

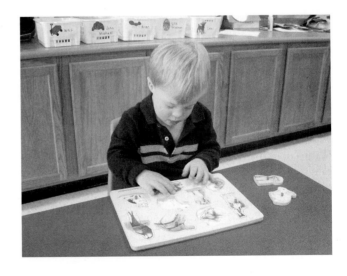

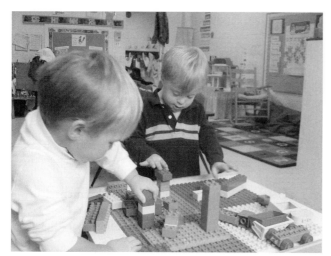

FIGURE 21-4 Important assessment data are gathered through structured observations of the child's play in his or her everyday environment.

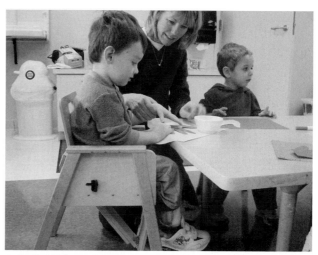

FIGURE 21-6 Adapted seating promotes good postural alignment for fine-motor play at a table.

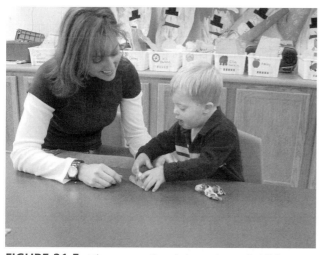

FIGURE 21-5 The occupational therapist and child use an activity to enhance fine-motor skills.

natural environments for a normally developing child of the same age. Some examples are a playgroup, mother's morning out program, childcare center, playgrounds, grocery stores, or fast-food restaurants (Figure 21-7).

Natural environments offer opportunities for therapists to coach parents and teachers to gain self-confidence and assume responsibility in the child's daily care. The key to successful intervention is collaboration between therapists and caregivers within the home or childcare setting. Intervention in natural environments includes using toys and materials that can be found in the natural environment and will remain available to the family on a consistent basis. Therapists who rely on clinical equipment, whether they bring it to home visits or use it in their centers, are trying to influence the child's

performance by using toys and equipment most comfortable for the therapist (Hanft & Pilkington, 2000). Suspended swings, therapy balls, or a child-sized table and chair may be optimal for a clinic-based program for addressing sensory or motor deficits but may not be available to families at home or in the absence of the therapist. It is equally important for the therapist in clinic settings to provide opportunities for the family and other caregivers to learn and practice the interactions and principles to promote generalization in the natural environment. Best practice in occupational therapy infers expanding direct treatment to include primary caregivers (parents, grandparents, childcare providers). This involves learning to accept and respect differences in philosophies, priorities, and practices (Hanft & Anzalone, 2001).

The Division of Early Childhood of the Council for Exceptional Children supports the philosophy of inclusion in natural environments with the following statement (DEC, 1993): "Inclusion, as a value, supports the right of all children, regardless of their diverse abilities, to participate actively in natural settings within their communities. A natural setting is one in which the child would spend time if he or she had not had a disability" (p. 4).

The philosophy of inclusion extends beyond physical inclusion to mean social and emotional inclusion of the child and family (Turnbull, Turnbull, & Blue-Banning, 1994). The implications for occupational therapists are that they provide opportunities for expanded and enriched natural learning with typically developing peers. Self-contained or segregated settings are more restrictive and do not prepare children for participating or being a part of their natural and spontaneous environment (Sheldon & Rush, 2001).

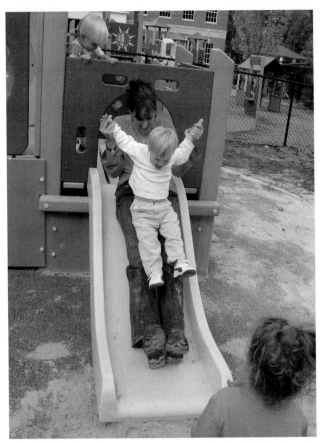

FIGURE 21-7 The therapist encourages a child to participate in sensory motor activities on the playground.

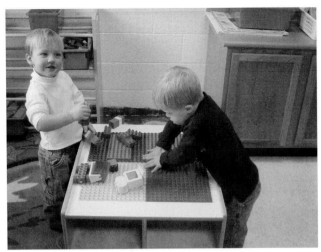

FIGURE 21-8 The occupational therapist uses preschool materials to achieve the child's fine-motor goals.

Advantages of Therapy in Natural Environments

"Therapy in natural environments occurs wherever a child and family choose to be and cannot be equated with setting up a therapy center in the home (e.g., a therapist schedules therapy in a child's home and then works with him or her alone in his or her bedroom because it is too noisy elsewhere in the house). Rather than think narrowly about selecting the natural environment, therapists should consider the key settings where a young child and family spend much of their time" (Hanft & Pilkington, 2000, p. 4). Natural learning environments are those where planned and unplanned, structured and unstructured, and intentional and incidental learning experiences occur (Dunst et al., 2001). Mothers' Morning Out or mother-infant playgroups exemplify a planned activity. Petting a puppy in the park is an unplanned activity. Hippotherapy or doing puzzles are structured activities, whereas playing on the playground is an unstructured one. Putting on one's clothes is an intentional task; falling into a pile of fall leaves is an incidental learning experience. Learning opportunities are composed of a variety of life experiences that make *activity setting* an apropos description for natural learning environments (Dunst, 2001). Literature on early intervention supports service delivery in natural environments and includes studies on natural intervention strategies, generalization of skills, inclusion, home-based services, and consultation with service providers (Sheldon & Rush, 2001).

Natural intervention strategies are those that use incidental learning opportunities that occur throughout the child's typical activities and interactions with peers and adults, follow the child's lead and use natural consequences. Researchers who studied acquisition of functional motor, social, and communication skills have supported intervention strategies that occur in real-life settings over those that take place in more contrived clinic-based settings (Bruder, 1993; Harris, 1997; McWilliam, 1996) (Figure 21-8). Segregated settings such as special preschools and pediatric therapy clinics in the past were seen as the only or preferred setting for children with disabilities to receive therapy services because inclusive opportunities were limited or did not exist. A resulting advantage of providing occupational therapy in natural environments is children tend to be more comfortable in familiar settings such as their home and are more apt to be responsive and interactive with the therapist.

Generalization of skills is the ability to respond appropriately under spontaneous and natural conditions such as responses to people, environments, objects, and stimuli. Generalization of skills and behaviors will occur more readily when the intervention setting is the same as the child's natural environment(s) (Figure 21-9). This requires the therapist's ingenuity to develop

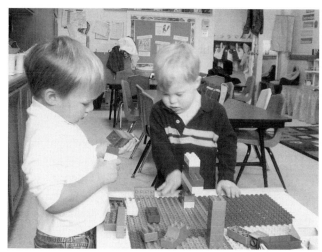

FIGURE 21-9 Peer play helps the child generalize newly learned skills.

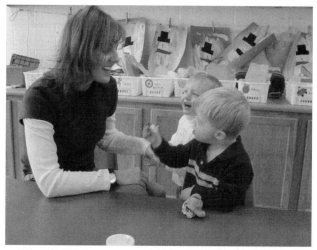

FIGURE 21-10 An occupational therapist uses a preschool peer to model, encourage, and support the child with developmental delays.

strategies that will be acceptable and supportive by the caregiver(s) (Hanft & Pilkington, 2000). Recognizing and accepting the family's uniqueness in cultural and child-rearing practices, therapists are able to facilitate the child's ability to generalize new skills to a variety of settings.

Inclusive early childhood programs provide opportunities for therapists to collaborate with primary caregivers including parents, grandparents, and childcare providers. Including siblings in therapy sessions can reinforce meaningful relationships between siblings who often feel left out during the care for their brother or sister with special needs. Inclusive settings provide a variety of enriching learning opportunities. Early childhood programs, for example, enhance opportunities for play and interactions with typically developing peers in real-life situations of the classroom. Therapists can benefit from collaborating with childcare providers through opportunities for peer role modeling and teaching (Figure 21-10). Participation in community programs gives the family common experiences for relating to friends and neighbors and helps them view their child as one with differing abilities rather than one with disabilities. To be successful, the inclusion program should ensure that (1) the child's individual needs are met with appropriate aids and support services, (2) the child with special needs benefits from the typical program, and (3) the needs of the typical children are not compromised.

Home-based services is another example of natural environment. Therapists have the benefit of seeing the child with special needs within the context of their family and activities of daily living and a multitude of interrelated roles (Hanft & Pilkington, 2000; Sheldon & Rush, 2001). Therapists are trained to be good observers, a skill that is a distinct advantage in natural environments. Home therapy programs designed during home-based visits tend to be more successful because therapists are

more realistic in suggesting goals that are based on the resources available, can problem-solve issues unique to the home environment, and can better individualize the program to meet the family's interests and needs.

Challenges to Implementing Therapy in Natural Environments

Providing therapy in natural environments presents several challenges from the perspective of therapy providers, families, and governing bodies (federal, state, and local agencies). The ability to collaborate and co-ordinate treatment objectives within a transdisciplinary service model is necessary. Therapists may engage in *role release* through coaching and support to caregivers within the child's natural environments, which requires developing effective communication skills (Sheldon & Rush, 2001). An intervention strategy that can only be implemented by a therapist and does not generalize to the child and family's routines is not meaningful or functional (Effgen & Chiarello, 2000).

Therapists must be able to work within multiple environments creatively and flexibly and take advantage of teachable moments. For example, the occupational therapist may have plans to use the playground for sensory integration strategies and the preschool classroom for addressing fine-motor skills, only to find it is a rainy day and the children cannot go outdoors. When she arrives at the classroom, the children are engaged in a rainy day activity of playing dressup. Being able to revise treatment requires quick thinking and creativity.

Providing services within natural environments requires therapists to travel. Travel time between cases can be lengthy due to traffic in urban settings and distances in rural settings resulting in increased mileage costs and lower caseloads.

Third-party payers (insurance companies, Medicaid, managed care organizations) may consider therapy in community settings as an indirect service which is not reimbursable (Hanft & Anzalone, 2001). Early intervention payers often reimburse only for direct or hands-on time with the child and generally will not reimburse for parent sessions, team meetings, or training of essential staff (Hanft & Pilkington, 2000).

Therapists must be familiar with state legislation related to early intervention and become advocates for their families. Early intervention therapists must be able to assume the role of political activist as legislation may be amended. Interpretations of the laws often differ from region to region and can affect service delivery.

Occupational therapy services are provided in various settings that represent a continuum from the most restrictive (e.g., hospital settings) to the least restrictive (e.g., community settings). The setting should reflect family preferences and should be consistent with the needs of the child and the goals identified on the IFSP. For example, one child with significant and acute medical problems may be best served in the hospital-based program, whereas another with similar problems may be best served in the home. One child with autism may function best in a preschool program with typically developing peers. Occupational therapy in this natural environment would focus on functional behaviors and skills such as facilitating transitions from one activity to another, engaging with and responding to peers and teachers, practicing activities of daily living, or participating in sensory or tactile activities (Figure 21-11). The occupational therapist can include the typical peers as role models and as partners in play (Figure 21-12). Another child with the same diagnosis may not be ready for a group environment and would be best seen in one-on-one therapy in an environment where there are fewer distractions, such as in a home. Early intervention

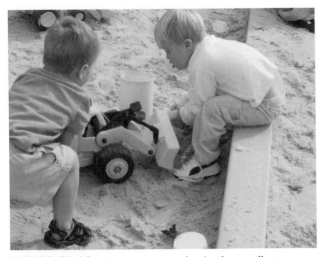

FIGURE 21-11 Sensory motor play in the sandbox.

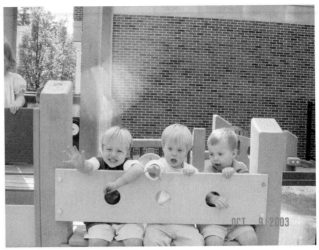

FIGURE 21-12 Children learn many skills through imitation of their peers.

legislation provides for interagency cooperation; thus, families can choose the most appropriate settings and services from either private or public providers.

Cultural Diversity

To provide appropriate intervention within the family-centered model, the occupational therapist must be aware of and respect differences in beliefs and values based on culture. "Perhaps no set of programs or services interacts with cultural views and values more than early intervention because of the focus on the very young child with a disability and the family" (Hanson, 1990, p. 116). The therapist who provides intervention in the home has an intimate view of such things as customs, eating habits, and childrearing practices that may vary among cultures. The family's beliefs and views of disability and its cause, their view of the health care system, and their sources of medical information affect their attitude toward early intervention. Based on individual cultural backgrounds, the family may view the therapist as either a helper or one who interferes.

Many of the areas in which occupational therapists provide intervention and suggestions involve caregiving and are closely tied to values and beliefs about parenting and cultural views of children. Practices regarding feeding, toileting, and bathing may vary among cultures. The therapist is urged to evaluate various health beliefs to determine whether the effects are beneficial, harmless, harmful, or uncertain before making recommendations for change (Hanson, 1998).

Early intervention legislation requires that the therapist administer assessments in the family's native language, if feasible, and conduct evaluation procedures in a manner that is not racially or culturally discriminatory (IDEA, 1990). Intervention methods and procedures should recognize and be sensitive to cultural differences. The following are some suggestions for the therapist (Vohs, 1989, p. 3):

- Learn about other cultures
- Learn how persons of other cultures view children with disabilities
- Invite members of minority cultures to become involved with your organization
- Learn at least a few words of the languages of your families
- Become familiar with your community and the cultures represented
- Examine ways to remove barriers to accessing services for minority groups
- Recognize that everyone has prejudices and believes that his or her values are right
- Be sensitive to problems of being a member of a minority

Planning

Occupational therapy intervention, as with other early intervention services, is based on identified concerns and expected outcomes in the IFSP. This document is family centered, with emphasis on intervention in the natural environment. It also specifies the various services to be provided; who the provider will be; the location of the services; the frequency, intensity, and duration of services; and the funding sources.

The occupational therapist in the early intervention setting focuses on outcomes from a family-centered perspective and identifies the child's occupational performance as it relates to daily family routines. An outcome is a statement of changes desired by the family that can focus on any area of the child's development or family life as it relates to the child (Kramer, McGonigel, & Kaufman, 1991). It reflects family priorities, hopes, and concerns in a broad statement which the whole team addresses.

Occupational therapists focus on child and family function and context (Cohn & Cermak, 1998). Outcomes should reflect performance areas and contexts rather than performance components. For example, it is not appropriate to write an outcome to "improve pincer grasp," but instead to link the problem to daily function of both the child and the family unit. Examples of outcomes are "to feed himself finger food" or "to play with toys." Often, outcome statements for children in early intervention are concerned with social participation. This includes those behaviors and skills needed to "fit in" and have been defined as "active engagement in typical activities available to and/or expected of peers in the same context" (Coster, 1998, p. 338). Typical outcome statements might be "to go to the grocery store with her parent" or "to play with other children." Other outcome statements are parent focused and might include learning strategies to support the child or validation and understanding of the role of a parent of a child with special needs.

When an outcome is developed, the next step is to describe what is happening now and what will happen when the outcome is achieved. Strategies are listed to address the outcome with people and resources that are needed. All relevant team members should be included. For example, if the outcome is "to feed himself finger food at a family meal," the current problems might be "unable to hold food in hand and bring to mouth, cannot sit at a table, cries during meals unless parent is feeding him." The team will recognize progress when the child can sit at the table independently and pick up and eat small pieces of food. In order to achieve this outcome a number of strategies are proposed. The physical therapist might address stability for sitting and the speech therapist might work on oral motor function, while the occupational therapist addresses sensory issues and hand use.

Approaches
Developmentally Appropriate

The occupational therapist plans and carries out therapy for the infant and child within the framework of developmentally appropriate play rather than the acquisition of isolated skills. For example, it would be inappropriate for the occupational therapist to concentrate on the development of precise fingertip prehension without consideration of how this skill contributes to the overall function of the child in the environment or how it fits into the developmental needs of the child.

Developmentally based curricula such as the HELP, the Activities-Based Intervention (AEPS for Infants and Children; Bricker, 1993), or Transdisciplinary Play Based Intervention (Linder, 1993b) provide activities matched to the developmental sequences within each domain. However, the therapist should guard against using a "cookbook" approach in intervention for specific developmental deficits.

A team whose members have overlapping functions can effectively address developmental needs (Figure 21-13). When the therapist identifies a need in a specific domain (e.g., fine-motor skills), he or she can implement activities that require a child to use fine-motor skills. To promote generalization of the fine-motor skills practiced in therapy, the therapist should employ play activities that involve the "just right" challenge to the child across domains (i.e., activities that include skill building in the cognitive and social domains). For example, stacking items such as blocks or rings on a stick is a motor task but also involves cognitive skills such as concept of size, shape, and dimension. The activities also could involve

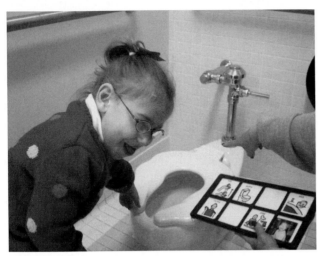

FIGURE 21-13 The occupational therapist integrates speech goals into toilet training.

social interaction, including give and take with another child or adult, eye contact, praise, and delight at successful attempts.

Family-Centered Intervention

In family-centered intervention the occupational therapist addresses the needs of the entire family rather than only concentrating on specific deficits in the child. The therapist should be guided by family concerns and the amount of involvement that various family members choose to have in the child's intervention program. One important way for the therapist to increase the effect of therapy is to make it relevant to the family's life style and time commitments. Activities should be those that target behaviors and skills that the child can generalize to his or her daily routines at home, school, and community. Parents vary in their ability to implement structured therapy activities with their children. Family demands and support networks are always considerations when discussing home programs with parents. One mother stated the following: "There are times when even an acceptable amount of therapy becomes too much—when your child needs time just to be a child, or when you need time to be with the rest of the family. It is okay to say 'no' at those times, for a while. Your instinct will tell you when" (Simons, 1985, p. 51).

Sometimes it is more important to support the role of parent than to assume that the parent can take on the role of the therapist. Daily routines in a family with a child who has a disability can take an excessive amount of time and energy, which does not allow for carrying out a therapy home program. Suggestions that the family can incorporate into the daily routine are the most successful. For example, the caregiver can provide tactile stimulation and range of motion at bath time; an older

sibling can encourage the infant to reach for toys while their mother cooks dinner.

Occupational therapists can provide support for families by listening to them, giving positive feedback regarding parenting skills, encouraging recreational activities for the family, and helping them access community resources (Case-Smith, 1998b). Often the therapist can help the family by providing intervention to make daily routines go more smoothly. Examples are suggestions for positioning and handling to make feeding more efficient or an adapted bath seat to make bathing less taxing.

Areas of Intervention

Hanft (1989) applied five practice perspectives to occupational therapy with infants and children: prevention, habilitation, remediation, compensation, and maturation (Table 21-2). The therapist can use these various perspectives at different times, depending on the child's needs and development. The therapist must determine the appropriateness of an approach at any given time. Regardless of the perspective, the therapist works in collaboration with the family and other professionals to develop functional abilities. The child is viewed in a holistic manner in enhancing development; however, the following are ones that occupational therapists have traditionally emphasized.

Development of Play

One of the most important areas of a child's development is involvement in play. Play is open-ended, self-initiated, self-directed, and unlimited in its variety. It gives the child the opportunity to develop and practice skills that will be the foundation for later occupational tasks, such as the ability to manipulate objects, problem-solve, and attend to tasks (Burke, 1998). Play can be exploratory, symbolic, creative, or competitive in nature (see Chapter 17).

Sometimes therapists are so intent on remediating certain deficits that they ignore the importance of play. A toy becomes only a motivator, or a diversion, so that the therapist can elicit a certain movement pattern (Burke, 1998). Although this may sometimes be necessary, the therapist must also facilitate play skills in the child and use play as a way of enabling the child to gain function and enhance development. To use play as intervention, the occupational therapist must be playful in interactions with the child. Whether it is a game of peek-a-boo or knocking down a pretend wall when pushed on a scooter board, the activity should elicit a sense of enjoyment and fun (Figure 21-14).

Children with special needs may not have developed play skills because of long hospitalizations or medical treatments or because of the limitations imposed by a physical impairment. Other children may experience

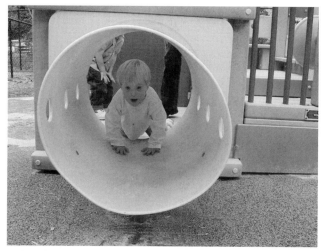

FIGURE 21-14 Exploratory, sensory motor play enhances body scheme, coordination, and a range of motor skills.

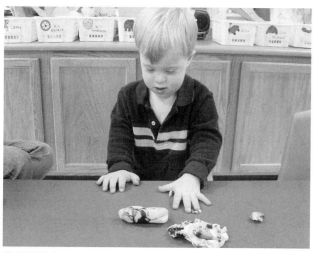

FIGURE 21-15 The occupational therapist uses preschool materials to assess fine-motor skills.

TABLE 21-2 Occupational Therapy Intervention for a 5-Month-Old Boy

Practice Perspective	Examples of Occupational Therapy Goals and Activities
Prevention (check the negative effect of developmental problems on future abilities)	■ Develop awareness of body parts through sensory input to prevent spatial orientation problems. ■ Increase attention and eye contact to enhance interaction with others.
Habilitation (promote developmental acquisition of future skills)	■ Develop child's head control through movement, neuromuscular facilitation, and positioning. ■ Enhance basic oral motor functions of breathing, sucking, and swallowing in preparation for speech.
Remediation (attempt to diminish dysfunction)	■ Decrease drooling through neuromuscular facilitation to mouth. ■ Enhance interaction through alerting techniques before play.
Compensation (substitute different skills for delayed ones)	■ Encourage mother and father to carry the infant in an infant carrier ("snugli") until the infant can move on his or her own. ■ Position child so pacifier remains in mouth.
Maturation (use child's own developmental schedule)	■ Provide appropriate toys to enhance visual attention in crib and play areas. ■ Offer finger foods during meals as child develops pincer grasp.

From Hanft, B. (1989). The changing environment of early intervention services: Implications for practice. In B. Hanft (Ed.), *Family-centered care: An early intervention resource manual.* Rockville, MD: American Occupational Therapy Association.

deficits in play because of cognitive limitations or difficulties in social interactions. The use of a play-based assessment can enable the occupational therapist to define the problem areas and plan intervention.

Fine-Motor and Manipulative Hand Function

The occupational therapist is often concerned with delayed function or atypical function in fine-motor skills. These skills include grasp and release of objects, bilateral manipulation, in-hand manipulation, hesitancy to touch and explore with the hands, lack of hand-to-mouth pattern, and other skills. Intervention begins with analyzing the quality of movement and determining underlying factors, such as tactile discrimination and kinesthetic awareness.

First, the therapist observes how functional a child is in a particular skill. When a skill such as stacking

blocks appears delayed or deficit, the therapist analyzes which underlying skills are interfering with performance (Figure 21-15). For example, the therapist notes the influence of muscle tone and proximal stability when the child attempts stacking 1-inch cubes. He or she must then determine the following:

■ Does muscle tone increase?
■ Are spasticity, tremor, or associated movements (mirroring) present?
■ Does total body tone change with effort?
■ Can the child stack the cubes while sitting unsupported on the floor?
■ Does the infant slump or demonstrate lack of postural stability?
■ Can the child easily disassociate the movement of the arm from the body?
■ Is the child's hand-eye coordination delayed?

- Does inattention or a lack of understanding interfere with performing the task?
- Does the child have difficulty with the motor planning needed for precise release of one block on top of another?
- Does tactile hypersensitivity cause the child to be reluctant to handle the block or result in flinging or throwing any object in his or her hand?

A child with autistic spectrum disorder or other dysfunction that interferes with the child's ability to interact with persons and things in the environment may be unable to imitate or follow directions for a task. Therefore inability to stack blocks may not reflect a deficit in fine-motor ability but rather inexperience or disinterest in the activity. The best indication of the child's fine-motor abilities may be through observation of spontaneous activity.

Stacking blocks is not an important functional skill, but it is important for developing sufficient hand skill for manipulating, placing, and releasing objects. These skills enable the child to use tools with control and with their arms unsupported. The occupational therapist uses various age-appropriate toys, games, sensorimotor experiences, and other strategies with the child to remediate underlying factors that interfere with the development of fine-motor skills.

Sensory Integration

Infants who have difficulty processing sensory information lack the ability to cope with environmental demands or achieve internal control. These infants may be irritable, cry frequently, be difficult to comfort, or have difficulty with changes in routine. The ability to cope "requires the ability to modulate incoming sensory information while engaged in feeding, face-to-face interactions with family, bathing, and diapering, or just being held" (Stallings-Sahler, 1998, p. 240).

The therapist must recognize and address sensory integrative dysfunction in the child because of its pervasive influence on all areas of development. The therapist should use appropriate tactile, vestibular, and proprioceptive input that elicits organized behavior and simple adaptive responses on the part of the child. For example, it was determined that a 1-year-old child displayed tactile sensitivity. He refused to hold toys, refused to bear weight on his arms, was irritable when held, pulled away from touch, and avoided exploring his environment. The occupational therapist planned intervention that included proprioceptive and tactile input and midline play with textured toys. She recommended to the mother that additional tactile stimulation be provided at bath time with water play, foamy soap, and terrycloth rubs. Soon the child was clapping his hands spontaneously—a skill he had not attempted before and a nice adaptive response (see Case Study 1).

Oral Motor Function and Feeding

Occupational therapists who work with infants and children often address problems in eating and feeding. Problem areas may include inadequate intake, excessive time for feeding, or oral motor problems associated with sucking, swallowing, and chewing (Glass & Wolf, 1998). Additional problems may center on behavioral issues such as refusals, overactivity, or messiness. Other concerns are in the area of self-feeding and drinking from a cup.

Addressing concerns in the area of feeding is also important for mother-child bonding. Glass and Wolf (1998) suggest three guiding principles of treatment for the infant:

1 Providing proper alignment of the trunk and neck
2 Providing proximal stability, especially in the head and jaw
3 Facilitating appropriate oral motor patterns through inhibitory and facilitation techniques (see Chapter 14).

Self-Help Skills

Occupational therapists have longstanding experience in the area of activities of daily living (ADL), also referred to as self-help skills. In children, the focus is on functional participation in eating and feeding, dressing, toileting, sleeping, and self-regulation. Problems may include physical difficulties such as bringing hand to mouth, chewing and swallowing food and liquids, or cooperating in dressing by extending arm or leg. Psychosocial behaviors that influence the acquisition of self-help skills are temperament, self-regulation, parent-child interaction, motivation, and adaptability. Sensory processing problems may cause aversive behaviors, such as the child with tactile hypersensitivity who gags on some foods or refuses to wear certain articles of clothing. The evaluation of self-help skills should occur in the natural environment in which the skills occur, such as the child's home, daycare, or preschool (Figure 21-16).

Adapted Equipment and Positioning

The occupational therapist in early intervention can make an important contribution to the overall functioning of children through the recommendation and provision of appropriate adapted equipment (Figure 21-17). A floor sitter may enable the child with cerebral palsy to play on the floor near his or her typically developing peers. An adapted insert for a chair may make it possible for a child to begin to use his or her hands for an art project or to self-feed. As the neurologically involved child approaches preschool age and is not yet ambulating, the parents may have to face the prospect of the need for a wheelchair. The occupational therapist can assist in

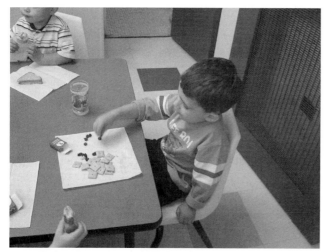

FIGURE 21-16 The therapist assesses feeding skills during the lunchtime routine in preschool.

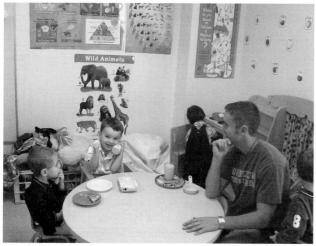

FIGURE 21-17 Adapted seating enables a child with postural instability to play with a peer at the table.

recommending appropriate equipment and in being sensitive to the effect that envisioning their child in a wheelchair may have on the family. The child with a neurologic impairment who can stay in an infant stroller or a highchair does not appear as different as the 3-year-old child who must have a wheelchair and special equipment.

SUMMARY

Occupational therapists use holistic approaches with children and their families that emphasize functional, developmentally appropriate approaches. By recognizing that children are part of a family system, the therapist designs programs that fit into the family's daily routine; consider sensory, motor (gross and fine), social, and cognitive

aspects of performance; and emphasize the child's occupations of physical and social play.

Case Study 1: Alex
Background

Alex's pediatrician referred him to occupational therapy at 11 months of age because of suspected sensory integrative problems. He had a diagnosis of developmental delay and had been receiving physical therapy because of gross-motor delays. Alex cried often in a distressful manner. Problem areas for Alex, as reported by his mother, included uncooperative behaviors, rages or temper tantrums, whining and fussing, feeding problems, fearfulness, poor balance, and a dislike for being on his tummy. Although he sat independently at 6 months of age, he did not reach and grasp an object until 8 months of age. He rolled from back to stomach at 9 months of age, and he was not yet crawling at 11 months of age.

Assessment

Alex was a pleasant infant who preferred not to be touched or held. He interacted with the examiner with caution after a brief period of ignoring her. His mother remained in the room and participated in the assessment. The examiner obtained a sensorimotor history by interview with Alex's mother. His mother had noticed that he had difficulty and pulled away when touched. Sometimes he stiffened and arched his back when held. Alex's mother reported that he was irritable when held and resisted having his hair or face washed. Alex seemed oversensitive to noises and was bothered by such things as a vacuum cleaner and hair dryer. Although his aversion to sound had improved, he remained apprehensive of toys with noises. Alex seemed to be fearful in situations with auditory and visual stimulation, such as a shopping mall. Alex enjoyed swinging and other movement stimuli.

The examiner administered the Test of Sensory Functions in Infants (Degangi & Greenspan, 1989) to Alex. Results showed deficiencies in reactivity to tactile deep pressure and adaptive motor functions, at-risk response to visual-tactile integration and ocular-motor control, and normal response to vestibular stimulation. Specifically, Alex exhibited a mildly defensive reaction to touch. He was not effective in his motor responses to tactile input, such as removing a mitt on his foot or a piece of tape on the back of his hand. He was more efficient using his right hand than his left. Visual-tactile response was better because he was able to locate the stimulus visually, although he could not plan the movement to remove it. However, visual tracking was delayed and inconsistent. Alex enjoyed the vestibular input as he was held and moved up and down or in circular motions. He also enjoyed upside-down positions.

The examiner observed that Alex avoided and resisted changing his body position (e.g., going from sitting to quadruped) and resisted the proprioceptive input of weight bearing on his upper extremities. Extensor muscle tone was increased with lower-extremity weight bearing, so much so that it was difficult to flex his hips passively for sitting. Alex went into plantar flexion and lower-extremity extension when bounced on his bare feet.

At a chronologic age of 11 months, Alex received an age equivalent of 9 months on the fine-motor subtest of the Peabody Developmental Motor Scales. He used his right hand more efficiently than his left but was able to bring his hands to midline to bang cubes. However, he resisted clapping his hands. Alex removed pegs from a pegboard and briefly manipulated a piece of paper. He was able to transfer a cube from his left hand to his right when the cube was placed in his left hand. Alex had difficulty removing rings from a stand. He also displayed difficulty in deliberately releasing cubes to give to the examiner or to put them in a cup.

Summary and Interpretation

Alex was a delightful infant who experienced significant difficulties in receiving and modulating sensory information. This was evident particularly in his irritability and intolerance to touch and auditory stimulation. Inadequate adaptive motor function seemed to be related to his hypersensitivity. Alex's tactile sensitivity probably contributed to his fine-motor delays. Given his hypersensitivity to touch, it is understandable that he was limited in his abilities to explore and manipulate objects, especially those that were new to him and in an unfamiliar environment.

Intervention

The team recommended weekly occupational therapy for Alex, which became part of his IFSP. The occupational therapist provided services in his child center once a week and at home once a month. The therapist used a sensory integrative approach with developmentally appropriate play with emphasis on increased functional hand use. Intervention included frequent brushing of the extremities and the back with a soft surgical brush followed by deep proprioceptive input. Treatment sessions included vestibular input, which Alex tolerated well, and proprioceptive and tactile input as tolerated. The therapist encouraged Alex to play with textured toys, use both hands for midline activities, and bear weight on his upper extremities. Alex's mother participated actively in each session and created additional opportunities for tactile exploration and play at home. The therapist provided his mother with reading material and a videotape to help her learn about sensory integration and understand how sensory processing affects behavior.

Alex responded well to the treatment approach and began to show indications of more efficient sensory processing and the ability to modulate sensory input. Within a few weeks, Alex began to mold to his mother when she held him and was less irritable and more relaxed in situations with auditory stimulation. After 3 months of therapy, Alex's mother reported increased cuddling and noticeable improvement in eating. He attempted a greater variety of foods and few aversions, feeding time was shorter, and it was no longer necessary to use the television as a diversion to get him to eat. Alex began to interact more with his siblings and explore his environment. Best of all, he no longer had temper tantrums when his mother left the room. His childcare provider reported that Alex tolerated the prone position and weight bearing on his hands; he had recently begun to crawl. Play skills and hand use also appeared to increase.

Case Study 2: Jeremy
Background

Jeremy's pediatric neurologist referred him for a transdisciplinary assessment at 18 months of age because of motor delays caused by his mitochondrial encephalopathy. An early intervention team, which consisted of an occupational therapist, a physical therapist, a speech-language pathologist, and an early childhood intervention specialist, assessed him in an arena assessment. Both parents participated in the assessment. Although Jeremy had received occupational therapy and physical therapy since he was 6 months old, his parents thought he would benefit from a small group in which he could receive his therapies and special instruction in an integrated manner.

Assessment

The team chose to administer the BDI and HELP. They administered the latter through observation, direct administration of test items, and interview with the parents. The team modified portions to accommodate for Jeremy's physical limitations. Most important, the therapists engaged him in play activities and used their interpretation of his interactions and movements to estimate his functional abilities.

Overall, Jeremy had very low muscle tone and poor physical endurance. He needed support for sitting and could only bear some of his weight when supported in standing. He was unable to roll or crawl. Head control was poor with head stacking in a supported sitting position and lack of head righting in the prone position. He used his left hand very well to play with toys when he was positioned appropriately but did not use his right hand and protested when the therapist attempted to evaluate passive range of motion. Jeremy was alert and interested but was reluctant to leave his mother's lap. Communication skills and cognition appeared to be on age level, whereas social skills seemed immature.

Intervention

Jeremy started in the summer session of a center-based early intervention program as part of a group of six children who met twice a week. He received occupational therapy, physical therapy, speech therapy, and special instruction in a small group format with close coordination and carry over of all skills throughout the 4-hour session. The team aimed all therapies and special instruction at helping Jeremy improve social interaction with peers, improve self-help skills, and develop physical abilities to the greatest extent possible. The team obtained adapted seating and eating utensils for him and modified group activities to enable him to participate actively and as independently as possible.

Individual Family Service Plan Review

After 6 months, the service coordinator, intervention team, and family members met to review the goals on Jeremy's IFSP and to update and modify it as needed. The family and the team were pleased with Jeremy's progress and thought that he was benefiting from his intervention program. However, they also discussed Jeremy's need to be around his normally developing peers and participate in community-based activities. Jeremy was gaining confidence in a small group, developing good social and communication skills, and no longer tiring as easily. When he reached 2 years of age, the team decided to add an inclusion program to his early intervention services.

Jeremy's service coordinator arranged for him to participate in a special grant program at a local childcare center. He was enrolled in a class for 2-year-old children that met a few hours a week and had the support of an assistant who had been trained to facilitate the inclusion of children with special needs in the typical childcare setting. Although this facilitator had several other children to work with and was not in Jeremy's class all the time, she was available at any time that he needed help or that the teacher had a question or concern. After a few months, Jeremy started attending this program two times a week; meanwhile, he continued to attend the early intervention program and receive his therapies.

Annual Reassessment

One year after entrance into the early intervention program, the intervention team reassessed Jeremy in preparation for the development of a new IFSP. They did not perform this assessment in a formal testing session but over a period of weeks as Jeremy participated in various activities with the group. In addition to the BDI, Jeremy's team also updated the HELP.

Results of the reassessment indicated a bright, happy, verbal 2-year-old child. Although he had gained in physical abilities, Jeremy needed a stroller-type wheelchair with special inserts for appropriate seating. The removable seat also acted as a floor sitter so that Jeremy could be close to the same level as his peers when they played on the floor. The teacher observed that Jeremy had shown considerable improvement in his play skills and that they were definitely more appropriate when he was positioned upright rather than lying on the floor. He demonstrated spontaneous interactions with his peers, he took turns with little prompting, and he began to share toys.

Jeremy continued to participate in the class at the childcare center, although the grant had ended and the facilitator was no longer there. Initially, the childcare center believed that it would be unable to take Jeremy without the facilitator's support. The occupational therapist and the physical therapist provided onsite consultation. Through a problem-solving approach with close cooperation among the family, childcare personnel, and therapists, strategies were developed that made it possible for Jeremy to remain in the class. These strategies included providing wheelchair access to the playground (they had been carrying him), teaching principles of lifting and carrying, and making the stroller available to transport him from room to room so that the teacher had her hands free to keep up with other active 2-year-old children.

Summary

Jeremy is an example of a child who was able to benefit from a combination of programming that included center-based early intervention and inclusion in a typical childcare setting. This required close cooperation among the family, early intervention personnel, and community resources. As Jeremy grows and develops, his parents plan to place him in a total inclusion program, but they believe that, at $2\frac{1}{2}$ years of age, he still needs the intense intervention that he gets in the center-based program. Meanwhile, they look forward to his graduation to the class for 3-year-old children and increasing his typical class time to 3 days a week. They have already visited the neighborhood school and hope that he will attend a regular kindergarten class when he is 5 years of age and will be supported by therapies at school. Jeremy is bright, and with the right kind of support and technology he should be able to grow up in the mainstream of society.

REFERENCES

Bailey, D.B. (1991). Building positive relationships between professionals and families. In M.J. McGonigel, Kaufmann,

R.K., & Johnson, B.H. (Eds.). *Guidelines and recommended practices for the Individualized Family Service Plan* (2nd ed., pp. 29-38). Bethesda, MD: National Early Childhood Technical Assistance System and Association for the Care of Children's Health.

Bayley, N. (1993). *Bayley Scales of Infant Development* (2nd ed.). San Antonio, TX: The Psychological Corporation.

Blackman, J.A. (2002). Early Intervention: A Global Perspective. *Infants & Young Children, 15* (2), 11-19.

Bricker, D. (Ed.). (1993). *AEPS measurement for birth to three years.* Baltimore: Brookes.

Brown, W., & Rule, S. (1993). Personnel and disciplines in early intervention. In W. Brown, S.K. Thurman, & L.K. Pearl (Eds.), *Family-centered early intervention with infants and toddlers and innovative cross-disciplinary approaches.* Baltimore: Brookes.

Bruder, M.B. (1993). The provision of early intervention and early childhood special education within community early childhood programs: Characteristics of effective service delivery. *Topics in Early Childhood Special Education, 13,* 19-37.

Bruder, M.B., & Bologna, T. (1993). Collaboration and service coordination for effective early intervention. In W. Brown, S.K. Thurman, & I.F. Pearl (Eds). *Family centered early intervention with infants and toddlers: Innovative cross-disciplinary approaches* (pp. 103-127). Baltimore, MD: Brookes.

Burke, J. (1998). Play: The life role of the infant and young child. In J. Case-Smith (Ed.), *Pediatric occupational therapy and early intervention* (pp. 189-206). Boston: Butterworth-Heinemann.

Buysse, V., & Wesley, P. (1993). The identity crisis in early childhood education: A call for professional role clarification. *Topics in Early Childhood Special Education, 13* (4), 418-429.

Case-Smith, J. (1998a). Assessment. In J. Case-Smith (Ed.), *Pediatric occupational therapy and early intervention* (pp. 49-82). Boston: Butterworth-Heinemann.

Case-Smith, J. (1998b). Defining the early intervention process. In J. Case-Smith (Ed.), *Pediatric occupational therapy and early intervention* (pp. 27-48). Boston: Butterworth-Heinemann.

Case-Smith, J., & Wavrek, B. (1998). Models of service delivery and team interaction. In J. Case-Smith (Ed.), *Pediatric occupational therapy and early intervention* (pp. 83-108). Boston: Butterworth-Heinemann.

Cohn, E.S., & Cermak, S.A. (1998). Including the family perspective in sensory integration outcomes research. *American Journal of Occupational Therapy, 52* (7), 540-546.

Coster, W. (1998). Occupation-centered assessment of children. *American Journal of Occupational Therapy, 52,* 337-344.

DeGangi, G.A., & Greenspan, S.I. (1989). *Test of Sensory Functions in Infants manual.* Los Angeles: Western Psychological Services.

Division of Early Childhood. (1993). DEC position statement on inclusion. *DEC Communicator, 19,* 4.

Dunst, C.J. (1991). Implementation of the individualized family service plan. In M.J. McGonigel, R. Kaufmann, & B. Johnson (Eds.), *Guidelines and recommended practices for the individualized family service plan* (2nd ed., pp. 67-78).

Bethesda, MD: Association for the Care of Children's Health.

Dunst, C.J., Trivette, C.M., Humphries, T., Raab, M., & Roper, N. (2001). Contrasting approaches to natural learning environment interventions. *Infants & Young Children, 14* (2), 48-63.

Effgen, S.K., & Chiarello, L.A. (2000). Physical therapist education for service in early intervention. *Infants & Young Children, 1* (4), 63-76.

Furuno, S., O'Reilly, K.A., Hosaka, C.M., Inatsuka, T.T., Allman, T.L., & Zeisloft, B. (1994). *Hawaii Early Learning Profile activity guide.* Palo Alto, CA: Vort.

Garbarino, J., & Ganzel, B. (2000). The human ecology of early risk. In J.P. Shonkoff & S.J. Meisels (Eds.) *Handbook of early childhood intervention* (2nd. ed., pp. 76-93). Cambridge, MA: Cambridge University Press.

Garland, C., & Linder, T.W (1994). Administrative challenges in early intervention. In L.J. Johnson, R.J. Gallagher, M.J. Montagne, J.B. Jordan, J.J. Gallagher, P.L. Hutinger, & M.B. Karnes (Eds.) *Meeting early intervention challenges: Issues from birth to three* (2nd ed., pp. 133-166). Baltimore, MD: Brookes.

Giangreco, M.F. (1986). Delivery of therapeutic services in special education programs for learners with severe handicaps. *Physical and Occupational Therapy in Pediatrics, 6,* 5.

Glass, R., & Wolf, L. (1998). Feeding and oral motor skills. In J. Case-Smith (Ed.), *Pediatric occupational therapy and early intervention* (pp. 127-166). Boston: Butterworth-Heinemann.

Greenspan, S.I. (1992). *Infancy and early childhood.* Madison, CT: International Universities Press.

Greenspan, S.I., & Meisels, S. (1994). Toward a new vision for the developmental assessment of infants and young children. *Zero to Three, 14* (6), 2-41.

Hanft, B. (1989). The changing environment of early intervention services: Implications for practice. In B. Hanft (Ed.), *Family-centered care: An early intervention resource manual.* Rockville, MD: American Occupational Therapy Association.

Hanft, B.E., & Anzalone, M. (2001). Issues in professional development: Preparing and supporting occupational therapists in early childhood. *Infants & Young Children, 13* (4), 67-78.

Hanft, B.E., & Pilkington, K.O. (2000). Therapy in natural environments: The means or end goal for early intervention? *Infants & Young Children, 12* (4), 1-13.

Hanson, M.J. (1990). Honoring the cultural diversity of families when gathering data. *Topics in Early Childhood Special Education, 10* (1), 112-131.

Hanson, M.J. (1998). Ethnic, cultural, and language diversity in intervention settings. In E. Lynch & M. Hanson (Eds.), *Developing cross-cultural competence* (2nd ed., pp. 3-22). Baltimore: Brookes.

Harbin, G.L., McWilliam, R.A., & Gallagher, J.J. (2000). Services for young children with disabilities and their families. In J.P. Shonkoff & S.J. Meisels (Eds.), *Handbook of early childhood intervention* (2nd ed., pp. 387-415). Cambridge, MA: Cambridge University Press.

Harris, S.R. (1997). The effectiveness of early intervention for children with cerebral palsy and related motor disabilities. In

M.J. Guralnick (Ed.), *The effectiveness of early intervention.* (pp. 327-347). Baltimore: Paul H. Brookes, 327-347.

Individuals with Disabilities Education Act of 1990 Amendments (P.L. 102-119), 20 USC et seq. 1400-1485.

Individuals with Disabilities Education Act of 1997 Amendments (P.L. 105-17), 20 U.S.C. et seq.

Klein, N.K., & Gilkerson, L. (2000). Personnel preparation for early childhood intervention programs. In J.P. Shonkoff & S.J. Meisels (Eds.), *Handbook of early childhood intervention* (2nd ed., pp. 454-485). Cambridge, MA: Cambridge University Press.

Kramer, P., & Hinojosa, J. (1999). *Frames of references for pediatric occupational therapy.* Philadelphia: Lippincott Williams & Wilkins.

Kramer, S., McGonigel, M., & Kaufman, R. (1991). Developing the IFSP: Outcomes, strategies, activities, and services. In M. McGonigel, R. Kaufmann, & B. Johnson (Eds.), *Guidelines and recommended practices for the individualized family service plan* (2nd ed.). Bethesda, MD: Association for the Care of Children's Health.

Linder, T.W. (1993a). *Transdisciplinary play-based assessment: A functional approach to working with young children.* Baltimore: Brookes.

Linder, T.W. (1993b). *Transdisciplinary play-based intervention: Guidelines for developing a meaningful curriculum for young children.* Baltimore: Brookes.

Mahoney, G., & Filer, J. (1996). How responsive is early intervention to the priorities and needs of families? *Topics in Early Childhood Special Education, 16* (4), 437-457.

McGonigel, M.J., & Garland, C.W. (1988). The individualized family service plan and the early intervention team: Team and family issues and recommended practices. *Infants and Young Children 1,* 10-21.

McGonigel, M.J., Woodruff, G., & Roszmann-Millican, M. (1994). *The transdisciplinary team: A model for family-centered early intervention* (pp. 95-132). Baltimore: Brookes.

McLean, M., & McCormick, K. (1993). Assessment and evaluation in early intervention. In W. Brown, S.K. Thurman, & L.K. Pearl (Eds.), *Family-centered early intervention with infants and toddlers and innovative cross-disciplinary approaches.* Baltimore: Brookes.

McWilliam, R.A. (1996). How to provide integrated therapy. In R. A. McWilliam (Ed.), *Rethinking pull-out services in early intervention* (pp. 49-69). Baltimore: Paul H. Brookes.

McWilliam, R.A., & Strain, P. (1993). Service delivery models. In S.L. Odom & M. McLean, *DEC recommended practices: Indicators of quality in programs for infants and young children with special needs and their families* (pp. 40-46). DEC Task Force on Recommended Practices: Council for Exceptional Children.

Miller, L.J. (1994). Journey to a desirable future: A value-based model of infant and toddler assessment. *Zero to Three, 14* (6), 23-26.

Miller, L.J., & Hanft, B.E. (1998). Building positive alliances: Partnerships with families as the cornerstone of developmental assessment. *Infants and Young Children, 11* (1), 49-60.

Newborg, J., Stock, J.R., Wnek, L., Guidubaldi, J., & Svinicki, J. (1988). *Battelle Developmental Inventory.* Chicago: Riverside.

Odom, S.L., & McLean, M. (Co-chairpersons). (1993). *DEC recommended practices: Indicators of quality in programs for infants and young children with special needs and their families.* DEC Task Force on Recommended Practices: Council for Exceptional Children.

Orelove, F.P., & Sobsey, D. (1991). *Educating children with multiple disabilities: A transdisciplinary approach.* Baltimore: Brookes.

Parks, S. (1992). *Inside HELP: Administration and reference manual for the HELP.* Palo Alto, CA: VORT Corporation.

Rosenbaum, P., King, S., Law, M., King, G., & Evans, J. (1998). Family-centered service: A conceptual framework and research review. *Physical & Occupational Therapy in Pediatrics, 18,* (1), 1-20.

Sheldon, M.L., & Rush, D.D. (2001) The ten myths about providing early intervention services in natural environments. *Infants & Young Children, 14* (1), 1-13

Shonkoff, J.P., & Meisels, S.J. (1990). Early childhood intervention: The evolution of a concept. In S.J. Meisels & J.P. Shonkoff (Eds.), *Handbook of early childhood intervention* (pp. 3-31). Cambridge, MA: Cambridge University Press.

Simeonsson, R.J., & Bailey, D.B. (1990). Family dimensions in early intervention. In S.J. Meisels & J.P. Shonkoff (Eds.), *Handbook of early childhood intervention.* Cambridge, MA: Cambridge University Press.

Simons, R. (1985). *After the tears.* New York: Harcourt Brace Jovanovich.

Stallings-Sahler, S. (1998). Sensory integration: Assessment and intervention with infants. In J. Case-Smith (Ed.), *Pediatric occupational therapy and early intervention* (pp. 309-341). Boston: Butterworth-Heinemann.

Teti, T.M., & Gibbs, E.D. (1990). Infant assessment: Historical antecedents and contemporary issues. In E.D. Gibbs & D.M. Teti (Eds.), *Interdisciplinary assessment of infants* (pp. 3-10). Baltimore: Brookes.

Trivette, C.M., Dunst, C.J., & Deal, A.G. (1997). Resource-based approach to early intervention. In S.K. Thurman, J.R. Cornwell, & S.R. Gottwald (Eds.), *Contexts of early intervention: Systems and settings.* Baltimore, MD: Brookes.

Turnbull, A.P., Turbiville, V., & Turnbull, H.R. (2000). Evolution of family-professional partnerships: Collective empowerment as the model for the early twenty-first century. In J.P. Shonkoff & S.J. Meisels (Eds.), *Handbook of early childhood intervention* (2nd ed., pp. 630-650). Cambridge, MA: Cambridge University Press.

Turnbull, A.P., Turnbull, H.R., & Blue-Banning, M. (1994). Enhancing inclusion of infants and toddlers with disabilities and their families: A theoretical and programmatic analysis. *Infants and Young Children, 7* (2), 1-14.

Vohs, J. (1989). Recommendations for working with families and children with special needs from diverse cultures. In J. Vohs (Ed.), *Organizational resources for understanding families from diverse cultures. Coalition Quarterly: Toward Multiculturalism, 6* (2 & 3), 23.

School-based Occupational Therapy

Jane Case-Smith ▪ Jan Rogers

KEY TERMS

Individuals with Disabilities Education Act (IDEA)
Least restrictive environment
Inclusion
Multidisciplinary evaluation

Related services
Individualized Education Program (IEP)
Collaboration
Integrated therapy models
Consultation

CHAPTER OBJECTIVES

1 Apply the principles and regulations of the Individuals with Disabilities Education Act to occupational therapy practice.
2 Explain the continuum of least restrictive environment.
3 Describe appropriate evaluation as defined in the Individuals with Disabilities Education Act.
4 Discuss the participation of students in special education in proficiency testing.
5 Explain a problem-solving approach to school-based occupational therapy evaluation.
6 Define the components of and process for developing a student's Individualized Education Program.
7 Describe how an integrated therapy model supports inclusion of students with disabilities.
8 Define and apply consultation models, methods, and styles.
9 Explain how occupational therapy consultation contributes to inclusive models of practice.

All children are required to spend considerable time in an educational setting in preparation for adult roles in life. Schools prepare students to enter the community and the work environment, enabling them to successfully contribute to society. Fullan (1993) explained that education has a moral purpose to make a difference in the lives of students regardless of background and to help produce citizens who can live and work productively in increasingly dynamically complex societies (p. 4). The occupational therapist that works in a school setting has the unique opportunity to help students become as functional as possible in their own environments. This chapter discusses schools as a context of occupational therapy practice and the roles and functions of therapists in educational settings.

IDEA PRINCIPLES AND IMPLICATIONS FOR OCCUPATIONAL THERAPISTS

The role of occupational therapists in the school system has roots in the concepts of equality and civil rights that evolved from monumental changes in philosophic and political thinking during the late part of the eighteenth century. Humanitarianism and moral treatment began to be part of the public consciousness, and over the past hundred years, the United States has enacted laws that reflect this philosophy (Hopkins, 1988). Although private institutions and organizations, such as churches and hospitals, provided ethical care and assistance to persons with disabilities, humanitarianism brought these concerns to the public. Soon Americans came to believe that ethical care of individuals with disabilities was a public responsibility and, over time, established care of, and accommodations for, individuals with disabilities as part of their civil rights.

Legislation that began in the 1930s (and continues to today) established public health programs that are available to all citizens. Federal laws have also established public education as a right of all children, regardless of privilege or power. Legal support of the right to education began with litigation related to racial desegregation then moved on to protect the rights of students with disabilities.

In the early 1970s, most states had statutes requiring educational services to be provided to certain children with disabilities. Although some states mandated services to all children with disabilities, inconsistencies were common across states and many children with disabilities were excluded from special education. At the time of enactment of the Education of the Handicapped Act (EHA) (1975), more than half of all children with disabilities in the United States did not receive appropriate educational services. In addition, more than one million children with disabilities were excluded from the public school system. Many families were forced to find services outside the public school system, often at great distance from their homes and at their own expense (EHA, 1975).

The EHA established six principles to guide the education of individuals with disabilities (Box 22-1). These principles have remained unchanged in subsequent amendments to the EHA, including the current version, the Individuals with Disabilities Education Act (IDEA).

Each of these concepts has significant implications for the public education system, for children with disabilities and their families, and for occupational therapists. A "free appropriate public education" refers to special education and related services that (1) are provided at public expense, (2) are under public supervision and direction, (3) meet the standards of the state educational agency, and (4) include an appropriate education at

preschool, elementary, or secondary levels. "Free" means at no cost to parents, but of course does not preclude the incidental fees that are normally charged to students without disabilities. The word "appropriate" is more difficult to define, because it does not necessarily refer to a grade level or the chronological age of a child. Appropriate is determined by the Individualized Education Program that is developed for each student by the educational team. This program is based on results of a comprehensive, multidisciplinary assessment. As part of the educational team, occupational therapists have essential roles in these processes.

In the regulations for Part B of IDEA, occupational therapy is defined as a related service that may be required to enable a student to benefit from special education. The services of an occupational therapist are, therefore, designed to enhance a student's abilities to participate in the educational process. The regulations of IDEA define occupational therapy as "(i) improving, developing or restoring functions impaired or lost through illness, injury or deprivation, (ii) improving ability to perform tasks for independent functioning when functions are impaired or lost, and (iii) preventing, through early intervention, initial or further impairment or loss of function" [34 C.F.R., §300.16(a)(5)].

The IDEA guarantees that each child with a disability be educated in the least restrictive environment. Children with disabilities are most appropriately educated with their peers who are not disabled. Whatever the disability, the first student placement that should be considered is to assign the child to a general-education classroom, with appropriate aids and supports (Heumann & Hehir, 1994). This policy is clearly stated in IDEA, the "removal of children with disabilities occurs only when the nature or severity of the disability of a child is such that education in regular classes with the use of supplementary aids and services cannot be achieved satisfactorily" (32 C.F.R., §612[5][A]).

The amount of support provided to these students varies from a full-time aide to periodic, consultative services by an occupational therapist or special educator. When a child cannot be educated in the regular classroom, an alternative placement is considered. Accordingly, schools are required by law to ensure that a continuum of alternative placements is available to meet the needs of children with disabilities. This continuum includes a range of alternative placements such as instruction in regular classes, special classes, special schools, home instruction, and instruction in hospitals and institutions. Most children with disabilities spend at least a portion of their day in regular-education classrooms.

Inclusion is a frequently used term to describe how "least restrictive environment" is implemented. *Full inclusion* refers to a child's access to and participation in all activities of the school setting. Supports and adaptations are provided as needed to enable the child with

---

BOX 22-1 **Principles of the Individuals with Disabilities Education Act (formerly EHA [PL. 94-142])**

1 *Free Appropriate Public Education* (FAPE). Every eligible child is entitled to an appropriate education that is free to families (supported by public funds).

2 *Least Restrictive Environment.* Children with disabilities are most appropriately educated with their nondisabled peers. Special classes, separate schooling, or other removal of children with disabilities from the regular educational environment is to occur only when the nature or severity of the disability of a child is such that education in regular classes with the use of supplementary aids and services cannot be achieved satisfactorily [Section 612 (a)(5)(A)].

3 *Appropriate Evaluation.* All children with disabilities must be appropriately assessed for purposes of eligibility determination, educational programming, and individual performance monitoring.

4 *Individualized Education Program.* A document that includes an annual plan is developed, written, and (as appropriate) revised for each child with disabilities.

5 *Parent and Student Participation in Decision Making.* Parents and families must have meaningful opportunities to participate in the education of their children at school and at home.

6 *Procedural Safeguards.* Safeguards are in place to ensure that the rights of children with disabilities and their parents are protected, and that students with disabilities and their parents are provided with the information they need to make decisions. In addition, procedures and mechanisms must be in place to resolve disagreements between parents and school officials.

disabilities to participate in activities with his or her peers. These services are typically provided in the child's neighborhood school. For example, Josh, a child with spina bifida and mild learning disabilities, attends his local, home elementary school in a rural community. Josh is in the regular classroom for the entire day, with a classroom aide assisting him with self-care tasks as needed. The school's special education teacher helps the classroom teacher in adapting Josh's assignments when needed.

Inclusion can consist of a variety of learning options. A student may spend a portion of the day in a resource room and a portion in regular-education classes. For instance, Brian, who is in the sixth grade, participates in the regular-education classroom for all of his classes, except math and reading. For these subjects, he receives instruction from the resource room teacher because his performance in these classes is significantly lower than his peers, and he requires a special curriculum to progress in these areas.

Modifications and accommodations are made to support Brian's learning needs so that he can participate in learning activities. Often the regular classroom teacher groups students for science and social studies projects so that each of the students is given a task that he or she can manage. Because Brian has difficulty with manipulation, the teacher gives manipulation tasks to the other students in the group and often selects Brian to search the Internet or oversee final-project assembly. Tests are read to Brian, and he is allowed to dictate his answers. Greg attends full-day, inclusive kindergarten with occupational therapy, physical therapy, and special education supporting his participation in the regular-education curriculum (Figures 22-1 and 22-2).

Inclusive experiences in regular education classrooms also serve social purposes. For example, Mary, a child with cerebral palsy and significant learning disabilities, participates in the regular half-day kindergarten class in the morning. During this time, the emphasis is placed on providing socialization experiences for Mary with the students in the typical class. Mary's day is extended, and in the afternoon she is instructed in her academic subjects in the resource room.

The model for implementing "least restrictive environment" can significantly affect the delivery of occupational therapy service. Integrated, or inclusive, classrooms and resource classrooms place different demands on the student. For example, a self-contained class of eight children with a special education teacher and an aide demands a different set of skills of each student than does a class of 25 students taught by one regular education teacher who may have minimal specialized training in educating students with disabilities. Occupational therapists must be adept in assessing the child's performance, the context in which the child is placed, and the effects of that context on the child's performance. Therapists need to consider the difference

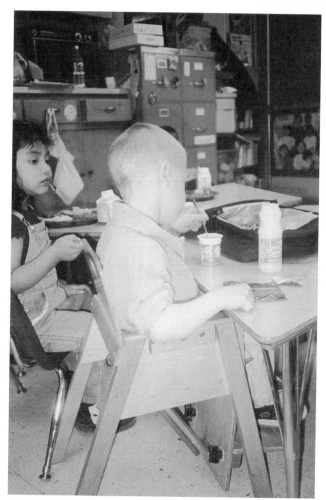

Figure 22-1 Greg participates in all of the kindergarten class activities with adapted equipment (e.g., Rifton chair) and modifications to the environment (e.g., placement of activities).

between special-education and regular-education models. Additionally, they must assess the teacher's level of expertise in working with a student and the level of support needed by the teacher. Other types of schools in which occupational therapists provide services are listed (Box 22-2). When serving students in these schools, therapists should make a specific effort to understand the mission, goals, and unique characteristics of each learning environment.

EVALUATION

IDEA has specific requirements for evaluation. States must comply with federal regulations and may adopt more restrictive requirements. For example, although the federal law requires that students are tested with "technically sound instruments," some states require that norm-referenced standardized tests are used in evaluation. The following section describes the requirements for evaluation defined in IDEA.

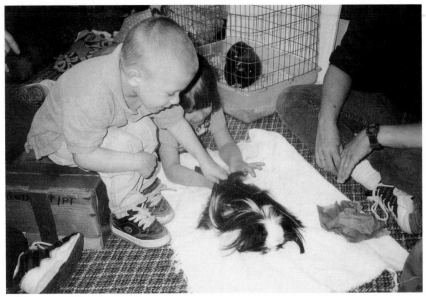

Figure 22-2 Kindergarten offers a multitude of social experiences, emphasizing socially appropriate behavior, responsibility, self-maintenance, and respect and caring of others (including pets).

BOX 22-2 Types of Schools in Which Occupational Therapists Provide Services

Occupational therapists provide services to students in private and parochial schools, charter schools, and alternative schools. When indicated, and when students are eligible for special education, they are entitled to services through IDEA. This is true even when the parents elect to enroll them in private, or nonpublic, schools (Federal Regulations, 34 C.F.R., §300.341). When it is determined to be the most appropriate environment for a child's education, occupational therapists may also provide educationally relevant services in the home or a residential center.

Charter schools are typically small, responsive schools that allow for the development of alternative curriculum, administration of their own budgets, and autonomous decision making. They are a departure from the large public school systems and tend to put curricular and programmatic decisions in the hands of parents. Charter schools are typically unique entities and tend to reflect the interests and needs of the community they serve. They are often developed with a particular educational emphasis such as math and science, foreign languages, or the arts. Many charter schools are designed to serve children at risk for learning disabilities or school problems (Zepeda & Langenbach, 1999). Therapists working in charter schools need to learn about the focus and direction of the school as well as the types of children and families who enroll in them. By understanding the school's mission and character, the therapist can work with administrators, teachers, and families successfully.

Alternative schools are typically administered by public schools. They may be "magnet" schools that provide enriched education based on programmatic themes such as math and science, the arts, or foreign languages. They may be schools that offer a last chance before expulsion, or they may provide remediation and rehabilitation to students with academic,

social, or emotional problems (Zepeda & Langenbach, 1999). Occupational therapists may provide services in both types of alternative schools. When working in a remediation and rehabilitative school, therapists should have skills and experience in psychosocial intervention and behavioral management. Many of these schools provide a curriculum and code of conduct, with structured rules and regulations to which the therapist must adhere for the safety of staff and students.

Vocational schools may be an option for students who plan to seek immediate employment after high school graduation. They also prepare the student for the option of attending a trade school after high school graduation. Vocational schools are generally separate schools that students attend after they have obtained some of their basic high school education requirements in their home school district. The students may choose one of several career paths that may include business, health care professions, computer technology, and various trades. The emphasis of these schools tends to shift the student from an academic to a vocational perspective. Students are generally provided with specialized skills that will make them employable upon graduation. Occupational therapists assist students in developing prevocational and vocational skills. They also help students to adapt to work environments.

Occasionally medically fragile or severely impaired students receive *home-based related services.* Although a child may have extensive medical needs, the role of the school-based occupational therapist is to provide educationally relevant services. Students may also receive home-based services when suspended or expelled from school. Students with Individualized Education Programs (IEPs), who have been suspended or expelled, are entitled to the full scope of their IEP, including occupational therapy services (Federal Regulations 34 C.F.R., §300.522).

Legal Requirement for Evaluation

The IDEA requires that a multidisciplinary team conduct a comprehensive evaluation to determine whether a child has exceptional educational needs that warrant special education services. This evaluation can be initiated by the parents or by the school team when either party notices particular problems in how the child learns or suspects that the child has a disability. This multidisciplinary evaluation is needed even when the child has an obvious disability (e.g., cerebral palsy, Down syndrome) and has received therapeutic services in the past (e.g., in an early intervention program).

Because most children with disabilities enter the school system without an educational diagnosis (or a diagnosis of developmental delay), a purpose of the initial evaluation is to give the child a specific educational diagnosis. In most states this diagnosis (e.g., orthopedic disability, learning disability, multiple disabilities) is required for the child to receive specific services. Box 22-3 lists categories of disability as defined in IDEA.

The phrase *child with a disability* for children aged 3 through 9 may, at the discretion of the state and LEA and in accordance with §300.313, include a child who is experiencing developmental delays, as defined by the state and as measured by appropriate diagnostic instruments and procedures, in one or more of the following areas: physical development, cognitive development, communication development, social or emotional development, or adaptive development; and who, by reason thereof, needs special education and related services (Authority: 20 U.S.C. 1401(3)(A) and (B); 1401(26)).

The 1997 Amendments to IDEA shifted the emphasis from evaluation as the basis of a diagnostic label to evaluation focused on identifying functional problems and goals. The specific questions to be answered by the initial evaluation are as follows:

1 What is the child's present level of educational performance?
2 What are the child's educational needs?

3 Does the child need special education and related services?
4 What additions or modifications, if any, are needed to the special education and related services to enable the child to meet annual goals in the Individualized Education Program (IEP) and to participate, as appropriate, in the general curriculum? [Section 614 (c)(2)(B)]

The results of the initial evaluation define the student's present levels of performance for purposes of writing the IEP. Therefore, evaluation findings need to relate to the curriculum as well as the student's developmental function.

Students with IEPs (i.e., those who receive special education services) are considered for reevaluation at least every three years to determine if they continue to need special education and related services. Through reevaluation, the IEP team decides if additions or changes need to be made to the special education and related services the child is receiving, to enable the child to meet IEP goals and to participate (as appropriate) in the general curriculum [IDEA, 20 U.S.C. 1400 et seq., §614 (c)(1)]. Reevaluation is not needed if sufficient information has been obtained during the course of the 3 years. The intent of this recent change in the law is to prevent unnecessary testing, such as repeated intelligence tests.

Based on current thinking and on language in IDEA, evaluation is a multidisciplinary, collaborative effort focused on function and the issues that appear to be impeding learning. Norm-referenced tests give standardized scores helpful in determining eligibility, but information from a norm-referenced test can be difficult to relate to functional performance in a classroom. Standardized assessments are most helpful when they are criterion referenced, with the performance of peers in the same grade and the curriculum used as the criteria. For example, does the student demonstrate the same ability to attend, persist in tasks, and organize his or her materials as the other students in the classroom? Although standardized tests offer an objective measure of abilities, informal observational assessment of the student in his classroom or other school environment is also important to establishing goals and objectives.

The other specific requirements for evaluation established by IDEA are listed in Box 22-4. These requirements place emphasis on using a variety of measures, including parent report, and using technically sound instruments. "Trained," "knowledgeable," and "qualified" personnel are to administer the evaluation methods; occupational therapists qualify to administer many of the evaluation methods used in schools. It is essential that assessment tools and strategies provide "relevant information that directly assists persons in determining the educational needs of the child" (Authority: 20 U.S.C. 1412(a)(6)(B), 1414(b)(2) and (3)).

BOX 22-3   Categories of Disability (IDEA regulations, 1997)

1 Mental retardation
2 Hearing impairment including deafness
3 Speech or language impairment
4 Visual impairment including blindness
5 Emotional disturbance
6 Orthopedic impairment
7 Autism
8 Traumatic brain injury
9 Other health impairment
10 Specific learning disability
11 Deaf-blindness
12 Multiple disabilities

BOX 22-4 Requirements for Appropriate Evaluation as Defined in IDEA

1 Tests and other evaluation materials used to assess a child under Part B must be
   a Selected and administered so as not to be discriminatory on a racial or cultural basis.
   b Provided and administered in the child's native language or other mode of communication, unless it is clearly not feasible to do so.
2 A variety of assessment tools and strategies are used to gather relevant functional and developmental information about the child, including information provided by the parent, and information related to enabling the child to be involved in and progress in the general curriculum (or for a preschool child, to participate in appropriate activities), that may assist in determining
   a Whether the child is a child with a disability under §300.7; and
   b The content of the child's IEP (the child's educational goals and expected outcomes).
3 When standardized tests are given to the child, they must be
   a Validated for the specific purpose for which they are used
   b Administered by trained and knowledgeable personnel in accordance with any instructions provided by the producer of the tests. If an assessment is not conducted under standard conditions, a description of the extent to which it varied from standard conditions must be included in the evaluation report.
4 Tests and other evaluation materials include those tailored to assess specific areas of educational need and not merely those that are designed to provide a single general intelligence quotient.
5 Tests are selected and administered so as best to ensure that if a test is administered to a child with impaired sensory, manual, or speaking skills, the test results accurately reflect the child's aptitude or achievement level or whatever other factors the test purports to measure, rather than reflecting the child's impaired sensory, manual, or speaking skills (unless those skills are the factors that the test purports to measure).
6 No single procedure is used as the sole criterion for determining whether a child has a disability and for determining an appropriate educational program for the child.
7 The child is assessed in all areas related to the suspected disability, including, if appropriate, health, vision, hearing, social and emotional status, general intelligence, academic performance, communicative status, and motor abilities.
8 In evaluating each child with a disability under §§300.531-300.536, the evaluation is sufficiently comprehensive to identify all of the child's special education and related services needs, whether or not commonly linked to the disability category in which the child has been classified.
9 The public agency uses technically sound instruments that may assess the relative contribution of cognitive and behavioral factors, in addition to physical or developmental factors.
10 The public agency uses assessment tools and strategies that provide relevant information that directly assists persons in determining the educational needs of the child (34 C.F.R., §300.532).

*Authority: 20 U.S.C. 1412(a)(6)(B), 1414(b)(2) and (3).

Occupational Therapy Evaluation

Occupational therapy evaluation in the school focuses on the child's ability to participate in functional school activities or for preschool children to participate in developmentally appropriate activities. A problem-solving approach is used to identify the issues that are relevant to the problem and to identify strategies that may help to resolve those issues. In the first step of a problem-solving approach to assessment, teacher and parent concerns are identified and primary functional problems are defined (Clark & Coster, 1998). Once the functional problems are identified, further assessment is carried out to identify the reasons for the problems and potential solutions. This process includes trial of potential solutions and intervention strategies to determine the likelihood that they will be effective. This trial helps to determine the level of change that can be expected.

A problem-solving model is circular: once decisions are made regarding intervention approaches, their effectiveness is monitored and periodically reevaluated to make adjustments, select alternative methods, or stay on course (see Clark & Coster, 1998, or Clark & Miller,

1996). As described in the following section, assessment begins by determining the degree to which a student *participates* in school; then it focuses on *performance* of specific school activities.

Student's Level of Participation

A goal of public education is that students participate in school activities to the maximum extent possible. It is expected that students demonstrate consistent progress in the curriculum or toward their individual educational goals. In addition to academic outcomes, students must demonstrate socially appropriate behaviors and functional performance that enables them to participate in nonacademic school activities (e.g., eating lunch, playing with peers on the playground). A typical lunchroom presents multiple challenges to children with disabilities (Figure 22-3). Occupational therapists often focus on functional performance in nonacademic areas in addition to providing support for academic performance. As a comprehensive assessment of function and participation, the *School Function Assessment* (SFA) (Coster, Deeney, Haltiwanger, & Haley, 1998) is a helpful initial

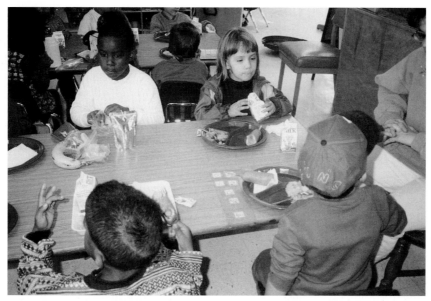

Figure 22-3   Lunchtime is relatively unstructured and presents multiple challenges to children with disabilities. Participation in the lunchroom may be limited by the stimulating environment, noise levels, fine-motor skills to open cartons and packages, and balance and mobility when carrying a lunch tray in a crowded environment.

evaluation of the child. Its three sections provide scales for identifying a child's level of participation, assessing need for task support, and evaluating performance in school activities. This criterion-referenced tool assesses the school functions that are primary domains of concern for occupational and physical therapists. The physical subscales identified in the SFA include travel, maintaining and changing positions, recreational movement, using materials, setup and cleanup, eating and drinking, hygiene, clothing management, written work, movement up and/or down stairs, and computer and equipment use. The cognitive and or behavioral subscales identified in the SFA include functional communication, memory and understanding, following social conventions, task behavior and completion, compliance with adult directives and school rules, positive interaction, behavior regulation, personal care awareness, and safety.

To rate the SFA, the child is judged in relationship to the performance of the other students in his or her grade level or classroom. A child's participation is understood through observation of how peers perform and function relative to the curriculum and environment and what level of participation the teacher expects. To thoroughly identify the problem and to complete the SFA, the teacher is interviewed. Through her everyday observations of the student, the teacher identifies the activities in which the student struggles or fails. Informal observation by the occupational therapist validates and augments the teacher's explanation of the problem and the student's level of participation. Based on the occupational therapist's observation, the child and the context become well understood, often leading to an interpretation of the problem that sheds new light on the child's behaviors.

These three methods (i.e., use of the SFA, informal observation, and teacher-parent interview) allow for accurate identification of the problem. Using different perspectives brings the problem(s) into focus and leads into the next steps of successful problem solving.

Assessment of Performance

Specific assessment of performance follows, using the problems observed in school functions as a basis for selecting evaluation tools. At this stage, the goal is to identify reasons for the student's difficulties. Standardized tools and structured observation are used. Survey research has identified the tests used by school-based occupational therapists (Burtner, McMain, & Crowe, 2002; Crowe, 1989). These studies indicate that occupational therapists predominately use tests that analyze performance. In a survey of school-based therapists in Northwestern United States, Crowe (1989) found that the Peabody Developmental Motor Scales (PDMS), the Bruininks-Oseretsky Test of Motor Proficiency (BOTMP), the Ayres Clinical Observations, the Developmental Test of Visual Motor Integration (VMI), and the Motor–Free Visual Perceptual Test (MVPT) were most frequently used. In a more recent survey of occupational therapists in Southwestern United States, Burtner et al. (2002) found similar results in that the most commonly used tests were the PDMS, the BOMPT, the VMI, and the MVPT. The surveys indicate the prevalence of using standardized assessments to analyze performance and indicate which performance areas are evaluated by occupational therapists. Typical areas of assessment—(1) *motor performance,* (2) *sensory responsiveness,* (3) *perceptual processing,* (4) *psychosocial and cognitive abilities,* and (5) *school environment,* and (6) *teacher and curricular expectation*—are described in the following sections.

Motor Performance. Children in school are expected to independently travel within the school and move safely within the classroom, playground, and hallways. They must manipulate their schoolbooks, writing and cutting tools, paper, and materials; use tools such as scissors; produce legible handwriting; eat and drink independently; and use a computer. Related to their self-maintenance, they must use the toilet, wash their hands, put on and take off their jackets, and demonstrate other hygiene skills. Standardized tests to measure motor performance include the *Peabody Developmental Motor Scales* (2nd ed.) (PDMS) (Folio & Fewell, 2000) and the *Bruininks-Oseretsky Test of Motor Proficiency* (BOTMP) (Bruininks, 1978) (see Chapters 7 and 8). Although both of these tests offer a method for evaluating a child's motor performance, the items do not necessarily relate to school function and, therefore, a cautious interpretation of the scores is needed. Visual motor tests (e.g., *Developmental Test of Visual-Motor Integration* [Beery, 1997]) that require paper and/or pencil skills relate to school functions, such as handwriting and tool use. These tests measure the child's skills in tracing and copying designs. The SFA has sections that measure physical performance, using a comprehensive representation of the movements and manipulation skills required to function at school.

Sensory Responsiveness. A child's sensory responsiveness can be assessed using standardized interviews, inventories, or observational tests. Inventories such as the *Sensory Profile* (Dunn, 1999) rate sensory responsiveness in natural situations. Standardized observational assessments of children's sensory responsiveness and sensory integration are used to supplement the parent's or teachers' report on the child's sensory responsiveness (e.g., *Sensory Integration Inventory— Revised, for Individuals with Developmental Disabilities* [Reisman & Hanschu, 1992]).

Perceptual Processing. Assessment of a child's visual perceptual processing is particularly important to his or her school function. Standardized instruments to measure visual perception include the *Developmental Test of Visual Perception* (2nd ed.) (DTVP-II) (Hammill, Pearson, & Voress, 1993) and the *Motor–Free Visual Perception Test—3* (Colarusso & Hammill, 2002). Aspects of visual perception that relate to school function (e.g., reading, handwriting) include spatial relations, figure-ground perception, and form constancy. Other perceptual skills important to understanding performance in school activities include body scheme and body awareness, orientation to time and place, and spatial awareness (see Chapter 12).

Psychosocial and Cognitive Abilities. Problem solving, organizational skills, attention, and appropriate interactions with peers and adults are essential performance areas of school function. The SFA Activity Scales rate behavior and cognition using 10 scales. Each has high relevance to a child's success in the school environment. Behaviors are often the focus of the IEP because they determine the child's ability to function in a structured environment (e.g., classroom), to attend, demonstrate responsibility, positively interact with others, cope with new situations, and fit into the social norms of the classroom. Socially appropriate behavior is highly related to the student's academic achievement and his or her ability to succeed in environments outside school (e.g., community, work). Important elements of behavior that are often the focus of occupational therapy are attention and persistence, task completion, compliance, self-esteem and self-image, peer and adult interaction, problem solving, and safety. Students frequently have difficulty transitioning from one activity to another and adapting to new situations. Adaptive behaviors are analyzed to determine the antecedents to aggressive or disruptive behaviors, or to withdrawal behaviors.

Occupational therapists are most involved in evaluation of behavior when the behaviors relate (at least in part) to the child's sensory processing. As in every other performance area, standardized tools are available. Examples include the *Behavior Evaluation Scale-2* (McCarney & Leigh, 1990) and the *Child Behavior Checklist* (Achenbach & Edelbrock, 1991). Interpretation of standardized results requires specific observations of in-classroom and out-of-classroom behaviors. It also requires the interpreter to conduct teacher and parent interviews. These interviews provide an understanding of behavioral expectations, suggest possible reasons for behaviors, define the extent of the problem, and determine desired functional outcomes.

School Environment. Evaluation of functional performance includes assessment of the school environment. All of the student's school environments should be examined, including the classrooms, cafeteria, playgrounds, gymnasium, and other spaces (Figure 22-4). For children in wheelchairs or walkers, the focus of this part of the assessment may be accessibility. For children with sensory processing problems, the focus may be the degree and types of sensory stimulation in the environment. Classrooms tend to be highly visually stimulating environments, and they can be disorganizing and overwhelming to students with sensory processing problems (Figure 22-5).

Teacher and Curricular Expectations. To analyze the extent and the basis for a student's performance problem, the expected performance (as defined by the teacher and curriculum) must be fully understood. When teachers expect neat, precisely aligned, and well-formed handwriting, a student with poor handwriting will have a significant problem in meeting that teacher's standard. As another example, some teachers show high tolerance for disruptive behaviors and allow students to move freely about the room. A student with a high activity level and sensory seeking behaviors would have greater success in a classroom where movement was allowed, rather than one where students were expected to remain in their seats. Often a student's goals and services are based more on the discrepancy between the student's performance and classroom-teacher expectations than on performance delays as determined by norms that reference the student's age.

Linking Assessment to Intervention

Evaluation of students is focused on the problems that seem to be affecting the child's ability to learn and function in school. Problem-based evaluation is focused and in depth; that is, relevant performance areas are thoroughly explored in various environments and situations to determine what strategies would be most helpful in improving performance. When possible, the initial evaluation (i.e., the evaluation completed before a written plan is developed) includes a trial of possible interventions and an assessment of their effectiveness. This part of the evaluation, sometimes termed *intervention-based assessment,* helps the therapist to contribute in an optimal way to the student's IEP.

Through evaluation of potential interventions, the therapist can judge the following:

1 The level or amount of change that can be expected in the course of the year (i.e., What goals should be established?)
2 The most appropriate intervention strategies
3 The most effective service-delivery models (e.g., integrated therapy, consultation)
4 Because the child's plan details each of these areas of concern, trials of intervention prepare the therapist

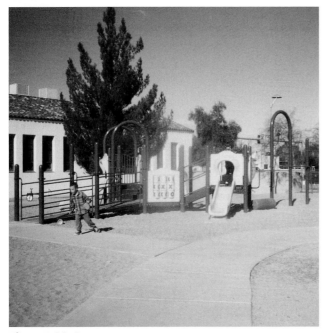

Figure 22-4 The playground is one environment to be evaluated, emphasizing accessibility and safety. Although schools are constructing playgrounds with wheelchair accessibility, many remain only partially accessible. Playgrounds should include equipment that requires a range of skills and a range of sensory input.

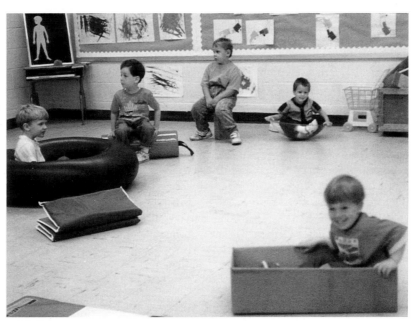

Figure 22-5 Preschool classrooms tend to have high levels of visual and auditory stimuli.

to offer valid contributions to the planning process. Intervention-based assessment prior to the IEP may preclude the need for therapy. Sometimes, simple interventions can be instituted that resolve the problem for which special education and related services were considered.

Reporting Progress

Assessment is ongoing and becomes the basis for reporting the child's progress at regular intervals. IDEA requires that regular progress reports for all children be given to parents. In the past, parents of special-education students rarely received regular reports from schools on their child's progress in achieving academic goals. The IDEA amendments of 1997 require reporting to parents at the same intervals for all students. The progress reports for students with IEPs should relate to the regular curriculum and to the student's specific individualized goals. The occupational therapist may send home a written progress report on the goals for which she or he is a listed related service.

Students in special education are now expected to meet the same academic standards as students in regular education. Based on the law, "No Child Left Behind" (2001), students with disabilities have the same right as all other children to be included in state standards, assessments, and accountability systems (Education Week, 2004). Accommodations and modifications may be needed for students in special education to participation in district and statewide proficiency testing. Often the occupational therapist provides consultation as to how testing can be modified for students with disabilities. Students may be allowed to take proficiency tests on the computer, may have scribes to write their answers, or may be allowed to take the test orally. Computer programs can provide a number of accommodations to students (e.g., tests can be scanned into the computer and displayed in large, high-contrast fonts on the screen or read to the student). Keyboarding can replace writing, and aids such as Co-Writer or Write Outloud may be allowed. Occupational therapists often identify technology that can enable a student to accomplish the mechanics of test taking. Each state determines the testing modifications and accommodations that are allowable. Some states have defined specific lists of acceptable modifications and accommodations while others allow the IEP team to determine what is the most appropriate for testing.

Some students who receive special-education services are unable to take proficiency tests even with accommodations or modifications. When taking a standardized proficiency test is not appropriate, the IEP team determines that alternative testing is necessary. The IEP team must justify why it is necessary and should recommend the most appropriate alternative testing methods. States

must develop guidelines for the participation of children with disabilities in alternate assessments. Examples of the types of alternative assessment that may be provided are (1) observing the student in classroom activities, (2) interviewing parents or family members about what the student does at home, (3) observing performance of a specific activity, (4) administering another assessment more developmentally appropriate, or (5) reviewing records. The team should identify methods that appear to match the purpose of the proficiency test. The results of alternative testing are reported to the public as are the results of proficiency testing. States are allowed to use alternative assessment on only a small percentage of their students. Occupational therapists may assist in identifying the most appropriate alternative assessment for students and may individualize a school-wide alternative assessment for one student. Despite the mandate to include virtually all students in statewide proficiency testing, eight in ten teachers believe that most special-education students should not be expected to meet the same standards as others their age, rather they should be expected to meet a separate set of academic standards (Education Week, 2004).

DEVELOPING INDIVIDUALIZED EDUCATION PROGRAMS

The collaborative planning procedure that begins the process of developing an IEP involves many steps. The first steps involve interpretation of the most recent evaluation of the child, consideration of the child's performance on any general state or district-wide assessment programs, and identification of the student's strengths and needs. It also involves discussion with the parents, educational team, and sometimes the student regarding priorities and proposed interventions. Additionally, this team considers what special factors, such as behavioral problems, issues of limited English proficiency, visual impairment needs, communication concerns and assistive technology devices or services, need to be addressed in the plan (Federal Register C.F.R., §300.346).

The IEP is a formal planning process that establishes the services and programs that will enable the student to participate in school and classroom activities and to receive an "appropriate education." The IEP developed through this process serves as a plan and a contract; it is a legal, written statement of the child's unique educational program and a delineation of what the school will provide to help the child meet his or her educational goals. It is developed, reviewed, and revised in a meeting in accordance with the guidelines of the IDEA. More than this, the IEP process also incorporates the following unique philosophical concepts (Council for Exceptional Children, 1999):

1 It values all students and respects their differences, supporting their integration into the school and community.

2 It looks broadly at the goals of education, beyond high school graduation, to establish a satisfying quality of life and a productive adulthood.

3 It acknowledges the primary importance of the family and its participation in every step of the process.

4 It emphasizes the role of community as an essential partner with family and school to help provide services and plan for the transition beyond high school.

5 It relies on a decision-making and planning process developed by a team, not by any individual person.

6 It strives to intervene early with services to prevent a student's difficulties from evolving into more stubborn and long-term problems.

7 It views special education as a set of supportive and individually designed services, not as a place to which a student is assigned.

Components of an IEP

The IEP is meant to be a comprehensive document with a number of interrelated components. The school-based occupational therapist contributes to many of those components when participating as a member of a student's IEP team. Although the exact components may vary from state to state, depending on the special education policies and procedures adopted by the state, the following items represent at least the minimum for all states since they are mandated as general requirements by the IDEA (Federal Register C.F.R., §300.347) (Table 22-1).

Each IEP must contain a statement of the child's present levels of performance that indicate how the child's disability affects his or her participation in the general curriculum (see Box 22-5). For a preschool student, consideration is given to whether the disability impacts participation in any activity appropriate for a preschooler. Typically, all team members participate in developing this statement that includes a summary of all evaluation results, thus giving a total picture of the student's performance. Occupational therapists contribute the results of their assessments, which are included in the student's present levels of performance. They should also document in this section how the student's performance on their testing indicates problems that will negatively impact the student's access to the general education curriculum. In the case of a preschool student, the therapist should document if the performance results suggest problems that will impact the student's access to typical preschool activities.

The IEP also includes annual goals and benchmarks or short-term objectives. The goals should be

TABLE 22-1 Elements of the Individualized Education Program

Component	Explanation
Present levels of educational performance	What are the student's strengths and weakness? What areas of skills need to be addressed? How does the child's disability affect his or her involvement and progress in the general curriculum?
Annual goals and short-term objectives	What educational goals are appropriate for the student, considering the areas of difficulty? What can the student reasonably accomplish in a year? (The goals must be annual and measurable and must relate to helping the child be "involved in and progress in the general curriculum.")
Special education and related services	What special education and related services are required to attain the annual goals? What supplementary aids and services are necessary to enable the student to be involved in the general curriculum, to participate in extracurricular activities, and to be educated and participate with other children?
Explanation of nonparticipation	The IEP* must include an explanation of the extent, if any, to which the child or youth will *not* be participating with nondisabled children in the regular education class, in the general curriculum, and in extracurricular and nonacademic activities; this requirement emphasizes the importance of deciding the most appropriate educational setting for each student on an individual basis.
Participation in assessments	A statement must be written that outlines the specific modifications that will be made to enable the student to participate in district-wide student achievement assessments.
Dates, frequency, location, and duration of services	A statement must be written that specifies when the student's special education and related services will begin, how long they will go on, how often they will be provided, and where he or she will receive those services.
Transition services	Beginning when the student is age 14 and every year thereafter, the IEP must include a statement of that student's transition service needs in his or her courses of study.
Measuring and reporting student progress	A statement must be written that outlines how the student's progress toward the annual goals and short-term objectives will be measured. The parents of the child will be kept regularly informed about their child's progress toward the annual goals listed in the IEP; they must be informed at least as often as the parents of nondisabled children.

IEP, Individualized education program.

measurable and attainable within one year and the benchmarks or short-term objective should be the steps in attaining the goals. Many states are linking their goals and objectives to their state curriculum content standards. This assures that the goals and objectives are directly related to the learning objectives mandated by each state's education agency (SEA) for all students.

Goal writing is a collaborative process and is completed at the IEP meeting with the input of all team members including the parents and in some cases the student. Student needs are prioritized and goals and objectives are selected based on identifying skills that are needed to progress in the general educational environment. Skills that the student needs to progress in the general education curriculum are considered a priority; team members, including occupational therapists, must relate their activities and recommendations to the general education curriculum. Each team member needs to be able to compromise and select goals and objectives that have the student's progress in the general education curriculum as the primary focus.

A statement of the special education, related services, supplemental aids and services, modifications, and supports to be provided by the school is included on the IEP. These pertain to the student's advancement toward the annual goals and access to the general education curriculum, as well as participation in nonacademic and extracurricular activities. If the occupational therapist is to provide services to the student, it must be noted specifically in this section. The occupational therapist may also participate in suggesting appropriate modifications and support based on the assessment results. As an example, the occupational therapist may suggest limiting the amount of information on the student's worksheets due to a student's poor visual figure ground processing. If the team were to agree to the recommendation, it would be documented on the IEP.

If a child will not be participating fully with children without disabilities in a regular classroom, nonacademic and extracurricular activities, there must be an explanation on the IEP as to the extent the child will not be participating. Additionally there must also be statements about the student's participation in state-mandated or district-wide assessments. If a student will not participate in the testing in the usual way, as other nondisabled students, then any individual modifications must be documented. The occupational therapist may contribute in the team discussion about appropriate testing modification. For example, the occupational therapist may suggest testing a student with sensory sensitivities in a separate room. For a student with motor limitations and difficulty with handwriting, the occupational therapist may suggest using an electronic text format of the test that would allow the student to use a keyboard. Each state determines the allowable modifications. If the student will not participate in the testing, which can only

be determined by a team decision, then a statement of why the assessment is not appropriate for the student and how the child will be assessed using an alternate assessment is documented on the IEP.

The projected date for initiating services, anticipated frequency, location, and duration of the services including occupational therapy services if warranted are documented in the IEP. A description of how the child's progress toward the annual goals will be measured is also included, as well as how often the parents will be informed of this progress. It should be noted that the frequency of reporting progress must be at least as often as the progress reports parents of nondisabled students receive. The actual progress attained toward the goals must be included. Occupational therapists are responsible for measuring progress toward annual goals and objectives when they are one of the services listed to support that student's goal. Often, several members of the IEP team share data keeping for a student's progress toward general education goals.

Transition is the process of beginning to plan for the student's completion of education and to begin to explore the plans the student has for the period of time following school. This may include vocational training, supported employment, independent living, work experience, community participation, or planning appropriate high school classes in preparation for college. Documentation of transition services is included on the IEP when a child reaches the age of 14 years or services may be initiated at an earlier age if determined by the IEP team. The transition statement should include a statement of the services needed and should clearly connect the student's goals for after-school life and a planned course of studies in high school. When the student reaches age 16, a statement of interagency responsibility is also included in the IEP. Occupational therapists may be involved in this process by providing input on the student's functional capabilities related to vocational planning and community living.

IEP Team Process

The IEP team is made up of individuals who are familiar with and knowledgeable about the child. The required team members at an IEP team meeting consist of at least one regular education teacher, at least one special education teacher, a local education agency representative (LEA), an individual to interpret evaluation results, parents, the student if age 14 or older and any other individuals who the parents or LEA representative feel have knowledge or expertise about the child. This may include related service personnel such as the occupational therapist (Federal Register C.F.R., §300.344).

IEP teams have characteristics that make them like other types of working teams, but there are also unique characteristics to IEP teams that need to be considered by the various members. It has been suggested that IEP teams differ from other teams in the following ways (Council for Exceptional Children, 1999):

1 There is a legal framework of required relationships among partners. Federal, state, and local laws and policies spell out in some detail who must participate and what they must do. This is especially true for the school district, which has many legal responsibilities regarding the education of students with disabilities.

2 The team members share both responsibility and accountability for the success of the student in meeting his goals.

3 The process is "results oriented," meaning that what matters is not how happy everyone is with the process, but the success of the student's educational program.

As a result of these differences, development of the IEP involves high levels of collaboration and, at times, negotiation and consensus building by all team members. The written IEP document is developed in a formal meeting, so the contents reflect the consensus of the team. Parents and other team members, including occupational therapists, contribute equally to the process. The team members discuss the student's strengths and needs and then develop goals, outcome statements, and plans through a collaborative process. By developing the student's IEP using a team process, the team assures the family that the IEP belongs to the student and is unique to that student's educational needs.

Educational Goals and Objectives

IEP goals reflect a holistic picture of the child, an understanding of what is required to function in the school environment, and knowledge of the curriculum. At times, the occupational therapist may feel that a particular skill is a priority for a child. However, when viewing the whole child, the team may not concur. If this is the case, some negotiation by IEP team members may be needed to select the priorities for the child so that appropriate goals and objectives can be developed for the student.

For years it was assumed that related service providers must have separate goals and objectives that are discipline specific; however, this idea conflicts with IDEA's requirement that IEP goals relate to the student's progress in the general curriculum. Bateman and Linden (1998) stated, "Most people have assumed related services must have goals and objectives. However, this is incorrect" (p. 44). They further stated, "If one assumes that a related service is being provided, as it should be, because it is necessary to enable a student to benefit from special education, then it follows logically that a goal that evaluates the effectiveness of special education also evaluates the supporting related service" (p. 45).

Additionally, they provided support with a letter from Office of Special Education Programs, 1994:

> [W]hile there is no Part B requirements that an IEP include separate annual goals of short-term instructional objective for related services, the goals and objectives in the IEP must address all of the student's identified needs that the IEP team has determined warrant the provision of special education, related services, or supplementary aids and services and must enable the team to determine the effectiveness of each of those services.
>
> For example, if the IEP team has determined that a student needs speech and language therapy services as a component of free and appropriate public education (FAPE), the IEP must include goals and objectives that address the student's need to develop and/or improve communication-related skills. It would not be necessary, however, to label the goals and objectives as "speech therapy" goals and objectives. Therefore, if the IEP includes goals and objectives which appropriately address the student's need to develop communication-related skills no additional or separate "therapy" goals and objectives would be required.

Swinth and Handley-More (2003) further encouraged therapists to consider the following: "IEP goals and objectives should be student-centered, identifying skill areas that are necessary for the student to succeed in the educational environment. Therapy centered goals that address therapy techniques or underlying skill deficits should be avoided" (p. 23). A description of how to develop goals is provided in Box 22-5.

OCCUPATIONAL THERAPY INTERVENTIONS IN THE SCHOOLS

School-based occupational therapy intervention focuses on the child's educational goals, and can support academic goals (e.g., handwriting and literacy) or functional goals (e.g., manipulating and organizing materials). Therefore, the role of the school-based occupational therapists is not to provide a full rehabilitation program but to support the child's efforts within the academic environment and only if necessary (Giangreco, 1995). In general, school-based occupational therapy services are not provided when a student has a temporary impairment (e.g., a fractured bone) or when an impairment does not interfere with the student's performance in school. For example, a bright first-grader had mild left hemiparesis cerebral palsy. This student participated in all aspects of the educational program, including physical education, with few adaptations. The disability did not interfere with the student's educational program. Therefore, she was not eligible for occupational therapy in school, despite the fact that she did not have the full use of her left hand (Figure 22-6).

Sometimes students with diagnoses such as attention deficit hyperactivity disorder are not eligible for special

BOX 22-5   Writing Goals and Objectives

Goals or objectives guide intervention and provide a measure of intervention efficacy. Goals should be developed through a collaborative process including the parents or caregivers, other significant adults such as teachers, the child, and the occupational therapy practitioner. The intervention goal reflects a specific, clear change in the child's behavior. The development of a goal must reflect the needs of the child within the demands of the environment. A well-written goal consists of three parts (Zimmerman, 1988):

1 A behavioral statement of what occupation or performance skill the child is expected to complete or perform
2 A criterion that stipulates the measure of the stated behavior; this is a statement of how well the child is expected to perform
3 The conditions for the performance of the stated behavior including such items as equipment, specific environments, social settings, or other people

Goals can be divided into two classifications: long-term and short-term goals. In some settings the word *goal* represents a *long-term goal* and the word *objective* represents a *short-term goal*. Long-term goals generally reflect a terminal behavior for the child and participation in life activities, such as in the areas of activities of daily living, instrumental activities of daily living, school-related tasks, social participation, play, and leisure activities (American Occupational Therapy Association [AOTA], 2002). As an example, here is a long-term goal developed by the IEP team for Salvador, a fourth-grader, addressing school-related tasks:

1 Salvador will accurately copy 12 math problems from the board (using a built-up pencil and slant board desktop) within 10 minutes by the end of the school year. Another long-term goal addresses Salvador's social participation within the educational setting. This goal was developed after a concern was raised about Salvador's limited social interaction with classmates. The classroom setting can provide opportunities to foster social skills.
2 Salvador will invite one classmate to join him to play a board game during class free time after one verbal prompt by the end of the second reporting period.

Short-term goals or objectives can be written as smaller steps that lead to the targeted occupation or focus on developing the underlying skills to be mastered to meet the demands of a specified occupation. A short-term goal addressing the underlying performance skills needed to achieve independence in self-feeding would state: *Vanessa will use a radial digital grasp to self-feed dry cereal within 2 weeks.* The focus of this goal is on the skill of grasp, not a step within the process of feeding. Another example of this type of short-term goal would be: *Vanessa will use lip closure on four-fifths spoonfuls of applesauce.* In this goal, the targeted behavior is not the occupation of feeding but instead on the performance skill of lip closure.

A long-term goal that identifies self-feeding as the desired outcome involves many underlying skills. Clinical reasoning is used to determine what performance skills or patterns should be addressed to support the desired occupation. The long-term goal that *by January, Vanessa will independently feed herself all meals* requires the therapist to consider several performance skills that may need to be addressed within the intervention plan to support the occupation of feeding. The following are examples of underlying performance skills that need to be addressed to meet a goal successfully:

1 The child will exhibit the fine-motor skills to handle utensils efficiently.
2 The child will exhibit the oral-motor skills necessary to eat various textures of foods.
3 The child will exhibit the ability to initiate and terminate the behavior appropriately.
4 The child will maintain attention on the meal.
5 The child will exhibit the postural control to maintain an upright sitting position.

Table 22-2 provides examples of behavioral statements that can be used to formulate long-term and short-term goals. For each statement the child's name would precede the behavior and a criteria and condition statement must be included.

A *condition* refers to the environmental situation in which the behavior will be performed. This includes the physical environment, the equipment necessary for completion of the task, and the social context for the performance of the specified behavior. Conditions must be stated to clarify the range of the child's behavior. An example of conditions for a task such as self-feeding includes the specific meal, the type of foods, the equipment used, or the social setting. These conditions dramatically alter the child's performance and must be included in every goal to clarify the extent of the child's performance. Examples of categories of conditions to be incorporated into a long- or short-term goal (Box 22-6).

Goals can be constructed easily by stating the specific behavior that the child will perform and selecting a measure of that behavior followed by the condition for performance. An example from the case of Salvador is the following: *In 4 weeks, Salvador will sign his name in cursive within 5 seconds staying on the line, using narrow-lined paper.* In this example, the behavior identified is *sign his name in cursive,* the criteria are a time limit of *5 seconds,* and the quality indicator is *staying on the line.* The condition is *using narrow-lined paper.* If Salvador were using unlined or wide-lined paper, it may alter his performance. The advantage of constructing clear, measurable goals can be seen when progress notes are required and the therapist can quickly identify whether the targeted behavior was observed.

Courtesy Pam Richardson and Winifred Schultz-Krohn.

education programs. However, these students may struggle to fully participate in classroom activities and often benefit from occupational therapy services. Occupational therapy in the schools can be provided to these students under Section 504 of the Title V of the Rehabilitation Act of 1973. Section 504 protects the rights of individuals with disabilities against discriminatory practices. The provisions of IDEA and Section 504 are compared in Table 22-3. Because the definition of disability is broader in this civil rights act, a child may be eligible for occupational therapy even when he or she is not eligible for special education services. Although school personnel are not required to develop IEPs for students served under the Rehabilitation Act, a team should develop a written plan that states goals, services, and accommodations needed to meet those goals (AOTA, 1997).

TABLE 22-2 Selected Behavioral Statements for Long- and Short-Term Goals

Long-term goal: Area of occupation	Short-term goal: A small step within the occupation	Short-term goal: Performance skills supporting the area of occupation
Dressing: Dress self in school uniform Dress self in pajamas Dress in gym clothes	Pull a T-shirt over head Pull socks over heels Fasten Velcro closures on shoes	**Motor skills:** Grasp patterns, reach, balance, and posture **Process skills:** Chooses correct clothing, initiates, sequences; organize or lay out clothes
Meal preparation and cleanup: Make microwave popcorn Make a sandwich	Open a juice box container Pour from a carton of milk into a glass Spread peanut butter with a knife	**Motor skills:** Graded grasp and release, bimanual manipulation skills, posture, and strength **Process skills:** initiates, sequences, attention, gathers necessary items **Communication/interaction skills:** Asks for desired items
Educational participation: Completes written assignments Participates in classroom discussions Copies assignments from the board	Write name on the top of a page Answer a question posed by teacher Talk to a classmate during cooperative learning exercises	**Motor skills:** Stabilizes paper when writing, uses a tripod grasp on a pencil, holds scissors correctly **Process skills:** Initiates work, sequences work, attends to class **Communication/interaction skills:** Engages in classroom activities, conforms to classroom rules
Social participation: Plays with peers Participates in community organizations (e.g., Scouts)	Play catch with friend Attend a children's fair Ask a friend to a play date	**Motor skills:** Mobility skills, coordination skills **Process skills:** Initiates, sequences, attention, adapts to environmental cues **Communication/interaction skills:** Shares personal information, conforms to social rules, respects others

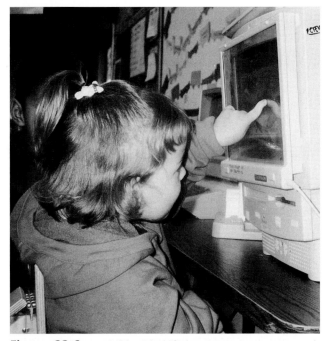

Figure 22-6 A child with left hemiparesis uses a touch window on the classroom computer. Despite her left-side motor impairments, she did not qualify for related services under IDEA because she was fully functional and met all standards for kindergarten performance.

BOX 22-6 Conditions to Be Incorporated into a Long- or Short-Term Goal

EQUIPMENT USED TO COMPLETE THE TASK
Specific positioning device
Specific adapted utensil
Modified classroom equipment such as slant boards or pencil grips

PHYSICAL ENVIRONMENT
Specific location (demands to eat in the classroom are different than in school cafeteria)

SOCIAL ENVIRONMENT
Specific persons are present (persons included in environment and social context; behavior demonstrated within structured classroom may not be exhibited in free play setting because of child's lack of organization)

Best practice models for related services define how occupational therapists and other related services support the primary tenets and the philosophical underpinnings of the IDEA (see Box 22-1). Principles to guide occupational therapy practice in school settings have been adopted and disseminated by The Association of Severely Handicapped (TASH) (1999) (see Box 22-7). In accordance with the principles of inclusion and least restrictive environment, many school-based therapists travel to neighborhood schools, serving as many as five to eight different schools during the week. Often services are provided in a regular education classroom. Although providing services within numerous schools and classrooms can place some hardships on occupational therapists, IDEA is clear in its mandate that, when possible, children attend their neighborhood schools and participate in regular education classrooms. To effectively support inclusion of children in regular education, occupational

TABLE 22-3   Comparison of IDEA and Section 504 of the Rehabilitation Act

	IDEA	Section 504
Funding for provisions	All states accept federal funding through IDEA. When federal funds are accepted, a state must comply with IDEA requirements.	Section 504 applies to all entities that receive federal financial assistance; however, Section 504 itself provides no funding. Therefore, all public schools are covered under Section 504. Private schools must follow Section 504 if they receive federal funds.
Eligibility	To be eligible for IDEA services, a student must be placed in one or more of the categories listed in Box 22-3. All categories other than speech and language impairment require that the child's disability adversely affect educational performance and require special education intervention.	Section 504 does not use categories for eligibility. Any student with an identified physical or mental disability that substantially limits a major life activity (e.g., learning) is entitled to protection. In contrast to IDEA, a student with a disability may qualify for special education or related services. Section 504 does not require that a student has special education in order to qualify for related services.
Evaluation and reevaluation	IDEA requires specific multidisciplinary evaluation procedures. See Box 22-4.	Section 504 requires that the school district establish evaluation procedures that are nondiscriminatory, use tests that are validated for their stated purpose, accurately reflect the child's ability, and incorporate information from a variety of sources.
Special education and related services	IDEA requires that all eligible students receive a free appropriate education, including special education and related services, necessary for a child to benefit from his or her education. IDEA regulations define the content of the Individualized Education Plan (Table 22-1).	Section 504 requires a free appropriate education designed to meet the child's individual needs as adequately as the needs of students without disabilities are met. Services can include specialized instruction, related services, or accommodation within the regular classroom.
Least restrictive environment	IDEA requires that the child, to the maximum extent appropriate, be educated with children who do not have disabilities. The child must be educated in the class that he or she would attend if he or she did not have a disability. The child must have access to the general curriculum.	Children with disabilities shall be educated to the maximum extent appropriate with children who do not have disabilities unless it is demonstrated that the education of the person in the regular environment with the use of supplementary aids and services cannot be achieved satisfactorily.
Procedural safeguards	Parents have a wide variety of detailed procedural rights. Parent rights include participating in all staffings, consenting to initial evaluation and placement in special education, proposing changes in placement or services, and requesting a due process hearing. Parents' rights for due process are specifically delineated.	Parents must be notified of actions regarding the identification, evaluation, or educational placement of their child. Section 504 provides for an impartial hearing but does not provide details as to how it should operate.

IDEA (1997) (www.ideapractices.org); Section 504 of the Rehabilitation Act of 1974 (as amended through 1988) (www.edlaw.net/public).

therapists use indirect and integrated therapy models (Giangreco, 1986, 1995, 1996). Integrated therapy models imply high levels of collaboration, therapy sessions within the classroom, and working directly with the teacher (e.g., co-teaching). When providing indirect services, occupational therapists use consultation and training of others to implement intervention strategies. These models are described in the following sections.

Integrated Therapy

In an integrated therapy model, the practitioner provides intervention in the child's natural environment (e.g., within the classroom, on the playground, in the cafeteria, on and off the school bus) emphasizing nonintrusive methods. The therapist's presence in the classroom benefits the instructional staff members, who observe the occupational therapy intervention. Working within the classroom benefits the therapist as he or she gains a thorough understanding of the classroom environment and the behavioral and achievement expectations of its students. This integrated model of therapy also allows the student to participate in the classroom activities, with therapy support. Integrated therapy ensures that the therapist's focus has high relevance to the performance expected within the student's classroom. It also promotes the likelihood that adaptations and therapeutic techniques will be carried over into classroom activities (York, Giangreco, Vandercook, & McDonald, 1992). Giangreco (1996) described an integrated therapy model

BOX 22-7   TASH Resolution on Related Services (1999)

Effective services provision requires that related services personnel do the following:

- Establish positive and respectful relationship with the person who has disabilities and with individuals who are significant in his or her life, working in a person-centered or family-centered manner such that self-determination is encouraged
- Determine appropriate services and supports based on an understanding of the desires and needs of the person and on assessment of participation in everyday activities and routines
- Collaborate with others who facilitate inclusive education and living for the person with disabilities to determine supports, adaptations, and interventions that optimize meaningful participation in typical home, school, and community life, both immediately and in the future
- Provide individualized services in real-life settings and teach others to provide specific and individualized support and intervention strategies to enhance participation in everyday activities and routines
- Evaluation effectiveness of services and supports through feedback from the person with disabilities and significant individuals in his or her life and through outcomes in real-life settings

From www.tash.org/resolutions.

as one in which teams that include related services (1) establish a shared set of goals and objectives, based on family priorities and participation in the general curriculum, (2) support the teachers' goals, and (3) provide a just-right level of related service support with guidance from the team. Occupational therapists are responsible for ensuring that their services are integral to the education program (Rainforth, 2002).

Educational proponents of inclusion who support integrated models of therapy suggest that pull-out services are only appropriate when students need to work on a skill that is far below the tasks presented to other students in the classroom or when the intervention activities cannot appropriately occur in a typical classroom (e.g., therapeutic use of equipment such as a swing). When intervention activities create a distraction that prevents other students from learning or the teacher from teaching, they should be performed outside the classroom (Elliot & McKenney, 1998). McWilliam (1995) cautions that pull-out therapy is less effective when compared to integrated services.

One method to promote integrated services is *block scheduling*, in which therapy sessions are scheduled in longer blocks of time than usual, so the therapist has time to work within the classroom setting during the times when meaningful activities occur (Rainforth & York-Barr, 1997). The overall total therapy time in a given month may remain the same, but the students are seen every other week rather than weekly. If several students are seen in the same classroom, the therapist may continue weekly services for each by combining the students' time. The therapist remains in the classroom for the entire morning, or afternoon, and moves between students during each of the activities presented. Block scheduling gives the therapist opportunities for *co-teaching* or *team teaching*. In this method, a therapist and classroom teacher jointly design and implement learning experiences within the classroom setting. The therapist's time is scheduled for the co-planned activities, rather than for individual sessions. Scott and McWilliam (2001) explained the benefits of working with young children in their classrooms.

> Working within classroom routines supports my intervention by allowing me to have a realistic perspective of the contexts in which the child is performing, giving me more opportunities to consult with teachers, increasing the chances of repetition and practice, and providing extra sources of motivation for the child to participate in whatever play and self-care routines have been identified. (p. 3)

Not only do the targeted students benefit from the interventions, but also the other students in the class benefit from the multidisciplinary input. For example, the classroom teacher and occupational therapist may co-plan a handwriting session. The session may include both the third-grade curriculum and practice of the mechanics of handwriting. Other examples of activities to promote fine-motor skills related to school functions are listed in Table 22-4. Activities to improve handwriting skills are listed in Table 22-5.

In integrated services, the occupational therapist may plan a program that involves specific activities for a student to be carried out with the help of other personnel (e.g., teaching assistant, aide). To enable the person who is chosen to implement the program, the therapist uses modeling and coaching as the child attempts the activities in his or her natural routine. The therapist may leave materials helpful for implementing the intervention (e.g., tongs to practice dynamic grasp, sensory bag, tweezers, clothespins) or help to adapt the environment so that the child can participate (e.g., establish a sensory corner, set up a tent, obtain bean bag chairs, therapy balls, prone standards). Regular contact is necessary to update programs and supervise the manner in which the activities are implemented. Examples of activities that the occupational therapist may initiate and then help staff to implement are positioning a student for written activities or implementation of assistive technology (e.g., adapted keyboard).

Consultation

Integrated therapy almost always involves consultation with the teacher, aides, or other therapists. In consultation, the therapist and teacher (or other professional)

TABLE 22-4   Recommended Fine-Motor Activities to Improve School Functions

Student Goal	Activities
Strengthening	Playdough, Silly Putty, clay
	Hide and then find tiny pegs, beads, marbles in Silly Putty or playdough
	Crumple paper or tissue paper to fill a bag
	Nuts and bolts
	Roll and pull taffy
	Build with magnets
	Use cloths pins on rope
Visual-motor/ eye-hand coordination	Cut shapes
	Lite Brite
	Make a necklace
	String macaroni
	Play Jenga
	Use a toy hammer and nails
	Draw with templates
	Use tweezers to pick up small objects
	Lacing projects
Manipulation skills	Place stickers on paper
	Use eye dropper to squirt colored water on paper; place dried peas in a small container with tweezers.
	Use a small musical keyboard
	Hold coins and place one at a time into slot
	Use turkey baster to blow ping-pong balls
	Use chop sticks to pick up marshmallows

Adapted from Fine/Visual Motor Activities and Developed by School Therapists, compiled by Deanna Iris Sava, 2004, retrieved on April 28, 2004, at www.otexchange.org. Fine Motor List.

TABLE 22-5   Activities to Prepare Children for Writing

Goal	Strategies/Activities
Improve posture	Adjust the seat and table height
	Recommend standing during writing work
	Use of a therapy ball with a stand
	Use of a "sit n'move" cushion
Improve hand dominance and grasping patterns	Practice cutting
	Use a nuts and bolts game
	Use a toy hammer and nails
	Lacing
	Stringing beads
	Drawing with templates and stencils
Improve use of appropriate force	Using clothes pins
	Hiding small objects in playdough
	Practice writing on NCR paper
	Practice writing on sandpaper
	Practice using a mechanical pencil without breaking the tip
Improve tripod grasp	Tweezer games
	Clothespin games
	Manipulation nuts and bolts
	Twisting on/off lids
	Using small crayons or small chalk
	Lacing
	Using a pencil grip
Improve letter forms	Use color codes to identify top and bottom of each line
	Have the student fill in missing parts of letters
	Practice dot-to-dot pictures and letters
	Draw letter in sand or sugar
	Print over tactile surfaces such as sand paper
Improve spacing and alignment	Use graph paper and ask the student to leave one box open as a space between words
	Use a popsicle stick between words
	Have student review his work and self correct
	Use paper with raised lines
	Use paper with different colors for each line (e.g., earth paper)
	Have child draw letters in small boxes

Amundson, S. (1999). *Tricks for written communication.* Homer, Alaska: OTKids, Inc; Ginsberg-Brown, C., & Schotzer, T. (2004). *Pre-referral form: Intervention strategies.* Retrieved on April 28, 2004, from www.otexchange.org.

form a cooperative partnership and engage in a reciprocal, problem-solving process. The goal is to enhance the skills of the consultee and to improve the targeted performance area of the students. At times the focus of consultation is enhancing the teacher's knowledge and skills. At other times the focus is more directly on implementation of a specific program for the student.

To provide effective consultation, the occupational therapist needs (1) in-depth knowledge and understanding of the problem, (2) knowledge of appropriate interventions, and (3) effective communication and interaction skills. The occupational therapist also must thoroughly understand the educational system so that the intervention strategies that he or she recommends are feasible within the system. Understanding the educational system also helps the therapist to ensure that appropriate classroom and student supports are identified. An understanding of the system and school policies is particularly important when the therapist identifies curricular or environmental modifications that would benefit the student's educational program.

Collaborative consultation emphasizes that the consultant and the consultee have equally important roles. The parties agree on and work toward common goals to make decisions. Although the consultant and consultee work jointly on an equal basis, they have different roles (Zins & Erchul, 1995). The consultant structures and guides the overall process, while the consultee provides information about the problem and the expectations. The consultee generally (1) retains responsibility for the student, (2) judges treatment acceptability, and (3) implements the intervention. Because the consultee implements the intervention, it is important that he or

TABLE 22-6 Intervention Strategies When Consulting

Intervention Strategies	Examples
Reframe the teacher's perspective	Explain the functional consequences of the perceptual problems observed in children with spina bifida.
	Identify that a child with autism is hypersensitive to tactile and auditory stimuli.
	Suggest that the reason that a child's difficulty in sitting quietly is related to his or her low arousal level and need for sensory input.
Improve the student's skills	Recommend that a student use carbon paper to monitor the amount of force applied with his pencil.
	Recommend that a student practice letter formation, using large-lined paper and beginning at the top of the letter.
	Recommend that a teacher provide standby assistance when the child practices carrying a lunch tray in the cafeteria.
Adapt the task	Recommend that a student begin to use a computer keyboard.
	Introduce compensatory methods for donning a jacket.
	Teach one-handed techniques during toilet training.
	Recommend that a student use earphones with music during written tests.
Adapt the environment	Establish a quiet area with a tent in which a student can hide and remove himself from the stimulating environment.
	Suggest that excess visual stimulation is removed from the wall in front of a student.
Adapt the routine	Recommend that a student have opportunities for exercise three times each day.
	Recommend that a student be given extra time to complete certain written assignments.
	Suggest that the student receive speech therapy after occupational therapy so that he or she is focused and attentive during the session.

she can accurately apply it, recognize the expected or desired response, and judge when modifications to the strategy are needed. It is the responsibility of the consultant to ensure that the consultee is well informed and sensitive to the issues. Therefore the consultant's responsibilities include (1) presenting a new or more in-depth understanding of the student's problem, (2) identifying and presenting interventions for possible implementation, (3) assisting in selecting the most appropriate and realistic solutions, and (4) developing an evaluation plan. These differing responsibilities suggest that a complementary, interdependent working relationship is needed (Zins & Erchul, 1995).

Hanft and Place (1996) described types of decision making required in the consultation role. The most appropriate intervention strategies are selected first. These decisions are based on (1) the student's and teacher's goals, (2) the student's problems, (3) the consultee's skills and interaction style, and (4) the flexibility and constraints of the environment. Examples of typical strategies recommended by occupational therapists are listed (Table 22-6).

With appropriate intervention strategies in mind, the occupational therapist selects a method for implementing the strategies. Methods range from very directive (e.g., modeling, teaching) to indirect strategies where the therapist primarily offers encouragement and support. The occupational therapist also provides specific information to help the teacher in problem solving. The method selected is based on the teacher's knowledge about and experience with children with disabilities, and his or her learning style. One teacher may be quite

experienced in working with children with physical disabilities and need little support; another teacher may have minimal experience in working with students with physical disabilities and need more support.

In each model, clarity, specificity, and accuracy of the information are important. Generally a combination of methods works best. For example, the therapist can model joint compression and hand massage before writing activities or one-hand techniques in dressing. Providing written handouts and verbal cues are also helpful in guiding the teacher's facilitation of student's performance. The therapist can ask the teacher to try intervention, to give the therapist feedback on its success, so that adjustments can be made or the strategies refined. Feedback is important to the success of the interventions over time; the student and the environment continually evolve.

The third decision that the therapist must make is selection of interaction style. The occupational therapist selects an interaction style that he or she believes will be most effective with the consultee. Interaction styles are defined using different parameters. Examples of interaction styles are achiever, analyst, supporter, and persuader (DeBoer, 1991).

These four styles reflect that individuals vary along a continuum of high to low people-orientation and of high to low risk-taking. Table 22-7 describes each style and the implication for consulting with an individual with each style.

As Hanft and Place (1996) have suggested, the consultant's style varies from being very directive to being primarily supportive, based on the consultee's needs and

TABLE 22-7 Consultation by Interaction Style

Style	Primary Characteristics of Consultee	Implications for a Consultant
Achiever	Consultee is directive, likes to make decisions, is a risk taker, likes to be in charge, needs an end goal, and may not be sensitive to personal issues in desire to accomplish a goal.	Consultant needs to be directive and assertive; should keep recommendations short, make measurable, achievable recommendations; allow the achiever to feel in charge; should be incisive.
Analyst	Consultee is precise, detail oriented, low in people orientation, and therefore satisfied to work on own; needs lots of data to act, and needs to know that solutions are correct. Consultee implements recommendations with high precision; not a risk taker.	Consultant needs to give detailed, precise directives, and have patience with the analyst's need for information. Consultant should not push this person into decisions, respect the person's analytical ability. Include data collection in the plan. Consultant should encourage decision making in a timely way. The consultant should minimize risks.
Persuader	Consultee is enthusiastic, good at influencing others, relates well to almost everyone.	This consultee is fun to consult with, but follow-up is necessary.
	Consultee is highly people oriented and is a high-risk taker; will sell solutions to the consultant.	Often this person will try whatever is readily available in the environment. Consultant needs to be aware that the consultee is easily influenced and may jump tracks midstream.
	Consultee does not need details—likes to take action.	Consultant should market ideas with enthusiasm and optimism.
Supporter	Consultee is encouraging and supportive of everyone, has high people-orientation skills and prefers that people get along rather than achieve specific goals.	Consultant's job is easy because this person is agreeable and flexible.
	Consultee is good at holding together a team; may not be efficient in implementing recommendations, because this person easily becomes overcommitted.	Consultant should listen attentively and make clear recommendations that include a rationale. It is important to be positive, since this consultee is often sensitive. Follow-up is needed, because often the supporter has taken on too much.
		Consultee may be slow to respond to recommendations because of other commitments.

Adapted from DeBoer, A. (1991). *The art of consulting.* Chicago: Arcturus.

style. Also the degree of specificity and detail depends on the consultee's preference and ability to generalize concepts and principles. It is important that the occupational therapist identify his or her own style, so he or she can recognize when styles may conflict and when changes in the predominant approach are needed.

Implementing Integrated Therapy into Regular Education Classrooms

When school-based therapists were surveyed, many believed that children were best served when they received a combination of the various service models, when therapy was integrated into the classroom, and when therapists consulted with teachers (Cable & Case-Smith, 1996). In the integrated therapy, described in the previous section, services are provided in the student's environment and focus on priority activities for that student. Therapists evaluate students within their natural environment; then they try the intervention strategies, solve implementation problems, modify programs, and model for and coach staff members who are with the student throughout the day. They also monitor progress and support other professionals with information to ensure that intervention occurs frequently throughout the day in the student's typical environments.

When school personnel frequently collaborate and share information, discipline-specific skills become difficult to discern among professions. With experience, professionals become more knowledgeable about the methods of other disciplines. For example, eating and feeding are often areas where both the occupational therapist and speech pathologist have experience. In some instances, the occupational therapist may take the primary responsibility for a student's feeding problem. In other instances, the speech pathologist may take the leading role. For most significant functional problems, a number of professionals become involved in intervention. Goals and objectives are more likely to be successfully met when the child has an opportunity to practice the skill across many different environments and with many different people. Rainforth (2002) recommends that a primary therapist model be used in which occupational and physical therapy services are provided by a single individual who spends more time with the student and has fewer students to manage. The primary therapist model has not been widely adopted, but it presents a number of advantages to children who can establish a stronger relationship with one consistent individual and to therapists who can focus their energies on fewer teams, children, and families. This model is only viable if occupational therapists and physical therapists spend

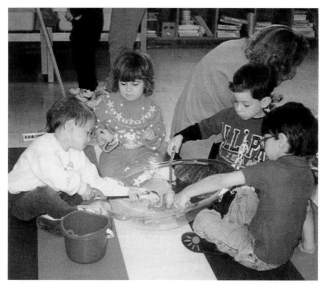

Figure 22-7 The occupational therapist may help the teacher establish learning centers for sensory exploration.

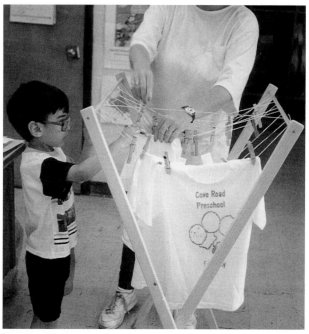

Figure 22-8 A fine-motor learning center may include hanging up T-shirts and pictures using clothespins.

time in ongoing consultation with and training of each other related to the needs of the students served.

When working with students in a regular-education classroom, the therapist needs to have a clear understanding of the classroom expectations. This includes knowledge of classroom rules, routines, and dynamics, as well as knowledge of the general-education curriculum and special education adaptations. Each classroom teacher has unique teaching and classroom-management styles. Intervention techniques conducted in the classroom that may be acceptable to one teacher may not be acceptable to another teacher; they may even be considered intrusive.

Griswold (1993) recommended that therapists offer interventions that fit the existing classroom structure and culture. For example, a teacher who values child-directed learning and hands-on learning centers may respond well to a therapist's suggestions for activities to be included in the learning centers (Figures 22-7 and 22-8). Another teacher, who uses a strong teacher-directed classroom, may prefer to engage in team-teaching activities with the therapist.

Therapists also need to be sensitive to the regular-education schedule and not disrupt the child's and the classroom schedule, if possible. Teachers may prefer to have the therapist in the classroom at certain times or on certain days. These preferences should be negotiated with the teacher before intervention, and attempts should be made to schedule times for providing services to the child that coincide with targeted goal areas. For example, handwriting interventions can be integrated into the student's language arts time and keyboarding skills can be addressed during a student's computer or business education class.

Finally, special education teachers provide valuable resources to related service personnel. Special education teachers are usually in school buildings on a daily basis, and they know the regular-education curriculum and classroom teachers. They often function as liaisons between the regular-education teacher and the occupational therapist. Because special education teachers generally understand therapy service and the regular-education curriculum, they can be important advocates for integrated therapy services.

The support that an occupational therapist provides within the school should make both the child and the teacher's jobs easier, without placing unreasonable burdens on either the student or teacher. Although the teacher and therapist's jobs are to support the child's role as a student, at times there is a mismatch between what teachers (and parents) want and what occupational therapists want. Conflicts in point of view can be minimized or avoided if consistent communication is maintained between teachers and support personnel. The responsibility for maintaining open pathways of communication rests equally on all members of the team.

PROCEDURAL SAFEGUARDS

According to IDEA, parents have rights in determining what services their child receives; in accessing information about their child's evaluation results, program, and progress; and in making decisions about placement. Parents are also given a mechanism for resolving disputes with the school system about services and programs for their child. The procedural safeguards defined in IDEA do not directly involve occupational therapists. However, it is important that therapists are knowledgeable about procedures, safeguards, and parental rights so that they follow correct procedures, accurately inform parents, and guide parents to appropriate resources when a concern arises. The procedural safeguards defined in IDEA are listed in Box 22-8. Safeguards are implemented in different ways in each state, and therapists should become knowledgeable as to how his or her state interprets the federal safeguards through state laws, regulations, policies, and procedures.

The procedural safeguards delineated in IDEA protect parents' rights and, at the same time, promote mediation rather than litigation. Mediation is an impartial system that brings the parties who have a dispute to confidentially discuss the disputed issues with a neutral party with the goal of resolving the disputes in a binding written agreement. IDEA provides for the option of mediation whenever a due process is requested and local education agencies are strongly encouraged to use mediation, rather than due process, to resolve disputes (U.S. Office of Special Education Programs, November 30, 2000). Although court cases have set important precedents for how IDEA is to be interpreted and implemented, they are costly to local and state educational agencies and

disruptive to school systems. Battles over placement and services are often painful for students, professionals, and their families. IDEA appropriately emphasizes mediation as the first and most helpful method for resolving conflicts between parents and school systems. Occupational therapists must fully acknowledge and respect parents' rights. When conflicts arise between parents and the school system, therapists should know the steps involved in mediation and encourage parents to seek mediation to resolve a conflict. The therapist's own skills in resolving conflict can be instrumental in helping the team and parents identify what is best for the student. These skills can also be important in negotiating what services and strategies will optimally serve the student.

PLANNING TO TERMINATE SERVICES

Termination of a student's occupational therapy program is often more difficult than initiation of services. It is the responsibility of the occupational therapist, in collaboration with the team, to make decisions regarding termination of services (Carver, 1998). It may be appropriate to discontinue occupational therapy when the following occurs:

1 The student has accomplished established intervention goals and objectives.
2 The student performs at a standard expected of his or her typical peers.
3 The student is no longer making significant progress on established objectives despite changes in intervention strategies or service-delivery models.
4 The student continues to make gains but there is no evidence that the occupational therapy interventions are related to the gains.
5 The identified priority skills are no longer a concern within the student's educational context.
6 The student expresses a desire to discontinue services.

Although these examples do not imply that occupational therapy should be automatically discontinued, these considerations warrant examining the appropriateness and value of continuing occupational therapy services. Occasionally, when students reach adolescence and become extremely concerned about forming and maintaining peer relationships, they begin to feel self-conscious about receiving special education services. Parents, the therapists, the teachers, and the student may need to examine the social, emotional, and educational costs and benefits of intervention when the student reaches adolescence.

A descriptive study (Long, 2003) examined the average duration of occupational therapy services for students who received direct weekly services. Using record review of a sample of 464 students from 11 districts in New York, Long found that the mean duration for weekly occupational therapy services was 29 months.

BOX 22-8 Implications of Procedural Safeguards for Occupational Therapists

PROCEDURAL SAFEGUARDS

Parents have the right to inspect and review all of their child's educational records.

Parents have the right to obtain an independent educational evaluation (IEE) of their child.

Parents have the right to request a due-process hearing on any matter with respect to the identification, evaluation, or placement of their child or the provision of free appropriate public education (FAPE).

Parents have the right to have a due-process hearing conducted by an impartial hearing officer, to appeal the initial hearing, and to bring civil action in court.

Parents must receive written notice about their rights and protections under law.

States must have a voluntary mediation process in place as a means of resolving disputes between local education agencies and parents of children with disabilities.

Parents must notify the local educational agency when they intend to remove their child from public school and place the child in a private school at public expense.

Parents must notify the local educational agency when they intend to file a due-process complaint.

Under certain circumstances, such as a child bringing a weapon to school, the child may be removed from his or her current educational placement and placed in an interim alternative education setting or suspended or expelled from school.

Attorneys' fees may, under certain circumstances, be reduced or denied.

The duration varied by diagnosis, and students who have multiple disabilities (42 months), mental retardation (36 months), traumatic brain injury (41 months), or autism (35 months) received the most services. In general, students with moderate degrees of disability received services longer than students with mild or severe disabilities, but intervention is generally discontinued after $2\frac{1}{2}$ years and rarely extends beyond 4 years.

The occupational therapist sometimes discontinues services for a period and then resumes services when the student reaches a new developmental level or must cope with new environmental demands. For example, occupational therapy services were terminated when a student with cerebral palsy functioned adequately in an elementary school environment. However, when this student entered middle school, physical growth, psychosocial issues associated with adolescence, and the stress of learning a new environment created several functional problems, and occupational therapy services were reinitiated.

When determining the appropriateness of terminating services, the student's needs, the context for performance, and the future needs of the student should be considered (Campbell & Bain, 1991). For example, should the therapist terminate services for a second-grade student who has achieved his handwriting goals at the end of the school year (with intensive therapy and teacher accommodation), knowing that in the third grade, the student will be expected to master cursive handwriting. When considering terminating services, the IEP team, including the parents, should be consulted. Often other team members contribute valuable insights as to why a student can benefit from continued therapy or what alternative supports should be provided when occupational therapy services are discontinued.

From the beginning of services with a student, the therapist should plan for discontinuation, by asking: How can this student become more independent so that occupational therapy support is not needed? Although students may receive occupational therapy for several years, it is helpful to discuss (with parents and the student's teachers) the scope of services, projected timelines, and expected outcomes at the time of annual review of the IEP. These discussions early in the year help the parent and the student's classroom teachers understand and appreciate that therapy services may not be appropriate for the child's entire school career.

Once the therapist recognizes that discontinuation of services is appropriate, he or she should begin to prepare the student and the family. Termination of occupational therapy is particularly difficult when therapists, students, and families have had longstanding relationships over several school years. Parents and students often look to the occupational therapist as the constant contact person from school year to school year, providing a sense of continuity and a watchful eye.

Families may rely on this unspoken aspect of therapy for emotional support, making its termination difficult. When possible the therapist should begin the transition months in advance to ease the sense of loss. When additional alternative supports are needed, these can also be planned for and arrangements can be made. This can help to make the actual termination a more agreeable and hopeful experience for students and families.

The following case studies illustrate the process of occupational therapy evaluation and intervention and provide examples of the range of services provided by occupational therapists.

Case Study 1: Alex

Alex was born prematurely and due to complications developed spastic diplegic cerebral palsy and chronic lung problems. Alex is ambulatory with a walker, but he also uses a wheelchair that he propels by himself and by others for longer distances. He needs assistance to manage most transfers safely. He has some significant difficulties with fine-motor coordination, motor planning, visual perception, and visual-motor skills. He also has difficulty managing some self-care tasks independently. At 9 years old, he is an outgoing young man who is easily able to communicate with others. He has a supportive family and many neighborhood friends.

School Services

Alex is a fourth-grade student whose category of eligibility for special education services is identified as other health impaired. This category of eligibility was selected by his assessment team after evaluating his abilities, school achievement, and functional skills within the school setting. Alex fully participates in a regular education classroom, including all grade-level curricula with some accommodations. He has a classroom aide who provides "as needed" assistance with setup and manipulation of classroom materials, as well as transfer and self-care assistance due to his difficulties with mobility and manipulation. School-based occupational therapy, as well as other related services including physical therapy and speech therapy, has been available to Alex since preschool. The focus of intervention and the participating team members has changed over the years as his classroom needs have changed. Currently Alex's IEP team consists of Alex, his parents, a district representative, the classroom teacher, classroom assistant, adapted physical education teacher, occupational therapist, and physical therapist.

School Performance

Recently the occupational therapist and classroom teacher became concerned about Alex's increasing difficulties in producing written assignments. Handwriting legibility has been a struggle for Alex throughout the years, and more recently he has struggled to keep up with the increasing volume of written work required in each passing school year. Additionally, Alex's already poor handwriting legibility became increasingly more illegible as he tried to write more quickly. This has occurred despite the individual interventions by the occupational therapist focused on improving his handwriting skills and developing typing skills using an AlphaSmart keyboard as an alternative to handwriting. Alex has also begun to express more dislike for writing activities, and when requested to produce a creative writing assignment, he often sits for long periods of time or begins to write and then repeatedly erases his work. Alex states, "Writing is just too difficult." Accommodations for written assignments have been made by the classroom teacher and attendant and include copying/scribing of notes that are written on the board or on the overhead, shortened written assignments, extended time to complete written assignments, dictation when longer test or assignment responses are required, providing graph paper to assist in aligning math problems, and the use of an AlphaSmart to type written responses.

Identifying Specific Critical School Skills

The team decided that it may be time to look for additional writing supports for Alex and that perhaps other types of assistive technology solutions may be a possibility. As a result, they decided to look in depth at the specific writing tasks that Alex would need to be able to complete to be successful in the fourth grade. They decided that the most critical need was to find a more efficient and independent way for Alex to participate in written work. The specific tasks required were as follows: he needs to be able to complete fill in the blank worksheets, answer true/false questions, align math problems appropriately, complete short answers, respond to essay questions, write reports with legibility and appropriate speed, and edit work efficiently.

The Role of IEP Team Members

Each of the team members was assigned specific areas to assess and it was agreed that the team would reconvene at a later date to share results and compile an assistive technology assessment of Alex's writing skills.

The occupational therapist and physical therapist were asked to work together to evaluate the student's seating and positioning to make sure that it was appropriate for writing needs. The occupational therapist agreed to gather baseline data on the student's typing skills using the AlphaSmart and to also gather information on the student's writing skills comparing handwriting and typing while the student is engaged in a variety of writing conditions (e.g., creative writing, copying task, fill-in-the-blank activity). The classroom teacher agreed to gather data on the student's effectiveness in writing under a variety of conditions while using a scribe.

IEP Team Members' Findings

The team reconvened to share evaluation results. The occupational therapist and physical therapist both concurred that the student's current seating was adequate for writing tasks. Alex is most comfortable and functional sitting at a regular classroom desk using a slant board that provides forearm and trunk support and places written materials at an angle that improves his visual tracking. He sits on an angled stool without back support that facilitates upright posture and assists in transfers. The occupational therapist found that Alex typed faster than he wrote and legibility and editing improved when using a typed text method; however, he was slower than same age peers in both methods of written production. When the creative writing was compared across handwritten, scribed, and typed methods, the classroom teacher and occupational therapist found that Alex had more difficulty organizing his thoughts when he was dictating to the scribe. The end result was that he produced more (legible and coherent) written work when typing than when he handwrote or used a scribe to complete creative writing assignments.

AT Features and Products

As a result of these findings, the team then generated a list of assistive technology features they hypothesized would be useful for this student. It seemed appropriate to encourage this student to use electronic text generation, as this was the student's fastest and most legible means of producing written text. The student currently uses an AlphaSmart. This device has worked well to help the student produce a legible product and to easily edit his work; however, alone the AlphaSmart was not efficient enough for Alex to keep pace with his same-age peers in producing written assignments. A laptop computer may be a better alternative so that additional software supports can be provided to help increase his speed. The occupational therapist suggested that Alex could benefit from software that would reduce the keystrokes needed to write words and phrases such as abbreviation/expansion software (e.g., Type-It-4-Me). This would help to increase the quantity of his text generation. Additionally the occupational therapist suggested word processing software that can easily be set up to create electronic worksheets/templates and could limit the quantity of material presented per screen, highlight important information, enlarge text, allow for color contrasts of foreground and background, and provide self-cueing of directions with voice output such as that found in a talking word processor (e.g., IntelliTalk II, Write:Outloud, Text Edit Plus). Software to help the student manage the visual demands of math problems with features such as color-coding and grid lines was also suggested (e.g., MathPad Plus, Access to Math).

Equipment trials were completed with the above-mentioned items, and Alex found all items to be useful. Use of the laptop with these features not only improved Alex's ability to produce a legible product within a reasonable time but also allowed Alex to work more independently. As Alex gained proficiency on his laptop computer, it also seemed to change his peer's perceptions of him and he quickly became the classroom computer expert and "go-to man" when the other students had questions about the classroom computers.

Ongoing Occupational Therapy Intervention

In this particular case study, the focus of the IEP team was in resolving some specific writing difficulties for Alex. The occupational therapist continued to have a significant role in providing ongoing support to this student when his assistive technology devices arrived. The occupational therapist assisted in training staff, the student, and his family in the use of the devices/software and assisted the classroom staff in modifying the student's lessons electronically as assignment types change. The occupational therapist also provided ongoing support in further developing Alex's word processing and typing skills.

Whereas Alex's fourth-grade classroom was self-contained, in the following school year Alex was scheduled to move to a middle school building where the students change classes. The new building and changing classes will likely present a whole new set of access issues for this student. The focus of occupational therapy interventions may again change to support Alex's ever-changing needs within school environments.

Case Study 2: Thomas

This case study demonstrates how occupational therapy services can benefit students in educational and life goals through effective problem solving, partnerships with other educational professionals and families, and application of intervention strategies well-grounded in theory.

Thomas was a 10-year-old child in the third grade. He had a diagnosis of autism and, at that time, attended school three partial days a week. He was placed in a classroom for children with multiple impairments without participation in a regular education classroom.

Participation: Overall Functional Level

Thomas's strengths were his mobility skills and self-care performance. He independently ate, including cutting meat and opening cartons. He dressed independently, including buttoning and zipping. He was also independent when using the toilet. In activities that required manipulation of materials, he efficiently used two hands together and manipulated small objects within his hand. Precise prehension using fingertips was accurate and consistent. Thomas had a number of behavioral issues that are described here. However, he consistently followed routines once he had learned them. He performed structured tasks that were familiar to him on a day-to-day basis.

Thomas's limitations were in the areas of sensory modulation, language, and social interactions. He had tremendous difficulty in communication and displayed echolalic speech most of the time. He had recently begun to use 1- to 2-word statements with meaning. However, he was not able to communicate using language consistently or fluidly. His receptive language was also severely delayed, and he did not demonstrate understanding of phrases with any consistency. Thomas also had difficulty engaging in an activity for more than 10 minutes at a time (other than routine activities, such as watching "his videos," swinging, or looking at books in his quiet space). He did not interact with peers or adults consistently or meaningfully. Behavioral issues included that he had difficulty making transitions or adapting to new environments. He often had tantrums when in a highly stimulating environment, such as a gymnasium.

Evaluation of Performance

The focus of the occupational therapist's performance evaluation was on sensory processing. Thomas's behavioral and social interaction and his motor skills were also examined.

Sensory Processing. As a preschooler, Thomas lacked tolerance of most activities with high sensory stimulation. He would scream and cry when students approached him quickly or unexpectedly. He was easily upset by common environmental noises. At the time of this evaluation, Thomas craved bouncing, rough play and wrestling, and swinging. He enjoyed watching videos and playing on the computer. His sensory needs seemed to fluctuate within a very short period of time. For example, one minute he withdrew and retreated to a quiet corner of the room, and the next minute he was sensory seeking (e.g., swinging, jumping, climbing).

Behavior and Social Interaction. Thomas did not interact with peers and adults appropriately. In preschool and kindergarten, he could not leave his mother's side. Even in the year prior to this evaluation, he screamed and cried for the first hour of every day. He became upset if anyone came near him or if a peer would play alongside him. By third grade, he was more tolerant of being near his peers. On occasion he initiated interaction with adults.

Motor. Gross-motor skills were an asset. Thomas had good balance and demonstrated the strength of a typically developing child. He could climb on playground equipment and easily get in and out of a swing. Fine-motor skills were also strengths, although he demonstrated some delays when compared to his peers. Although he had mastered buttoning and zipping, he continued to struggle with tying. This problem may have related to difficulty in understanding the steps involved in the process, rather than with the actual motor skill involved in tying.

Priorities

The functional priorities for Thomas were language, communication, and socialization. Another focus was improving his ability to make transitions and to change activities and environments. The team decided on the following annual goals for his Individualized Education Program: Thomas would do the following:

1 Demonstrate understanding of and answer simple "wh" questions without prompting.
2 Demonstrate appropriate social skills in the classroom, such as greeting adults and peers.
3 When given visual cues and prompts, transition to a new environment or a new activity without outbursts.
4 Recognize and regulate his sensory needs by requesting time out or specific sensory input.

Occupational Therapy Intervention

The occupational therapist recognized Thomas's need for organized sensory input and encouraged play activities that involved jumping, hopping, and climbing. Through assessing his response to these activities, she determined that proprioceptive and vestibular input helped to calm and organize Thomas and seemed to promote his ability to attend to other activities. Using these insights, she designed a sensory diet with the teacher, incorporating sensory activities into the day's routine at points when they could occur without major interruption to the other students. Together, they developed a schedule that included two to three sessions of "motor time" for Thomas, primarily implemented by the classroom aide. At these times, he and his aide visited a motor room next to the classroom, which contained swings and balls. He spent 10 to 15 minutes on the equipment, preferring rhythmical swinging and spinning. He also participated in outdoor recess, preferring to climb, jump, slide, run, and swing. He was also allowed to visit his quiet space in the classroom when needed. In the space was his rocking chair, his headset playing quiet, rhythmical music, and his videos and VCR with monitor. Initially Thomas was led to his space when he had an outburst. However, he quickly determined when and for how long he needed his space.

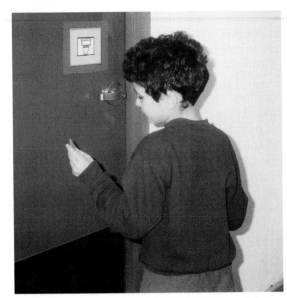

Figure 22-9 Thomas is holding his picture card indicating time for a restroom break. The picture on the card matches the one on the door.

The occupational and speech therapists developed a picture schedule of his daily activities, so Thomas had a visual reminder of what came next (Figure 22-9). When an activity was completed, he took the picture of the activity off his activity board and placed it in a box. Then Thomas pointed to the activity that came next, and his aide or the therapist talked to him about "what comes next." This visual cueing system worked well in helping him adjust to transitions and in helping him end one activity and transition to the next.

Strategies for Teamwork

These strategies were incorporated into Thomas's daily schedule, and the teacher informed the occupational therapist about the success of the various strategies once a week. Success was measured by Thomas's behavior in the classroom and his participation in classroom activities. Thomas's speech therapist discussed how these strategies appeared to be helpful to his development of communication skills and suggested modifications. The teacher felt that the sensory diet and picture board for transitioning helped Thomas do several things: tolerate school activities that were stimulating, pay attention to tasks, sit in his desk and perform academic skills, and work on task while near his peers. His negative behaviors decreased, and when he began to feel agitated, Thomas expressed the need to visit the motor room or his quiet space.

The speech therapist noted how Thomas's attention and spontaneous speech increased after participating in sensory modulating activities. His focus on other's verbalizations was greater, and his responses were more frequent when he had adequate sensory input that day. The strategies, therefore, appeared to positively influence the team's primary goals of communication and social interaction.

Case Study 3: William

This case study emphasizes teamwork and consultation with a student preparing to enter high school. William was 13 years old and in middle school. He was the oldest of three children and loved nothing more than being with his younger brother and sister. At age 2, William had suffered a severe traumatic brain injury when he was in a car accident. He emerged from a 3-week coma with no movement on his right side and no speech. Although he regained some function in his right arm and leg, his movement remained quite impaired. William demonstrated partial range in his right shoulder and elbow but was unable to move his wrist and fingers. He used a one-hand drive wheelchair for mobility and could stand with assistance and take several steps. However, independent ambulation was not a goal.

William was essentially nonverbal in preschool. However, by age 13 he used 2- and 4-word phrases appropriately. He impulsively responded to every query by saying "no" when he generally meant "yes," and he required a long time to think of words. The words he could produce were quite simple, his cognitive limitations were severe, and learning required many repetitions. William's primary asset was his social nature. He was friendly and cheerful; he offered everyone a smile. He tried new activities, even when they caused him discomfort. Staff in the school and his peers reported that they enjoyed being around William.

Participation in the School Environment

Information about William's level of participation at school was gathered from his mother and teacher. His mother reported that he was easy-going and happy. At times he demonstrated some frustration, because he had become more aware that he was different from other children. His mother's greatest concerns related to his judgment. He did not seem to understand when he was in danger and when he could hurt someone else. His mother reported that he had begun to develop some peer relations. In the past, he would spend time at school by himself. However, in middle school he had established some friends and spent more time interacting with his peers.

William's teacher reported that he was a "doll, as sweet as he could be." His academic work was at a low level, and he required extra time to complete all work. However, he had made steady, slow progress in his reading and writing.

His teacher was concerned with his safety. She worried about his judgment, particularly outside the classroom.

Currently his reading program emphasized safety words and concepts.

William had great difficulty in handling his school materials. He printed with cueing. However, his letters were poorly formed. He used a keyboard, also with verbal prompts. He independently turned on the computer and operated preschool-age storybook programs. Most of his work required assistance to keep him focused and to read difficult words. Both handwriting and keyboarding required great amounts of time and effort.

Performance in School Activities

Self-Maintenance. William ate independently in the cafeteria after his cartons were opened and his food was cut up. Eating was a favorite activity. He required minimal assistance to don his jacket, because he continued to neglect his right arm and only dressed his left side. William required assistance during two-hand activities and needed minimal assistance in transferring from his wheelchair to the toilet.

Manipulation of Materials and Writing. William required intermittent assistance to manage his school materials. He tended to neglect materials on his right side, and activities needed to be placed on his left side. He was unable to use scissors or other tools that required two hands. To help him write, William's paper was stabilized on his desk with a clipboard and dycem. In writing, his letters were large and poorly formed. He copied letters but did not compose.

Posture and Mobility. William's posture had deteriorated in the previous year; he leaned to the right with a rounded trunk. Poor posture had begun to interfere with eye-hand coordination and his ability to move his left arm. In addition, the occupational therapist was concerned about the potential of developing scoliosis.

Behaviors. William was cooperative and pleasant. He followed instructions, although at times he did not attend well to classroom instructions. In addition, William continued to need one-on-one supervision for many activities, primarily due to his low cognitive level and his difficulty in problem solving the steps of a task. However, he initiated social interaction and consistently responded to others. He was motivated to try new activities and demonstrated persistence, particularly in one-on-one situations. Judgment remained a problem and seemed to relate to his impulsiveness and deficits in problem solving.

Occupational Therapy Services

The occupational therapist contributed to all of these performance issues. She worked with William in a small group of his peers, generally on computing skills and functional mobility within the school environment. She used several typing programs that could be easily graded for beginners. William's favorite was "Slam Dunk," because he was an avid basketball fan. His family also purchased this program for practice at home.

The occupational therapist adapted William's wheelchair to improve his posture by moving his tray to a higher position and recommending a new strapping system that included a chest strap. A lateral pad on the right was tried, but it was not effective when he slumped forward in trunk flexion.

Once a month, William's therapy group planned and completed a community outing. A variety of field trips were planned, including a trip to a restaurant, a movie, a shopping trip, as well as a visit to a nearby factory and the post office. The purpose of these field trips was to increase William's ability to function in the community. Safety concepts were practiced and reinforced, including crossing the street, mobility around stairs and escalators, and care of his right arm. Appropriate social interactions with strangers and service persons were practiced. Basic concepts regarding handling money, ordering food and service, and requesting assistance were also emphasized.

These community outings were extremely helpful in identifying issues that would need to be addressed in the coming years, when William's ability to function in the community would become an important goal. Transition into community living and vocation are addressed at age 14, and these experiences helped the team establish realistic goals for the next year's IEP.

SUMMARY

School-based practice offers many challenges and many rewards. The Individuals with Disabilities Education Act, which defines the legal aspects of school-based therapy, frames this practice arena of occupational therapy. Although this education law establishes the scope of occupational therapy practice in the schools, the rich diversity, complexity, and significance of services provided by occupational therapists in schools extends well beyond legal definitions. Occupational therapists within schools have the potential to positively influence and enhance the lives of children by becoming part of their everyday lives and their natural environments.

Integrating therapy services into a child's natural environment and routine requires ingenuity and adaptability. The therapist must identify the student and teacher's priorities and decide which strategies are most important to that student's ability to participate in school. Effectiveness in school-based practice relates to the therapist's ability to analyze performance, solve problems, develop effective interventions, and to partner with families, teachers, and other professionals. The occupational therapist also advocates for children to increase their ability to participate in school and to promote the reality of schools that include all children.

STUDY QUESTIONS

1 For a child with autism, such as Thomas (described in the case study), what intervention should be carried out in the classroom? What intervention strategies should be implemented outside the classroom?

2 Give one example of an occupational therapy evaluation tool used with children that appears to have a degree of cultural bias. What items appear to be culturally biased? What adaptations to (a) items and (b) administration procedures should be considered when using this test with a student from a minority group?

3 The primary teacher is a good resource for information concerning a child's participation in the classroom. Name other persons who may be important to interview to assess a child's overall ability to participate in school activities. Explain the benefits of using multiple informants when identifying a student's problems.

4 Using William (described in the case study), write two ecological goals for his transition to high school.

5 Explain a situation in which expert consultation would be the most appropriate model to implement. Describe a situation in which collaborative consultation would be the most effective model.

6 Given the scope and focus of occupational therapy and the curriculum for third-grade children, describe an appropriate topic for team teaching with a regular-education teacher. What therapist-teacher instructional activities could be implemented to build the students' skills related to this topic?

7 Review Alex's case, then answer the following three questions:

  a What issues of access might become a factor in a move to a different school building?

  b What issues of access may become an issue for this student given change from a self-contained regular education class to a building where students are expected to change several classes in a school day?

  c What should the occupational therapist do to prepare the student, family, and receiving fifth-grade teachers for the student's arrival?

REFERENCES

Achenbach, T.M., & Edelbrock, C.S. (1991). *Child Behavior Checklist*. Burlington, VT: University of Vermont.

American Occupational Therapy Association (1997). *Occupational therapy services for children and youth under the*

Individuals with Disabilities Education Act. Bethesda, MD: American Occupational Therapy Association.

American Occupational Therapy Association (AOTA) (2002). Occupational practice framework: Domain and process. *American Journal of Occupational Therapy, 56,* 609-639.

Bateman, B.D., & Linden, M.A. (1998). Better IEPs: *How to develop legally correct and educationally useful programs* (3rd ed.). Longmont, CO: Sopris West.

Beery, K.E. (1997). *Beery Development Test of Visual MotorI-integration* (4th rev.). Cleveland, OH: Modern Curriculum Press.

Bruininks, R.H. (1978). *Bruininks-Oseretsky test of motor proficiency.* Circle Pines, MN: American Guidance Service.

Burtner, P., McMain, M.P., & Crowe, T.K. (2002). Survey of occupational therapy practitioners in southwestern schools: Assessments used and preparation of students for school-based practice. *Physical and Occupational Therapy in Pediatrics, 22* (1), 25-39.

Cable, J., & Case-Smith, J. (1996). Perceptions of occupational therapist regarding service delivery models in school based practice. *Occupational Therapy Journal of Research, 13,* 23-43.

Campbell, T.F., & Bain, B.A. (1991). How long to treat: A multiple outcome approach. *Language, Speech and Hearing Services in Schools, 22,* 271-276.

Carver, C. (1998, July/August). Crossing thresholds: School based occupational therapists discuss how they move young clients into—and out of—therapy programs. *OT Practice, 3* (7), 18-21.

Clark, G., & Coster, W. (1998). Evaluation/problem solving and program evaluation. In J. Case-Smith (Ed.), *Occupational therapy: Making a difference in school system practice.* Bethesda, MD: AOTA.

Clark, G., & Miller, L. (1996). Providing effective occupational therapy services: Data-based decision making in school based practice. *American Journal of Occupational Therapy, 50,* 701-708.

Colarusso, R.P., & Hammill, D.D. (2002). *Motor-Free Visual Perception Test-3 (MVPT-R).* Novato, CA: Academic Therapy Publications.

Coster, W., Deeney, T., Haltiwanger, J., & Haley, S. (1998). *School Function Assessment.* San Antonio: Psychological Corporation.

Council for Exceptional Children. (1999). *IEP team guide.* Arlington, VA: Council for Exceptional Children.

Crowe, T.K. (1989). Pediatric assessments: A survey of their use by occupational therapists in northwestern school systems. *Occupational Therapy Journal of Research, 9,* 1-14.

DeBoer, A.L. (1991). *The art of consulting.* Chicago: Arcturus Books.

Dunn, W.W. (1999). *Sensory Profile.* San Antonio, TX: Psychological Corporation.

Education of the Handicapped Act (1975). 20 U.S.C., §1400 et seq.

Education Week (January 8, 2004). *Special needs, common goals.* Retrieved on April 26, 2004, at www.edweek.org/sreports.

Elliot, D., & McKenny, M. (1998). Four inclusion models that work. *Teaching Exceptional Students, 30* (4), 54-58.

Federal Register. (1998). C.F.R., 34, Parts 300 to 399.

Folio, R., & Fewell, R. (2000). *Peabody Developmental Motor Scales* (2nd ed.). Austin, TX: Pro-Ed.

Fullan, M. (1993). *Change forces: Probing the depths of educational reform.* New York: The Falmer Press.

Giangreco, M.F. (1986). Delivery of therapeutic services in special education programs for learners with severe handicaps. *Physical and Occupational Therapy in Pediatrics, 6* (2), 5-15.

Giangreco, M.F. (1995). Related services decision-making: A foundational component of effective education for students with disabilities. *Physical amd Occupational Therapy in Pediatrics, 15* (2), 47-67.

Giangreco, M.F. (1996). *Vermont interdependent services team approach: A guide to coordinating education support services.* Baltimore: Paul H. Brookes.

Griswold, L. (1993). Ethnographic analysis: A study of classroom environments. *American Journal of Occupational Therapy, 48,* 397-402.

Hammill, D.D., Pearson, N.A., & Voress, J.K. (1993). *Developmental Test of Visual Perception* (2nd ed.) Austin, TX: Pro Ed.

Hanft, B.E., & Place, P.A. (1996). *The consulting therapist: A guide for OTs and PTs in Schools.* San Antonio, TX: Therapy Skills Builders.

Heumann, J.E., & Hehir, T. (1994). *OSERS memorandum to Chief State School Officers: Questions and answers on the least restrictive environment requirements of the Individuals with Disabilities Education Act.* Washington, DC: U.S. Department of Education.

Hopkins, H.L. (1988). A historical perspective on occupational therapy. In H.L. Hopkins & H. Smith (Eds.), *Willard & Spackman's occupational therapy* (7th ed.). Philadelphia: J.B. Lippincott.

IDEApractices (2004). *Regulations for IDEA Amendments (1997).* Retrieved on March 15, 2004, at www.ideapractices.org/law/regulations/

Individuals with Disabilities Education Act Amendments of 1990. 20 U.S.C., §1400-1485.

Long, D. (2003). Predicting length of service provision in school-based occupational therapy. *Physical and Occupational Therapy in Pediatrics, 23* (4), 79-93.

McCarney, S.G., & Leigh, J.E. (1990). *The Behavior Evaluation Scale—2.* Columbia, MO: Educational Services.

McWilliam, R.A. (1995). Integration of therapy and consultative special education: A continuum in early intervention. *Infants and Young Children 7* (4), 29-38.

NICHCY (1999). *Office of Special Education Programs' IDEA 1997 training packet.* www.nichcy.org

Rainforth, B. (2002). The primary therapist model: Addressing challenges to practice in special education. *Physical and Occupational Therapy in Pediatrics, 22* (2), 29-51.

Rainforth, B., & York-Barr, J. (1997). *Collaborative teams for students with severe disabilities: Integrating therapy and educational services* (2nd ed.). Baltimore: Brookes.

Rehabilitation Act of 1973, 29 U.S.C., §706 (8) and §794.

Reisman, J., & Hanschu, B. (1992). *Sensory Integration Inventory—Revised, for individuals with developmental disabilities.* Hugo, MN: PDP Products.

Scott, S., & McWilliam, R.A. (2001). Integrating therapy into the classroom: Integrating occupational therapy. In

Individualizing inclusion in child care (p. 3). Chapel Hill, NC: Frank Porter Graham Child Development Center.

Swinth, Y., & Handley-More, D. (2003). Update on school-based practice. *OT Practice 8* (15), 22-24.

TASH. (1999). *TASH Resolution on Related Services.* Retrieved on April 30, 2004, at www.tash.org/resoluations.

U.S. Office of Special Education Program. (2000). *OSEP memorandum "Questions and Answers on Mediation"* (November 30, 2000). Retrieved on April 29, 2004, at www.direction-services.org/cadre/vet_Qaonmediation.cfm.

York, J., Giangreco, M.F., Vandercook, T., & McDonald, C. (1992). Integrating support personnel in the inclusive class-room. In S. Stainback & W. Stainback (Eds.), *Curriculum considerations in inclusive classrooms: Facilitating learning for all students* (pp. 101-116). Baltimore: Paul H. Brookes.

Zepeda, S.J., & Langenback, M. (1999). *Special programs in regular schools: Historical foundations, standards, and contemporary issues.* Needham Heights, MD: Allyn & Bacon.

Zimmerman, J. (1988). *Goals and objectives for developing normal movement patterns.* Rockville, MD: Aspen Publishing.

Zins, J.E., & Erchul, W.P. (1995). Best practice in school consultation. In A. Thomas & J. Grimes (Eds.), *Best practices in school psychology—III* (pp. 651-660). Washington, DC: The National Association of School Psychologists.

Recommended Web Sites

EARLY CHILDHOOD

The National Early Childhood Technical Assistance Center

www.nectac.org

A technical assistance effort that supports programs for young children with disabilities and their families under IDEA

National Center on Educational Outcomes (NCEO)

http://education.umn.edu/nceo

The NCEO offers information on assessments, accountability policy and practices, national and state data collection programs, and standards setting for all students, including those with disabilities.

EMOTIONAL AND BEHAVIORAL PROBLEMS AND DISORDERS

Center for Effective Collaboration and Practice (CECP)

http://cecp.air.org

The CECP identifies promising programs and practices for children with serious emotional disturbance, promotes the exchange of useful and useable information, and facilitates collaboration among stakeholders at federal, state, and local levels.

National Information Center for Children and Youth with Disabilities (NICHCY)

www.nichcy.org

An information and referral center that provides information on disabilities and disability-related issues. The focus is on education and children and youth, ages birth to 22 years.

IDEA '97

Association of Service Providers Implementing IDEA Reforms in Education (ASPIIRE)

www.ideapractices.org

ASPIIRE brings together teachers and related services providers to help educational programs implement the requirements of IDEA '97. The ASPIIRE project is under the leadership of the Council for Exceptional Children (ASPIIRE's primary partner).

Families and Advocates Partnership for Education (FAPE)

www.fape.org

This project aims to inform and educate families and advocates about the Individuals with Disabilities Education Act of 1997 and promising practices. The FAPE partnership is under the leadership of the PACER Center.

MINORITIES

National Center for Culturally Responsive Educational Systems (NCCRESt)

www.nccrest.org

NCCRESt provides technical assistance and professional development to close the achievement gap between students from culturally and linguistically diverse backgrounds and their peers and reduce inappropriate referrals to special education. The project targets improvements in culturally responsive practices, early intervention, literacy, and positive behavioral supports.

Project LASER (Linking Academic Scholars to Educational Resources)

www.coedu.usf.edu/laser

LASER's mission is to enhance the capacity of faculty and graduate students in minority institutions to engage in research that impacts children from minority or low-income backgrounds.

The Alliance Project

www.alliance2k.org

The Alliance Project's mission is to address the increasing demand for and declining supply of personnel from historically underrepresented groups for special education and related services.

Parents Engaged in Education Reform (PEER)

www.fcsn.org/peer

PEER provides opportunities for parents, parent organizations, and professionals to learn from each other about school restructuring efforts.

Technical Assistance Alliance for Parent Centers— The Alliance

www.taalliance.org

The Alliance provides technical assistance for establishing, developing, and coordinating Parent Training and Information Projects under the Individuals with Disabilities Education Act.

PROFESSIONS AND PROFESSIONAL DEVELOPMENT

National Clearinghouse for Professions in Special Education

www.special-ed-careers.org

The clearinghouse gathers, organizes, and disseminates information for recruiting, preparing, and retaining those interested in or currently serving children with disabilities.

Access Center: Improving Outcomes for All Students K-8

www.k8accesscenter.org

The Access Center is a national technical assistance (TA) center funded by the U.S. Department of Education's Office of Special Education Programs (OSEP) to improve educational outcomes for elementary and middle school students with disabilities. It works to build the capacity of state educators, TA systems, districts, schools, and individuals to help students with disabilities engage in and learn from the general education curriculum.

Center on Positive Behavioral Intervention and Supports (PBIS)

www.pbis.org

The Technical Assistance Center on PBIS has been established to give schools capacity-building information and technical assistance for identifying, adapting, and sustaining effective school-wide disciplinary practices. The center focuses on disseminating PBIS technology to schools, families, and communities and demonstrating at the level of individual students, schools, districts, and states the feasibility and effectiveness of school-wide PBIS.

Federal Resource Center for Special Education (FRC)

http://dssc.org/frc

The FRC supports a nationwide technical assistance network to respond to the needs of students with disabilities, especially students from underrepresented populations.

National Research Center on Learning Disabilities (NRCLD)

http://smarttogether.org/nrcld

The NRCLD engages in research, develops recommendations, and provides training to help administrators, teachers, parents, and policy makers address the complex issues surrounding the proper identification of students with learning disabilities who need special education services.

TECHNOLOGY AND CAPTIONING

Center for Communicative and Cognitive Disabilities

www.edu.uwo.ca/cccd/index.html

The center researches computer technology and special-education resources for students with disabilities.

Descriptive Video Service

http://main.wgbh.org/wgbh/access/dvs

This national service makes visual media accessible to people who are blind or visually impaired.

LINK-US

www.startechprogram.org/stech/startechprogram.html

LINK-US guides urban schools in their quest to access and effectively utilize information and support about the use of technology for students with disabilities.

Make It Happen!

www.edc.org/FSC/MIH

Make It Happen! is an approach that improves middle school education for students with diverse learning abilities. Interdisciplinary teams of teachers design and implement inquiry-based I-Search Units and integrate technology into these units in meaningful ways to benefit students.

TRANSITION

National Center on Secondary Education and Transition (NCSET)

www.ncset.org

The National Center on Secondary Education and Transition seeks to increase the capacity of national, state, and local agencies and organizations to improve secondary education and transition results for youth with disabilities and their families.

National Transition Alliance for Youth with Disabilities (NTA) http://ici.umn.edu/ncset/publications/nta/default.html

NTA has promoted the transition of youth with disabilities toward desired postschool experiences.

Transition Research Institute

www.ed.uiuc.edu/SPED/tri/institute.html

The institute identifies effective practices and provides technical assistance activities on the successful transition of youth with disabilities from school to adult life.

Services for Children with Visual or Auditory Impairments

Elizabeth Russel ■ Patricia S. Nagaishi

Conductive hearing
  loss
Sensorineural hearing
  loss
Hearing impairment
Sign language
Total communication
American Sign
  Language
Auditory
  training/learning

Visual impairment
Legal blindness
Low vision
Neurologic visual
  impairment (cortical
  visual impairment)
Orientation and
  mobility training
Braille
Low-vision training

CHAPTER OBJECTIVES

1 Explain the implications of hearing impairment and visual impairment in the occupations of activities of daily living, education/learning, play, social performance, and preparation for work.

2 Describe special techniques and strategies that can be used with children with hearing and visual impairments.

3 Discuss the evaluation of a child with hearing and visual impairment, as well as assessments that are helpful in the development of intervention plans.

4 Define terms related to visual and hearing impairment.

5 Discuss the possible effects of visual and hearing impairments on a child's development.

6 Describe intervention strategies for children with auditory and visual impairments that promote their participation in activities and occupations.

7 Illustrate principles of evaluation and intervention with case studies.

Hearing and vision allow us to understand what is happening in the world around us. Those with normal sensory function cannot truly understand the experience of being hearing or visually impaired. However, participating in sensory awareness activities can increase understanding of the difficulties associated with hearing or vision loss. Such sensory awareness activities include eating a meal blindfolded or listening to recordings that simulate what songs sound like to an individual with a certain type of hearing loss.

However, sensory awareness activities do not give the total picture of what it is like to have a hearing- or vision-related disability, because individuals with normally functioning senses have a vast wealth of visual and auditory memories to call upon that are not available to children with hearing or vision impairments, most of whom have congenital conditions. As with other aspects of development, the development of hearing and vision (i.e., making sense of the sights and sounds around us) is experience dependent.

The sense organs (e.g., eyes, ears, skin, nose, tongue) are all extensions of the brain. The brain's primary function is to receive information, or sensory stimuli, from the world for processing and coding. This information is integrated and associated with past experiences. Because the nature and intensity of stimulation to the sense organs vary greatly, one experience may take precedence over others. If a particular sense organ is not working properly, the others do not totally compensate for the loss. However, a sensory system may take precedence over a weak or damaged system; for example, vision may take precedence in the child with auditory impairment.

Ayres (1972) developed a multifaceted systems approach to sensory perceptual development that aids understanding of sensory impairments. The senses develop and work in an interactive manner. They do not perform in isolation, but rather in the internal and external contexts of the developing child. The *vestibular* and *tactile* (touch) systems are the foundations of sensation.

The vestibular system gives information about the body's position in space, movement or lack of movement through space, and direction of movement. It is thought that the auditory system evolved from the more primitive vestibular system (Ayres, 1972; Behrman, Kliegman, & Jenson, 2000). The receptors for the vestibular system are located in the inner ear (Figure 23-1).

Visual and auditory sensations are received by the brain against a constant background of tactile stimuli and the body's position in space. It is important to think about the level of alertness required by the brain for auditory and visual perceptual processes to occur. The vestibular system and the reticular activating system have a great influence on this level of alertness. Being either overly alert or insufficiently alert can have detrimental effects on visual and auditory perceptions.

Vision is the sense we use for understanding the relationships between people and objects. It puts the environment in perspective and is an efficient integrator of multisensory information that contributes to the development of perceptual abilities and concept formation. We use vision to scan the environment (e.g., obtain information about distance, movement, spatial relations) and to discriminate features of objects and symbols (e.g., the size, shape, color, and orientation of letters). Children with visual impairment often have delayed language because it is more difficult for them to grasp relationships and associations between people and objects. In a discussion of vision, it is important to differentiate between *sight,* the ability to discriminate small objects, which is measured as visual acuity, and *vision,* the process of taking in, processing, and integrating visual and other sensory information to form a perception. Vision includes eyesight, oculomotor skills, eye teaming, focusing, depth perception, color vision, peripheral vision, visual processing, and visual perception (Titcomb, Okoye, & Schiff, 1997). Impairment can occur at any or all components, and it can occur in varying degrees in components.

In addition to its function as the building block for speech and language, *audition* is the sense that conveys sound. Sound gives information on distance and direction. For example, we can hear a dog bark and, without seeing the dog, judge where and how far away it is. *Auditory perception* is the attachment of meaning to sound patterns. Sound has qualities of *tone* and *pitch* that make up auditory acuity.

As with vision, impairment can occur at the level of acuity, processing, integration, awareness, and/or perception. Although language development appears to be the most serious problem for a child with a hearing loss, the situation is much more complex, because language is a force in the socialization and development of the child's inner logic. The capacity for language is innate, but it requires environmental stimulation to trigger its development (Chomsky, 1993; Ling, 1989; Pinker, 1994). As the child learns language, he or she can exert greater control over this environment.

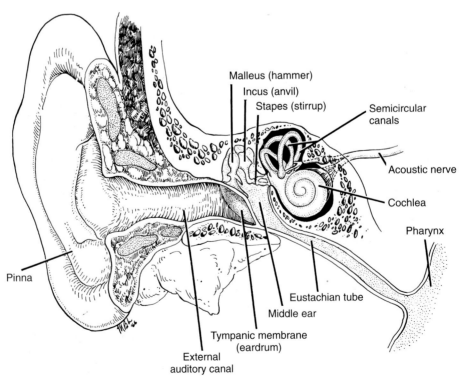

FIGURE 23-1   Cross section of the ear. (From Ingalls, A.J., & Slalerno, M.C. [1983]. *Maternal and child health nursing* [5th ed.]. St. Louis: Mosby.)

Children with visual or hearing impairments can experience substantial difficulties that affect their development and learning. Although these children face many shared difficulties, the differences are striking. For this reason, this chapter deals separately with children with hearing impairment, visual impairment, and multisensory impairment. Occupational therapists provide critical services for the associated functional problems incurred by these children. Services may be provided to individual children and families, entire classrooms, programs or agencies, or in residential settings. The occupational therapist may incorporate one or more intervention approaches, from establishing or restoring skills and abilities, to compensation or adaptation, to prevention of barriers to performance. The occupational therapist implements these approaches through therapeutic use of occupations and activities, consultation, and/or education.

Occupational therapy services often promote activities of daily living (e.g., feeding, dressing, toileting), education/learning, play, social participation, and preparation for work. In addition, occupational therapists also help children achieve performance skills, including sensory processing and perceptual skills, gross motor skills and postural control, and fine motor coordination and dexterity. The goal of occupational therapy services is to help the child and family engage in typical occupations. These activities need to have meaning and purpose to the child and his or her family, and they need to occur in the natural contexts the child and family experience. Consultation with parents, teachers, and caregivers is provided as part of the child's overall developmental and educational plan (and in conjunction with the professionals primarily involved with the child who has visual and/or hearing impairment).

In the provision of occupational therapy for children with sensory loss, the importance of play cannot be overemphasized. Play is the means by which the child learns how to solve problems, to cope with the environment, to face the unknown, and to adapt by changing behaviors (Gitlin-Weiner & Michelman, 1971; Parham & Fazio, 1997; Sandgrund & Schaefer, 2000). For children whose distance senses and perceptions of the environment are limited, the development of play skills, particularly active play involving use of the vestibular and proprioceptive systems, should be the highest priority (see Chapter 17 for a full discussion of play).

VISUAL IMPAIRMENT

Because the effects of visual impairment are evident in the acquisition of early milestones for mobility and manipulation, children with visual impairments are often referred for developmental evaluation and intervention by pediatricians. Therefore many of these children are identified in the first year of life and begin to receive services from local early intervention programs. The majority of students with visual impairment receive services through departments of education (84%); others receive services through residential schools (8%), rehabilitation centers (5%), and programs for children with multiple impairments (3%) (Kelley, Sanspree, & Davidson, 2000). Diagnostic information, identification of children with visual impairment, common pediatric eye disorders, and other specialists who may be involved in these cases are presented in Appendix 23-A.

Just as do children with other disabilities or impairments, children with visual impairment demonstrate a wide range of abilities and functional outcomes. The picture becomes more complex when the developing child with visual impairment has other associated problems or is multi-impaired. Therefore it is important that the etiology, age of onset, degree of visual impairment, and the presence of co-existing conditions be taken into consideration when occupational therapy assessment and intervention services are provided.

In a national collaborative study that examined the developmental trajectories of a group of 186 children with visual impairment, Hatton, Bailey, Burchinal, and Ferrell (1997) found that children with visual impairment and co-occurring disabilities (e.g., mental retardation [MR] or developmental delay [DD]) had lower developmental age scores, as measured by the Battelle Developmental Inventory (BDI), and showed a slower rate of development compared to children with visual impairment who did not have MR/DD, regardless of the levels of visual functioning demonstrated by the children. However, the level of visual function was highly related to the presence of MR/DD in that more than half of the children with severe vision loss also had MR/DD, whereas children with mild to moderate vision loss did not, which suggests that a more severe underlying central nervous system disorder was responsible both for the visual impairment and for MR/DD in these children. When they compared the development of the children with the least vision and no MR/DD with that of the children with the most vision and no MR/DD, these investigators found significantly lower BDI scores across all domains and slower rates of motor and personal-social development in those with the least vision. The degree of visual impairment, therefore, is a factor in the development of these children, and those with better vision are more likely to have favorable developmental outcomes (Hatton et al., 1997).

However, the degree of visual impairment is only one variable that must be considered in the individual child's developmental trajectory. Based on the variability in functional performance of children with visual impairment, Warren (1994, 2000) argued that an individual differences approach is more meaningful for studying visual impairment in young children than is a comparative approach that relies on chronologic age norms for sighted children. Some children with visual impairments function at least within the average range or even at the high end of developmental age norms for sighted children. Therefore the evaluation of development in relation to the demands (i.e., expectations and challenges) of the environment in which the child with visual impairment functions and how these interactions change over time is presented as a more useful framework (Warren, 2000). This perspective is consistent with the transactional model of early intervention (Sameroff & Fiese, 2000) and with the person-environment-occupation (PEO) framework of occupational therapy discussed in Chapter 3. Whether the child with a visual impairment is singly impaired or multi-impaired, occupational therapists view the child and family in relation to their ability to participate and engage in occupations and activities that are meaningful to their everyday lives.

Developmental Considerations and the Impact of Visual Impairment

It is important that an occupational therapist understand the development of the visual system, as well as the development of visual functioning, in order to assess the ability of children to engage in age-appropriate occupations and to design appropriate interventions. Vision is a quick, efficient integrating sense that allows immediate feedback and appreciation of both near and distant information in multiple locations about the environment (Kelley et al., 2000; Teplin, 1995). By 23 to 24 weeks' gestation, the major structures of the eye and the visual pathway to the level of the visual cortex are in place, but the eyelids are fused and the visual system is still immature (Glass, 1995, 2002). Therefore infants born extremely premature are at high risk for retinopathy of prematurity, because the retina and visual cortex undergo further maturation during the last trimester of pregnancy (Glass, 1995). By 24 to 28 weeks the eyelids are no longer fused and an immature visual response emerges, but the awake and sleep states are not well differentiated. By 30 to 34 weeks, sleep and awake states become differentiated, the eyes may open, and brief visual fixation may occur. By 36 weeks, the visual evoked response is similar to that of a full-term infant, and the awake state can be sustained for longer periods (Glass, 2002).

The maturation of the visual system in typical infants continues after birth and is a function of the transactions that occur between the infant and the environment and concurrent changes in the synaptic density of the visual cortex and other parts of the brain (Glass, 2002). Vision enables an infant to explore the environment and negotiate space, to learn about the properties of objects, to interact and communicate with caregivers, and to develop visual-perceptual skills needed for more complex activities such as reading and writing and for play and self-care occupations. In addition, vision is a major contributor to praxis, which allows an individual to organize ideas and actions and to anticipate, monitor, and

adapt to the demands of the environment (Smith Roley & Schneck, 2001). Because many of the conditions that affect vision are congenital or have a prenatal etiology, a major system for processing and interpreting information is compromised at birth, and this has a substantial impact on the child's development in all areas. The following discussion focuses on areas relevant to occupational therapy, except for visual perception, which is discussed in Chapter 12.

Participation in Co-Occupations of Caregiving

Through engagement in the daily caregiving activities and routines of feeding, bathing, sleep, and playful interactions, the infant and caregiver co-regulate their signals and responses, and each actively participates in these interactions. Also, through these interactions the infant and caregiver develop their relationship, and infant behaviors, such as eye gaze and visual regard of faces, and the mother's interpretations of these behaviors, are seen as important to this process. However, according to Warren (2000), the basic infant behaviors that elicit caregiver responses, such as smiling and vocalizing, do not depend on vision, and vision is not required for infants to perceive the caregivers' responsive behaviors, such as vocalizing, cuddling, or feeding. In their study of mothers' interpretations of their infants' behaviors, Baird, Mayfield, and Baker (1997) found that their sample of infants with visual impairments engaged in similar proportions of facial expressions that were considered meaningful by their mothers as did sighted infants, and smiling was the predominant facial expression interpreted.

Indeed, positive and strong attachment relationships can occur in infants with visual impairment (Warren, 1994). A caregiver who is coping with learning that his or her infant has a visual impairment may have difficulty responding to the infant's cues, but at the same time, the infant may display fewer behaviors that elicit positive responses from the caregiver, setting up a cycle of interactions that are out of sync or not mutually and emotionally satisfying. Vision loss itself is not necessarily a causal factor, but it may create a condition of risk for early social-emotional development and attachment (Warren, 2000).

Exploration and Play

As discussed previously in the study by Hatton (1997), many children with visual impairment demonstrated delayed achievement of certain milestones, such as crawling and walking. In a survey of 200 families with children with visual impairment in Virginia, Celeste (2002) found that the total sample demonstrated delayed gross motor development for nearly every milestone, but that the greatest delays occurred for milestones related to locomotion, such as cruising around furniture, walking independently, and negotiating stairs. Among the subgroups in the sample, children with the least vision (i.e., light perception or no light perception) had the poorest motor outcomes, followed by children with visual impairments who were born prematurely. However, the author indicated that further research is needed to disentangle the effects of prematurity from the effects of visual impairment.

Warren (2000) suggested that lack of vision may have an indirect rather than a direct effect on locomotion, because studies have shown significant variance among infants with vision impairment, with some achieving milestones for crawling and walking well within the normal range. He suggests that vision may serve as a motivator for infants to explore interesting sights out of reach, and that perhaps more important is the extent to which infants are provided with opportunities and encouragement to explore. Other studies have shown no difference in the performance of auditory and verbal tasks between preschool children with vision and those without vision; however, the children with vision impairment had difficulty with tasks that involved manipulation of objects and spatial components (Kelley et al., 2000). Even so, some children with blindness due to congenital conditions showed typical or above average performance on spatial tasks, which suggests that variables other than vision affect the development of spatial task performance.

Use of Information from Other Sensory Systems

It is a common belief that children with visual impairment are able to compensate for the loss of vision through increased use or heightened performance of the remaining senses. Infants who are visually impaired do make sensory associations to form perceptions through their experiences, and if the remaining sensory systems are working well and the infant is otherwise healthy, the capacity to become competent and independent in performing meaningful occupations can be realized (Smith Roley & Schneck, 2001). Furthermore, the research suggests that visual impairment does not have a negative impact on early development of tactile and auditory perception in that infants with visual impairment demonstrate basic discrimination abilities similar to those of sighted infants (Warren, 2000). As Glass (2002) noted, infants with visual impairment may have a heightened behavioral response to auditory stimuli. In addition, normal newborns respond differentially to sound of a given intensity, depending on the intensity of the corresponding light level (visual input).

Although infants with visual impairment are able to discriminate and thus respond accordingly to caregivers' voices or touch, their ability to connect auditory input to signify external objects in a specific location and to use this information to reach for objects appears to take longer to develop (Warren, 2000). It is not a simple matter for an infant to know that a sound goes with an object that would be desirable to play with and that it can easily be located. Ross and Tobin (1997) contended that an infant may expend energy trying to interpret sounds at the expense of exploratory motor behavior, and infants who have limited interactions with the physical environment experience less information about the nature of that environment.

The development of fine motor skills depends on visual monitoring, and loss or distortion of visual input makes it more difficult for children to acquire these skills, although information from the tactile system can offer some compensatory strategies (Smith Roley & Schneck, 2001). Children with visual impairment can manipulate objects to detect their form and shape, therefore their concepts of objects are developed using haptic perception. In addition, their ability to coordinate reaching with sound depends on precise tactile system perception used for exploration and concept development (Lampert, 1998), as well as the use of audition to locate an object in space. Although object concept behaviors in children with visual impairment are similar to those of sighted infants through the first year and a half, performance on tasks that involve complex spatial displacements that cannot easily be tracked by audition or touch is more difficult, therefore spatial understanding may be more of a problem than object conceptualization for children with visual impairment (Warren, 2000).

The use of remaining sensory systems does not substitute for the efficiency of the visual system in integrating the child's sensory experiences, therefore the child with a visual impairment takes longer to develop his or her conceptual understanding of the world (Recchia, 1997). Although the child may gain specific information about an object's unique properties, the remaining senses do not necessarily provide him or her with sufficient information about the contexts in which the actions take place while he or she engages in the action (Smith Roley & Schneck, 2001). For example, a child may learn about the cup he uses for drinking but may not come to understand for years that his plastic tumbler, his father's coffee mug, and the crystal wine glass used for special occasions all are variations of a class of objects used for drinking, especially if he has not had direct tactile experience with these items. If a child has limited experiences and does not have a systematic introduction to objects in context, he or she will have a narrow range of schemes to work with, and these available schemes may not be fully validated by others (Recchia).

Children with visual impairment may have restricted interactions with the environment and fewer typical motor and manipulative experiences that allow them to develop the postural control, gross and fine motor skills, and praxis at similar levels of competence and quality as those of typical sighted children for engagement in object manipulation and play, self-care, and learning activities.

Sensory Modulation

Children with visual impairment and blindness often are described as demonstrating stereotypic or repetitive behaviors, such as hand flapping, eye poking, or self-rocking. However, occupational therapists need to be mindful that these behaviors are also seen in children with other conditions, such as autistic spectrum disorder, severe or profound mental retardation, and other developmental disabilities. Therefore the presence of these behaviors (with the exception of eye poking) may not be due to blindness per se but rather to the underlying cause of the blindness, particularly in children with multiple disabilities. These stereotypic behaviors have been hypothesized to be sensory-seeking activities that may compensate for the vision loss, but another explanation may be that the behaviors emerge as a result of the severely limited repertoires of movement and behavior available to children with visual impairment (Smith Roley & Schneck, 2001).

Some children with visual impairment also present with behaviors that suggest tactile defensiveness, postural instability, or gravitational insecurity. That is, a child may withdraw his or her hand from an object or art media, may object to being touched, may be fearful of moving through space, or may be afraid to get on playground equipment, such as swings or the jungle gym. The intensity of the child's responses in these situations varies, as does the degree to which the responses interfere with the child's ability to engage in everyday occupations. It therefore becomes important for the occupational therapist to evaluate the child's behaviors carefully. For example, a child who may appear to demonstrate tactile hypersensitivity may not truly have a sensory modulation disorder or generalized hypersensitivities, but rather may need additional cues and strategies for managing new tactile experiences. The child may tolerate other tactile experiences, such as being held or wearing clothing made of different fabrics, and once the child becomes familiar with the object or material, the "defensive" reactions no longer occur. This is different from a child who consistently demonstrates tactile hypersensitivity even to familiar tactile experiences or who exhibits strong reactions to tactile stimuli beyond what could be attributed to caution or hesitance.

Children with visual impairment whose motor experiences are limited may be fearful about moving through open space (e.g., crawling across the room, walking across the playground), moving on equipment such as tricycles or swings, or climbing on play structures or going down a slide. In addition, caregivers (e.g., parents, day care staff, teachers) who are concerned about safety may become overprotective and prevent or restrict children from engaging in movement and exploratory activities and experiencing the bumps and bruises that go with them, thus transmitting their fear to the child. Without vision, the child must use vestibular, proprioceptive, and auditory information to get accurate information about spatial orientation and alignment against gravity and to use equilibrium and righting reactions for adaptive postural adjustments during the performance of these activities (Smith Roley & Schneck, 2001). To gain this information, the child must have opportunities to actively engage in and experience movement in a variety of situations.

Activities of Daily Living

Children with visual impairment may also have difficulty performing activities of daily living such as dressing and self-feeding. The impact of vision impairment on the development of locomotion, gross and fine motor skills, and praxis for play may also affect the child's ability to stand and lift his or her leg to put on a pair of pants, or to direct the spoon to the plate to scoop up food, or to get in and out of the bathtub. In addition, if tactile hypersensitivity is present, the child's ability to engage in dressing, grooming, and toileting activities may be limited, or if oral hypersensitivity is present, the progression to more textured foods and to eating a variety of foods may be problematic. These reactions can have a disruptive impact on the daily caregiving routine for both the child and the caregivers, and negative associations with these activities can have long-lasting effects on the relationship.

Social Participation and Communication

According to Warren (2000), the basis for verbal communication is established with the development of preverbal and nonverbal communication long before words and sentences are used. He also emphasized that the patterns of interaction for young children with visual impairment and their caregivers differ from those of sighted children, although much of preverbal and nonverbal communication continues to occur in the absence of full functional vision. Again, it is the nature of the experiences that appears to be the key factor in the development of children with visual impairment.

As children grow older, the complexity of social interactions increases, and the contextual aspects of language and communication become important. Vision plays a significant role in the interpretation of facial expressions and body language and in the initiation and sustaining of the give and take of these interactions. According to Smith Roley and Schneck (2001), making eye contact, imitating facial gestures, shifting gaze, and perceiving the contextual perception of visual images are often not part of the repertoire or experience of children who have vision loss at an early age. The English language has many visual references that describe images, and Western culture expects individuals with visual impairment to communicate using the language of those who have sight, as if they have shared experiences in common.

Children with congenital visual impairment cannot "see" many features or qualities of objects using the other sensory channels, such as a "red" button or "green" grass, nor can they see "a beautiful sunset" or "that one over there"; consequently, they can only try to imagine what is meant when such descriptors or phrases are used (Smith Roley & Schneck, 2001). In addition, children with visual impairment may not demonstrate the animation and nuances of facial expression, because they have not experienced seeing and imitating these expressions. Because they need to concentrate on what is being said when there is other activity and noise in the surroundings, they may be perceived as not paying attention to the speaker or as being bored or unfriendly.

As can be seen, then, not only do difficulties such as delayed motor skills or limited range of manipulative interactions and play with objects affect the ability of children with visual impairment to engage in play activities with peers or to participate in social activities, such as eating lunch; but social communication skills are also limited. These difficulties affect the child's ability to develop friendships or to fit in with the social demands and expectations of his or her peer group.

Occupational Therapy Evaluation and Intervention

Evaluation

In many respects occupational therapy evaluation of the occupational performance of children with visual impairment encompasses the same components as evaluation of children with other disabilities. Participation in play, self-care, and school occupations and preparation for work are areas of focus for evaluation, depending on the age and needs of the child. Evaluation of the performance skills (e.g., motor, process, and communication/interaction skills) that support or limit the child's ability to engage in specific activities in these areas, as well as the activity demands, client factors, and contexts in which the child performs these activities, is also part of a comprehensive assessment. For example, a toddler with a visual impairment who has difficulty playing with toys may need evaluation of fine motor skills, tactile and proprioceptive processing, and postural control in sitting, with observations conducted in the home as well as in day care or early intervention settings.

Standardized assessment tools for evaluating overall development in major domains (e.g., the Bayley Scales of Infant Development [BSID-II] [Bayley, 1993] or the Peabody Developmental Motor Scales [PDMS-2] [Folio & Fewell, 2000]) should be used with caution because these measures were not standardized on children with visual impairment and the administration procedures do not include adaptations for this group. Therefore comparison of performance to sighted peers and use of the standard scores based on the normative sample is not appropriate. A few tools, such as the Battelle Developmental Inventory (BDI) (Newborg, Stock, Wnek, Guidubaldi, & Svinicki, 1988), are both standardized and criterion referenced and include administration instructions for children with motor or sensory impairments.

In light of Warren's individual difference perspective (Warren, 1994, 2000), criterion-referenced measures such as the Hawaii Early Learning Profile (HELP) (Parks, 1999) or play-based assessment tools such as the Transdisciplinary Play-Based Assessment (TPBA) (Linder, 1993) may be more useful because they yield a profile of individual strengths and limitations or concerns that can be used to formulate an intervention plan. In addition, tools such as the Oregon Project Skills Inventory (fifth edition) (Anderson, Boigon, & Davis, 1986) take into consideration what is known about the unique developmental trajectories of certain skills (e.g., walking independently, reaching to sound) in children with visual impairment. Other assessment tools specifically designed for children with visual impairment or that evaluate visual skills are described in Appendix 23-A.

Skilled observation and parent or caregiver questionnaires can be useful for gathering information about the child's temperament, self-regulation capacities, and sensory processing and sensory modulation behaviors, as well as caregiver-child interactions. In addition, interviews with the parents, teachers, or other caregivers can provide information about the daily routines, contexts, and expectations and resources available to support the family's as well as the child's participation in activities. As children get older, in addition to the relevant areas and skills discussed previously, the focus of evaluation for the occupational therapist may involve collaboration with the special education or regular education teacher, as well as vision specialists (e.g., orientation and mobility specialist, developmental optometrists), to assess barriers in school and play settings and determine the need for adaptations for performing classroom activities or organization of desk space or the use of assistive technology (Porr, 1999). In addition, the occupational therapist may evaluate functional independence in all areas of activities of daily living at home and at school. In adolescence, the occupational therapist, in collaboration with teachers, vision specialists, and the family, may evaluate the individual's ability to travel in the school, community, or work setting, in addition to leisure interests and activities, levels of school functioning, functional

BOX 23-1 Signs and Symptoms of Vision Problems

If a child shows the following signs or symptoms, a referral to an eye care specialist is indicated:

- Eyes shake or randomly wander.
- Eyes are not able to follow the face of the parent.
- Pupils of the eyes are excessively large or small.
- Pupils of the eyes are not black; a cloudy film appears to be present.
- Eyes are not in alignment (e.g., they are crossed or turn outward).
- Child frequently rubs eyes.
- Child turns or tilts head when looking at detail.
- Child covers or closes one eye when looking at detail.
- Child squints frequently.
- Child complains of tired eyes.
- Child does not appear to focus with central vision.
- Day vision is markedly different than night vision.
- Child responds significantly better to objects on one side of the body than on the other.
- Child sits excessively close to the television.
- Child avoids or becomes tired after close work.
- Child appears clumsy, or frequently bumps into objects when walking and running.

From Dr. Bill Takeshita, Center for the Partially Sighted, Santa Monica, CA.

independence in activities of daily living, and level of work skills and behaviors.

In some instances a child who presents with developmental delays or difficulties may be referred for occupational therapy evaluation but has not yet been diagnosed with a visual impairment. If a child shows signs or symptoms of a vision problem (Box 23-1) and a visual impairment is suspected, the occupational therapist can assist in the diagnostic process through screening or evaluation of oculomotor skills (e.g., visual tracking, fixation, shifting gaze), focusing skills (e.g., shift from near to far), and eye teaming. or binocularity (e.g., strabismus), as well as describing the child's visual perceptual skills (e.g., visual discrimination, visual spatial relations) and visual motor integration, as appropriate for the child's age and the impact on the child's performance of activities. Some developmental measures (e.g., BSID-II) include items that involve visual attention, visual tracking, visual memory, and other vision-related areas; specific visual perception and visual-motor tests are also available (see Chapter 13).

Case Study 1: Kevin

Kevin is a 5-year, 5-month-old boy who has been diagnosed with optic nerve hypoplasia with septo-optic dysplasia, nystagmus, and developmental delays. He lives with his parents and three siblings, ages 2, 7, and 10 years. Kevin's mother reported that she had regular prenatal care and an uneventful pregnancy. Labor and delivery were uncomplicated, and Kevin weighed 6 pounds, 8 ounces and was 20 inches long at birth.

When Kevin was about 2 months old, his mother became concerned that he did not appear to be tracking moving objects. Kevin's pediatrician referred Kevin to an ophthalmologist, who diagnosed bilateral optic nerve hypoplasia.

Kevin's early development was delayed. His mother reported that Kevin began to vocalize when he was about 3 years old and that he said his first word at 5 years. He sat alone at $1\frac{1}{2}$ years and walked alone at 2 years. He needed a great deal of assistance with self-care tasks. He held a cup to drink at 4 years of age and began to feed himself using his fingers when he was $4\frac{1}{2}$ years old. He was able to remove his shoes and socks at the age of 3 years and cooperated in dressing at the age of 4 years. He does not yet demonstrate toileting skills. He was described as an affectionate, happy infant, and he currently does not have any serious behavior difficulties.

Questions to consider:

1 What areas of occupation would you address in your evaluation of Kevin?
2 What performance skills would you assess? Why?
3 What methods of evaluation and assessment tools would you use to assess the areas of occupation and performance skills you identified?
4 In what context or contexts would you conduct your evaluation?
5 With whom should you collaborate to conduct your evaluation?

Occupational Therapy Intervention

The overall outcome of occupational therapy intervention for children with visual impairments is engagement in occupations to support participation in the contexts in which they function on a daily basis. Occupational therapy approaches typically include establishing skills and abilities; maintaining performance capabilities; using compensatory strategies, adaptations, or modifications; and preventing barriers to occupational performance. For example, for a 6-month-old premature infant with retinopathy of prematurity, the occupational therapist may focus on establishing oral-motor skills for feeding and self-soothing strategies for calming; he or she may also recommend positioning strategies for feeding and caregiver-infant interactions and may aid the caregiver in selecting toys that enhance the use of available vision, as well as auditory and tactile channels. For a 10-year-old who has cerebral palsy with spastic hemiparesis and is legally blind, the school-based occupational therapist may focus on maintaining self-care skills; establishing organizational skills for using desk space and completing assignments; devising strategies that support the use of low-vision aids; and promoting social participation in games with peers with modifications and adaptations.

Occupational therapy models of practice that are particularly useful for evaluation and intervention with children who have visual impairments include sensory integration, motor acquisition and motor learning, visual information processing/visual perception, and person-environment-occupation (PEO) frameworks. Neurodevelopmental and biomechanical models of practice may also be useful, particularly for children with multiple disabilities. All types of occupational therapy interventions—therapeutic use of self; therapeutic use of occupations and activities; consultation; and education—may be incorporated in different combinations and at different points during intervention in a dynamic process that changes based on the needs of the child and family; the progress and response to intervention; and the demands of the contexts involved. The occupational therapist may be the primary interventionist for children who have visual impairments with other conditions; however, if the visual impairment is the primary or sole condition, it is more likely that a vision specialist will be the primary interventionist, and the occupational therapist may provide consultation as needed. Generally, the occupational therapist is a member of a team of professionals (e.g., teacher, orientation and mobility specialist, speech therapist, low vision or visual impairment specialist) who, along with the family, collaborate to identify the child's and family's needs and to develop an intervention program to address those needs, with one or more individuals providing services.

The occupational therapist often provides services to support the following goals:

- *Develop self-care skills.* The therapist can consult with and educate those who work with the child to identify skills levels and explain problems in the child's development of self-care skills. The occupational therapist may work collaboratively with the family and the team to incorporate behavioral or learning strategies; suggest adaptations or modifications to the environment; recommend seating or other equipment; and incorporate cues that support independence (e.g., placing a tactile cue in specific areas of clothing to distinguish front from back or to identify color; using a divided plate or the clock orientation to serve food items).
- *Enhance sensory processing, sensory modulation, and sensory integration.* Developmentally age-appropriate activities and materials that provide tactile, auditory, proprioceptive, and vestibular input can benefit the child with visual impairment and enhance or promote the development of body concept, postural control, and tactile discrimination for recognizing and manipulating objects; self-regulation; spatial relation perceptions; and grasp, release, bilateral hand use, and praxis. Swings, scooterboards, tilt boards, obstacle courses, and other movement or balance equipment are useful, but it is also important to provide

interventions using playground equipment (e.g., slides, jungle gyms, tricycles, swings) in the natural settings in which the child will be required to function (Figure 23-2). It is important, however, that safety be maintained in the use of equipment and that, as appropriate, the child be allowed to control the movement and amount of input within his or her range of adaptive responses.

The child with visual impairment does not see the approach of people and objects and may therefore exhibit hypersensitivity to touch. In many instances children who have some or variable vision may have more difficulty with this than children with total blindness because children with some functional vision receive unpredictable visual input from light patterns and movements. For children with total blindness, the visual input is essentially consistent. Firm touch generally is better than light touch, which can be interpreted as painful or aversive. The child is more comfortable and less defensive when a verbal cue accompanies or precedes the tactile cue. Strategies to help children modulate their reactions to tactile input include activities that encourage the child to explore and play with various materials using graded textures (e.g., sand, dried lentils, beans, and rice); activities that include vibration or proprioceptive input; and incorporation of a sensory diet at home and in the classroom.

Preparatory activities can be included prior to art time, sand play, or eating, for example, and recommendations for clothing, sleepwear, and linens can be offered. In addition, if oral sensory defensiveness is a factor, strategies such as graded introduction of food and liquid textures and tactile/proprioceptive activities involving the mouth (e.g., games involving making faces; using straws with thickened liquids;

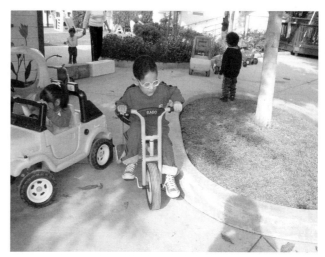

FIGURE 23-2 Child with low vision tracking around a curb on a playground tricycle. (Courtesy Jill Brody, OTR/L, Blind Children's Center, Los Angeles, CA.)

blowing activities with bubbles or whistles) can be implemented. It is important for the child to experience contingent responses to his or her behaviors, taking into consideration individual needs and preferences, rather than to be a passive recipient of adult actions (noncontingent experiences) (Chen, 1999). A child should not experience tactile stimulation in isolation (e.g., rubbing of different textured cloths on the arm); rather, the tactile experiences should be provided in the context of real life activities (e.g., using a nubby towel to dry oneself after a bath) so that the child associates tactile experiences with actions and events.

■ *Enhance postural control and movement in space.* Providing a variety of movement experiences throughout the daily routines early in life is important. Caregivers can be encouraged to use different carrying positions or carriers while engaging in everyday activities so that infants experience movement (and vestibular and proprioceptive input) under secure conditions. Instead of passive positioning in prone, in which motivation to the lift the head is minimal with significant visual impairment, caregivers can be encouraged to engage in games that include tilting the child toward and away from them while talking and having fun with the child (Porr, 1999). The occupational therapist and orientation and mobility specialist can work closely to facilitate and establish the child's ability to move through space through the use of push toys, riding toys, and moving over surfaces of different heights, density or firmness, and textures (Figure 23-3). Occupational therapists may also use neurodevelopmental facilitation techniques to help the child use trunk rotation instead of moving in straight planes, develop balance and righting reactions on unstable equipment,

and improve transitional movements. In addition, motor learning strategies may be incorporated to provide children with opportunities to practice a variety of movement strategies during different play activities, with feedback on their performance and the results of their actions.

■ *Develop body awareness and spatial orientation.* Many of the activities described above can also help the child develop body awareness and directionality. Obstacle courses can teach the child how large his or her body is in relation to other objects, as well as spatial concepts such as left-right, up-down, over-under, in-out, beside, around, and behind. It is important to describe the movement or direction the child experiences to help him or her establish the associations that will give meaning to the spatial concepts. Body awareness and spatial awareness are important for children with visual impairment if they are to develop mobility and language skills (Sanspree, 2000).

■ *Develop tactile-proprioceptive perceptual abilities.* The child with visual impairment needs to maximize tactile discrimination abilities to learn about the features and properties of objects, to adjust grasp according to the size, shape, and weight of an object, and to grade the amount of pressure, force, or speed needed to manipulate toys or use tools. Tactile discrimination is also important for learning to read Braille. Finger painting, finding and identifying objects hidden in sand or beans, and experiencing gradations of textures among everyday objects and materials, clothing, and surfaces are examples of activities that increase tactile awareness. In addition, providing multiple opportunities to manipulate objects, to operate or use toys functionally (e.g., pushing buttons on a toy phone, playing with shape sorter toys), and to combine objects in familiar and new ways helps children use tactile-proprioceptive information.

■ *Improve manipulation and fine motor skills.* At first, the world has to come to the child. A variety of toys and objects should be maintained within reach (e.g., tied to the crib or tabletop). By assessing the sensory features of the toys or objects, the therapist can select objects appropriate for the child's ability to process the information and for his or her skill level. For example, objects may vary in texture, or in texture and sound, or may have multisensory features (e.g., sound, texture, and flashing lights). Providing opportunities for the child with visual impairment to practice in-hand manipulation with activities that involve rotation and translation of small objects can dynamically improve the use of tools. Some of the activities described previously (e.g., that address sensory integration and tactile hypersensitivity) can also be used for sensory preparation of the hands prior to manipulation of objects. Toys, objects, and materials should also be placed or used at different locations or heights

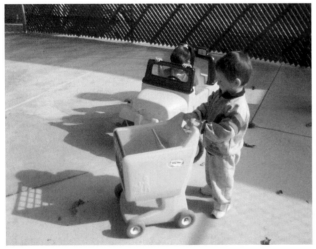

FIGURE 23-3 Child with severe visual impairment using a push toy as a mobility aid. (Courtesy Jill Brody, OTR/L, Blind Children's Center, Los Angeles, CA.)

(e.g., on the floor, on the table, inside, outside), and the child should be encouraged to engage in activities with these materials in different positions (e.g., sitting, kneeling, standing).

- *Maximize use of residual vision.* The occupational therapist should always facilitate the child's use of whatever vision is available to him or her during intervention and everyday activities. The more a child uses visual pathways, the better vision develops (Baker-Nobles & Rutherford, 1995). Visual awareness and discrimination activities, such as color or shape recognition and matching, are important for children with functional vision. Activities, such as use of a flashlight in a darkened room, may also improve visual skills. The occupational therapist also can support the use of low-vision aids recommended by the vision specialists, such as large print books or magnifiers, as well as any other assistive technology that may be appropriate (e.g., closed circuit TV, computers with special software).

All these goals require the occupational therapist to educate and consult with family members. Family members should be encouraged to handle the child with visual impairment as they would an infant without disability. Verbal and physical interaction should also be encouraged, because the child may not always demonstrate behaviors that elicit interaction.

The family should be informed about the importance of early intervention and their options for services. Occupational therapists may consult with parents on ways to create a safe environment in which the child can play independently and make recommendations for adapting the environment to optimize independent functioning of the child.

Additional team goals to which the occupational therapist contributes include the following:

- *Encourage socially acceptable behaviors.* Children with visual impairments are at a disadvantage in social situations, particularly at school, where typical children are active and often participate in a variety of physical games. It is difficult for children with visual impairment to signal their interest in playing with peers, and reliance on others to help them with these interactions limits their ability to experience social competence (Kelley et al., 2000). It is important to provide the child with real life activities with specific instruction in symbolic play, perhaps with one other child at first and introducing other children as the child gains skills. Role playing, turn taking, and use of exaggerated facial expressions are strategies that can be used to facilitate social interaction. The child should be encouraged to face people when they speak, to smile, and to maintain an upright posture with his or her head in the midline. He or she must learn to determine how others are reacting based on voices rather than gestures, facial expressions, or body language.

- *Encourage language and concept development.* The child must consciously be taught to develop cognitive schemes that the sighted child picks up in a relatively casual manner. This is done with verbalization and use of the child's intact sensory systems. Those things that cannot be touched or heard (e.g., clouds) need to be described and explained.

- *Strengthen cognitive skills, such as object permanence, cause and effect, object recognition, and ability to match and sort.* A variety of toys are available to help infants and toddlers develop these skills. For older children, these goals can be accomplished through games and many simple craft activities. The unique abilities and limitations of the child must be considered when addressing academic goals.

- *Maximize auditory perceptual abilities.* The child with visual impairment must learn to identify sounds and their meanings and react to them appropriately. Sounds come from several basic sources: toys, speech, and the environment. Active, rather than passive, listening should be emphasized. Helpful activities include locating a variety of sounds in the environment, identifying sounds, and following directions from persons and recordings.

Case Study 1 (Continued): Kevin

The following observations and findings were obtained through an evaluation conducted by the team assigned to Kevin's case, which included an occupational therapist:

- Kevin demonstrated a limited repertoire of movement patterns and limited motivation to explore his environment actively. His posture and movement are influenced by the presence of hypotonia, decreased strength and endurance, and blindness. He also has had limited experience engaging in a variety of movement activities.

- Kevin maintained an erect posture when sitting in a chair, but when sitting on the floor or a mat, he tended to relax after a brief period and sat more on his sacrum, with a very rounded back. He ambulated with a slightly wide base and tended to shift his weight from side to side, with very little trunk rotation. He locked his knees with each step and kept his arms close to his body. He took one step up a set of stairs, holding on to both rails. He needed encouragement to continue up the remaining steps. He took one step down, then scooted down the rest of the way in a sitting position.

- Kevin did not appear to have a hand preference. He was beginning to use his hands to interact with objects. He generally exhibited a decreased level of interest in manipulating objects and toys. However, he did demonstrate accurate use of auditory and kinesthetic information to locate objects on the tabletop in front of him. When presented with a block that made noise when shaken, he accurately reached toward it with his left hand and made contact, even when the position was changed. However, he did not grasp it. If the examiner attempted to place the block in his hand, he withdrew it. Although he did not grasp objects presented, he reportedly does grasp familiar objects such as a cup or a sock, and he likes being hugged and kissed.

- Kevin demonstrated good auditory attention: he listened intently to each examiner's unfamiliar voice and turned accurately toward the voice. He was less consistent with other auditory stimuli, such as the sound of a bell. Kevin is said to enjoy vestibular activities (e.g., bouncing, swinging, rocking, and movement through space), but during this evaluation he preferred passive movement and usually did not generate his own movement through space.

- Kevin exhibited some self-stimulatory behaviors: he turned himself around in a circle, he sometimes waved his hands, and he engaged in repetitive vocalizations. He also reportedly does some eye pressing. He was observed to do some of the above during this assessment, usually when there was a break in the pace of the assessment and if left to himself. However, Kevin was easily redirected and could be encouraged to engage in other activities.

- Kevin demonstrated limited problem-solving abilities. Mouthing, banging, and some manual exploration of objects were observed. He searched for displaced objects, but if he did not locate the desired item on the first attempt when an auditory cue was given, he did not persist in his search. However, verbal encouragement and auditory cues (i.e., tapping an object) were successful in eliciting prolonged searching behavior. During structured activities one on one with an adult, Kevin's attention span ranged from 3 to 5 minutes.

Questions to consider:

1. What areas of strength does Kevin demonstrate?
2. What participation and activity limitations can you identify?
3. What occupational therapy models of practice would be useful for you to develop your intervention plan?
4. Identify three primary goals or outcomes that you will address with occupational therapy intervention.
5. What approaches, methods, techniques, or strategies will you incorporate into your intervention for Kevin?
6. What additional recommendations might be appropriate for Kevin and his family?

Special Techniques and Strategies

Children with severe visual impairments may rely on Braille and talking books for their education. Braille is a system of six raised dots arranged in a cell to represent the letters of the alphabet, numbers, and words. It is produced on a special slate or on a machine called a Braillewriter. The system was developed by a young, blind French student, Louis Braille, in 1824, and was found to be more efficient than attempting to read the raised Roman alphabet. Advances in technology now make it possible to use computer software and tools that incorporate Braille.

For the young child who will eventually use Braille in school, the importance of early tactile perceptual training cannot be overemphasized (Figure 23-4). Braille can be written in three levels, or grades, depending on the degree of contraction used. It is read left to right with one or two hands. Usually the index finger is used with a light touch. Reading speeds for Braille vary, but 104 words per minute is the average, making it useful in the educational setting.

Talking books on a wide variety of topics and for any age level are also available for individuals with visual impairment. The development of attentive listening can be encouraged during short story-telling sessions, and adults should carefully monitor the child's attention to promote good listening skills. Scratch-and-sniff books and tactile books are also available to help in early story telling. Those who can discriminate a large typeface can read large print books, and enlarged letters and contrasting colors are accessible through most computer programs.

Various types of lenses are available for individuals with visual impairment, from the relatively common ones used to correct refractive errors to telescopic and microscopic lenses that are used as low-vision aids for certain types of blindness. There are also projection and magnifying devices, such as the opticon, which converts ink print into a readable vibrating tactile form.

Optometrists provide vision therapy using various lenses, prisms, occlusion (patching), and other low-vision

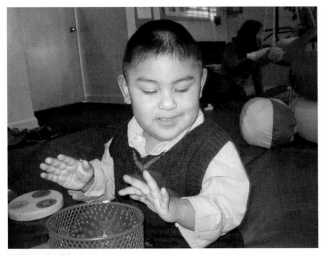

FIGURE 23-4 Child working on tactile defensiveness in preparation for Braille training.

aids (Chaikin & Downing-Baum, 1997; Scheiman, 1997). The purpose of this vision therapy is to provide devices and activities to increase visual efficiency and visual information processing skills. Occupational therapists often team with optometrists to reinforce these goals.

Mobility training teaches techniques such as the use of guide dogs and of long canes (Lampert, 1998). The techniques of echo detection, trailing, and body protection are also important. Sighted guides usually walk a half step in front of the person with visual impairment. The visually impaired individual holds the guide's arm just above the elbow, with fingers inside (next to guide's body) and the thumb outside. A small child can hold the guide's wrist. With a sighted guide, body movement on uneven surfaces and changes of direction are easily perceived. Should the person with visual impairment need to change sides, the guide gives a verbal clue and the guided person slides over, tracing a finger along the back of the guide's waist. He or she then switches hands and grasps the guide's opposite elbow. In going through a narrow passage, the guide puts the opposite elbow behind his or her waist as a clue. The person with visual impairment then falls back a full step behind the guide, with the elbow straight and more directly in back rather than to the side.

For stairs, the sighted guide gives a verbal indication of stairs ahead and whether they are up or down, as well as information on rail availability and placement. One technique for navigating stairs requires the guide to pause and turn at a right angle to the person with visual impairment. They take each step one at a time in a foot-to-step fashion with the guide one step ahead of the person with visual impairment. Another technique involves using the rail, if available. In this case, the guide goes up or down the stairs without turning at a right angle, one step ahead of the guided person. Cane technique is also a specialized procedure that requires training from a professional.

As a rule, the orientation and mobility specialist is the one who teaches trailing and body protection. However, occupational therapists who work with individuals with visual impairment should learn the basic techniques. *Trailing* is the use of a wall as a guide for walking. The hand closest to the wall is extended at hip level until the outside of the little finger touches the wall; then the backs of the fingertips are used to guide the person in walking.

In the *body protection* technique, the upper arm is held at shoulder height and parallel to the floor with the palm facing out to meet any obstacle before the body does. The lower arm is extended downward and forward with the palm facing out. Another protection technique, which can be used when bending down to retrieve a dropped object, is to extend the arm palm out in front of the head. The child with visual impairment can search for a lost object by touching the ground to establish a beginning point and then searching in an ever-widening concentric circle pattern.

A technique for exploring a room involves searching the parameters of the room first, then mentally dividing it into grids to be searched methodically. This method can be used to introduce the child with vision loss to a new classroom or new home setup. The use of landmarks and clues (e.g., the grass at the edge of the sidewalk) is important for independent movement.

Some occupational therapists are involved in low-vision training (Baker-Nobles, 1997; Gentile, 1997; Hyvarinen, 1995; Lampert & Lapolice, 1995). The basic premise of low-vision training is that a child with poor visual acuity can be taught to use his or her residual vision. Because visual acuity, by itself, is not the most important part of visual ability, planned stimulation can help a visually impaired child increase his or her visual efficiency.

Often light is used initially to increase focusing ability. Once fixation is achieved, the child can learn to discriminate global aspects of an image . When this happens, the child can move on to analyze discrete elements and finally to identify form, outline, and other aspects of an image. Although this method does not work with all children with visual impairment, it does have good results with some of them, particularly when combined with a good overall program to heighten the child's levels of perception.

With increasing use of sophisticated electronics and compact components, positive outcomes for the visually impaired are possible. For example, a light sensor can be used to train a child with low vision to detect variable light intensities. Specific training in the detection of light can improve function at school or work (Schaefer & Specht, 1979).

Other advances that give individuals with visual impairment access to computers include voice-activated software and keys with Braille. Computers can increase the amount and quality of written output, and if equipped with voice and sound capabilities, they can provide opportunities for interactive learning. Given the versatility and increasing capacity of computers, this technology holds great promise for individuals with visual impairments.

Preparation for Adulthood

The adolescent who is visually impaired faces a great challenge in selecting an appropriate occupation (Lampert, 1998), although with the current technology, many more opportunities are available than in the past (Sanspree, 2000). Unfortunately, visual impairment is often associated with unemployment or underemployment. However, an appropriate fit between the personality and talent areas of the adolescent can result in a successful and enduring career. Lack of exposure to many vocational options is a problem the occupational therapist can address, through community orientation and various activities, to give the child more prevocational experiences.

Certain mannerisms and behaviors often interfere with optimal social interaction in the work environment. Behaviors the occupational therapist and all professionals involved with the adolescent should work to modify include the following:

- Standing in the personal space of others
- Rocking the body
- Blinking, rubbing, or rolling the eyes
- Stamping or shuffling the feet
- Lack of eye contact with the person who is speaking

Daily living skills, such as cooking, cleaning, and recreation, become increasingly important as the child with visual impairment reaches adolescence. The American Foundation for the Blind provides a comprehensive list of aids and appliances that can help the visually impaired perform these skills. Devices such as a sugar meter that dispenses one half a teaspoon of sugar at a time and an elbow-length oven mitt that helps protect against accidental burns are extremely useful. Kits for marking canned goods are also available, as are self-threading needles and tools with marking gauges. Recreational activities, such as games with Braille cards and low-vision cards and table games (e.g., Scrabble and Monopoly) with Braille markings are available.

Self-care can be facilitated by careful organization of the wardrobe and tactile cues for clothing color. Handling money and shopping can be difficult tasks for the visually impaired and require training and assistance.

Leisure activities are important for well-rounded adulthood. Exercise groups, weightlifting, dance classes, and bowling are all excellent physical activities that should be encouraged, because many adults with severe visual impairments lead sedentary lives. Individuals with visual impairment can play ball sports with sound balls and can run or jog with minimal track guidance aids.

HEARING IMPAIRMENT

The occupational therapist encounters children with hearing impairment in neonatal intensive care units or later in hospitals, clinics, early intervention programs, and community and school settings. Prematurity increases the risk of hearing impairment (Steinberg & Knightly, 1997), and often infants leave the neonatal unit with a suspected hearing loss. Most states have programs for screening newborn hearing using risk criteria developed by the Joint Committee on Infant Hearing of the American Academy of Pediatrics (1995). Universal hearing screening of all newborns has also been proposed

(Northern & Downs, 2002). Hearing loss also is often identified through developmental testing in the clinic or is later discovered in school.

With the emphasis on least restrictive environments and natural environments, the percentage of children with hearing impairment who have been integrated into regular education classrooms has markedly increased, whereas the percentage attending residential schools has decreased (Moores, 2001; Northern & Downs, 2002). However, a small number of children with hearing impairments (particularly those with severe hearing loss or multisensory handicaps) continue to attend these schools.

In education programs, the occupational therapist has a strategic role in supporting students' activities of daily living, education/learning, play, social participation, and preparation for work. The increasing number of early intervention programs and earlier identification of hearing impairment allow for more therapist involvement in intervention for young children with hearing impairments and in the all-important parent-child interaction process. Just as do children with visual impairment, the child with hearing impairment demonstrates a wide range of abilities and functional outcomes. It is important that factors such as age of onset, degree and type of loss, and presence of co-existing conditions be taken into consideration when occupational therapy assessment and intervention services are provided.

Developmental Considerations and the Impact of Hearing Impairment

To the occupational therapist, the most important characteristic of the child with hearing impairment is the lack of early language development and the profound problems this delay causes in all other areas of development (Ling, 1989; Marschark, 1993; Meadow-Orlans, 1990; Moores, 2001; Northern & Downs, 2002; Nowell & Marshak, 1994; Scheetz, 2001). What at first appears to be a fairly simple problem becomes complicated when one considers the importance language plays in our society. Without language, social participation and communication at all levels are disrupted.

Researchers believe that if intervention is delayed until 3 or 4 years of age, the most important formative period of language development has been lost and the child's full potential is lessened (Ling, 1989; Meadow, 1980; Northern & Downs, 2002; Paul, 2001). Indeed, most research now indicates that the first 18 months of life are the most critical for the development of language (Coplan, 1999). Hearing loss decreases stimulation of neural connections and results in subsequent loss of available auditory synapses used to develop auditory perception/language skills in the young child. Physiologic measurements of the infant's critical synapses have found that "mapping" of auditory input is complete by the end of the first year (Kuhl, 1988). If the child is denied cortical stimulation by organic means (because of impaired auditory stimuli), he or she may need to conceptualize by other means (e.g., visual, experiential, tactile). Unfortunately, despite the emphasis on early identification, the average age for diagnosis and the subsequent beginning of intervention is 18 to 30 months (Goldberg, 1996; Kramer & Williams, 1993).

Babbling is an early indicator of language development and has been researched with hearing and hearing-impaired babies. Babbling is vocal play that uses the vocal cords and muscles of the mouth, tongue, and larynx; all children do this. Children who are able to hear receive the stimulus of hearing themselves and their parents' vocalized responses. In contrast, children with hearing impairment get insufficient feedback, and babbling does not progress to language development. The infant with deafness generally babbles normally until approximately 5 months of age (Stoel-Gammon & Otomo, 1986). However, after 5 months, as the typically developing infant develops a growing repertoire of sounds, the child with hearing impairment begins to demonstrate language delay.

Whether by auditory or visual means, language assists in environmental manipulation and gives the child labels for objects and concepts. Language allows children to share their thoughts and ideas with others. Children with hearing impairment can have difficulty learning abstract concepts and multiple meanings of words. Language also plays a critical role in socialization and in adult-child and child-child interactions (Easterbrooks & Baker, 2002; Lederberg, 2002). With peers, age-appropriate social skills, such as turn taking and the ability to control impulsivity, can be affected by a lack of language skills.

The co-occupations of caregiving between mother and child also can be affected. For example, the typically developing infant smiles and quiets to the sounds of his or her mother, whereas the infant with a hearing impairment does not respond to his or her mother's soft voice (Marschark & Clark, 1993). Parental communication is limited because the child needs to be close to and visually focused on the mother to hear her. Strong and positive attachments can occur, but the mother may have to learn coping techniques to gain the child's attention. As with the visually impaired child, the infant and/or mother may display fewer behaviors that elicit positive responses, setting up a cycle that can lead to interactions that are out of sync and not emotionally satisfying.

Researchers have found differences in mother-child interactions when both mother and child have hearing impairments and when a hearing mother has a hearing-impaired child (Easterbrooks & Baker, 2002; Meadow, 1980; Meadow-Orlans, 1990). Ease of communication was significantly different in these two groups. When both mother and child had hearing impairments, signing was a natural method of communication, done in a rich and fluent manner. In contrast, hearing mothers of children with hearing impairments often struggled, not only with adjusting to the knowledge that her child had a disability but also with learning an entirely new language. Given the decrease in deafness caused by hereditary factors, fully 90% of children with hearing impairments now have hearing parents (Lederberg, 1993). The mismatch in communication skills in these dyads becomes a pivotal issue in the mother-child relationship. Mohay (2000) discussed strategies that parents with hearing impairments use to communicate with their children with hearing impairments and suggested that these strategies, (e.g., using touch to gain the child's attention, breaking the child's line of gaze with movements of the body or hands) can be taught to hearing parents to facilitate communication.

Social participation and communication are also affected by the fact that hearing impairment causes the loss of knowledge associated with the "incidental" reception of sound. Aside from direct communication with others, a great deal of social and environmental information is gained from this incidental or background sound. Sound prompts us to look. Many think the child with hearing impairment can compensate for the loss of hearing with the use of vision. However, it is important to note that if the child is communicating using signing, lipreading, and/or cued speech, visual attention must be closely focused on the individual communicating with the child, which eliminates the ability to use vision for other individuals and aspects of the physical environment. Also, as noted above, the individual wishing to communicate must first obtain the child's visual attention to be successful.

Occupational Therapy Evaluation and Intervention
Evaluation

As with the child with visual impairment, occupational therapy evaluation of the child with hearing impairment encompasses the occupational performance areas and performance skills of the child that either support or limit the child's ability to participate in home, community, and school settings. Activity demands, client factors, and contexts in which the child performs these are also part of a comprehensive evaluation. For example, a child with a hearing impairment who has difficulty playing with toys may need evaluation of process skills related to how to choose appropriate toys for his or her age and skill level, how to use the toys appropriately, and how to heed directions and ask for help.

Given the later average age of identification of hearing impairment, compared with that for visual impairment, and the difficulty differentiating hearing loss (especially at lower levels of loss) from other behavioral and cognitive impairments, the occupational therapist may identify a mild problem that may previously have gone undiagnosed. For example, when a pediatrician or other referral source recommends evaluation of a child who is showing problems with attention deficit, distractibility, delayed language, or behavioral issues, a hearing loss may be identified.

Although each child's language development is unique, certain findings indicate the possibility of hearing loss and suggest referral to appropriate professionals (Box 23-2). Any finding of decreased socialization and interaction, although indicative of other difficulties, may also be a subtle indication of hearing loss (Kenna, 1999).

In most cases the parents are the keenest observers of their infants. Special attention should be given to a child whose mother or father reports that he or she does not awaken to loud noises, respond when called, or attend to noisy toys or who turns up the sound on a television or computer. In addition, it is important to follow up a parental report that a child gestures to communicate wants, to the exclusion of words. Therapists should attend to the parent's complaints (e.g., the child's distractibility, inattention to commands, lack of feedback to the mother or father, inappropriate responses to verbal stimuli) and recommend testing or referral to hearing specialists. Referral is also appropriate when a child with a history of recurrent ear infections or upper respiratory infections presents with a possible conductive hearing loss. Although many difficulties can be attributable to other causes, hearing impairment should be considered.

With some adaptation in instructional methods, developmental assessments of fine motor, gross motor, visual motor, sensory integration, and self-care skills can be administered to children with hearing impairments. The therapist can use norm-referenced and criterion-referenced developmental assessment instruments (e.g., the Battelle Developmental Inventory [BDI], the revised Bayley Scales of Infant Development [BSID-II], or the Hawaii Early Learning Profile [HELP]) as part of a comprehensive evaluation of the child with hearing impairment. However, the language areas of these tests must be modified, and standard scores should not be used. If reported, scores must acknowledge any modifications made to the test. If the child is using a hearing aid, cochlear implant, lipreading, or sign language, the therapist should understand the implications of these specialized devices and/or techniques. If the child uses sign language and the therapist testing the child is unable to give the commands using the type of sign the child uses, the test results should include that information. In some instances, it is necessary to use a registered interpreter to test a client with hearing impairment accurately. A functional developmental assessment, such as the Transdisciplinary Play-Based Assessment (TPBA), is helpful in determining the child's strengths and limitations (Linder, 1993) and avoids problems with test validity. The TPBA can be very useful with the child with hearing impairment, because the assessment setting is natural, and standard responses are not expected. In this assessment the play facilitator should be skilled in the communication system used by the child. This allows other team members, who are not skilled in the communication system used by the child, to observe the testing and request that the facilitator attempt to obtain certain information. Another advantage of TPBA is that viewing a video recording of the session afterward allows the assessment team to pick up emerging signs and beginning language and/or communication attempts that may be too subtle to be noted initially.

Skilled observation and parent and caregiver questionnaires can be useful for gathering information about the child's temperament, self-regulation capacities, sensory processing, and sensory modulation behaviors, as well as caregiver-child interactions. Interviews with parents, teachers, and other caregivers can provide information about daily routines, contexts, expectations, and resources available to support the child's participation in activities. As the child gets older, the focus of evaluation may be participation in school and education/learning, with various educational task assessments used. However, written instructions should be used only if the child has the appropriate level of written comprehension,

---

BOX 23-2   Findings that Indicate the Possibility of Hearing Loss

Possible hearing impairment must be considered in the following instances:

- A newborn does not awaken to sounds as expected.
- A newborn does not exhibit a startle *(Moro)* reflex in response to a sharp clap 3 to 6 feet away.
- A 3-month-old child has not developed auditory orienting responses, as indicated by not becoming alert to noises made by certain toys.
- An 8- to 12-month-old child does not turn to a whispered voice.
- An 8- to 12-month-old child does not turn to sounds, such as a rattle, 3 feet to the rear.
- A 1-year-old child does not understand a variety of words, such as "bye-bye" and "doggie."
- A 2-year-old child is not using words.
- A 2-year-old child is unable to identify an object with a verbal cue alone, such as, "Show me the ball."
- A 3-year-old child has largely unintelligible speech.
- A 3-year-old child omits final consonants.
- A 3-year-old child does not use two- and three-word sentences.
- A 3-year-old child mainly uses vowel sounds.
- A child of any age speaks in a voice that is too loud, too soft, of poor quality, or of a quality that does not fit his or her age and gender.
- A child always sounds as if he or she has a cold.

and consideration of the language demands of any written test is important to interpretation of the results. The results of testing should also note the method of communication used (i.e., oral, sign, and/or pantomime). In adolescents, the occupational therapist, in collaboration with the educator and vocational counselor, may evaluate the individual's ability to participate in activities of daily living, such as driving and communicating with others with no knowledge of signing, as well as work skills and behaviors.

Diagnostic information and a description of specialized tests and interventions for children with hearing impairment can be found in Appendix 23-B.

Case Study 2: Tori

Tori is a 4-year-old girl who developed a hearing loss at 2 years of age after having bacterial meningitis (streptococcal pneumonia). At that time she was hospitalized for 2 weeks. Her mother's pregnancy and delivery, as well as Tori's early development, were described as normal. Tori has no other disabilities. She lives with a single mother and a sibling age 6 years in an apartment in an urban environment.

Initial testing indicated a moderate to severe flat loss bilaterally. Tori first received hearing aids at 2 years, 9 months, but because they did not fit appropriately, little speech was being received. She also had recurring middle ear problems, including negative pressure, fluid, and ear wax buildup. Testing when she began preschool indicated a more profound loss, with better thresholds in the left ear. She currently shows a severe-profound sensorineural loss and wears bilateral behind-the-ear aids. She is awaiting insurance approval for a cochlear implant. She also uses an FM system in the classroom 4 days a week. She currently attends a preschool program specifically for hearing impaired children with an auditory-verbal focus. The classroom includes typical children.

She is described by her mother and staff members at the preschool as a pleasant, somewhat reserved child who is distractible and has a short attention span. She is secure in her attachment to her mother, who reports no behavioral issues except in the area of feeding/eating.

Questions to consider:

1 What areas of occupation would you address in your evaluation of Tori?
2 What performance skills would you assess? Why?
3 What methods of evaluation and which assessment tools would you use to assess the areas of occupation and performance skills you have identified?
4 In what contexts would you conduct your evaluation?
5 What difficulties might you expect to see relative to Tori's performance in the classroom?
6 With whom should you collaborate to conduct your evaluation?

Occupational Therapy Intervention

The overall outcome of occupational therapy intervention for children with hearing impairment is engagement in occupations to support participation in the contexts in which they function on a daily basis. Approaches include establishing skills and abilities; maintaining performance capabilities; using compensatory strategies, adaptations, or modifications; and preventing barriers to occupational performance. For example, with a 16-year-old with severe hearing loss and mild mental retardation (MR), the occupational therapist may address communication and interaction skills, such as using appropriate gestures to gain attention and adaptations for obtaining needed information. For a 9-month-old who is rejecting the placement of hearing aids, the early intervention occupational therapist may focus on sensory processing and modulation skills and use various desensitization techniques. With an 8-year-old with profound hearing loss who shows difficulty with fine motor coordination, the school occupational therapist may address the motor performance skills and also process skills (e.g., attention to task and temporal organization) to improve the child's signing abilities.

Occupational therapy models of practice that are particularly useful in the evaluation and intervention process with children who are hearing impaired are sensory integration, visual information processing/visual perception, PEO, cognitive, and psychosocial (coping and social skills development) frameworks.

The occupational therapist's goals must be well coordinated with the goals of those involved with the child, including the parent, early infant specialist, special educator, speech therapist, and audiologist. Generally, the occupational therapist is not the primary participant in intervention for the child with hearing impairment, therefore the treatment goals for the child with hearing impairment are embedded in the team's goals for the child. As with any other child, the occupational therapist incorporates use of self and selects activities to encourage participation in occupations meaningful to the child and family. However, with the child with hearing impairment, the type of communication system chosen by the parents and educators may affect the focus and nature of the type of activities selected to facilitate this participation. Because of the frequent delay in diagnosis until the age of 18 to 30 months (Kramer & Williams, 1993), all intervention, including occupational therapy, may well need, at least initially, to focus on developing and/or improving performance skills that are lagging as a result of auditory language deprivation.

Examples of typical occupational therapy objectives include the following:

- *Enhance sensory processing, sensory modulation, and sensory integration.* The child with hearing impairment must learn to use all available sensory stimulation to the fullest. Problems in sensory processing, sensory modulation, and sensory integration can greatly interfere with function. The therapist can enhance kinesthetic, tactile, and visual processing through multisensory activities. Sensory integrative techniques are useful for developing the kinesthetic system (Figure 23-5). The tactile and proprioceptive systems are important in the use of sign language. Tactile activities, such as having the child locate objects hidden in sand or identify objects behind a shield, are among many that can be used. Tracking exercises, perceptual-motor activities, and many games and crafts can enhance the visual system.

- *Maximize use of residual hearing.* The child with hearing impairment is denied normal cortical stimulation by auditory channels and needs to learn to maximize the auditory stimulation available, as well as to increase auditory awareness, processing, and perception skills Auditory games and auditory input accompanying other activities (especially active rather than passive activities) can facilitate maximum use of available auditory abilities.

- *Encourage age-appropriate self-care skills.* Often the occupational therapist acts as a consultant, recommending strategies for improving the child's self-care independence. Of special importance for the child with hearing impairment is inserting and removing, caring for, and maintaining the hearing aid or cochlear implant. Adapted techniques or assistive devices may be needed. At times self-care skills involve concepts that require concrete cues the child must learn. For example, the idea of left shoe and right shoe can be shown visually with color coding.

- *Enhance fine motor coordination skills.* The movements of the hands of a fluent signer require opposition, finger and thumb flexion and extension, and finger and thumb abduction and adduction. These movements are performed by isolated digits and in total patterns, but they are all done in rapid succession and with remarkable coordination (Figure 23-6). The hand's coordination seems to be related to its sensory abilities, particularly tactile discrimination. This skill does not always come naturally to a child with hearing loss and therefore has to be learned. Occupational therapy's emphasis on hand skills can do much for the child with hearing loss, particularly for children who have an identified delay in fine motor skills.

- *Maximize visual processing, integration, and perception.* A child with hearing loss relies on the visual system to some degree to perceive communication. Children with no usable hearing must rely totally on vision for perception of sign language and finger spelling. Children using auditory methods of communication rely on vision for lipreading and/or cued speech. It is important that scanning and figure-ground perception be well developed. The child must learn to attend simultaneously to multiple sources of visual input (see Chapter 12 for discussion of visual perception).

- *Encourage socialization and peer interaction.* This part of occupational therapy intervention cannot be done in isolation and is of utmost importance to the child with hearing impairment. Involving the child in group activities with his or her peers encourages socialization. A child with a hearing impairment may not be aware of or may not process all the nuances of spoken language. Hearing impairment is not a visible disability. A child with hearing impairment can be mistaken as being rude if he or she does not answer questions or respond to social overtures, when in fact the child has simply not received the correct stimuli. Therefore development of the child's ability to adapt to the

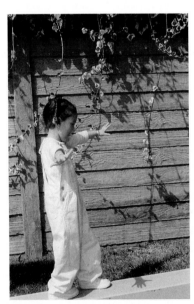

FIGURE 23-5 Child with behind-the-ear aids working on balance and equilibrium skills. (Courtesy Beth Jacobs, OTR/L, John Tracy Clinic, Los Angeles, CA.)

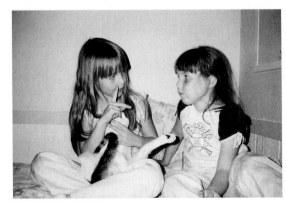

FIGURE 23-6 Sisters communicating using sign language, discussing playing with their pet cat—a favorite shared occupation.

environment and understand social interaction and communication should also be stressed.

- *Maximize oral-motor coordination.* The motor skills necessary for eating (e.g., jaw control, tongue lateralization, and lip closure) are similar to those needed for speech (Figure 23-7). The child with limited speech use may have decreased oral-motor coordination, strength, and endurance. The occupational therapist, in conjunction with the educator and speech therapist, can use various oral-motor games and activities to facilitate the development of oral-motor skills, as well as oral language if this a program goal.

Case Study 2 (continued): Tori

The following observations and findings were obtained through a team (including occupational therapist) evaluation utilizing the Gesell Preschool Test, the Transdisciplinary Play Based Assessment (TPBA; Linder, 1993) and the Leiter International Performance Scale. Observations were also done in the home, classroom, and play area.

- Tori demonstrated a full repertoire of age-appropriate motor skills. She was able to walk, run, and climb well. She engaged in rapid running and jumping inside and outside, apparently attempting to integrate stimuli. She preferred W-sitting with frequent postural changes and frequently engaged in head shaking as a form of sensory self-stimulation.
- Tori exhibited a definite right preference and used a neat pincer grasp and age-appropriate pencil grasp. She sorted objects by color and shape. She

enjoyed puzzles, drawing, and art activities. Her attention to task was limited secondary to visual and physical distraction.

- Tori appeared to understand multiple commands. She used gesturing, some signing, and physical prompting for expression but seemed resistant to initiate conversation with verbal speech. She was predominantly at the single word phrase linguistically and struggled with questioning techniques and conversational turn taking.
- Tori undressed herself with minimal assistance, removed her own shoes and attempted to put them on. She inserted her hearing aids and turned them on with minimal assistance. She was toilet trained and predominantly independent in this task. She fed self with fork and spoon but often preferred to be fed by her mother.
- Tori demonstrated difficulty chewing hard foods and bi-textured foods, gagging and spitting out pieces. She was a very slow eater, frequently needing cues to continue, and did not want to try new foods. Her diet was limited to soft and carbohydrate-type foods. She demonstrated low oral motor tone with open mouth posture, decreased tone in the upper lip and cheeks, low tone in the jaw affecting chewing skills, as well as oral hypersensitivity to touch. She had low chewing endurance.
- Tori adjusted to new situations with relative ease, often sought out attention from other children, usually engaged in interactive and pretend play but had definite preferences. She appeared to struggle with integrating intense stimuli, especially when fatigued.

Questions to Consider

1 What areas of strength does Tori have?
2 What participation and activity limitations can you identify?
3 What occupational therapy model or models of practice would be useful to you to develop your intervention plan?
4 Identify three primary goals or outcomes that you would address with occupational therapy intervention?
5 What approaches, methods, techniques, or strategies will you incorporate in your intervention with Tori?
6 What additional recommendations might be appropriate for Tori and her family?
* Special thanks to Beth Jacobs, MA, OTR/L for her contributions to this case study.

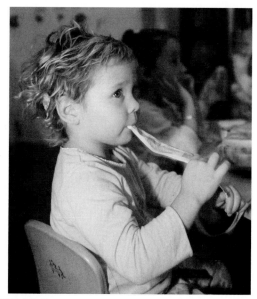

FIGURE 23-7 Child with a cochlear implant participating in an oral-motor group to facilitate oral language skills. (Courtesy Beth Jacobs, OTR/L, John Tracy Clinic, Los Angeles, CA.)

Special Techniques and Strategies

The therapist who works with a child with a hearing impairment becomes intimately involved with the special techniques and/or equipment used with that child (e.g., sign language, lipreading, hearing aids, and cochlear implants). In the field of hearing loss, a battle traditionally has been waged between the *oralists* (i.e., oral language only, through the use of lipreading, auditory training/learning, and speech therapy) and the *sign language users,* or *manualists* (Chamberlain, Morford, & Mayberry, 2000; Hull, 1997; Paul, 2001). Many advocate total communication, which involves the use of all avenues of communication simultaneously (e.g., oral speech, lipreading, auditory training/learning, sign language, finger spelling, gesture, and body language).

Sign language and total communication proponents argue that sign encourages communication and language development and that the child with hearing impairment needs sign for early concept development (Moores, 2001). These experts believe that children demonstrate earlier development of linguistic skills and better interpersonal relationships and understanding of self and environment with this approach. The *bilingual-bicultural* approach entails using sign until well established and then introducing English later, as a second language (Steinberg & Knightly, 1997). Oralists maintain that if a child is taught sign, he or she may never learn to use oral language successfully as the primary mode of communication.

The decision on what techniques and equipment will be used with a child is the prerogative of the child's family and educational system. It is important that the occupational therapist realize and understand the theory behind the decision and that he or she know how best to facilitate the use of the techniques or equipment chosen.

At first glance, teaching the child *speech reading* (lipreading) would seem to be a good choice. However, only one third of speech sounds are visible to the speech reader. In addition, many of the sounds made in English look alike. For example, *p*, *m*, and *b* are all made with the same lip movement (i.e., lips together). Another example of look-alike movements would be *f* and *v*, which both are formed with the teeth to the lower lip. *Cued speech* is a system of hand signs and positions designed to help speech readers distinguish between sounds that look the same on the lips (Ling, 1989).

Another option, sign language, is not easily understood, and it involves many different methods. For example, in the United States, finger spelling, or *dactylology*, is done with one hand, and each configuration represents a letter in the English alphabet. Finger spelling is used by itself or in conjunction with other forms of sign language. Although it is not too difficult for the hearing person to learn to finger spell, when receiving, or listening, the tendency is to see the individual letters and not the words. With finger spelling, it is important that the hand be close enough to the face so that the person with hearing impairment can see both the lip movements and the finger spelling at the same time. For fluency and readability, the hand must be held in a comfortable position, not stiffly.

Sign language can be divided into two categories, American Sign Language (ASL), and *Signing Exact English* (SEE) and other related systems (Bornstein, Saulnier, & Hamilton, 1983; Gustafson & Zawalkow, 1990; Humphries & Padden, 1994; Paul, 2001; Wilbur, 1987). ASL, or Ameslan, is a language in itself and is not directly translatable to English. ASL has many abbreviations and phrases contained in a single sign, and it does not conform to the structure of English. ASL is a spontaneous visual language developed by individuals with hearing impairment at American schools for the deaf, and it is an integral part of the "deaf culture," serving as its native language (Nowell & Marshak, 1994; Scheetz, 2001; Vernon & Andrews, 1990). There is no written language associated with ASL. However, SEE does conform to the structure and form of the English language and is purported to facilitate reading and writing skills in children with hearing impairments.

Many arguments have been made for and against ASL, SEE, and other types of sign. If sign is used, it is important that the therapist become as fluent as possible in the particular system used by the child. Many occupational therapists learn only the simplest and most frequently used words and phrases. However, the more the therapist knows of the child's sign system, the more effective the communication/interaction will be and consequently the more effective the intervention. Many good texts are available on the different types of sign. However, it is best to attend a class or practice with a friend who knows sign, because it often is difficult to interpret the configuration and movement patterns of the hands correctly.

The occupational therapist is sometimes involved with the child during the initial stages of learning sign. In this case, it is best to select the first signs to be taught from those that represent familiar objects, real life situations, and familiar actions. The adult should begin with what is available to the child (i.e., things to feel, handle, or do) and provide parents with a likes-dislikes checklist to determine what is appropriate for the individual child. Often a food item is used first because of its value as a reward. The adult should work at the eye level of the child, obtain eye contact, make the sign, and then physically manipulate the child's hands through the sign. Some basic suggestions for the use of total communication are listed in Box 23-3.

An occupational therapy perspective, in addition to the education perspective, can add to the process of learning sign language. Occupational therapy's emphasis on occupation can assist the team by ensuring that the child and family are taught signs that label the activities that have particular meaning and purpose to them; that

BOX 23-3 Suggestions for Use of Total Communication

- Face the child squarely at eye level.
- Position yourself so that the child can easily see your face and hands at the same time.
- Make sure you have the child's attention.
- Avoid backlighting. If the child has to look into the light, he or she may be unable to see your lips.
- Use a normal tone of voice. Do not exaggerate mouth movements, because this practice tends to confuse the lip reader.
- Speak the word and give the sign at the same time rather that in sequence.
- Use appropriate pauses between words, especially when finger spelling is used.
- Sit close to the child rather than across the room.
- Keep instruction simple and to the point.
- Be consistent, especially with a young child.
- Talk to the child. He or she needs to receive the same amount of input as a hearing child.
- Check to make sure the auditory equipment is working properly.

is, their occupations. An occupational therapy profile can be used to gain an understanding of the child's and family's occupational experiences, patterns of daily living, interests, values, and needs and may add to the team's knowledge of the child and family and the language that is uniquely important to them.

The occupational therapist may also be involved in the initial stages of hearing aid use. Often a history shows that the child had a hearing aid but rejected it. This sometimes can be traced to the lack of professional support for the parents and child during the difficult adjustment period, or it can be traced to the professional's lack of familiarity with the aid. The occupational therapy perspective on sensory processing, modulation, and integration can be useful in addressing these issues in the wearing of hearing aids.

Hearing aids can be of great assistance to children with hearing impairment, depending on the type and severity of hearing loss. They are of great help in auditory training/learning and can assist the child sound awareness/recognition, sound localization, and speech perception. However, they do not allow the child to hear normally. Hearing aids cannot restore hearing as glasses can restore vision. They amplify all the sounds in the environment, which leads to distortion and interference with auditory perception and differentiation of sound. Because of this interference the following situations may present difficulties:

- Environments with excessive background noise
- Groups of three or four people speaking at the same time
- Reamplification (e.g., listening to a television or tape recorder)

- Distance listening

The newer, digital aids, however, are much more sophisticated than analog models and actually decrease reception of noise that may interfere with speech perception.

Despite the shortcomings of hearing aids, they are extremely valuable for providing auditory input, and it is regrettable when an instrument that can be of help to a child is not used simply because it is not perfect. The therapist should help the parents and child by clarifying realistic expectations about the hearing aid and explaining what it can and cannot do for the child.

Because the head is one of the most sensitive parts of the body, one of the main problems found in children with new aids is tactile sensitivity. However, the child must learn to think of the aid as a piece of clothing that is put on automatically in the morning, along with shoes and socks. The earlier an aid is fitted to a child and put into use, the better the chances for language development (Ling, 1989).

Children who use hearing aids need to adjust to the feel of the aid and recognize its importance. It usually is best for the child to begin wearing the aid during a quiet activity that involves just one person speaking. The maximum benefit from an aid is obtained in relatively quiet settings.

The hearing aid is a sensitive piece of equipment with several parts, and it can often need repair. It is estimated that as many as 50% of hearing aids used by school-age children are not working properly (Ross, Brackett, & Maxon, 1991). Everyone involved with the child should be aware of some of the common problems, because an improperly working aid is useless to the child. Four common problems are (1) dead batteries, (2) improperly placed or corroded batteries, (3) squeal (check for looseness of the earmold), and (4) impaction of the earmold with wax, which must be cleared.

The type of hearing aid prescribed for a particular child depends on the degree and configuration of the loss (Chase & Gravel, 1996; Northern & Downs, 2002). Two types of hearing aids are widely used, the *in-the-ear* type and the *behind-the-ear* type. The in-the-ear aid is used only for mild losses and has no external wires. The behind-the-ear aid is used for mild to profound losses and is the most popular type of aid. It is a small unit, made up of a microphone, amplifiers, and receiver. These components are located together behind the ear and are connected by a short tube to a silicone earmold that has been custom formed to the shape of the child's external auditory canal. The earmold is seated directly in the ear (Figure 23-8, *A*). The microphone picks up the sound waves and converts them to electric signals. The amplifiers then increase the strength of the signal, and the receiver changes the electric signals back to sound waves that are sent to the earmold. A *monaural aid* refers to

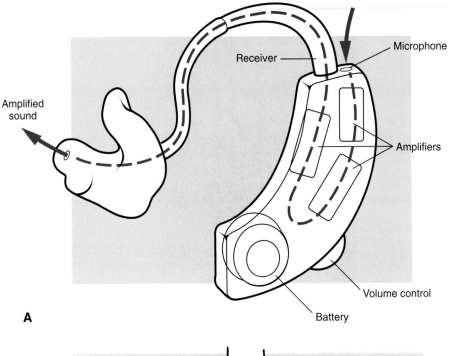

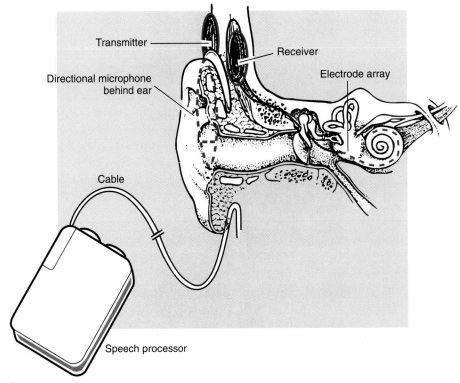

FIGURE 23-8 **A,** Diagram of a behind-the-ear hearing aid. **B,** Diagram of a cochlear implant.

the use of just one aid, and *binaural aid* refers to the use of two separate aids.

Cochlear implants (Figure 23-8, *B*) are devices that can be surgically implanted in the cochlea of individuals with severe to profound hearing losses (Kreton & Balkany, 1991; Nevins & Chase, 1996; Steinberg & Knightly, 1997; Tye-Murray, 1992). They have been used in children since the early 1980s and are becoming much more common in this age group. Cochlear implants create possibilities for auditory input for those who could not benefit from traditional hearing aids. These devices provide the sensation of sound by acting as substitutes for hair cells in the organ of Corti; they provide direct stimulation to the auditory nerve and thus are able to detect all speech sounds. Cochlear implants can now be fitted in children as young as 12 months, but only after the child has gone through a trial period with a traditional hearing aid.

The implant has four components: (1) a receiver seated in the temporal bone, (2) an external microphone attached to a transmitter, (3) a speech processor that records and electronically codes incoming sounds, and (4) an electrode array implanted in the cochlea itself. The external transmitter is held in place on the head by a magnet that attracts a magnet in the receiver embedded in the temporal bone. The receiver is attached to the electrode array in the cochlea, and a cord connects the transmitter and microphone to the speech processor. The cord is usually run under the child's clothing, and the speech processor is contained in a fanny pack worn at the waist. Alternatively, many children now are wearing behind-the-ear speech processors.

Sound flows from the microphone to the speech processor, where it is converted into an electrical signal. The coded signal is sent back to the transmitter and then to the receiver, where it is decoded and delivered to the actual electrodes in the cochlea. The electrodes bypass the damaged hair cells and directly stimulate the nerve fibers in the cochlea.

Although this technique brings state-of-the-art technology to the child's functional hearing ability, the degree of hearing improvement is variable. Most children are able to hear at least environmental sounds immediately and by 6 months can understand some speech and respond to their names (Christiansen & Leigh, 2002). Like a hearing aid, the implant does not restore normal hearing, but it does allow many children to perceive open-set speech; that is, speech without context. However, it is difficult to hear in groups and noisy environments, as well as individuals whose speech patterns are unfamiliar to the child (Christiansen & Leigh, 2002). Also, as with the hearing aid, the best results are achieved if the device is worn consistently. Mapping, or programming, of the speech processor is a complex process upon which the success of the implant depends. How much benefit the child obtains from the implant depends a great deal on auditory training of discrimination abilities, neural survival of synapses, and parental involvement. Research indicates that the earlier the implantation, the better the results (Christiansen & Leigh, 2002). There has been much debate in the deaf culture over whether the device should be implanted in young children before they are able to understand and take part in the decision making, but for the most part, the positive results appear to outweigh the negatives. Padden (1996) discusses a shift from deaf culture to bicultural orientation that seems to be occurring more rapidly with the advent of the cochlear implant.

Therapists must be aware of the external equipment and its location during motor activities with the child.

The equipment is expensive, and components worn on the child's body can be damaged by water, rough physical activity, or electrostatic discharge. Electrostatic discharge (ESD) is of special concern to the occupational therapist, because various pieces of therapy equipment can interfere with the mapping of the speech processor and damage the implant. For these reasons, the external components should be removed before activities involving such therapy equipment or activities. If the occupational therapist has any question about engaging the child in a specific activity, it is best to check with the parent, audiologic professional, or primary service provider.

Like hearing aids, cochlear implants have external components and may cause problems with tactile defensiveness; therefore desensitization can be an appropriate goal for therapists working with children who have been fitted with these devices. As part of the intervention team, the occupational therapist can help by providing feedback to the audiologists on the types of sounds the child appears to hear.

As with the hearing aid, the key to success with the cochlear implant is use. All adults working with the child need to check that the equipment is in good working order and that the child is spoken to frequently. A normal tone of voice should be maintained, and speech volume and tones should be the same as those used with any other child during therapy activities. In addition, language should be kept at age level and within the context of the situation.

In school settings, FM systems are often used with children with hearing impairments. With an FM system, the teacher wears a microphone and wireless transmitter to speak directly into the child's FM system, hearing aid, or cochlear implant. This device helps control the level of background noise in the classroom, because the teacher's voice can be amplified for the students who have hearing loss without disturbing other students in the classroom.

Preparation for Adulthood

The adolescent with hearing impairment may struggle to blend into a hearing world. Universal recognition of the importance of inclusion and required accommodations in school and work settings has afforded more opportunities, and the growing technology of communication has improved future prospects. For most adolescents, an important task is learning to drive a car. Adolescents with hearing impairment can receive special driving training. These students are taught to constantly visually scan the environment while driving.

Another important aspect of interacting with the hearing world is the use of a daily communication device often taken for granted—the telephone. Some hearing aids have a telephone setting. However, if amplification alone is not sufficient to allow the wearer to understand conversation, the Telecommunication Device for the Deaf (TDD) is available. The TDD is a communication device that uses the telephone lines with a keyboard to "talk" and a printout device to receive the conversation. In addition, the telephone ring is replaced with a flashing light or a fan that moves back and forth to indicate an incoming call. The obvious disadvantage of the TDD is that both ends of the line must be equipped with this system. E-mail and text-messaging pagers can also be used as alternative, and increasingly available, forms of communication by individuals with hearing impairment.

Watching television provides another aspect of daily life. The frequency of closed-captioned programs has increased, and all televisions manufactured after 1995 are required to have a built-in decoding device. The individual with hearing impairment uses this decoding device to view captioned versions of programs.

Occupational choice has always been difficult for young adults with hearing impairment. Fortunately, today many universities offer programs designed to integrate students with hearing loss into the general student population by providing special services, such as interpreters, computer assisted real time captioners (CART), and note takers. The Americans with Disabilities Act (ADA) (1990) requires that all public education programs provide interpreters, CART, or note takers for individuals with hearing impairment when it is determined that they are required.

When an individual with hearing impairment enters a work environment, he or she is likely to miss a great deal of information transmitted in conversation, as well as environmental sounds (Steinberg & Knightly, 1997). Other factors that historically have adversely affected occupational choice for individuals with hearing loss include (1) differences that affect self-perception and perception of others, (2) a restricted life space, which adversely affects knowledge of areas other than the immediate social or geographic area, and (3) limited sociocultural understanding (Hull, 1997; Schein & Delk, 1975). Adolescents with a hearing impairment may lack work-related experiences, role models, exploration of their talents and interests, effective interpersonal skills, and knowledge of work behaviors needed for vocational success (Scheetz, 2001).

Occupational therapists are aware of how important meaningful and purposeful activity is in the life and health of an individual. As part of an interdisciplinary team, therapists can help address many of the above issues and prepare the child with hearing impairment for transition to work and fuller participation in work.

MULTISENSORY IMPAIRMENT

A combination of sensory losses creates significant challenges, and the interaction of problems associated with the various disabilities must be considered. A common challenge for the occupational therapist is the child whose primary problem is a physical disability or mental retardation but who also has visual or hearing deficits, or both. Sometimes a child's visual impairment may be the primary focus of intervention and education, and other sensory or learning impairments may go undetected; on the other hand, a child with obvious multiple disabilities may have visual or hearing impairments that are not identified (Teplin, 1995).

Diagnostic Information

Although the majority of individuals with vision impairment have some degree of functional vision, about one third of children with partial sight and two thirds of children with blindness also have other developmental disabilities (Miller, Menacker, & Batshaw, 2002). Whenever a developing brain incurs injuries, the chances of multiple impairments are significantly greater. For instance, about 32% of children with cerebral palsy have severe visual impairments, and 30% have some form of hearing, speech, and language impairment (Pellegrino, 2002). The incidence of visual and auditory deficits is also high for children with mental retardation. With both of these diagnoses, accurate assessment of acuity, awareness, and perception often is difficult, because these children do not always give the examiner reliable feedback.

Embryologic studies show that the timetables for development of the eye and ear are similar (Jones, 1997), therefore a number of diagnoses involve both systems (e.g., cytomegalovirus infection, maternal rubella, toxoplasmosis, congenital syphilis, Hurler's syndrome, Waardenburg's syndrome, and Goldenhar's syndrome). Meningitis is a leading cause of noncongenital hearing and visual impairment in children.

Other Services

As mentioned earlier, a team of professionals may be involved with children who have multiple sensory disabilities. Orthopedists, neurologists, and cardiologists are a few medical specialists whose expertise is often needed. Given the multiple needs of these children, it is highly likely that the occupational therapist will become involved. He or she may be a major team member, especially with the physically impaired child who has visual deficits, or with the child who is both visually and hearing impaired. Often the occupational therapist's first contact with visual or hearing impairment is through a child with multiple disabilities.

Occupational Therapy Evaluation and Intervention

A primary consideration and focus in the care and management of visual impairment in children with multiple disabilities is to provide individualized plans for helping the child to use his or her residual vision (Zambone, Ciner, Appel, & Garboyes, 2000). Many of the behaviors and occupational performance concerns discussed previously also apply to children with multisensory impairment. Children with both visual and hearing impairments may show extreme tactile defensiveness. Consider how frightening it must be for a child who has two sensory channels that are unavailable or that provide information that is out of focus or indistinct. These children may not like anything new or different, and changes of any type often are not well accepted. Oral hypersensitivity may also be present, and the change from smooth to textured foods is difficult. Neuromotor function often is affected by hypotonicity and hypermobility of the joints or by spasticity. Some children learn to walk, but they may remain cautious about giving up support.

Children who are visually and hearing impaired often have had difficult infancy periods, including negative reactions to parental handling that can lead to less and less parental handling. Stimuli may not make sense to children who are visually and/or hearing impaired, therefore they ignore them or respond in a defensive manner (Chen, 1999). Stereotypic behaviors may be observed, and these may be confused with signs of autistic spectrum disorder. As discussed previously, the presence of stereotypic behaviors does not automatically indicate a diagnosis of autism, because these behaviors may be seen in other conditions. Conversely, it cannot be assumed that atypical or stereotypic behaviors in children with multiple disabilities are primarily attributable to their sensory impairment.

Every child is different and may manifest these behaviors to a different degree. The occupational therapist can be a key member of the treatment team, assisting in the diagnostic process through evaluation and description of the child's occupational performance in relation to age, developmental level, and severity of impairment. The therapist also can interpret behaviors and can offer hypotheses that could help tease out whether, for example, sensory processing or modulation difficulties, or other underlying factors, are contributing to those behaviors.

With the child who has visual and hearing impairment, as well as physical or cognitive disabilities, it is important for occupational therapists to remember that consistent repetition often is needed for the child to learn skills in everyday contexts and situations and that progress can be made but frequently is slow. For example, a simple task, such as learning the hand-to-mouth motor pattern necessary for self-feeding, may require years of practice with multiple cues and much consistency. Hand-over-hand guidance frequently is used during activities with children with multiple and severe disabilities. However, this approach takes control away from the child and may actually lead to passivity or over-reliance on the adult. An alternative approach is hand-*under*-hand guidance, with the child's hand on top of the adult's. Although facilitating movement from underneath the hand can be a more difficult maneuver for the therapist, it is easier for the adult subtly to remove the support, promoting the child's independence in the activity.

Campbell, McInerney, and Cooper (1984) found that functional patterns of movement were achieved at faster rates when children with multiple disabilities were able to practice the desired movement patterns more frequently. Other studies have found that orientation and mobility training for infants and toddlers is beneficial for children with visual and additional impairments and that parents can effectively implement premobility programs to help children develop the needed skills (Kelley et al., 2000). Training of caregivers and school staff, therefore, becomes extremely important. The orientation and mobility specialist and the occupational therapist should assess the child and identify specific tasks or movements to be targeted, determine the appropriate intervention strategies, and instruct others in how to carry out the tasks or movements with accuracy.

As discussed previously, the role of the occupational therapist often is that of consultant. Consultation and monitoring to promote self-care skills, such as dressing, require that the therapist develop rapport with those doing the training and develop the ability to encourage and reward others to help them follow the program correctly. Diagrams or pictures with clearly written directions can be helpful guides to caregivers for carrying out self-care programs with their children. The therapist monitors the self-care programs by observing others implement a technique and also by directly implementing the technique with the child to receive direct feedback about the child's performance.

Evaluation

Developmental scales can be used for assessment and treatment planning for children with visual and hearing impairments. Of special interest are the prehension and tactile processing abilities, because almost everything has to be taught using manual guidance strategies. Play- and occupation-based assessments, along with skilled observations, are useful and can provide a comprehensive description of levels of function in all areas of development or occupational performance. Play and social skills, activities of daily living, arm and hand skills, and community living are often key areas to address. The child should be observed in structured and unstructured settings, and significant others should be consulted about the child's skills. The occupational therapist, along with other members of the team, analyzes the findings and observations, arrives at hypotheses about the degree to which functional limitations can be attributed to various factors, and designs appropriate interventions. The occupational therapist's PEO perspective is valuable in identifying and addressing the child's and family's ability to engage in meaningful occupations. Indeed, a top-down approach is preferred to a traditional developmental approach in the assessment of children with dual sensory impairments or multiple disabilities, because the focus is on identifying the skills needed to perform life tasks rather than on sequential skill acquisition. Building sequential developmental skills may further delay the child's participation in activities, given that slow progress is likely (Porr, 1999).

Intervention Goals and Methods

Intervention goals depend on the individual assessment of the child and his or her identified levels of functioning, but interventions should build on all the skills and remaining sensory channels available to the child (Porr, 1999). Although goals can vary from child to child, some typical goals of occupational therapy intervention include the following:

- *Promote or establish self-feeding skills.* Feeding is often a problem for children who have multiple disabilities. They frequently have several medical problems that require long periods of non-oral feeding. Occupational therapy intervention with the infant should focus on obtaining good sucking skills (good rhythm and appropriate strength) and decreasing oral-facial hypersensitivity. Later, problems such as tongue thrust, fatigue during feeding, and poor coordination of mouth movements sometimes occur. Learning to accept textured foods and chewing usually requires intervention, and physically moving the child through self-feeding and cup placement often is necessary. Hypersensitivities and resistance to change are two major difficulties that can be intensified with the presence of increased tone and reflex patterns. Strategies need to be developed for the child who remains on a bottle or extensively drinks a high-caloric food supplement. The transition from bottle feeding to drinking from a glass and eating table foods is a long process, possibly taking several years to achieve. To increase independence, adaptive equipment often is required (e.g., a large wheelchair tray with raised edges or a scoop bowl with suction cups).
- *Promote or establish self-care skills.* Achieving as much independence as possible should be the goal for each child. Toileting is often a problem because of resistance to the task and difficulty understanding what is required. For the child who has physical disabilities in addition to visual and auditory impairments, adapted toilet seats and scheduling techniques may be needed. Dressing and hygiene skills are also often difficult, requiring adaptation and physical guidance or assistance.

- *Promote or establish play skills.* It is important that children with multiple sensory and other impairments be provided a variety of experiences and opportunities to engage in play with objects, toys, and other children so that they can learn about their world and learn how to interact with objects and people. Because they have multiple impairments that affect their ability to engage in interactions, these children are at risk of becoming isolated, therefore they need many opportunities to participate in daily activities, including play. Additional interventions address the underlying performance skills needed to engage in play, self-care, and learning activities.

- *Promote tactile awareness, enhance tactile processing, and promote adequate sensory modulation of tactile experiences.* Because acceptance of touch is basic to any interaction, integration of the tactile system often is an initial goal. The child should be gradually introduced to a variety of tactile experiences in the context of everyday activities and encouraged to reach out and explore independently. Use of vibration and proprioceptive input may also be helpful.

- *Provide adequate positioning and postural alignment.* The child with multiple sensory disabilities often is fearful of moving through space independently. In addition, habitual postural patterns may develop that could affect the alignment of the body. For these reasons, adequate positioning of the child to allow interaction with the environment and to prevent contractures and deformities is extremely important. Functional positioning to ensure that the child can use his or her strongest sensory systems is the aim of a considerable proportion of treatment. With children who cannot move by themselves, it is important that the occupational therapist teach the caretakers and education staff different positions and encourage them to change these positions often. Engaging the children in vestibular-proprioceptive activities, at the level they can tolerate, often is helpful.

- *Promote postural control and facilitate normal movement patterns.* The occupational therapist may use facilitation and handling techniques to work on postural control and movement with a child. However, engaging these children in active movement interactions, as much as is possible, is critical for moving them toward independence. When a new movement pattern is introduced, practice time should be allowed and new activities introduced gradually. Activities on tilt boards, swings, and bolsters are useful, but more important is movement activities in natural or authentic settings, with peers and family.

- *Provide family members with support and education.* Family members need information about appropriate levels of stimulation and effective strategies for interaction with the child. Support groups, or parents of children with similar disabilities, can become a greatly valued resource for the parents.

As a team member, the occupational therapist may also assist with the following goals when working with children with visual and hearing impairments:

■ *Develop a sense of mastery or competence.* Children with multiple impairments need to be able to experience control and mastery at whatever level in a variety of contexts and situations. Young children need to learn about cause-and-effect relationships and that their actions have an effect on others and the environment. Many switch-activated toys (e.g., toys that have a switch a child can press to activate a fan or vibrator) provide sensory input that is pleasurable and motivating to these children and can help them learn that they can make something work. This sense of mastery and competence must be promoted continually as the child grows older.

■ *Develop socially acceptable behaviors.* Children with multiple impairments who have stereotypic behaviors need to be taught more acceptable and functional strategies for meeting their sensory needs (e.g., the behaviors serve a sensory-seeking purpose) or communicative needs (e.g., the child does not have a means to convey wants or needs). If the behavior is simply extinguished, without the underlying problem being addressed or an alternative provided, the child may find another, still unacceptable way to fulfill the need. Rather than viewing the child as a "behavior problem," the therapist should evaluate the behaviors in the context in which they occur and arrive at possible hypotheses for why they occur, which can lead to strategies or alternatives that are meaningful to the child. In addition, the child needs consistency and continuity, with clear expectations. If tactile signs are used, they should be simple initially and consistent from one person to the next. The development of interpersonal and play skills is also crucial.

Special Techniques and Strategies

Many of the specialized techniques used with children with multiple impairments deal with the development of some form of communication (Hyvarinen, Gimble, & Sorri, 1990) and mobility (Huebner, Prickett, Welch, & Joffe, 1995). Children with multiple sensory disabilities have a slower pace of development. Therefore task analysis and breaking down a task into its smallest component parts can be useful in setting realistic goals for therapy and in establishing objectives for the individualized education program (IEP).

Task analysis can be especially useful in daily living and vocational skills activities. For example, in teaching a child with multiple sensory disabilities to butter a piece of bread, the total task can be broken down into steps, which then can be repeated in backward or forward order (i.e., chaining). In *backward chaining,* all steps are performed for the child except the last, which is the first taught, then the next to last, and so on. In *forward chaining,* the first step is taught until it is mastered, then the second, and so on. Regardless of the instructional direction used, it is important to fade out assistance but still give as much as is needed to help the child master the task in its entirety.

Another useful approach with children who have multisensory impairment is *behavior modification.* This is a systematic approach to altering the child's behavior through environmental programming. In behavior modification, reinforcement is often used and detailed records of the child's responses are kept. Often a positive trait (e.g., urinating when placed on the toilet) needs to be reinforced, or a negative trait (e.g., eye poking) needs to be discouraged. The therapist charts the behaviors, and the correct response is provided. Although being ignored is negative reinforcement for many children, children who have multiple sensory disabilities are often happy to be left alone. Therefore this technique may not have the desired effect.

For the child with multisensory impairment and severe physical and mental challenges, the occupational therapist often focuses on safety, survival, or self-care skills. These skills, even if they are learned in a rote manner and require extremely specific environmental cues to elicit, are important to the child's ability to function. If possible, carryover should be sought. However, after all factors have been weighed, clinical judgment may indicate that concentrating on specific skills is most important to function.

Preparation for Adulthood

The child with multiple sensory disabilities and severe physical or mental impairment is usually prepared for supported employment rather than for independent living. For the most part, supported employment activities may be repetitive and involve manipulative skills; they can include folding, stamping, collating, counting, gluing, bending, sorting, assembling, wrapping, stuffing, filing, measuring, stapling, and clipping. If the individual has abilities that can be supported through use of a job coach in a work setting, the occupational therapist can assist with evaluating the skills that can be matched to the job, as well as any accommodations or modifications that may be needed in the work place.

Several key behaviors the adolescent needs to develop for more self-sufficient living are (1) communication of basic emergency and survival words, such as "Stop," "Eat," "More," "No," and "Finish"; (2) social skills; (3)

self-care skills; (4) telling time; (5) cooking and shopping skills; (6) home management; (7) travel and mobility; and (8) housekeeping. Supported living and group home settings with supervision available are possible options for some individuals with multiple disabilities.

If the child has remained at home with the family through school, adolescence often is when a move must be made to a residential setting. Both the family members and the child must be prepared for this. Also, the child's emerging sexuality must be dealt with at the level of his or her understanding.

SUMMARY

This chapter provided an overview of occupational therapy services with the child with visual and/or hearing impairment. Occupational therapy assessment emphasizes how the child's development and function are affected by loss of one or both of these senses. General intervention goals have been presented, stressing provision of activities and experiences that allow the child to develop adaptive behaviors. Brief explanations of specialized techniques used with these children have also been provided, including the use of hearing aids, cochlear implants, sign language, Braille, and low-vision aids. Occupational therapists use their knowledge of adaptation, task and activity analysis, and developmental sequence to help children who have visual and/or hearing impairments engage in meaningful and purposeful occupations.

REFERENCES

American Academy of Pediatrics. (1995). Joint Committee on Infant Hearing: 1994 Position statement. *Pediatrics, 95,* 152-156.

American Academy of Pediatrics. (2003). Eye examination in infants, children, and young adults by pediatricians. *Pediatrics, 111,* (4 Pt 1), 902-907.

American Foundation for the Blind. (2000). *Statistics and sources for professionals.* Retrieved August 7, 2003, from http://www.afb.org/info_document_view.asp?documented=1367

Anderson, K.L., & Matkin, N.D. (1991). *Relationship of degree of long term hearing loss to psychosocial impact and educational needs.* Los Angeles: John Tracy Clinic.

Anderson, S., Boigon, S., & Davis, K. (1986). *Oregon Project Skills Inventory* (5th ed.). Medford, OR: Jackson Education Service District.

Association for Retinopathy of Prematurity and Related Diseases. (2003). *What is retinopathy of prematurity?* Retrieved August 26, 2003, from http://www.ropard.org/what_is.shtml

Ayres, A.J. (1972). *Sensory integration and learning disorders.* Los Angeles: Western Psychological Services.

Baird, S.M., Mayfield, P., & Baker, P. (1997). Mothers' interpretations of the behavior of their infants with visual and other impairments during interactions. *Journal of Visual Impairment and Blindness, (September-October),* 467-483.

Baker-Nobles, L. (1997). Pediatric low vision. In M. Gentile (Ed.), *Functional visual behavior: A therapist's guide to evaluation and treatment options* (pp. 375-401). Bethesda, MD: American Occupational Therapy Association.

Baker-Nobles, A., & Rutherford, A. (1995). Understanding cortical visual impairment in children. *American Journal of Occupational Therapy, 49,* 899-911.

Bayley, N. (1993). *Bayley Scales of Infant Development Manual* (2nd ed.). San Antonio, TX: Psychological Corporation.

Behrman, R.E., Kliegman, R.M., & Jenson, H.B. (2000). *Nelson textbook of pediatrics* (16th ed.). Philadelphia: W.B. Saunders.

Bernbaum, J.C. (1999). Follow-up of the high-risk infant. In F.D. Burg, E.R. Wald, J.R. Ingelfinger, & R.A. Polini (Eds.), *Gellis and Kagan's current pediatric therapy* (16th ed., pp. 332-336). Philadelphia: W.B. Saunders.

Blind Babies Foundation. (2003). *Cortical visual impairment pediatric visual diagnosis fact sheet.* Retrieved July 17, 2003, from http://www.tsbvi.edu/Outreach/seehear/fall98/cortical.htm

Bluestone, C.D., & Klein, J.O. (2001). *Otitis media in infants and children* (3rd ed.). Philadelphia: W.B. Saunders.

Bornstein, H., Saulnier, K., & Hamilton, L. (1983). *A comprehensive signed English dictionary.* Washington, DC: Gallaudet College Press.

California Deaf-Blind Services. (2003). *Neurological visual impairment.* Fact Sheet #022. Retrieved August 26, 2003, from http://www.sfsu.edu/~cadbs/Eng022.html

Campbell, P.H., McInerney, W.F., & Cooper, M.A. (1984). Therapeutic programming for students with severe handicaps. *American Journal of Occupational Therapy, 38,* 594-602.

Celeste, M. (2002). A survey of motor development for infants and young children with visual impairment. *Journal of Visual Impairment and Blindness (March),* 169-174.

Chaikin, L.E., & Downing-Baum, S. (1997). Functional visual skills. In M. Gentile (Ed.), *Functional visual behavior: A therapist's guide to evaluation and treatment options.* Bethesda, MD: American Occupational Therapy Association.

Chamberlain, C., Morford, J.P., & Mayberry, R.I. (2000). *Language acquisition by eye.* Mahwah, NJ: Erlbaum.

Chase, P.A., & Gravel, J.S. (1996). Hearing aids for children. In R.A. Goldberg (Ed.), *Hearing aids: A manual for clinicians.* Philadelphia: J.B. Lippincott.

Chen, D. (1999). Interactions between infants and caregivers: The context for early intervention. In D. Chen (Ed.), *Essential elements in early intervention: Visual impairment and multiple disabilities* (pp. 22-54). New York: AFB Press.

Chomsky, N. (1993). *Language and thought.* Wakefield, RI: Moyer Bell.

Christiansen, J.B., & Leigh, I.W. (2002). *Cochlear implants in children.* Washington, DC: Gallaudet University Press.

Coplan, J. (1999). Voice, speech and language disorders. In F.D. Burg, E.R. Wald, J.R. Ingelfinger, & R.A. Polini (Eds.), *Gellis and Kagan's current pediatric therapy* (16th ed., pp. 425-429). Philadelphia: W.B. Saunders.

Dickens, C.J., & Hoskins, H.D. (1989). Developmental glaucoma. In S.J. Isenberg (Ed.), *The eye in infancy.* Chicago: Year Book.

Easterbrooks, S.R., & Baker, S. (2002). *Language learning in children who are deaf and hard of hearing.* Boston: Allyn & Bacon.

Erhardt, R.P. (1990). *Developmental visual dysfunction: Models for assessment and management.* San Antonio, TX: Therapy Skill Builders.

Folio, M.R., & Fewell, R.R. (2000). *Peabody Developmental Motor Scales examiner's manual* (2nd ed.). Austin, TX: Pro-Ed.

Gentile, M. (1997). *Functional visual behavior: A therapist's guide to evaluation and treatment options.* Bethesda, MD: American Occupational Therapy Association.

Gitlin-Weiner, Sandgrund & Schaefer (2000). Introduction, emergence, and evaluation of children's play as a focus of study. In K. Gitlin-Winer, A. Sandgrund, & C. Schaefer (Eds.), *Play diagnosis and assessment* (2nd ed., pp. 12). New York: John Wiley.

Glass, P. (1995). Development of visual function in preterm infants: Implications for early intervention. *Infants and Young Children, 6,* 11-20.

Glass, P. (2002). Development of the visual system and implications for early intervention. *Infants and Young Children, 15,* 1-10.

Goldberg, D. (1996). Early intervention. In F. Martin & J.C. Clark (Eds.), *Hearing care for children.* Boston: Allyn & Bacon.

Groenveld, J., Jan, J.E., & Leader, P. (1990). Observations on the habilitation of children with cortical visual impairment. *Journal of Visual Impairment and Blindness (January),* 11-15.

Gustafson, G., & Zawalkow, E. (1990). *Signing exact English.* Los Alamitos, CA: Modern Signs Press.

Hartmann, E.E. (2000). Visual functioning in pediatric populations with low vision. In B. Silverstone, M.A. Lang, B.P. Rosenthal, & E.E. Faye (Eds.), *The Lighthouse handbook on vision impairment and vision rehabilitation: Vol. 1. Vision impairment* (pp. 225-247). New York: Oxford University Press.

Hatton, D.D., Bailey, D.B., Burchinal, M.R., & Ferrell, K.A. (1997). Developmental growth curves of preschool children with vision impairments. *Child Development, 68,* 788-806.

Heydt, K., Clark, M.J., Cushman, C., Edwards, S., & Allon, M. (1992). *Perkins Activity and Resource Guide: A handbook for teachers and parents of students with visual and multiple disabilities.* Watertown, MA: Perkins School for the Blind.

Hiles, D.A., & Hered, R.W. (1989). Disorders of the lens. In S.J. Isenberg (Ed.), *The eye in infancy.* Chicago: Year Book.

Hiskey, M.S. (1983). The development, administration, scoring, and interpretation of the Hiskey-Nebraska Test of Learning Aptitude. In C.R. Reynolds & J.H. Clark (Eds.), *Assessment and programming of young children with low incidence handicaps.* New York: Plenum Press.

Huebner, K.M., Prickett, J.G., Welch, T.R., & Joffe, E. (Eds.). (1995). *Hand in hand: Essentials of communication and orientation and mobility for your students who are deaf-blind.* New York: AFB Press.

Hull, R.H. (1997). *Aural rehabilitation: Serving children and adults* (3rd ed.). San Diego: Singular.

Humphries, T., & Padden, C. (1994). *A basic course in American Sign Language.* Silver Spring, MD: T.J. Publishers.

Hyvarinen, L. (1995). Considerations in evaluation and treatment of the child with low vision. *American Journal of Occupational Therapy, 49,* 891-897.

Hyvarinen, L., Gimble, L., & Sorri, M. (1990). *Assessment of vision and hearing of deaf-blind persons.* Melbourne, Australia: Royal Victorian Institute for the Blind.

Individuals with Disabilities Education Act (IDEA). (1997). Individuals with Disabilities Education Act Amendments of 1997. Public Law No. 105-17.

Isenberg, S.J. (Ed.). (1989). *The eye in infancy.* Chicago: Year-Book.

Johnson, D.J. (1999). *Deafness and vision disorders.* Springfield, IL: Charles C. Thomas.

Jones, K.L. (1997). *Smith's recognizable patterns of human malformation* (5th ed.). Philadelphia: W.B. Saunders.

Kelley, P.A., Sanspree, M.J., & Davidson, R.C. (2000). Vision impairment in children and youth. In B. Silverstone, M.A. Lang, B.P. Rosenthal, & E.E. Faye (Eds.), *The Lighthouse handbook on vision impairment and vision rehabilitation: Vol. 2. Vision rehabilitation* (pp. 1137-1151). New York: Oxford University Press.

Kenna, M.A. (1999). Hearing loss. In F.D. Burg, E.R. Wald, J.R. Ingelfinger, & R.A. Polini (Eds.), *Gellis and Kagan's current pediatric therapy* (16th ed., pp. 1019-1021). Philadelphia: W.B. Saunders.

Kramer, S.J., & Williams, D.R. (1993). The hearing-impaired infant and toddler:

Identification, assessment, and intervention. *Infants and Young Children, 61,* 35-39.

Kreton, J., & Balkany, T.J. (1991). Status of cochlear implantation in children. *Journal of Pediatrics, 118,* 1-7.

Kuhl, P.K. (1988). Auditory perceptions and the evolution of speech. *Human Evolution, 3,* 19-43.

Lampert, J.L. (1998). Working with students with visual impairment. In J. Case-Smith (Ed.), *Occupational therapy: Making a difference in school system practice.* Bethesda, MD: American Occupational Therapy Association.

Lampert, J.L., & Lapolice, D.J. (1995). Functional considerations in evaluation and treatment of the client with low vision. *American Journal of Occupational Therapy, 49,* 885-890.

Lederberg, A.R. (1993). The impact of deafness on mother-child and peer relationships. In M. Marschark & M.D. Clark (Eds.), *Psychological perspectives on deafness* (pp. 93-119). Hillsdale, NJ: Erlbaum.

Linder, T.W. (1993). *Transdisciplinary play-based assessment.* Baltimore: Brookes.

Ling, D. (1989). *Foundations of spoken language for hearing impaired children.* Washington, DC: A.G. Bell Association.

Marschark, M. (1993). Origins and interactions in social, cognitive, and language development of deaf children. In M. Marschark & M.D. Clark (Eds.), *Psychological perspectives on deafness* (pp. 7-26). Hillsdale, NJ: Erlbaum.

Marschark, M., & Clark, M.D. (1993). *Psychological perspectives on deafness.* Hillsdale, NJ: Erlbaum.

Martin, F. (1991). *Introduction to audiology.* Englewood Cliffs, NJ: Prentice-Hall.

Martin, F., & Clark, J.G. (1996). *Hearing care for children*. Boston: Allyn & Bacon.

Meadow, P. M. (1980). *Deafness and child development*. Berkeley: University of California Press.

Meadow-Orlans, P.M. (1990). Research on developmental aspects of deafness. In D.F. Moores, K.P. Meadow-Orlans (Eds.), *Educational and developmental aspects of deafness* (pp. 283-320). Washington, DC: Gallaudet University Press.

Mervis, C.A., Boyle, C.A., & Yeargin-Allsopp, M. (2002). Prevalence and selected characteristics of childhood vision impairment. *Developmental Medicine and Child Neurology, 44*, 538-541.

Michelman, S. (1971). The importance of creative play. *American Journal of Occupational Therapy, 25*, 285-290.

Miller, M.M., Menacker, S.J., & Batshaw, M.L. (2002). Vision: Our window to the world. In M.L. Batshaw (Ed.), *Children with disabilities* (5th ed., pp. 165-192). Baltimore: Brookes.

Mohay, H. (2000). Language in sight: Mothers' strategies for making language visually accessible to deaf children. In P.E. Spencer, C.J. Erling, & M. Marschark (Eds.), *The deaf child in the family and at school: Essays in honor of Kathryn P. Meadow-Orlans* (pp. 151-166). Mahwah, NJ: Erlbaum.

Moores, D.F. (2001). *Educational and developmental aspects of deafness*. Boston: Houghton Mifflin.

Nevins, M.E., & Chase, P.M. (1996). *Children with cochlear implants in educational settings*. San Diego: Singular.

Newborg, J., Stock, J.R., Wnek, L., Buidubaldi, J. & Svinicki, J. (1988). *Battelle Developmental Inventory: Examiner's manual*. Chicago, IL: Riverside.

Newby, H.A., & Popelka, G.R. (1985). *Audiology* (5th ed.). Englewood Cliffs, NJ: Prentice-Hall.

Northern, J.L., & Downs, M.P. (2002). *Hearing in children* (5th ed.). Baltimore: Lippincott Williams & Wilkins.

Nowell, R.C., & Marshak, L.E. (1994). *Understanding deafness and the rehabilitation process*. Boston: Allyn & Bacon.

Oyler, R., Oyler, A., & Matkin, N. (1998). Unilateral hearing loss: Demographics and educational impact. *Language, Speech and Hearing in Schools, 19*, 201-210.

Padden, C. (1996). From the cultural to the bicultural. In I. Parasnic (Ed.), *Cultural and language diversity and the deaf experience* (pp. 79-98). New York: Cambridge University Press.

Parham, L.D., & Fazio, L.S. (1997). *Play in occupational therapy for children*. St. Louis: Mosby.

Parks, S. (1999). *Inside HELP: Administration and reference manual for the Hawaii Early Learning Profile (Birth-3)*. Palo Alto, CA: Vort.

Paul, P.V. (2001). *Language and deafness* (3rd ed.). San Diego, CA: Singular.

Pellegrino, L. (2002). Cerebral palsy. In M. L. Batshaw (Ed.), *Children with disabilities* (5th ed., pp. 443-466). Baltimore: Brookes.

Pelton, S.I. (1999). Otitis media. In F.D. Burg, E.R. Wald, J.R. Ingelfinger, & R.A. Polini (Eds.), *Gellis and Kagan's current pediatric therapy* (16th ed., pp. 1021-1024). Philadelphia: W.B. Saunders.

Pinker, S. (1994). *The language instinct*. New York: Morrow.

Porr, S.M. (1999). The visual and auditory systems. In S.M. Porr & E.B. Rainville (Eds.), *Pediatric therapy: A systems approach* (pp. 241-266). Philadelphia: F.A. Davis.

Recchia, S. (1997). Play and concept development in infants and young children with severe visual impairments: A constructionist view. *Journal of Visual Impairment and Blindness, (July-August)*, 401-406.

Reynell, J., & Zinkin, P. (1979). *Reynell-Zinkin Developmental Scales for Young Visually Handicapped Children*. Windsor, England: NFER.

Roid, G.H., & Miller, L.J. (1997). *General instructions for the revised Leiter International Performance Scales*. Wood Dale, IL: Stoelting.

Rosenthal, B.P., & Fischer, M.L. (1997). Optometric assessment of low vision. In M. Gentile (Ed.), *Functional visual behavior: A therapist's guide to evaluation and treatment options* (pp. 345-373). Bethesda, MD: American Occupational Therapy Association.

Ross, M., Brackett, D., & Maxon, A. (1991). *Assessment and management of mainstreamed hearing impaired children*. Austin, TX: Pro-Ed.

Ross, S., & Tobin, M.J. (1997). Object permanence, reaching, and locomotion in infants who are blind. *Journal of Visual Impairment and Blindness (January-February)*, 25-32.

Sameroff, A.J., & Fiese, B.H. (2000). Transactional regulation: The developmental ecology of early intervention. In J.P. Shonkoff & S.J. Meisels (Eds.), *Handbook of early childhood intervention* (2nd ed., pp. 135-159). Cambridge: Cambridge University Press.

Sanspree, M.J. (2000). Pathways to habilitation: Best practices. In B. Silverstone, M.A. Lang, B.P. Rosenthal, & E.E. Faye (Eds.), *The Lighthouse handbook on vision impairment and vision rehabilitation: Vol. 2. Vision rehabilitation* (pp. 1167-1182). New York: Oxford University Press.

Schaefer, K.J., & Specht, M.A. (1979). A light probe adapted for use in training the blind. *American Journal of Occupational Therapy, 33*, 640-643.

Scheetz, N.A. (2001). *Orientation to deafness*. Boston: Allyn & Bacon.

Scheiman, M. (1997). *Understanding and managing vision deficits: A guide for occupational therapists*. Thorofare, NJ: Slack.

Schein, J.D., & Delk, M.T. (1975). *The deaf population of the United States*. Silver Spring, MD: National Association for the Deaf.

Schepens Retinal Foundation (2003). Retinopathy of prematurity. Retrieved August 26, 2003 from: http://www.schepens.com/retinopathy of prematurity.htm.

Smith Roley, S., & Schneck, C. (2001). Sensory integration and visual deficits, including blindness. In S. Smith Roley, E.I. Blanche, & R.C. Schaaf (Eds.), *Understanding the nature of sensory integration with diverse populations* (pp. 313-344). San Antonio, TX: Therapy Skills Builders.

Steinberg, A.G., & Knightly, C.A. (1997). Hearing: Sounds and silences. In M.L. Batshaw (Ed.), *Children with disabilities* (4th ed.). Baltimore: Brookes.

Stoel-Gammon, C., & Otomo, K. (1986). Babbling development of hearing-impaired and normally hearing subjects. *Journal of Speech and Hearing Disorders, 51*, 33-41.

Teplin, S.W. (1995). Visual impairment in infants and young children. *Infants and Young Children, 8*, 18-51.

Titcomb, R.E., Okoye, R., & Schiff, S. (1997). Introduction to the dynamic process of vision. In M. Gentile (Ed.), *Functional visual behavior: A therapist's guide to evaluation and treatment options* (pp. 3-54). Bethesda, MD: American Occupational Therapy Association.

Trief, E., Duckman, R., Morse, A.R., & Silberman, R.K. (1989). Retinopathy of prematurity. *Journal of Visual Impairment and Blindness (December),* 500-504.

Tye-Murray, N. (1992). *Cochlear implant and children: A handbook for parents, teachers, and speech and hearing professionals.* Washington, DC: A.G. Bell.

Verloed, M.P.J., Hamers, J.H.M., van Mens-Weisz, M.M., & Timmer-Van de Vosse, H. (2000). New age levels of the Reynell-Zinkin Developmental Scales for young children with visual impairments. *Journal of Visual Impairment and Blindness (October),* 613-624.

Vernon, M.C., & Andrews, J.F. (1990). *The psychology of deafness: Understanding deaf and hard-of-hearing people.* New York: Longman.

Warren, D. (1994). *Blindness in children: An individual differences approach.* New York: Cambridge University Press.

Warren, D. (2000). Developmental perspectives. In B. Silverstone, M.A. Lang, B.P. Rosenthal, & E.E. Faye (Eds.), *The Lighthouse handbook on vision impairment and vision rehabilitation: Vol. 1. Vision impairment* (pp. 325-337). New York: Oxford University Press.

Wilbur, R. (1987). *American Sign Language: Linguistics and applied dimensions* (2nd ed.). Boston: Little, Brown.

Zambone, A.M., Ciner, E., Appel, S., & Garboyes, M. (2000). Children with multiple impairments. In B. Silverstone, M.A. Lang, B.P. Rosenthal, & E.E. Faye (Eds.), *The Lighthouse handbook on vision impairment and vision rehabilitation: Vol. 1. Vision impairment* (pp. 451-468). New York: Oxford University Press.

DIAGNOSTIC INFORMATION

Definitions and Prevalence

Estimates vary on the number of children in the United States with visual impairment (i.e., blindness or low vision), depending on the definitions used and the source of the data. The legal and federal education definition of *blindness* is central visual acuity of 20/200 or worse in the better eye with the best possible correction, as measured on a Snellen vision chart, or a visual field of 20 degrees or less (Individuals with Disabilities Education Act [IDEA], 1997; American Foundation for the Blind, 2000). Children with *low vision* (partially sighted) have visual acuity better than 20/200 but worse than 20/70 with correction (Miller, Menacker, & Batshaw, 2002).*

According to the American Foundation for the Blind (2000), 93,600 students (birth through 21 years) with visual impairments or blindness received special education services in the United States in 1998. Of these, 10,800 were deaf-blind. A population study of 6- to 10-year-old children who were blind, conducted in Atlanta, Georgia, arrived at a prevalence rate of 10.7 per 10,000 children (Mervis, Boyle, & Yeargin-Allsopp, 2002). Estimates of the overall incidence of blindness in children are low, ranging from 0.4 per 1,000 (Porr, 1999) to 1 per 1,000 (Hatton, Bailey, Burchinal, & Ferrell, 1997) to 3 per 1,000 (Miller et al., 2002). The range of functional vision generally is described in four groups: total blindness, some light perception, performance of visual tasks with poor efficiency, and ability to read large type (Miller et al.).

Visual System

As with the auditory system, it is important that the occupational therapy practitioner have a basic knowledge of the anatomy and physiology of the visual system in order to understand visual impairment. The reader should review the anatomy of the eye in Chapter 12 (also see Titcomb, Okoye, & Schiff, 1997; Glass, 2002; Miller et al., 2002). The visual system is complex, and one that

we rely on to give us information about the world quickly and efficiently. Although the visual system components are functional at birth, allowing newborns to see high-contrast lines and slow-moving objects or to follow horizontal movement in the first few months, the visual system is the least mature functionally (Glass, 2002; Miller et al.). That is, *vision* is more than *seeing*.

Causes of Blindness

Childhood blindness has many causes. The impairment can occur in the structure of the eye itself or in some part of the visual pathways or processing centers in the brain. Congenital causes include intrauterine infections, such as toxoplasmosis, herpes, and cytomegalovirus, as well as malformations of the visual system, such as colobomas, optic nerve hypoplasia, and brain malformations (Porr, 1999; Miller et al., 2002). Many of the children seen by occupational therapists have visual impairment as a result of other causes, such as retinopathy of prematurity (ROP), traumatic brain injury, tumors, or other conditions. Visual impairment may also be caused by an inherited disorder, such as albinism. Although blindness can occur as a single disability, visual impairment in children often is associated with other conditions, such as cerebral palsy, Down syndrome, or other developmental disabilities.

Identifying Children with Visual Impairment

Guidelines for eye examinations and for vision assessment of young children have been established by the American Association for Pediatric Ophthalmology and Strabismus, the American Academy of Ophthalmology, and the American Academy of Pediatrics. It is recommended that eye examination and age-appropriate vision assessment begin in the newborn period and continue at all subsequent well child visits (American Academy of Pediatrics [AAP], 2003). *Visual acuity,* or *central vision,* can be measured in children using a number of tests. When the child is capable of understanding verbal directions, visual acuity most often is tested using the Snellen chart. This procedure tests central acuity with letters, numbers, or symbols in graded sizes that are drawn to Snellen measurements. Each size is labeled with the

---

* All references cited in this appendix can be found under the References list at the end of Chapter 23.

distance from which it can be seen by the normal eye. The child stands 20 feet from the chart and indicates to the examiner what he or she sees, line by line. Eye report terms include *OD* (refers to the right eye), *OS* (refers to the left eye), and *OU* (refers to both eyes).

The legal definition of blindness, therefore, means that the child who is legally blind can see an object clearly at 20 feet that a child with normal vision can see at 200 feet. The *peripheral vision*, the second part of the definition, means that the child can see only in a field of 20 degrees, whereas a child with normal vision can see in a field of over 180 degrees. Box 23A-1 lists generally accepted gradations of acuity with correction. Other acuity tests include the Tumbling E, or the HOTV Test (Matching Test) for children who may be unable to identify letters or numbers. Tests such as the Allen Cards and LH Symbols (LEA Symbols) use flash cards that contain figures (e.g., a truck, house, and telephone, or a house, apple, circle, and square, respectively). Visual acuity scores or values are calculated based on the distance at which the figures or symbols can be accurately identified using standard criteria specific to the test.

Other tests of visual function do not rely on verbal responses or recognition of symbols but rather require higher technology to assess different aspects of visual function. These include optokinetic nystagmus, preferential looking, and electrophysiologic tests. Optokinetic nystagmus is an involuntary response that is present soon after birth and is elicited by rotating a black and white–striped drum in front of the child's eyes. Visual acuity also may be assessed by progressively varying the width of the stripes. However, absence of optokinetic nystagmus may not necessarily mean that visual impairment is present, because other factors, such as inattention, the distance at which the drum is held, and the speed of drum rotation, can affect the child's response.

For the preferential looking (PL) test, a set of cards is presented to an infant or a young child at a specified distance; the cards have a pattern of black and white stripes or gratings and a blank gray target that is equally luminous. Infants preferentially fixate on the striped pattern, and the examiner observes the visual response through a

small peephole in the center of each card. The widths of the stripes are progressively thinner with each card presented. Visual acuity can be determined, but the PL test generally is not used for this purpose; it is more useful for assessing visual improvement in children with amblyopia or for detecting differences in vision between eyes (Miller et al., 2002). The PL test requires a trained observer, sufficient responsiveness or cooperation from the child, and a distraction-free environment. Some developmental tests (e.g., the Bayley Scales of Infant Development II) have incorporated a variation of the PL test to assess visual fixation or attention, which can provide valuable information about early visual function. Because occupational therapists are often among the first to evaluate development in infants and young children, if vision impairment is suspected, a referral can be made to the appropriate eye specialist.

Two electrophysiologic tests, the electroretinogram (ERG) and the visual evoked potential (VEP), are used to determine whether a vision problem is due to a retinal impairment or to an impairment in the visual pathway between the eye and the brain (Miller et al., 2002; Rosenthal & Fischer, 1997). Electrodes are used in both tests, and the results are analyzed by a computer. Sedation of the child may be necessary to administer the ERG. If visual function is poor but the retina looks normal on examination, an ERG may be indicated. If the retina is functioning normally, a VEP may be considered, especially if cortical visual impairment is suspected. The VEP may also be used to assess visual acuity in infants and children with severe disabilities.

Common Pediatric Eye Disorders

As stated previously, visual impairment can occur within the structures of the eyeball, at the retina, along the nerve pathway to the brain, and in the brain itself. Refractive errors arise when deviation occurs in the course of the light rays as they pass through the eye, preventing sharp focus on the retina. Scheiman (1997) identified myopia and hyperopia as the most common refractive errors.

- A child with *myopia*, or nearsightedness, sees most clearly at close range and much less efficiently at a distance. The eyeball is too long or refractive power is too strong, therefore the focus point is in front of the retina. This causes the child to have blurred vision, and external strabismus is possible when the individual is looking at a distance. The child often holds printed material close to the eyes.
- A child with *hyperopia*, or farsightedness, has blurred vision and may experience headaches when trying to focus on near images (e.g., when reading). The eyeball is too short and underdeveloped, the refractive power is too weak, and the focus point is behind the retina. This child sees most clearly at a distance,

BOX 23A-1   Gradations of Acuity with Correction

- 20/20 to 20/70: Normal to slightly defective vision
- 20/70 to 20/100: Mild visual limitation or good partial vision
- 20/100 to 20/200: Moderate visual impairment or fair partial vision
- 20/200 to 20/1,000: Legally blind with severe impairment
- Over 20/1,000: Finger counting ability; form perception; hand movement; light perception (i.e., sees light and can tell where it is); light perception (i.e., sees light but cannot locate it)

and with constant effort to focus at close range, his or her eyes become fatigued.

Although these refractive errors usually can be corrected with lenses, if left undiagnosed or untreated during early school years, they can have a significant impact on the child's development in all areas.

Cataracts are often a congenital condition that can result in poor vision or visual loss (Hiles & Hered, 1989; Porr, 1999). A cataract occurs when the lens of the eye changes from clear to cloudy or opaque. After removal of the lens, the child must wear corrective lenses. Although often the result of heredity, childhood cataracts can be associated with juvenile diabetes, Down syndrome, or Hallermann-Streiff syndrome.

Glaucoma is another visual problem that can occur in childhood (Dickens & Hoskins, 1989; Porr, 1999). Glaucoma is an increase in the intraocular pressure of the eyeball, resulting in hardening of the eye and damage to the cornea. Congenital glaucoma occurs in the first year of life as a result of blockage of fluid outflow from an abnormal membrane that covers the meshwork; acquired glaucoma may occur secondary to intrauterine infection, ROP, ocular inflammation, or eye trauma (Miller et al., 2002). Surgery is necessary for congenital glaucoma, whereas medications alone often can be used successfully to treat the acquired form.

Neurologic visual impairment (NVI), the preferred term for the condition formerly known as cortical visual impairment (CVI), is a common cause of visual impairment in children (California Deaf-Blind Services, 2003). NVI includes CVI, delayed visual maturation, and cortical blindness, depending on the area of the brain affected. NVI occurs when damage to the brain results in impairment of the brain's ability to process visual information even through the eye itself is normal.

Cortical visual impairment (CVI) may be temporary or permanent and arises when a disturbance or abnormality occurs in the posterior visual pathways and/or the occipital lobes of the brain (Baker-Nobles, 1997; Blind Babies Foundation, 2003). The child demonstrates impaired visual functioning, but the ophthalmologic examination essentially is normal. The degree of neurologic and visual impairment, which depends on the time of onset and the location and intensity of the insult, ranges from severe visual impairment to total blindness.

The proportion of children with CVI has increased as a result of (1) advances in neonatal care; (2) higher survival rates for infants with hypoxic ischemic encephalopathy that results in CVI; and (3) a simultaneous decrease in blindness from treatable causes as a result of advances in ophthalmology (Miller et al., 2002). Children with CVI often show variability in the degree of functional vision (Baker-Nobles, 1997; Groenveld, Jan, & Leader, 1990), but improvement usually is seen over time, possibly because of the brain's ability to compensate for inefficient or damaged areas. This is why early intervention is so critical for young children with this condition.

Retinopathy of prematurity (ROP), a condition affecting the light-sensitive membrane in the back of the eye, is seen in premature, low birth weight infants. Abnormal growth of retinal blood vessels may occur toward the center of the eye, rather than along the back wall of the retina toward the front, forming a ridge. The abnormal blood vessels die and scar tissue forms, which constricts and can pull on the retina and could result in complete retinal detachment (Association for Retinopathy of Prematurity and Related Diseases, 2003; Schepens Retinal Foundation, 2003). Because the growth and maturation of retinal blood vessels occur in the fourth month of gestation and continue to the ninth month, infants born at 28 weeks or earlier or who weigh 1,500 g or less should be screened for ROP. It once was thought that the high levels of oxygen given to premature infants contributed to ROP; however, oxygen administration is not the sole cause, and it now is believed that ROP is a multifactorial disease of unknown origin (Hartmann, 2000). The key factors are birth weight, gestational age, and duration of administration of oxygen (Trief, Duckman, Morse, & Silberman, 1989).

ROP is described in terms of five stages relative to the progression of the abnormal growth of blood vessels and three zones relative to the location in the eye (zone 1 is the most centrally located area where damage occurs; zone 2 is the intermediate area where growth of blood vessels often stops; and zone 3 is the peripheral area of the retina where vessels are absent) (Hartmann, 2000; Schepens Retinal Foundation, 2003). Stage 1 or stage 2 ROP may not require treatment, but treatment is required (usually laser, or cryotherapy) with stage 3 disease. Stage 4 ROP involves partial retinal detachment, and surgical procedures such as scleral buckle or vitrectomy may be performed. Stage 5 ROP is the end stage of the progression, marked by complete retinal detachment, and surgery (i.e., open-sky vitrectomy) usually is performed. Visual outcomes in children with ROP, which vary, may include low vision, light perception only, or total blindness (Trief et al., 1989).

The following are other eye conditions and common optical terms (Isenberg, 1989; Miller et al., 2002):

- *Amblyopia:* A condition of diminished visual acuity, sometimes called *lazy eye*, that usually cannot be relieved by lenses. The child may have depth perception problems and may tilt his or her head.

- *Astigmatism:* Unequal curvature of the refractive surfaces of the eye that may result in distorted images. This may cause focusing problems, because light is not sharply focused on the retina but spread over a more or less diffuse area.

- *CHARGE association:* A group of abnormalities, including coloboma, heart malformations, atresia of the nasal passage, retardation, genital abnormalities, and ear abnormalities.

- *Coloboma:* A congenital defect of the eye caused by failure of complete growth in the affected area (usually the iris, choroids, or ciliary body).
- *Microphthalmos:* An abnormally small eyeball.
- *Nystagmus:* Rapid involuntary movement of the eyes. This condition may be hereditary and may result in inability to fixate accurately and constantly. The movement is repetitive and may be lateral, vertical, rotary, or mixed.
- *Optic atrophy:* Degeneration of the optic nerve fibers.
- *Optic nerve hypoplasia:* Failure of the optic nerve to develop fully.
- *Ptosis:* Drooping of the eyelid caused by weak or absent muscle. This condition usually does not interfere with vision.
- *Retinoblastoma:* A malignant tumor of the retina and eye orbit that is either unilateral or (more often) bilateral.
- *Strabismus:* Squint or cross-eyes. Failure of the eyes to converge properly on an image, or a condition in which both eyes are not directed at the same point. Strabismus is often caused by muscle imbalance and frequently results in double vision. With *esotropia* the eye turns inward; with *exotropia* the eye turns outward; with *vertical strabismus* the eye turns up or down.
- *Toxoplasmosis:* A parasitic disease, which may be congenital or acquired from household pets, that causes scarring, usually on the retina and choroids.

OTHER SERVICES

In addition to the occupational therapist, children with visual impairment often receive treatment from other professionals. Those most often involved include the following:

- *Ophthalmologist:* A physician who specializes in the diagnosis and treatment of defects and diseases of the eye. He or she performs surgery when necessary and prescribes other types of treatment, including corrective lenses.
- *Optometrist:* A licensed specialist in vision (OD) who is trained in the art and science of vision care. This specialist examines the eyes and preserves and restores vision through optometric means; he or she also measures refractive error and assesses for eye muscle disorders.
- *Optician:* An individual who grinds lenses, fits them into frames, and adjusts the frames to the wearer.

In addition to the above professionals, the following specialists may be involved in providing services to children with visual impairments:

- *Behavioral or developmental optometrist:* A specialist in an area of optometry based on the philosophy that vision is a complex process that involves learned skills and that takes into account the brain-behavior relationships. Behavioral optometrists perform a behavioral vision analysis and, in addition to prescribing corrective lenses and pharmaceuticals, provide vision therapy to address visual skill dysfunctions.
- *Neuro-optometrist:* Neuro-optometrists, practitioners of a subspecialty of optometry, conduct diagnostic testing to identify acquired visual dysfunctions and provide interventions such as prisms, lenses, and visual therapy.
- *Orientation and mobility specialist:* An individual who specializes in orientation and mobility training of the visually impaired. *Orientation* is the process of using the remaining senses to establish one's position and relationship to all other significant objects in one's environment. *Mobility* is the ability to move safely and efficiently from one point to another in the environment.

SPECIALIZED ASSESSMENT TOOLS

Several assessment tools have been developed specifically for children with visual impairment.

- *Reynell-Zinkin Developmental Scales for Young Visually Handicapped Children* (Reynell & Zinkin, 1979). Similar to the Bayley Scales of Infant Development, the Reynell-Zinkin test has two parts, one covering mental development and one assessing motor development. The mental scales include sections on social adaptation, sensorimotor understanding, exploration of the environment, response to sound and verbal comprehension, expressive language, and communication. The motor scales cover hand function, locomotion, and reflexes. A profile type of scoring is used, and standard scores are not available. However, age equivalents are given for children (with and without visual impairment) from birth to 5 years of age. A study that described new developmental age levels based on a sample of Dutch children and psychometric properties of this measure provides some recommendations for use of the Reynell-Zinkin scales and interpretation of scores (Verloed, Hamers, van Mens-Weisz, & Timmer-Van de Vosse, 2000).
- *Oregon Project Skills Inventory* (Anderson, Boigon, & Davis, 1988). This inventory was developed as an assessment for the child with visual impairment up to 6 years of age and for writing educational and intervention objectives. It covers the areas of cognitive, language, social, vision, compensatory, self-help, and fine and gross motor development. Teaching activities are suggested for each area. The inventory also takes into account the vast difference in degrees of visual impairment by indicating items that are acquired at a later age or that may not be appropriate for children with total vision loss.

- *Perkins Activity and Resource Guide* (Heydt, Clark, Cushman, Edwards, & Allon, 1992). This resource guide includes developmental checklists and developmental activities and resources for the areas of language and cognition, social development, motor development, functional academics, vocational training, daily living skills, independent living skills, and sensory integration.
- *Erhardt Developmental Vision Assessment (EDVA)* (Erhardt, 1990). This observational assessment measures the development of ocular-motor skills that typically occurs from birth to 6 months. It is divided into two sections, one covering primarily involuntary visual patterns (i.e., eyelid reflexes, pupillary reactions, and doll's eye responses), and the other covering voluntary patterns (i.e., fixation, localization, ocular pursuit, and gaze shift). The EDVA is designed to evaluate visual function in children with developmental disabilities and can be helpful to the occupational therapist in determining the child's developmental level of functional ocular-motor abilities.

Observation of the young child's functional vision is important. In addition to a physical examination, observation of the child's use of objects and toys often provides important information (Hyvarinen, 1995; Lampert & Lapolice, 1995). The subjective description of functional vision from the parent, teacher, or therapist can also add greatly to the physician's assessment.

Several intelligence tests have been adapted for use with the visually impaired, including the Binet and the Wechsler tests. Other oral tests are easily adaptable. The American Foundation for the Blind publishes a comprehensive listing of psychologic, vocational, and educational tests appropriate for use with the visually impaired.

WEB SITES FOR ADDITIONAL INFORMATION

American Foundation for the Blind (AFB)
www.afb.org
A resource for professional materials on blindness and low vision, the AFB is the home of the Helen Keller Archives. The organization publishes the *Journal of Visual Impairment and Blindness* and *AccessWorld: Technology and People with Visual Impairments*.

Lighthouse International
www.lighthouse.org
A resource for information on prevention, treatment, research, and rehabilitation. The organization publishes a newsletter, *En Vision*.

American Printing House for the Blind (APH)
www.aph.org
The APH is a source for educational and daily living aids. It publishes books and magazines on topics related to visual impairment.

American Council of the Blind
www.acb.org
The ACB is a source of information on Braille, guide dogs, and large print material. It is the distributor of the *Braille Forum*.

Blind Children's Center
www.blindchildrenscenter.org
A resource for information about children with visual impairments, including list of publications, toll-free number, telephone assistance, and programs.

Hearing Impairment

DIAGNOSTIC INFORMATION

The estimates of children with hearing impairment vary with the criteria applied. Bernbaum (1999)* reported incidence rates of sensorineural hearing loss in premature infants of 1% to 3%. Among infants in general, it is estimated that 3 in 1,000 are born with a significant hearing loss, and another 3 in 1,000 develop significant loss in childhood (Northern & Downs, 2002). Thirteen of 1,000 school-age children are estimated to have a hearing loss of 26 dB or greater (Behrman, Kliegman, & Jenson, 2000). However, total deafness is rare and usually occurs only with aplasia, failure of the inner ear to develop, or a disease process (e.g., bacterial meningitis) severe enough to destroy all hearing. Unfortunately, hearing loss is very difficult for the pediatrician to identify in the course of a typical physical examination (Coplan, 1999), which highlights the importance of an early hearing screening and developmental history.

A person with *deafness* is one whose hearing is so severely impaired that he or she must depend primarily on visual communication, such as writing, lipreading, manual communication, or gestures. The Conference of Executives of American Schools for the Deaf has designated deafness as a hearing loss of 70 dB or greater in the better ear, and hard of hearing as 35 to 69 dB in the better ear (Northern & Downs, 2002). Almost all children who are deaf have some residual audition that can be used for environmental awareness (Northern & Downs), as well as speech perception when properly aided.

Anatomy of the Ear

To properly examine the subject of hearing loss, the occupational therapist must have a basic understanding of the nature of sound and the anatomy of the ear. Sound sets up a disturbance in the air. Air consists of more than 400 billion particles per cubic inch. As a person speaks or makes a sound, these particles are set in motion, hitting against each other and forming a wave of sound energy.

The ear acts as a receiver, amplifier, and transmitter and is composed of three sections (see Figure 23-1 in the chapter text). The outer ear includes the visible part *(pinna)* and the external auditory canal extending to the eardrum *(tympanic membrane)*. The function of the outer ear is to collect the sound, or acoustic energy, and channel it to the eardrum, which vibrates with the sound wave and changes the acoustic energy to mechanical energy.

The middle ear consists of three small bones (the *hammer,* or *malleus; the anvil,* or *incus;* and the *stirrup,* or *stapes*), which conduct vibrations from the eardrum to the inner ear. The stapes is inserted into the oval window, beyond which is the fluid-filled vestibule of the inner ear. This fluid-filled vestibule, along with the semicircular canals found in the inner ear, make up the organs of equilibrium. The motions of the bones of the middle ear result in an increase of the mechanical energy of sound so that by the time sound travels from the eardrum to the oval window, it has been intensified many times.

The inner ear is composed of the hearing organ, the *cochlea,* which coils off the vestibule and the *acoustic nerve* (eighth cranial nerve). The cochlea transforms the mechanical energy of the sound waves into neural energy for reception by the auditory nerve.

HEARING LOSS

The two types of hearing loss are *conductive hearing loss* and *sensorineural hearing loss.* The type of loss a child has depends on the part of the ear that has been damaged or is underdeveloped. Hearing loss can also be unilateral or bilateral. In conductive hearing loss, the problem lies in the sound-transmitting portions; that is, the outer or middle ear. Conductive hearing loss most often is caused by otitis media (Bluestone & Klein, 2001). Some common causes of conductive loss are infection, wax build-up, puncture of the eardrum, or inability of the middle ear bones to move properly.

Humans hear by bone conduction as well as by air conduction, and the relationship of these two functions provides diagnostic information about the location of the hearing loss. Diagnoses marked by permanent conductive hearing loss include *Treacher-Collins syndrome,* a hereditary underdevelopment of the external canal and

---

*All references cited in this appendix can be found under the References list at the end of Chapter 23.

middle ear, and *otosclerosis,* a progressive condition that occurs as early as late adolescence (Steinberg & Knightly, 1997). Fortunately, when detected early, many conductive losses are temporary and can be corrected by medical or surgical means, such as antibiotics, removal of ear wax, myringotomies, or placement of *pressure equalization (PE)* tubes. Unfortunately, considerable impairment of the developmental process (e.g., poor articulation, delayed speech development, and poor school performance) can occur before the child's hearing loss is detected. Of special note is recurrent otitis media, which can result in sporadic hearing loss that is very detrimental to language, behavior, and social development (Kenna, 1999; Pelton, 1999).

In sensorineural hearing loss, or *nerve loss,* the problem occurs in the inner ear, with damage to the cochlear hair cells, the acoustic nerve (the eighth cranial nerve), or the brain stem. A nerve loss generally is not correctable by medical or surgical means and requires the use of hearing aids or cochlear implants. This type of loss often produces problems with loudness and distortion of sound. Sensorineural hearing loss often is associated with genetic syndromes, hypoxia, cytomegalovirus (CMV) infection, toxoplasmosis, meningitits, hyperbilirubinemia, unstable blood pressure, and environmental noise; it also can be a sequela of ototoxic drugs such as gentamicin and streptomycin (Bernbaum, 1999; Behrman et al., 2000). Drugs used in the neonatal intensive care unit (NICU) and in early infancy to save lives can have a toxic effect on the hearing organs.

Of the infections, CMV is the most common congenital cause of sensorineural hearing loss. A genetic etiology is found in as many as 50% of cases of sensorineural hearing loss, with genetic syndromes often involving other systems (Behrman et al., 2000). Other diagnoses include tumors of the auditory nerve. These tumors are most usually unilateral, with the exception of von Recklinghausen's disease, in which they are bilateral. Trauma, especially repeated exposure to loud noise, can also be a factor in hearing loss later in the child's life (Steinberg & Knightly, 1997). In general, the etiology of permanent hearing loss is estimated to be one third genetic, one third acquired, and one third of unknown cause (Coplan, 1999).

It is common to have a mixed hearing loss, with both conductive and sensorineural loss present. The conductive loss must be medically treated as efficiently as possible to minimize the total effect of the loss. Generally, if a hearing loss is measured in the "marked loss" range, it is likely to include sensorineural components. In addition to being sensorineural, conductive, or mixed, hearing loss can be of a gradual or sudden onset, stable or progressive, fluctuating or permanent.

Unilateral hearing loss is also of note because it results in weaker sound input and difficulty localizing the source of a sound. Children with unilateral hearing loss may exhibit no speech or language difficulties in early years, but research has shown a significantly higher percentage of academic failure (over 25%) in these children (Oyler, Oyler, & Matkin, 1988). This can be attributed to the developmental switch in context involved when the child goes from home, with its close parental contact, to school, with its more distant instructional form; school therapists may find this an important contributing factor in behavioral, social, and educational difficulties.

Usher's syndrome, a medical problem of adolescents with hearing loss, deserves particular consideration (Johnson, 1999). Usher's syndrome is a genetic disease that affects 3% to 6% of all individuals with congenital deafness. It is marked by the progressive blindness of retinitis pigmentosa and degeneration of the retina, which progresses from impaired night vision to gradual constriction of the visual field (with loss of peripheral vision, to blindness, usually by 20 to 30 years of age). Different types of Usher's syndrome have been identified based on symptoms and the age of onset of symptoms (Johnson, 1999). Because Usher's syndrome influences the education and vocational choices available to adolescents already dealing with hearing loss, emphasis is placed on early screening.

Measurement of Hearing Loss

The occupational therapist working with a child with hearing impairment must have an understanding of the measurement of hearing loss. This includes knowledge of the severity of the loss and its practical meaning to the child. The most commonly used measuring device is the *audiogram* (Figure 23B-1). An audiogram uses a grid to record the child's response to auditory stimuli and has a vertical axis that measures decibels. The decibel level is an indication of the loudness or intensity of the sound or sound pressure; it goes from 0 dB (the point at which

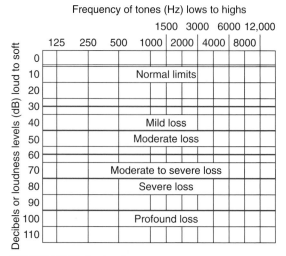

FIGURE 23B-1 Audiogram.

sound is first perceived by typically hearing people) to 140 dB (the point, or threshold, of pain of typically hearing people).

The horizontal axis of the audiogram is the *hertz* (Hz) level. This is a measure of the frequency or number of sound vibrations per second—the pitch or tone of sound. *Pitch*, or *frequency*, ranges from a low of 125 Hz to a high of 18,000 Hz on the audiogram. The range of 250 to 4,000 Hz is most important because it encompasses most speech sounds. On the audiogram, scores are plotted on the graph, beginning with the hearing threshold level (where the child first begins to hear sounds). In addition, the left and right ears are differentiated by use of colors or symbols (e.g., a circle for right and an X for left).

The decibel level is related to the distance a sound moves an air particle; it is measured by a particular standard or norm, such as the 1969 American National Standards Institute (ANSI) norm. Although it varies slightly with the norm used, a hearing level of 0 to 25 dB is considered within normal limits. Typical loss is classified according to loudness or to decibel loss and the respective therapy-education effects, which are general in nature and, of course, vary somewhat for each child and program (Anderson & Matkin, 1991). However, these measurements give the occupational therapist an idea of what to expect with a certain level of hearing loss (Table 23B-1).

Functional Implications and Intervention

A hearing aid can be used with mild hearing loss. However, the greatest benefit is derived when the hearing aid is used with a loss of up to 90 dB. Beyond that point, the loss is so severe that only partial help can be obtained. If hearing aids have been tried for a time with little or no success, individuals with a severe or profound loss may receive cochlear implants.

The frequency at which a child's loss occurs also has implications for his or her particular hearing loss. A child may have limitation in the sound frequency that helps him or her to produce particular speech sounds. This, in turn, affects hearing and language development. The hair cells inside the cochlea respond best to varied levels of frequency, depending on location, with the innermost hairs responding best to the low-tone frequencies. Depending on the location and extent of damage, there may be high-tone loss, low-tone loss, or flat loss. Frequency limitations can adversely affect syllable discrimination and understanding of speech.

A high-frequency loss means that the child can hear most of the vowel sounds (because they have a lower frequency) but misses the consonants. Because the consonant sounds carry most of the information needed to understand speech, receptive language is seriously impaired. This is because, unlike with vowels, if the

TABLE 23B-1 Therapy and Education Implications of Typical Hearing Loss Classifications

Classification	Implications
Mild loss (25 to 40 dB)	May have difficulty hearing faint or distant speech; needs favorable seating and lighting in therapy or school settings; may need speech therapy, special attention to vocabulary, or aid in some instances
Moderate loss (40 to 55 dB)	Can understand face-to-face conversational speech at a distance of 3 to 5 feet; may miss as much as 50% of group discussion if voices are low or not in the direct line of vision; may show limited vocabulary and speech anomalies; needs hearing aid evaluation and training, speech therapy, help in vocabulary and reading, and favorable seating and lighting; may need special class placement or lipreading training
Moderate to severe loss (55 to 70 dB)	Has increasing difficulty in group discussions; shows limited vocabulary and is likely to have speech anomalies and be delayed in language use and comprehension; needs special education services, speech therapy, lipreading instruction, special help with language skills, and hearing aids; needs to be encouraged in therapy-education settings to pay attention to visual and auditory input at all times; use of sign language may increase understanding
Severe loss (70 to 90 dB)	May hear loud voices about 1 foot from ear and may be able to identify environmental sounds (e.g., vacuum cleaner); may have speech difficulties, with some ability to discriminate vowels but not all consonants; if loss is present before 1 year of age, will not develop spontaneous language; needs special education services, support services, hearing aid and/or cochlear implant; needs a comprehensive program that emphasizes language and concept development, speech, lipreading, and sign language
Profound loss (90 dB or more)	May hear some loud sounds (e.g., car horn) that are very close but is aware of vibrations more than tonal patterns; must rely on vision rather than hearing as primary means of communication; sign language often the primary means of communication; deficient in speech, which does not develop spontaneously if loss is present before 1 year of age; needs special education on a comprehensive, intensive basis. (*Note:* Shouting, talking loudly, or exaggerating mouth movements and distorted speech are not helpful techniques for increasing understanding.)

consonants are deleted from words, the words are impossible to understand.

With a low-frequency loss, the child misses vowels but hears many consonants. Voices sound weak and thin, but they are understandable if the child is close enough to the speaker. A flat loss means that all frequencies are evenly affected. Voices sound far away, and certain strong vowels, such as the *a* in father, are heard best.

Although the audiogram gives information on both the decibel and hertz loss of a particular child (Martin, 1991; Newby & Poploka, 1985), the therapist should consult with the family and other professionals involved to understand how the hearing loss affects the child's functional performance.

With the increase in hearing screening programs for infants and the decrease in severe hearing loss incurred through infections subsequent to the use of antibiotics and vaccines, the focus now has switched to children with milder impairments. According to estimates by Northern and Downs (2002), compared with statistics from 20 years ago, the number of children identified with severe to profound hearing loss has decreased 50%, and the number identified with mild to moderate hearing loss has increased tenfold.

OTHER SERVICES

Often many professionals provide services to a particular child with hearing impairment. Those who specialize in hearing loss include the following:

- *Otolaryngologist* (ear, nose, and throat specialist): A physician who specializes in the anatomy, physiology, and pathologic conditions of the head and neck, including the ears, nose, and throat, and uses medical and surgical treatment techniques.
- *Otologist:* A physician who specializes in the anatomy, physiology, and pathologic conditions of the ear and uses medical and surgical treatment techniques.
- *Audiologist:* A specialist in the study of hearing who performs hearing tests and provides rehabilitation and treatment, including hearing aids, for those whose impairment cannot be improved by medical or surgical techniques.
- *Audiometrist:* A technician trained to test and measure hearing ability.
- *Auditory-verbal therapist:* A teacher of the deaf, audiologist, or speech-language pathologist who has achieved advanced practice in auditory learning.
- *Speech-language pathologist:* A specialist in the study of speech and language.

SPECIALIZED ASSESSMENT TOOLS

In the area of psychologic testing, several tests are used with children with hearing impairment. They include the following:

- *Hiskey Nebraska Test of Learning Abilities* (Hiskey, 1983). A test developed and standardized for hearing impaired children 2 to 17 years of age. It consists of subtests selected to cover a broad span of intellectual abilities without language; subtests include bead patterns, picture associations, puzzle blocks, completion of drawings, and memory for digits. The test is given in an untimed fashion.
- *Leiter International Performance Scale* (Roid & Miller, 1997). A widely used, individual IQ test administered without language for children 2 to 16 years of age. The Leiter scale is a performance test that was developed as a nonverbal counterpart to the Stanford-Binet test. It is used with children with hearing impairment, as well as others (e.g., those who do not speak English). Directions are pantomimed, and the test is not timed. Administration begins with items below the child's estimated skill level so that the child has an opportunity to become accustomed to the testing procedure. The Leiter scale has numerous subtests, which include items such as matching colors, number discrimination, pattern completion, similarities, classification of animals, and spatial relationships.
- *Kaufman Assessment Battery for Children (K-ABC)* (Kaufman & Kaufman, 1983). This test has a nonverbal scale with instructions that can be pantomimed. It is used for children 4 through $12\frac{1}{2}$ years of age, and the results provide useful information on educational recommendations for the child with hearing impairments.

Audiologic testing is a complicated and involved process (Martin, 1991; Martin & Clark, 1996; Newby & Popelka, 1985). The occupational therapist should consult the professional administering the test on details of testing with the individual child. The most common method of testing requires the use of earphones and placement of the child in a soundproof testing booth. The child indicates when he or she hears a sound.

Other forms of behavioral testing are used with children who are unable to follow the specific instructions in a standardized test. Behavioral observation audiometry (BOA) is often used with young children. In BOA, the parent holds the child in his or her lap, and the audiologist notes different behavioral responses to sounds at different levels. Another test, visual reinforcement audiometry (VRA), teaches the child to orient to a sound source reinforced with light or a visual stimulus, such as an animated lighted toy. VRA can be used for infants over 6 months of age who are normally developing to accurately assess thresholds of hearing (Kramer & Williams, 1993). Tangible reinforcement operant conditioning audiometry (TROCA) uses a token or piece of candy for reinforcement when sounds are identified. In play audiometry, the child does a certain task, such as putting a cube in a bucket, when the sound is heard.

With infants and young children who cannot be tested adequately by other means, measurement of physiologic responses is helpful in the diagnosis of hearing impairment. Auditory brain stem response (ABR) is a noninvasive procedure often done in high-risk infant follow-up programs with infants under 6 months of age or unresponsive children. It uses a type of electroencephalograph machine and a computer. Earphones are placed on a sedated or quiet child, and a series of clicks or tone bursts are played into the ears. The computer records the brain wave responses and supplies information about the auditory nerve's response to sound.

Tympanometry does not measure hearing per se but is a reliable and objective way to assess eardrum mobility or detect fluid in the middle ear. This technique requires placement of a probe in the ear canal and can be difficult to perform on an uncooperative child. The acoustic reflex measurement is tested with the same instrument as the tympanogram, but it measures the response of the two middle ear muscles to the presentation of sound.

Otoacoustic emissions (OAE) is another physiologic method useful for infants and other children who cannot be tested by behavioral means. OAE measures the responses of the middle ear and cochlea. Sound is put into the ear and is emitted back if the child has a healthy middle ear and cochlea. OAE responses are absent if the child has a middle ear problem, such as otitis media. A fail, therefore, indicates the need for further testing. Technologic advances continue to improve the efficiency and validity of audiologic testing.

WEB SITES FOR ADDITIONAL INFORMATION

National Association for the Deaf
www.nad.org
A source of books, periodicals, and videos on sign language. The organization distributes the *Deaf American Monograph Series* (deaf culture and history).

Alexander Graham Bell Association for the Deaf and Hearing Impaired
www.agbell.org
A resource center for information on hearing loss and the spoken language approach. The organization publishes the *Volta Review* (cochlear implants, hearing aids, and cued-speech; auditory verbal learning).

Registry of Interpreters for the Deaf
www.rid.org
A national organization of professionals who provide sign language interpretation/transliterating service. The organization distributes the *Journal of Interpretation*.

American Speech-Language and Hearing Association
www.asha.org
A resource for information on anatomy and etiology, assessment, and treatment of auditory impairment.

American Annals of the Deaf
www.gupress.gallaudet.edu/annals
This journal is dedicated to quality education and related services for the hearing impaired.

Journal of Deaf Studies and Deaf Education
www.deafed.oupjournals.org
A journal that integrates and coordinates basic and applied research (culture, development, linguistics, and education).

CHAPTER 24 Hospital Services

Laura Crooks ■ Barbara Marin Wavrek

CHAPTER OBJECTIVES

1 Understand the characteristics of children's hospitals.
2 Explain the roles and functions of occupational therapists in pediatric hospitals.
3 Describe occupational therapy intervention in intensive-care units and acute-care units.
4 Explain outpatient intervention models.
5 Describe hospital-based occupational therapy services for children with burns, bone marrow transplants, and failure to thrive.

Intervention with children in hospitals presents the occupational therapist with a unique set of challenges. The demands of the evolving health care system, the varied medical conditions of the children, family dynamics, and the hospital's milieu all impact occupational therapy practice. This chapter describes occupational therapy services to pediatric patients within the hospital setting. It illustrates the medical model of service delivery and explains the roles and function of hospital-based occupational therapy practitioners.

CHARACTERISTICS OF HOSPITALS AND MEDICAL SYSTEMS

Hospitals, by definition, are institutions where individuals who are ill or injured receive medical care designed to diagnose and treat the presenting problem. Over time, however, hospitals have greatly expanded their roles in the provision of health care, offering both inpatient and outpatient services for the ill and injured, as well as prevention or wellness programs designed to decrease the need for future hospitalizations and treatment. Hospitals in which pediatric patients are served generally fall into three categories: general hospitals, trauma centers, and pediatric hospitals.

General hospitals serve the needs of the community in which they are located. A wide variety of patients can be served in this type of hospital, including patients crossing the entire lifespan from infant to geriatrics. The therapist working in the general hospital setting may have the challenge of serving both adult and pediatric patients. General hospitals may have some special units dedicated to serving the needs of pediatric populations; however, the numbers of pediatric patients are not as great as found in the other two types of hospitals.

Trauma centers are hospitals certified to treat patients with more acute life-threatening injuries. Whereas general hospitals are able to serve most patients within the community, patients taken to trauma centers may have extensive injuries requiring multiple specialists. As in the general hospital setting, the occupational therapist working in the trauma center may serve patients of a variety of ages and injuries. Evaluations and treatments may initially be directed toward supporting the initial medical care of the patient, such as splinting, positioning, and evaluating oral motor skills for initial feeding. As the patient becomes more stable, additional types of interventions, such as activities of daily living (ADL) training and developmental play, can be implemented. In addition to the stress on the family of having their child in the trauma center, there may be additional family members receiving care, or families may be some distance from their homes. Therapists need to be sensitive to the stress that the families experience when their children are in these centers. Once patients are stabilized and treatment has been established, patients in the trauma centers may receive ongoing care in that particular hospital, or they may be transferred to the general hospital in their community. Therapists may be required to see patients for initial evaluations, establish some treatment plan, and then transition services to a new therapist.

Pediatric hospitals are specialty hospitals that offer a full range of inpatient and outpatient services for infants, children, and adolescents. A wide range of pediatric diagnoses are evaluated and treated, and length of stay may be longer than in a general hospital. The therapist working with children in a pediatric hospital may also have exposure to children with diseases rarely seen with limited information on treatment protocols or outcomes. For this reason, the therapist working in the pediatric hospital must have good communication skills to obtain information from medical team members of various specialties, and she or he must have a solid medical treatment foundation from which to draw treatment plan ideas. Because of the high volume of patient activity in hospitals, hospital personnel have the opportunity to gain experience in evaluation and treatment of medical conditions. In addition, these health care professionals learn to recognize individual differences in children's responses to similar medical problems. Therapists providing services within this setting type need to provide medically based intervention that is developmentally appropriate for each child.

Services provided to children in hospitals, whether general or specialized, tend to differ from the services provided to adults. Provision of medical intervention to children tends to be more labor intensive than provision of medical intervention to adults. "Sick children need more nursing care and therapy than sick adults, and children's care is about 30% more labor intensive" (Considine, 1994, p. 84). Not only must the therapist address the complications of the medical condition of the child, but he or she must also address the developmental process that has been disrupted. The therapist may not only be responsible for occupational therapy treatment planning but may also help other team members assess the impact of hospitalization on the child and develop age-appropriate strategies. Because the family is an integral part of the health care team, clear communication about the child's care plan and coordination of efforts are essential (Lindeke, Leonard, Presler, & Garwick, 2002).

Region Served

Hospitals that provide services to children may also differ in the size and location of their service regions. Children's hospitals, as specialized health care institutions, tend to serve a broader geographic region than general hospitals. This has several implications.

First, a child may be hospitalized a significant distance from home, increasing the sense of separation from family, peers, and familiar environment. Second, the distance between the home and the hospital may affect the family's ability to visit the child and remain in contact with the health personnel caring for the child. Frequently only one family member may be available to remain with the child. This can pose additional challenges for the family of not only the financial burden and psychological strains of having a child in the hospital, but the distance among family members may produce additional pressures. Third, the size of the service area, as well as the part of the country in which it is located, may mean

greater cultural diversity and socioeconomic variation among those served by the hospital. Diversity in clientele requires the medical team to be sensitive to the cultural beliefs and practices of the patient and family (Watkins, 2003). Finally, the broader geographic region served by most children's hospitals usually requires hospital personnel to interact with a great number of organizations and programs in the community to plan for services after hospital discharge (Gilkerson, Gorski, & Panitz, 1990). This distance can pose challenges for the hospital-based occupational therapist to communicate with community-based therapists regarding changes to the child's function.

Health Care Costs

An issue of concern facing hospitals that provide service to children is the cost of health care. In recent years, heath maintenance organizations (HMOs) and preferred provider organizations (PPOs) have proliferated, and between 75% and 90% of all those insured are in a managed care plan (Gabel et al., 2002; Keisler, 2000). These organizations have had a huge impact in how services are delivered and reimbursed, because they control costs by limiting consumers' options regarding services to in-network providers (Christiansen, 1996).

The prospective payment system, introduced through Medicare legislation in 1983, has also had a strong impact on reimbursement for services. This system uses pre-established rates of reimbursement for almost 1900 diagnostic groups and using more than 8000 Current Procedural Terminology (CPT) codes (Appold, 2003; Guske, 2003; Tarantino, 2002). Although this does not have as great an implication for the pediatric population as it does for the adult patient, payers do take these guidelines into consideration when authorizing care for inpatient stays. The therapist must remain aware of payment limitations when providing care and clearly communicate with families when establishing treatment plans, including equipment needs and ongoing outpatient service needs (O'Hara, 2003).

Other managed-care strategies are also designed to contain costs while maintaining quality of care. Examples of cost containment strategies include requirements for patients to obtain certification or second opinions prior to obtaining desired medical intervention (Christiansen, 1996). Managed-care strategies may result in shorter hospital stays, provision of fewer services, or limited reimbursement for services provided. One result of shorter hospital stays is the increased emphasis on outpatient diagnostic and treatment services (Buchanan, Rumpel, & Hoenig, 1996; Welch, 2002).

In addition to government-sponsored institutions, hospitals may be classified as private, nonprofit institutions or private, for-profit institutions. Each of these individual types of institution has constraints and financial limitations within their particular classification that the therapist must keep in mind when providing services. With the increasing costs and decreasing reimbursement rates or coverage for families, therapists must remain creative in their recommendations and funding options for additional services for children seen in the hospital settings.

Critical Pathways

An external force that affects the provision of occupational therapy services for children is the development of *critical pathways* for decisions regarding the most appropriate care based on a child's diagnosis. Critical pathways are diagnosis-specific protocols that define essential medical care to be provided, or actions to be taken, within identified timelines to achieve optimal outcomes for the client (Abreu, Seale, Podlesak, & Hartley, 1996; Williams, 1996).

These written documents often prescribe specific day-by-day caregiving, medical, and therapeutic procedures, from onset of the diagnosis (admission) to discharge. Ideally, critical pathways are designed to maintain the quality of patient care while increasing efficiency in the use of available resources. One area of concern is that adherence to critical pathways may decrease use of resources, thereby containing costs at the expense of quality of patient care.

Family-Centered Care

Family-centered care when a child is hospitalized means that the family has an integral role in their child's health care (Eckle & Maclean, 2001). To implement family-centered care, the family must be valued as a member of the health care team and take an active part of the decision making required to develop a treatment plan for the child. The occupational therapist working in the hospital setting where family-centered care has been adopted for the pediatric clientele must use clear descriptions to communicate evaluation results to the family, seek input from the family on which intervention outcomes for the child have priority, and come to a mutually agreed upon treatment plan. As evaluations are completed and team meetings established, caregivers are an integral part of the health care decision-making team. They, in collaboration with other team members, use the information they have learned about the child to develop care plans and a direction for treatment that involves input from all members.

Health Care Trends

Health care trends have the potential to affect the occupational therapy services provided to children. For example, affiliating children's hospitals may compare productivity statistics and quality improvement strategies among occupational therapy departments, or they may share program development information.

Hospitals are governed by internal policies and procedures that are usually designed to assist the institution in meeting standards of external, private accrediting agencies, government agencies, and insurance providers. Organizations such as the *Joint Commission for the Accreditation of Health Care Organizations (JCAHO)* and the *Commission for the Accreditation of Rehabilitation Facilities (CARF)*, as well as government agencies, such as the *Occupational Safety and Health Administration (OSHA)*, have set standards regarding hospital operations. These include standards for providing professional services, documenting patient care activities, patient and employee safety, and quality improvement activities (Commission for the Accreditation of Rehabilitation Facilities [CARF], 2003; Joint Commission for the Accreditation of Health Care Organizations [JCAHO], 1994).

Employee education regarding safety practices (when there is risk of exposure to patient blood or body fluids) or to hazardous materials is also mandated (Occupational Exposure to Blood-Borne Pathogens, 1991). Also of particular importance when working with pediatric populations in the hospital setting is the inclusion that occupational therapists are mandated reporters of child abuse. They are required to report any suspicion of abuse to designated personnel within the hospital setting, who, when appropriate, contact community support services such as law enforcement personnel or Child Protective Services (CPS). Specific training in each institution regarding reporting protocols must be established and provided to the therapists in these settings. These safety and protective measures are included in the occupational therapy department policies, procedures, and service delivery.

One trend among hospitals has been the affiliation of similar institutions, offering opportunities for consolidation of information and equipment, achievement of common goals, and program development. Hospitals are generally part of medical systems directed by a single administration and linking facilities that share certain resources and specialized personnel. One system offers patients are spectrum of placement options including acute, subacute, rehabilitation, outpatient, skilled nursing facilities, and home health care.

Trends in managed care that result in shorter hospital stays and limited reimbursement have the potential to restrict occupational therapy services and to shift the emphasis to provision of outpatient services. As part of the current trend toward decentralization of hospital-based services, many pediatric facilities have established outpatient satellite centers in the community, which may provide both medical and therapy services (Cheng, Greenberg, Loeser, & Keller, 2000; Gipe, 2000; Jordan, 2001).

HOSPITAL-BASED SERVICES

Gilkerson (1990) identified the preservation of life as the most important function in a hospital and suggested that life-threatening conditions take priority in the scheme of hospital activities. Hospitals offer a range of hospital-based-services designed to provide medical care to children with acute or chronic illness, traumatic injury, or special needs. The method of service delivery varies according to the needs of the patient and the nature of the medical care required. For patients with burns, patients undergoing oncology treatment, or those who require bone marrow transplants, the hospital environment is designed to minimize the risk of infection to patients who are especially susceptible, while enabling the completion of the medical protocol.

Acute care, intensive and critical care, special care, medical or surgical care, ambulatory or *outpatient services, and teaching and research* are just some of the hospital-based services with which occupational therapists should be familiar. Many children enter and leave the hospital system at different points along this continuum of services; others experience the full range of services. Therapists must be familiar with the treatment implications at each stage of the service delivery.

A child with severe burns, for example, may initially be admitted to an intensive care unit (ICU) because of the life-threatening nature of the injury. Once the child's medical condition stabilizes, he or she may be transferred to a special unit for children with burns for continuation of treatment. When hospitalization is no longer necessary, the child is discharged but may be asked to return to the outpatient clinic for occupational therapy, physical therapy, or for follow-up visits with physicians, therapists, and other hospital personnel.

Most patient-care activity in hospitals is acute care. Acute care refers to short-term medical care provided during the acute phase of an illness or injury, when the symptoms are generally the most severe. Just as there are degrees of severity that categorize illnesses and injuries, there are also levels of acute care designed to meet these varied needs. The occupational therapist providing services to pediatric patients during this phase must consider the long-term implications of the illness or injury while addressing the acute needs of the patient. Families may experience increased stress during this phase and therefore may require that the information be repeated or may need more time to process the results from testing. The therapist should involve the family in treatment planning, including discharge planning. Because hospital stays are short, available outpatient treatment options need to be considered early and caregivers given this information to facilitate continuity of services from inpatient to outpatient settings.

Critically ill patients who require continuous monitoring and frequent medical attention, and patients who often need special equipment to maintain or monitor vital functions, are admitted to *intensive care units (ICUs)* or *critical care units (CCUs)*. Hospitals may have several intensive-care units, each of which is designated for a specific patient population or purpose. *Neonatal intensive-care units (NICUs), pediatric intensive-care units (PICUs)* for older children, and *surgical intensive-care units (SICUs)* are examples of intensive care units that may be found in hospitals. Personnel who provide care for patients in ICUs receive special training to enable them to respond quickly and effectively to meet the needs of medically unstable patients in this challenging environment. Families are generally in closer contact during this time, and it is imperative that the therapist keeps family caregivers apprised of the ongoing treatment plan and implications during this stage. Therapists must also have clear communication with other medical personnel working with the patient on these units, particularly with the intensive-care nurse caring for the child.

A child whose illness or injury results in hospitalization, but who does not need the continuous attention, high technology, and specialized care of an ICU, may be admitted to a *medical* or *surgical acute-care unit*. Medical and surgical units also tend to be designated for specific types of patients. For example, patients requiring neurosurgical services may be cared for on one unit, whereas patients requiring orthopedic-related treatment may be served on another. Within the designation of these units, patients may also be grouped according to age. Grouping children by age can facilitate developmentally appropriate care and allow for environments that are designed to match children and youth's age-based interests.

Although patients in a critical-care unit may share a common diagnosis, they may be at different points in their treatment and recovery. By contrast, patients with infectious conditions may have a variety of diagnoses that require treatment under isolation conditions. If this is the case, these patients are often placed in *special-care units*. Three conditions that require a child to be treated in a special care unit are (1) *acute burns,* (2) *infectious diseases,* and (3) *bone marrow transplantation.*

Medical intervention for chronically ill patients may also be provided in hospitals that emphasize acute care. Often, chronically ill patients are admitted for an acute exacerbation of their illnesses or for treatment of complications. Diabetes, asthma, cystic fibrosis, and cancer are examples of chronic illnesses occurring in children that may require periodic hospitalization. Patients who have progressive illness may also be seen for acute issues relating to the next stage of the disease process. For example, a youth diagnosed with Duchenne's muscular dystrophy may experience a decrease in oral motor skills and subsequently be admitted for aspiration pneumonia. The therapist must not only be aware of ongoing disease process but also take into consideration maximal quality of life when establishing treatment strategies for these patients.

In some instances, chronically ill patients who are medically fragile may receive long-term care in an acute hospital setting. This long-term care may be required because the family is unable or unwilling to care for the child at home and a special placement elsewhere in the region is not readily available. DeWitt, Jansen, Ward, and Keens (1993) found that children who required ventilator assistance often remained in the hospital for nonmedical reasons after becoming medically stable. Two factors that significantly delayed hospital discharge were difficulty arranging either out-of-home placement or financial assistance to enable care in the home. Although a growing number of pediatric specialized subacute settings are available for these patients, they often cannot meet the numbers of patients who would benefit from such a setting. Despite the shortage of subacute facilities, there continues to be an increasing emphasis on arranging return to home or community placement as quickly as possible, including the use of medical foster care placement (Committee on Early Childhood, Adoption, and Dependent Care, 2002; Leslie, Kelleher, Burns, Landsverk, & Rolls, 2003; Smith, 2002).

Ambulatory and outpatient services or programs are designed for patients who require medical services but whose conditions do not require hospitalization. These services may also include visits to clinics (for continuity of care after discharge from the hospital) or special services, such as outpatient occupational therapy or physical therapy. Therapists may see pediatric patients in conjunction with other subspecialty health care providers to provide the family with new or ongoing information and help formulate a plan of care and support for additional services needed in the community. Occupational therapists may see pediatric outpatients for one-time evaluations, such as for equipment recommendations to support community providers, or for ongoing outpatient treatment, such as for the pediatric patient who underwent hand surgery.

Although most hospital services are directed toward providing medical care to the ill or injured, many hospitals also include teaching and research as part of their missions. The hospital, as a teaching institution, provides clinical education experiences for medical students, interns, residents, nursing students, and students from other health-related professions. As a research institution, a hospital often provides resources and opportunities for clinical research to advance medical knowledge and practice. In training and research hospitals, occupational therapists can access many different educational opportunities, including access to many different health care professionals. Continual education and teaching within these settings, not only for the occupational therapy student but also for students of other health professions, is important. Another benefit to the occupational therapist working in a teaching institution is the access to the latest intervention strategies and clinical trials to facilitate new medical interventions. A therapist may participate in research or provide information to a researcher conducting a study, making it important for that therapist to understand the hospital's policies on informed consent, confidentiality, and protection of research participants.

MEDICAL MODEL AND TEAM INTERACTION

In most medical systems, the physician is considered the leader of the medical team for a given child, although leadership may shift to other team members during the course of the child's stay (Case-Smith & Wavrek, 1998). The child's *care manager* is often a registered nurse or other medical professional whose services have been formally requested by the physician. The parents who are also members of the team are also responsible for the child's care.

Three factors that often affect the parents' participation in the child's care are (1) the distance between the family's home and the hospital, (2) the parents' other obligations including work and child care, and (3) cultural values. These factors may limit the parents' ability to visit the hospital and may limit their ability to interact with the professionals caring for their child. This is particularly true when the child is experiencing a prolonged hospital stay. When parents are limited in their ability to participate, the therapist must find alternative ways to facilitate communication regarding evaluations and treatment plans. Cultural implications may also influence family participation including experiential influences. For family members, there may be beliefs or previous situations that lead to preconceived ideas of what will happen during the hospital stay. This can lead to a feeling of discomfort with medical personnel and situations. The therapist must reflect on his or her own belief systems and attitudes and refrain from passing judgement of parents who have different obligations, attitudes, beliefs, in order to foster open communication and thus enhance the therapy intervention process.

Another significant characteristic of medical teams is their dynamic nature. Because the health care disciplines represented in a specific case depend on the patient's needs, the medical team is continually changing. For example, a child with a feeding disorder who is failing to grow and gain weight may have a physician, nurses, an occupational therapist, a dietitian, and a social worker as members of his or her medical team. However, a child hospitalized with multiple injuries resulting from a motor vehicle accident may have several physicians, nurses, an occupational therapist, a physical therapist, a speech pathologist, a dietitian, a respiratory therapist, and a social worker as members of his or her medical team. In addition, the team within one child's hospitalization may change. For example, the child admitted to the hospital for pneumonia may initially be seen by the pulmonary physician and perhaps social worker, along with nursing, later to have the occupational therapist and speech pathologist involved when aspiration is suspected and later a physician from gastroenterology involved when it is discovered reflux is the culprit. As a potential member of multiple medical teams within one hospital, the occupational therapist must communicate and collaborate with professionals from many different health-related fields. Frequently, the therapist may be required to continually redefine or explain the role of the occupational therapist to other team members, as well as to develop an understanding of the ways in which different team members' roles complement each other in the provision of services to children. With the trend toward "hospital systems," described previously, occupational therapists employed by hospitals may face the more complex challenges of defining their roles in several different settings within one integrated system of care and participating in interdisciplinary medical teams across the spectrum of care (Treloar & Graham, 2003).

Communication of hospital team members is dependent on a number of factors. One significant factor is the limited availability of team members for scheduled meetings. Communication tends to occur *formally* through documentation in the patient's chart and *informally* during telephone calls or chance meetings throughout the day. "What appear as unplanned interactions are actually an accepted and effective way of doing business in a setting where time is at a premium, needs are immediate, and staff schedules can change daily" (Gilkerson et al., 1990, pp. 453-454).

Communication with the patient or parent occurs at separate times for most team members. Regular team meetings, although ideal, are often not feasible in a hospital setting because of the multiple demands on hospital personnel and the likelihood of schedule changes.

SPECIAL NEEDS OF CHILDREN IN HOSPITALS

Hospital services, including occupational therapy, must take into consideration the child's developmental level and needs, the impact of illness or injury and hospitalization on development, and the coping strategies and needs of the family in relation to the child's medical condition. Hospitalized children are placed in a situation filled with unknowns and events over which they have little control. Sources of stress for the child include separation from family and the home environment, the unfamiliarity of the hospital, the increased dependency that often is associated with illness or injury and hospitalization, the unfamiliar and frequently changing

hospital caregivers, and the often painful medical procedures that may be required (Board & Ryan-Wenger, 2002).

Realization of potential disability or disfigurement and boredom may also add to the child's stress. The child may experience anxiety, withdrawal, regression, increased demand for parental attention, and a need for behavioral management (Knudson-Cooper, 1982; Suhr, 1986). For very young children, this is complicated by their limited ability to understand the purpose or need for the hospitalization and the anxiety produced by separation from parents or other caregivers (Rennick, Johnston, Dougherty, Platt, & Ritchie, 2002; Wilson & Broome, 1989).

The fears provoked by hospitalization may be exacerbated by a diminished ability to cope (Gohsman, 1981). Consequently, the illness or injury and the stress of hospitalization may result in developmental regression, or it may hinder developmental progress. Petrillo and Sanger (1980) suggested that the child's successful adaptation to the overwhelming stresses of illness and hospitalization relates to his or her ability to achieve a sense of mastery over the situation.

The occupational therapist's knowledge of age-appropriate developmental tasks and understanding of the importance of purposeful activity can help the child achieve a sense of control in the foreign environment of the hospital. The occupational therapist can also help other members of the medical team understand the developmental issues of concern and suggest strategies to caregivers and family members that support typical development and help the child better cope with hospitalization. In addition, the occupational therapist may work closely with the child life specialist to help develop coping strategies within the functional abilities of the child.

CHARACTERISTICS OF HOSPITAL-BASED OCCUPATIONAL THERAPY

Many of the evaluation and treatment strategies used by occupational therapists are not unique to hospital-based practice. Instead, they tend to be the same approaches used with children in other settings. However, the diagnoses seen in hospitals challenge the occupational therapist to adapt intervention to meet specific, often acute, needs, and they require the therapist to utilize multiple intervention approaches to achieve goals.

Examples of diagnoses and problems referred to occupational therapy include developmental delay, feeding disorders, orthopedic disorders, traumatic brain injury, neurological problems, neuromuscular diseases, or congenital syndromes resulting in medical complications. Specific diagnoses the occupational therapist working with pediatric patients may encounter may include burns, cancer, renal disease, cardiac defects, endocrine disorders, traumatic brain injury, muscular dystrophy, and encephalitis or meningitis, to name a few. The occupational therapist must have a thorough understanding of the diagnosis, prognosis, contraindications, and other implications of the child's illness, injury, or medical treatment.

For most children, services are provided in a relatively brief period, requiring the occupational therapist to be highly efficient. This brief treatment requires the therapist to establish realistic treatment priorities appropriate for the patient's projected length of stay in the hospital (Freda, 1998). To do this, the evaluation process must be streamlined, and occupational therapists must prioritize treatment goals as they are identified. When possible, discharge plans are articulated as part of the initial evaluation (Freda, 1998). Rausch and Melvin (1986) suggested, "A target skill for the acute-care therapist is the ability to integrate evaluation, treatment, and patient instruction into each therapy session" (p. 321).

In a children's hospital, the broad range of diagnoses requires that occupational therapists have expertise in a wide range of assessment, modalities, and interventions. However, the need for a broad range of skills does not mean a lack of specialization. "Occupational therapy services tend to be highly specialized in a pediatric facility and well-developed in specialty areas (e.g., neonatal care, upper-extremity anomalies, and burns)" (Case-Smith & Wavrek, 1998, p. 84).

Occupational therapy services for the hospitalized child vary according to the type of facility, the child's diagnosis, and the length of stay. For a child with a short or acute stay, the emphasis of occupational therapy tends to be on assessment, with program planning, recommendations for follow-up after discharge, and equipment provision or fabrication occurring as needed. The initial evaluation may be the only contact the therapist has with the child before discharge, and thus the therapist must quickly determine additional outpatient needs or home instructions for patients and families.

A child hospitalized for a long time may have the benefit of receiving occupational therapy services one or two times daily, depending on the child's needs. A longer stay also provides the occupational therapist with more opportunities to interact with the family, provide parent education, and plan for discharge cooperatively with the family and other team members. Children with extended acute phases of illness or injury (e.g., those with burns, traumatic brain injury, or encephalitis), often require different and more comprehensive services than chronically ill children (e.g., those with cancer, cystic fibrosis, or diabetes) who are hospitalized frequently for exacerbations of their illness. The longer lengths of stay allow time for teams to meet to coordinate services and to collaborate in developing discharge plans.

In some instances, services for children with acute illness or injury may be limited to provision of a piece of adaptive equipment, such as a protective helmet for a patient with neurosurgical needs or a bath bench for a patient undergoing limb lengthening of their lower extremity. For patients with chronic conditions who receive occupational therapy in the community, occupational therapy services in the hospital may focus on provision of equipment or completion of evaluations that are not readily available to the occupational therapist in the community.

For example, a child with a severe developmental disability who is hospitalized with pneumonia resulting from the aspiration of food might be referred to the hospital radiology, occupational therapy, and speech pathology departments for an evaluation of feeding. This evaluation would include a videofluoroscopic swallowing study (Figure 24-1). In situations of this type, close communication between the hospital- and community-based occupational therapists is essential and can result in better total care for the child and family.

SCOPE OF OCCUPATIONAL THERAPY SERVICES

Pediatric patients are admitted to the hospital setting for several different reasons, and they can move through these categories as symptoms stabilize or effects become more apparent.

- Patients may be admitted for acute care of their illnesses. The therapist must perform an initial assessment of the patient and provide caregivers and the patient with instructions, home programs, or follow-up outpatient services. This can also include those patients admitted for diagnostic reasons that then need to be transitioned to outpatient services.
- Patients may be admitted for rehabilitation services. The child may initially be admitted for acute care reasons, then require more extensive and comprehensive therapy interventions. In this case, the therapist must evaluate the level of functioning of the child, develop a treatment plan, and involve the family in implementation of treatment goals and objectives that lead to increased function and independence in order to discharge from the hospital.
- Patients with chronic illnesses may be admitted for exacerbation of symptoms or for complications resulting from illnesses. These patients may be seen for modified continuation of their outpatient therapy already established, or they may need to be evaluated to provide information regarding changing levels of function.

In each case, occupational therapy intervention may differ according to the patient's needs and the length of stay. In some instances, level of service may be affected by staff shortages, which result in prioritizing which patients receive occupational therapy services (Rausch & Melvin, 1986). Payers may also dictate length of stay for

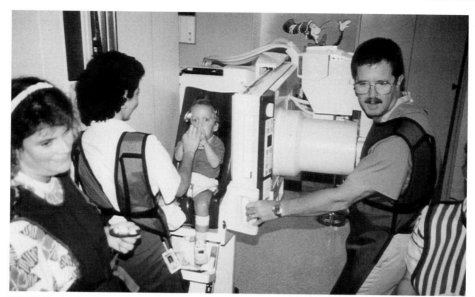

FIGURE 24-1 An interdisciplinary team uses videofluoroscopy to assess a client's swallowing and risk for aspiration.

the patient, and shortened stays necessitate streamlined service delivery.

The patient with a single injury (e.g., a hand injury) or a single episode of illness tends to have a short hospital stay with a predictable course of treatment. Some patients admitted for an acute illness or injury may require extended rehabilitation, depending on the severity of the injury and resulting complications. Traumatic brain injury and spinal cord injury are two examples of injuries that require both initial acute treatment and long-term rehabilitation. The length of the hospital stay for this type of patient during the acute phase of illness or injury tends to vary because the potential for complications is greater and these patients must be relatively medically stable before transferring to the rehabilitative service.

The chronically ill patient is hospitalized periodically for acute episodes of an illness or complications of an illness. Children with diabetes, cancer, or cardiac conditions fall into this category. The length of hospital stay for these patients is also variable. Children hospitalized for diagnostic testing or adjustment of medications can expect a comparatively short hospital stay. Consequently, the occupational therapist may be involved in evaluation and treatment planning that may transfer to community providers. Occupational therapy evaluation in acute-care services focuses on the child's developmental or functional status within the context of the illness or injury that has resulted in hospitalization. Completion of the assessment may present a challenge for the occupational therapist, because the length of hospital stay is often short and other hospital services are competing for the patient's time. Evaluations completed by the occupational therapist may also be used as a screen to rule out

other illnesses or processes (e.g., in a child with pneumonia, an evaluation for aspiration can lead to an eventual diagnosis of reflux).

Evaluation may begin with a chart review to obtain information about the child's medical status, the current course of medical care and goals, contraindications or precautions that may have an impact on the occupational therapy services provided, and the patient's functional level before the hospitalization. Information concerning family structure, birth history, and the child's past developmental course may also contribute to the occupational therapist's understanding of the child and family's needs. An interview with the parents, if possible, is often the source of valuable information regarding the child's current status and reveals the parents' priorities for the child.

Before completing a functional or developmental evaluation, the occupational therapist establishes a rapport with the child and family. Increasing the comfort level of the child and family is particularly important because of the stressful and frightening nature of the hospital environment. A positive relationship between the child and therapist serves to foster cooperation, decrease the child's anxiety about the evaluation process, and enable the therapist to obtain results that reflect the child's actual functional abilities. Tiberius, Sackin, Tallett, Jacobson, and Turner (2001) completed a study in which medical students were given the opportunity to talk informally with parents of medically ill children. They found that this interaction not only decreased the anxiety of the parents and the child, but enhanced the provision of services by allowing more honest and complete information sharing between caregivers, namely the parents and the medical student, establishing a foundation for

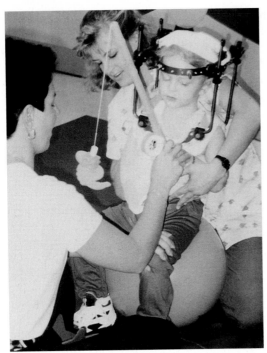

FIGURE 24-2 An occupational therapist and physical therapist collaborate on a client evaluation.

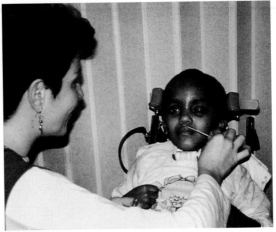

FIGURE 24-3 An occupational therapist evaluates oral-motor skills before feeding a client.

communication and trust within the stressful hospital environment.

The choice of evaluation tools and methods depends on the child's age, diagnosis, and the protocol of the occupational therapy department. For example, a 10-year-old child with a serious hand injury might be referred for evaluation of strength, sensation, fine coordination, passive and active range of motion, independence in self-care, and the need for a splint to assist function or prevent deformity. By contrast, a 2-year-old child referred for developmental delay (secondary to chronic illness) may receive a developmental assessment that includes administration of a standardized test, such as the Bayley Scales of Infant Development, revised (BSID-II), evaluation of motor function (e.g., muscle tone, automatic postural responses, or coordination), daily living, and play skills.

An evaluation of this type is often performed in collaboration or cooperation with professionals from other disciplines, such as physical therapy and speech pathology (Figure 24-2). In both instances, the occupational therapist is concerned with occupational performance areas, skills, and contexts in relation to the child's age and development.

In some cases, the child's medical condition, a short length of stay, or a stressful and restrictive environment (e.g., an ICU) may prohibit the administration of a standardized evaluation. In these instances, the therapist's clinical observations of key performance areas and components may be the best alternative (Figure 24-3).

Finally, assessment in acute care also includes evaluation of the need for specialized equipment, both for use in the hospital and for use after discharge. Specialized equipment may include adapted utensils for self-feeding for a patient with a spinal cord injury, an adapted bath seat for a patient with cerebral palsy, a pressure garment to prevent hypertrophic scarring for a patient with burn injuries, a protective helmet for a patient with a skull fracture, or splints for a patient with juvenile rheumatoid arthritis. In some instances, the therapist and child may need to experiment with different pieces of equipment to determine which is best for the child's use. Therapists must also be cautioned when recommending equipment for children whose families have limited funding or resources. The occupational therapist must have knowledge of the payer durable medical equipment (DME) benefits and discuss potential financial obligations of equipment to families. Therapists should offer families options for obtaining needed equipment. This may include lower-cost alternatives, such as using piping insulation for built-up handles rather than prefabricated ones or accessing "loner closets" for obtaining or renting used equipment, such as bath equipment or lifts.

INTENSIVE CARE UNIT SERVICES

Occupational therapy services may be initiated with a patient at any point during the course of hospitalization. However, they usually occur once a patient has achieved sufficient medical stability to initiate rehabilitation. In the intensive care unit, the child is often evaluated and treated at bedside because of the critical nature of the illness or injury and the need for constant monitoring of the child's medical status.

Occupational therapy intervention in intensive care supports the medical team's priorities and goals for the child. It is also essential that the therapist be knowledgeable about the child's diagnosis and resulting potential precautions as well as the implications of medical procedures, the use of life-support or monitoring equipment, and contraindications for certain activities or positions. The occupational therapist is responsible for constant monitoring of the child's status during the time he or she is with the patient, making it imperative for the therapist to understand the significance of changes in the patient's vital signs, respiratory function, appearance, or symptoms as a result of the intervention being completed.

There are three categories of problems related to the intensive care environment and child's status that affect both the child and intervention. These are (1) immobility and the need for bed rest, (2) sensory deprivation and stress, and (3) extended mechanical ventilation (Affleck, Lieberman, Polon, & Rohrkemper, 1986; Morrison, Haas, Shaffner, Garrett, & Fackler, 2003).

Prolonged bed rest and immobility often occur as a result of the critical nature of the illness, the use of high-technology equipment, or the need for restraints for the child's safety and care. The average length of stay for a child in the ICU is 4 to 6 days. However, it may be extended if the illness or injury is severe. The potential impact of extended immobility includes decreased endurance, potential for contractures, generalized weakness, and poor tolerance for sitting. As part of an occupational therapy program, graded activities are presented and the child's participation is solicited to improve endurance and strength and to enhance functional performance. It is important the therapist collaborate with family caregivers and other health care providers to establish a treatment plan. The therapist may have goals of increasing participation, independence, and endurance for the child, while the nurse may feel more rest is required. Discussing goals and outcomes including balancing the medical needs can facilitate a team approach to accomplishing the desired outcome for the patient. Establishment of a routine, including regular therapy times within the constraints of the intensive care unit, can also help with orientation for the patient and help facilitate regular participation. Family members or other caregivers are also often involved in carrying out treatments, such as range of motion, throughout the day. This provides them the opportunity to become more involved in the care of their child during this portion of their hospitalization (Tomlinson, Swiggum, & Harbaugh, 1999; Tomlinson, Thomlinson, Peden-McAlping, & Kirschbaum, 2002).

"Elements of activities that can be graded include time required to complete the task, amount and speed of active movement, level of assistance given, adaptive aids, and position and postural support. The most important parameter in grading a task is a patient's physiological response. The patient's level of activity can be upgraded only when vital signs, symptoms, and respiratory function are acceptable at the existing level of activity" (Affleck et al., 1986, p. 324).

In addition to a program of graded activity, occupational therapy intervention may include positioning recommendations or splints to preserve range of motion and prevent deformity, and specialized equipment to facilitate function. A plan for wear or use should be established with the family and other care providers to ensure compliance. Caregivers should also be instructed on any potential side effects, such as pressure areas with splints, so plans can be modified as needed.

Sensory deprivation and stress resulting from the intensive care environment may also complicate a child's illness and recovery. The lack of privacy, immobility, and the continuous sounds and lights of the intensive care unit provide the child with an atypical sensory experience. If the child is hospitalized within the intensive care unit for a prolonged period, ICU psychosis may ensue, in which the child may have altered mental status (Granberg, Engberd, & Lundberg, 1999; Hewitt-Taylor, 1999). In addition, there are few indicators to orient the child to changes in time and day. Occupational therapy intervention may help counteract the effects of stress and sensory deprivation by fostering the establishment of a routine for the child and providing purposeful activities to facilitate cognitive, psychosocial, and motor functions (Affleck et al., 1986). Positive social interaction and the use of entertainment and play activities may be especially helpful for reducing stress and promoting development of young children in the ICU.

To summarize, the occupational therapist providing services in the ICU must have a thorough understanding of the patient's condition, the purpose of intensive care, the medical priorities for the patient, and the importance of monitoring the patient's physiologic status before, during, and after occupational therapy. Two important emphases for the occupational therapist working with children in intensive care are (1) provision of graded, meaningful activities (e.g., play activities, self-care activities) to improve endurance, strength, and functional abilities (e.g., cognition, psychosocial function, and motor abilities) and (2) provision of specialized equipment, splints, and positioning recommendations as needed (Figure 24-4).

Case Study: Intervention for Child in the Intensive Care Unit
Presenting Information

Michael is a 6-year-old boy admitted to the intensive care unit with a diagnosis of necrotizing fasciitis with sepsis. He was initially seen at the general hospital in his community, approximately 2 hours distance from the pediatric hospital in the area. On initial examination, Michael was found to have decreased sensation with decreased circulation to both fingers and toes. In addition he had

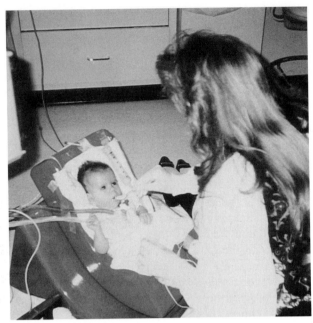

FIGURE 24-4 An occupational therapist assesses oral motor and feeding abilities in a client requiring ventilator assistance for respiration.

a high fever (104.7° F) and was lethargic. He was airlifted to the pediatric center, and en route he began experiencing organ failure, including a cardiac arrest. His mother was able to accompany him in the airlift, but his father was required to drive due to space constraints.

Background Information

Prior to his hospitalization, Michael was a typically developing young boy. He resided on a reservation with both of his parents. He attended first grade at the local elementary school, achieving average grades for his age. He also took pride in participating in the Native American Dance Troupe associated with his tribe and had been participating in exhibits nationally with his troupe since age 3.

Michael had been playing in the park near his home with friends when he fell out of a tree and was cut by a branch. He did not return home right away, but once he did return, his mother noted that the area was red and slightly warm. She cleaned the area with soap and water and placed a Band-Aid. The next day, Michael was noted to have a slight fever and was complaining of generalized discomfort. By the second day, he was increasing in his complaints, would not let anyone touch his arm, and his fever had increased, even with medication and home remedies. He was taken to his family physician. By the time he was seen in the physician's office, Michael had increased lethargy, was in and out of consciousness, and had a high fever. He was subsequently airlifted to the local pediatric hospital due to his quickly advancing deterioration.

Medical and Occupational Therapy Intervention

Upon arriving at the pediatric hospital, Michael had required ventilation support, and his medical status continued to deteriorate. Evaluation revealed staphylococcal sepsis with intravascular coagulopathy and he was admitted to the intensive care unit. During the first 48 hours, Michael continued to deteriorate, with continued organ failure. He required continuous medical interventions including dialysis, ventilation support, and surgical intervention for increasing necrotizing digits including amputation of toes and fingers.

Occupational therapy was consulted early in his care to provide positioning and maintain range of motion for those joints not affected. The occupational therapists fabricated splints for both his hands and feet, and he was placed on a schedule that required him to wear them at all times except when dressing changes. His parents were also instructed on simple range of motion techniques they could carry out to maintain his range and to participate in his care.

Although Michael's condition initially continued to deteriorate, necessitating amputation on one leg above knee, the other at the ankle, and all but two fingers, his family held out hope that he would come through this devastating illness. The parents pulled in the assistance of their tribal leaders to provide guidance and use tribal medicine to enhance Western medicine techniques. Leaders were granted permission to visit Michael within the intensive care unit, with clear guidelines on acceptable interventions.

During this time, the occupational therapist continued to monitor positioning and range of motion. The therapist collaborated with nursing personnel to help with positioning both Michael and his medical devices to enable his mom to rock him in a chair at bedside. As his medical condition stabilized, endurance and strengthening activities were introduced. This included adaptive devices to enable him to begin basic bedside ADL. His physical therapist gave Michael a wheelchair, and gloves were adapted to ease the use of his hands when he propelled the chair to and from the nurses' station. As he continued to increase his strength and function, he was eventually discharged from the intensive care unit and transferred to the pediatric rehabilitation unit where he continued to increase his functional performance.

BURN UNIT

One of the specialty ICUs found in larger hospitals is the *burn unit*. The cause of the burn injury, the depth of the burn (e.g., partial to full thickness), the percentage of total body surface area (TBSA) affected, the location of the burn, and the age of the patient are factors considered in classifying a burn according to severity. Medical treatment for burns varies according to the severity. However, in general, burn wounds are treated with a local application of an antibacterial agent and, if needed, surgeries to remove burned tissue and cover the affected area with skin grafts (Rivers & Jordan, 1998).

Parenteral hyperalimentation is often administered to maintain adequate nutrition during the early recovery periods. Major burns result in a 40% to 100% increase in energy expenditure, and good nutrition is essential for healing (Murphy, Purdue, Hunt, & Hicks, 1997). The long, often painful recovery process and the potential for lasting disfigurement and disability challenge the child and family's coping skills. For these reasons, occupational therapy with the burned child presents a special challenge.

Rivers and Jordan (1998) described three stages in the burn-injury recovery process: (1) the acute-care stage, (2) the surgical and postoperative stage, and (3) the rehabilitation stage.

The medical focus of the acute-care stage is the replacement of lost body fluids, stabilization of the patient, and care of the burn wounds. Daily wound débridement and dressing changes are needed. Occupational therapy intervention during this phase may include prevention of the loss of joint mobility, strength, and endurance; self-care activities; and education of the child and family regarding the rehabilitation process (Rivers & Jordan, 1998).

Surgical removal of burned tissue, skin grafts, and postoperative recovery characterize the surgical and postoperative stage. Immobilization of the affected area through positioning or splints is required for approximately 3 to 7 days after surgery. In addition to the fabrication of splints and provision of positioning recommendations, serial splint placement may be used to gradually increase range of motion. The occupational therapist may provide adaptive devices to assist with ADL or other activities (Biggs, de Linde, Banaszewski, & Heinrich, 1998; Ho, Chan, Ying, Cheng, & Wong, 2001).

During the rehabilitation stage, wound healing continues. The patient is susceptible to scarring and contracture formation during this period. Although the rehabilitation phase begins during hospitalization, it often continues after discharge on an outpatient basis and through home programs until the patient's scars are mature. This process may take up to 2 years. Scarring, especially hypertrophic scarring, can significantly interfere with a patient's functional recovery. Hypertrophic scars tend to be thick, inflexible, and red. If they cross joints, these scars can impair joint mobility because of tightening of the skin.

Elastic wraps (e.g., Jobst garments), tailor-made to conform to the child's body, decrease the formation of hypertrophic scarring. Constant pressure through these

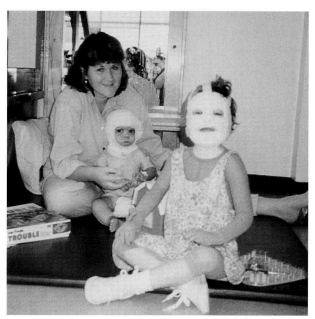

FIGURE 24-5 Face masks and custom-fabricated pressure garments assist in scar management for children with severe burns.

Jobst garments, elastomer inserts, and facial masks is applied 24 hours a day for 6 to 24 months to obtain an optimal cosmetic result (Murphy et al., 1997). (See Figure 24-5.)

Occupational therapists contribute to the following desired outcomes:

Occupation Level
1 Enable the child to return to his or her prior level of independence in school and the community
2 Return the child to developmentally appropriate levels of play and daily living skills
3 Support and, when needed, improve the child's social participation.

Client Factors
4 Assist in the prevention of deformity, contracture, and hypertrophic scar formation
5 Maintain full active range of motion and strength

The following case study illustrates the complexity of intervention with a child admitted to the burn unit of a hospital.

Case Study: Intervention for Child with Burn Injuries
Presenting Information

Katie was a 20-month-old girl who was admitted with 65% TBSA flame burns.

Background Information

Katie was a typically developing toddler prior to her burns. She lived in a ranch-style home with her mother and maternal grandfather and several animals. Katie was described as an outgoing, active child. The family had been fumigating the home, and on the evening of the house fire, candles were burning to decrease some of the smells. One candle was inadvertently left burning too close to a curtain in the bedroom shared by Katie and her mother, and the curtain caught fire. Her mother discovered the fire, and her grandfather ran in to get Katie, whose bed had caught fire at that point. Neither Katie's mother nor her grandfather was injured in the incident.

Occupational Therapy and Medical Intervention

Katie was initially seen in the emergency room where she was diagnosed with 65% total body surface area partial and full thickness burns. Initial upper extremity escharotomies were performed, and she was transferred to the burn intensive care unit. She continued to have complications from her burns, requiring bilateral upper and lower extremity escharotomies, decompressive laparotomy, debridement of burns, grafting, with nonburned skin areas used as donor sights. Integra was also used for grafting as Katie did not have enough viable donor skin to cover burned areas. She required initial pinning of her left hand with metacarpophalangeal (MCP) joint flexion and interphalangeal (IP) extension. She subsequently required additional pinning of her right hand in the same manner. Throughout her initial course, Katie remained on mechanical ventilation with transcutaneous parenteral nutritional support. She was heavily medicated to provide sedation throughout the initial period.

Occupational therapy was consulted for positioning and splinting while Katie was in the ICU. Initial splinting included bilateral resting hand splints and lower extremity foot drop splinting. She required positioning to keep bilateral axilla areas open, with stockinette used as a sling over the bed frame. Once Katie was stable, a range-of-motion program was instituted. She required multiple revisions of her splints as her swelling decreased and some of her grafts became stable. She was transferred from the ICU to the burn unit when she became more stable and less sedation was required. Serial casting of her elbows and wrists was also completed. During this time, her family was taught to begin some of her stretching program. Once her grafts were stable, pressure garments were measured and obtained.

Of particular concern for Katie was her scarring. She developed hypertrophic scarring on the dorsal surfaces of both hands, with ligamentous tightening on her left hand despite stretching and splinting efforts. These required surgical release and additional grafting. Lotion was applied to skin to keep grafts supple and for scar massage. She was placed in pressure garments, including face mask, for 23 hours per day.

Katie also experienced delays in her ADL and play occupations and in motor skills as a result of her burns and her prolonged hospitalization. She lost previously mastered milestones and required distraction and encouragement to bear weight on her feet due to pain from burns. Child life therapists were involved to help Katie develop coping mechanisms during painful procedures through play and relaxation techniques such as music and therapeutic touch. Her family was shown play techniques to allow Katie to slowly increase her independence and play skills. Adaptive utensils for eating and eventually for writing/coloring were used, first with the use of a universal cuff and then with built-up handles. Over time, as her range of motion increased, she was able to eliminate the use of adaptations and use standard tools (utensils, markers, crayons).

Once Katie was medically stable, she was transitioned to an outpatient program, with therapy (occupational therapy and physical therapy) three times per week. Therapy goals included maintaining range of motion, further increase of her strength and endurance, developmental therapy, and monitoring splinting and pressure garment needs. During her outpatient program, Katie required a revision of her left hand, with additional pinning needed. This limited some of her advancement in bilateral activities; however, once pins were removed, she was able to resume her play skills. Katie was eventually transitioned to a child developmental center where her rehabilitation continued to focus on mastering sensory motor skills, age appropriate play, and ADL.

ONCOLOGY AND BONE MARROW TRANSPLANT UNITS

Another type of highly specialized acute-care service is the *oncology unit*, which may include a bone marrow transplant unit. Patients served on these two units may include those diagnosed with various types of cancer, immunodeficiency disorders, hemophilia, and aplastic anemia. These two units may be housed close together and share some resources including staff or may be located in separate areas within the hospital setting.

The staff on the oncology unit provides care for those pediatric patients who are newly diagnosed with cancer and are undergoing induction chemotherapy, are receiving chemotherapy courses that require close monitoring, may have complications from their treatments, such as fever with neutropenia, or may have undergone tumor resections. The occupational therapist working with these patients may encounter patients and families in different stages of the diagnostic and treatment continuum. Because of the chronic nature of illness for patients located on this unit, the therapist may have time to develop relationships with the child and family. Children may come in and out of the hospital throughout their treatment, and the therapist may see the child for both inpatient and outpatient therapy or may coordinate with outpatient therapists to continue care while the patient experiences an extended inpatient stay. Patients may also vary greatly in their ability to participate in treatments, even from morning to afternoon. Coordinating therapy with other medical interventions may enhance therapy benefits by providing interventions when the child's energy is highest.

The bone marrow transplant unit has certain similarities to the oncology unit, with intensified therapies and additional toxic agents used as life-saving treatments. Bone marrow transplants are used as part of a medical treatment protocol for a number of life-threatening childhood illnesses, including leukemia, aplastic anemia, immunodeficiency syndromes, and tumors (Furman & Feldman, 1990; Williams, 1990; Williams & Safarimaryaki, 1990). Because of the complications of the treatment, the therapist must be aware of the stages the child is in during the transplant process and must strictly adhere to any precautions required (Diaz de Heredia, Moreno, Olive, Iglesias, & Ortega, 1999; Rogers et al., 2000; Shaw, 2002).

Oncology Treatment

During the initial phase of treatment for cancer, pediatric patients undergo a series of evaluations to determine type of cancer type and staging, which includes determining if the cancer has metastasized. Patients generally receive a permanent line placement through which they receive their chemotherapy. They are initially hospitalized for their induction chemotherapy, which is the initial course, and may be quite intense for some children. Hospitalization is required initially to assess effects of chemotherapy and to watch for any complications. Children frequently decrease their oral intake during treatment, so nutrition needs to be carefully monitored as well.

As treatment progresses, children are often discharged from the inpatient setting and are monitored between chemotherapy sessions in outpatient visits. If the child does not have a negative reaction, or if the agents given do not have high levels of toxicity, the patient may receive chemotherapy on an outpatient basis. Patients receiving chemotherapy are often at high risk for infections and are susceptible to contagious diseases; therefore, they need to take precautions, particularly if they are neutropenic, which affects their ability to fight off disease. This is a frequent cause for admissions between chemotherapy sessions and can mean patients are readmitted multiple times throughout their treatment.

The occupational therapist working with these patients should be aware of the cancer types and have general knowledge of chemotherapy drugs and their complications, as well as general oncology knowledge. All personnel must adhere to infection control procedures. The therapist may focus on strengthening, range of motion, endurance, ADL, feeding, or play activities with patients, depending on their needs. Patients and families frequently develop a close relationship with the therapist because of the physical aspects of treatment, along with the normalcy and expectation of survival that families can perceive with everyday activities.

Occasionally, cure is not an option for patients, and focus of treatment may change to be palliative in nature. The therapist working with the dying child and his or her family must respect the cultural beliefs of the family, along with grief processes. The occupational therapist can assist with suggesting energy conservation techniques to enable the patient to continue to play and interact with family members. Positioning becomes particularly important as the patient develops increased weakness, difficulty with breath support, or pain, and the therapist can help families problem-solve alternative positioning to be close to their child when comfort is of utmost importance (Drake, Frost, & Collins, 2003). It is also important the therapist respect family and patient wishes for withdrawal or continuation of services. Some may wish to discontinue therapy intervention, choosing to narrow the circle of support, others develop a closeness with the therapist throughout the treatment and want to continue contact. The therapist needs to look at his or her own support systems, beliefs, and feelings around end-of-life issues to assist the patient and family during this difficult time (Vincent, 2001).

Transplant Procedure, Sequela, and Intervention

The procedure for bone marrow transplant involves chemotherapy, radiation, or both before the transplant. This is followed by intravenous infusion of the bone marrow taken from a compatible donor or from the patient before the pretransplant regimen of chemotherapy and radiation. Those patients who are undergoing treatment for disease processes that do not invade the bone marrow may be eligible to undergo stem cell transplant (Sanders, 1997). This involves the harvest of stem cells throughout their initial chemotherapy treatment while in the remission stage. Although bone marrow and stem cell transplants both involve intense chemotherapy and radiation, patients who receive a stem cell transplant experience lower rejection rates and fewer complications from graft versus host disease. The intense chemotherapy or radiation before the transplant and the underlying disease processes cause severe immunosuppression in patients, making them highly susceptible to life-threatening infections until the new bone marrow is established and the patient's immuno-hematopoietic system is once again functioning effectively (Lenarsky, 1990; Zander & Aksamit, 1990). Continued long-term effects are also a complication of transplant. Chronic graft versus host disease (GVHD), abnormal neuroendocrine function, secondary malignancies, and avascular necrosis are a few of the complications seen in pediatric patients (Sanders, 1991). Stretching, extremity weight bearing, and general endurance exercises improve function in children experiencing these GVHD complications (Beredjiklian et al., 1998).

Because these children have significant compromise of their immune systems, the hospital environment is carefully designed to significantly reduce the risk of infection. Common strategies to protect bone marrow transplant patients include room isolation, reverse isolation, and laminar airflow in a clean or sterile environment (Lenarsky, 1990). Additionally, persons having access to the unit may be limited. Those staff and visitors who have flu or virus related symptoms may not be allowed onto units serving these severely compromised patients.

Another issue of concern is the *psychosocial stress* for the patient and family. Sources of stress include the child's life-threatening illness, the risks of bone marrow transplantation, the painful or uncomfortable medical procedures and extended period of isolation that the child must endure, and concern about the cost of the treatment. In addition, the transplant may occur at a hospital distant from the family's home, creating an additional burden for family members (Williams, 1990), or access to family may be limited during treatments. Patients may be limited to phone contact with extended family members and friends when undergoing treatment or transplant. Family members may become bone marrow donors in some instances. This further increases stress levels for family members while the donor is recovering from surgery, and all are waiting for engraftment to occur for the patient. The cost of the complicated treatments and ongoing care needs, along with possible additional housing needs if families are treated some distance from their home community, can place a significant financial burden on families. They may complete fund raisers to help raise finances to support the coverage offered by insurers, or they may rely on community entities such as churches or businesses for additional support.

The many complex needs of the patient and family emphasize the importance of a collaborative team approach. The physician, nurses, occupational therapist, physical therapist, pharmacist, clinical social worker, psychologist, dietitian, chaplain, child life specialist, and a hospital-based teacher may all serve as members of a team caring for the bone marrow transplant patient and the patient's family (Spruce, 1990). The efforts of such a large team work well when care is coordinated and communication with the family is consistent.

Intervention may include a pretransplant assessment of the child's development and functional abilities, as well as identification of limitations or problems caused by the underlying disease process. After the transplant, the occupational therapist's goals may be to (1) promote age-appropriate play, daily living, and social participation occupations; (2) enhance coping and interaction skills; and (3) develop a plan for follow-up in the community. The following case study describes a child from initial diagnosis and chemotherapy through the transplant process and posttransplant intervention.

Case Study: Intervention for Child with Cancer
Presenting Information

Danielle was a 16-month-old girl who was initially seen at a general hospital near her home when she experienced a decrease in standing and sitting balance and was subsequently admitted to a pediatric tertiary care center approximately 400 miles from her community. Initial examination and imaging revealed a neuroblastoma in her spinal cord. Danielle was immediately placed on the pediatric oncology unit, a peripherally inserted central catheter (PICC) line was placed, and chemotherapy induction was initiated. At initial presentation, both parents flew in with Danielle, although they had been separated just prior to diagnosis.

Background Information

Danielle had been a typically developing 16-month-old girl prior to diagnosis. She had not yet learned to walk independently, but she was cruising between furniture and was able to stand without support for extended periods of time. Danielle was initially described as a reserved, cautious child. She resided with her mother, and her father had moved out just 1 month prior to her diagnosis. They lived in a small village, with many community friends available for support. Her parents had moved from a large city prior to conceiving Danielle to "obtain a simpler lifestyle." Upon hearing the diagnosis, further stress was revealed when it was discovered the maternal grandfather had died of a glioblastoma just 1 year previously.

Medical and Occupational Therapy Intervention: Oncology Phase of Treatment

Danielle was initially referred to occupational therapy immediately after diagnosis. She was having initial complications coping with the increased noise and the number of caregivers, along with decreased performance. She was also seen by a child life specialist for developmentally appropriate coping strategies such as creating a calming environment and play to facilitate release of emotions. Danielle was not able to sit independently on initiation of treatment and her arm strength was diminished.

Danielle was given chemotherapy to shrink the tumor, and because of its location, resection was not recommended. Stem cell transplant was discussed at initiation of treatment as the best course of possible cure for her cancer. Thus, the medical plan was to reduce her tumor size, obtain remission, harvest stem cells, and prepare Danielle for transplant. She was placed on a chemotherapy protocol recommended for her tumor type, and the family was informed of all complications, side effects, and statistical outcome possibilities.

In an initial assessment, the occupational therapist evaluated Danielle's performance skills and strength. She also completed family interviews to learn about the child's previous skill levels, occupations, and particular interests. A plan was made in conjunction with the parents and the nurse for a daily schedule, including times when Danielle could receive therapy. She was moved to a corner room to decrease noise, and times were posted when curtains were to be drawn to allow the family private time. Pictures of caregivers, including therapists, primary nurses, and physicians, were posted for reference for both Danielle and her parents.

Ongoing communication was established among all team members through the use of progress notes, team rounds, and a care book placed at Danielle's bedside where information and questions could be posted to further facilitate communication between both parents and medical personnel. In addition, care conferences were held weekly where all team members, including parents, could get together to discuss treatment planning.

Occupational therapy treatment consisted of age-appropriate strengthening activities, play opportunities, and basic ADL. Her family, along with the nurses, was instructed on position strategies to increase Danielle's function and thus participation. Her medical treatment made Danielle's ability to participate in regular sessions difficult, not only due to nausea but also due to neutropenic compromise resulting in additional weakness and lethargy. During particularly difficult periods, treatment sessions were limited to gentle range of motion or were canceled.

As medical intervention, including chemotherapy, progressed, Danielle experienced an increase in function. Her occupational therapy treatment plan was continually revised to reflect increased strength and independence. As a result of her chemotherapy, Danielle began to decrease her oral intake. Strategies were implemented to maintain oral motor skills and optimizing oral intake.

Danielle was eventually transitioned to outpatient care, where both her oncology treatment and her occupational therapy continued. Because of behavior challenges, family requests, and training expertise, direct physical therapy was discontinued. Instead, a collaborative approach of consultation with the occupational therapist at regular intervals to facilitate ambulatory and lower extremity skills was established. Her parents also divided care, with one parent returning to their home

community, and alternating times when parents would be present.

Prior to transplant, Danielle regained her motor skills, and 2 days before the transplant she was able to walk for the first time. She was able to complete age-appropriate ADL and participate in developmentally appropriate play activities. Medications were given between chemotherapy courses to facilitate stem cell production and were then harvested.

Once the transplant regime was initiated, Danielle was hospitalized for an extended stay. She underwent intensive chemotherapy and radiation to ablate her current marrow and subsequently receive a stem cell transplant. During her initial stages, Danielle experienced a significant decrease in her strength and developmental skills. She had toxicity-related complications including sluffing of her skin and mouth sores, which made participation in activities difficult. As an added complication, Danielle also experienced life-threatening pulmonary complications that required ventilation support and necessitated a 2-week stay in the intensive care unit.

Family stresses throughout this portion of her treatment were enormous, and Danielle's mother asked Danielle's maternal grandmother, who lived in France, to come for support. Once here, interpreters translated necessary information as the parents desired. Danielle eventually achieved slow engraftment, and transplant-related complications diminished.

As engraftment progressed, Danielle quickly regained her play and daily living skills, including ambulation. She was transferred to outpatient services and continued to receive occupational therapy intervention to address decreased strength and delayed motor skills. She was discharged back to her community, once she had completed her 90-day posttransplant evaluation, and engraftment was clear. She continued to receive ongoing occupational therapy in her community to help facilitate progress in her development.

GENERAL ACUTE-CARE UNIT

General acute-care units tend to be designated by medical specialty. For example, patients of various ages, with different types of orthopedic conditions and treatment, may be served in the same acute-care unit. Similarly, patients requiring different types of surgery may be admitted to the same general surgical unit for preoperative and postoperative care. Designating units in this manner enables physicians and other members of the medical team to use their patient-care time and equipment more efficiently. This system of designation also results in increased opportunities for formal and informal communication between team members regarding each child's care.

General acute-care units differ from ICUs in several ways. Patients tend to be more medically stable and less dependent on life-sustaining equipment as part of their medical treatment. The less serious nature of their medical conditions may enable them to receive greater benefit from occupational therapy and permit them to leave the unit for occupational therapy or other services (although services may be provided at bedside, if necessary).

Occupational therapists may be responsible for patients on one or more acute-care units, requiring them to be familiar with the procedures of each unit, the types of patients admitted to the different units, and the nurses and other hospital personnel who provide services. Patients admitted directly to an acute-care unit of this type also tend to have a shorter hospital stay than those who progress from ICU to another type of unit. Consequently, the occupational therapist often has less opportunity to develop a relationship with both the patient and the family.

Case Study: Intervention for a Child on the General Medicine Service
Presenting Information

Jacobi was a 13-month-old girl who was admitted for surgical intervention and subsequent casting for a dislocated hip. She was admitted to the orthopedic service immediately following surgery.

Background Information

Jacobi was born weighing 9 pounds, 10 ounces at 41 weeks gestation. After going through a complicated course of 28 hours of labor, Jacobi was born via natural birth. Initially she could move all of her limbs, but did appear to have initial discomfort in her right lower extremity. Jocobi's parents were instructed on positioning techniques to increase their daughter's comfort and were instructed to follow up with their pediatrician. They did so, and Jacobi was closely monitored for possible dislocation. At 9 months of age, Jacobi was still not sitting independently and had not shown any interest in crawling. She was seen by an orthopedist who diagnosed a right dislocation, with soft tissue tightening. Jacobi was placed in a hip spica splint to assist with positioning. Surgery was discussed at that time. She continued to display a lag in her motor skills, with decreased range in her hips, and surgery was scheduled for release and positioning of hip joint.

Medical and Occupational Therapy Intervention

Following release of hip adductor muscles including the gracilis, she was placed in a hip spica cast that encompassed her right leg to the ankle and her left leg to above the knee, placing her hips in abduction and slight flexion at her right knee. She spent the night in the hospital following the surgery so that her status could be monitored and her pain controlled.

Prior to discharge, an occupational therapist was consulted because Jacobi could not fit in her car seat. When placed in the seat, the front portion of her hip spica would push in against her belly, causing discomfort and a decreased ability to breathe. The therapist first attempted to obtain an alternative car seat for Jacobi, a hip spica seat; however, none were immediately available. The car seat coalition in her state was contacted to determine what modifications could safely be made. A foam positioning device was fabricated to fit just behind the cast, with side supports to keep it forward when sitting. The occupational therapist instructed the family on positioning and how to monitor Jacobi in the vehicle during transport. The therapist recommended a local vendor where the parents could obtain a modified car seat. Jacobi was then discharged.

This example illustrates the challenge of creative thinking required by the occupational therapist when working in the general acute medicine service in a pediatric setting. In attempting to assist the patient and family, different functional and logistical obstacles may arise. The therapist has to be able to meet the needs of the patient and family while taking medical needs and complications into consideration. Community resources, such as the restraint coalition in this example, may need to be accessed to determine the safest course of action to meet these needs. Often the therapist has limited time prior to discharge and must act immediately to check on or obtain resources.

FAILURE TO THRIVE

Failure to thrive (FTT) is a diagnosis given to children, frequently infants and young children, who fail to grow or gain weight. FTT may be designated as *organic,* arising from a diagnosable physical cause, or as *nonorganic,* which denotes impaired growth without apparent physical cause (Frank, 1985). Children with FTT often require hospitalization for acute care and can have additional complications including immune deficiencies, generalized weakness, and developmental delay due to their malnutrition.

Although organic FTT can be attributed to a specific physical disorder, nonorganic FTT is primarily (but not exclusively) associated with psychosocial factors. Disturbances in parent-child interaction and development of attachment early in life, difficult infant temperament and behavior, maternal social isolation, and financial difficulties within the family are some of the variables associated with nonorganic FTT (Bithoney & Newberger, 1987; Mantymaa et al., 2003; Piazza et al., 2003).

In some instances, FTT may be attributed to both organic and nonorganic factors. Frank (1985) suggested that children with nonorganic FTT may still have biologic risks. She identified three categories of risk: (1) *perinatal,* (2) *toxic and immunologic,* and (3) *neurodevelopmental.*

Perinatal risk refers to the potential for FTT in infants who are considered low birth weight, possibly as a result of prematurity or intrauterine growth retardation. Toxic and immunologic risks arise from significant nutritional deficiency, which has the potential to increase vulnerability to infection and increase susceptibility to lead toxicity. Neurodevelopmental risk results from effects of inadequate nutrition on the developing nervous system. Although toxic and immunologic risks are generally reversible through medical treatment, treatment may not fully reverse the neurodevelopmental consequences.

The complexity of factors implicated in FTT emphasizes the need for a coordinated team approach that offers medical, nutritional, developmental, and psychosocial intervention. As a member of the hospital-based team, the occupational therapist may contribute to both the diagnosis and the treatment of the child with FTT. A comprehensive occupational therapy assessment provides the medical team with information regarding the infant's developmental status, feeding behaviors, infant-caregiver interactions during play and feeding, and infant interactions with nonfamily members (e.g., the occupational therapist). Children may require enteral nutrition or a nasogastric tube for nutritional support during the initial phases of evaluation and treatment. A more permanent gastric tube for feeding may be required if it is suspected additional nutritional support may be needed for an extended period.

Denton (1986) differentiated between FTT in infants and children around 2 years of age, suggesting that 2-year-old children who fail to thrive present with poor feeding skills that may be the result of behavioral issues. Infant assessment emphasizes interactional issues with the caregivers, while the assessment of older children focuses more on behaviors in the feeding situation and attempts to differentiate between environmental factors and neuromotor difficulties that may be affecting feeding. A developmental and feeding history obtained from the parent is a valuable component of the occupational therapy assessment of all children with FTT.

Occupational therapy intervention goals with a child who fails to thrive may include improving oral-motor and feeding skills and facilitating development. Promoting positive parent-child interaction may also be emphasized, using strategies that help the parent understand infant behavioral cues and engage the child in positive, developmentally appropriate play experiences. This emphasis on positive parent-child interaction also encourages parents to develop behavioral expectations consistent with the child's level of functioning. Ongoing outpatient therapy is needed following discharge to support goals established on the inpatient stay and to foster typical feeding behaviors.

Case Study: Intervention for a Child with FTT

Presenting Information

Kevin was a 3-month, 7-day-old boy transferred from a community hospital to a regional children's hospital by helicopter after suffering a seizure. He was intubated en route. Initial diagnoses included rule-out abuse, severe nonorganic FTT, anemia, rule-out sepsis and bacteremia, hyponatremia, dehydration, and seizures.

On examination, Kevin was noted to have bruising above both knees and over his right buttocks. He was also observed to have diaper rash and wasting of the left hip and extremities. Because he demonstrated poor oral feeding, the PICU attending physician referred Kevin to occupational therapy on the third day of hospitalization.

Background Information

Kevin's parents brought him to the referring hospital's emergency room after a home visit by a Child Protective Services worker. He was left at the emergency room, and his parents did not visit during his 14-day hospitalization at the children's hospital. His maternal great aunt visited occasionally, and she expressed interest in adopting him.

Kevin was born at term and weighed 5 pounds 12 ounces. He went home after a 48-hour hospital stay. He was hospitalized at 2 months of age for FTT, upper respiratory tract infection, and otitis media. He was discharged to his parents with home health nursing, a Child Protective Services referral, and pediatrician follow-up. Kevin's parents missed all follow-up appointments until they brought him to the emergency room.

Medical and Occupational Therapy Intervention

A pH probe showed severe gastroesophageal reflux. An upper gastrointestinal series was performed and ruled out anatomic abnormality. Stool samples were analyzed and showed malabsorption, reducing substances, increased fatty acids, and *Giardia lamblia,* all of which combined to reduce his level of nutrient absorption and increase fluid loss. As a result, Kevin was severely underweight and lethargic. Medical treatment for the reflux included positioning on an elevated wedge, thickened feeds, and medications.

Kevin was evaluated by occupational therapy using clinical observations for his oral-motor, feeding, and developmental skills. He demonstrated intact oral structures and sensation, with functional oral skills for safe oral feeding. He had small sucking pads with a weak suck and fair coordination of suck-swallow-breathe. His suck and coordination improved with support at his jaw and cheeks. Kevin's developmental skills were delayed, and he demonstrated poor state control with high irritability.

It was the therapist's impression that Kevin's weak suck, poor feeding, and irritability were from overall weakness, malnutrition, and recent intubation, rather than from a neurologic deficit.

The occupational therapist developed a bedside plan of specific facilitation techniques to be used during feeding. These included jaw and cheek support, external tongue stimulation, flexion swaddling, decreasing external stimulation, upright and well-aligned feeding positioning, limiting oral feeding to 30 minutes, and turning off the continuous pump, feeding Kevin through a nasal gastric tube.

After implementation of occupational therapy recommendations by nursing staff, Kevin's oral intake increased dramatically over the next 3 days, with the occupational therapist feeding him once daily to monitor progress. Once the acute feeding issues were resolved, occupational therapy emphasis switched to interaction skills, with the focus on developmental activities to improve self-calming, visual tracking, and social interactions.

Kevin was referred for outpatient occupational therapy and early intervention services before discharge. Children's Protective Services assumed custody of Kevin, and he was discharged to a foster home with a weight increase of 2.4 pounds (follow-up weekly weight checks were scheduled with his pediatrician). The occupational therapist provided the foster parents with a home program, including positioning, feeding, and activities to promote Kevin's play development.

OUTPATIENT SERVICES

Outpatient services are important components of the total spectrum of hospital care and may be provided at the hospital, at a hospital satellite center, or as part of an interdisciplinary hospital-based clinic (e.g., arthritis clinic, feeding clinic, or cerebral palsy clinic). Outpatient occupational therapy is generally provided for one of three purposes: (1) as part of a diagnostic assessment, (2) to provide needed intervention after hospital discharge, or (3) to provide occupational therapy intervention for individuals with disabilities or other medical conditions not requiring hospitalization (Figure 24-6).

In general, the referral base for outpatient services may extend beyond the hospital's medical staff. Patients may be referred for outpatient occupational therapy by their attending physicians in the hospital, by a community-based physician (e.g., pediatrician or family practi-

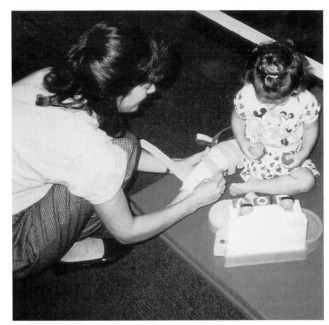

FIGURE 24-6 An occupational therapist fabricates a splint for a young client with juvenile rheumatoid arthritis.

tioner), or by a physician in a hospital-based specialty clinic. As with inpatient services, a referral from a physician determines the services to be provided.

Provision of inpatient occupational therapy services differs from provision of outpatient services in a number of ways. Services are usually provided to outpatients less frequently (e.g., one to three times per week) and may continue for weeks or months. The longer duration provides a greater opportunity for the occupational therapist to get to know the child's family and develop a collaborative relationship. In addition, it may provide the therapist a chance to observe the natural progression of some conditions, including healing progression, in order to better predict outcomes for patients. Children seen on an outpatient basis are medically stable, as opposed to children who are hospitalized for an acute or transient illness.

One disadvantage of outpatient therapy is the limited opportunity for collaboration and communication with other professionals who provide services to the child. In most cases, the child served as an outpatient does not have a medical team with members who meet to discuss and coordinate services. If the therapist is part of a larger hospital therapy department, he or she may draw on the experience of fellow therapists within the working group to help guide practice. The therapist must also take the initiative to collaborate with other community professionals by participating in the care of the child when appropriate. These may include the primary care provider, school physical or occupational therapists, or educators. The occupational therapist must be diligent in obtaining consents for the sharing or releasing of information according to the standard established by the Health Insurance Portability and Accountability Act of 1996 (HIPAA).

Outpatient services provided as part of an interdisciplinary specialty medical clinic usually have a specific focus (e.g., feeding clinic, behavioral disorders clinic). Occupational therapy services in specialty clinics are limited, as children typically attend only one to two times a year. In some instances, the occupational therapist functions as a consultant, completing an assessment, then making recommendations to the physician. In other cases, the occupational therapist is an integral part of the decision-making team and may be involved in patient assessment, treatment or equipment recommendations, or the provision of splints and adaptive equipment.

DOCUMENTATION OF OCCUPATIONAL THERAPY SERVICES

Documentation of patient care is an essential and time-consuming component of occupational therapy service provision in hospitals. Occupational therapy evaluation reports, treatment plans, patient progress notes, and discharge summaries are used to communicate occupational therapy intervention to the physician, other members of the medical team, the patient and family, and reimbursement agencies.

Format and frequency of documentation are determined by the policies and procedures of the hospital and occupational therapy department. Accreditation guidelines regarding documentation are provided to institutions by agencies such as the JCAHO and the CARF. Agencies that reimburse services, such as Medicaid or private insurance, also have requirements for documentation with which occupational therapists must comply.

Documentation of services to hospitalized patients through evaluation reports with accompanying treatment plans, progress notes, and discharge summaries occurs in the patient's medical chart. Because the medical chart remains on the unit or accompanies the patient when he or she receives services elsewhere in the hospital, information is readily available to other health professionals. The increasing use of information technology such as online charting has also facilitated access of information and documentation that is readily available to all providers. Documentation of occupational therapy intervention with outpatients may take a different form, because reports are often sent to referring physicians or other agencies in the community. Copies of these outpatient reports are also retained in the patient's hospital medical record. Documentation of services in clinics may follow a different format because each clinic may have a medical chart for the patient. However, regardless of the format, documentation of services must meet the criteria established by accrediting and reimbursement agencies (Jongbloed & Wendland, 2002).

SUMMARY

The provision of occupational therapy services to children in hospitals is a specialized and challenging area of practice. Occupational therapists in hospitals must have a thorough understanding of the characteristics of health care systems; the numerous factors and trends that affect hospitals, including legal and accreditation requirements; and the specialized needs of hospitalized children and their families. The occupational therapist must also understand the roles of others involved in the care for patients to accomplish both medical and functional goals of the hospitalized child. Occupational therapists who are employed in hospitals have the opportunity to gain expertise in assessment and treatment of children of various ages with many different diagnoses, within a dynamic, fast-paced environment. As hospitals broaden their range of services in response to a changing health care system, hospital-based occupational therapists will have opportunities to broaden their areas of expertise, apply different models of service delivery, and develop new practitioner roles.

STUDY QUESTIONS

1 Consider the various hospital settings in which the occupational therapist may serve pediatric patients. List the types of patient care specialized to each type of hospital.

2 What are the major roles and functions of the occupational therapist working with children on the oncology unit? How do these roles change as the care turns palliative in nature?

3 List three roles of the occupational therapist with a child who has received severe burns. Give examples of occupational therapy activities at each phase of recovery (i.e., acute, surgical, and rehabilitation).

4 Describe the characteristics of occupational therapy services in a medical model. Compare these characteristics with those of occupational therapy in education settings (Chapter 22). What are advantages and disadvantages of each model of service delivery?

REFERENCES

Abreu, B., Seale, G., Podlesak, J., & Hartley, L. (1996). Development of critical paths for postacute brain injury rehabilitation: Lessons learned. *American Journal of Occupational Therapy, 50*, 417-427.

Affleck, A.T., Lieberman, S., Polon, J., & Rohrkemper, K. (1986). Providing occupational therapy in an intensive care unit. *American Journal of Occupational Therapy, 40,* 323-332.

Appold, K. (2003). Meeting the challenges of compliance. *Clinical Leadership & Management Review, 17,* 53-55.

Beredjiklian, P.K., Drummond, D.S., Dormans, J.P., Davidson, R.S., Brock, G.T., & August, C. (1998). Orthopaedic manifestations of chronic graft-versus-host disease. *Journal of Pediatric Orthopeadics, 18* (5), 572-575.

Biggs, K.S., de Linde, L., Banaszewski, M., & Heinrich, J.J. (1998). Determining the current roles of physical and occupational therapists in burn care. *Journal of Burn Care & Rehabilitation, 19,* 442-449.

Bithoney, W.G., & Newberger, E.H. (1987). Child and family attributes of failure-to-thrive. *Developmental and Behavioral Pediatrics, 8,* 32-36.

Board, R., & Ryan-Wenger, N. (2002). Long-term effects of pediatric intensive care unit hospitalization on families with young children. *Heart & Lung: Journal of Acute & Critical Care, 31,* 53-66.

Buchanan, J.L., Rumpel, J.D., & Hoenig, H. (1996). Charges for outpatient rehabilitation: Growth and differences in provider types. *Archives of Physical Medicine and Rehabilitation, 77,* 320-328.

Case-Smith, J., & Wavrek, B.B. (1998). Models of service delivery and team interaction. In J. Case-Smith (Ed.), *Pediatric occupational therapy and early intervention* (2nd ed. pp. 83-107). Boston: Butterworth-Heinemann.

Cheng, T.L., Greenberg, L., Loeser, H., & Keller, D. (2000). Teaching prevention in pediatrics. *Academic Medicine, 75,* S66-S71.

Christiansen, C. (1996). Nationally speaking—managed care: Opportunities and challenges for occupational therapy in the emerging systems of the 21st century. *American Journal of Occupational Therapy, 50,* 409-416.

Commission for the Accreditation of Rehabilitation Facilities. (2003). *2003 CARF standards manual.* Tucson, AZ: CARF.

Committee on Early Childhood, Adoption, and Dependent Care: American Academy of Pediatrics (2002). Health care of young children in foster care. *Pediatrics, 109,* 536-541.

Considine, W.H. (1994). Children's needs: A health care reform priority. *Hospital and Health Networks, 68,* 84.

Denton, R. (1986). An occupational therapy protocol for assessing infants and toddlers who fail to thrive. *American Journal of Occupational Therapy, 40,* 352-358.

DeWitt, P.K., Jansen, M.T., Ward, S.L., & Keens, T.G. (1993). Obstacles to discharge of ventilator-assisted children from the hospital to home. *Chest, 103,* 1560-1565.

Diaz de Heredia, C., Moreno, A., Olive, T., Iglesias, J., & Ortega, J.J. (1999). Role of the intensive care unit in children undergoing bone marrow transplantation with life-threatening complications. *Bone Marrow Transplantation, 24,* 163-168.

Drake, R., Frost, J., & Collins, J.J. (2003). The symptoms of dying children. *Journal of Pain & Symptom Management, 26,* 594-603.

Eckle, N., & MacLean, S.L. (2001). Assessment of family-centered care policies and practices for pediatric patients in nine US emergency departments. *Journal of Emergency Nursing, 27,* 238-245.

Frank, D.A. (1985). Biologic risks in "nonorganic" failure to thrive: Diagnostic and therapeutic implications. In D. Drotar (Ed.), *New directions in failure to thrive* (pp. 17-26). New York: Plenum Press.

Freda, M. (1998). Facility-based practice settings. In M.E. Neistadt & E.B. Crepeau (Eds.), *Willard & Spackman's occupational therapy* (9th ed., pp. 803-809). Philadelphia: Lippincott Williams & Wilkins.

Furman, W.L., & Feldman, S. (1990). Infectious complications. In F.L. Johnson & C. Pochedly (Eds.), *Bone marrow transplantation in children* (pp. 427-450). New York: Raven Press.

Gabel, I., Levitt, L., Holve, E., Pickreign, J., Whitmore, H., Dhoni, K., Hawkins, S., & Rowland., D. (2002). Job-based health benefits in 2002: Some important trends. *Health Affairs, 21* (5), 143-151.

Gilkerson, L. (1990). Understanding institutional functional style: A resource for hospital and early intervention collaboration. *Infants and Young Children, 2,* 22-30.

Gilkerson, L., Gorski, P., & Panitz, P. (1990). Hospital-based intervention for preterm infants and their families. In S. Meisels & J. Shonkoff (Eds.), *Handbook of early childhood intervention* (pp. 445-468). Cambridge, MA: Cambridge University Press.

Gipe, B.T. (2000). The cost and quality of hospitalists. *Cost & Quality, 6,* 20-23.

Gohsman, B. (1981). The hospitalized child and the need for mastery. *Issues in Comprehensive Pediatric Nursing, 5,* 67-76.

Granberg, A., Engberg, I.B., & Lundberg, D. (1999). Acute confusion and unreal experiences in intensive care patients in relation to the ICU syndrome, part II. *Intensive & Critical Care Nursing, 15,* 19-33.

Guske, P. (2003). Follow the codes. *Rehab management, 16,* 58-60.

Health Insurance Portability and Accountability Act of 1996. 45 CFR, Subtitle A, Subchapter C, part 160.

Hewitt-Taylor, J. (1999). Children in intensive care: Physiological considerations. *Nursing in Critical Care, 4,* 40-45.

Ho, W.S., Chan, H.H., Ying, S.Y., Cheng, H.S., & Wong, C.S. (2001). Skin care in burn patients: A team approach. *Burns, 27,* 489-491.

Joint Commission on the Accreditation of Health Care Organizations. (1994). *1995 comprehensive accreditation manual for hospitals.* Oakbrook Terrace, IL: JCAHO.

Jongbloed, L., & Wendland, T. (2002). The impact of reimbursement systems on occupational therapy practice in Canada and the United States of America. *Canadian Journal of Occupational Therapy, 69,* 143-152.

Jordan, W.J. (2001). An early view of the impact of deregulation and managed care on hospital profitability and net worth. *Journal of Healthcare Management, 46,* 161-171.

Keisler, C.A. (2000). The next wave of change for psychology and mental health services in the health care revolution. *American Psychologist, 55,* 481-487.

Knudson-Cooper, M. (1982). Emotional care of the hospitalized burned child. *Journal of Burn Care and Rehabilitation, 3,* 109-115.

Lenarsky, C. (1990). Technique of bone marrow transplantation. In F.L. Johnson & C. Pochedly (Eds.), *Bone marrow transplantation in children* (pp. 53-67). New York: Raven Press.

Leslie, L.K., Kelleher, K.J., Burns, B.J., Landsverk, J., & Rolls, J.A. (2003). Foster care and Medicaid managed care. *Child Welfare, 82,* 367-392.

Lindeke, L.L., Leonard, B.J., Presler, B., & Garwick, A. (2002). Family-centered care coordination for children with special needs across multiple settings. *Journal of Pediatric Health Care, 16,* 290-297.

Mantymaa, M., Puura, K., Luoma, I., Salmelin, R., Davis, H.J., Tsiantis, J., Ispanovic-Radojkovic, V., Paradisiotou, A., & Tamminen, T. (2003). Infant-mother interaction as a predictor of child's chronic health problems. *Child: Care, Health & Development, 29,* 181-191.

Morrison, W.E., Haas, E.C., Shaffner, D.H., Garrett, E.S., & Fackler, J.C. (2003). Noise, stress, and annoyance in a pediatric intensive care unit. *Critical Care Medicine, 31,* 113-119.

Murphy, J.T., Purdue, G.F., Hunt, J.L., & Hicks, B.A. (1997). In D.L. Levin & F.C. Morris (Eds.), *Essentials of pediatric intensive care* (2nd ed.). New York: Churchill Livingstone.

Occupational Exposure to Blood-Borne Pathogens, 56 Fed. Reg. 64175-64182 (1991).

O'Hara, K. (2003). Plenty of CPT changes for 2003, latest on additions, revisions, and deletions. *Journal of AHIMA, 74,* 80-82.

Petrillo, M., & Sanger, S. (1980). *Emotional care of hospitalized children.* Philadelphia: J.B. Lippincott.

Piazza, C.C., Fisher, W.W., Brown, K.A., Shore, B.A., Patel, M.R., Katz, R.M., Sevin, B.M., Gulotta, C.S., & Blakely-Smith, A. (2003). Functional analysis of inappropriate mealtime behaviors. *Journal of Applied Behavior Analysis, 36,* 187-204.

Rausch, G., & Melvin, J.L. (1986). Nationally speaking: A new era in acute care. *American Journal of Occupational Therapy, 40,* 319-322.

Rennick, J.E., Johnston, C.C., Dougherty, G., Platt, R., & Ritchie, J.A. (2002). Children's psychological responses after critical illness and exposure to invasive technology. *Journal of Developmental & Behavioral Pediatrics, 23,* 133-144.

Rivers, E.A., & Jordan, C.L. (1998). Skin system dysfunction: Burns. In M.E. Neistadt & E.B. Crepeau (Eds.). *Willard & Spackman's occupational therapy* (9th ed., pp. 741-755). Philadephia: Lippincott Williams & Wilkins.

Rogers, M., Weinstock, D.M., Eagan, J., Kiehn, T., Armstrong, D., & Sepkowitz, K.A (2000). Rotavirus outbreak on a pediatric oncology floor: Possible association with toys. *American Journal of Infection Control, 28,* 378-380.

Sanders, J.E. (1991). Long term effects of bone marrow transplantation. *Pediatrician, 18,* 76-81.

Sanders, J.E. (1997). Bone marrow transplantation for pediatric malignancies. *Pediatric Oncology, 44* (4), 1005-1020.

Shaw, P.J. (2002). Suspected infection in children with cancer. *Journal of Antimicrobial Chemotherapy, 49,* 63-7.

Smith, J.M. (2002). Foster care children with disabilities. *Journal of Health & Social Policy, 16,* 81-92.

Spruce, W.E. (1990). Supportive care in bone marrow transplantation. In F.L. Johnson & C. Pochedly (Eds.), *Bone marrow transplantation in children* (pp. 69-86). New York: Raven Press.

Suhr, M.A. (1986). Trauma in pediatric populations. *Advances in Psychosomatic Medicine, 16,* 31-47.

Tarantino, D. (2002). Making the most of DRGs. *Physician Executive, 28,* 50-52.

Tiberius, R.G., Sackin, H.D., Tallett, S.E., Jacobson, S., & Turner, J. (2001). Conversations with parents of medically ill children: A study of interactions between medical students and parents and pediatric residents and parents in the clinical setting. *Teaching & Learning in Medicine, 13,* 97-109.

Tomlinson, P.S., Swiggum, P., & Harbaugh, B.L. (1999). Identification of nurse-family intervention sites to decrease health-related family boundary ambiguity in PICU. *Issues in Comprehensive Pediatric Nursing, 22,* 27-47.

Tomlinson, P.S., Thomlinson, E., Peden-McAlping, C., & Kirschbaum, M. (2002). Clinical innovation for promoting family care in pediatric intensive care: Demonstration, role modeling and reflective practice. *Journal of Advance Nursing, 38,* 161-170.

Treloar, C., & Graham, I.D. (2003). Multidisciplinary cross-national studies: A commentary on issues of collaboration methodology, analysis, and publication. *Qualitative Health Research, 13,* 924-932.

Vincent, J.L. (2001). Cultural differences in end-of-life care. *Critical Care Medicine, 29,* N52-5.

Watkins, P. (2003). Ethnicity and clinical practice. *Clinical Medicine, 3,* 197-198.

Welch, W.P. (2002). Outpatient encounter data for risk adjustment: Strategic issues for Medicare and Medicaid. *Journal of Ambulatory Care Management, 25,* 1-15.

Williams, M. (1996). Three alternative methods of developing critical pathways cost and benefits. *Best Practices & Benchmarking in Healthcare, 1,* 126-128.

Williams, T.E. (1990). Ethical and psychosocial issues in bone marrow transplantation in children. In F.L. Johnson & C. Pochedly (Eds.), *Bone marrow transplantation in children* (pp. 497-504). New York: Raven Press.

Williams, T.E., & Safarimaryaki, S. (1990). Bone marrow transplantation for treatment of solid tumors. In F.L. Johnson & C. Pochedly (Eds.), *Bone marrow transplantation in children* (pp. 221-242). New York: Raven Press.

Wilson, T., & Broome, M.E. (1989). Promoting the young child's development in the intensive care unit. *Heart & Lung, 18,* 274-281.

Zander, A.R., & Aksamit, I.A. (1990). Immune recovery following bone marrow transplantation. In F.L. Johnson & C. Pochedly (Eds.), *Bone marrow transplantation in children* (pp. 87-110). New York: Raven Press.

CHAPTER OBJECTIVES

1 Describe the types of children who are commonly treated within hospital-based pediatric rehabilitation units and those who typically receive specialized outpatient clinic and therapy services.
2 Discuss existing research of pediatric rehabilitation programs and of specific interventions for children with common diagnoses.
3 Identify and describe collaborative relationships with other providers in interdisciplinary and transdisciplinary practice settings.
4 Propose and apply a prioritization system for assessment and intervention planning that guides the selection of therapy goals and intervention approaches.
5 Emphasize teaching strategies as an integral component of therapy designed to optimize occupational performance.
6 Describe frames of reference commonly used in pediatric rehabilitation and apply them in a complementary manner in treatment planning.
7 Recognize opportunities for family involvement and explain levels of family participation.
8 Discuss the elements of a plan for transition of care from the hospital setting to home and the community.

In the past, children who required pediatric rehabilitation often experienced long-term hospital stays or fre-

quent hospitalizations. For some children, the hospital and staff members nearly took on the roles of a home and family. These environments addressed medical care and rehabilitative intervention and often branched into programs addressing socialization, education, and vocation (Burkett, 1989; Edwards, 1992). Currently, most pediatric therapy practice is delivered through school systems. This shift in policy, along with advances in medical care and rehabilitation practice, has changed the role of hospital-based pediatric rehabilitation. In general, most hospital-based programs now focus on acute-onset problems and provision of specialized services for children and adolescents with disabilities that are of low occurrence but high complexity. Hospital-based programs are continuing to evolve, aiming to address known and newly identified health threats in a way that emphasizes a partnership with the child and family and resources in their local community.

This chapter describes the scope of occupational therapy services provided as part of hospital-based pediatric rehabilitation services. As a context for occupational therapy practice, the organization of rehabilitation services is outlined and the types of children treated in these settings are discussed. The chapter emphasizes interdisciplinary care, with the child and family as central participants in goal setting and decision making. Case studies are used to illustrate the role of the occupational therapist (OT) in family-based evaluation, goal setting, and intervention processes. This chapter stresses strategies used by occupational therapists to address activities of daily living (ADLs), instrumental ADLs (IADLs), and other occupations of children, which include participation in school and other community activities. Specific techniques that reduce impairment and minimize disability are prioritized to support the child's requisite and desired performance goals within the environment that he or she regards as home and community.

A primary concept in the practice of pediatric rehabilitation is the differentiation of *habilitation* and *rehabilitation*. For children, *habilitation* is the term most often used to denote attention to the child's acquisition of expected age-level skill and function. *Rehabilitation* is the classic term used to reflect the process of an individual working to regain skills and functions that had been established but subsequently lost. For most practi-

[1] I wish to thank the children and families involved with Children's Hospital and Regional Medical Center, Seattle, Washington, for their willingness to share their experiences. I also want to acknowledge the advice and help of colleagues from the same institution in preparation of this chapter.

tioners in pediatrics, the term *rehabilitation* is used to encompass both concepts. This is true because disability, whether new or chronic, creates ongoing challenges to current function and future demands that evolve as part of growth and development. In this chapter, the term *rehabilitation* is used to express both concepts.

Children who experience injuries, diseases or illnesses, and complications from chronic disorders often experience the loss of existing functions for which rehabilitation of previous skills becomes the primary goal. Nevertheless, ongoing development of age-specific skills throughout childhood, adolescence, and young adult years necessitates frequent reappraisal and shifts in rehabilitation goals and programming to address new skill needs. Gans (1993) has cautioned that some physical medicine and rehabilitation specialists incorrectly think of children as small adults. Orientation to the developmental needs of children and an appreciation for intensive involvement with families are critical to working within hospital-based pediatric rehabilitation programs.

Pediatric rehabilitation might be distinguished as a planned approach involving any type and number of providers, who specify a mission to focus on functional and psychosocial needs of children and their families. More formally, rehabilitation services in pediatrics may be received within one or more levels of care that have evolved as part of the health care delivery system. In general, these interdisciplinary services are designed to address the management of acute disabling conditions, the prevention of secondary complications, the recovery or enhancement of function, and a return to home, school, and community participation. Outcomes from pediatric rehabilitation can be difficult to predict because of the complexity of factors shaping performance. The severity of impairments and spontaneous recovery, developmental changes and maturation, use of specific rehabilitation approaches, and characteristics of families and their environments combine to influence outcomes. Rehabilitation care should always be perceived as an ongoing process that is best carried out as a partnership between the family, community, school, and the hospital's specialized programs.

LEVELS OF SERVICE

Levels of rehabilitation services are subacute, acute, and outpatient or ongoing care. Reviewing typical programs of care and contrasting different purposes within and across settings illustrate this range.

Subacute Rehabilitation

Subacute rehabilitation services are typically organized within skilled nursing facilities (SNFs) or other long-term care settings. Such programs are designed for children and adolescents who are too medically fragile or dependent to be cared for at home but who are not yet able to tolerate or benefit from the intensive efforts of acute rehabilitation (Grebin & Kaplan, 1995). After initial hospitalization, children and adolescents with moderate to severe head injury, multitrauma, or other systemic illnesses may be admitted to an SNF with subacute rehabilitation services. In these settings, they may receive daily therapy to prevent secondary complications and work toward goals of greater independent function. This interdisciplinary care may culminate in admission to an acute rehabilitation program or a planned discharge to an organized home- and community-based service system of care.

Acute Rehabilitation

Acute rehabilitation is characterized by inpatient hospital units and services. Three types of programs are included in this category. The most common are dedicated rehabilitation units within children's hospitals. Another form of organization is the specification of beds and services for pediatric patients within a large rehabilitation hospital, or an entire hospital devoted to pediatric rehabilitation. A third setting involves the designation of pediatric beds in a large rehabilitation unit that is part of a comprehensive hospital system. Adolescents 15 years of age or older may also be admitted to rehabilitation units that commonly serve adults and older adults. Children and adolescents are admitted to acute rehabilitation from other acute or transitional care medical services within the hospital, other local hospitals, or subacute rehabilitation settings. Children and adolescents who are admitted to trauma centers may be regularly screened to identify the need for transfer to children's hospitals or other rehabilitation units. Some children are also admitted to acute rehabilitation directly from community care providers or through the hospital's outpatient clinics and services. Overall, admission to pediatric rehabilitation and length of inpatient stay is largely based on the child's or youth's level of function (DeNise-Annunziata & Scharf, 1998).

Essential to acute rehabilitation programs is the presence of a broad range of services, including occupational therapy. The mixture and intensity of services are planned to meet systematically developed goals. Such programs are characterized as meeting three types of needs (Tables 25-1 to 25-3):

1 Organize and implement a planned approach for the management of recovery and rehabilitation of children with rapid-onset disorders.

2 Redirect care after onset of complications in children with chronic disorders.

3 Provide an environment for specialized medical or surgical procedures that involves specific care regimens and protocols.

Table 25-1 Rapid Onset

Type of Onset	Examples
Accidental injury	Traumatic brain injury (e.g., closed head injury)
	Skull fracture or penetrating head injury
	Burns and smoke inhalation
	Multitrauma
	Near drowning
	Spinal cord injury
Violence	Multitrauma
	Traumatic brain injury (e.g., gunshot wound)
	Burns, iron burns, cigarette burns, and scalding
Disease processes	Central nervous system infection (e.g., encephalitis and meningitis)
	Transverse myelitis
	Guillain-Barré syndrome
	Cancer

Table 25-2 Complications in Children with Chronic Disorders

Type of Onset	Examples
Neurologic	Spina bifida
	Cerebral palsy
	Mental retardation
Orthopedic	Juvenile rheumatoid arthritis
	Congenital amelia and dwarfism
	Arthrogryposis multiplex congenital
Muscular	Muscular dystrophy
Pulmonary	Bronchopulmonary dysplasia

Table 25-3 Special Medical Procedures

Type of Procedure	Examples
Clinical procedure	Selective dorsal rhizotomy
	Continuous intrathecal baclofen
	Ilizarov
Medical technology	Ventilator dependence

Children and adolescents who sustain a sudden illness or injury are the most common type of admission in acute rehabilitation. Table 25-1 indicates the common problems that affect a typically developing child who experiences injury from accidents, violence, or rapid-onset disease. Acquired injuries or diseases represent a substantial health threat to children (Moront & Eichelberger, 1994; Rodriquez & Brown, 1990). Injuries are the leading cause of death and disability among children older than 1 year of age. Traumatic brain injuries (TBIs), including closed head injury, skull fracture, and penetrating brain injuries, are an ongoing concern for children and adolescents due to transportation-related crashes, falls, recreational injury, and vio-lence (Mazzola & Adelson, 2002). Such causes are also associated with children who sustain spinal cord injury (SCI) and multitrauma. Environmental hazards, accidents, and abuse are also implicated among children who experience burns, near drowning, smoke inhalation, carbon monoxide poisoning, or drug overdose.

Aside from known hazards, children also develop infections that involve the central nervous system (CNS); they may sustain cerebrovascular accidents or get other neurological disorders such as transverse myelitis or Guillain-Barré syndrome. Cancer and its treatment may cause children and adolescents to develop problems that necessitate acute rehabilitation. All of these disorders are characterized by typical development and an acute health crisis that causes a severe loss of function, a likelihood of prolonged recovery with residual disability, and chronic health complications associated with disability. For such children and their families, the purpose of rehabilitation is to prevent further deterioration or the development of complications, as well as to organize and implement an approach to initial and long-term management that optimizes function in family and community life.

Children with congenital or chronic disorders may also require acute rehabilitation (see Table 25-2). Many youths with genetic disorders or other congenital abnormalities, or those who experience chronic disease, often have delayed or atypical patterns of functional skill development. These children are also at risk for complications that can create a gradual or critical loss of function. Episodes of respiratory complications, bony fractures and dislocations, skin breakdown, or other systemic complications may be associated with functional deterioration. Children with cerebral palsy, spina bifida, or other types of congenital defects are included in this at-risk group. Likewise, children with congenital limb deficiency or arthrogryposis multiplex congenital syndrome may have reconstructive surgery necessitating acute rehabilitation. Children with osteogenesis imperfecta may have episodes of curtailed functional gains after injury and require acute rehabilitation services. Juvenile rheumatoid arthritis and systemic disorders can be associated with periods of rapid decline in function. For these children, the goals of rehabilitation are to limit or prevent further losses and facilitate reacquisition of skills consistent with the pattern of functional progression that was previously shown.

The third major group of children who receive acute rehabilitation services are those who are hospitalized for treatment with special medical, surgical, or technologic procedures (see Table 25-3). For children with cerebral palsy, casting procedures and uses of new medical interventions such as selective dorsal rhizotomy, continuous intrathecal baclofen, or other neurosurgical techniques to reduce spasticity may involve admission to acute rehabilitation (Fleet, 2003). Ilizarov procedures, the surgical technique of increasing congenital limb length or repairing severe orthopedic injury, may also be associated with acute rehabilitation (Karger, Guile, & Bowen, 1993; Mosca, 1991). Children with severe pulmonary complications or those who are ventilator dependent may be admitted for acute rehabilitation to assist families in learning how to perform care procedures and use medical technology (Buschbacher, 1995), for which long-term outcomes can be positive (Gilgoff & Gilgoff, 2003). These interventions often involve the therapists in following specific evaluation and treatment protocols designed to optimize functional outcomes.

A key feature of all types of admissions to acute rehabilitation is an emphasis on the planning and facilitation of community-based care plans. Discharge planning typically begins at referral to rehabilitation. School and other community-based providers are invited to participate in discharge arrangements to ease the transition from hospital to home and school settings. Often the hospital's outpatient services or clinics are recommended to monitor care and serve as an ongoing resource to the family and local care providers who implement the greater part of rehabilitation that takes place in home and school settings.

Outpatient and Ongoing Rehabilitation

Another major component of pediatric rehabilitation exists within specialized outpatient services and clinics that provide ongoing care. Typically, as part of children's hospitals or rehabilitation hospitals, interdisciplinary outpatient clinics are organized to provide monitoring and interventions with children who experience particular types of chronic health risks and disabilities. Occupational therapists often provide follow-up and follow-along attention to children and families after hospitalization, but many of these children are never hospitalized. Therapists who work at these clinics most often focus on the child or adolescent's health status and development, emphasizing functional progress and participation in home, school, and community activities.

Clinic programs that most commonly involve occupational therapists are displayed in Table 25-4. Such clinic programs may be scheduled weekly, monthly, quarterly, or even annually as needed. Sometimes these programs are conducted away from the hospital facility at community sites such as schools. Often the therapists offer consultation and recommendations to the family and local therapists who know the particular child well but have limited experience with a specific disorder or type of specialized intervention. For example, school personnel may have limited experience with children who have arthrogryposis, limb deficiency, or various forms of muscular dystrophy, whereas the hospital clinic therapists would have regular (e.g., weekly) experiences with these disabilities. Rapid developments in assistive technology (AT) also limit the likelihood that all schools or local

Table 25-4 Outpatient Clinics and Programs Often Served by Occupational Therapists

Clinic Title	Example of Clients or Services
Congenital disorders	Spina bifida
Neuromuscular disorders	Cerebral palsy
Developmental disabilities	Down syndrome
	Fetal alcohol syndrome
Rheumatology	Juvenile rheumatoid arthritis
	Systemic lupus erythematosus
Craniofacial abnormality	Cleft lip and palate
Orthopedic	Traumatic hand injury
	Congenital limb deficiency
Rehabilitation	Traumatic brain injury
	Spinal cord injury
Muscular dystrophy	Duchenne's muscular dystrophy
	Spinal muscle atrophy
Limb deficiency	Congenital amelia
	Traumatic amputation
Cystic fibrosis	Cystic fibrosis
Assistive technology	Seating and positioning
	Wheelchair control
	Augmentative communication
	Computers and information technology
	Environmental controls

programs can remain current and effective in applying new systems and approaches. Therapists who work in specialized hospital programs are provided with unique exposure to otherwise uncommon diagnoses and clinical procedures and can pass this experience on to other families and therapists as a conduit of information and new ideas. Specific study and preparation for consultation is suggested for entry-level therapists and can be an important skill for the therapist to develop as part of pediatric rehabilitation (Dudgeon & Greenberg, 1998).

Therapists also provide outpatient services in the form of individualized assessment and therapy trials at the hospital, home-based programs, or free-standing outpatient clinics. Outpatient services often occur concurrently with the child's return to school and school-based therapy; the former is organized around medical needs, whereas the latter addresses educational performance.

Efforts to augment function beyond the child's current development are also represented by efforts to apply uses of AT (see Chapters 18 and 19). The therapist may plan outpatient services to permit intensive evaluation and trials in the use of aided and augmentative communication systems, computer access and use of information technologies, therapeutic seating, powered mobility, or other technologies that enable environmental access and control. These applications of special procedures or AT devices are characterized by preplanned and often short trials leading to prescription of devices. Efforts culminate in intensive family training and transitions to follow-up in the community, often as a partnership with local providers in the environments in which AT devices are used.

Residential or intensive day-treatment programs characterize another form of outpatient pediatric rehabilitation service. Interdisciplinary services are most often organized for children and adolescents with brain injury. These extended care programs are geared toward direct assistance with community reentry and participation. Simulated or actual environments become the training site for skills that enable community participation and effective performance toward goals of independent living, education, and work activities.

Accrediting Agencies

Pediatric rehabilitation advocates and service providers have both influenced and been shaped by accreditation processes. For example, the Centers for Medicare and Medicaid Services (CMS) designate requirements for services that are organized and paid to provide "medical rehabilitation." To meet CMS guidelines for rehabilitation, rules are placed on such systems that mandate specific program emphasis, dedicated space and personnel, admission and discharge procedures, service intensity, goal setting, and monitoring of progress toward goals. Most rehabilitation programs also pursue voluntary accreditation by groups such as the Joint Commission on Accreditation of Healthcare Organizations (JCAHO) and the Commission on Accreditation of Rehabilitation Facilities (CARF). These organizations assign additional mandates that also shape program characteristics. Such guidelines may include integrated planning with community-based services and continuous quality improvement procedures. Every few years, accreditation standards and procedures based on JCAHO and CARF shift emphasis and specification of essential requirements. Generally, after initial accreditation, reaccreditation reports or visits are scheduled every 3 years, and programs may be subject to periodic interim review and reporting about their overall performance.

Reimbursement for Services

Inpatient pediatric rehabilitation services are typically funded by a combination of private insurance carriers, Medicaid or special programs within a state, and under some circumstances by Medicare. Preadmission review and authorization are generally required. For adults, as part of the Balanced-Budget Act of 1997, inpatient rehabilitation units are now required to use a prospective payment funding system (Cotterill & Gage, 2002). This mechanism is based on case-mixed groups, patterned after functional independence measure-function-related groups (FRGs) (Centers for Medicare and Medicaid

Services, 2003; Stineman, 2002). Pediatric rehabilitation costs are generally regarded as difficult to predict, and the development of appropriate prospective payment systems for such services is pending. Occupational therapy has typically been recognized as a service that is reimbursed within inpatient medical rehabilitation, home health care, and less commonly in outpatient services. Medicare guidelines are generally universal across different states. However, each state's Medicaid rules and regulations, and local insurance companies, have differing provisions related to funding of occupational therapy services and supplies or assistive devices that may be used or recommended. Local regulations must be reviewed to ensure that appropriate levels of reimbursement are available and that families are informed about service options.

Lengths of stay for acute pediatric rehabilitation are varied, from as short as a few days, to weeks, or perhaps months. Like adult rehabilitation units and all inpatient hospitals, third-party payers and other regulators strive to control costs by seeking shortened lengths of stay and by transferring clients more quickly to less costly skilled nursing facilities, home care, outpatient, or school-based services. Changes within and across treatment settings can be problematic, often creating confusion among families about entitlements and expectations for services. Clearly stated goals and time frames for outcomes in each care setting are desired. Case managers, who are familiar with funding rules and regulations, work with families and rehabilitation teams to coordinate services and prepare the family for transitions among care settings.

REHABILITATION TEAM

Hospital-based rehabilitation permits the child and family to benefit from a wide range of medical care specialists and services that they can access as needed. Pediatric rehabilitation teams also include various providers with differing expertise. Such teams are most often led by physicians who are trained as pediatricians and in other arenas of practice, such as neurology, orthopedics, or developmental medicine. Leadership and commitment in pediatric rehabilitation has come primarily from pediatricians jointly certified in the practice of physiatry (rehabilitation medicine) (Sneed, May, Stencel, & Paul, 2002).

The rehabilitation team places an emphasis on interdisciplinary teamwork, with each discipline having particular capabilities or areas of focus. Sometimes the team uses a transdisciplinary model so that only one or two professionals work directly with a particular child or family. Specific roles for each discipline within acute rehabilitation have been described for teams consisting of physicians, nurses, occupational therapists, physical therapists, speech-language pathologists, therapeutic recreational specialists, psychologists, social workers, educators, and other specialists (Blatzheim, Edberg, & Lacy, 1987; Eigsti, Aretz, & Shannon, 1990; Gardner & Workinger, 1990). In larger programs, specialty teams may develop so that the same personnel treat children grouped by diagnosis (e.g., TBI or SCI).

Team Interaction

Interdisciplinary care within pediatric rehabilitation is common and mandated by most regulatory mechanisms. The success of such collaboration often depends on a shared mission that focuses the team's energy and creativity. Team conferences that involve the family are typical. The team holds family conferences on admission, at key decision points during the hospitalization, and at discharge to ensure communication and clarification of care recommendations with the family and local care providers. In addition, the team conducts weekly rounds to review the progress of each child and discuss any changes in treatment plans that are designed for each problem.

The occupational therapy practitioner's holistic concerns related to health, function, and participation necessitate and are enriched by the collaborative relationships among team members of multiple disciplines. Partnerships between OTs and occupational therapy assistants can broaden the scope and timeliness of services. Need for frequent reevaluation and trials with new strategies necessitate dynamic and shared interventions. Team efforts are the rule rather than the exception in pediatric rehabilitation. For example, occupational and physical therapists often take a joint interest in addressing a child's gross- and fine-motor skills related to positioning, transfers, wheelchair seating, and functional mobility. The therapists can evaluate feeding and swallowing and augmentative communication and plan interventions in cooperation with speech-language pathologists. Nursing and occupational therapy personnel typically have collaborative roles dealing with skills such as grooming, dressing, and bathing and training in special-care routines of toileting and skin care. Occupational therapists may work together with therapeutic recreation specialists to provide adaptive play and socialization through activity and community outings.

A primary goal with children is to improve their participation and performance in educational programs. Acute rehabilitation programs and children's hospitals typically have teachers on staff. In conjunction with occupational therapists and other team members, these educators and developmental specialists can address skills and special needs that the child will have upon returning to school. Psychologists and those who specialize in neuropsychology also provide suggestions for school placement and may work with occupational therapists to adapt learning strategies for the child as he or she returns to the classroom. Social workers typically address issues of adjustment and coping with the child and family. All team members strive to be sensitive and supportive when educating family members to assume new duties as care providers. Recommendations should seek a realistic balance within the family culture, established roles, and new responsibilities for care.

Families

The therapist must recognize that many families are dealing with tragic events or at least unexpected complications that seriously affect their life processes. The children and adolescents are also challenged to deal with changes, and this process can be further complicated by their own cognitive or behavioral impairments (Donders, 1993). An educational model may provide a helpful perspective. Recognizing that family members have a short amount of time to learn a great deal about caring for their family member who is faced with new disabilities, rehabilitation team members also need to devote their time and attention to understanding the family's priorities and learning preferences. In all cases, the normal routines of the family are severely altered by hospitalization and residual disability (Rivara, 1993). This often creates worry, grief, and financial hardships that necessitate a transformation of relationships (Guerriere & McKeever, 1997). Families function in different ways, and variations in styles appear to have a lot to do with effective coping (Rivara et al., 1996). Healthy and resilient families may show exceptional caring, open communication, balancing of family needs, and positive problem-solving abilities. Families with limited coping skills may need increased support and help in identifying resources to meet immediate needs and in coping with problems that they will face during transitions back to managing the child at home. In either case, the needs of families often change during the rehabilitation process, requiring ongoing attention to maintain a collaborative partnership that can achieve the best outcomes for the child.

Transition from Rehabilitation to the Community

To facilitate continuity of care when the child is discharged from a pediatric rehabilitation hospitalization, the team and family should develop a comprehensive plan of transition. The child's transition from hospital to home is successful when both the sending and receiving agencies coordinate the transition (Case-Smith & Wavrek, 1998). Often a child with a TBI requires special education services after discharge from the medical center, and readiness to return to school may be particularly problematic due to social-behavioral challenges (Bedell, Haley, Coster & Smith, 2002). Team and family activities and communication need to focus on the transition from rehabilitation to school and community as soon as discharge is considered. Transition activities include interagency team meetings at which school and rehabilitation team members are represented. Ideally, at least one interagency meeting occurs in the rehabilitation unit and at least one in the school. By sharing where the meeting is hosted, team members get a realistic picture of the child's environments. When the meeting is at the team's home site, most, if not all, team members who worked with the child can be involved. By meeting the child and family before discharge and learning about the child's condition and needs, the school personnel can begin to plan and prepare an educational program. Visits by the medical team to the school at which the child will receive follow-up services can promote continuity of care.

Therapists from the hospital and school should share information related to concerns, priorities, and results of intervention approaches (what worked and what did not). The child's rehabilitation team can help problem-solve issues in the school's accessibility and possible modifications to the classroom and curriculum. Visits to the child's classroom can help identify accommodations that need to be in place. During these visits, the rehabilitation team can present information to the other students in the class about the child's disability, his or her rehabilitation, and the types of changes that they may expect in their peer. An inservice about the injury is most important when a child returns to his or her preinjury classroom, because the student's peers have preset expectations about his or her behavior and personality or, in the case of severe burns, about the student's appearance. In addition, before discharge the child should visit his or her home, school, and other important environments to determine what accommodations will need to be made. Visits followed by a return to the hospital can allow both school and hospital teams to address the issues proactively.

The rehabilitation team often monitors the child's progress during the first few months after discharge. The child may continue with outpatient services while initiating school-based services. Duplicate services can be beneficial during the period of transition as the child continues to make rapid progress while struggling to adapt to new environments. The consistent individuals in the transition are the family members, who ultimately support the child through the transition to the home. In support of this, the teams involved should provide the parents with comprehensive information about the special education system in their community, their rights as parents of a child who newly qualifies for special education services, and other community programs, supports, and resources that they can access. (See resources: www.familyvillage.wisc.edu/index.htmlx.)

RESEARCH ON EFFICACY OF PEDIATRIC REHABILITATION PROGRAMS

ADL and IADL status, discharge placement, health-related quality of life, and well-being are some of the typical measures used to document the rehabilitation outcomes (Fuhrer, 1987, 2000). Over the past 20 years, increasing emphasis has been placed on outcomes and ways to use research outcomes in evidence-based decision making (Bury & Mead, 1998). For adults, inpatient rehabilitation program outcomes have been assessed based on a variety of factors. Context of care and transition to different services have been appraised and questions have been asked about relative costs and functional gains made when receiving inpatient, outpatient or home-based services. Overall, dedicated units for some diagnoses are favored (Cardenas, Haselkorn, McElligott, & Gnatz, 2001), but it remains unclear if an advantage exists for one context of care over another. These findings, and other kinds of evidence, are reported in the Cochrane Library (www.update-software.com/Cochrane), where systematic reviews on these and other topics are collected and updated, or other sources of review including the *Bandolier Journal* (www.jr2.ox.ac.uk/bandolier).

In evidence-based-decision making, occupational therapy practitioners use research studies that describe medical and functional sequelae, validity of assessment tools related to diagnostic problem solving, and effectiveness of specific treatment strategies or techniques (Tickle-Degnen, 2000). O'Donnell and Roxborough (2002) recognize the challenge for therapists to find current research relevant to their practices. They offer guidelines on seeking evidence in pediatric rehabilitation. Researchers can now find systematic reviews (e.g., The Cochrane Library), seek topical reviews (e.g., *Bandolier Journal*), or pursue a precise search of research literature through electronic information sources (e.g., PUBMED, CINAHL).

Whereas adult inpatient rehabilitation programs have received considerable attention, comparable benefits to similar programs designed for children appear to be lacking. So far, most research about inpatient pediatric rehabilitation outcomes has described residual disability (Haley, Dumas, & Ludlow, 2001; Jaffe, Okamoto, & Lemire, 1986). Particular attention is usually paid to the most common diagnostic groups treated in these settings. For example, Dumas, Haley, Ludlow, and Rabin (2002) have reported functional gains demonstrated by children with TBI undergoing inpatient pediatric rehabilitation. The greatest gains were made in mobility, but also in social function and self-care for all ages of children. But after TBI, an extended period of recovery is expected. Boyer and Edwards (1991) reviewed outcomes of 220 children and adolescents with TBI who were admitted to a comprehensive pediatric rehabilitation program. They reported continued progress in mobility, ADLs, and education and cognition for up to 3 years after the injury. Physical recovery was greatest in the first year, and cognitive and language gains generally occurred later. Researchers have also studied complications from TBI by following children identified in trauma registries (Coster, Haley, & Baryza, 1994; DiScala, Osberg, Gans, Chin, & Grant, 1991). Jaffe and others conducted a thorough follow-up of children with head injury (Fay et al., 1994; Jaffe, Fay et al., 1993; Jaffe, Massaglio et al., 1993; Jaffe, Polissar, Fay, & Liao, 1995). In this series, researchers developed an age-matched cohort to provide a careful appraisal and monitoring of sequelae from mild, moderate, and severe classifications of TBI. Among these children who were 6 to 15 years of age at the time of injury, many with moderate and most with severe injury evidenced persisting and widespread cognitive, language, academic, behavioral, and functional deficits.

Some outcomes of pediatric rehabilitation have also been addressed by describing both inpatient and outpatient rehabilitation needs of specific populations. Massagli and Jaffe (1990) have described rehabilitation approaches for children with SCI, and Garcia, Gaebler-Spira, Sisung, and Heinemann (2002) reported that children with various SCI characteristics all made functional gains during inpatient rehabilitation. Dudgeon, Massagli, and Ross (1997) reported the follow-up of a series of children returning to school. Children with a primary brain tumor who received rehabilitative care have been reported to show improved management of residual disability (Philip, Ayyangar, Vanderbilt, & Gaebler-Spira, 1994). Rehabilitative needs of other children have also been demonstrated, including those with burns (Herndon, Rutan, & Rutan, 1993; Latenser & Kowal-Vern, 2002), osteogenesis imperfecta (Binder et al., 1993), spina bifida (Watson, 1991), asthma (Strunk, Mascia, Lipkowitz, & Wolf, 1991), pulmonary disorders (Buschbacher, 1995), and other disorders (Heery, 1992; Russman, 1990). Assessment practices in pediatric rehabilitation are also getting more attention (see the discussion under "Evaluation"). Specific assessment tool developments are under way to more effectively appraise function and residual function and participation challenges (Hotz, Helm-Estabrooks, & Nelson, 2001).

Evidence regarding efficacy of specific intervention strategies is known to be lacking because it is tremendously difficult and costly to conduct research that analyzes the application of particular techniques or rehabilitation strategies. Experimental research of rehabilitation effectiveness is particularly difficult to conduct because of the heterogeneity of participants and ethical conflicts encountered by suspending or withholding services to specific children. Randomized clinical trials are particularly problematic and alternate research strategies are being proposed (Ottenbacher & Hinderer, 2001) with an emphasis on humanistic elements as part of therapeutic practice (Halstead, 2001) and client's views about process and outcomes (Armstrong & Kerns, 2002; Kramer, 1997). However, a specific analysis of different priorities within pediatric rehabilitation, mixtures of service providers, or contrasts with less intensive subacute or outpatient services have not been reported. Routine appraisal of client benefits and overall program effectiveness are being mandated by professional organizations, the insurance industry, and governmental agencies involved in regulation and reimbursement of rehabilitation programs and services. Therefore, further research of pediatric rehabilitation program outcomes of common diagnostic groups should be anticipated in coming years.

OCCUPATIONAL THERAPY SERVICES

Functions of Occupational Therapists

The primary focus of the occupational therapy practitioner within pediatric rehabilitation is on ADLs and other instrumental tasks associated with independent living, education, and community participation. Therapists use many frames of reference to develop insights about the child's function, establish priorities for treatment, and guide the organization of treatment goals with the child, family, and local care providers. In most forms of rehabilitation, the therapist follows a prioritization system that first focuses on prevention of problems associated with major trauma or disability, then resumption of the able self, and finally restoration of lost skills and functions. A key concept in rehabilitation is the recognition that many therapeutic outcomes relate to learning (Schwartz, 1991). Thus, therapists employ behavioral and cognitive learning principles and attend to the teacher-pupil relationship. The therapist blends his or her technical competency with personal caring and mutuality of goals and efforts with children and families.

Task, activity, and occupation analyses form another universal strategy that therapists use to determine the skill requirements of functional tasks and the therapeutic uses of occupation to improve skills. Such analysis breaks down tasks into performance skills and factors, such as demands placed on body structures and functions, as well as motor, process, and communication and interaction strategies used in functioning. The therapist can reorganize or adapt activities so that certain skills are substituted or emphasized over those that are missing or in deficit. Specific intervention techniques used to achieve priority goals combine biomechanical, sensorimotor, perceptual-cognitive, and rehabilitative treatment approaches (see Chapters 9 to 12).

A critical component of all treatment planning is also the occupational therapy practitioner's attention to goal setting (Kielhofner & Barrett, 1998). A collaborative process with families is essential in specifying goals and sometimes has as much to do with outcomes as any particular therapeutic techniques that are used (Bower, McLellan, Arney, & Campbell, 1996).

Prevention

Primary prevention is a term used to denote efforts that decrease the likelihood of accidents, violence, or disease for everyone. *Secondary* and *tertiary prevention* refer to specific interventions, arrangement of care systems, and environmental modifications to prevent the onset of problems among at-risk populations. Children admitted to pediatric rehabilitation units are typically at risk for developing a number of secondary disabilities. The therapist, along with other team members, has a responsibility to be familiar with such risks. Included are concerns for safety in positioning and movement, risks of aspiration in swallowing, provision of orientation, and appropriate measures to reduce stresses experienced in an unfamiliar environment and to prevent self-injurious behaviors. The therapist must be aware of risks and avoid involving the child in occupations that would be harmful or would perpetuate impaired habits that could hamper recovery. Complications from immobilization, abnormal muscle tone, and other neuromuscular abnormalities often necessitate careful attention to maintaining range of motion, strength, and general fitness (Figure 25-1). Concern for wound healing and protection of neurogenic skin are also essential to the early planning

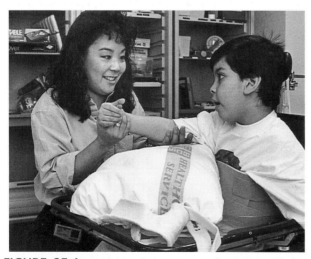

FIGURE 25-1 Active assistive range of motion exercises are performed several times each day to prevent joint and muscle contractures with this boy who sustained a severe closed head injury. Stretch is also applied to existing contractures, along with other joint mobilization techniques.

and ongoing achievement of goals, interventions, and education of the child and his or her family.

Resumption

The second level of priority for occupational therapy is a focus on resuming the use of available skills and independence in easily accomplished tasks. Emphasizing the able self provides the individual child with an opportunity to resume doing tasks on his or her own, or at least to have a say about how he or she is assisted. Such an approach may be important in preventing the child or adolescent from developing dependent behaviors or learned helplessness. The latter has been commonly described in adults who are admitted to institutional-like settings in which supervision is abundant (Raps, Peterson, Jonas, & Seligman, 1982). Efficiency demands placed on nursing may often result in the child becoming a passive recipient of care. The therapist should provide the child with sufficient time to perform activities on his or her own. Early emphasis on providing children with opportunities to make choices about the types of assistance they receive or activities they pursue should help them develop confidence in their returning abilities.

Restoration

Lost skills and function follow in priority, with efforts to restore abilities. The therapist uses biomechanical, sensorimotor, perceptual-cognitive, and rehabilitative approaches in various combinations to restore function. Such approaches may necessitate extensive retraining or complex adaptation. When performance is severely impaired, reacquisition of skill is often initiated during acute rehabilitation with continuation of training as part of outpatient and ongoing rehabilitative care.

Each prioritization level may capitalize on treatment strategies drawn from frames of references that directly address performance skills and factors. For example, biomechanical and sensorimotor techniques are designed to improve skills and factors such as strength, range of motion, postural control, skilled movements, and coordination. Such approaches include the use of therapeutic activities and exercise, splinting and positioning, physical handling, and the use of biomedical devices like functional electric stimulation. Other physical agent modalities such as superficial heat or cold may be used, whereas deep-heating techniques such as ultrasound are often avoided because children's bone epiphyseal (growth plates) areas may be damaged (Michlovitz, 1996). Children with perceptual and cognitive difficulties often go through retraining or are taught to go through methods of adaptation.

The occupational therapist often helps the client practice activities that selectively challenge individual's skills or factors with the expectation that these will then transfer or generalize to occupational performance areas.

Rehabilitative approaches contrast with biomechanical and sensorimotor techniques that are designed to address underlying performance skills and factors. In the rehabilitation approach, therapists teach clients compensatory techniques that use existing skills to maintain or restore occupational performance. In rehabilitative approaches, therapists teach clients to use adapted routines and AT devices and modify environments to promote optimal function. Initial training and the use of AT devices to enable manipulation, mobility, cognition, and communication are part of restoration. Client outcomes are optimal when occupational therapy practitioners use complementary strategies to improve the child's skills, adapt functional activities, and modify environmental contexts.

Evaluation

In nearly all instances, occupational therapy services in hospital-based pediatric rehabilitation are initiated through physician's orders. Often required by law or regulatory guidelines, therapists respond to initial orders and negotiate as necessary with the physician to add specific elements to assessment and intervention activities. Most commonly, initial orders to occupational therapy involve a focus on ADLs and performance skills and factors that support function.

Multiple sources for data are available within the pediatric rehabilitation setting. Review of medical records and discussions with other providers may form the initial basis for evaluation. In general, evaluation consists of asking (e.g., clinical interview), looking (e.g., clinical observation), touching (e.g., physical examination), and testing (e.g., using standardized assessments). Most often, the therapist uses clinical interview and observation to initiate the assessment process. Observed areas of concern may necessitate a more thorough evaluation through physical examination and direct observation with the use of standardized tests. Such measures help in the diagnostic process. Impairments in performance components are likely to be implicated as causes of difficulties in areas of occupation. Once the therapist makes the hypotheses and initiates intervention plans, the repeated use of clinical examination and standardized tests serves as objective measures of skill improvement. For diagnostic purposes, the therapist judges a child's performance against normed scores, but for evaluative purposes, the therapist judges a child's scores on reassessment against his or her previous performance. Selection of a specific measure should be based on its reliability, sensitivity, and appropriateness given the child's age and diagnosis.

Evaluation of ADL and IADL skills helps prioritize which performance skills and factors may be impaired and require the use of more specific assessments. After the child's ability to participate in functional activities has been evaluated, the therapist analyzes performance skills and factors to determine those that may be targeted in intervention and the types of adaptations that may be warranted. The child's contexts affect occupational performance and require careful analysis and modification.

The therapist may organize assessment of ADL and IADLs around checklists or other reporting tools that specify activities and methods of rating the individual's level of skill. For example, the Functional Independence Measure (FIM) was developed as part of a Uniform Data System for Medical Rehabilitation for use in client-specific as well as program monitoring and outcome evaluation systems (Keith, Granger, Hamilton, & Sherwin, 1987). The FIM is generally for individuals 7 years of age and older. A pediatric version of this tool, called the Wee-FIM, has been developed for children of developmental age 6 months to 7 years (Msall, DiGaudio, & Duffy, 1993), and validity studies have been completed (Ottenbacher et al., 2000). Eighteen specific ADL tasks, including communication and social cognition, are rated for dependence based on the individual's need for adaptation and assistance from a helper.

Another tool that the therapist can use for rating and describing function in children is the Pediatric Evaluation of Disability Inventory (PEDI) (Haley, Coster, Ludlow, Haltiwanger, & Andrellos, 1992). Based on a combination of interview and observation, the PEDI specifies discrete levels of skills in domains of self-care, mobility, and social function. A description of needs for care provider assistance and reliance on AT devices is included with the measure. Both the FIM and PEDI are used for individualized assessment and planning; and both can also be used as part of program evaluation. The PEDI and Wee-FIM have been shown to measure similar constructs (Ziviani et al., 2001). Although these tools focus directly on daily functional tasks, the use of additional broad-based measures that assess play- and school-related performance is also encouraged in rehabilitation settings (Johnston & Granger, 1994).

Following these functional assessments, the therapist has specific needs to pursue an analysis of performance skills and factors. Tools and methods to evaluate performance skills and factors are described in Chapters 7 and 8. Careful appraisal of motor, process, and communication skills helps to identify intervention goals and plans. Performance contexts can enable or hinder function. Cultural, spiritual, and social contextual factors influence the selection of intervention strategies and styles of communicating and interacting.

Determining Intervention Goals

As stated throughout this text, goals for services must be explicitly stated, measurable, and functionally relevant. A goal to "increase ADL skills" is not adequate. For the child, family, and third-party payers, the therapist must specify clearer targets for functional outcomes. The therapist should write long-term goals to reflect the outcomes expected during the child's length of stay (e.g., acute rehabilitation admission). The therapist specifies short-term goals as interim steps toward reaching long-term goals. Goals describe specific tasks that the child will perform, conditions of performance, and the type and frequency of assistance needed. Component skills that are emphasized by the therapist may be described as goals if they are appropriately linked to meaningful functional outcomes (e.g., achieve eye-hand coordination and manipulation skills sufficient for desktop activities and writing at school).

Functional goals must include specification of skills and the level of independence that is being sought. Levels of *independence* describe varying degrees of dependence on personal assistance, adaptive environments, and the use of AT devices. In many cases, ADL goals describe how the child or adolescent will manage personal care assistants to achieve a self-managed dependence. On most ADL scales, level of independence is rated as the amount of physical and cognitive assistance needed as a proportion of the task (e.g., moderate assist = 50% assistance of the amount of time required for partial task, whole task, and task transition assistance by a care provider). However, when concerned with the integration of an individual back into his or her home, the concept of *interdependence* among family members may be a more important consideration. Given the negative value associated with dependence in the Anglo-American culture, a more positive term to express shared needs between family members is interreliance.

In pediatric rehabilitation, the selection of specific goals is influenced by various factors. Goals based on the family's priorities are likely to garner the best participation and support. Priorities for function are individualized and may differ from those presumed by therapists. The child or adolescent's ability to restore skills in personal ADLs and important everyday occupations helps restore a sense of well-being. However, institutional and insurance directives also influence the selection of goals. A reduction of dependence makes care possible in progressively less restrictive and less costly environments. Intervention goals most often focus on functional skill acquisition that enables the child to be discharged from inpatient hospital settings to services provided within long-term care, home health care, outpatient care, and eventually to use of non-medical community support systems.

Intervention
Preventing Secondary Disability and Restoring Performance Skills

The prevention of secondary disability and the reduction of existing complications is of the highest priority in a treatment plan. The therapist typically addresses neuro-muscular and musculoskeletal complications by using programs designed to help the client maintain or regain normal passive range of motion. Through the use of special handling techniques, the occupational and physical therapists carry out daily programs that can involve slow stretch and joint mobilization. The therapists can correct existing limitations by using a combination of these techniques and specialized positioning and splinting. The therapist may apply splints for various purposes, including maintaining positions (e.g., resting hand splint), increasing range of motion (e.g., drop-out splints, dynamic splints with spring tension forces, or serial casting), or promoting function (e.g., wrist cock-up, tenodesis splints) (Figure 25-2).

The therapist facilitates improved movement and strength by using activities and exercises that are most often incorporated into play. For children and adolescents with musculoskeletal and lower motor neuron or motor unit disorders, the use of progressive exercise and activity routines may be appropriate. For those with TBI causing upper motor neuron dysfunction, muscle tone and voluntary motor control are addressed. The therapist can use various sensorimotor techniques to manage muscle tone, with the goal of promoting agonist and antagonist balance as a basis for movement (see Chapters 9 and 10).

A second major concern of pediatric rehabilitation is skin care. Pressure areas from bed positioning, static sitting, and the use of orthosis and splints call for routine skin monitoring. The child must often develop a tolerance to new positioning strategies and splint applications over several days, with skin tolerance being a critical issue in decisions to change bed positions, increase sitting time, and use splints or other orthotic devices.

Individuals often experience perceptual, cognitive, and behavioral dysfunction after TBI. With a prevention emphasis, programs to ensure safety in movement and

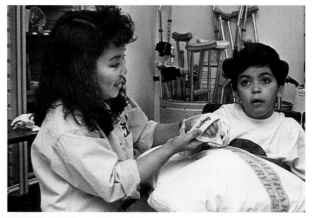

FIGURE 25-2 Splints are used to prevent or reduce contractures. The use of serial static splints requires regular monitoring and clear instructions for use to family members and other care providers.

with manipulation of objects are critical. Environmental modifications are made to ensure the child's safety. The therapist also implements methods to alleviate stresses of disorientation and memory loss, although restricted environments and restraints may be necessary initially. The placement of family pictures and other familiar items from home may create a stimulating and more comforting environment. When the child is more alert and aware of his or her surroundings, the therapist may use an educational approach coupled with behavioral interventions. The therapist should inform the child of unit rules, post such rules, and emphasize strict adherence to them. The therapist may carry out reinforcement programs structured through a team and family approach to shape behaviors (Silver, Boake, & Cavazos, 1994). The therapist can also use daily orientation programs and memory books to ease the burden of confusion. It is important to teach the family about the child's perceptual and cognitive impairments and programs in place to ensure safety and comfort.

Resuming and Restoring Occupational Performance

Once the therapist negotiates goals for ADL performance, he or she determines what the child needs to learn, how such learning will take place, and how training can best be organized within the clinical care setting. Through natural learning, the child or adolescent may discover, in one or more sessions, simple strategies to resume activity performance. If these techniques are safe and efficient, the therapist need only guide the child in determining appropriate means to achieve consistent performance. However, many times the child is unable to make natural adaptations to achieve performance. Therapists can then guide new learning by instructing the child or adolescent and other care providers in the principles of adaptation and engage them in joint problem solving to determine the most effective methods of performance.

Once the therapist determines what the child needs to learn, he or she organizes specific and desired routines for learning. In guided learning, some form of instruction takes place through a combination of directions and the use of instructional aids. For initial instruction of new or adapted tasks, the therapist may demonstrate the task to be learned and have the child copy that demonstration. The therapist may also use verbal or manual guidance cues to assist learning (Figures 25-3 and 25-4). For some tasks, predetermined scripts or learning materials are available (Pedretti & Early, 2001; Trombly & Radomski, 2002).

When the therapist has determined a particular task sequence, he or she selects methods to achieve repetition, generalization, and development of new skills (Figure 25-5). For example, the therapist may help the

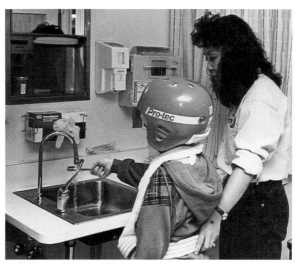

FIGURE 25-3 The occupational therapist provides the child with cues and performance feedback while he carries out an adapted personal ADL sequence. A helmet is required to protect the head because of an open skull fracture.

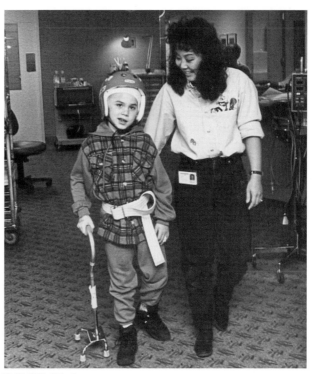

FIGURE 25-4 Mobility is a fundamental part of ADL routines. After completing a morning care routine, this child walks to breakfast with assistance from the occupational therapist for safety and technique.

child memorize a routine so that the child can guide his or her own performance using verbal, visual, or tactile feedback. If the child cannot memorize a routine, the therapist can use other training tools. A therapist can prepare written instructions, pictorial step cues, and

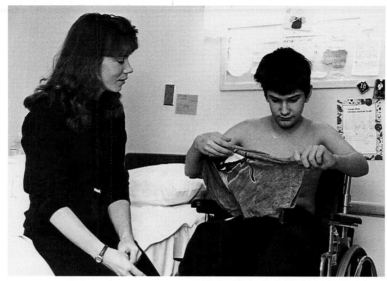

FIGURE 25-5 Adapted dressing routines are developed to achieve success and ease learning. For this boy, who has perceptual and cognitive deficits after brain injury, the occupational therapist cues him in a repetitive sequence of steps that accomplish the task.

audiotapes with specific directions. Whole-task instruction and the use of forward- or reverse-step sequence training are common methods. The therapist can implement training over several days that capitalizes on the times when tasks are routinely performed (e.g., dressing in the morning and at night or before and after swimming). As training progresses, the therapist gradually reduces the extent of external cueing from a person or instructional aids so that only a minimal amount of such support is required for safe and efficient performance. Often the team and family plan for the gradual withdrawal of aides and assistance after the child is discharged from the inpatient hospital setting. Strategies that will continue to promote the child's participation in daily activities, including school, form the basis of family or care provider training.

The environment used for ADL therapy sessions is also important. Most therapists agree that children prefer familiar environments. However, except in home health care service delivery, environments must be simulated in hospital rooms or clinics. Generalization of performance from one setting to another can be difficult because familiar settings may provide unrecognized prompts that are not present in simulated settings. Home visits with the child and family to survey and collaborate in planning for organizational changes, equipment needs, and architectural modifications can facilitate the necessary transition. Day or weekend home passes for the child are desirable when possible. The therapist often develops specific goals, and feedback from the family about the time at home can be important to prioritizing goals, equipment, and family educational needs.

Adaptations for ADL Skills

Basic principles apply to adapted performance of ADL skills, and these are described in Box 25-1. New learning is generally more difficult and more energy consuming than old habit patterns, but change is often necessary. Safety in performance and the avoidance of abnormal or unsafe movements are essential. Principles of joint protection and work simplification are commonly used, and performance is geared toward functioning in a barrier-free environment with the use of familiar conveniences. Adaptations of a routine are aimed at reducing complexity, ensuring safety, and minimizing complications if errors occur.

Adaptive methods of ADL and IADL skills may include the use of different strategies and devices (see Box 25-1). A client's reliance on AT devices may be temporary or permanent. The early use of devices can increase safety or immediate function during recovery. The permanent use of devices is also common when the individual exhibits residual impairments necessitating adaptation. When selecting devices, therapists often choose to adapt existing equipment that is already familiar to them. If such adaptation is not desirable or practical, the therapist may direct the family toward purchase of items with features that are more compatible with the child's or adolescent's special needs through standard shopping sources. If needs cannot be met, specialized rehabilitation devices are purchased through medical and rehabilitation equipment vendors. AT devices are generally designed to accommodate or substitute for skill limitations in gross movement, reach, prehension and

BOX 25-1 Basic Rehabilitation Strategies

Occupational therapists use several strategies for specific types of dysfunctions to adapt activities for children with functional limitations. In addition to these suggestions, ADL and IADL adaptations have been described (see Chapter 15) along with the uses of assistive technology (AT) that should be reviewed (see Chapters 18 and 19).

MOTOR LIMITATIONS
Limited Range of Motion

Reduced range of motion in the neck, trunk, and proximal and intermediate joints of the limbs limits ability to reach all parts of the body and objects within the immediate environment. Limitations of hand motion can reduce holding and handling of objects. To substitute for reach, the child should use extended and specially angled handles (e.g., long-handled spoon or fork, bath brush, dressing stick, or shoe horn) or devices that are more specialized, such as reachers. If a child is unable to use devices that extend reach, the therapist employs other strategies to permit function. Mounting objects on the floor, wall, or table and bringing the body part to the device (e.g., boot tree for removing shoes, friction pad on floor for socks, hook on the wall to pull pants up or down, or sponges mounted in the shower to wash) prove useful. For some tasks, devices may replace any reach requirement, such as the use of a bidet for hygiene after toileting or manual or electric feeders operated by microswitches to bring food to the mouth.

When motion of the hand is limited, the therapist can assist holding and manipulating of objects by providing enlarged or differently styled handles that reduce the grasp requirement (e.g., T-handled cup). The therapist can replace holding functions by the use of universal cuff or C-shaped handles. Friction surfaces may provide more secure grasp. When forearm rotation is limited, swivel spoons or angled utensils may assist bringing food to the mouth.

Limited range of motion also reduces gross-motor movements, such as in bed mobility and elevation changes (moving from sitting to standing and performing transfers in bathing and toileting). The therapist typically changes surface levels (i.e., raised or lowered) to limit the extent of elevation change required. The therapist may lower the bed height to allow ease in wheelchair transfers or raise it to ease in coming up to standing from sitting. Raised chairs, toilet seats, and bath benches reduce extreme changes in elevation required in transfers.

Decreased Strength and Endurance

Strength and endurance limitations are common among children who are acutely ill or injured. The goals of adaptation are to reduce the effects of gravity by the use of lightweight objects, movements in the horizontal plane, reduced friction, and, when possible, the use of body mechanics for leverage and gravity to assist movement. Electrically powered devices may meet goals of work simplification. Efficiency of movement is essential. Similar to limited range of motion, weakness can cause inability to reach body parts or make elevation changes. Extended handles may be necessary; however, increased weight and the forces required to handle and apply leverage can increase difficulty.

A major goal with activity adaptation for decreased strength is to limit the need to sustain static postures and prolonged holding. The therapist can use surfaces to support posture and proximal limb positions in various ways (e.g., bed positioning, seating adaptations, and the use of armrests and table surfaces). The therapist reduces the need for sustained holding by mounting devices or stabilizing devices with friction

(e.g., Dycem or spike board) or using an enlarged lightweight object. Universal cuffs or C-cuffs are also common to limit demands for grasp. Manipulation may be impaired and necessitate the use of hooks and loops on clothing and adaptation of fasteners by the use of Velcro, zippers, enlarged buttons, or elastic shoelaces. Less complex movement and reduced force is required to manipulate lever handles on faucets, doors, and appliances. The therapist helps the child reduce movement against gravity in transfers by changing the heights of surfaces and using devices such as sliding boards, springs, or hydraulic lifts to aid movement.

For children with cardiac or pulmonary disorders, progression of ADL performance may be based on estimated metabolic equivalents levels or by direct monitoring. The therapist should schedule and pace tasks, simplify work, and use rest breaks within tasks.

Incoordination

Incoordination primarily causes difficulty with manipulation skills. The extent to which incoordination influences performance is determined by the range of movement required, weight and resistance of objects being handled, and positioning of the body in relation to objects. A primary concern is to achieve proximal stability when executing movements. Stabilizing the trunk and head while making movements of the arm and hand is thought to improve skilled movements. Likewise, the therapist should stabilize the proximal segments of the limb while manipulating the hand (e.g., resting the elbow and forearm on the table while using the wrist and fingers to manipulate objects). Friction surfaces and containers that hold objects being manipulated may also be suggested for stabilization of the limb (e.g., friction pad plate or nonslip cup).

Another common strategy is to determine if increased weight dampens exaggerated movements and tremor. The therapist may select heavier objects or add weight to objects. The therapist can attach a weight to the arm or apply resistance to movement by placing devices across joints (e.g., elastic sleeves, friction feeder) to determine if more precise movements can be achieved. When such methods are inadequate, other techniques employed are similar to those for reduced range of motion and strength, including mounting devices on stable surfaces and bringing the body to these devices using gross movements.

One-Handed Techniques

When a child has to perform most activities with one hand, the barriers to be overcome typically involve replacing the stabilization function of the other limb, improving the skills of the hand being used, and adapting tasks that require alternating movements of two hands. Generally, the child can accomplish many tasks easily with the use of one hand. If the hand being used was not previously the preferred or dominant hand, skilled movements may take a greater amount of time to develop. For those with perceptual and cognitive impairments, learning to use one hand may be particularly difficult. For children with hemiplegia, various dressing routines have been scripted that follow the rules of dressing the affected limb first and avoiding the use of abnormal postures. The stabilization function of the impaired limb may not be entirely lost, although the child may need to learn how to assist movement in placing or positioning the limb to effectively stabilize objects. To entirely replace the stabilization function of the impaired or lost upper limb, the therapist may use mounting or friction surfaces. Some two-handed tasks require the use of

Continued

BOX 25-1 Basic Rehabilitation Strategies—*cont'd*

specially designed devices or methods. For example, the therapist can provide the child with a rocker-knife or cutting-edged fork to help him or her cut with a knife and fork, a button hook to aid in buttoning, a special lacing technique to aid in shoe tying, and a one-handed keyboard arrangement and training program to aid in typing.

PERCEPTUAL AND COGNITIVE LIMITATIONS

Sensory, perceptual, and cognitive impairments alone pose various challenges to ADL performance but are most often associated with other physical disorders previously described. If retraining of performance skills is ineffective and dysfunction continues, the therapist should consider substitution for impaired skills by using more intact sensory, perceptual, or cognitive skills (e.g., using a bell on the hemiplegic arm to draw attention if being neglected tactually or visually). Compensation techniques may also be planned that modify the activity sequence and environment to enable the child to accomplish the challenging task.

Perceptual and Cognitive Deficit

Perceptual and cognitive deficits affect ADL skill routines and school performance. To compensate for perceptual or cognitive deficits, the therapist can design step-by-step routines with cueing systems and repeat them in training. The therapist

employs work simplification principles and uses substitution strategies. Children with these deficits may rely on memorizing and reciting a verbal routine or follow audiotaped instruction. They may also rely on written instructions or pictorial cues. With impaired visual perception, the child may need to learn reliance on tactile feedback cues. At times, the therapist specially selects materials used in ADL to compensate for impairments. The therapist may use color-contrasted clothing, texture, or color-coding cues with objects. Sometimes the therapist can encourage the use of mirrors to give the child feedback about his or her performance.

Visual Impairment

Blindness or severe visual impairment requires that the therapist employ strategies to substitute for vision by the use of other sensory skills and cognitive routines. Consistent organization of the environment and storage of items is necessary. The therapist may use tactile identifiers on objects such as raised letters and locations of more transient items described by a companion or a standard technique such as analog clock location. The therapist can build sound feedback into some items to aid in orientation or search. Mobility specialists instruct individuals to use techniques such as long canes or guide dogs for ambulation or wheelchair guidance and to use a leader's arm for guidance in walking.

---

manipulation, sensation, or perception and cognition. The use of devices should reduce task difficulty and complexity, although initial learning and use may seem awkward.

SUMMARY

Hospital-based pediatric rehabilitation services play a unique role in the overall management of children and adolescents with a new or chronic disability. In addressing acute and chronic problems, the emphasis of practice is nearly always on function and participation in life's events at home, at school, and in the community. Both new and established impairments and disabilities pose risks for further complications, which necessitate a prevention prioritization through subacute, acute, and outpatient or ongoing rehabilitation interventions.

Services are medically oriented and delivered within constraints imposed by accreditation and regulatory agencies and third-party payers. Collaboration with school- and community-based services is critical to effective intervention and transition. The challenge of pediatric rehabilitation is to address the acute problems while considering the overall development of the individual and the priorities of the family.

Using strategically placed guiding questions, the following case descriptions promote the student's ability to use clinical reasoning. Students should respond to the questions after each section before reading the next.

Case Study 1: Stephen

Physician prescription: 8-year-old boy with mild R hemiplegia 2° traumatic brain injury, skull fracture

Precautions: Dysphagia, aphasia, falls

Treatment objectives: Evaluate and train ADL skills, Passive Range Of Motion (PROM) with Right Upper Extremity (RUE), facilitate the use of RUE, evaluate and intervene for visual/perceptual and cognitive skill deficits

1 Given this prescription, what would you do next?
2 What information would you collect before seeing Stephen?
3 Which frames of reference would you use and why?

Referral History

Stephen is an 8-year-old boy from a two-parent, three-sibling home in a small coastal town. Family members describe Stephen as being energetic and well-liked. In October, he was a passenger on a three-wheel all-terrain vehicle when it rolled over. Stephen was not wearing a helmet and was reported to have struck his head. He was initially alert but soon experienced diminished wakefulness and was unresponsive when paramedics arrived. At the trauma center, Stephen was found to have a left basilar skull fracture, and a computed tomography (CT) scan showed bilateral frontal punctate lesions and an apparent left temporal-parietal focal lesion. Three days after the injury, Stephen became more responsive, but he demonstrated minimal movement of his right arm and leg, no vocalizations, and dysphagia. He continued to show gradual improvement in his level of consciousness and was evaluated for transfer to acute rehabilitation. His injury was classified as moderate. Twelve days after the accident, Stephen was transferred to the local children's hospital.

1 Given this information, identify your initial priorities for evaluation.
2 What specific evaluation activities do you suggest? Specify an assessment sequence and time period for evaluations.
3 Based on your evaluation activities, what are your intervention priorities?

Clinical Findings

On admission to rehabilitation, Stephen was following simple one-step commands and attempting to verbalize, but word finding was difficult. He was noted to be fatigued and difficult to engage for more than a few minutes at a time. He was also regarded as quiet, reserved, and fearful of being separated from his mother, who stayed with him nearly full-time during the day and evenings. Diminished alertness, easy distraction, and disorientation to place and time were also noted. These dysfunctions caused Stephen to become anxious during evaluation and treatments. Swallowing was judged safe from aspiration, although one-to-one supervision was recommended because of Stephen's tendency to over-stuff food and poorly sequence his intake of fluids and solids.

During grooming and dressing tasks, Stephen was observed as being disorganized. In part because of his age, he showed poor ability to make natural adaptations to hemiplegia. Continual verbal cues were needed to initiate, set up, and proceed with grooming, dressing, and bathing tasks. Physical demonstration and cues were needed to teach adapted sequences. No perceptual deficits were found by observation or by the use of standardized tests.

Further observations showed mild right hemiplegia, characterized by effortful movements of both upper and lower limbs. Little spontaneous use of his right arm was seen, and Stephen showed characteristic synergy patterns and increased muscle tone when he attempted to grasp objects on command. Passive range of motion was normal. In sensory testing, Stephen showed impaired proprioception and localization to touch in distal portions of the arm and leg. Stephen did not ambulate but had partial weight bearing in stance with foot drop when he tried to walk. The physical therapist initiated the use of a right ankle-foot orthosis (R-AFO) and a cane.

1 Based on these evaluation findings, identify specific priorities to address in interventions.
2 Suggest at least three long-term treatment goals that could be negotiated with family.

3 Specify frames of reference, intervention activities, and treatment time planning to address each goal.
4 Identify appropriate strategies to meet Stephen's cognitive and behavioral needs
5 Suggest teaching and training methods for ADLs.
6 Plan strategies to promote fine-motor function.

Intervention Activities

The therapist initiated the use of an orientation board in Stephen's room, regular reminders provided by staff and his mother, written schedules, and a memory book that Stephen completed after each treatment session. The therapist planned consistent routines for personal ADLs, sequenced daily therapies, and structured play activities. The therapist used familiar play items, pictures of family, his own clothes, his favorite music, and art supplies to enhance comfort and provide memory cues and prompts for orientation. The therapist organized visits by other family members and friends from school and included them as part of scheduling and memory book entries.

The therapist scheduled Stephen for one-to-one therapy sessions twice each day and planned morning personal ADL training and afternoon therapeutic activities. In addition to structured ADL routines and orientation-memory programs, the therapist also engaged Stephen in selected activities to facilitate the use of his right arm and provide cognitive challenge in organizing steps, following sequences, and sustaining engagement in both familiar and novel tasks (Figure 25-6). The therapist taught Stephen self-daily range-of-motion and whole-body stretches to maintain normal range and facilitate symmetric trunk and limb use.

Spontaneous use of his right arm improved, but poor recovery of his right hand resulted in Stephen attempting to perform activities using his nondominant left hand. Such attempts proved to be awkward and

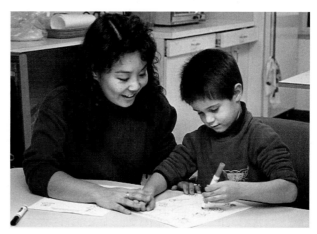

FIGURE 25-6 The occupational therapist promotes the use of the hemiparetic arm to hold the paper while the child carries out a drawing and writing activity.

unsuccessful. The therapist trained Stephen and cued him to use both hands together (Figure 25-7), using the right hand as an assist to the left hand. This strategy improved his personal ADL performance so that the therapist discontinued use of adaptive devices such as a button-aid and a rocker knife after 2 weeks. Handwriting with either the right or left hand was not satisfactory for schoolwork because of language disorders, illegibility, and slow speed. The therapist introduced a computer keyboard and initiated supplementary handwriting activities to facilitate movement and augment function. The therapist judged Stephen's physical management of other school-related tasks to be adequate, although communication and cognitive impairments posed major challenges to his return to school. Three weeks after admission, Stephen was ambulatory with the use of an AFO. He continued to show evidence of topographic disorientation, getting lost between the hospital room and the clinic, but otherwise he was thought to be a safe ambulator, even on uneven surfaces and stairs. He groomed, dressed, and bathed with supervision for initiation and safety. Stephen appropriately initiated toileting, and his mother judged his hygiene after bowel movements to be adequate.

1 Determine discharge training needs with Stephen, his family, and school personnel.
2 Specify follow-up plans and extension of pediatric rehabilitation services.

Discharge Follow-up Plan

Discharge planning included home program suggestions for Stephen and his family. In addition to organizing ADL routines for Stephen to use at home, the therapist wrote activities to promote fine-motor skills and reviewed them with Stephen's mother. The team held meetings with school personnel to address academic program needs and potential benefits from school-based therapy services. The team attempted to determine

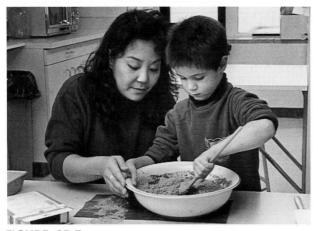

FIGURE 25-7 The therapist provides guidance in using both arms while participating in a cookie-baking activity.

eligibility for special education and used age/gender-normed tests that the school system would accept in its review. The team scheduled interim school visits by the hospital neuropsychologist to occur after Stephen's return to a half-day school program 2 weeks after discharge. The team scheduled a rehabilitation medicine outpatient clinic follow-up visit to include occupational therapy in 6 weeks, with a plan for regular follow-along clinic visits at 2-month intervals during the next 6 months.

Case Study 2: Lydia

Physician prescription: 9-year-old girl with 2-month history of pneumonia; recent left fibular fracture; secondary diagnosis includes cerebral palsy with spastic quadriplegia, developmental delay, and seizure disorder

Precautions: Dysphagia, osteoporosis, pain, declining ADL function

Treatment objectives: Evaluate skills and retrain adaptive ADL routines with family

1 Given this prescription, what would you do next?
2 What would you do before seeing Lydia?
3 Which frames of reference may you use? (State assumptions about the use of each intervention.)

Referral History

Lydia's mother brought her to the emergency room the previous spring because of severe pulmonary distress attributed to viral pneumonia. Lydia was intubated with a tracheostomy and did well with medications and respiratory therapy. Extubation was performed, but she soon experienced another episode of pulmonary distress that required reintubation and the use of a ventilator for about 1 week. Her respiratory problems dramatically altered her participation in school and her regular routines for more than 8 weeks. Lydia refused her mother's attempts to resume walking, and she had apparent swelling and pain in her left ankle. Orthopedic consultation determined that Lydia had developed a stress fracture of her distal fibula. Her ankle was casted, but she was free to bear weight. Late in her second hospitalization, she was evaluated for admission to acute rehabilitation. Transfer was determined to be necessary because of Lydia's deterioration in gross-motor function, oral motor function, and ability to perform ADLs compared with her baseline skills when seen through the neuromuscular clinic and from school records. A short-term rehabilitation program was planned to ensure safety and adequate nutrition by oral feeding and to retain functional short-distance ambulation by instructing Lydia to use bilateral plastic AFOs and a walker, crawl up and down stairs, and use a long-distance wheelchair for mobility. In addition, the program was planned to promote upper extremity endurance, to resume a routine of assisted dressing and supervision with feeding and hygiene and family use of adaptive equipment for safety in transfers, to improve speech intelligibility to preinfection status, and to facilitate Lydia's transition back to school and an extended school-year program.

1 State a plan for evaluation priorities and methods.
2 Goals for the admission have been stated. Elaborate on likely ADL and performance issues that would need to be addressed in intervention.

Clinical Findings

Through an interview with the family, prior therapists, and direct observation, the following information was gathered. Viewed by parents as an imaginative girl, Lydia enjoys various games and activities. She was reported to be cooperative and could normally express needs in short words and phrases, although picture books for communication in some ADL and therapy routines had been developed. She had also used task-specific communication boards at school. Lydia was observed to pull her hair, bite her hands, and use her wheelchair to collide with objects; these behaviors were believed to be signs of frustration and fatigue. The therapy team chose to follow Lydia's school and home behavior routine, including giving her a short-term timeout, acknowledging her emotions, and then redirecting her to a new activity. Lydia's mother reported a prior level of ADL function in which Lydia ate and dressed with minimal help but received a great deal of assistance with toileting and bathing. With setup help and supervision for quality, Lydia brushed her teeth and enjoyed other grooming tasks. While hospitalized, Lydia had indicated her need to toilet but had been assisted for the most part with all functions and had not initiated any personal care. Lydia had much more difficulty eating, and her communication attempts had diminished.

1 Consider collaborations with other rehabilitation team members to address overall admission goals.
2 Determine likely discharge goals for ADL performance and other occupational needs.
3 Outline intervention plans, including frequency and length of visits and activities to be addressed.

Intervention Activities

In addition to collaborative sessions with other team members, Lydia was seen in hour-long therapy sessions that included weekday morning ADL training and afternoon gross-motor and fine-motor activities. Occupational therapy focused on Lydia's use of sequenced routines of dressing and hygiene with the nursing staff. In conjunction with the speech pathologist, a swallowing evaluation showed microaspirations that required a change in Lydia's foods to a dysphagia mechanical diet with thick liquids. One-to-one supervision was needed to cue for bite size and complete chewing before swallow. The speech pathologist gave Lydia oral exercises to increase strength and coordination of her tongue, lips, and jaw for purposes of speech and the oral phase of feeding. Therapeutic recreation involved Lydia in play activities such as group puppet shows and construction of posters. The occupational therapist emphasized strengthening her arms through therapeutic activities emphasizing aerobic tolerance. The therapists also stressed wheelchair propulsion, wheelchair pushups for pressure relief, and crawling to help Lydia recover her baseline abilities in the use of her upper extremities. The therapists noted fatigue in fine-motor tasks, although skilled movements appeared similar to her prior status. The therapists stressed endurance with tabletop tasks of writing and the use of manipulatives.

Lydia's mother was infrequently involved with therapy sessions because of her job responsibilities. Care provider instruction emphasizes assisted bathtub and car transfers, increasing Lydia's participation in assisted routines of bathing and toileting and organization and planning for supervision in eating, hygiene, and dressing activities. Lydia and her mother had previously developed a fast-paced care routine that allowed Lydia few opportunities to participate in or influence her care. The occupational therapist placed emphasis on having Lydia and her mother develop and follow simplified written routines, which enabled Lydia to direct more of her own care. This was thought to be important to her mother but also essential for use with other care providers like Lydia's father, with whom she stayed every other month for a weekend. Lydia's admission to acute rehabilitation lasted 12 days. Her tolerance of bracing returned, and she was able to use a walker for up to 25 yards. She continued to need contact guarding in wheelchair-to-floor transfers and was able to crawl up and down seven carpeted steps. Manual wheelchair propulsion was limited to 100 yards on smooth and level surfaces. No complaints of arm fatigue were noted with activities of 15 minutes' duration. Lydia advanced to a regular diet, although the therapists instructed her mother to follow precautions that included the use of an upright posture while eating and drinking, a slow eating pace, and avoidance of foods with stringy texture that were difficult for Lydia to manage as a bolus and during the pharyngeal phase of swallowing.

1 Suggest follow-up or follow-along services to recommend.

Discharge Follow-up

The therapists made plans with the school for an extended school-year program to complete the work missed during Lydia's long absence. At discharge, follow-up clinic visits for orthopedics and pulmonary disorders were scheduled, and Lydia was scheduled to see her physiatrist as part of her routine neurodevelopmental clinic visit in 2 months.

Case Study 3: Kyle

Physician prescription: 14-year-old male adolescent with congenital limb deficiencies, undergoing second-stage orthopedic surgery to rotate and lengthen left leg

Precautions: Falls, Ilizarov protocol

Therapeutic objectives: Evaluation of ADLs and retraining with adaptive techniques and AT

1 Consider plans and actions to follow before seeing Kyle.
2 Specify frame of references likely to be used in interventions.

Referral History

Kyle has a long history of involvement with rehabilitation specialists. He was born with a unique combination of limb deficiencies. His right upper extremity amelia resulted in the equivalent of a right shoulder disarticulation, and his left upper extremity hemimelia resulted in a short above-elbow residual limb. His left lower extremity had femoral and tibial shortening with ankle and foot deformity. Kyle's right lower limb was comparatively normal. Multiple limb abnormalities resulted in Kyle being followed for several years through a specialized clinic for children with limb deficiency. Several attempts at prosthetic fit for his left leg proved expensive and nonfunctional. Kyle developed good use of his right foot for prehension and used his left foot as an assist. As a teenager, Kyle had good family support, attended school with his same-aged cohort in his hometown, and was a good student.

At that time, Kyle was considered a good candidate for left leg surgery to correct a rotation deformity and lengthen the limb by the Ilizarov procedure. Kyle's balance had begun to deteriorate with growth. His leg length discrepancy became more pronounced, causing severe problems when barefoot and not using his large shoelift, which was also viewed as unsightly. Although he could walk, run, and use his lower limbs well for many ADL skills, it was believed that he would benefit from the surgical procedure, which would add approximately 6 cm of length to his left tibia. Anticipated benefits included better single-leg balance in functional mobility and reduced need for extensive lifts on his left shoe.

Two stages were planned for the surgical correction. The first included a left distal femoral wedge osteotomy to correct the rotation deformity of his knee and a heel cord release at the ankle. The second procedure would involve tibial lengthening with the Ilizarov technique. Kyle underwent the first part of this series with mixed results. Because of his upper limb deficiency, the use of traditional crutches was not possible, and he required a

lengthened period of rehabilitation to learn to walk again. He experienced several falls and complained of ankle pain. Because his running skills decreased after the first surgery, he became reticent about the second procedure. Kyle showed anxiety and depressive reactions, and referrals were made for more extensive assessment and treatment. It was determined that both Kyle and his family needed more information about the surgery and the expected course of recovery.

In planning his second surgery, which was expected to have an even longer recovery time, the team carefully assessed Kyle's rehabilitation needs, including his mobility and the use of his lower limbs in personal ADLs and IADLs. A prosthetist developed a crutch device that molded to the axilla for weight bearing through the ribs and the latissimus muscle and had a detachable post modified from a Loftstrand design (Mosca, Okumura, & Jaffe, 1993). Kyle learned to use the crutch quickly. During the summer he underwent the second procedure and was admitted to acute rehabilitation. Goals after his surgery were to restore safe mobility and, before returning home, reestablish desired independence in feeding, grooming, bathing, dressing, and written communication skills all of which he did with his feet. The admission also provided an opportunity to more directly evaluate and explore options for the skills that Kyle had been inconsistent in performing.

1 Identify Kyle's options to increase his reach and prehension and techniques used with ADL tasks.
2 Propose options to explore in terms of AT for purposes of communication and environmental control.
3 Discuss how Kyle's psychosocial needs can be addressed during this admission.

Clinical Findings

External fixation of the tibia created some difficulty when Kyle attempted to use his left foot to assist in daily living tasks. An occupational therapist saw Kyle twice per day to address further adaptation of functional skills. The therapist recruited Kyle to participate in problem solving, and Kyle willingly tried new techniques. He resumed feeding by using his regular routine of his right foot over his left thigh and handling utensils to bring food to his mouth from a specially positioned plate. He continued to have difficulty opening packaged foods because of his left foot immobility.

Intervention Activities

The occupational therapist introduced adaptations to Kyle's usual AT devices that allowed him to resume independence in grooming and bathing tasks. The therapist configured a dressing board similar to the one Kyle used at home to provide him with independence in donning and doffing his clothes by the use of specially placed stationary hooks. Kyle also resumed right-foot writing and computer operation using a miniature keyboard and other adaptive interface features with the Windows operating system. The therapist introduced Kyle to Internet access and arranged it as an evening activity, along with custom access devices for video games. The therapist also explored driving with Kyle and scheduled a referral to the local adaptive drivers' training program for a time after healing and before his 16th birthday. The physical therapist engaged Kyle in ambulation training and specific muscle strengthening of the left lower extremity. At discharge he was able to walk with his crutch for distances up to 300 feet and bear approximately 80% of his body weight over his left leg. Transfers from seated surfaces and standing were independent, but he continued to require assistance to get up from the floor.

1 Recommend home program activities.
2 Suggest further options to address pediatric rehabilitation needs.

Discharge Follow-up Plan

Kyle's admission to acute rehabilitation lasted 3 weeks, with additional community-based physical therapy planned. Continued visits to the limb deficiency program at the rehabilitation clinic were scheduled, along with referral to adaptive driving program and AT clinics. These systems would address with Kyle and his family his progression in needs or transitions in school, independent living, and vocational exploration.

STUDY QUESTIONS

1 For a child with traumatic injury, suggest reasons why acute rehabilitation would be recommended. How would recommendations differ from care in subacute or outpatient rehabilitation settings? How would this differ for a child with a congenital onset disorder?
2 Considering the intensive yet comprehensive nature of acute rehabilitation, suggest types of program outcomes that would reflect the contribution of occupational therapy in this setting.
3 For a new admission to acute rehabilitation, describe how assessment and treatment planning would be prioritized. Consider how the family is involved in the process of setting goals and selecting treatment strategies.
4 For teaching adaptive methods that may involve the use of assistive technology devices, suggest three alternatives for providing such instruction.
5 Short of independence, suggest long-term goals for acute rehabilitation that would be relevant to the child's function at home, at school, and in other community settings.

REFERENCES

Armstrong, K., & Kerns, K.A. (2002). The assessment of parent needs following paediatric traumatic brain injury. *Pediatric Rehabilitation, 5*, 149-160.

Bedell, G.M., Haley, S.M., Coster, W.J., & Smith, K.W. (2002). Participation readiness at discharge from inpatient rehabilitation in children and adolescents with acquired brain injuries. *Pediatric Rehabilitation, 5*, 107-116.

Binder, H., Conway, A., Hanson, S., Gerber, L.H., Marini, J., Berry, R., & Weintraub, J. (1993). Comprehensive rehabilitation of the child with osteogenesis imperfecta. *American Journal of Medical Genetics, 45*, 265-269.

Blatzheim, L.L., Edberg, A., & Lacy, L. (1987). Operationalizing primary nursing in the pediatric rehabilitation setting. *Journal of Pediatric Nursing, 2*, 434-437.

Bower, E., McLellan, D.L., Arney, J., & Campbell, M.J. (1996). A randomised controlled trial of different intensities of physiotherapy and different goal-setting procedures in 44 children with cerebral palsy. *Developmental Medicine and Child Neurology, 38*, 226-237.

Boyer, M.G., & Edwards, P. (1991). Outcome 1 to 3 years after severe traumatic brain injury in children and adolescents. *Injury, 22*, 315-320.

Burkett, K.W. (1989). Trends in pediatric rehabilitation. *Nursing Clinics of North America, 24*, 239-255.

Bury, T., & Mead, J. (1998). *Evidence-based healthcare: A practical guide for therapists.* Boston: Butterworth-Heinemann.

Buschbacher, R. (1995). Outcomes and problems in pediatric pulmonary rehabilitation. *American Journal of Physical Medicine and Rehabilitation, 74*, 287-293.

Cardenas, D.D., Haselkorn, J.K., McElligott, J.M., & Gnatz, S.M. (2001). A bibliography of cost-effectiveness practices in physical medicine and rehabilitation, AAPM&R white paper. *Archives of Physical Medicine and Rehabilitation, 82*, 711-719.

Case-Smith, J., & Wavrek, B. (1998). Models of service delivery and team interaction. In J. Case-Smith (Ed.), *Pediatric occupational therapy and early intervention* (pp. 83-108). Boston: Butterworth-Heinemann.

Centers for Medicare and Medicaid Services (2003, August 1). Medicare program; changes in the inpatient rehabilitation facilities prospective payment system and fiscal year 2004 rates. Final Rule. *Federal Register, 68* (148), 45673-45728.

Coster, W.J., Haley, S., & Baryza, M.J. (1994). Functional performance of young children after traumatic brain injury: A 6-month follow-up study. *American Journal of Occupational Therapy, 48*, 211-218.

Cotterill, P.G., & Gage, B.J. (2002). Overview: Medicare postacute care since the Balanced Budget Act of 1997. *Health Care Financing Review, 24* (2), 1-6.

DeNise-Annunziata, D.K., & Scharf, A.A. (1998). Functional status as an important predictor of length of stay in a pediatric rehabilitation hospital. *Journal of Rehabilitation Outcomes Measurement, 2*, 12-21.

DiScala, C., Osberg, J.S., Gans, B.M., Chin, L.J., & Grant, C.C. (1991). Children with traumatic head injury: Morbidity and postacute treatment. *Archives of Physical Medicine and Rehabilitation, 72*, 662-666.

Donders, J. (1993). Bereavement and mourning in pediatric rehabilitation settings. *Death Studies, 17*, 517-527.

Dudgeon, B.J., & Greenberg, S.L. (1998). Preparing students for consultation roles and systems. *American Journal of Occupational Therapy, 52,* 801-809.

Dudgeon, B.J., Massagli, T.L., & Ross, B.W. (1997). Educational participation of children with spinal cord injury. *American Journal of Occupational Therapy, 51,* 553-561.

Dumas, H.M., Haley, S.M., Ludlow, L.H., & Rabin, J.P. (2002). Functional recovery in pediatric traumatic brain injury during inpatient rehabilitation. *American Journal of Physical Medicine and Rehabilitation, 81,* 661-669.

Edwards, P.A. (1992). The evolution of rehabilitation facilities for children. *Rehabilitation Nursing, 17,* 191-195.

Eigsti, H., Aretz, M., & Shannon, L. (1990). Pediatric physical therapy in a rehabilitation setting. *Pediatrician, 17,* 267-277.

Fay, G.C., Jaffe, K.M., Polissar, N.L., Liao, S., Rivara, J.B., & Martin, K.M. (1994). Outcome of pediatric traumatic brain injury at three years: A cohort study. *Archives of Physical Medicine and Rehabilitation, 75,* 733-741.

Fleet, P.J. (2003). Rehabilitation of spasticity and related problems in childhood cerebral palsy. *Journal of Paediatrics and Child Health, 39,* 6-14.

Fuhrer, M.J. (1987). *Rehabilitation outcomes, analysis and measurement.* Baltimore: Brookes.

Fuhrer, M.J. (2000). Subjectifying quality of life as a medical rehabilitation outcome. *Disability Rehabilitation, 22,* 481-489.

Gans, B.M. (1993). Rehabilitation of the pediatric patient. In J.A. Delisa (Ed.), *Rehabilitation medicine, principles and practice* (2nd ed.). Philadelphia: J.B. Lippincott.

Garcia, R.A., Gaebler-Spira, D., Sisung, C., Heinemann, A.W. (2002). Functional improvement after pediatric spinal cord injury. *American Journal of Physical Medicine and Rehabilitation, 81,* 458-463.

Gardner, J., & Workinger, M.S. (1990). The changing role of the speech-language pathologist in pediatric rehabilitation/habilitation. *Pediatrician, 17,* 283-286.

Gilgoff, R.L., & Gilgoff, I.S. (2003). Long-term follow-up of home mechanical ventilation in young children with spinal cord injury and neuromuscular conditions. *Journal of Pediatrics, 142,* 476-480.

Grebin, B., & Kaplan, S.C. (1995). Toward a pediatric subacute care model: Clinical and administrative features. *Archives Physical Medicine Rehabilitation, 76* (12 Suppl.), SC16-20.

Guerriere, D., & McKeever, P. (1997). Mothering children who survive brain injuries: Playing the hand you're dealt. *Journal of the Society of Pediatric Nurses, 2,* 105-115.

Haley, S.M., Coster, W.J., Ludlow, L.H., Haltiwanger, J.T., & Andrellos, P.J. (1992). *Pediatric Evaluation of Disability Inventory.* San Antonio: Psychological Corporation.

Haley, S.M., Dumas, H.M., & Ludlow, L.H. (2001). Variation by diagnostic and practice pattern groups in the mobility outcomes of inpatient rehabilitation programs for children and youth. *Physical Therapy, 81,* 1425-1436.

Halstead, L.S. (2001). The John Stanley Coulter lecture. The power of compassion and caring in rehabilitation healing. *Archives of Physical Medicine and Rehabilitation, 82,* 149-154.

Heery, K. (1992). Restoring childhood through rehabilitation. *Rehabilitation Nursing, 17,* 193-195.

Herndon, D.N., Rutan, R.L., & Rutan, T.C. (1993). Management of the pediatric patient with burns. *Journal of Burn Care and Rehabilitation, 14,* 3-8.

Hotz, G., Helm-Estabrooks, N., & Nelson, N.W. (2001). Development of the pediatric test of brain injury. *Journal of Head Trauma Rehabilitation, 16,* 5, 426-440.

Jaffe, K.M., Fay, G.C., Polissar, N.L., Martin, K.M., Shurtleff, H.A., Rivara, J.B., & Winn, H.R. (1993a). Severity of pediatric traumatic brain injury and neurobehavioral recovery at one year—a cohort study. *Archives of Physical Medicine and Rehabilitation, 74,* 587-595.

Jaffe, K.M., Massagli, T.L., Martin, K.M., Rivara, J.B., Fay, G.C., & Polissar, N.L. (1993b). Pediatric traumatic brain injury: Acute and rehabilitation costs. *Archives of Physical Medicine and Rehabilitation. 74,* 681-686.

Jaffe, K.M., Okamoto, G.A., & Lemire, C. (1986). Inpatient pediatric rehabilitation: A five year review. *Rehabilitation Literature, 47,* 286-289.

Jaffe, K.M., Polissar, N.L., Fay, G.C., & Liao, S. (1995). Recovery trends over three years following pediatric traumatic brain injury. *Archives of Physical Medicine and Rehabilitation, 76,* 17-26.

Johnston, M.V., & Granger, C.V. (1994). Outcomes research in medical rehabilitation: A primer and introduction to a series. *American Journal of Physical Medicine and Rehabilitation, 73,* 296-303.

Karger, C., Guile, J.T., & Bowen, J.R. (1993). Lengthening of congenital lower limb deficiencies. *Clinical Orthopedics and Related Research, 291,* 236-245.

Keith, R.A., Granger, C.V., Hamilton, B.B., & Sherwin, F.S. (1987). The functional independence measure: A new tool for rehabilitation. *Advances in Clinical Rehabilitation, 1,* 6-18.

Kielhofner, G., & Barrett, L. (1998). Meaning and misunderstanding in occupational forms: a study of therapeutic goal setting. *American Journal of Occupational Therapy, 52,* 345-353.

Kramer, A.M. (1997). Rehabilitation care and outcomes from the patient's perspective. *Medical Care, 35* (6 Suppl.), JS48-57.

Latenser, B.A., & Kowal-Vern, A. (2002). Paediatric burn rehabilitation. *Pediatric Rehabilitation, 5,* 3-10.

Massagli, T.L., & Jaffe, K.M. (1990). Pediatric spinal cord injury: Treatment and outcome. *Pediatrician, 17,* 244-254.

Mazzola, C.A., & Adelson, P.D. (2002). Critical care management of head trauma in children. *Critical Care Medicine, 30* (Suppl.), S393-S401.

Michlovitz, S.L. (1996). *Thermal agents in rehabilitation* (3rd ed.). Philadelphia: F.A. Davis.

Moront, M., & Eichelberger, M.R. (1994). Pediatric trauma. *Pediatrics Annals, 23,* 186-191.

Mosca, V.S. (1991). The Ilizarov method: Orthopedic and rehabilitation management. *Physical Medicine and Rehabilitation Clinics of North America, 2,* 951-970.

Mosca, V.S., Okumura, R., & Jaffe, K.M. (1993). Prosthetic crutch for a patient with congenital bilateral, upper extremity deficiencies undergoing lower extremity lengthening by the Ilizarov method. *Journal of the Association of Children's Prosthetic-Orthotic Clinics, 28,* 19-20.

Msall, M.E., DiGaudio, K.M., & Duffy, L.C. (1993). Use of functional assessment in children with developmental disabilities. *Physical Medicine and Rehabilitation Clinics of North America, 4,* 517-527.

O'Donnell, M.E., & Roxborough, L. (2002). Evidence-based practice in rehabilitation. *Physical Medicine and Rehabilitation Clinics North America, 13,* 991-1005.

Ottenbacher, K.J., & Hinderer, S.R. (2001). Evidence-based practice: methods to evaluate individual patient improvement. *American Journal of Physical Medicine and Rehabilitation, 80,* 10, 786-796.

Ottenbacher, K.J., Msall, M.E., Lyon, N., Duffy, L.C., Ziviani, J., Granger, C.V., & Braun, S. (2000). Functional assessment and care of children with neurodevelopmental disabilities. *American Journal of Physical Medicine and Rehabilitation, 79,* 114-123.

Pedretti, L.W., & Early, M.B. (Eds.). (2001). *Occupational therapy: Practice skills for physical dysfunction* (5th ed.). St. Louis: Mosby.

Philip, P.A., Ayyangar, R., Vanderbilt, J., & Gaebler-Spira, D.J. (1994). Rehabilitation outcome in children after treatment of primary brain tumor. *Archives of Physical Medicine and Rehabilitation, 75,* 36-39.

Raps, C.S., Peterson, C., Jonas, M., & Seligman, M.E. (1982). Patient behavior in hospitals: Helplessness, reactance, or both? *Journal of Personality and Social Psychology, 42,* 1036-1041.

Rivara, J.B. (1993). Family functioning following pediatric traumatic brain injury. *Pediatric Annals, 23,* 38-43.

Rivara, J.B., Jaffe, K.M., Polissar, N.L., Fay, G.C., Liao, S., & Martin, K.M. (1996). Predictors of family functioning and change 3 years after traumatic brain injury in children. *Archives of Physical Medicine and Rehabilitation, 77,* 754-764.

Rodriquez, J., & Brown, S.T. (1990). Childhood injuries in the United States, Division of Injury Control, Center for Environmental Health and Injury Control, Center for Disease Control. *American Journal of Diseases of Children, 144,* 627-646.

Russman, B.S. (1990). Rehabilitation of the pediatric patient with a neuromuscular disease. *Neurology Clinics, 8,* 727-740.

Schwartz, R.K. (1991). Educational and training strategies, therapy as learning. In C. Christiansen & C. Baum (Eds.), *Occupational therapy: Overcoming human performance deficits* (pp. 664-698). Thorofare, NJ: Slack.

Silver, B.V., Boake, C., & Cavazos, D.I. (1994). Improving functional skills using behavioral procedures in a child with anoxic brain injury. *Archives of Physical Medicine and Rehabilitation, 75,* 742-745.

Sneed, R.C., May, W.L., Stencel, C., & Paul, S.M. (2002). Pediatric physiatry in 2000: A survey of practitioners and training programs. *Archives of Physical Medicine and Rehabilitation, 83,* 416-422.

Stineman, M.G. (2002). Prospective payment, prospective challenge. *Archives of Physical Medicine and Rehabilitation, 83,* 1802-1805.

Strunk, R.C., Mascia, A.V., Lipkowitz, M.A., & Wolf, S.I. (1991). Rehabilitation of a patient with asthma in the outpatient setting. *Journal of Allergy and Clinical Immunology, 87* (3), 601-611.

Tickle-Degnen, L. (2000). Gathering current research evidence to enhance clinical reasoning. *American Journal of Occupational Therapy, 54,* 102-105.

Trombly, C.A., & Radomski, M.V. (Eds.). (2002). *Occupational therapy for physical dysfunction* (5th ed.). Baltimore: Williams & Wilkins.

Watson, D. (1991). Occupational therapy intervention guidelines for children and adolescents with spina bifida. *Child: Care, Health, and Development, 17,* 367-380.

Ziviani, J., Ottenbacher, K.J., Shepard, K., Foreman, S., Astbury, W., & Ireland, P. (2001). Concurrent validity of the Functional Independence Measure for Children (WeeFIM) and the Pediatric Evaluation of Disabilities Inventory in children with developmental disabilities and acquired brain injuries. *Physical and Occupational Therapy in Pediatrics, 21,* 91-101.

SUGGESTED READINGS

Molnar, G.E., & Alexander, M.A. (Eds). (1999). *Pediatric Rehabilitation* (3rd ed.), Philadelphia: Hanley & Belfus.

Rosenthal, M., Kreutzer, J.S., Griffith, E.R., & Pentland, B. (Eds.) (1999). *Rehabilitation of the adult and child with traumatic brain injury* (3rd ed.). Philadelphia: F.A. Davis.

Wallace, H.M., Biehl, R.F., MacQueen, J.C., & Blackman, J.A. (Eds.). (1997). *Mosby's resource guide to children with disabilities and chronic illness.* St. Louis, Mosby.

INTERNET RESOURCES

The Bandolier Journal: www.jr2.ox.ac.uk/bandolier
CARF Commission on Accreditation of Rehabilitation Facilities: www.carf.org/
The Cochrane Library: www.update-software.com/Cochrane
Family Village: www.familyvillage.wisc.edu/
Joint Commission on Accreditation of Healthcare Organizations: www.jcaho.org

Karen C. Spencer ■ Susan O'Daniel

CHAPTER OBJECTIVES

1 Describe the federal legislative mandate for transition services.
2 Describe an ecologic approach for transition-age students.
3 Identify the role of occupational therapy in the transition process including evaluation, intervention (planning, implementation, review), and outcomes.
4 Compare types of occupational therapy interventions that support transition: direct, therapeutic use of occupation and activity; consultation processes; and education processes.
5 Describe collaborative teamwork as it applies to the school-to-adult life transition process.
6 Describe the interagency linkages needed for positive transition outcomes.

Individuals with disabilities may spend from 12 to 18 years receiving a public education. Public education is viewed as a way for these young people to develop the knowledge, skills, and experiences necessary to participate in a variety of adult roles and activities. Upon exiting school, young adults with disabilities can face a dizzying array of options including postsecondary education, paid employment, volunteer work, establishing a home, and participating in meaningful relationships. Navigating the transition to adult life with all of its choices and decisions can be challenging. When a person has a disability, this transition can be particularly difficult and may require variety of supports and services.

Occupational therapists are well qualified to be key players in the school-to-adult life transition process. With a large proportion of OTs already working in public schools, the opportunity exists for OTs to significantly contribute to the design and delivery of transition-related services for students with disabilities who are enrolled in secondary level programs. For those OTs who enjoy teens and young adults and who understand the challenges faced by youth as they move toward adult roles and responsibilities, transition can be an exciting and rewarding area for employment and professional growth. This chapter introduces the legislative and policy contexts surrounding transition services provided by the public schools and describes recommended transition practices from an occupational therapy perspective.

LEGISLATIVE BACKGROUND

Since passage of Public Law 94-142, the Education for All Handicapped Children Act of 1975 (EHA), special education and related services have been made available through the public education system to the nation's children and youth who have disabilities. The EHA and its subsequent amendments (Individuals with Disabilities Education Act [IDEA], 1990, 1997) guarantee a free and appropriate education for all children with disabilities. An appropriate education is one in which children with disabilities acquire, to the maximum extent possible, the skills, knowledge, and behaviors that will ultimately help them function successfully as adults. Occupational therapy was described in the EHA and its subsequent amendments as a *related service* intended to help children and youth with disabilities benefit from their individualized special education program (Box 26-1).

When the Education for All Handicapped Children Act was amended in 1990, its name was changed to the Individuals with Disabilities Education Act (IDEA, P.L. 101-476). In addition to a name change, the act mandated for the first time that schools provide a coordinated set of outcome-oriented transition services to youth with disabilities who are preparing to exit the public schools.

BOX 26-1 Related Services and Transition Services

RELATED SERVICES

"[R]elated services means transportation and such developmental, corrective, and other supportive services as are required to assist a child with a disability to benefit from special education, and includes speech-language pathology and audiology services, psychological services, physical and occupational therapy, recreation, including therapeutic recreation, early identification and assessment of disabilities in children, counseling services, including rehabilitation counseling, orientation and mobility services, and medical services for diagnostic or evaluation purposes. The term also includes school health services, social work services in schools, and parent counseling and training" (34 C.F.R. §300.24[a]).

TRANSITION SERVICES

"[T]ransition services means a coordinated set of activities for a student with a disability that—(1) is designed with an outcome-oriented process, that promotes movement from school to post-school activities, including postsecondary education, vocational training, integrated employment (including supported employment), continuing and adult education, adult services, independent living, or community participation; (2) is based on the individual student's needs, taking into account the student's preferences and interests; and (3) includes instruction, related services, community experiences, the development of employment and other post-school adult living objectives and if appropriate, acquisition of daily living skills and functional vocational evaluation. Transition services for students with disabilities may be special education, if provided as specially designed instruction, or related services, if required to assist the student with a disability to benefit from special education" (34 C.F.R. §300.29).

Research had revealed that previous well-intended programs of special education and related services had largely failed to prepare these youth for productive adult life in the community. In fact, upon leaving high school, large numbers of young adults with disabilities were experiencing unemployment, poverty, isolation, and dependency on family and public assistance (Blackorby & Wagner, 1996; Wagner et al., 1994). These and other poor postschool outcomes fueled needed changes in special education law (Rusch, Destefano, Chadsey-Rusch, Phelps, & Szymanski, 1992; Ward, 1992).

In 1997, IDEA was reauthorized and amended (P.L. 105-17). Key changes in the law included the addition of a general education focus, expansion of transition planning requirements, and the use of educationally relevant evaluation. These three changes are discussed next.

Amendments to IDEA added a powerful new general education focus. Though controversial, the law now required students receiving special education to participate in and make progress in the general education curriculum alongside their age peers without disabilities. Adding a general education focus significantly raised educational expectations for the nation's children and youth with disabilities. It challenged previous practices of separate special and general education programs and curricula. Furthermore, students with disabilities were now required to participate in district and statewide accountability efforts to measure student progress and performance related to general education standards. The 1997 amendments clearly intended for children with disabilities to gain greater access to the general education curriculum and, in doing so, acquire knowledge and skills that would allow them to function to the maximum extent possible as literate, productive citizens.

For special and general educators as well as related service personnel, the new focus on helping students achieve within the general curriculum created new opportunities and challenges. For example, the 1997 amendments to IDEA required justification for services provided outside the general education environment to students with disabilities (34 C.F.R. §300.347). By requiring justification, the central importance of the general curriculum in a student's overall education was demonstrated. Although this may seem like a small change in the law, it has profound implications for special educators, general educators, and related services personnel. It means that general education teachers are becoming the teachers for *all* children and the general classroom is the place where much of this education is to occur (Orelove & Sobsey, 1996). Special educators and related service personnel were now needed to support a student's access to and participation in the general education environment (Downing, 1996; Tomlinson, 2001). Not surprisingly, isolated pullout services delivered by related service personnel or others have come into question (Swinth & Hanft, 2002; Tomlinson, 2001). The focus on the general curriculum does not mean, however, that all students must spend all of their school time attending general classes. This is particularly true for students receiving transition services who may participate in a variety of work-study experiences, internships, service-learning projects, independent living training, or other programs within the school or the community. A variety of community-based opportunities are particularly important for students who learn best through doing and who need direct practice and feedback in order to build needed knowledge and skills that will translate to adult life (Benz, Lindstrom, & Yovanoff, 2000; Rainforth & York-Barr, 1997) (Figures 26-1 and 26-2).

As with previous versions of the Individuals with Disabilities Education Act (IDEA), the 1997 amendments reaffirm that students receiving special education must have an *Individualized Education Program* (IEP) that is developed by a team of people (34 C.F.R. §§300.29 and 300.347). The IEP is a written plan and a legal document that describes the specially designed instruction including related services and transition services that will

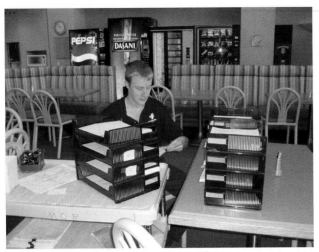

FIGURE 26-1 Transition student gaining work experience at a community job site.

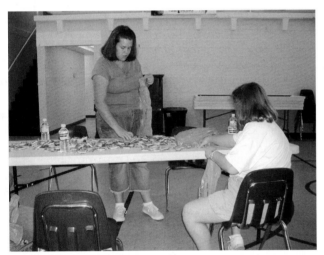

FIGURE 26-2 Students volunteer at the food bank to learn job skills.

be provided to meet the unique needs of the student. By law, an IEP must address the following:

1 How a student's disability affects his or her involvement and progress in the general curriculum
2 The student's annual education goals and short-term objectives or benchmarks
3 A statement of special education and related services to be provided
4 A statement of the extent to which the student will participate in the regular classroom and general education activities
5 A statement of any modifications in the administration of state or district-wide assessments
6 A projected date for the initiation of services or modifications
7 A statement of how the student's progress will be measured and how parents will be informed

8 A statement of transition needs when the student is 14 years old and commencement of specific transition services by the age of 16. Transition needs identification and specific transition services may begin even earlier if the team feels this is necessary.

Decisions regarding a student's eligibility for special education and the nature of a student's educational program including related services rest with the IEP team. The IEP team for a transition-aged student is comprised of the student, school personnel (administrators, teachers, related services, and others as needed), and the student's parents or guardians. When needed, representatives from community agencies may attend and contribute to planning and intervention efforts. The student's presence at the IEP meeting encourages him or her to actively participate in planning and decision making. According to a growing body of research, providing students who have disabilities with opportunities to participate in planning and decision making can promote self-determination as an adult (Wehmeyer, Palmer, Martin, Mithaug, & Martin, 2000; Wehmeyer & Schwartz, 1997). In addition to providing an opportunity to learn skills in self-determination, student participation in the transition-focused IEP requires that all other team members pay close attention to their own communication to create a comfortable, positive, and respectful environment that allows the student to participate to the maximum extent possible. Examples of transition-related IEP goals and the characteristics of services needed to address goal areas are provided in Table 26-1.

From an occupational therapy perspective, the 1997 amendments to IDEA significantly affected how services are designed and justified. The IEP requirement specifying how a child's disability affects his or her participation in the general education curriculum requires occupational therapists to understand the general curriculum including academic, nonacademic, and extracurricular components. The general curriculum, in large part, constitutes the occupational performance context for students with disabilities. Most school districts and states have established and published general education "standards." These standards are an essential resource for occupational therapists who are becoming informed about general education expectations for different age groups.

IDEA requires educationally relevant evaluations to be conducted by all members of the IEP team. Evaluation must focus on critical discrepancies between the student's current performance and the performance expectations established by the general education environment (including community-based learning opportunities). Educationally relevant evaluation completed by an OT must focus on the extent to which the student can access and participate in available education-related activities (American Occupational Therapy Association

---

TABLE 26-1   Transition-Related IEP Goals and Characteristics of Services

The following transition-related IEP goals and services were developed by the IEP team for a 17-year-old student with emotional and behavioral disabilities.

Goal 1: By the end of the school year and following a supported job search process to locate construction-related positions near public transportation, Jonathon will successfully complete two 15-hour work-study experiences with intermittent job coach support.

Goal 2: By the end of the semester Jonathon will independently balance his checkbook using an online check balancing program as measured by 3 out of 3 consecutive and successful attempts.

CHARACTERISTICS OF SERVICES

Service to Be Provided	Location	Beginning Date	Frequency	Anticipated Duration
Special education teacher and paraprofessional job coach	Classroom and community	September 15	3 times per week during vocational course block	School year
Vocational education teacher	Classroom	September 15	2 times per week during wood shop class	1 semester
Occupational therapy consult and direct	Classroom and community	September 15	Registered occupational therapist (OTR)—2 hours/month occupational therapy assistant (OTA)—1 hour/week	4 months

---

[AOTA], 1999) and identify the student's need for support, services, adaptations, or accommodations that could maximize that performance. Among the performance contexts an OT may use during evaluation are the student's classroom, the school lunchroom, other school environments frequented by the student, the physical education program, community work and recreation sites, public transportation available to the student, and other relevant performance contexts. An occupational therapist must, therefore, analyze the student's occupational performance within available school and community contexts and then convey findings to the IEP team in a way that helps the team plan special education and related services.

Recommended Transition Practices

Consistent with general occupational therapy practices, federally mandated transition services are outcome and performance oriented. The student's educational program (IEP) delineates goals and services that will help the student move toward the performance of desired and necessary occupations in a variety of environments. Effective transition services are evaluated based on the extent to which students and young adults exiting the schools actually achieve meaningful work roles, live in the community, engage in chosen recreation activities, and have ongoing positive social relationships. Accountability for these types of outcomes rests to a large extent with the student's IEP team. How well a student actually performs in transition-related areas provides critical feedback for teachers and related service personnel alike. What follows is a description of three recommended school-to-adult life transition practices:

1 The use of collaborative teaming among professionals, agencies, the student, and family members (AOTA, 1999; Giangreco, 1996; Mostert, 1998; NICHCY, 2001; Pugach & Johnson, 1995; Rainforth & York-Barr, 1997; Snell & Janney, 2000; Swinth & Hanft, 2002)

2 The use of an *ecologic curriculum* that focuses on the interactions between the student and his or her current or anticipated performance environments (Benz, Yovanoff, & Doren, 1997; Kennedy, Shukla, & Fryxell, 1997; Rainforth & York-Barr, 1997)

3 The establishment and use of interagency linkages to facilitate the smooth transfer of support and training from the school to adult and community agencies when the student exits public schools (Benz et al., 2000; Benz et al., 1997; Everson & McNulty, 1992; NICHCY, 1999)

Collaborative Teaming

Rainforth and York-Barr (1997) described collaboration within an educational context as "an interactive process in which individuals with varied life perspectives and experiences can join together in a spirit of willingness to share resources, responsibility, and rewards in creating inclusive and effective educational programs and environments for students with unique learning capacities and needs" (p. 18). For transition-aged students, collaboration is viewed as an effective way for a team to help the student achieve his or her goals related to future adult living. The primary team member is the student. Other team members may include the student's family, friends, classmates, teachers, related service professionals, representatives of adult service agencies, and others.

The collaborators on the team must have a shared sense of purpose that is driven not only by the student, but also by the student's unique interests, abilities, and needs. Central to effective collaborative teamwork is each team member's ability to share responsibility for student outcomes and not work solely from their discipline's singular perspective. For example, the occupational therapist, teacher, and paraprofessional may all work with a student who has significant physical limitations toward the goal of completing written classroom assignments. This would be an appropriate transition goal because it is grounded in the general education curriculum; it is based on the student's anticipated need for literacy as an adult and on the student's aspirations for postsecondary education. The occupational therapist may oversee and coordinate an assessment of the student's technology-related needs and abilities, followed by the selection of specific hardware and software for adapted computing. With the technology in place, the occupational therapist may spend time working with the student, teacher, and paraprofessional who will be involved in the day-to-day use of the technology in the classroom. Therefore, a collaborative working relationship is established, with the team sharing responsibility for meeting the *student's* goal of completing written work. It is inappropriate to develop separate, discipline-specific goals to guide each member of the team (AOTA, 1999; Council for Exceptional Children, 2000).

Collaboration requires a commitment on the part of the different team members to teach and learn from each other across traditional professional boundaries (Giangreco, 1996; Mostert, 1998; NICHCY, 2001; Snell & Janney, 2000). For example, the occupational therapist may share or exchange roles with the speech pathologist in training a student to use augmentative communication to order in a restaurant. Collaboration is born of necessity when services are delivered in functional, real-life and often complex situations (Rainforth & York-Barr, 1997). Occupational therapists most frequently work with the students in the classroom where other students are also engaged in written work. Although evaluation of the student's need for technology and any initial technology training may have occurred outside of the general classroom, the goal is to transfer writing as quickly as possible back into the student's typical performance context (the classroom) where instruction and support are available from the teacher.

In addition to the need for collaboration among the team members at the student's school, there is a need for collaboration between the school and other community agencies related to transition (NICHCY, 1999). As students with disabilities approach the end of their school careers, many will need ongoing supports or services (Figure 26-3). These services may help the young adult

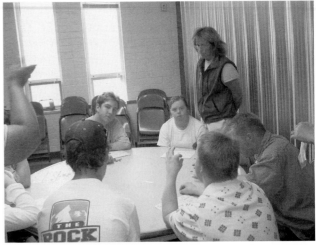

FIGURE 26-3 Students meet to discuss and practice skills needed in a work environment.

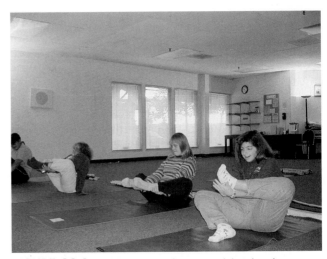

FIGURE 26-4 Transition students participating in a community yoga class.

obtain and maintain community employment, live in the community, and participate in social and recreational activities (Figure 26-4). To achieve a smooth transition from the supports and services of the schools to the supports and se rvices of other external community agencies requires extensive communication and collaboration. It is therefore critical to include community agencies in the transition planning process. These agencies are also potential providers of some transition services while the student is still enrolled in school. Community agencies often involved in transition services are the state vocational rehabilitation agency, mental health or developmental disability agencies, independent living centers, and the Social Security Administration (NICHCY, 1999).

Collaborative teamwork can clearly benefit transition-aged students when a team's diverse perspectives and resources can be brought together to create effective services and to solve challenging problems. Team members themselves can also benefit, because collaboration promotes the establishment of cooperative and caring relationships among team members characterized by communication, shared responsibility, and mutual support (Giangreco, 1996; Rainforth & York-Barr, 1997).

Ecologic Curriculum

For the purposes of this chapter, the term "curriculum" refers to carefully selected and sequenced activities used primarily by teachers to guide classroom teaching. General education curricula reflect the "standards" that have been adopted by a school, a school district, or a state. For students enrolled in special education, the general curriculum serves as an overarching framework within which individualized education programs (IEPs) are designed and implemented (IDEA, P.L. 105-17, 1997).

The general education curriculum in most states has a strong academic focus on areas such as language arts, math, science, geography, and history. Though information rich, this curriculum and the associated teaching methods may require adjustment or adaptation for many students with disabilities. In addition to academically strong classroom-based teaching and learning, students with disabilities often benefit from participating in a variety of real-life, contextual, and experientially based learning opportunities. These "ecologic" opportunities are developed by a team and documented in the student's IEP.

Brown and others (1979) first described a broad ecologically oriented curricular model for students with significant disabilities. It addressed student performance in essential life domains: domestic (home), vocational, community, and leisure (Figures 26-5 and 26-6). These domains were later expanded to include school (York & Vandercook, 1991), where children and youth spend a great deal of time. This domain-based curriculum is highly relevant for transition-aged students because it focuses the efforts of teachers and related service personnel on enhancing student performance in areas that are essential for productive and meaningful adult life (NICHCY, 1999). It considers each student as a unique individual who must function in a variety of school and community contexts.

A domain-based curriculum for transition-aged youth specifies to some extent how and where transition services should be delivered. According to Rainforth and York-Barr (1997), the *how* aspect of service delivery relates to the use of collaborative teaming and the use of highly relevant learning materials and activities. The *where* aspect of service delivery relates to the team's use

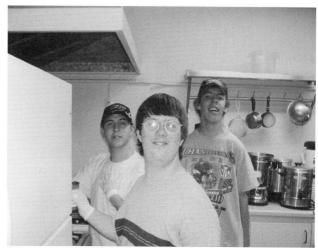

FIGURE 26-5   Students prepare chili for a parent banquet.

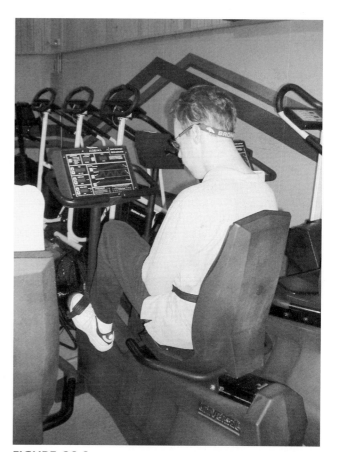

FIGURE 26-6   Transition student working out at a community recreation center and learning how to access community resources.

of highly relevant teaching and learning contexts to include the school, home, and assorted community environments. Taken together, the *how* and *where* aspects of a transition curriculum may be termed *ecologic*, focusing on the interaction between the student and the environments in which he or she participates.

An effective ecologic curriculum for transition-aged students is based fundamentally on the belief that *all* students can learn to assume meaningful and valued roles within their communities. Furthermore, effective transition services must be based on some core principles that are shared by all members of a student's educational team, including the occupational therapist. These principles include the following:

1 The student is included in classrooms and activities with same-age peers with and without disabilities.
2 Teachers and related service professionals coordinate their efforts on behalf of the student.
3 Functional, educationally relevant and contextual evaluation is applied.
4 The student is actively involved in planning and decision making.
5 The student is instructed in a variety of relevant school and community environments.
6 Students' achievement of targeted transition outcomes is evaluated.

Age-appropriate placement of students with disabilities in educational activities alongside their chronologic age peers, with and without disabilities, represents the intent of IDEA and is considered optimal practice (Giangreco, Cloninger, & Iverson, 1998; Tomlinson, 2001). The inclusion of students who have disabilities in typical educational activities and environments is believed to promote student performance, offer rich opportunities for learning, provide age-appropriate role modeling, increase awareness among all students of diverse learning styles and abilities, and provide opportunities for relationship building that is so important during adolescent development (McGregor & Vogelsberg, 1998). Age-appropriate placement does not mean that students with disabilities are simply placed in a typical class or at a community job site. Appropriate support services and resources that facilitate the student's full inclusion and maximum participation in the environment must accompany these placements. Despite research demonstrating the benefits of inclusion for secondary-level students with disabilities (Kennedy, Shukla, & Fryxell, 1997), implementation has proved challenging. Based on a systematic review of the literature, Stodden, Galloway, and Stodden (2003) identified a need for professional development among general and special educators to achieve successful inclusive practices for secondary level students.

Coordination between education and related services brings members of the team together to address a student's goals. Responsibility for serving students with disabilities in a variety of contexts and alongside their chronological age peers cannot fall solely on the teacher. It must be shared among different members of the student's educational team. The occupational therapist may work in the classroom or on a job site with the teacher, paraprofessional, employer, or student. The services provided by the occupational therapist or occupational therapy assistant may include, for example, engaging the student in contextually relevant activities such as learning to ride public transportation, consulting with the teacher or employer to build his or her capacity to independently supervise a student who is nonverbal, or educating a student's peers and paraprofessional about wheelchair safety in anticipation of a class field trip. A coordinated approach involving different school personnel can best be explained through an example:

Amelia is an 18-year-old student who wants to live in the community after she completes high school. At her IEP meeting, a transition goal to use neighborhood services was developed. Amelia has significant cognitive, communication, and mobility limitations that currently interfere with her ability to access and use services and businesses in her neighborhood. To meet her transition goal, the team identified the need for Amelia to begin to participate in purchasing needed food and personal items at her neighborhood grocery store. A coordinated approach was developed involving the teacher, speech-language pathologist, and occupational therapist. Amelia's special education teacher developed strategies with Amelia that allowed her to shop from a pictured list of items. Amelia's speech-language pathologist worked with Amelia at the grocery store, teaching her to initiate a transaction and communicate with grocery store employees. The occupational therapist, addressing the same goal, worked with Amelia to devise a way for her to carry grocery items and move safely around the store. In addition to their own specific responsibilities, each professional worked with Amelia in the grocery store environment and communicated what occurred to the other team members so that efforts were overlapping, complementary, and reinforcing.

Functional, educationally relevant and contextual evaluation is considered an essential feature of effective transition-related practices (Giangreco, 1996; Rainforth & York-Barr, 1997; Spencer & Sample, 1993; Woolcock, Stodden, & Bisconer, 1992). The purpose of an ecologic approach is to identify student performance needs and abilities in the environments that he or she currently uses or is expected to use as an adult. For example, if the team seeks to identify the student's interests, needs, and abilities as they relate to future employment, the assessment must take place, to a large extent, in actual employment settings. Systematic and careful observation of the student's performance during actual work tasks is completed to identify discrepancies between the demands of the job and the student's current performance level. Services are subsequently designed to reduce these discrepancies as the student acquires context-specific work skills, therefore increasing his or her level of participation in the work task. Because of the highly individual nature of transition planning, services, and environments for any given student, traditional discipline-specific assessments are not recommended (Council for Exceptional Children, 2000; Giangreco et al., 1998; Rainforth & York-Barr, 1997). Collaboration among team members during an ecologic assessment process will yield the most valid and useful information for designing or adjusting services and supports.

A student's *active involvement in planning and decision making* is considered an important aspect of effective transition services (Sands & Wehmeyer, 1996; Ward, 1992; Wehmeyer & Sands, 1998; Wehmeyer & Schwartz, 1997). The ultimate goal of education according to Ward (1992) is for students to actively participate in and fully manage their own lives: "Professionals can facilitate the development of self-determination skills by involving youth with disabilities in the transition planning process. . . . The goal is for students to assume control over their transition program, and identify and manage its various components" (p. 389).

For a student to actively participate, thoughtful attention is needed by the professional members of the education/transition team. The format of the IEP meeting may need adjusting to facilitate student involvement. For example, the student (with or without support) may prepare the agenda, introduce team members, or chair the meeting. To assume these functions, it is likely that the student would need help, possibly from the OT, in preparing for and participating in the meeting. This preparation should include some discussion of possible transition goals, activities, and timetables. During the IEP meeting, the attending professionals must follow the student's lead and keep discussions constructive by focusing primarily on the student's strengths and abilities.

Effective transition services require the delivery of *instruction in a variety of relevant, school and community environments* (Benz et al., 2000; Giangreco et al., 1998). In many cases, students with disabilities, particularly those with severe disabilities, have difficulty learning needed skills. This problem, combined with the associated challenge of identifying optimal learning styles and teaching approaches, requires the attention of both education and related service professionals. In addition to difficulty with learning, students with significant disabilities may not readily generalize learning to new environments or situations. For these reasons, it is best to provide education and related services in the actual performance contexts that the student will be using.

Implementation of an ecologic approach requires periodic *evaluation of the extent to which students are achieving targeted transition outcomes* (AOTA, 2002; Hasazi, Hock, & Cravedi-Cheng, 1992). Given the focus of an ecologic curriculum on preparing students to function in five major life domains (domestic, school, community, leisure, and vocational), recommended practices would suggest the need for ongoing evaluation of the extent and quality of student performance in each domain. Without periodic evaluation of the overall effectiveness of transition services, decisions regarding local educational practices and policies will be misguided. Outcome evaluation must occur at the individual, local, and national levels to account for the expenditure of public resources on transition efforts.

Transition outcomes that may be tracked by school districts include the extent to which students are (1) employed in the community, (2) living in the community, (3) satisfied with their lives, (4) using community services, (5) socially connected, and (6) participating in chosen leisure activities. These outcome data can be helpful to the members of the educational team who are responsible for designing and implementing individualized transition services. Occupational therapists, as members of educational transition teams, can specifically benefit from feedback regarding the contribution of occupational therapy toward student performance.

Larger scale evaluations of transition effectiveness are also needed. To this end, a national longitudinal transition study (NLTS2) was funded by the U.S. Department of Education in 2000 to provide a "national picture of experiences and achievements of young people that will guide future educational policy and programs" (SRI International, 2003). The NLTS2 was preceded by an earlier nationwide study that completed data collection in 1987. Comparisons between the two studies will help document large-scale changes over time and the extent to which transition-age youth are actually achieving targeted transition outcomes.

Interagency Linkages

Although transition services mandated by IDEA are to be initiated by the school on behalf of students with disabilities, Congress did not intend for schools to have sole responsibility for the transition process. The need for *interagency linkages* became a part of the law in 1990, indicating the expectation for shared responsibility across local education agencies and adult or community programs such as the state vocational rehabilitation agency (NICHCY, 1999). The interagency linkages envisioned by Congress also included shared financial responsibility for the cost of needed transition services.

Implementing the vision from Congress of interagency linkages and shared resources is, without a doubt, challenging. This task is viewed as an administrative responsibility that should not fall solely on already overextended teachers and related-service personnel (NICHCY, 1999). Education and related-service personnel responsible for the implementation of transition services must know, however, who the other transition "players" and agencies are and must be prepared to invite them to participate fully in the transition process. The potential benefits of clear interagency linkages, however difficult to implement, are many.

Establishing such interagency linkages can be of enormous benefit to students planning for transition. As students with disabilities leave the public education system at the age of 21, their entitlement to school sponsored educational, vocational, and other services ends. In the place of one lead agency (the school system), there may be a confusing array of service providers (e.g., the state vocational rehabilitation agency, the state department of mental health and developmental disabilities, and the Social Security Administration). Individuals with disabilities who are no longer eligible for the school's services become responsible for identifying where to obtain the ongoing services they need and for demonstrating their eligibility to receive the services. Before students with disabilities leave the public schools, it is critical to identify relevant adult service providers, establish eligibility to receive adult services, and clearly state interagency responsibilities and linkages in the IEP in order for the student to experience a smooth transition from school to adult life (NICHCY, 1999). Failure to initiate and formalize these connections while the student is still in school can result in the student being left out of services, sitting for extended periods on waiting lists, or losing skills because of lost opportunities to participate in active and supported learning. The importance of strong interagency linkages cannot be overstated.

OCCUPATIONAL THERAPISTS' ROLES IN TRANSITION

The ultimate purpose of transition services is to enable students with disabilities to engage in a variety of occupations that support their participation in everyday contexts. Occupational therapy services provided to support a student's transition from school to adult life follow the same overall processes as OT services delivered in other service systems and with different populations. The OT process includes three distinct phases that overlap and interact: *evaluation, intervention* (including planning, implementation, and ongoing review), and outcome assessment (AOTA, 2002). Next, this OT process will be expanded and applied to school-to-adult life transition services.

Evaluation Tied to Future Performance Outcomes

Keeping in mind that transition services must be collaborative and closely tied to the student's current and anticipated performance contexts, any OT evaluation effort must be similarly focused. It is also strongly recommended that before conducting specific evaluations, the student, family, occupational therapist, and other members of the educational team work together to identify what would constitute a desirable future (performance outcomes) for the student. This requires considering the student in the five major life domains: domestic, school, vocational, community, and leisure. Often the student and the team will envision a future that includes having a home in the community, use of assorted community services and amenities, some sort of job or productive activity, ongoing relationships, and participation in chosen recreational or leisure activities. Not surprisingly, these are things that most people, with or without disabilities, envision for themselves.

In addition to clarifying a positive vision for the student's future, the team must discuss the student's anticipated long-term needs for resources and supports that will allow the vision to become reality. For example, a young adult with significant disabilities may require long-term job support in the form of a job coach who provides on-the-job training and other support needed to maintain employment. Another individual may require in-home support with personal hygiene, dressing, and meal preparation to live in the community.

Focused evaluation activities follow the establishment of a vision of a high-quality life in the community *and* the team's identification of areas in which the student is likely to need support (Giangreco, 1996). The occupational therapist and others on the team then assess the extent to which the student can currently achieve this vision based on existing skills and experience. The team also identifies discrepancies between the level at which the student needs to be performing and his or her current level of performance. Evaluation, therefore, must include observation of the student's performance in the actual situations and environments he or she is likely to encounter as a young adult. To conduct this type of ecologic evaluation, the team does the following:

1 Specifies the environments in which the student will participate (domestic, school, vocational, community, and leisure).

2 Prioritizes the performance environments considered to be most essential in the short term and those that will become more important over time.

3 Identifies the activities that occur naturally in the selected, prioritized environments. The student's actual performance of relevant activities in relevant environments provides essential information from which the team can plan and make decisions.

4 Divides the responsibility for conducting different parts of the assessment among members of the educational team. Family members as well as professionals may share responsibilities during the assessment process.

5 Conducts the assessment by actually observing student performance during activities in the selected environments. Based on careful observation, discrepancies between the environment and activity demands and the student's ability to perform should be noted. This type of *discrepancy analysis* forms the heart of the assessment and guides planning and decision making.

6 Records the evaluation findings for the purposes of communicating with all members of the educational team, including the student and his or her parents. It is recommended that a consistent recording format be used, such as the one presented in Figure 26-7 (Spencer, Murphy, Bean, & Schelly, 1991).

7 Presents the findings to the team during the IEP meeting. With all the needed information before

them, the team can proceed with planning transition services using an ecologic model.

The following is an example of a transition-related assessment process conducted by an occupational therapist:

Ron is 16 years of age and is enrolled in his neighborhood high school. He is about to attend his IEP meeting, and his team has already discussed what a desir-

Student: _____

Date and time of assessment: _____

Persons involved and roles: _____

_____

Domain: ___ Domestic
           ___ School
           ___ Vocational
           ___ Community
           ___ Recreation

Environment observed (describe general environment along with physical, social, and cultural attributes):

Activities observed in this environment:
1.
2.
3.

STUDENT PERFORMANCE

Strengths/interests	Supports needed/barriers
Activity:	
add pages as needed	

Summary:

FIGURE 26-7   Ecologic assessment. (Modified from Spencer, K., Murphy, M., Bean, G., & Schelly, C. [1991]. Vocational needs assessment: A functional, community-referenced approach. In K. Spencer [Ed.], *From school to adult life: The role of occupational therapy in the transition process* [pp. 185-213]. Fort Collins, CO: Office of Transition Services Department of Occupational Therapy, Colorado State University.)

able future for Ron would look like. Ron's desired future includes living in the community with other people that he chooses, shopping at his neighborhood grocery store, and having a few ongoing and close friendships. Ron is very sociable, enjoys music, communicates with a combination of sign language and words, and walks slowly with a walker. Ron has cerebral palsy and severe mental retardation.

In preparation for the IEP, members of the team have been assigned to gather information about Ron's current performance in domestic, vocational, school, community, and recreational domains. An ecologic assessment format was chosen with different members of the team coordinating assessment activities in each domain. The occupational therapist, with specific skills in assessing personal and instrumental activities of daily living in the home environment, coordinated an assessment of Ron's performance in the domestic domain. This involved a trip to Ron's home, an interview with Ron and his mother, and direct observation of Ron during dressing, meal preparation, and eating activities. Evaluation findings are presented, in part, in Figure 26-8.

The occupational therapist also collaborated with the teacher to evaluate Ron's use of public transportation. While the teacher evaluated Ron's ability to follow a bus schedule, identify correct stops, pay, and communicate with the bus driver, the occupational therapist focused on the physical barriers that interfered with Ron's ability to ride the bus. This type of shared responsibility for an aspect of the assessment reflects collaborative teamwork.

Intervention
Planning

The mechanism for planning transition services is the IEP. Members of the team come together with assessment findings to discuss the student's identified abilities, interests, and needs. Sample and others (1990) developed a useful way to approach the development of an IEP for transition. Specifically, an IEP meeting is held and the student and team members who know the student well and who have information to contribute to the planning effort are in attendance. One member of the team facilitates the meeting and guides discussion around five questions:

1 What are the dreams for the student when he or she leaves school? The team records these dreams as *transition goals.*
2 What is the student able to do now? The team records current student abilities as *current levels of function.*
3 What does the student need? Needs relate to the discrepancies between what the student is able to do now in all five performance domains (domestic, school, vocational, community, and leisure) and the level of performance needed for an effective transition. *Student needs* also encompass the types of services and supports needed to maximize performance in the different transition domains.

4 What is the student going to do this year? The team records this year's plan as *annual goals.*
5 Who, what, when, where, and how? Responsibility for implementation of the transition plan is assigned to members of the team and recorded as *characteristics of services.* In addition to the delegation of responsibility, the nature of services is determined and must be consistent with an ecologic approach.

A useful way to organize and summarize transition planning during the IEP meeting is to write main points on a blackboard or flip chart for all team members to see. The five questions previously listed serve as headings (Figure 26-9). This type of recording allows all members of the team to follow the process and to actively participate in decisions.

The role of the occupational therapist during transition service planning is to contribute information (based on evaluation results) and to share ideas for service delivery (goals, learning activities, and learning environments) that will ultimately help the student achieve his or her transition goals. The occupational therapist may contribute information about the student in all domains or in one or two domains, depending on the areas evaluated and on how the team has divided the responsibilities. It is important to remember that transition and annual goals belong to the student and not to the members of the educational team. Effective transition planning requires collaboration and respect for input provided by the student, family members, teachers, and related service personnel.

Intervention Implementation

Following evaluation, an ecologic approach is recommended for transition-related occupational therapy services. The student's IEP for transition, specifically the student's transition goals, should determine to what extent OT will be involved in the delivery of services. These services will likely include a combination of the following strategies depending on the needs of the student and the resources of the team (AOTA, 2002; NICHCY, 2001):

1 *Direct service* may be provided by the occupational therapist or occupational therapy assistant to the student. Direct service requires the OT to use his or her personality, insights, and interaction skills in a therapeutic manner that will engage the student. Additionally, the OT will use purposeful, occupation-based activity during intervention. This activity should naturally occur within the student's performance context and must relate to the student's transition goals. Following the delivery of direct service, the OT may turn over the day-to-day delivery of service to another member of the team. When this occurs, the OT assumes a *monitoring role* where the OT continues to

Student: Ron Hunt

Date and time of assessment: October 3, 1994, 7:30AM-9:00AM

Persons involved and roles: Ron Hunt, student; Marie Hunt, mother; Sara Clark, occupational therapist

Domain: __X__ Domestic
           ____ School
           ____ Vocational
           ____ Community
           ____ Recreation

Environment observed (describe general environment along with physical, social, and cultural attributes):

The assessment took place at Ron's home, which is located in a quiet, older residential neighborhood with large trees and off-street sidewalks. The single-level, three bedroom house has five steps up to the entrance. Ron lives with his mother and a younger sister who is 13 years old. Assessment activities took place in the well-equipped kitchen and in Ron's bedroom and bathroom.

Activities observed in this environment:
1. Clothing selection, dressing, grooming
2. Breakfast preparation and eating
3. Lunch preparation/packing

STUDENT PERFORMANCE

Strengths/interests	Supports needed/barriers
Activity: Clothing selection, dressing, grooming. Ron selected a matching shirt and pants from his closet that were appropriate for the cool season.	Ron's mother, Marie, does Ron's clothes shopping and buys clothes in basic colors and styles that can be mixed and matched. Clothes are washed and hung in the closet by Marie.
Ron located socks and shoes, which he put on independently while sitting down.	Ron's shoes have velcro closures.
Ron combed his hair while looking in the mirror in the bathroom.	Marie verbally directed Ron to comb his hair. She also "touched up" his hair combing job. Marie schedules Ron's haircuts with the local barber.
Ron located his toothbrush and opened and squeezed a small amount of toothpaste onto his toothbrush. He brushed his teeth while receiving verbal guidance from his mother.	Marie verbally reminded Ron to brush his teeth. During the activity she verbally cued him to "brush the back teeth, top teeth," etc.
Ron independently located his wallet and pocket comb and put these in his rear pants pocket.	
Ron and Marie "talked" about plans for the day as Ron got ready. Ron used gestures, basic sign language, and "yes" and "no" to communicate. Ron initiated communication by saying "Mom!" loudly.	Marie communicates primarily by asking Ron "yes" and "no" questions, or she asks Ron to "show me."

FIGURE 26-8 Example of ecologic assessment.

Question #1	Question #2	Question #3		Question #4	Question #5
Transition goals	Current levels of function	Student learning needs	Support/ training needs	Annual goals	Characteristics of services

FIGURE 26-9   Form to record a transition plan.

maintain primary responsibility for student outcomes and maintains regular contact with the student and the person(s) carrying out service.

2 *Consultation may* be provided to members of the student's educational team, including the student, teachers, family members, other school personnel and representatives from community agencies. During consultation, the OT's focus is on enabling others to identify problems, create solutions, and intervene. If consultation is done well, the OT builds the capacity of others to assume responsibility and more independently address student needs (Schein, 1999).

3 *Educating or teaching* may be the focus of OT intervention and involvement. It involves disseminating knowledge or information to others about a student's characteristics and abilities, the overall transition process, and areas of occupation and activity as they interact with a student's school-to-adult life transition. Frequently, occupational therapists educate students in using new assistive technology and adults in supporting students to operate the technology.

To illustrate direct service approaches for transition-aged students, some examples are useful. Consider a student with limited movement caused by severe and persistent spasticity. Direct occupational therapy services for this student may include selecting and setting up a wheelchair positioning system to allow her to maintain an upright seating position needed to complete school assignments and to eventually work in the community. Direct occupational therapy services may also include teaching the student how to independently use a wheelchair mounted switch that operates the telephone, unlocks and open doors, turns lights on and off, and controls the television or radio. Direct occupational therapy services during a student's school lunch may include training in the use of adapted eating utensils. In general, direct services should be paired with consultation or educational approaches to assure that others understand what the student is doing and can support or enhance the intervention.

At some point, the OT may determine that day-to-day service provision can be turned over to another member of the service team. When this occurs, the OT can take on a monitoring role. The occupational therapist's responsibility for service outcomes continues despite delegating the day-to-day implementation of the program to another such as a teacher, paraprofessional, or anyone who has regular, daily contact with the student. Before monitoring begins, it must be determined that the person identified to implement the services is sufficiently skilled and available. The occupational therapist must provide training and supervision to ensure that the services being delivered are those that are needed.

The following example describes direct service paired with monitoring, which can be an effective service strategy for a student with learning disabilities who needs to complete written school assignments.

After a thorough assessment of the student's assistive technology needs and the acquisition of an adapted laptop computer and software, the occupational therapist and the student used the student's English assignments as the focus of intervention. This provided an opportunity for the student to learn how to use his new computer technology while engaging in meaningful activity. Direct OT services enabled the student to learn to use scanning and reading software plus word prediction. The occupational therapist then taught the English teacher and paraprofessional how to use the computer programs and how they could support the student's participation in English. Once the teacher and parapro-fessional demonstrated proficiency with the assistive technology, the occupational therapist then reduced involvement to occasional monitoring visits to assess the student's progress and staff comfort with the assistive technology. If the student failed to make expected progress toward independent completion of written assignments using the computer, the occupational therapist would reevaluate and redesign the intervention.

Direct services followed by monitoring can be an effective way to deliver transition-related services. It requires an intensive, upfront investment of time followed by decreased involvement from the occupational therapist. When monitoring is effective, the people who work most frequently with the student acquire the skills needed to implement occupational therapy recommendations throughout the student's day. This infusion of occupational therapy into the student's overall education program is an efficient way to use services to optimize the student's outcomes (Giangreco, 1986).

Consultation differs from direct service or direct service with monitoring. It requires excellent listening, observing, and communication skills. Consultation fits well within a collaborative team framework where information is readily shared with team members and where no one team member is viewed as having ultimate "authority" or decision-making responsibility (Pugach & Johnson, 1995). Consultation may occur when a job coach approaches the OT with concerns about the student's unreliable and inconsistent performance on the job. Through questioning and observation, the OT gathers more information to gain a full understanding of the situation. Subsequently, the OT would work with the job coach and the student to help them clearly define the problem that needs to be solved. Once the problem has been clearly identified, the consultant, job coach, and student contribute to finding a workable solution. Using this sort of process consultation model (Schein, 1999), the consultant has passed on problem identification and problem-solving skills to the people most involved: the job coach and the student. In the process, these people have gained strategies that can help them solve similar problems in the future. When consulting, it is important to note that the OT is not directly responsible for the outcome of the intervention (AOTA, 2002).

Consider a 16-year-old student who was working on community job skills as a part of his transition program. The student had a work-study position in the laundry area of the local hospital. The teacher and job coach recognized that the student could not perform some of the required job tasks despite his strong motivation to work. To address the student's difficulties on the job, the team requested consultation from the school's occupational therapist. After observing the student's job performance and interviewing the employer, the student, and the job coach, the occupational therapist met with the other team members for discussion and joint problem solving. Together, the team clarified the problem and determined that the student lacked the coordination and strength to safely push the heavily loaded laundry carts. Additionally, the student consistently lost track of the number of towels he had folded and was frequently overstocking the clean laundry carts, causing linens to fall to the floor. On the positive side, team members recognized that the student was skillful at folding towels and small linens, locating supplies, asking for help, and interacting with coworkers in a friendly way. During a consultation session, the occupational therapist helped the team reach a decision about how to solve the problems. They elected to approach the employer to try to renegotiate the student's job description to include more towel folding and linen cart stocking instead of pushing the large laundry carts. Next, the OT helped the job coach solve the problem of overstocking the laundry cart. Consultation with the job coach helped her come up with a system that would allow the student to consistently and accurately load the correct number of towels. The system devised by the job coach included a stiff cardboard box placed at the student's work station and sized to hold exactly eight folded towels. Through trial and error with the student, the job coach determined that by first filling the box with folded towels then transferring the stack to the cart, the student was able to stock the correct number and keep clean towels from falling on the floor. When it was determined that the job coach and student had worked out an effective system, the occupational therapy consultation ended.

Educating others is another type of OT intervention that can be used to benefit transition-aged students with disabilities as illustrated in the following example:

Renee is a 20-year-old student participating in a transition program at her high school. Renee sustained a severe brain injury when she was a sophomore. She is now applying for a part-time job stocking and cleaning shelves at a small, local sporting goods store and has completed an application and interview. Renee really wants this job because it is within walking distance of her home and has good hours. If she gets the job, Renee hopes to keep it after she completes high school with ongoing support provided by the state vocational rehabilitation agency. Renee's prospective employer has indicated that while he liked Renee, he is uncertain about having a person with a disability working at his store. Furthermore, he indicated that he is uncertain about what Renee can do and if she would be a productive employee. The occupational therapist, who knows Renee and understands the demands of the job, decided to visit the job site to meet with the employer. With permission from Renee and her parents, the OT met with the employer over a cup of coffee to share information about brain injury and how a brain injury can impact a person's performance of everyday activities. The OT also shared examples of effective strategies used by other employers to help employees who had disabilities similar to Renee's. The OT also took the opportunity to educate the employer about "supported employment," a service that would be available to Renee and her employer. After a half hour meeting, the OT thanked the employer, provided him with her business card, and encouraged him to call with any other questions or concerns. The next day, Renee received a phone call from the employer offering her the position.

In this situation, the OT's well-timed sharing of information and resources helped reassure a prospective employer. The employer's knowledge was expanded, allowing him to ultimately make the decision to hire Renee. The OT also used an educational approach to positively "reframe" the employer's perception of disability by sharing positive contributions made by people with disabilities and job support strategies that are realistic and effective.

Transition Stories
Sam

Sam entered the school district's Transition Services program at age 18. He was a personable, social young man who had cerebral palsy and used a manual wheelchair. At the age of 18, Sam's plans for the near future included an office job, living at home with his parents, and continuing his role as assistant manager for a Special Olympics basketball team. Cognitive and perceptual disabilities prevented Sam from learning to read or write. The OT at Transition Services worked as Sam's case manager overseeing transition-related evaluation, planning, and services. She worked with Sam, his family, his job coaches and other staff who provided direct services to Sam in a variety of community settings. With ongoing support from Transition Services staff, Sam maintained paid employment at a real estate company near his home. His job duties included stamping return addresses on envelopes and doing some filing. To meet the demands of the job, Transition Services staff provided Sam with a "jig" that organized his work area and correctly positioned the envelopes to be stamped. A job coach trained Sam how to file and also trained Sam's coworkers so they could provide Sam with ongoing supervision and support for filing. During Sam's last year with Transition Services, the real estate company where Sam worked moved to a different location and Sam's job ended. Sam, his family, and his OT case manager explored a variety of vocational options for Sam, which eventually led to a new office-type job. In addition to supporting the job search process, the OT case manager coordinated the transfer of responsibility for Sam's transition services from the school district to the local developmental disability service agency, which could provide ongoing vocational and residential support to Sam after he turned 22. On Sam's 22nd birthday, he was no longer eligible for transition services through the school district.

Janna

When Janna was 18, she entered the Transition Services program offered by her school district. By law, Janna would be eligible for transition services until she turned 22. With support from her case manager (an occupational therapist), the Transition Services team focused on several of Janna's critical performance areas: learning to use the public bus system, being safe in the community, using and handling money, homemaking skills, social/interpersonal skills, and building job experience. With support, Janna eventually began working at a major grocery store as a courtesy clerk. This job began with the full-time help of a job coach. As Janna became more proficient and confident on the job, the job coach provided less and less support. During her time with Transition Services, Janna changed from being rather shy to being a confident, socially active young adult. At the time of graduation from Transition Services and the public schools, Janna was working part time with the hope that she would increase her hours to full time. This happened when she transferred to another store in the same chain. At graduation, Janna was continuing to live with her parents but expressed interest in eventually moving into a more independent setting. Now at age 24, Janna is working full time and has recently moved into an apartment near work. Janna independently travels to and from work and prepares all her own meals. Her supportive parents continue to provide intermittent assistance at home and are committed to helping Janna solve problems that occur in her new living situation. Janna also receives some services from the local developmental disability service system, which is prepared to increase their support if Janna and her family need it.

SUMMARY

What happens to people with disabilities after they complete 12 to 18 years of public education? This question has received a great deal of attention from legislators, researchers, teachers, and related service personnel, including occupational therapists, over the years. Public education is often viewed as an investment in the future of society and specifically in youth. As with all investments, there is a desire to obtain a positive and profitable return. The return on the education investment for children and youth with disabilities relates to their eventual and successful transition from school to a productive and meaningful adult life.

Responsibility for the delivery of transition services clearly rests with all members of the IEP team, including occupational therapy personnel (Brollier, Shepherd, & Markley, 1994; Spencer, Emery, & Schneck, 2003;

Spencer & Sample, 1993). The ability of occupational therapists and occupational therapy assistants to focus on the needs of youth in the context of their approaching adult roles and performance environments adds strength to an educational team charged with designing and implementing transition services. Occupational therapy evaluation and intervention related to a student's participation during school, activities of daily living, work, and recreation are consistent with the transition services mandated in federal law and are essential components of effective transition planning and service delivery.

STUDY QUESTIONS

1 Consider the school-to-adult life transition process for a student with significant disabilities. How would this be similar or different from your own transition from high school to new and different adult roles?

2 What does an occupational therapist bring to the transition process for students with disabilities? How would you describe the occupational therapist role to a high school teacher? A transition-aged student? A transition-aged student's parent?

3 Explain how the role of occupational therapy may be affected by the requirement to work within the framework of the general education curriculum.

4 What skills do you have that will help you work as a collaborative team member? What skills do you think you will need to develop?

5 What would an ecologic assessment have looked like for you during your initial transition from high school to the adult world?

REFERENCES

American Occupational Therapy Association. (1999). *Occupational therapy services for children and youth under the Individuals with Disabilities Education Act* (2nd ed.). Bethesda, MD: American Occupational Therapy Association.

American Occupational Therapy Association. (2002). Occupational therapy practice framework: Domain and process. *American Journal of Occupational Therapy, 56,* 609-639.

Benz, M.R., Lindstrom, L., & Yovanoff, P. (2000). Improving graduation and employment outcomes of students with disabilities: Predictive factors and student perspectives. *Exceptional Children, 66,* 509-529.

Benz, M.R., Yovanoff, P., & Doren, B. (1997). School-to-work components that predict postschool success for students with and without disabilities. *Exceptional Children, 63,* 151-165.

Blackorby, J., & Wagner, M. (1996). Longitudinal postschool outcomes of youth with disabilities: Findings from the national longitudinal transition study. *Exceptional Children, 62* (5), 399-413.

Brollier, C., Shepherd, J., & Markley, K. (1994). Transition from school to community living. *American Journal of Occupational Therapy, 48,* 346-353.

Brown, L., Branston-McLean, M.B., Baumgart, D., Vincent, L., Falvey, M., & Schroeder, J. (1979). Using the characteristics of current and future least restrictive environments in the development of curricular content for severely handicapped students. *American Association for Education of the Severe and Profound Handicapped Review, 4* (4), 407-424.

Council for Exceptional Children. (2000). Developing educationally relevant IEPs: A technical assistance document for speech language pathologists. Reston, VA: The Council for Exceptional Children.

Downing, J.E. (1996). Including students with severe and multiple disabilities in typical classrooms: Practical strategies for teachers. Baltimore: Paul H. Brookes.

Education of All Handicapped Children Act of 1975 (Public Law 94-142). 20 U.S.C., 1400, et seq.

Everson, J., & McNulty, K. (1992). Interagency teams: Building local transition programs through parental and professional partnerships. In F. Rusch, L. Destefano, J. Chadsey-Rusch, L.A. Phelps, & E. Szymanski (Eds.), *Transition from school to adult life: Models, linkages, and policy* (pp. 342-351). Pacific Grove, CA: Brooks/Cole.

Giangreco, M. (1986). Effects of integrated therapy: A pilot study. *Journal of the Association for Persons with Severe Handicaps, 11* (3), 205-208.

Giangreco, M. (1996). Vermont interdependent services team approach: A guide to coordinating educational support services (VISTA). Baltimore: Brookes.

Giangreco, M.F., Cloninger, C.J., & Iverson, V.S. (1998). Choosing outcomes and accommodations for children: A guide to educational planning for students with disabilities (2nd ed.). Baltimore: Brookes.

Hasazi, S., Hock, M., & Cravedi-Cheng, L. (1992). Vermont's post-school indicators: Using satisfaction and post-school outcome data for program improvement. In F. Rusch, L. Destefano, J. Chadsey-Rusch, L.A. Phelps, & E. Szymanski (Eds.), *Transition from school to adult life: Models, linkages, and policy* (pp. 485-506). Pacific Grove, CA: Brooks/Cole.

Individuals with Disabilities Education Act Amendments of 1990 (Public Law 101-476). 20 U.S.C., 1400 et seq.

Individuals with Disabilities Education Act Amendments of 1997 (Public Law 105-17). 20 U.S.C., 1400 et seq.

Kennedy, C.H., Shukla, S., & Fryxell, D. (1997). Comparing the effects of educational placement on the social relationships of intermediate school students with severe disabilities. *Exceptional Children, 64,* 31-48.

McGregor, G., & Vogelsberg, R. T. (1998). *Inclusive schooling practices: Pedagogical and research foundations.* Baltimore: Paul H. Brookes.

Mostert, M. P. (1998). *Interprofessional collaboration in schools.* Boston: Allyn & Bacon.

NICHCY: National Information Center for Children and Youth with Disabilities. (1999). *Transition planning: A team effort.* Washington, DC: NICHCY. Retrieved November 25, 2003, from www.nichcy.org.

NICHCY: National Information Center for Children and Youth with Disabilities. (2001). *Related Services.*

Washington, DC: NICHCY. Retrieved November 25, 2003, from www.nichcy.org.

Orelove, F.P., & Sobsey, D. (1996). Educating children with multiple disabilities: A transdisciplinary approach (3rd ed.). Baltimore: Paul H. Brookes.

Pugach, M.C., & Johnson, L.J. (1995). *Collaborative practitioners, collaborative schools.* Denver: Love Publishing.

Rainforth, B., & York-Barr, J. (1997). Collaborative teams for students with severe disabilities: Integrating therapy with educational services (2nd ed.). Baltimore: Brookes.

Rusch, L. Destefano, J. Chadsey-Rusch, L.A. Phelps, & E. Szymanski (1992). *Transition from school to adult life: Models, linkages, and policy.* Pacific Grove, CA: Brooks/Cole.

Sample, P., Spencer, K., & Bean, G. (1990). *Transition planning: Creating a positive future for students with disabilities.* Fort Collins, CO: Office of Transition Services, Department of Occupational Therapy, Colorado State University.

Sands, D.J., & Wehmeyer, M.L. (1996). *Self-determination across the life span.* Baltimore: Brookes.

Schein, E.H. (1999). Process consultation revisited: Building the helping relationship. Reading, MA: Addison Wesley.

Snell, M.E., & Janney, R. (2000). *Collaborative teaming.* Baltimore: Paul H. Brookes.

Spencer, J.E., Emery, L.J., & Schneck, C.M. (2003). Occupational therapy in transitioning adolescents to post-secondary activities. *American Journal of Occupational Therapy, 57,* 435-441.

Spencer, K., Murphy, M., Bean, G., & Schelly, C. (1991). Vocational needs assessment: A functional, community-referenced approach. In K. Spencer (Ed.), *From school to adult life: The role of occupational therapy in the transition process* (pp. 185-213). Fort Collins, CO: Office of Transition Services Department of Occupational Therapy, Colorado State University.

Spencer, K., & Sample, P. (1993). Transition planning and services. In C. Royeen (Ed.), *Classroom applications for school-based practice* (pp. 6-48). Rockville, MD: American Occupational Therapy Association.

SRI International. (2003). National Longitudinal Transition Study-2 (NLTS2) Update. Retrieved from www.nlts2.org/pdfs/NLTS2_news_spring_4_1.pdf, November 25, 2003.

Stodden, R.A., Galloway, L.M., & Stodden, N.J. (2003). Secondary school curricular issues: Impact on postsecondary students with disabilities. *Exceptional Children, 70,* 9-25.

Swinth, Y., & Hanft, B. (2002). School-based practice: Moving beyond 1:1 service delivery. *OT Practice, 7* (16), 12-20.

Tomlinson, C.A. (2001). *How to differentiate instruction in mixed ability classrooms* (2nd ed.). Alexandria, VA: Association for Supervision and Curriculum Development.

Wagner, M., Newman, L., D'Amico, J., Butler-Nalin, P., Marder, C., & Cox, R. (1994). What happens next? Trends in post-school outcomes of youth with disabilities. Menlo Park, CA: SRI International.

Ward, M. (1992). Introduction to secondary special education and transition issues. In F. Rusch, L. Destefano, J. Chadsey-Rusch, L.A. Phelps, & E. Szymanski (Eds.), *Transition from school to adult life: Models, linkages, and policy* (pp. 387-389). Pacific Grove, CA: Brooks/Cole.

Wehmeyer, M.L., Palmer, S.B., Martin, A., Mithaug, D., & Martin, J. (2000). Promoting causal agency: The self-determined learning model of instruction. *Exceptional Children, 66,* 439-453.

Wehmeyer, M.L., & Sands, D.J. (1998). Making it happen: Student involvement in education planning, decision making, and instruction. Baltimore: Brookes.

Wehmeyer, M.L., & Schwartz, M. (1997). Self-determination and positive adult outcomes: A follow-up study of youth with mental retardation or learning disabilities. *Exceptional Children, 63,* 245-255.

Woolcock, W., Stodden, R., & Bisconer, S. (1992). Process- and outcome-focused decision making. In F. Rusch, L. Destefano, J. Chadsey-Rusch, L.A. Phelps, & E. Szymanski (Eds.), *Transition from school to adult life: Models, linkages, and policy* (pp. 219-244). Pacific Grove, CA: Brooks/Cole.

York, J., & Vandercook, T. (1991). Designing an integrated education for learners with severe disabilities through the IEP process. *Teaching Exceptional Children, 23* (2), 22-28.

RESOURCES

IDEA Partnerships Projects: www.ideapractices.org

National Dissemination Center for Children with Disabilities: www.nichcy.org

Transition Guide: www.nichcy.org/transitn.asp#ts10

Related Services: www.nichcy.org/ideapubs.asp#nd16

National Longitudinal Transition Study 2: www.nlts2.org

National Center on Secondary Education and Transition: www.ncset.org

Index